TC Fifth Edition

JEAN GRAY, BSC, MD, FRCPC, EDITOR

Therapeutic Choices

PUBLISHED BY:
Canadian Pharmacists Association
Ottawa, Ontario, Canada
www.pharmacists.ca

Published by:
Canadian Pharmacists Association
1785 Alta Vista Drive
Ottawa, ON K1G 3Y6
Canada
Tel: (613) 523–7877 or 1–800–917–9489
Fax: (613) 523–0445
Website: www.pharmacists.ca

The editors wish to acknowledge the assistance of Irina Karagodina and Kristin McCulloch in the preparation of this edition.

e-Therapeutics provides web access to *Therapeutic Choices* and e-CPS, the on-line version of the *Compendium of Pharmaceuticals and Specialties*. To subscribe to e-Therapeutics go on-line to www.e-therapeutics.ca. For multi-user licences or more information contact us at sales@pharmacists.ca.

Printed in Canada by:
Webcom, Toronto, ON, Canada

Library and Archives Canada has catalogued this publication as follows:

Therapeutic Choices.

Once every 2 to 3 years.

[1st ed.]-

ISSN 1495-9208

ISBN 978-1-894402-32-3 (5th edition)

1. Therapeutics — Handbooks, manuals, etc. I. Canadian Pharmacists Association

RM121.5.T44 615.5 C00-301973–X

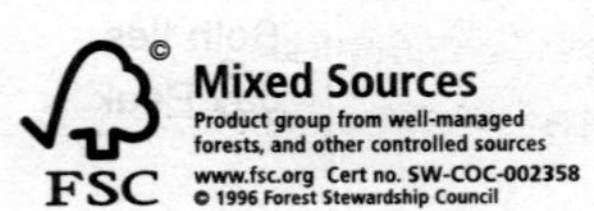

Table of Contents

Genitourinary Disorders

Sexual Health

Musculoskeletal Disorders

Skin Disorders

Blood Disorders

Fluid and Electrolyte Disorders

Infectious Diseases

Cancer Chemotherapy Toxicity

Symptom Control

Appendices

Reviewers

Editor

Jean Gray, BSc, MD, FRCPC
Professor Emeritus, Medical Education, Medicine and Pharmacology
Dalhousie University
Halifax, NS

Reviewers

David R. Anderson, MD, FRCPC
Queen Elizabeth II Health Sciences Centre
Halifax, NS

Jennifer Blake, BSc, MD, FRCSC
Women's College Hospital
University of Toronto
Toronto, ON

P. Joan Bobyn, BSP, PhD
College of Pharmacy and Nutrition
University of Saskatchewan
Saskatoon, SK

Gary Butterworth, BScPharm, OD
Winnipeg, MB

Sharon E. Card, MD, MSc, FRCPC
Royal University Hospital
Saskatoon, SK

John Conly, MD, FRCPC, FACP
Calgary Health Region
Calgary, AB

Paul Daeninck, MSc, FRCPC
St. Boniface General Hospital
Winnipeg, MB

Allison Dekker, BSP
The Hospital for Sick Children
Toronto, ON

Mario L. de Lemos, BSc(Pharm), MSc (Clin Pharm), PharmD, MSc (Oncol)
BC Cancer Agency
Vancouver, BC

John M. Esdaile, MD, MPH, FRCPC
Mary Pack Arthritis Centre
Vancouver, BC

Barb Evans, BSP, MSc, FCSHP
Royal University Hospital
Saskatoon Health Region
Saskatoon, SK

David Gardner, BScPharm, PharmD, MSc
Capital Health
Mental Health Services
Halifax, NS

Alfred S. Gin, BScPharm, PharmD
Health Sciences Centre
Winnipeg, MB

David Goldbloom, DPsy, FRCPC
Addiction and Mental Health Centre
Toronto, ON

Henry Haddad, MD, CSPQ, FRCPC
Professor Emeritus, Faculty of Medicine
University of Sherbrooke
Sherbrooke, QC

Antony J. Ham Pong, MBBS, FRCPC
Children's Hospital of Eastern Ontario
Ottawa, ON

Bill Hodge, MD, MPH, PhD
University of Ottawa Eye Institute
The Chalmers Evidence Based Practice Centre &
The Ottawa Health Research Institute
Ottawa, ON

Shinya Ito, MD, ABCP, FRCPC
Hospital for Sick Children
Department of Pediatrics
Toronto, ON

Jeffrey A. Johnson, BSP, MSc, PhD
Institute of Health Economics
University of Alberta
Edmonton, AB

David N. Juurlink, BPhm, MD, PhD, FRCPC
Clinical Pharmacology & Toxicology and Clinical Epidemiology
Sunnybrook and Women's College Health Sciences Centre
Toronto, ON

Heather Kertland, PharmD
St. Michael's Hospital
Toronto, ON

Sandra Knowles, BScPhm
Drug Information Centre
Sunnybrook and Women's College Health Sciences Centre
Toronto, ON

Anisha Lakhani, BSc(Pharm), PharmD
Fraser Health Authority
Surrey Memorial Hospital
Surrey, BC

Shallen Letwin, BScPharm, PharmD, FCSHP
Fraser Health Authority
Langley, BC

Michael Libman, MD, FRCPC
Department of Microbiology & Division of Infectious Disease
McGill University Health Centre
Montreal, QC

Mark J. Makowsky, BSP, PharmD, ACPR
EPICORE Centre/COMPRIS, Division of Cardiology
University of Alberta
Edmonton, AB

Anne Massicotte, BPharm, MSc
Drug Information Centre
The Ottawa Hospital
Ottawa, ON

Doreen Matsui, MD, FRCPC
London Health Sciences Centre
University of Western Ontario
London, ON

P.J. McLeod, MD, FRCP, FACP
McGill University
Montreal General Hospital
Montreal, QC

Michelle Mezei, BSc(Pharm), MDCM, FRCPC
Division of Neurology
University of British Columbia
Vancouver, BC

Scott Murray, MD, FRCPC
Division of Dermatology
Dalhousie University
Halifax, NS

Tania Mysak, BSP, PharmD
University of Alberta Hospital
Edmonton, AB

J. Stuart Oake, MD, FRCSC, DABU
Riverside Professional Centre
Ottawa, ON

Rakesh V. Patel, MD, MSc, PharmD
Department of Critical Care Medicine
The Ottawa Hospital
University of Ottawa
Ottawa, ON

C. Jane Richardson, BSP, PhD, FCSHP
Clinical Pharmacy Services
Saskatoon Health Region
College of Pharmacy & Nutrition
University of Saskatchewan
Saskatoon, SK

Neil Skjodt, MD, MSc, FRCPC, FCCP, D, ABSM
Respiratory & Critical Care Medicine
University of Alberta
Edmonton, AB

Kathryn Slater, BScPhm, PharmD
Department of Medicine, Division of Infectious Diseases
Victoria General Hospital
Halifax, NS

Nese Yuksel, BScPharm, PharmD
University of Alberta
Edmonton, AB

Alice Yuk-Yan Cheng, MD, FRCPC
Department of Medicine
Credit Valley Hospital
Mississauga, ON

Authors

Sueda Akkor
University of British Columbia
Vancouver, BC

Fred Y. Aoki
University of Manitoba
Winnipeg, MB

Benoit Bailey
Hôpital Ste-Justine
Montreal, QC

Rosemary Basson
Vancouver Hospital & Health Sciences Centre
Vancouver, BC

C. Laird Birmingham
St. Paul's Hospital
Vancouver, BC

David Birnie
University of Ottawa Heart Institute
Ottawa, ON

Edith M. Blondel-Hill
Dynacare Kasper Medical Lab
Edmonton, AB

Mark A. Boctor
Professor Emeritus, Faculty of Medicine
University of Saskatchewan
Saskatoon, SK

Anna M. Borowiec
University of Alberta
Edmonton, AB

Susan K. Bowles
Dalhousie University
Halifax, NS

Vivian P. Bykerk
Mount Sinai Hospital
Toronto, ON

Piera Calissi
St. Paul's Hospital
Saskatoon, SK

Norm R. C. Campbell
University of Calgary
Calgary, AB

Bruce Carleton
BC Children's and Women's Hospital
Vancouver, BC

Hugh Chaun
St. Paul's Hospital
Vancouver, BC

Terry Chisholm
Queen Elizabeth II Health Sciences Centre
Halifax, NS

Anthony W. Chow
Vancouver Hospital Health Sciences Centre
University of British Columbia
Vancouver, BC

Victoria J. Cook
BC Centre for Disease Control
Vancouver, BC

Robert Côté
Montreal General Hospital
McGill University
Montreal, QC

Amie J. Cullimore
St. Joseph's Healthcare
Hamilton, ON

Paul Davis
Heritage Medical Research Centre
Edmonton, AB

Simon de Denus
Montreal Heart Institute
Montreal, QC

Jean-Pierre DesGroseilliers
SCOHS Elisabeth-Bruyère Health Centre
Ottawa, ON

P.J. Devereaux
McMaster University
Hamilton, ON

Virginia Devonshire
UBC Hospital
Vancouver, BC

Orna Diav-Citrin
The Israeli Teratology Information Service
Jerusalem, Israel

Simon Dobson
Children's & Women's Health Centre
Vancouver, BC

Paul Dorian
St. Michael's Hospital
Toronto, ON

David Duperé
Queen Elizabeth II Health Sciences Centre
Halifax, NS

Beata S. Eisfeld
University Health Network
Toronto, ON

Jean Éthier
Centre Hospitalier de l'Université de Montréal-Hotel-Dieu
Montreal, QC

Brian G. Feagan
London Health Sciences Centre
London, ON

Richard N. Fedorak
University of Alberta
Edmonton, AB

Laura A. Finlayson
IWK Health Centre
Halifax, NS

J. Mark FitzGerald
Vancouver Hospital & Health Sciences Centre
Vancouver, BC

Jonathan A.E. Fleming
University of British Columbia
Vancouver, BC

Pierre Fortin
Grand River Regional Cancer Centre
Kitchener, ON

Susan R. Fryters
Capital Health
Royal Alexandra Hospital
Edmonton, AB

Stan P. George
Nova Scotia Eye Centre
Halifax, NS

Glenn H. Gill
Cariboo Memorial Hospital
Williams Lake, BC

G. Barry Gilliland
Saskatoon District Health Board
Saskatoon, SK

Fabian P. Gorodzinsky
Children's Hospital of Western Ontario
London, ON

Michelle M. Graham
University of Alberta Hospital
Edmonton, AB

Gillian Graves
IWK Health Centre
Halifax, NS

Laurence D. Green
McGill Centre for Tropical Diseases
Montreal General Hospital
Montreal, QC

Peter Green
Dalhousie University
Halifax, NS

David A. Grimes
University of Ottawa
Ottawa, ON

Ruby E. Grymonpré
University of Manitoba
Winnipeg, MB

Gord Gubitz
New Halifax Infirmary
Halifax, NS

Lyn Guenther
Guenther Dermatology Research Centre
London, ON

David A. Hanley
University of Calgary
Health Sciences Centre
Calgary, AB

John G. Hanly
Queen Elizabeth II Health Sciences Centre
Dalhousie University
Halifax, NS

Marianne Harris
St. Paul's Hospital
Vancouver, BC

Geralynn Hirsch
Capital District Health Authority
Halifax, NS

L. John Hoffer
SMBD Jewish General Hospital
Montreal, QC

Blair Jarvis
Canadian Pharmacists Association
Ottawa, ON

David W. Johnson
Alberta Children's Hospital
Calgary, AB

Jeffrey A. Johnson
Institute of Health Economics
Edmonton, AB

Gary I. E. Joubert
London Health Sciences Centre
London, ON

Angela Juby
University of Alberta
Edmonton, AB

Suneil Kapur
The Ottawa Hospital
University of Ottawa
Ottawa, ON

James R. Kennedy
St. Paul's Hospital
Vancouver, BC

Sidney H. Kennedy
University Health Network
Toronto General Hospital
University of Toronto
Toronto, ON

Tammy M. Keough-Ryan
Queen Elizabeth II Health Sciences Centre
Halifax, NS

J. S. Keystone
Centre for Travel & Tropical Medicine
Toronto General Hospital
Toronto, ON

James Kissick
Palladium Sports Medicine & Physiotherapy
Kanata, ON

Sandra Knowles
Sunnybrook Health Sciences Centre
Toronto, ON

Gideon Koren
The Hospital for Sick Children
Toronto, ON

Gunnar Kraag
The Ottawa Hospital (Riverside)
Ottawa, ON

Anne-Louise Lafontaine
Montreal General Hospital
Montreal, QC

Joanne M. Langley
Dalhousie University
IWK Health Centre
Halifax, NS

Mark R. Lesk
Maisonneuve-Rosemont Hospital
Montreal, QC

Duane Lichtenwald
Midtown Medical Centre
Saskatoon, SK

Heather Lochnan
University of Ottawa
Ottawa, ON

Timothy P. Lynch
Children's Hospital of Western Ontario
London, ON

Catherine MacLean
Dalhousie University
Queen Elizabeth II Health Sciences Centre
Halifax, NS

J. Dick MacLean
McGill Centre for Tropical Disease
Montreal General Hospital
Montreal, QC

W. Stuart Maddin
Vancouver Hospital Skin Care Centre
Vancouver, BC

Elizabeth Mann
Queen Elizabeth II Health Sciences Centre
Dalhousie University
Halifax, NS

Thomas J. Marrie
University of Alberta
Edmonton, AB

Cindy Marshall
Family Health Group
Lower Sackville, NS

David G. McCormack
London Health Sciences Centre
London, ON

James McCormack
St. Paul's Hospital
Vancouver, BC

R. Andrew McIvor
McMaster University
Hamilton, ON

Peter J. McLeod
Montreal General Hospital
Montreal, QC

Heather Milliken
Queen Elizabeth II Health Sciences Centre
Halifax, NS

Nicole Mittman
Sunnybrook Women's College Health Sciences Centre
Toronto, ON

Julio S.G. Montaner
St. Paul's Hospital
Vancouver, BC

Valentina Montessori
St. Paul's Hospital
Vancouver, BC

Mark Montgomery
Alberta Children's Provincial General Hospital
Calgary, AB

D. William Moote
London Health Sciences Centre
London, ON

Tania Mysak
University of Alberta Hospital
Edmonton, AB

Lynne Nakashima
BC Cancer Agency
Vancouver, BC

Lindsay E. Nicolle
Health Sciences Centre
Winnipeg, MB

Richard W. Norman
Dalhousie University
Halifax, NS

Richard I. Ogilvie
Toronto Western Hospital
Toronto, ON

Sagar V. Parikh
University Health Network
Toronto Western Hospital
Toronto, ON

Kevork M. Peltekian
Dalhousie University
Halifax, NS

Stephen J. Phillips
New Halifax Infirmary
Halifax, NS

Michael J. Potter
University of British Columbia
Vancouver, BC

Natasha Press
St. Paul's Hospital
Vancouver, BC

William Pryse-Phillips
Memorial University
St. John's, NF

R. Allan Purdy
Queen Elizabeth II Health Sciences Centre
Halifax, NS

Wayne Putnam
Dalhousie University
Halifax, NS

Paul Rafuse
Department of Ophthalmology and Visual Sciences
Dalhousie University
Halifax, NS

Edward D. Ralph
London Health Sciences Centre
London, ON

Jeffrey P. Reiss
PsycHealth Centre
Winnipeg, MB

Steven C. Reynolds
Vancouver Hospital Health Sciences Centre
University of British Columbia
Vancouver, BC

Kenneth Rockwood
Dalhousie University
Halifax, NS

Ghislaine O. Roederer
Institut de recherches cliniques de Montréal
Montreal, QC

Alana Rosenthal
North York General Hospital
Ottawa, ON

Coleman Rotstein
Hamilton Health Sciences
(Henderson)
Hamilton, ON

André Roussin
CHUM — Notre-Dame Hospital
Montreal, QC

Sheila Rutledge Harding
College of Medicine
University of Saskatchewan
Saskatoon, SK

R. Mark Sadler
Halifax Infirmary
Halifax, NS

Lindy Samson
Children's Hospital of Eastern
Ontario
Ottawa, ON

Peter Selby
The Hospital for Sick Children
Toronto, ON

Eldon A. Shaffer
Health Sciences Centre
University of Calgary
Calgary, AB

Arya M. Sharma
Hamilton General Hospital
McMaster University
Hamilton, ON

Neil H. Shear
Sunnybrook & Women's College
Health Sciences Centre
Toronto, ON

Robert Sheldon
Calgary General Hospital
Calgary, AB

Mathieu Simon
Hôpital Laval
Sainte-Foy, QC

Kurt Skakum
PsycHealth Centre
Winnipeg, MB

David P. Speert
University of British Columbia
BC Research Institute for
Children's & Women's Health
Vancouver, BC

Howard Stein
(deceased)
formerly University of British
Columbia
Vancouver, BC

Robert Strang
Public Health Services
Halifax, NS

Mark G. Swain
University of Calgary
Calgary, AB

R.P. Swinson
St. Joseph's Hospital
Hamilton, ON

Stephen R. Tan
Indiana University School of
Medicine
Indianapolis, IN USA

W. Grant Thompson
University of Ottawa
Ottawa, ON

Alan B.R. Thomson
University of Alberta
Edmonton, AB

Eldon Tunks
Chedoke Rehabilitation Centre
Hamilton, ON

Alexander G.G. Turpie
Hamilton General Hospital
Hamilton, ON

Joseph V. Vayalumkal
Ottawa, ON

Adil Virani
University of British Columbia
Burnaby, BC

David Warren
Children's Hospital of Western Ontario
London, ON

Walter Watral
Cancer Care Manitoba
Winnipeg, MB

C. Peter N. Watson
University of Toronto
Toronto, ON

Miriam Weinstein
Hospital for Sick Children
Toronto, ON

Michel White
Montreal Heart Institute
Montreal, QC

Sharon Whiting
Children's Hospital of Eastern Ontario
Ottawa, ON

Pearce Wilcox
St. Paul's Hospital
Vancouver, BC

William L. Williams
University of Ottawa Heart Institute
Ottawa, ON

W.L. Wobeser
Queen's University
Kingston, ON

James M. Wright
University of British Columbia
Vancouver, BC

Practitioner Review Board

Susan Beresford, BScPharm
Community Pharmacist
Kinburn Pharmasave
Mahone Bay, NS

Thomas Barry, MD, CCFP, FCFP
Family Practitioner
New Maryland, NB

Antony Gagnon, PharmD, CDE, CAE, FASCP
Clinical Pharmacist
Hamilton Family Health Team
Hamilton, ON

Roland Grad, MD, MSc, CCFP, FCFP
Family Practitioner
Herzl Family Practice Centre
Montreal, QC

Giselle McMurray, RN
Nurse Practitioner
Sudbury, ON

Shannan Neubauer, BSP, PharmD
Hospital Pharmacist
Yorkton Regional Health Centre
Yorkton, SK

Margaret Anne Woodside, BSc, MD
Family Practitioner
Frame Lake Family Physicians
Yellowknife, NT

Glossary of Abbreviated Terms

5-ASA	5-aminosalicylic acid
5HT	5-hydroxytryptamine
6-MP	6-mercaptopurine
AA	Alcoholics Anonymous
AAN	American Academy of Neurology
AAP	American Academy of Pediatrics
ABC	airway, breathing, circulation
ABG	arterial blood gases
AC	before meals
ACA	anticentromere antibodies
ACE	angiotensin-converting enzyme
ACEI	angiotensin-converting enzyme inhibitor
ACLS	advanced cardiac life support
ACT	assertive community treatment
AD	Alzheimer's disease
ADA	American Dental Association
ADH	antidiuretic hormone
ADHD	attention deficit hyperactivity disorder
ADL	activities of daily living; aids to daily living
ADR	adverse drug reaction
AE	adverse effect
AED	antiepileptic drug
AF	atrial fibrillation
AFB	acid fast bacilli
AFP	alpha-fetoprotein
AGEP	acute generalized exanthematous pustulosis
AHCPR	Agency for Health Care Policy and Research
AIDS	acquired immunodeficiency syndrome
AIMS	Abnormal Involuntary Movement Scale
AIN	acute interstitial nephritis
ALP	alkaline phosphatase
ALS	amyotrophic lateral sclerosis
ALT	alanine transaminase
AMD	age-related macular degeneration
AMS	acute mountain sickness
ANA	antinuclear antibody
ANC	acid neutralizing capacity
Anti HBe	antibody to HBeAg
Anti HCV	antibody to HCV
anti-TPO	antithyroid peroxidase
AOM	acute otitis media
AP	anteroposterior
APACHE	Acute Physiology and Chronic Health Evaluation
APSAC	anisoylated plasminogen streptokinase activator complex
aPTT	activated partial thromboplastin time

ARB	angiotensin receptor blocker
ARDS	acute respiratory distress syndrome
ARV	antiretroviral
ASA	acetylsalicylic acid
ASOT	antistreptolysin-o titer
AST	aspartate transaminase
AUA	American Urological Association
AUC	area under the concentration curve
AV	atrioventricular
AWS	alcohol withdrawal syndromes
BAC	benzalkonium chloride
BAL	bronchoalveolar lavage
BAS	Barnes Akathisia Scale
BCG	bacillus Calmette-Guérin
BDZ	benzodiazepine
BFHI	Baby-Friendly Hospital Initiative
BID	two times per day
BM	bowel movement
BMD	bone mineral density
BMI	body mass index
BMR	basal metabolic rate
BP	blood pressure
BPD	budesonide dipropionate
BPH	benign prostatic hyperplasia
BPM	beats per minute
BSA	body surface area
BSO	bilateral salpingo-oophorectomy
BSS	bismuth subsalicylate
BUN	blood urea nitrogen
C&S	culture and sensitivity
CABG	coronary artery bypass graft
CAD	coronary artery disease
CAM	complementary and alternative medicine
cAMP	cyclic adenosine monophosphate
CAP	community-acquired pneumonia
CBASP	Cognitive Behavioral Analysis System of Psychotherapy
CBC	complete blood count
CBT	cognitive behavioural therapy
CBZ	carbamazepine
CCB	calcium channel blocker
CCES	Canadian Centre for Ethics in Sport
CD	Crohn's disease
CDA	Canadian Diabetes Association; Canadian Dental Association
CDC	Centers for Disease Control (US)
CFC	chlorofluorocarbon
CFGHE	*Canada's Food Guide to Healthy Eating*
CFS	chronic fatigue syndrome
cfu/L	colony-forming units/litre

cGMP	cyclic guanosine monophosphate
CHD	coronary heart disease
CHF	congestive heart failure
CI	contraindication
CIN	chemotherapy-induced nausea
CK	creatine kinase
ClCr	creatinine clearance
CMV	cytomegalovirus
CNIB	Canadian National Institute for the Blind
CNS	central nervous system
CNV	choroidal neovascular membrane
COH	controlled ovarian hyperstimulation
COPD	chronic obstructive pulmonary disease
COXIB	cyclooxygenase-2 inhibitor
CPAP	continuous positive airway pressure
CPhIS	Canadian Pharmacist Intervention Study
CPK	creatine phosphokinase
CPR	cardiopulmonary resuscitation
CR	controlled release
CRP	C-reactive protein
CRPS	complex regional pain syndrome
CSF	cerebrospinal fluid
CSII	continuous subcutaneous insulin infusions
CT	computed tomography
CTD	connective tissue disease
CV	cardiovascular
CVA	cerebrovascular accident
CVD	cardiovascular disease
CVP	central venous pressure
CXR	chest x-ray
CYP2D6	cytochrome P450 2D6
DCCT	Diabetes Control and Complications Trial
ddI	didanosine
DEET	diethyltoluamide
DHA	dihydroxyacetone; docosahexaenoic acid
DHE	dihydroergotamine
DHEA	dehydroepiandrosterone
DHT	dihydrotestosterone
DHP	dihydropyridine
DI	drug interaction
DIC	disseminated intravascular coagulation
DIN	drug-induced nausea
DKA	diabetic ketoacidosis
DM	dextromethorphan; diabetes mellitus
DMARD	disease-modifying antirheumatic drug
DNA	deoxyribonucleic acid
DO	Doctor of Osteopathy
DOT	directly observed therapy
DOTS	directly observed therapy – short course

DRE	digital rectal examination
DSM-IV	*Diagnostic and Statistical Manual of Mental Disorders*, fourth edition
DTs	delirium tremens
DU	duodenal ulcer
DVT	deep vein thrombosis
DXA	dual energy x-ray absorptiometry
E3G	estrone-3-glucuronide
EAC	external auditory canal
EC	emergency contraception
ECF	extracellular fluid
ECFV	extracellular fluid volume
ECG	electrocardiogram
ECL	enterochromaffin-like
ECP	emergency contraceptive pill
ECT	electroconvulsive therapy
ED	erectile dysfunction
EDTA	ethylenediaminetetraacetic acid
EE	ethinyl estradiol
EEG	electroencephalogram
EF	ejection fraction
EGD	esophagogastroduodenoscopy
EHT	endoscopic hemostatic therapy
ELISA	enzyme-linked immunosorbent assay
EM	ethambutol
EMLA	eutectic mixture of local anesthetics
ENT	ear, nose and throat
EPA	eicosapentoenoic acid
EPS	extrapyramidal symptoms
ERCP	endoscopic retrograde cholangiopancreatography
ESR	erythrocyte sedimentation rate
ESRD	end stage renal disease
ESRS	Extrapyramidal Syndrome Rating Scale
ETEC	enterotoxinogenic *Escherichia coli*
ETS	environmental tobacco smoke
FA	fluorescein angiography
FAE	fetal alcohol effects
FAQ	functional assessment questionnaire
FAS	fetal alcohol syndrome
FCC	Food Chemical Codex
FCH	familial combined hyperlipidemia
FDA	Food and Drug Administration (USA)
FEV	forced expiratory volume
FEV_1	forced expiratory volume in one second
FHTG	familial hypertriglyceridemia
FiO_2	fraction of inspired oxygen
FIP	International Pharmaceutical Federation (France)
FNAB	fine needle aspiration biopsy
FP	fluticasone propionate

FSH	follicle-stimulating hormone
fT3	free triiodothyronine
fT4	free thyroxine
FVC	forced vital capacity
G6PD	glucose-6-phosphate dehydrogenase
GABHS	group A beta-hemolytic streptococcus
GAD	generalized anxiety disorder
GalU	galactose units
GBS	group B streptococcus
GCA	giant-cell arteritis
G-CSF	granulocyte colony-stimulating factor
GERD	gastroesophageal reflux disease
GFR	glomerular filtration rate
GGT	gamma glutamyl transpeptidase
GI	gastrointestinal
GM-CSF	granulocyte-macrophage colony-stimulating factors
GnRH	gonadotropin-releasing hormone
GnRH-a	gonadotropin-releasing hormone analogue
GPA	gastroprotective agent
GPC	giant papillary conjunctivitis
GTN	nitroglycerin
GTT	glucose tolerance test
GU	genitourinary, gastric ulcer
h	hour/s
H_2RA	H2-receptor antagonist
HAART	highly aggressive antiretroviral therapy
HACE	high-altitude cerebral edema
HAPE	high-altitude pulmonary edema
HAV	hepatitis A virus
HBeAg	hepatitis B antigen
HBIG	hepatitis B immune globulin
HBsAg	hepatitis B surface antigen
HBV	hepatitis B virus
HCG	human chorionic gonadotropin
HCV	hepatitis C virus
HDL-C	high-density lipoprotein cholesterol
HDV	hepatitis D (delta) virus
HEMA	hydroxyethyl methacrylate
HEPA	high efficiency particulate air
HEV	hepatitis E virus
HFA	hydrofluoroalkane
hFH	heterozygous familial hypercholesterolemia
Hgb	hemoglobin
HGPRT	hypoxanthine-guanine phosphoribosyl transferase
HH	hiatus hernia
HIT	heparin-induced thrombocytopenia
HIV	human immunodeficiency virus
HLA	human leukocyte antigen
HPN	high-potency neuroleptic

HPO	hypothalamic-pituitary-ovarian
HPV	human papillomavirus
HRQOL	health-related quality of life
HRT	hormone replacement therapy
HS	bedtime
HSDD	hypoactive sexual desire disorder
HSE	herpes simplex encephalitis
HSG	hysterosalpingogram
HSV	herpes simplex virus
HTN	hypertension
HZ	herpes zoster
hzFH	heterozygous familial hypercholesterolemia
IBCLC	International Board Certified Lactation Consultant
IBD	inflammatory bowel disease
IBS	irritable bowel syndrome
IBW	ideal body weight
I/C	imipenem/cilastatin
ICD	implantable cardioverter/defibrillator
ICF	intracellular fluid
ICG	indocyanine green
ICP	intracranial pressure
ICS	inhaled corticosteroids
ICU	intensive care unit
IDL	intermediate-density lipoproteins
IFNa	interferon alfa
IHD	ischemic heart disease
IL-1	interleukin-1
ILC	interstitial laser coagulation
ILI	influenza-like illness
IM	intramuscular
INH	isoniazid
INR	International Normalized Ratio
IOP	intraocular pressure
IPT	interpersonal psychotherapies
ISA	intrinsic sympathomimetic activity
ISD	intrinsic sphincter deficiency
ISDN	isosorbide dinitrate
ISG	immune serum globulin
IU	international unit
IUCD	intrauterine contraceptive device
IUD	intrauterine device
IUI	intrauterine insemination
IUS	intrauterine system
IV	intravenous
IVF-ET	in vitro fertilization – embryo transfer
IVIG	intravenous immune globulin
IVP	intravenous pyelogram
J	joule
JVP	jugular venous pressure

KSC	keratonconjunctivitis sicca
LABA	long-acting beta$_2$-agonist
LADA	latent autoimmune disease in adults
LBBB	left bundle branch block
LBP	low back pain
LCD	liquor carbonis detergens
LCR	ligase chain reaction
LDH	lactic dehydrogenase
LDL-C	low-density lipoprotein cholesterol
LES	lower esophageal sphincter
LET	lidocaine, epinephrine, tetracaine mixture
LFT	liver function test
LH	luteinizing hormone
LLQ	left lower quadrant
LMWH	low-molecular-weight heparin
LP	lumbar puncture
LPN	low-potency neuroleptic
LRTI	lower respiratory tract infection
L-T_4	sodium levothyroxine
LTBI	latent tuberculosis infection
LTRA	leukotriene receptor antagonist
LUNA	laparoscopic uterosacral nerve ablation
LV	left ventricular
LVEF	left ventricular ejection fraction
LYG	life year gained
MAC	*Mycobacterium avium* complex
MALT	mucosa-associated lymphoid tissue
MAO	monoamine oxidase
MAOI	monoamine oxidase inhibitor
MCV	mean corpuscular volume
MDD	major depressive disorder
MDI	metered-dose inhaler
MDS	myelodysplastic syndrome
MEE	middle ear effusion
MEN	multiple endocrine neoplasia
MER	meropenem
METS	metabolic equivalents
MH	malignant hyperthermia
MI	myocardial infarction
min	minute/s
MMI	methimazole
MMSE	mini-mental status exam
mo	month/s
MODS	multiple organ dysfunction syndrome
MODY	maturity-onset diabetes of the young
MOFS	multiple organ failure syndrome
MOH	medication-overuse headache; medical officer of health
MPA	medroxyprogesterone acetate
MRA	magnetic resonance angiography

MRI	magnetic resonance imaging
MRSA	methicillin-resistant *S. aureus*
MS	motion sickness; multiple sclerosis
MSG	monosodium glutamate
MSK	musculoskeletal
MSU	monosodium urate monohydrate
MTP	metatarsophalangeal (foot joint)
MTX	methotrexate
NA	Narcotics Anonymous
NAPA	N-acetylprocainamide
NAPRA	National Association of Pharmacy Regulatory Authorities
NDHP	nondihydropyridine
NDSAC	National Drug Scheduling Advisory Committee
NE	norepinephrine
NEC	necrotizing enterocolitis
NERD	nonerosive esophagitis disease
NG	nasogastric
NIH	National Institutes of Health
NMS	neuroleptic malignant syndrome
NRTI	nucleoside reverse transcriptase inhibitor
NNRTI	non-nucleoside reverse transcriptase inhibitor
NO	nitric oxide
NPT	nocturnal penile tumescence
NRT	nicotine replacement therapy
NS	normal saline
NSAID	nonsteroidal anti-inflammatory drug
NSTEMI	non-ST segment elevation myocardial infarction
NTD	neural tube defect
NTG	nitroglycerin
NUD	nonulcer dyspepsia
NYHA	New York Heart Association
N&V	nausea and vomiting
OA	osteoarthritis
OANV	opioid-associated nausea and vomiting
OC	oral contraceptive
OCD	obsessive-compulsive disorder
OCP	oral contraceptive pill
ODD	oppositional defiant disorder
OE	otitis externa
OI	opportunistic infections
OME	otitis media with effusion
ORS	oral rehydration solution; oculorespiratory syndrome
ORT	oral rehydration therapy
OTC	over-the-counter
PAD	peripheral arterial disease
PANV	pregnancy-associated nausea and vomiting
PASI	psoriasis area and severity index
PC	after meals
PCA	patient-controlled analgesia

PCI	percutaneous coronary intervention
PCNV	postchemotherapy nausea and vomiting
PCP	phencyclidine
PCR	polymerase chain reaction
PD	panic disorder
PDA	panic disorder with agoraphobia
PDE5	phosphodiesterase type 5
PDT	photodynamic therapy
PE	pulmonary embolism; premature ejaculation
PEEP	positive end-expiratory pressure
PEF	peak expiratory flow
PEFR	peak expiratory flow rate
PFAPA	periodic fever, aphthous stomatitis, pharyngitis and adenopathy
PFMT	pelvic floor muscle training
PFT	pulmonary function test
PG	prostaglandin
PG inhibitors	prostaglandin synthetase inhibitors
PGE_1	prostaglandin E_1
PHN	postherpetic neuralgia
PI	protease inhibitor
PID	pelvic inflammatory disease
PJP	*pneumocystis jirovecii* pneumonia
PKU	phenylketonuria
PMDD	premenstrual dysphoric disorder
PMMA	polymethylmethacrylate
PMN	polymorphonucleocyte
PMS	premenstrual syndrome
PO	by mouth
PONV	postoperative nausea and vomiting
POTS	postural orthostatic tachycardia syndrome
PPD	purified protein derivative
PPI	proton pump inhibitor
PR	rectally
PRCA	pure red cell aplasia
PRN	when necessary
PRP	primary Raynaud's phenomenon; planned replacement program
PRPP	phosphoribosyl pyrophosphate
PRSP	penicillin-resistant *S. pneumoniae*
PSA	prostate specific antigen
PSC	primary sclerosing cholangitis
PSN	presacral neurectomy
PT	prothrombin time
P/T	piperacillin/tazobactam
PTCA	percutaneous transluminal coronary angioplasty
PTH	parathyroid hormone
PTSD	post-traumatic stress disorder
PTT	partial thromboplastin time

PTU	propylthiouracil
PUD	peptic ulcer disease
PUVA	psoralen-ultraviolet light
PV	vaginally
PVCs	premature ventricular contractions
PVD	peripheral vascular disease
pVL	plasma viral load
PZA	pyrazinamide
QALY	quality adjusted life year
QHS	each bedtime
QID	four times per day
RA	rheumatoid arthritis
r-AFS	revised American Fertility Society classification
RAIU	radioactive iodine uptake
RAST	radio-allergosorbent testing
RAU	recurrent aphthous ulcers
RBC	red blood cell
RDA	recommended daily allowance
RE	retinol equivalents
REM	rapid eye movement
RGP	rigid gas permeable
rhv CNTF	recombinant human variant ciliary neurotrophic factor
RICE	rest, ice, compression, elevation
RIMA	reversible inhibitors of monoamine oxidase A
RL	Ringer's lactate
RLQ	right lower quadrant
RNA	ribonucleic acid
RNI	recommended nutrient intake
RP	Raynaud's phenomenon
RSV	respiratory syncytial virus
rt-PA	recombinant tissue plasminogen activator (alteplase)
RUQ	right upper quadrant
SABA	short-acting beta$_2$-agonists
SAC	seasonal allergic conjunctivitis
SAD	seasonal affective disorder
SAH	subarachnoid hemorrhage
SAM-e	S-adenosyl-methionine
SAS	Simpson Angus Scale
SBP	spontaneous bacterial peritonitis
SBT	serum bactericidal titer
SC	subcutaneous
SD	standard deviation; single dose; sexual dysfunction
sec	second/s
SHARP	swelling, heat, ache, redness, pus (signs of infection)
SIADH	syndrome of inappropriate antidiuretic hormone
SIDS	sudden infant death syndrome
SJS	Stevens-Johnson syndrome
SK	streptokinase
SL	sublingual

SLE	systemic lupus erythematosus
SLR	straight leg raise
SLS	sodium lauryl sulfate
SMBG	self-monitored blood glucose
SNRI	serotonin and norepinephrine reuptake inhibitor
SOGC	Society of Obstetricians and Gynaecologists of Canada
SPF	sun protection factor
SR	sustained release
SRP	secondary Raynaud's phenomenon
SPS	sulfasalazine
SSRI	selective serotonin reuptake inhibitor
SSSS	staphylococcal scalded skin syndrome
STI	sexually transmitted infection
STEMI	ST segment elevation myocardial infarction
SVT	supraventricular tachycardia
TAC	tetracaine, epinephrine, cocaine mixture
TBSA	total body surface area
TC	total cholesterol
TCA	tricyclic antidepressant
TD	tardive dyskinesia
TEN	toxic epidermal necrolysis
TENS	transcutaneous electrical nerve stimulation
TFPI	tissue factor pathway inhibitor
TG	triglycerides
TIA	transient ischemic attack
TIBC	total iron binding capacity
TID	three times per day
TIMI	Thrombolysis in Myocardial Infarction
TIPS	transjugular intrahepatic portosystemic shunt
TLESR	transient lower esophageal sphincter relaxation
TM	tympanic membrane
TMP/SMX	trimethoprim/sulfamethoxazole
TMT	tympanic membrane thermometer
Tn	troponin
TN	trigeminal neuralgia
TNF	tumor necrosis factor
TPN	total parenteral nutrition
TSH	thyroid-stimulating hormone
TSS	toxic shock syndrome
TST	tuberculin skin testing
TTH	tension-type headache
TTKG	transtubular K^+ concentration gradient
TUIP	transurethral incision of the prostate
TUMT	transurethral microwave thermotherapy
TUNA	transurethral needle ablation of prostate
TURP	transurethral resection of the prostate
TZD	thiazolidinediones
UA	unstable angina
UBT	urea breath test

UC	ulcerative colitis
UDCA	ursodeoxycholic acid
UFH	unfractionated heparin
UGI	upper gastrointestinal
UGIB	upper gastrointestinal bleeding
UK	urokinase
UP	ulcerative proctitis
USP	United States Pharmacopoeia
UTI	urinary tract infection
UVA	ultraviolet-A
UVB	ultraviolet-B
UVC	ultraviolet-C
VAS	vasoactive substances
VATS	video-assisted thoracic surgery
VDRL	Venereal Disease Research Laboratories
VED	vacuum erection device
VF	ventricular fibrillation
VLCD	very-low calorie diet
VLDL	very low-density lipoprotein
VMO	vastus medialis obliquus
VMS	vasomotor symptoms
VON	Victorian Order of Nurses
VSC	volatile sulfur compounds
VSST	visual sexual stimulation tests
VT	ventricular tachycardia
VTE	venous thromboembolism
VVS	vulvar vestibulitis
VZV	varicella zoster virus
WBC	white blood cell
WC	waist circumference
WHI	Women's Health Initiative
WHO	World Health Organization
wk	week/s
WOCN	wound, ostomy and continence nurse
y	year/s

Glossary of Microorganism Abbreviations

Abbreviation	Full Name
Bacteria	
B. forsythus	*Bacteroides forsythus*
B. fragilis	*Bacteroides fragilis*
C. jejuni	*Campylobacter jejuni*
C. pneumoniae	*Chlamydia pneumoniae*
C. trachomatis	*Chlamydia trachomatis*
C. difficile	*Clostridium difficile*
C. diphtheriae	*Corynebacterium diphtheriae*
E. aerogenes	*Enterobacter aerogenes*
E. cloacae	*Enterobacter cloacae*
E. faecalis	*Enterococcus faecalis*
E. coli	*Escherichia coli*
F. necrophorum	*Fusobacterium necrophorum*
F. nucleatum	*Fusobacterium nucleatum*
G. vaginalis	*Gardnerella vaginalis*
H. influenzae	*Haemophilus influenzae*
H. pylori	*Helicobacter pylori*
K. pneumoniae	*Klebsiella pneumoniae*
L. acidophilus	*Lactobacillus acidophilus*
L. vaginalis	*Lactobacillus vaginalis*
L. pneumophila	*Legionella pneumophila*
L. monocytogenes	*Listeria monocytogenes*
M. furfur	*Malassezia furfur*
M. catarrhalis	*Moraxella catarrhalis*
M. lacunata	*Moraxella lacunata*
M. tuberculosis	*Mycobacterium tuberculosis*
M. pneumoniae	*Mycoplasma pneumoniae*
N. gonorrhoeae	*Neisseria gonorrhoeae*
N. gonorrhoeae subsp	*Neisseria gonorrhoeae* subspecies
N. kochii	*Neisseria kochii*
N. meningitidis	*Neisseria meningitidis*
N. asteroides	*Nocardia asteroides*
P. acnes	*Propionibacterium acnes*
P. gingivalis	*Porphyromonas gingivalis*
P. intermedia	*Prevotella intermedia*
P. mirabilis	*Proteus mirabilis*
P. stuartii	*Providencia stuartii*
P. aeruginosa	*Pseudomonas aeruginosa*
S. typhi	*Salmonella typhi*
S. marcescens	*Serratia marcescens*
S. aureus	*Staphylococcus aureus*
S. epidermidis	*Staphylococcus epidermidis*

Abbreviation	Full Name
S. saprophyticus	*Staphylococcus saprophyticus*
S. pneumoniae	*Streptococcus pneumoniae*
S. mutans	*Streptococcus mutans*
S. pyogenes	*Streptococcus pyogenes*
S. viridans	*Streptococcus viridans*
U. urealyticum	*Ureaplasma urealyticum*
V. cholerae	*Vibrio cholerae*
Blood Parasites	
P. falciparum	*Plasmodium falciparum*
P. malariae	*Plasmodium malariae*
P. ovale	*Plasmodium ovale*
P. vivax	*Plasmodium vivax*
Fungi	
C. albicans	*Candida albicans*
C. glabrata	*Candida glabrata*
C. neoformans	*Cryptococcus neoformans*
E. floccosum	*Epidermophyton floccosum*
T. mentagrophytes	*Trichophyton mentagrophytes*
T. rubrum	*Trichophyton rubrum*
Protozoa/Parasites	
C. cayetanesis	*Cyclospora cayetanesis*
C. parvum	*Cryptosporidium parvum*
E. histolytica	*Entamoeba histolytica*
E. vermicularis	*Enterobius vermicularis*
G. lamblia	*Giardia lamblia*
P. jirovecii	*Pneumocystis jirovecii*
S. stercoralis	*Strongyloides stercoralis*
T. gondii	*Toxoplasma gondii*
T. vaginalis	*Trichomonas vaginalis*
Viruses	
CMV	Cytomegalovirus
HAV	Hepatitis A virus
HBV	Hepatitis B virus
HCV	Hepatitis C virus
HIV	Human immunodeficiency virus
HPV	Human papillomavirus
HSV	Herpes simplex virus
RSV	Respiratory syncytial virus
VZV	Varicella-zoster virus

Foreword

Welcome to the fifth edition of *Therapeutic Choices*. Much has happened since the fourth edition was published in 2003. *Therapeutic Choices* is now available electronically as part of an ambitious CPhA program of electronic publishing titled *e-Therapeutics*. The electronic format permits frequent revisions as new information becomes available and allows users to download tables of pharmacologic choices to their personal digital assistants. The availability of links to relevant information in *CPS* and other CPhA publications, to content references, government web sites and a commercially available drug interactions program enhances the information available to the user. This innovation was made possible by a generous contribution from the Primary Health Care Transition Fund of Health Canada.

CPhA has also taken a different approach to the editorial aspects of *Therapeutic Choices*. The Editorial Board has been replaced by a large network of reviewers from both medicine and pharmacy. Authors have been very accommodating in ensuring that their content is up to date and in incorporating revisions recommended by the reviewers. As with previous editions, there is a cadre of new authors in this edition and several new topics. The input of our Practitioner Review Board has been invaluable in ensuring that *Therapeutic Choices* is relevant for community-based practitioners of both medicine and pharmacy.

Carol Repchinsky is CPhA's Editor-in-Chief; she is supported by a strong group including clinical editors Alka Bhalla, Karen Fortin, Blair Jarvis, Barbara Jovaisas and scientific editor Sonal Acharya. In addition, the contributions of Kristina Allsopp and, more recently, Sylvie Brûlé as editorial managers, have been most appreciated. My personal gratitude to you all.

We continue to insist on an evidence-based approach to medical practice and hope that the fifth edition of *Therapeutic Choices* serves you well. Please let us know of any innovations or changes you would like to see in *Therapeutic Choices* as we continue the process of creating both electronic and print versions of the content in a format that we hope meets the needs of practitioners in Canada.

Jean Gray

How To Use *Therapeutic Choices*

The fifth edition of *Therapeutic Choices* includes 120 chapters and 3 appendices. Each chapter presents essential therapeutic information organized in easily readable algorithms and tables. The table(s) of drug choices appear at the end of each chapter. Chapters are referenced; citations to the literature follow the Suggested Readings section.

Drug therapy is discussed using generic drug names. Brand name inclusion in the chapters is not intended as an endorsement of that brand name. Many Canadian brand names are listed in the tables to the chapters. These are not all inclusive and are not listed in any order of preference.

The true cost of a specific therapy involves a number of elements including the manufacturer's list price, the mark-up and the dispensing fee, the length of drug therapy and costs related to drug administration. Prices used to determine cost of therapy in this book are the acquisition costs in Ottawa at the time of writing. The drug costs in the tables do not involve a dispensing fee or mark-up.

Costs shown are relative and are indicated by the $ symbol; actual costs are shown occasionally. For most conditions, calculations were made with the cost of the lowest priced product at the usual dosage for a given period. The treatment period selected for most chronic conditions is 30 days. However, treatment periods vary, and the legend accompanying each table should be consulted.

Readers of *Therapeutic Choices* requiring more detailed information on pediatric therapy should consult specialized texts.

Appendix I addresses dosage adjustment in patients with compromised renal function. In the tables, a small icon (❥) appears after the drug name if dosage adjustment should be considered.

The use of drugs during pregnancy and lactation is the subject of Appendix II.

Selected chapters include pharmacoeconomic considerations. They appear in shaded text following each of these chapters. General principles of pharmacoeconomics are discussed in Appendix III.

Description and Limitations of Information

Therapeutic Choices contains the best available evidence on selected topics. The authors, reviewers and editors have tried to ensure the accuracy of the information at the time of publication. Users of *Therapeutic Choices* should be aware that the text may contain information, statements and dosages for drugs different from those approved by the Therapeutic Products Directorate, Health Canada. The manufacturers' approval has not been requested for this information. Users are advised that the information presented in *Therapeutic Choices* is not intended to be all inclusive. Consequently, health care professionals are encouraged to seek additional and confirmatory information to meet their practice requirements and standards as well as the information needs of the patient.

Errata

In spite of the rigorous review process, should a major error occur, it will be corrected immediately on www.e-therapeutics.ca and posted on www.pharmacists.ca. All errors will be corrected in the next print edition.

CHAPTER 1
Acute Agitation

Kurt Skakum, MD, FRCPC and
Jeffrey P. Reiss, MD, MSc, FRCPC

Acute agitation is a dangerous condition, with a prevalence of 10–20% in hospitalized acutely ill patients.[1] It is essential to the well-being and safety of patients and staff that agitated patients be treated quickly, effectively and safely. To achieve this, the underlying cause of agitation must be determined and treated where possible.

Acute agitation is defined as a "state of anxiety accompanied by motor restlessness."[2] Aggression, defined as a "behaviour leading to self assertion,"[2] is often mislabelled as agitation, though it can occur in association with acute agitation. Although agitation occurs in many clinical settings, this chapter will focus on the emergency room, psychiatric and medical/surgical ward.

Agitation can be associated with delirium from any cause, including infection, neurologic conditions (e.g., trauma, seizure, stroke or tumor), intoxication, drug withdrawal (see Chapter 9), adverse drug reactions (e.g., toxicity, allergy or akathisia), endocrine disorders, blood sugar irregularities, cardiovascular problems and electrolyte disturbances. Agitation is also frequently associated with dementia. Psychiatric conditions that can cause agitation include psychosis, mania, depression, anxiety and personality disorders.

Goals of Therapy

- Create a safe environment for the treatment of the agitated patient and other patients
- Keep the work environment safe for staff
- Ameliorate the agitated state
- Prevent further episodes of agitation/aggression

Investigations

- Obtain history from the patient and descriptions of the patient's behaviour from staff and other collateral sources. Include:
  - triggers for the behaviour
  - previous episodes of agitation
  - description of the nature of the agitation
- Review medications and concomitant medical conditions
- Determine whether the agitation is accompanied by other symptoms such as confusion, clouded consciousness, cognitive impairment or physical symptoms such as fever, hypoxia or pain

- Mental status examination, a complete physical examination and relevant laboratory investigations are essential to the diagnosis

Therapeutic Choices (Figure 1)

Nonpharmacologic Choices

Give special attention to safety when encountering an acutely agitated/aggressive patient. This includes safety of the agitated patient and of other patients and staff in the environment. Often, both nonpharmacologic and pharmacologic interventions will be necessary. Address patients in a calm and reassuring yet confident tone of voice. There should be no hesitancy to have additional staff nearby. Direct patients to attempt to control their behaviour and reassure them that the environment is safe and that they have no reason to be fearful. Ask what the problem is and how it can be resolved. If necessary, patients can be asked to take medication to help decrease their distress.

If verbal approaches are unsuccessful, patients may need to be physically restrained or secluded. Details on the application of restraint and seclusion are not addressed in this chapter.

Pharmacologic Choices

Delirium

Delirium is a condition in which an acute onset of impairment in consciousness and cognition is associated with a medical/physical cause. The impairment typically fluctuates over the course of the day.

The first step is to determine and remove the medical cause of delirium. If the cause is removed or cannot be found and agitation persists, it may be necessary to treat the patient pharmacologically. Antipsychotics are first-line medications in these instances (Table 1). **Haloperidol** is the most studied and effective medication for decreasing agitation in delirious patients. It is available orally and for intramuscular and intravenous injection. Small, regularly scheduled doses are preferred over "as needed" dosing. The mid-potency first-generation antipsychotic **loxapine** and second-generation ("atypical") antipsychotics such as **olanzapine**, **risperidone** and **quetiapine** have also been used to treat delirium.[3] When used for several weeks to months, antipsychotics have been associated with an increased risk of stroke and death in elderly patients. Accordingly, their use in the elderly for managing acute confusional states with agitation or aggression should be done only when the benefits clearly outweigh the risks.[4,5]

Benzodiazepines should be reserved for cases where symptoms are attributed to alcohol withdrawal (see Chapter 9).

Dementia

Patients with various forms of dementia frequently exhibit agitation. These behaviours can be disruptive to the care environment and potentially dangerous. First, document the occurrence, frequency and nature of the behavioural disturbance and any recognizable triggers. If medications are necessary they should be prescribed following the "start low, go slow" principle.

Because of their more favourable side effect profile, atypical antipsychotics are being increasingly used over first-generation antipsychotics.[6] **Risperidone** has been shown in several studies[7] to have a favourable effect on the agitation and other behavioural symptoms (total behaviour, aggression and psychosis) associated with Alzheimer's disease. Risperidone at doses of 0.5, 1 and 2 mg per day is beneficial; the higher dosage may offer an efficacy advantage but does so at the risk of increased side effects including falls. **Olanzapine** 5 to 10 mg per day reduces aggressiveness, anxiety and euphoria.[7] There is little evidence on the use of **quetiapine** in the control of agitation and aggression in patients with dementia. A recent large, randomized, double blind, controlled trial of atypical antipsychotics in Alzheimer's disease patients showed that the chance of benefiting from treatment is equal to the chance of being harmed by the same treatment.[8] Considering the potential increased risks of treatment (e.g., stroke, death) and the limited tolerability and benefit in many patients, the decision to use an antipsychotic in the intermediate to long-term treatment of agitation or aggression in patients with dementia needs to be made on an individual patient basis and with caregiver support and consent.[5,8]

Haloperidol is effective in reducing aggression in patients with dementia but not in reducing other manifestations of agitation such as wandering and crying out.[9]

Other medications have also been studied, including **trazodone**, **cholinesterase inhibitors** and **benzodiazepines**. Data on trazodone are limited but it may be useful because of its sedative effects and minimal side effect profile.[10] A recent study suggests that cholinesterase inhibitors (e.g., donepezil) may reduce behavioural disturbances associated with Alzheimer's disease.[11] Benzodiazepines can be useful and effective for treating acute anxiety and agitation.[12] Care must be taken in prescribing this class of medications because of an increased risk of falls and impaired cognition. **Lorazepam** and **oxazepam** are the benzodiazepines of choice in this setting because they have no active metabolites and their metabolism is minimally affected by aging.

Brain Injury

Many medications from different classes have been used in this setting, though conclusive evidence is lacking. Give priority to minimizing the potential side effects when choosing a treatment in these patients. A recent review of the treatment of agitation and aggression in patients with acquired brain injury[13] found that **beta-adrenergic antagonists** are supported by the best evidence. In studies where **propranolol** has been found to be effective in reducing the incidence of aggression, high doses have been used. Antiepileptic drugs such as **carbamazepine** and

divalproex are also used. There is concern about paradoxical disinhibition when **benzodiazepines** are used in brain-injured patients. Antipsychotics seem to have a generally anti-aggressive effect regardless of the etiology.

There have been small studies of several other medications, including **tricyclic antidepressants**, **selective serotonin reuptake inhibitors**, **amantadine**, **buspirone**, **stimulants** and **lithium** in this patient population, though the evidence is not strong enough to recommend their use as first-line agents.

Mental Illness–associated Agitation

Psychosis

With acutely psychotic individuals, short-acting parenteral formulations of **antipsychotics** either alone or in combination with a parenteral **benzodiazepine** are recommended. Intramuscular olanzapine should *not* be combined with benzodiazepines because of the associated cardiac and respiratory complications. Rapidly dissolving or liquid formulations of the atypical antipsychotic medications with or without benzodiazepines are an effective alternative to intramuscular medications.[16,17] **Risperidone** is available in liquid and rapidly dissolving tablet preparations. **Olanzapine** is available in a rapidly dissolving wafer form. Several first-generation antipsychotics are also available in oral liquid formulations.

Mania

The acute control of severe agitation related to patients with mania involves both short-term treatment and initiation of longer term mood stabilizers. Initially, atypical antipsychotics (**risperidone**, **olanzapine** or **quetiapine**) are effective in establishing control of agitated behaviour. If oral medications cannot be administered, intramuscular administration is an effective alternative. Either intramuscular olanzapine *alone* or a first-generation antipsychotic with a benzodiazepine can be used.[18] Initiation of a mood stabilizer should also be undertaken in the acute phase of treatment (see Chapter 6).

Situational or Characterologic Agitation/Aggression

Agitation and aggression not attributable to any of the previously discussed causes is a common occurrence in emergency rooms. There is a relative lack of well-studied interventions in this setting. Nonpharmacologic interventions are essential. The most common medications used are **first-generation antipsychotics** along with a **benzodiazepine**, either by oral administration or intramuscular injection. Emerging evidence supports the use of atypical antipsychotics in this setting.[19]

Therapeutic Tips

- As a general rule, use lower doses of antipsychotics in older patients.
- Implement measures to *prevent* delirium (and any attendant agitation) in hospitalized patients (e.g., aids to remaining orientated such as

clocks and calendars, early mobilization following surgery, prevention of sleep deprivation, eyeglasses/hearing aids to optimize functioning and communication).

Figure 1: **Management of Acute Agitation**

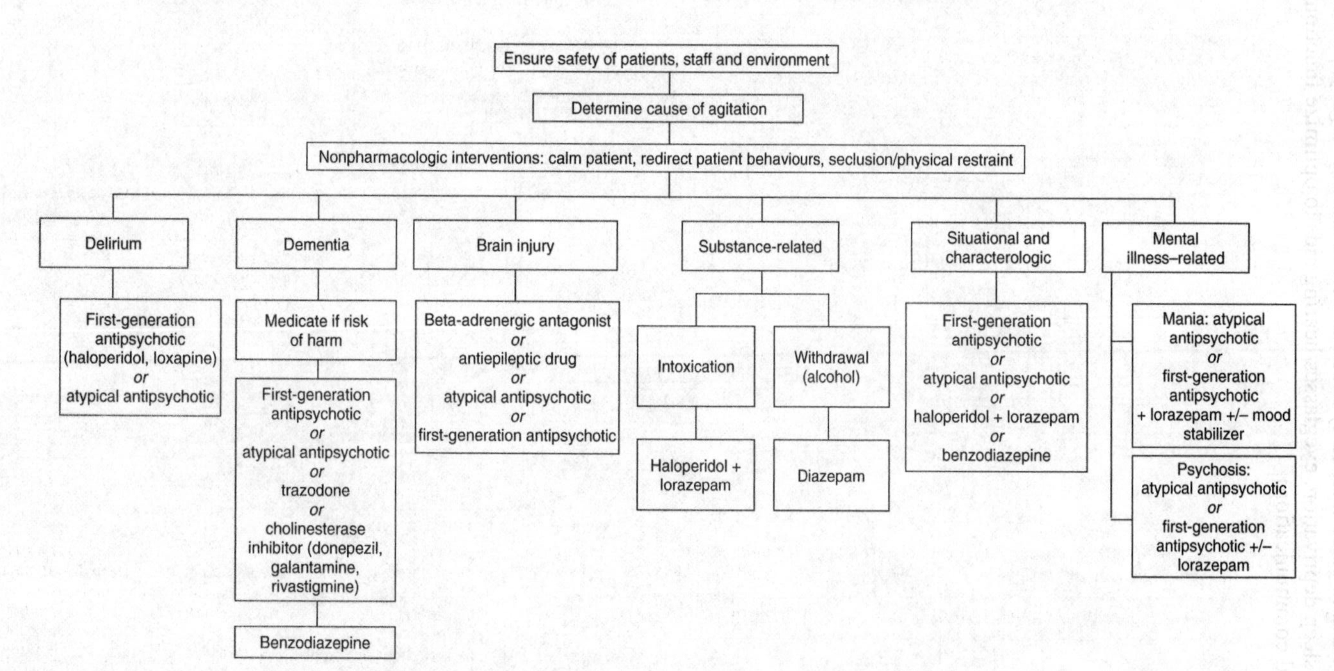

Table 1: **Drugs Used for the Management of Acute Agitation**

Class	Drug	Dose	Adverse Effects	Drug Interactions	Cost[a]
First-generation Antipsychotics	*haloperidol* generics	Delirium: 0.5–2.5 mg po/im BID Dementia: 0.5–1 mg po BID Psychosis: 5–10 mg/day po/im Mania: 5–10 mg/day po/im	Sedation, parkinsonism, akathisia, acute dystonia, neuroleptic malignant syndrome.	Additive effects with other CNS depressants, antagonism of dopamine agonists.	$
	loxapine generics	Delirium: 12.5–50 mg/day po Psychosis: 25–50 mg/day po	See haloperidol.	See haloperidol.	$
	zuclopenthixol, intramuscular Clopixol-Acuphase	Psychosis: 50–150 mg im; duration of action 2–3 days	See haloperidol.	See haloperidol.	$$$-$$$$
Atypical Antipsychotics	*risperidone* Risperdal, Risperdal M-Tab, generics	Delirium: 0.5–2 mg/day po Psychosis: 2–8 mg/day po Dementia: 0.5–2 mg/day po Mania: 2–3 mg/day po	Akathisia, dizziness, neuroleptic malignant syndrome.	Additive sedation with CNS depressants; antagonism of dopamine agonists; may potentiate antihypertensive drug effects.	$
	olanzapine, oral Zyprexa, Zyprexa Zydis	Delirium: 5–10 mg/day po Dementia: 2.5–5 mg/day po Psychosis: 10–30 mg/day po Mania: 5–20 mg/day po	Anticholinergic effects, akathisia, dizziness, neuroleptic malignant syndrome.	Additive sedation with CNS depressants; antagonism of dopamine agonists; may potentiate antihypertensive drug effects.	$–$$$

(cont'd)

Table 1: **Drugs Used for the Management of Acute Agitation** *(cont'd)*

Class	Drug	Dose	Adverse Effects	Drug Interactions	Cost[a]
	olanzapine, intramuscular Zyprexa Intramuscular	Delirium or mania: 2.5–10 mg im; repeat in 2 h and 6 h PRN to a max of 30 mg/24 h Use max of 2.5 mg/dose in debilitated patients, 5 mg in elderly	See olanzapine, oral.	See olanzapine, oral. Should **not** be administered simultaneously with parenteral benzodiazepines due to reports of cardiac and respiratory problems including deaths.	$$$-$$$$
	quetiapine Seroquel	Delirium: 25–100 mg/day po Dementia: 12.5–50 mg/day po Psychosis: 300–800 mg/day po Mania: start with 100 mg/day po; increase by 100 mg/day as needed to 300–600 mg/day divided BID	Sedation, dizziness, neuroleptic malignant syndrome.	Additive sedation with CNS depressants; antagonism of dopamine agonists; may potentiate antihypertensive drug effects.	$-$$
Benzodiazepines	*lorazepam* Ativan, generics	Dementia: 0.5–1 mg Q6–8H Mania/psychosis, adjunctively with antipsychotics: 1–2 mg po/im	Sedation, dizziness, cognitive impairment; rarely, respiratory depression can occur in this setting.	Additive sedation and possibly cardiorespiratory depression with other CNS depressants.	$
	oxazepam generics	Dementia: 10–15 mg po TID	See lorazepam.	See lorazepam.	$
	clonazepam Rivotril, generics	Mania: 0.25–0.5 mg po BID–TID	See lorazepam.	See lorazepam.	$

Class	Drug	Dose	Adverse Effects	Drug Interactions	Cost[a]
$Beta_1$-adrenergic Antagonists	*propranolol* generics	Brain injury: 20–40 mg po daily; increase by 20 mg/day Max: 640 mg/day Monitor heart rate and blood pressure	Bradycardia, hypotension, heart block, sedation.	Additive hypotension with other antihypertensives; additive sedation with other CNS depressants.	$
Antiepileptic Drugs	*carbamazepine* Tegretol, generics	Mania: 800–1200 mg/day po in 2 to 4 divided doses Target serum levels: 17–50 μg/L Brain injury: 200–300 mg po BID–TID	Rash, cognitive impairment, sedation, hyponatremia.	Induces cytochrome P450 enzymes; decreases clearance of many other drugs such as oral contraceptives, lovastatin, meperidine, morphine, nifedipine, oxycodone, trazodone.	$
	divalproex sodium Epival, generics	Brain injury: 250–500 mg po TID Target serum level 400–700 μmol/L	Nausea, tremor, sedation; rarely, edema.	Inhibits glucuronidation; may decrease clearance of other drugs such as lamotrigine and lorazepam.	$
Antidepressants	*trazodone* Desyrel, generics	Brain injury 25–50 mg po HS Max: 200 mg HS Dementia (for sedation): 25–100 mg/day po	Sedation, nausea, headache, dry mouth, priapism (rare).	May potentiate effects of other CNS depressants and augment hypotensive effects of antihypertensives.	$
Combination Therapy	*haloperidol/lorazepam*	Situational/characterologic agitation: haloperidol 5 mg po/im + lorazepam 2 mg po/im	See haloperidol. See lorazepam.	See haloperidol. See lorazepam.	$/for both

[a] Cost of 1-day supply; includes drug cost only.
Legend: $ < $5 $–$$ < $5–15 $$ $5–15 $–$$$ < $5–25 $$$ $15–25 $$$-$$$$ $15– >25 $$$$ > $25

Suggested Readings

Marder SR. A review of agitation in mental illness: treatment guidelines and current therapies. *J Clin Psychiatry* 2006;67(Suppl 10):13-21.

Nassisi D, Korc B, Hahn S et al. The evaluation and management of the acutely agitated elderly patient. *Mt Sinai J Med* 2006;73(7):976-84.

[No authors listed]. Practice guideline for the treatment of patients with delirium. American Psychiatric Association. *Am J Psychiatry* 1999;156(5 Suppl):1-20.

References

1. Trzepacz PT. Delirium. Advances in diagnosis, pathophysiology and treatment. *Psychiatr Clin North Am* 1996;19(3):429-48.
2. Dorland WAN. *Dorland's illustrated medical dictionary*. 27th ed. Philadelphia (PA): Saunders; 1988.
3. American Psychiatric Association Steering Committee on Practice Guidelines. *Practice guideline for treatment of patients with delirium*. 1999. Available from: http://www.psych.org/psych_pract/treatg/pg/DeliriumPG_05-15-06.pdf Accessed May 24, 2007.
4. Caine ED. Clinical perspectives on atypical antipsychotics for the treatment of agitation. *J Clin Psychiatry* 2006;67(Suppl 10):22-31.
5. Herrmann N, Lanctot KL. Atypical antipsychotics for neuropsychiatric symptoms of dementia: malignant or maligned? *Drug Saf* 2006;29(10):833-43.
6. Alexopoulos GS, Jeste DV, Chung H et al. The expert consensus guideline series. Treatment of dementia and its behavioral disturbances. Introduction, methods, commentary, and summary. *Postgrad Med* 2005;Spec No:6-22.
7. Ballard C, Waite J. The effectiveness of atypical antipsychotics for the treatment of aggression and psychosis in Alzheimer's disease. *Cochrane Database Syst Rev* 2006;(1):CD003476.
8. Schneider LS, Tariot PN, Dagerman KS et al., Effectiveness of atypical antipsychotic drugs in patients with Alzheimer's disease. *N Engl J Med* 2006;355(15):1525-38.
9. Lonergan E, Luxenberg J, Colford J. Haloperidol for agitation in dementia. *Cochrane Database Syst Rev* 2002;(2):CD002852.
10. Martinson-Torres G, Fioravanti M, Grimley EJ. Trazodone for agitation in dementia. *Cochrane Database Syst Rev* 2004;(4):CD004990.
11. Cummings JL, McRae T, Zhang R et al. Effects of donepezil on neuropsychiatric symptoms in patients with dementia and severe behavioral disorders. *Am J Geriatr Psychiatry* 2006;14(7):605-12.
12. American Psychiatric Association Steering Committee on Practice Guidelines. *Practice guideline for the treatment of patients with Alzheimer's disease and other dementias of late life*. Arlington (VA): American Psychiatric Association; 1997. Available from: http://www.psych.org/psych_pract/treatg/pg/AlzheimersPG_05-15-06.pdf Accessed May 24, 2007.
13. Fleminger S, Greenwood RJ, Oliver DL. Pharmacological management for agitation and aggression in people with acquired brain injury. *Cochrane Database Syst Rev* 2006;(4):CD003299.
14. Battaglia J, Moss S, Rush J et al. Haloperidol, lorazepam, or both for psychotic agitation? A multicenter, prospective, double-blind, emergency department study. *Am J Emerg Med* 1997;15(4):335-40.
15. Srisurapanont M, Kittiratanapaiboon P, Jarusuraisin N. Treatment for amphetamine psychosis. *Cochrane Database Syst Rev* 2001;(4):CD003026.
16. American Psychiatric Association Steering Committee on Practice Guidelines. Practice guideline for the treatment of patients with schizophrenia. Arlington (VA): American Psychiatric Association; 2004. Available from: http://www.psych.org/psych_pract/treatg/pg/Schizophrenia2ePG_05-15-06.pdf Accessed May 24, 2007.
17. Canadian Psychiatric Association. Clinical practice guidelines. Treatment of schizophrenia. *Can J Psychiatry* 2005;50(13 Suppl 1):7S-57S.
18. Yatham LN, Kennedy SH, O'Donovan C et al. Canadian Network for Mood and Anxiety treatments (CANMAT) guidelines for the management of patients with bipolar disorder: consensus and controversies. *Bipolar Disord* 2005;7(Suppl 3):5-69.
19. Rund DA, Ewing JD, Mitzel K et al. The use of intramuscular benzodiazepines and antipsychotic agents in the treatment of acute agitation or violence in the emergency department. *J Emerg Med* 2006;31(3): 317-24.

CHAPTER 2
Anxiety Disorders

R.P. Swinson, MD, FRCPsych, FRCPC, FCPA

Goals of Therapy

- Eliminate or decrease symptomatic anxiety
- Eliminate or decrease anxiety-based disability
- Prevent recurrence
- Treat comorbid conditions

Investigations

- Thorough history with attention to:
  - nature of symptoms and onset
  - nature and extent of disability
  - presence of comorbid medical or psychiatric conditions

Note: Treat comorbid mood disorders, especially depression, as the primary condition.

- Interview questions assist in obtaining an accurate diagnosis (Table 1, Table 2)
- Physical examination to exclude endocrine or cardiac disorders and to look for signs of substance use
- Laboratory tests:
  - CBC, liver function tests, gamma-glutamyl transpeptidase (GGT), thyroid indices (supersensitive TSH), ECG

Note: Treat physical disorders of recent onset before making a definitive diagnosis of an anxiety disorder.

Table 1: **Classification of Anxiety Disorders**[1]

Panic disorder with or without agoraphobia
Agoraphobia without history of panic disorder
Social anxiety disorder (social phobia)
Specific phobia
Obsessive-compulsive disorder
Post-traumatic stress disorder
Acute stress disorder
Generalized anxiety disorder
Anxiety disorder due to a general medical condition
Substance-induced anxiety disorder
Anxiety disorder not otherwise specified

Table 2: **Interview Questions to Establish Specific Anxiety Diagnosis[a]**

Questions	Further Inquiry
Do you have sudden episodes of intense anxiety?	Establish nature of attack.
Do you have difficulty going to places to which you used to be able to go?	Inquire about crowded places, line-ups, movies, highways, distance from home.
Do you have difficulty talking to people in authority or speaking in public?	Establish situations (one-on-one or groups).
Are you afraid of blood, small animals or heights?	Establish precise feared situation.
Do you repeat actions that you feel are excessive?	Ask about washing, counting, checking and hoarding.
Do you have thoughts that keep going in your mind that you can't stop?	Ask nature of thoughts (illness, harm, sex).
Have you experienced any emotionally stressful events?	Establish the nature (accident, sexual, torture) and timing of the trauma.
Do you worry a lot of the time?	Ask about worries related to health, family, job and finances.

[a] The order of asking the questions can be varied. The order represented in Table 2 reflects the sequence in the Diagnostic and Statistical Manual of Mental Disorders[1] in which panic attacks are diagnosed first, followed by phobic disorders, obsessive-compulsive disorder, post-traumatic stress disorder and generalized anxiety disorder. Anxiety disorders that do not fit into the above categories are atypical. Accurate diagnosis is recommended before instituting treatment.

Therapeutic Choices (Figure 1)

Relatively mild anxiety states in response to life circumstances are frequently time-limited, and many patients respond to anxiety management strategies without medication. Support, problem-solving and relaxation techniques may be helpful as the environmental crisis resolves. However, specific anxiety or mood disorders may develop as a consequence of the original stressor.

Nonpharmacologic Choices

- Caffeine or other stimulant use should be reduced and controlled.
- Alcohol use should be minimal; it should not be used to control anxiety.
- Reduce the "as-needed" use of short-acting benzodiazepines as much as possible; ideally, such use should *not* be continued for longer than four days.
- Stress reduction, including relaxation training and time management, is often helpful initially.
- Specific *cognitive behavioural therapy* (CBT) may be required; a psychiatric consultation is recommended for any patient who does not improve with trials of two separate antidepressants.

Pharmacologic Choices (Table 3)

The role of drug therapies varies among anxiety disorders. For some, drug treatment is not standard (e.g., specific phobia) and for others, drug therapy represents the most common intervention, especially when intensity of symptoms and disability are moderate to severe.

Panic Disorder

Antidepressants

The selective serotonin reuptake inhibitors (SSRIs) **citalopram**, **escitalopram**, **fluoxetine**, **fluvoxamine**, **paroxetine** and **sertraline** are all effective in reducing panic attacks. **Venlafaxine**, a serotonin-norepinephrine reuptake inhibitor (SNRI) has also demonstrated efficacy in repeated double-blind, placebo-controlled trials. SSRIs and SNRIs have become first-choice agents in treating panic disorder with or without agoraphobia.[2] There is usually a delay in response to these agents that may be accompanied by initial agitation. Combining the SSRI or SNRI with a brief course of low-dose benzodiazepine augmentation therapy (i.e., no longer than eight weeks) can increase adherence to medication and produce a more rapid response than with antidepressants alone.[3]

The tricyclic antidepressants (TCAs) **imipramine**, **desipramine** and **clomipramine** have been shown to reduce the frequency and severity of panic attacks[4] and are inexpensive. The side effect profiles of TCAs and SSRIs differ and are used to guide treatment choice. **Mirtazapine** has been effective in open-label trials.[5,6] The older monoamine oxidase inhibitors (MAOIs) **phenelzine** and **tranylcypromine** are also effective but more difficult to use.[7]

The dose requirements and length of treatment are the same as for major depression (see Chapter 5). However, the initial dose should be as low as possible (e.g., 10 mg daily of the TCAs or fluoxetine) and then increased, as tolerated, to the usual antidepressant dose range. If a higher starting dose is used, patients may become extremely agitated and discontinue treatment abruptly. Determining the duration of drug treatment is of great importance; medication is usually required for months or years. There is evidence that a majority of patients suffer relapse after benzodiazepines or antidepressants are discontinued.[8]

Benzodiazepines

Pharmacologic treatment of panic disorder is determined by the acuity of the disorder at presentation. Low doses of high-potency benzodiazepines can be used to abort initial panic attacks and may control high-frequency attacks later in the development of the disorder. **Alprazolam** 0.25 mg TID or QID or **clonazepam** 0.25 to 0.5 mg BID frequently makes panic attacks more manageable. **Lorazepam** and **diazepam** can also be used.

Although there is considerable evidence for the efficacy of benzodiazepines as monotherapy for panic disorder, they are best reserved for those cases where SSRI/SNRI treatment has not been successful or where there is need for augmentation of an antidepressant response.

Benzodiazepines are best used short term. Many patients have been maintained on stable low doses for years, and the potential benefits of discontinuation of benzodiazepines (i.e., decreased risk of sedation/falls, dependence/withdrawal) should be weighed against the frequent increase in panic frequency or severity on benzodiazepine discontinuation.[8]

Panic Disorder with Agoraphobia

The pharmacologic treatment of panic disorder with agoraphobia is the same as for panic disorder. However, much of the disability in panic disorder with agoraphobia arises from the avoidance behaviour rather than the panic attacks. This can be addressed with *cognitive behavioural therapy* (CBT), even if medication reduces or eliminates panic attacks. CBT can be more effective alone than when it is combined with medication.[8] However, access to specialized CBT is often limited.

Social Anxiety Disorder (Social Phobia)

This excessive fear of being criticized or negatively evaluated by others presents as shyness, avoidance of social contact or difficulty dealing with authority figures. The disorder may be present from childhood and often becomes noticeable in adolescence. It is particularly important to rule out comorbid major depression and alcohol use. *CBT* or other psychotherapy may be necessary to deal with significant social anxiety, even when medication is used.

SSRI and SNRI antidepressants are the mainstay of medical treatment for this condition. These agents are effective for generalized social anxiety and for milder cases manifesting as stage fright or fear of public speaking. **Escitalopram**,[9,10] **fluvoxamine**,[11,12] **paroxetine**,[13,14] **sertraline**[15,16] and **venlafaxine**[17] have demonstrated efficacy in repeated studies. Simple stage fright or fear of public speaking may respond to low-dose **propranolol** (10 mg) taken 30 minutes before the event, but in generalized social anxiety disorder propranolol is usually ineffective.[18,19]

Moclobemide has shown varying results but may be effective, particularly in higher doses.[20] At doses above 600 mg/day, moclobemide loses its isoenzyme specificity for MAO-A and as such, caution is needed regarding consumption of tyramine-rich foods such as aged cheeses, smoked meats, beer and red wine.

There is some evidence to support a trial of **gabapentin**[21] or **pregabalin**[22] in patients not responding to first-line measures. Benzodiazepines, particularly **clonazepam**,[23] are effective but should be used with the same restrictions as with other anxiety disorders (i.e., short-term use of lowest effective dose).

Specific Phobia

There is usually no indication for medication to treat the specific fear of heights, animals, injections or other common triggers. As little as six hours of CBT is often successful in producing marked, enduring change.

Obsessive–Compulsive Disorder

A chronic disorder that often begins in childhood or adolescence, obsessive–compulsive disorder can be extremely disabling. *CBT* is the psychotherapy of choice. Drug therapy is more easily available and is indicated for many patients. The SSRIs **fluoxetine**, **fluvoxamine**, **paroxetine** and **sertraline**, in the usual antidepressant dosing range, are recommended as first-line treatment in the Canadian Clinical Practice Guidelines for anxiety disorders.[25] It may take six to eight weeks to produce significant change in symptoms;[26] a trial at full dosages for at least six weeks is required to assess the effect of each SSRI used. There is no strong evidence to suggest that SSRIs vary in efficacy, but patients may respond to or tolerate one drug better than others in the same class. Second-line options include **clomipramine**, **venlafaxine**, **citalopram** and **mirtazapine**. SSRIs/SNRIs may be better tolerated than clomipramine, but agitation experienced early in therapy may cause some patients to discontinue the medication.

Treatment, if successful, may continue for years. Augmentation of SSRIs with atypical antipsychotics has been shown to increase the response in obsessive–compulsive disorder.[27] There is most evidence for the use of **risperidone** in this setting.

Benzodiadepines alone are not usually helpful in treating obsessive–compulsive disorder.

Post-traumatic Stress Disorder

Post-traumatic stress disorder (PTSD) presents following exposure to a traumatic event in which there is overwhelming anxiety and the threat or occurrence of injury or death to someone. PTSD may have its onset soon after the triggering event or may be delayed for years. The primary symptoms fall into three clusters of (i) persistent re-experiencing of the trauma, (ii) avoiding reminders of the events and numbing and (iii) persistent autonomic arousal (e.g., hypervigilance, enhanced startle reaction). Medication is one element of a multimodal treatment program that depends on the nature, severity and frequency of the trauma.

SSRI and SNRI antidepressants have been shown to reduce the severity of all the component symptoms of PTSD. Specifically, **fluoxetine**, **paroxetine**,[28] **sertraline**[29] and **venlafaxine**[30] are first-line options. Other antidepressants with evidence of efficacy include **fluvoxamine**,[31] **mirtazapine**,[3233] **moclobemide**[34] and **phenelzine**.[35,36] Additionally, the atypical antipsychotics **risperidone**[37] and **olanzapine**[38] have been shown to be effective augmenters of antidepressants in PTSD.

Monotherapy with benzodiazepines is not recommended due to their effects on disinhibition and the high rates of substance use disorders in those affected by PTSD.

There is some evidence that **propranolol** given within a few hours of an initial traumatic episode may help to prevent the onset of PTSD. Large-scale studies have not yet confirmed these early findings.[39]

Generalized Anxiety Disorder

Generalized anxiety disorder is characterized by excessive and uncontrollable worry related to everyday-life concerns, such as safety of family members, financial and job security and health. Patients with generalized anxiety disorder frequently exhibit depressed mood and other anxiety symptoms. *CBT* is the most effective psychosocial treatment but often takes 20 or more sessions to be effective.[40]

SSRIs and SNRIs have become established as first-line drug treatment for generalized anxiety disorder. The use of **escitalopram**,[41,42] **paroxetine**,[43] **sertraline** or **venlafaxine**[44] is supported by multiple efficacy studies. Because of its side effects and safety concerns in overdose, **imipramine**, an effective agent in generalized anxiety disorder, is usually reserved for when first-line choices are not effective. **Bupropion**[45] is a further choice, as is **pregabalin**.[46,47]

Low-dose benzodiazepines (e.g., **alprazolam**, **bromazepam**, **diazepam**, **lorazepam**) can be used for several weeks at a time for symptom relief, but attention must be paid to the risk of dependence and discontinuation symptoms.

Buspirone, an azapirone, has low abuse potential and is less sedating than benzodiazepines. Like antidepressants, it is relatively slow to have effect. In switching from long-term benzodiazepine therapy to buspirone, it is important not to discontinue the benzodiazepine abruptly; because there is no cross-tolerance between benzodiazepines and buspirone, benzodiazepine withdrawal symptoms could be precipitated.

Therapeutic Tips

- Short-term interventions (i.e., psychological therapies, relaxation techniques, benzodiazepines) may be effective.
- If one antidepressant is not effective in adequate dosage and after adequate time, switch to another antidepressant, which can be from the same class.
- If the second antidepressant is not effective in adequate dosage and after an adequate period of time, switch to one from another class.
- Restrict benzodiazepines to very short-term use (six to eight weeks) to assist with SSRI/SNRI-related agitation.

Figure 1: **Management of Anxiety Disorders**

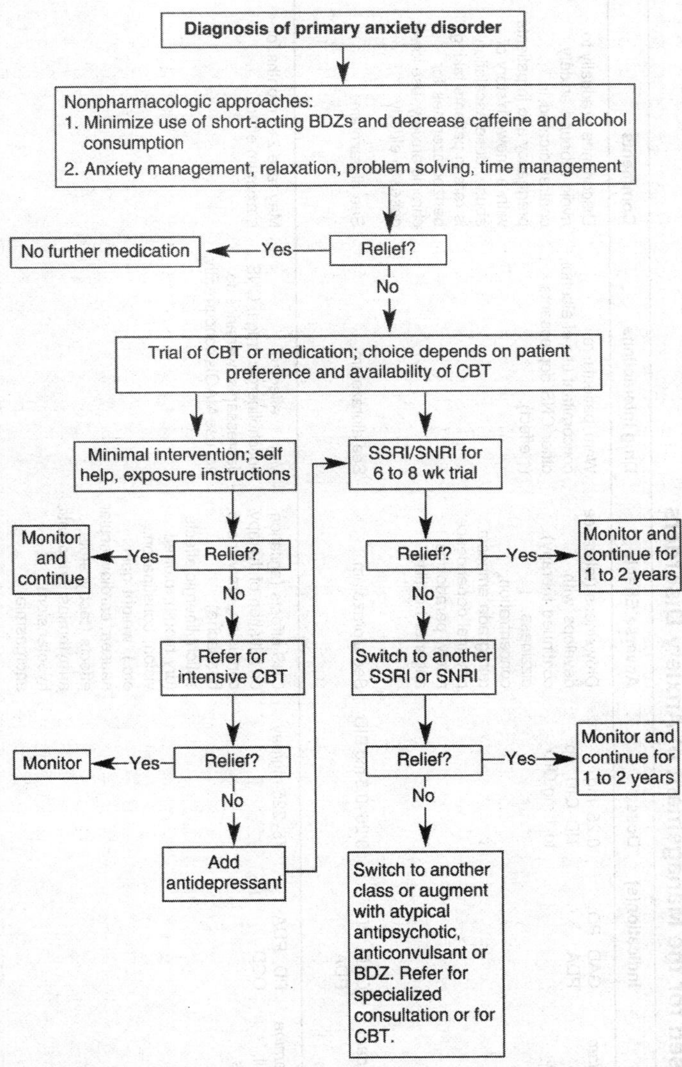

Abbreviations: BDZ = benzodiazepine; CBT = cognitive behavioural therapy; SSRI = selective serotonin reuptake inhibitor; SNRI = serotonin norepinephrine reuptake inhibitor.

Table 3: **Drugs Used for the Management of Anxiety Disorders**

Class	Drug	Indication(s)	Dose	Adverse Effects	Drug Interactions	Comments	Cost[a]
Benzodiazepines	*alprazolam* Xanax, generics	GAD, PD, PDA	0.25 mg TID–QID, up to 1 mg QID	Drowsiness (tolerance develops with continued therapy), dizziness, ↓ concentration, retrograde amnesia, physical dependence; rarely, paradoxical anger or hostility.	Warn patients re: concomitant use of alcohol, other CNS depressants (↑ effect).	Discontinue gradually to avoid rebound anxiety; contraindicated in pregnancy and in patients with a known history of abuse; dose escalation is rare in patients taking benzodiazepines for chronic anxiety; use lower doses in elderly.	\$–\$\$
	clonazepam Rivotril, generics	GAD, PD, PDA	0.25–0.5 mg BID	See alprazolam.	See alprazolam.	See alprazolam.	\$
Antidepressants, tricyclic	*clomipramine* Anafranil, generics	PD, PDA, OCD	75–225 mg/day	CNS effects (agitation on initiation of therapy, confusion, drowsiness, headache), anticholinergic effects (dry mouth, blurred vision, constipation, etc.), weight gain, nausea, cardiovascular effects (tachycardia, arrhythmias, orthostatic hypotension), anorgasmia.	May ↑ effect of anticholinergic drugs, CNS depressants, warfarin; do not use MAOIs concurrently.	May take 2–3 months for maximum effect.	\$–\$\$\$

Class	Drug	Indication(s)	Dose	Adverse Effects	Drug Interactions	Comments	Cost[a]
	desipramine Norpramin, generics	PD, PDA, GAD	75–300 mg/day	See clomipramine.	See clomipramine.	See clomipramine.	$–$$$
	imipramine Tofranil, generics	PD, PDA, GAD	75–300 mg/day	See clomipramine.	See clomipramine.	See clomipramine.	$-$$
Selective Serotonin Reuptake Inhibitors	*citalopram* Celexa, generics	PD, PDA, OCD, PTSD, SAD	20–60 mg/day	Agitation (on initiation of therapy), nausea, anorgasmia, insomnia, diarrhea, ↑ risk of GI bleeding.	Serotonin syndrome with MAOIs (hypertension, tremor, agitation, hypomania); ↑ risk of GI bleeding with NSAIDs; SSRIs are substrates and inhibitors of several cytochrome P450 isoenzymes, resulting in many potential interactions.	May take 2–3 months for maximum effect. Discontinue gradually.	$$–$$$
	escitalopram Cipralex	PD, PDA, GAD	10–20 mg/day	See citalopram.	See citalopram.	See citalopram.	$$-$$$
	fluoxetine Prozac, generics	PD, PDA, OCD, PTSD, SAD	20–80 mg/day	Agitation (on initiation of therapy), nausea, anorgasmia, insomnia, headache, ↓ appetite, diarrhea, ↑ risk of GI bleeding.	See citalopram.	See citalopram.	$$–$$$$$

(cont'd)

Table 3: **Drugs Used for the Management of Anxiety Disorders** *(cont'd)*

Class	Drug	Indication(s)	Dose	Adverse Effects	Drug Interactions	Comments	Cost[a]
	fluvoxamine Luvox, generics	PD, PDA, OCD, PTSD, SAD	150–300 mg/day	Agitation (on initiation of therapy), nausea, anorgasmia, anticholinergic effects, sedation, ↑ risk of GI bleeding.	See citalopram.	See citalopram.	$$–$$$$
	paroxetine immediate-release Paxil, generics	PD, PDA, OCD, PTSD, SAD	20–60 mg/day	Agitation (on initiation of therapy), nausea, anorgasmia, anticholinergic effects, sedation, ↑ risk of GI bleeding.	See citalopram.	See citalopram.	$$–$$$
	paroxetine controlled-release Paxil CR	PD, PDA, OCD, PTSD, SAD	12.5–37.5 mg/day	See paroxetine, immediate-release.	See citalopram.	See citalopram.	$$$-$$$$$
	sertraline Zoloft, generics	PD, PDA, OCD, PTSD, SAD	50–200 mg/day	Agitation (on initiation of therapy), nausea, anorgasmia, insomnia, diarrhea, ↑ risk of GI bleeding.	See citalopram.	See citalopram.	$$–$$$
Serotonin-Norepinephrine Reuptake Inhibitors	*venlafaxine extended-release* Effexor XR, generics	GAD, SAD	37.5–225 mg/day	Nausea, insomnia, dizziness, asthenia.	Do not use with MAOIs.	May take 2–3 months for maximum effect. Discontinue gradually.	$$–$$$$$

Class	Drug	Indication(s)	Dose	Adverse Effects	Drug Interactions	Comments	Cost[a]
Noradrenergic and Specific Serotonergic Antidepressants	*mirtazapine* Remeron, , Remeron RD, generics	OCD, PTSD	15–45 mg/day, at bedtime	Somnolence, increased appetite/weight gain, dizziness.	Do not use with MAOIs; additive sedation with other CNS depressants such as alcohol, benzodiazepines; substrate of CYP1A2, 2D6 and 3A4—caution with inhibitors or inducers of these isoenzymes.		$
Monoamine Oxidase Inhibitors	*phenelzine* Nardil	PD, PDA, OCD (refractory)	45–90 mg/day	Insomnia, dizziness, orthostatic hypotension, edema, sexual dysfunction.	Concurrent use with sympathomimetics may ↑ BP; do not use with SSRIs, TCAs; levodopa may ↑ effects and side effects; do not use with meperidine (agitation, hyperpyrexia, circulatory collapse may occur).	Dietary restrictions (tyramine-containing foods) are necessary.	$$–$$$
	tranyl-cypromine Parnate	PD, PDA, OCD (refractory)	20–60 mg/day	See phenelzine.	See phenelzine.	See phenelzine.	$–$$$
Reversible Inhibitors of Monoamine Oxidase-A (RIMAs)	*moclobemide* Manerix, generics	SAD	300–600 mg/day	Nausea, insomnia.	Do not use with meperidine, TCAs, SSRIs.	Dietary restrictions are not required at usual doses.	$–$$
Azapirones	*buspirone* Buspar, generics	GAD	5 mg BID–TID, up to 60 mg/day	Nausea, headache, dizziness, restlessness/insomnia.	Avoid use with MAOIs.	Onset of effect not as rapid as with benzodiazepines.	$$–$$$$$

(cont'd)

Table 3: **Drugs Used for the Management of Anxiety Disorders** *(cont'd)*

Class	Drug	Indication(s)	Dose	Adverse Effects	Drug Interactions	Comments	Cost[a]
$Beta_1$-adrenergic Antagonists	*propranolol* generics	SAD (specific task-related anxiety)	10 mg 30 min before task PRN	Hypotension.	Caution re: ↑ bradycardia with amiodarone.	For occasional use in situations such as public speaking, performing; not useful in generalized social anxiety disorder.	$
Antiepileptics	*gabapentin* Neurontin, generics	SAD	Initial: 300 mg/day Usual: 900–1800 mg/day in 2 divided doses	Somnolence, dizziness, ataxia, vision changes.	Magnesium- and aluminum-containing antacids may decrease the absorption of gabapentin.	Not a first-line agent; may be useful in patients not responding to first-line measures.	$$-$$$$$
	pregabalin Lyrica	SAD	Initial: 150 mg/day in 2–3 divided doses May be increased to 150 mg BID after 1 wk if necessary	Dizziness, sedation, peripheral edema.	No known significant drug interactions.	See gabapentin.	$$$$$

Class	Drug	Indication(s)	Dose	Adverse Effects	Drug Interactions	Comments	Cost[a]
Antipsy-chotics, atypical	*risperidone* Risperdal, generics	OCD, PTSD	Initial: 1 mg daily. Titrate gradually to desired effect, usually 1–2 mg daily. May need to increase to a max of 4 mg daily.	Insomnia, headaches, weight gain, orthostatic hypotension, rhinitis, anxiety, dose-related hyperprolactinemia and extrapyramidal effects.	Additive sedation with CNS depressants; may potentiate antihypertensive drug effects; inhibitors of CYP3A4 (e.g., clarithromycin, erythromycin, grapefruit juice, ketoconazole, prednisone) may ↑ risperidone levels; inducers of CYP3A4 (e.g., carbamazepine, phenytoin, rifampin) may ↓ risperidone levels.	Used as augmentation therapy with first-line agents in PTSD.	$-$$
	olanzapine Zyprexa, Zyprexa Zydis	PTSD	Initial: 2.5 mg daily. Titrate gradually to desired effect, usually 2.5 to 5 mg daily. May need to increase to a maximum of 10 mg per day.	Weight gain, dizziness, sedation, anticholinergic effects, hepatic transaminase elevation, orthostatic hypotension, ↑ risk of diabetes and dyslipidemia, extrapyramidal effects (especially akathisia).	Sedation with CNS depressants; may potentiate antihypertensive drug effects; inhibitors of CYP1A2 or CYP2D6 (e.g., diltiazem, fluvoxamine, paroxetine) may ↑ olanzapine levels; inducers of CYP1A2 or CYP3A4 (e.g., barbiturates, carbamazepine, phenytoin, rifampin) may ↓ olanzapine levels.	See risperidone.	$$$-$$$$$

[a] Cost of 30-day supply; includes drug cost only.

Dosage adjustment may be required in renal impairment; see Appendix I.

Abbreviations: MAOI = monoamine oxidase inhibitor; SSRI = selective serotonin reuptake inhibitor; TCA = tricyclic antidepressant; PD = panic disorder; PDA = panic disorder with agoraphobia; GAD = generalized anxiety disorder; OCD = obsessive–compulsive disorder; PTSD = post-traumatic stress disorder; SAD = social anxiety disorder

Legend: $ < $25 $-$$ < $25–50 $$ $25–50 $–$$$ < $25–75 $$–$$$ $25–75 $$$ $50–75 $$–$$$$ $25–100 $$$$ $75–100 $$–$$$$$ $25–>100 $$$-$$$$$ $50– >100 $$$$$ > $100

Suggested Readings

Antony MM, Swinson RP. Pharmacological and physical approaches. In: Antony MM, Swinson RP. *Phobic disorders and panic in adults: a guide to assessment and treatment.* Washington (DC): American Psychological Association; 2000. p. 265-86.

Baldwin DS, Anderson IM, Nutt DJ et al. Evidence-based guidelines for the pharmacological treatment of anxiety disorders: recommendations from the British Association for Psychopharmacology. *J Psychopharmacol* 2005;19(6):567-96.

Bandelow B, Zohar J, Hollander E et al. World Federation of Societies of Biological Psychiatry (WFSBP) guidelines for the pharmacological treatment of anxiety, obsessive-compulsive and posttraumatic stress disorders. *World J Biol Psychiatry* 2002;3(4):171-99.

Barlow DH, editor. *Anxiety and its disorders: the nature and treatment of anxiety and panic.* 2nd ed. New York (NY): Guilford Press; 2002.

Canadian Psychiatric Association. Clinical practice guidelines. Management of anxiety disorders. *Can J Psychiatry* 2006;51(8 Suppl 2):9S-91S.

References

1. American Psychiatric Association. Task Force on DSM-IV.*Diagnostic and statistical manual of mental disorders: DSM-IV-TR.* Washington (DC): American Psychiatric Association; 2000.
2. Boyer W. Serotonin uptake inhibitors are superior to imipramine in alleviating panic attacks: a meta-analysis. In: Darcourt G, editor. *Current therapeutic approaches to panic and other anxiety disorders.* New York (NY): Karger; 1994.
3. Goddard AW, Brouette T, Almai A et al.. Early coadministration of clonazepam with sertraline for panic disorder. *Arch Gen Psychiatry* 2001;58(7):681-6.
4. Mavissakalian MR, Perel JM. Long-term maintenance and discontinuation of imipramine therapy in panic disorder with agoraphobia. *Arch Gen Psychiatry* 1999;56(9):821-7.
5. Boshuisen ML, Slaap BR, Vester-Blokland ED et al. The effect of mirtazapine in panic disorder: an open label pilot study with a single-blind placebo run-in period. *Int Clin Psychopharmacol* 2001;16(6):363-8.
6. Sarchiapone M, Amore M, De Risio S et al. Mirtazapine in the treatment of panic disorder: an open-label trial. *Int Clin Psychopharmacol* 2003;18(1):35-8.
7. Buigues J, Vallejo J. Therapeutic response to phenelzine in patients with panic disorder and agoraphobia with panic attacks. *J Clin Psychiatry* 1987;48(2):55-9.
8. Marks IM, Swinson RP, Basoglu M et al. Alprazolam and exposure alone and combined in panic disorder with agoraphobia. A controlled study in London and Toronto. *Br J Psychiatry* 1993;162:776-87.
9. Kasper S, Stein D, Loft H et al. Escitalopram in the treatment of social anxiety disorder: randomised, placebo-controlled, flexible-dosage study. *Br J Psychiatry* 2005;186:222-6.
10. Lader M, Stender K, Burger V et al. Efficacy and tolerability of escitalopram in 12- and 24-week treatment of social anxiety disorder: randomised, double-blind, placebo-controlled, fixed-dose study. *Depress Anxiety* 2004;19(4):241-8.
11. Davidson J, Yaryura-Tobias J, DuPont R et al. Fluvoxamine-controlled release formulation for the treatment of generalized social anxiety disorder. *J Clin Psychopharmacol* 2004;24(2):118-25.
12. Westenberg HG, Stein DJ, Yang H et al. A double-blind placebo-controlled study of controlled release fluvoxamine for the treatment of generalized social anxiety disorder. *J Clin Psychopharmacol* 2004;24(1):49-55.
13. Baldwin D, Bobes J, Stein DJ et al. Paroxetine in social phobia/social anxiety disorder. Randomised, double-blind, placebo-controlled study. Paroxetine Study Group. *Br J Psychiatry* 1999;175:120-6.
14. Liebowitz MR, Stein MB, Tancer M et al. A randomized, double-blind, fixed-dose comparison of paroxetine and placebo in the treatment of generalized social anxiety disorder. *J Clin Psychiatry* 2002;63(1):66-74.
15. Liebowitz MR, DeMartinis NA, Weihs K et al. Efficacy of sertraline in severe generalized social anxiety disorder: results of a double-blind, placebo-controlled study. *J Clin Psychiatry* 2003;64(7):785-92.
16. Van Ameringen MA, Lane RM, Walker JR et al. Sertraline treatment of generalized social phobia: a 20-week, double-blind, placebo-controlled study. *Am J Psychiatry* 2001;158(2):275-81.

17. Rickels K, Mangano R, Khan A. A double-blind, placebo-controlled study of a flexible dose of venlafaxine ER in adult outpatients with generalized social anxiety disorder. *J Clin Psychopharmacol* 2004;24(5):488-96.
18. Falloon IR, Lloyd GG, Harpin RE. The treatment of social phobia. Real-life rehearsal with nonprofessional therapists. *J Nerv Ment Dis* 1981;169(3):180-4.
19. Liebowitz MR, Schneier F, Campeas R et al. Phenelzine vs atenolol in social phobia. A placebo-controlled comparison. *Arch Gen Psychiatry* 1992;49(4):290-300.
20. Stein DJ, Cameron A, Amrein R et al. Moclobemide is effective and well tolerated in the long-term pharmacotherapy of social anxiety disorder with or without comorbid anxiety disorder. *Int Clin Psychopharmacol* 2002;17(4):161-70.
21. Pande AC, Davidson JR, Jefferson JW et al. Treatment of social phobia with gabapentin: a placebo-controlled study. *J Clin Psychopharmacol* 1999;19(4):341-8.
22. Pande AC, Feltner DE, Jefferson JW et al. Efficacy of the novel anxiolytic pregabalin in social anxiety disorder: a placebo-controlled, multicenter study. *J Clin Psychopharmacol* 2004;24(2):141-9.
23. Otto MW, Pollack MH, Gould RA et al. A comparison of the efficacy of clonazepam and cognitive-behavioral group therapy for the treatment of social phobia. *J Anxiety Disord* 2000;14(4):345-58.
24. Stein MB, Liebowitz MR, Lydiard RB et al. Paroxetine treatment of generalized social phobia (social anxiety disorder): a randomized controlled trial. *JAMA* 1998;280(8):708-13.
25. Canadian Psychiatric Association. Clinical practice guidelines. Management of anxiety disorders. *Can J Psychiatry* 2006;51(8 Suppl 2):9S-91S.
26. Zohar J, Judge R. Paroxetine versus clomipramine in the treatment of obsessive-compulsive disorder. OCD Paroxetine Study Investigators. *Br J Psychiatry* 1996;169(4):468-74.
27. McDougle CJ, Epperson CN, Pelton GH et al. A double-blind, placebo-controlled study of risperidone addition in serotonin reuptake inhibitor-refractory obsessive-compulsive disorder. *Arch Gen Psychiatry* 2000;57(8):794-801.
28. Marshall RD, Beebe KL, Oldham M et al. Efficacy and safety of paroxetine treatment for chronic PTSD: a fixed-dose, placebo-controlled study. *Am J Psychiatry* 2001;158(12):1982-8.
29. Brady K, Pearlstein T, Asnis GM et al. Efficacy and safety of sertraline treatment of posttraumatic stress disorder: a randomized controlled trial. *JAMA* 2000;283(14):1837-44.
30. Seedat S, Stein DJ, Ziervogel C et al. Comparison of response to a selective serotonin reuptake inhibitor in children, adolescents, and adults with posttraumatic stress disorder. *J Child Adolesc Psychopharmacol* 2002;12(1):37-46.
31. Escalona R, Canive JM, Calais LA et al. Fluvoxamine treatment in veterans with combat-related post-traumatic stress disorder. *Depress Anxiety* 2002;15(1):29-33.
32. Connor KM, Davidson JR, Weisler RH et al. A pilot study of mirtazapine in post-traumatic stress disorder. *Int Clin Psychopharmacol* 1999;14(1):29-31.
33. Davidson JR,Weisler RH, Butterfield MI et al. Mirtazapine vs. placebo in posttraumatic stress disorder: a pilot trial. *Biol Psychiatry* 2003;53(2):188-91.
34. Neal LA, Shapland W, Fox C. An open trial of moclobemide in the treatment of post-traumatic stress disorder. *Int Clin Psychopharmacol* 1997;12(4):231-7.
35. Frank JB, Kosten TR, Giller EL et al. A randomized clinical trial of phenelzine and imipramine for posttraumatic stress disorder. *Am J Psychiatry* 1988;145(10):1289-91.
36. Kosten TR, Frank JB, Dan E et al. Pharmacotherapy for posttraumatic stress disorder using phenelzine or imipramine. *J Nerv Ment Dis* 1991;179(6):366-70.
37. Bartzokis G, Lu PH, Turner J et al. Adjunctive risperidone in the treatment of chronic combat-related posttraumatic stress disorder. *Biol Psychiatry* 2005;57(5):474-9.
38. Stein MB, Kline NA, Matloff JL. Adjunctive olanzapine for SSRI-resistant combat-related PTSD: A double-blind, placebo-controlled study. *Am J Psychiatry* 2002;159(10):1777-9.
39. Pitman RK, Sanders KM, Zusman RM et al. Pilot study of secondary prevention of posttraumatic stress disorder with propranolol. *Biol Psychiatry* 2002;51(2):189-92.
40. Borkovec TD, Ruscio AM. Psychotherapy for generalized anxiety disorder. *J Clin Psychiatry* 2001;62(Suppl 11):37-42.
41. Davidson JR, Bose A, Korotzer A et al. Escitalopram in the treatment of generalized anxiety disorder: double-blind, placebo controlled, flexible-dose study. *Depress Anxiety* 2004;19(4):234-40.
42. Goodman WK, Bose A, Wang Q. Treatment of generalized anxiety disorder with escitalopram: pooled results from double-blind, placebo-controlled trials. *J Affect Disord* 2005;87(2-3):161-7.
43. Pollack MH, Zaninelli R, Goddard A et al. Paroxetine in the treatment of generalized anxiety disorder: results of a placebo-controlled, flexible-dosage trial. *J Clin Psychiatry* 2001;62(5):350-7.
44. Davidson JR, DuPont RL, Hedges D et al. Efficacy, safety, and tolerability of venlafaxine extended release and buspirone in outpatients with generalized anxiety disorder. *J Clin Psychiatry* 1999;60(8):528-35.
45. Bystritsky A, Kerwin L, Eiduson S, Vapnik T. A pilot controlled trial of bupropion vs. escitalopram in generalized anxiety disorder (GAD). *Neuropsychopharmacol* 2005;30(Suppl 1):S101.
46. Rickels K, Pollack MH, Feltner DE et al. Pregabalin for treatment of generalized anxiety disorder: a 4-week, multicenter, double-blind, placebo-controlled trial of pregabalin and alprazolam. *Arch Gen Psychiatry* 2005;62(9):1022-30.

47. Feltner DE, Crockatt JG, Dubovsky SJ et al. A randomized, double-blind, placebo-controlled, fixed-dose, multicenter study of pregabalin in patients with generalized anxiety disorder. *J Clin Psychopharmacol* 2003;23(3):240-9.

CHAPTER 3
Attention-Deficit Hyperactivity Disorder

Adil Virani, BSc(Pharm), Pharm D, FCSHP

Attention-deficit hyperactivity disorder (ADHD), the most common neuropsychiatric disorder in school-aged children, is characterized by three hallmark symptoms—inattention, hyperactivity and impulsivity—the presence and severity of which vary among individuals.[1,2] Those affected by ADHD have impairment in behavioural, cognitive, academic, emotional and/or social functioning.[3] ADHD symptoms present before the age of seven and may persist throughout one's life.[2,3] There are three subtypes of ADHD:[3] predominantly inattentive (10–20%), predominantly hyperactive/impulsive (5–10%) and combined inattentive and hyperactive (70–80%).[3,4]

Goals of Therapy

- Eliminate or significantly decrease core ADHD symptoms
- Improve behavioural and academic performance
- Improve self-esteem and social functioning
- Minimize adverse effects of medications

Investigations

- Currently, there are no objective tests that unequivocally diagnose ADHD
- The diagnosis of ADHD is based on evidence of six or more specific behaviours/symptoms listed in Table 1
- Interview the patient, family/caregivers, teachers/assistants and psychologists (where applicable) to identify:
  - nature and duration of ADHD symptoms
  - impact of symptoms on functioning
  - age of onset
  - social interactions with family and peers
  - situations that exacerbate or ameliorate symptoms
  - symptoms suggestive of other potentially comorbid disorders such as oppositional defiant disorder, conduct disorder, mood/anxiety disorders, tic disorders and/or learning disabilities
- Various assessment/rating scales can be used to collect the above information and assess progress; see http://www.caddra.ca/english/phys_guide.html to find the most appropriate assessment vehicles and treatment suggestions for individual patients[5]

- Physical examination/medical history to assess hearing, vision, thyroid function, neurologic status, cardiac function, history of dysmorphic disorder (e.g., Down syndrome) or anemia
- Birth/prenatal history including in utero exposure to substances and premature birth[6]
- Baseline blood pressure, heart rate, height and weight (especially if stimulants are likely to be used)

Table 1: DSM-IV-TR Criteria for Diagnosing ADHD

A. Either (1) or (2):

(1) Six (or more) of the following symptoms of *inattention* have persisted for at least 6 months to a degree that is maladaptive and inconsistent with developmental level:

a. Often fails to give close attention to details or makes careless mistakes in schoolwork, work, or other activities.
b. Often has difficulty sustaining attention in tasks or play activities.
c. Often does not seem to listen when spoken to directly.
d. Often does not follow through on instructions and fails to finish schoolwork, chores, or duties in the workplace (not due to oppositional behaviour or failure to understand instructions).
e. Often has difficulty organizing tasks and activities.
f. Often avoids, dislikes, or is reluctant to engage in tasks that require sustained mental effort (such as schoolwork or homework).
g. Often loses things necessary for tasks or activities (e.g., toys, school assignments, pencils, books, or tools).
h. Is often easily distracted by extraneous stimuli.
i. Is often forgetful in daily activities.

(2) Six (or more) of the following symptoms of *hyperactivity-impulsivity* have persisted for at least 6 months to a degree that is maladaptive and inconsistent with developmental level:

a. Often fidgets with hands or feet or squirms in seat.
b. Often leaves seat in classroom or in other situations in which remaining seated is expected.
c. Often runs about or climbs excessively in situations in which it is inappropriate (in adolescents or adults, may be limited to subjective feelings of restlessness).
d. Often has difficulty playing or engaging in leisure activities quietly.
e. Is often "on the go" or often acts as if "driven by a motor."
f. Often talks excessively.
g. Often blurts out answers before questions have been completed.
h. Often has difficulty waiting for his/her turn.
i. Often interrupts or intrudes on others (e.g., butts into conversations or games).

B. Some hyperactive-impulsive or inattentive symptoms that cause impairment were present *before age 7 years*.

C. Some impairment from the symptoms is *present in two or more settings* (e.g., at school [or work] and at home).

(cont'd)

Table 1: **DSM-IV-TR Criteria for Diagnosing ADHD** *(cont'd)*

D. There must be clear evidence of clinically significant impairment in social, academic, or occupational functioning.

E. The symptoms do not occur exclusively during the course of a pervasive developmental disorder, schizophrenia, or other psychotic disorder and are not better accounted for by another mental disorder (e.g., mood disorder, anxiety disorder, dissociative disorder, or a personality disorder).

Adapted with permission from the *Diagnostic and Statistical Manual of Mental Disorders*, Fourth Edition, Text Revision. Copyright 2000. American Psychiatric Association.

Therapeutic Choices (Figure 1)

Evidence suggests that a combination of pharmacologic and nonpharmacologic therapies (e.g., behaviour modification programs) constitutes the best treatment strategy for children with ADHD.[7,8] Stimulant medications and atomoxetine are the most effective treatment for the core symptoms of ADHD.[5,8,9] Behavioural therapies play an important role in improving social interactions, self-esteem and the common behaviours seen in ADHD.[8,10]

Nonpharmacologic Choices

Despite high-quality evidence supporting the role of stimulants for ADHD, and the lack of high-level evidence for nonpharmacologic therapies, some clinicians, parents and/or patients have expressed a preference for approaches such as behaviour management, dietary changes, physical exercise, psychotherapy, neurofeedback (EEG biofeedback) and hypnosis.[11,12,13] When compared to stimulants, these nonpharmacologic options are less effective at reducing the core symptoms of ADHD.[4,8,10]

- *Behavioural therapies* are designed to minimize negative behaviours and promote positive ones by teaching parents (and sometimes teachers) techniques to improve a child's behaviours.[2] The Multimodal Treatment Study of ADHD (MTA) is one of the largest (597 children aged 7–9 with the combined subtype of ADHD) and longest randomized controlled trials comparing behavioural therapy with pharmacologic therapy and combined behavioural/pharmacologic therapy. This trial found that behavioural therapy alone was inferior to pharmacologic therapy alone at reducing core ADHD symptoms.[8] Combined behavioural/pharmacologic therapy was shown to be more effective at reducing oppositional behaviours and anxiety while improving social interactions and self-esteem when compared to either treatment strategy alone.[8] Another randomized controlled study, involving 103 children aged 7–9 years, confirmed the greater benefit of stimulant medications over behavioural strategies on core ADHD symptoms, and demonstrated a sustained benefit over a 2-year period.[10]
- The elimination of certain foods from the *diet* in an effort to minimize ADHD symptoms is not based on evidence from clinical trials, but rather on observations that some children exhibit more severe

hyperactive behaviours in association with certain sugars, dyes or preservatives.[11]

- Mind-body therapies such as *neurofeedback* or *hypnosis* are geared toward training the patient's mind (by modifying brainwave activity) to influence physical responses to ADHD symptoms.[13] Though some interesting research has been conducted in this area, well-designed trials are still required to confirm the efficacy of these strategies in reducing core ADHD symptoms.[12,13]

Pharmacologic Choices

Psychostimulants

Stimulant medications (**methylphenidate**, **dextroamphetamine**, **mixed salts amphetamine**) have been considered first-line agents for treating ADHD for decades.[2,4,9] Their efficacy at reducing core ADHD symptoms has been demonstrated in a wide range of patients aged 6 years to adult.[5,9] Controlled trials consistently demonstrate that at least 70% of patients receiving stimulant therapy will have a clinically significant decrease in core ADHD symptoms.[2,4,8,9]

No clinical predictors of who will benefit from which stimulant have been identified; therefore, the choice of agent will depend on patient and physician preferences.[9] Patients who do not tolerate or respond to one stimulant after two to three weeks of therapy should be switched to an alternative stimulant.[9]

Though methylphenidate sustained-release tablets (e.g., Ritalin SR) and dextroamphetamine sustained-release spansules (Dexedrine) have a longer duration of action (up to 8 hours) than their immediate-release counterparts (see Table 2), they often require more than once-daily dosing.

Long-acting stimulant formulations such as Concerta, Biphentin and Adderall XR (see Table 2) are as effective as appropriately dosed shorter-acting stimulants.[9] These formulations have a duration of action of 8 to 12 hours. Advantages of these long-acting products include single daily dosing, potential for improved adherence, avoidance of the need for medication administration at school, decreased abuse potential and decreased risk of rebound hyperactivity. Given these advantages, authors of recent Canadian guidelines on the treatment of ADHD recommend that long-acting agents be used as first-line treatment of ADHD.[5]

In 2006, Health Canada and regulatory agencies in other countries alerted health care providers and patients to concerns regarding the possible association of stimulants (and atomoxetine) with cardiovascular risks such as sudden cardiac death in those with underlying cardiac anomalies, and with adverse psychiatric symptoms such as hallucinations and irritability.

Though **modafinil** is a central nervous system stimulant that promotes wakefulness in the treatment of narcolepsy, it is less effective than other psychostimulants in ADHD and is not often used. It is not approved for use in ADHD. There is some evidence from double-blind trials in children and adults that modafinil (170–425 mg/day) is superior to placebo in decreasing core symptoms of ADHD.[14,15]

Atomoxetine

Atomoxetine, a norepinephrine reuptake inhibitor not classified as a stimulant, is indicated in children ≥ 6 years of age, adolescents and adults with ADHD. Its efficacy and tolerability have been studied in several well-designed trials.[16,17,18,19,20,21,22] Atomoxetine is not a controlled substance. Randomized, controlled trials confirm that after 6–12 weeks of treatment, atomoxetine reduces core ADHD symptoms by at least 25–30% in 60–70% of individuals.[17,20,22] The efficacy of atomoxetine approaches that of psychostimulants and may be appropriate for those who have either not responded to or not tolerated an adequate trial of stimulant medications. It should also be considered for those with ADHD and comorbid substance abuse disorder or depression.[9,23]

Antidepressants

In general, antidepressants are considered less effective than stimulants in the management of ADHD in children; hence, they are considered as second- or third-line options or as adjunctive therapy.[2,5,9] Antidepressants may benefit patients with comorbid conditions such as depression, anxiety, enuresis or tic disorders.[16]

Bupropion, a norepinephrine and dopamine reuptake inhibitor, has been found to be moderately effective for the treatment of ADHD in both children and adults.[16,25,26,27,28] Some evidence suggests **venlafaxine,** a serotonin and norepinephrine reuptake inhibitor, may be helpful in the management of ADHD.[9,23,31] To date, there is insufficient evidence from randomized, double-blind trials to recommend its use in the treatment of ADHD.

Many controlled trials have examined the effects of TCAs such as **desipramine**, **imipramine** and **nortriptyline** in the short-term treatment of ADHD.[24] TCAs are less effective than stimulants at reducing the core symptoms of ADHD. Despite the fact that most TCA studies have significant design flaws (e.g., open label, not randomized), the benefits of TCAs may outweigh their risks in some patients who cannot take stimulants, atomoxetine or bupropion.[6,9,16,24]

$Alpha_2$-Adrenergic Agonists

$Alpha_2$-adrenergic agonists, such as **clonidine**, are used as second- or third-line agents for ADHD.[2,9,30] They primarily reduce symptoms of aggression, impulsivity, overarousal and hyperactivity, and have minimal benefit on symptoms of inattention or poor concentration.[30] When used concurrently with stimulants, they often target sleep disruptions, aggression, impulsivity, comorbid oppositional defiant disorder and tics.[6,16]

Antipsychotics

Low doses of atypical antipsychotics (e.g., **risperidone**) may be moderately effective for the behavioural symptoms seen in hyperactive and impulsive children when stimulants alone are ineffective or not tolerated;[5] they have little effect on inattention. Atypical antipsychotics are also sometimes initiated to decrease behaviours seen in children with comorbid conduct disorder, oppositional defiant disorder, autistic disorders, impulse control disorders and Tourette's syndrome.

Some of these agents may negatively affect cognition in patients with ADHD. A systematic review of the role of atypical antipsychotics (primarily risperidone) could not identify a benefit of these agents in patients with ADHD.[29]

Natural Health Products

Though evidence from well-designed randomized trials is sparse, various natural health products (e.g., herbs, vitamins or nutritional supplements) have been tried on the basis of their traditional uses. For example, agents with possible anxiolytic, sedative or hypnotic effects (e.g., chamomile, valerian, melatonin) have been used in children who are restless, anxious or having sleep difficulties.[11] These herbs may play a role in calming a hyperactive child or promoting sleep in children with ADHD and insomnia. Other agents of interest include antioxidants such as blue-green algae, various B vitamins, ginkgo biloba, pycnogenol and evening primrose oil (essential fatty acids). In general, concerns regarding efficacy and quality of natural health products make it difficult to support their use in place of existing prescription medications; however, after evaluating potential drug interactions and clinical risks, it may be possible to use some of these products safely in conjunction with approved therapies.

Therapeutic Tips

- When selecting an appropriate pharmacologic regimen, consider the child's daily schedule, predominant ADHD symptoms, likelihood of adherence, patient preferences (including medication cost) and risk of adverse effects.
- Although more common with methylphenidate sustained-release (e.g., Ritalin SR), a small portion of patients prescribed long-acting stimulants such as Concerta, Biphentin or Adderall XR may require additional immediate-release stimulants in the afternoon to help with homework and control of early evening symptoms.
- Sustained-release or long-acting stimulant *tablets* cannot be crushed or chewed. Adderall XR, Dexedrine spansules and Biphentin capsules can be opened and sprinkled on soft foods (e.g., yogurt, applesauce). This may be helpful for younger children unable to swallow certain medications.
- Children taking stimulants should be monitored for potential growth suppression by recording their weight and height at baseline and

monthly during their stimulant therapy. These measurements can be compared with established norms for a given child's age/gender and plotted on growth charts.

- Extended "drug holidays" (e.g., several months over the summer holidays) from stimulants are generally not recommended in children with moderate-to-severe ADHD symptoms who are doing well on the stimulant. The return of symptoms and resultant effects on behaviour and self-esteem do not typically outweigh the risks of taking the medication. Drug holidays (at times of low environmental stresses), may be useful when adverse effects associated with stimulants (e.g., growth suppression or weight loss > 10% of initial body weight) are present or when attempting to assess the continued benefit of the stimulant.
- Some clinicians raise concerns about the risk of substance abuse with stimulants. Though this can occur, trials evaluating substance abuse in those with ADHD have found that adequately treated children with ADHD have a lower risk of substance abuse later in life when compared to those who are untreated.[30]

Figure 1: **Management of Attention-Deficit Hyperactivity Disorder[9]**

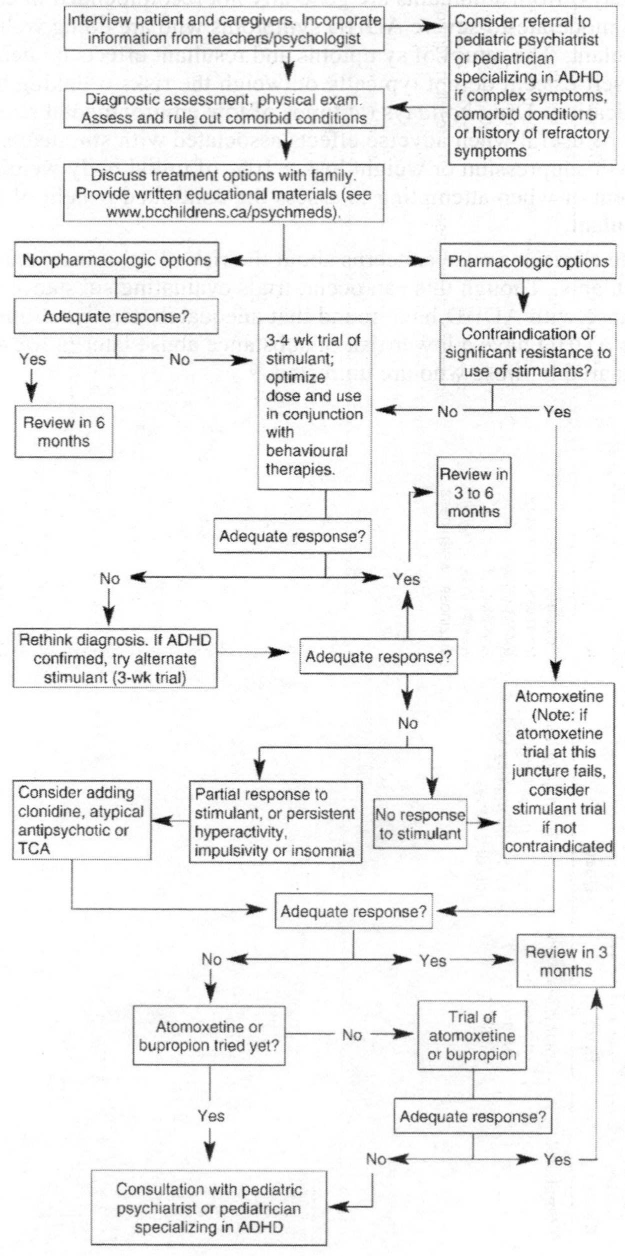

Table 2: Drugs Used in Attention-Deficit Hyperactivity Disorder

Class	Drug	Dose	Adverse Effects	Drug Interactions	Comments	Cost[a]
Stimulants	*methylphenidate immediate-release tablets* Ritalin, generics	Initial: 0.3 mg/kg/day Usual: 0.15–1 mg/kg/day **or** 10–60 mg/day in 1–3 divided doses	**Common, usually transient—continue therapeutic trial:** anorexia, insomnia, weight loss, irritability, dizziness, weepiness, headache, abdominal pain. **Transient—stop and re-evaluate:** zombie-like effects, psychotic reactions (e.g., hallucinations), agitation, tachycardia, hypertension, growth failure, rebound hyperactivity, leukopenia, blood dyscrasias. **Overdose symptoms—stop and retitrate:** "glassy eyes," insomnia, hyperactivity. **Significant:** sudden cardiac death reported; neurologic symptoms; exacerbation of tics; avoid in patients with a history of cardiovascular	*Stimulants:* Avoid concurrent use with MAOIs (phenelzine, tranylcypromine) and linezolid. Concurrent use of moclobemide can increase hypertensive effect of stimulant. Concurrent use of sibutramine may cause hypertension and tachycardia. Concurrent use of theophylline may ↑ risk of tachycardia, palpitations, dizziness, weakness. *Methylphenidate:* May ↑ plasma levels of phenytoin, TCAs, phenobarbital. Carbamazepine: ↓ plasma levels of methylphenidate. ↓ metabolism of warfarin, increased INR.	Last daily dose should be given before 4 p.m. to avoid insomnia. Doses greater than 60 mg/day usually do not result in additional efficacy in children. Pharmacokinetics reflect wide individual variations; strict weight-based dosing may not be predictive of clinical effect; titrate dose against response. Potential for abuse; use cautiously, especially in adolescents.	$$

(cont'd)

Table 2: **Drugs Used in Attention-Deficit Hyperactivity Disorder** *(cont'd)*

Class	Drug	Dose	Adverse Effects	Drug Interactions	Comments	Cost[a]
			conduction disturbances, hypertension, acute psychotic episodes and hyperthyroidism. If seizures occur, or if frequency increases in patient with controlled epilepsy, stop and re-evaluate.			
	methylphenidate sustained-release tablets Ritalin SR, generics	20 mg/dose, given 8 hours apart	See methylphenidate immediate-release.	See methylphenidate immediate-release.	See methylphenidate immediate-release.	$
	methylphenidate controlled-release capsules Biphentin	10–60 mg once daily in a.m.	See methylphenidate immediate-release.	See methylphenidate immediate-release.	See methylphenidate immediate-release. Capsule contents can be sprinkled on soft food such as applesauce, ice cream or yogurt.	$$$$
	methylphenidate bilayer controlled-release tablets Concerta	18–54 mg once daily in a.m.	See methylphenidate immediate-release.	See methylphenidate immediate-release.	See methylphenidate immediate-release. Consult product monograph for dosage conversion from other methylphenidate formulations.	$$$$$

Class	Drug	Dose	Adverse Effects	Drug Interactions	Comments	Cost[a]
	dextroamphetamine immediate-release tablets Dexedrine	0.15 mg/kg/day **or** 2.5–40 mg/day in 1–3 divided doses	See methylphenidate immediate-release.	See methylphenidate immediate-release. *Dextroamphetamine:* Acidifying agents (e.g., fruit juices, ascorbic acid) can ↓ absorption and ↓ elimination of dextroamphetamine. Alkalinizing agents (e.g, sodium bicarbonate) can ↑ absorption and ↑ elimination of dextroamphetamine.		$$
	dextroamphetamine sustained-release spansules Dexedrine	0.15 mg/kg **or** 10–40 mg once daily in a.m.	See methylphenidate immediate-release.	See methylphenidate immediate-release. See dextroamphetamine immediate-release.	Capsule contents can be sprinkled on soft food such as applesauce, ice cream or yogurt.	$$$$
	mixed salts amphetamine extended-release capsules Adderall XR	10–30 mg once daily in a.m.	See methylphenidate immediate-release.	See methylphenidate immediate-release.	Capsule contents can be sprinkled on applesauce and eaten immediately without chewing; doses should not be divided or stored.	$$$$$

(cont'd)

Table 2: **Drugs Used in Attention-Deficit Hyperactivity Disorder** *(cont'd)*

Class	Drug	Dose	Adverse Effects	Drug Interactions	Comments	Cost[a]
Norepinephrine Reuptake Inhibitors	*atomoxetine* Strattera	Children ≤ 70 kg: 0.5 mg/kg/day × 10 days, then 0.8 mg/kg/day × 10 days, then 1–1.2 mg/kg/day > 70 kg: 40 mg/day x 10 days, then 60 mg/day x 10 days, then increase to target of 80 mg/day if necessary Administer as one dose in a.m. or 2 divided doses in a.m. and late afternoon. Max 100 mg/day	Headaches, rhinorrhea, upper abdominal pain, nausea, sedation, vomiting, decreased appetite, dizziness, fatigue, emotional lability and small increases in heart rate and blood pressure. Significant: suicidal ideation, sudden cardiac death, liver toxicity, exacerbation of tics.	Inhibitors of CYP2D6 such as paroxetine, fluoxetine or quinidine can ↑ plasma levels. Some "slow metabolizers" (e.g., some Asian populations) may have extended elimination half-lives. Concurrent use of salbutamol may ↑ heart rate.	Dosing based on patient's weight. Requires 3–4 weeks to see beneficial effects.	$$$$$
Antidepressants, Atypical	*bupropion* Wellbutrin SR, generics	Initial: 2–3 mg/kg/day Usual: 200–300 mg/day in 2 divided doses. Single doses should not exceed 150 mg	Agitation, dry mouth, insomnia, headache, constipation, nausea, vomiting, nervousness, dizziness, sweating, hypertension and tachycardia. Significant: suicidal ideation, seizures (0.5–1% incidence). Avoid in patients with a history of seizure disorders, eating disorders or significant head injury. Seizure risk ↑ with doses > 300 mg/day.	Inducers of CYP2D6 or CYP3A4 (e.g., carbamazepine, phenytoin, rifampin) may ↓ plasma level of bupropion and ↑ level of hydroxybupropion (active metabolite). Plasma concentration of venlafaxine or TCAs such as imipramine, desipramine and nortriptyline may ↑ due to inhibition of CYP2D6 by bupropion. Avoid use with MAOIs; may cause mania, excitation, hyperpyrexia.	It may take 2–4 weeks before effects on ADHD symptoms are seen. Be vigilant for initiation of other medications that can decrease the seizure threshold (e.g., chloroquine, theophylline, tramadol, ciprofloxacin).	$$$$

Class	Drug	Dose	Adverse Effects	Drug Interactions	Comments	Cost[a]
Tricyclic Antidepressants	*desipramine* Norpramin, generics	6–12 y: 10–20 mg/day in 3–4 divided doses Adolescents: 30–50 mg/day in 3–4 divided doses Usual max 150 mg/day	Postural hypotension, anticholinergic effects (dry mouth, constipation, urinary retention), dizziness, nausea, drowsiness, weakness, tremor, weight gain, asymptomatic ECG changes and tachycardia. Significant: arrhythmias (potential for fatal arrhythmias in overdose). Where possible, avoid in patients with a history of cardiovascular conduction disturbances, urinary retention, seizure disorders, hyperthyroidism.	Avoid with MAOIs—may cause mania, excitation, hyperpyrexia. Inducers of CYP2D6 or CYP3A4 (e.g., carbamazepine, phenytoin, rifampin) may ↓ effect. Inhibitors of CYP2D6 or CYP3A4 (e.g., clarithromycin, erythromycin, grapefruit juice, fluoxetine, paroxetine) may ↑ effect and toxicity.	May require 3–4 weeks to see beneficial effects.	$$
	imipramine Tofranil, generics	6–12 y: 10–20 mg/day in 3–4 divided doses Adolescents: 30–50 mg/day in 3–4 divided doses Usual max 150 mg/day	See desipramine.	See desipramine.	See desipramine.	$

(cont'd)

Table 2: **Drugs Used in Attention-Deficit Hyperactivity Disorder** *(cont'd)*

Class	Drug	Dose	Adverse Effects	Drug Interactions	Comments	Cost[a]
	nortriptyline Aventyl, generics	6–12 y: 10–20 mg/day in 3–4 divided doses Adolescents: 30–50 mg/day in 3–4 divided doses Usual max 150 mg/day	See desipramine.	See desipramine.	See desipramine.	$
Alpha$_2$-adrenergic Agonists	*clonidine* Catapres, Dixarit, generics	Initial: 0.05–0.1 mg/day Usual: 3–10 µg/kg/day (0.05–0.4 mg/day), once daily or in divided doses	Hypotension, sedation and dizziness common initially; dry mouth; could exacerbate depression.	Avoid concurrent use with tricyclic antidepressants. Additive effects with other CNS depressants such as ethanol.	Caution in patients with cardiovascular disease or depression.	$$
Antipsychotics, atypical	*risperidone* ❥ Risperdal Preparations, generics	Initial: 0.25–0.5 mg at bedtime; increase at weekly intervals by 0.5 mg/day in 2 divided doses as needed Usual maintenance dose 0.75–1.5 mg/day	Weight gain, drowsiness, headache, orthostatic hypotension, dyspepsia, dose-related extrapyramidal effects; hyperprolactinemia.	Inhibitors of CYP2D6 or CYP3A4 (e.g., clarithromycin, erythromycin, grapefruit juice, fluoxetine, paroxetine) may ↑ effect and toxicity; inducers of these isoenzymes (e.g., carbamazepine, phenytoin, rifampin) may ↓ effect.	Oral liquid should not be mixed with cola or tea; may be mixed with water, orange juice or low-fat milk.	$$

[a] Cost of 30-day supply of mean dosage; based on 35 kg body weight; includes drug cost only.
❥ Dosage adjustment may be required in renal impairment; see Appendix I
Abbreviations: TCAs = tricyclic antidepressants; MAOIs = monoamine oxidase inhibitors
Legend: $ < $15 $$ $15–30 $$$ $30–45 $$$$ $45–60 $$$$$ > $60

Suggested Readings

Canadian Attention Deficit Hyperactivity Disorder Resource Alliance (CADDRA). *Canadian ADHD practice guidelines*. Toronto (ON): CADDRA; 2006. Available from: http://www.caddra.ca/english/phys_guide.html Accessed March 14, 2007.

Jensen PS, Hinshaw SP, Swanson JM et al. Findings from the NIMH Multimodal Treatment Study of ADHD (MTA): implications and applications for primary care providers. *J Dev Behav Pediatr* 2001;22(1):60-73.

Pliszka SR, Crismon ML, Hughes CW et al. The Texas Children's Medication Algorithm Project: revision of the algorithm for pharmacotherapy of attention-deficit/hyperactivity disorder. *J Am Acad Child Adolesc Psychiatry* 2006;45(6):642-57.

Rappley MD. Clinical practice. Attention deficit-hyperactivity disorder. *N Engl J Med* 2005;352(2):165-73.

References

1. [No authors listed]. Clinical practice guideline: diagnosis and evaluation of the child with attention-deficit/hyperactivity disorder. American Academy of Pediatrics. *Pediatrics* 2000;105(5):1158-70.
2. American Academy of Pediatrics. Subcommittee on Attention-Deficit/Hyperactivity Disorder and Committee on Quality Improvement. Clinical practice guideline: treatment of the school-aged child with attention-deficit/hyperactivity disorder. *Pediatrics* 2001;108(4):1033-44.
3. American Psychiatric Association. Task Force on DSM-IV. *Diagnostic and statistical manual of mental disorders: DSM-IV-TR*. Washington (DC): American Psychiatric Association; 2000.
4. Rappley MD. Clinical practice. Attention deficit-hyperactivity disorder. *N Engl J Med* 2005;352(2):165-73.
5. Canadian Attention Deficit Hyperactivity Disorder Resource Alliance (CADDRA). *Canadian ADHD practice guidelines*. Toronto (ON): CADDRA; 2006. Available from: http://www.caddra.ca/english/phys_guide.html Accessed March 14, 2007.
6. Linnet KM, Dalsgaard S, Obel C et al. Maternal lifestyle factors in pregnancy risk of attention deficit hyperactivity disorder and associated behaviors: review of the current evidence. *Am J Psychiatry* 2003;160(6):1028-40.
7. Daley KC. Update on attention-deficit/hyperactivity disorder. *Curr Opin Pediatr* 2004;16(2):217-26.
8. [No authors listed]. A 14-month randomized clinical trial of treatment strategies for attention-deficit/hyperactivity disorder. The MTA Cooperative Group. Multimodal Treatment Study of Children with ADHD. *Arch Gen Psychiatry* 1999;56(12):1073-86.
9. Pliszka SR, Crismon ML, Hughes CW et al. The Texas Children's Medication Algorithm Project: revision of the algorithm for pharmacotherapy of attention-deficit/hyperactivity disorder. *J Am Acad Child Adolesc Psychiatry* 2006;45(6):642-57.
10. Abikoff H, Hechtman L, Klein RG et al. Symptomatic improvement in children with ADHD treated with long-term methylphenidate and multimodal psychosocial treatment. *J Am Acad Child Adolesc Psychiatry* 2004;43(7):802-11.
11. Chan E. The role of complementary and alternative medicine in attention-deficit hyperactivity disorder. *J Dev Behav Pediatr* 2002;23(1 Suppl):S37-45.
12. Bernard-Bonnin A. The use of alternative therapies in treating children with attention deficit hyperactivity disorder. Canadian Paediatric Society Position Statement. *Paediatrics & Child Health* 2002;7(10):710-8. Available from: http://www.cps.ca/english/statements/PP/pp02-03.htm Accessed March 14, 2007.
13. Fox DJ, Tharp DF, Fox LC. Neurofeedback: an alternative and efficacious treatment for attention deficit hyperactivity disorder. *Appl Psychophysiol Biofeedback* 2005;30(4):365-73.
14. Biederman J, Swanson JM, Wigal SB et al. Efficacy and safety of modafinil film-coated tablets in children and adolescents with attention-deficit/hyperactivity disorder: results of a randomized, double-blind, placebo-controlled, flexible-dose study. *Pediatrics* 2005;116(6):e777-84.
15. Biederman J, Swanson JM, Wigal SB et al. A comparison of once-daily modafinil in children with attention-deficit/hyperactivity disorder: a randomized, double-blind, and placebo-controlled study. *J Clin Psychiatry* 2006;67(5):727-35.
16. Banaschewski T, Roessner V, Dittman RW et al. Non-stimulant medications in the treatment of ADHD. *Eur Child Adolesc Psychiatry* 2004;13(Suppl 1):102-16

17. Michelson D, Faries D, Wernicke J et al. Atomoxetine in the treatment of children and adolescents with attention-deficit/hyperactivity disorder: a randomized, placebo-controlled, dose-response study. *Pediatrics* 2001;108(5):e83.
18. Biederman J, Heiligenstein JH, Faries D et al. Efficacy of atomoxetine versus placebo in school-age girls with attention-deficit/hyperactivity disorder. *Pediatrics* 2002;110(6):e75.
19. Michelson D, Allen AJ, Busner J et al. Once-daily atomoxetine treatment for children and adolescents with attention deficit hyperactivity disorder: a randomized, placebo-controlled study. *Am J Psychiatry* 2002;159(11):1896-901.
20. Spencer T, Heiligenstein JH, Biederman J et al. Results from 2 proof-of-concept, placebo-controlled studies of atomoxetine in children with attention-deficit/hyperactivity disorder. *J Clin Psychiatry* 2002;63(12):1140-7.
21. Michelson D, Adler L, Spencer T et al. Atomoxetine in adults with ADHD: two randomized, placebo-controlled studies. *Biol Psychiatry* 2003;53(2):112-20.
22. Kelsey DK, Sumner CR, Casat CD et al. Once-daily atomoxetine treatment for children with attention-deficit/hyperactivity disorder, including an assessment of evening and morning behavior: a double-blind, placebo-controlled trial. *Pediatrics* 2004;114(1):e1-8
23. Bezchlibnyk-Butler KZ, Virani AS, editors. *Clinical handbook of psychotropic drugs for children and adolescents*. Cambridge (MA): Hogrefe & Huber; 2004.
24. Spencer T, Biederman J, Wilens T et al. Pharmacotherapy of attention-deficit hyperactivity disorder across the life cycle. *J Am Acad Child Adolesc Psychiatry* 1996;35(4):409-32.
25. Casat CD, Pleasants DZ, Van Wyck Fleet J. A double-blind trial of bupropion in children with attention deficit disorder. *Psychopharmacol Bull* 1987;23(1):120-2.
26. Barrickman LL, Perry PJ, Allen AJ et al. Bupropion versus methylphenidate in the treatment of attention-deficit hyperactivity disorder. *J Am Acad Child Adolesc Psychiatry* 1995;34(5):649-57.
27. Kuperman S, Perry PJ, Gaffney GR et al. Bupropion SR vs. methylphenidate vs. placebo for attention deficit hyperactivity disorder in adults. *Ann Clin Psychiatry* 2001 Sep;13(3):129-34
28. Wilens TE, Spencer TJ, Biederman J et al. A controlled clinical trial of bupropion for attention deficit hyperactivity disorder in adults. *Am J Psychiatry* 2001;158(2):282-8.
29. Einarson TR, Iskedjian M. *Novel antipsychotics for patients with attention-deficit hyperactivity disorder: a systematic review*. Ottawa (ON): Canadian Coordinating Office for Health Technology Assessment (CCOHTA); 2001.
30. Wilens TE, Faraone SV, Biederman J et al. Does stimulant therapy of attention-deficit/hyperactivity disorder beget later substance abuse? A meta-analytic review of the literature. *Pediatrics* 2003;111(1):179-85.
31. Motavalli Mukaddes N, Abali O. Venlafaxine in children and adolescents with attention deficit hyperactivity disorder. *Psychiatry Clin Neurosci* 2004;58(1):92-5.

CHAPTER 4
Dementia

Kenneth Rockwood, MD, FRCPC and
Terry Chisholm, MD, FRCPC

Dementia is a syndrome of acquired global impairment of cognitive function sufficient to interfere with normal activities. The most common causes are Alzheimer's disease, vascular dementia, a mixture of the two, Lewy body dementia and frontotemporal dementia. Dementia is also recognized as a complication of Parkinson's disease. Dementias are progressive, deteriorating illnesses in which treatment options are different at different stages of the illness (see Table 1).

Table 1: **Stages of Dementia**

Stage	Characteristics	Corresponding FAST rating[a]
Preclinical	Subjective complaints accompanied by very mild objective complaints; functioning is unimpaired. This stage has considerable overlap with normal aging and may or may not progress to dementia.	3
Mild	Impaired instrumental activities of daily living (IADL), e.g., driving, medication use, finances, use of telephone and housekeeping	4
Moderate	In addition to IADL impairment, personal activities of daily living (PADL) such as bathing, feeding, dressing and toileting can be done only with prompting	5
Severe	PADL cannot be done even with prompting	6
Terminal	Patients must be fed and become immobile and mute	7

[a] Included because many jurisdictions use the Functional Assessment Staging Tool (FAST)[1] in adjudicating reimbursement for dementia medications.

Goals of Therapy

- Alter the natural disease progression to meet patients' and caregivers' goals
- Treat cognitive, behavioural and psychological symptoms
- Alleviate caregiver burden
- Minimize medication side effects

Investigations

Dementia

- Thorough history with attention to memory impairment and potentially reversible causes. Cognitive impairment can be assessed using the Mini-Mental State Examination (MMSE);[2] functional disability is measured with tools such as the Disability Assessment for Dementia[3] or the Functional Assessment Staging Tool (FAST)[1]

- Medication history to rule out drug-induced cognitive impairment, e.g., anticholinergics
- Physical examination to identify the cause, which is rarely reversible[4]
- Laboratory tests: CBC, electrolytes, kidney function, TSH, calcium, blood glucose. Homocysteine is increasingly recognized as a marker of dementia risk, but its routine assessment is not yet recommended
- CT scan for young patients (< 60 years), new onset, rapid progression, post-head injury, focal or lateralizing signs, history of cancer, use of anticoagulants, early urinary incontinence and gait disorder or unusual cognitive symptoms

Behavioural and Psychological Symptoms (Figure 1)

Behavioural and psychological symptoms (BPS) are seen in three contexts:

- they can be part of the illness. These problems usually occur predictably, according to the stage of dementia. In Alzheimer's disease, for example, depression and apathy often occur early, when the dementia is mild. In contrast, psychosis and agitated behaviour tend to occur in the moderate to later stages. If agitation is seen early, more aggressive medical investigation is warranted.
- they can be related to psychiatric problems that predate the dementia, such as depression, anxiety, psychosis and personality issues. Elicit a careful psychiatric history; psychiatric syndromes that occurred earlier in the patient's life may recur and can guide treatment.
- they can have a delirium-like presentation, which usually indicates a medical and/or environmental precipitant[6] (Figure 1). The diagnostic approach in the setting of delirium includes:
  - history of concomitant symptoms, environmental precipitants or medication changes
  - examination for focal or lateralizing signs or meningismus; both sets of signs will usually be absent. Toxic or metabolic causes should be evaluated, as well as signs of infection or congestive heart failure.
  - laboratory tests: CBC, electrolytes, urea, creatinine, glucose, urinalysis, chest radiograph

Note: It is unusual for delusions or hallucinations to occur early. When this happens, it can indicate that the person is suffering from Lewy body dementia, which means that antipsychotics should be avoided, as they can precipitate an antipsychotic sensitivity syndrome.

Therapeutic Choices

Nonpharmacologic Choices

- Nonpharmacologic approaches are first-line therapy for behavioural symptoms of dementia, especially agitation; they are often sufficient to make a noticeable improvement in the target symptoms. Strategies include:
  - clear and respectful communication
  - changes to the physical environment such as ensuring safe places to wander
  - caregiver strategies such as distraction, avoiding confrontation and providing stimulation and structure
  - a multidisciplinary approach with involvement of services such as Psychology and Recreation Therapy, which can decrease agitation through activity programs and other behavioural interventions
- Involve family and other caregivers in all nonpharmacologic therapy.
- Before disease progression hampers competence, establish advance health care directives and durable powers of attorney.
- Because individuals with dementia are at increased risk for accidents (falls, burns), remove environmental hazards.
- Counsel patients against driving after the initial stages of disease.
- Caregiver stress is common and should be anticipated. Support groups, such as those coordinated by the Alzheimer Society of Canada (www.alzheimer.ca), can be helpful in mitigating feelings of burden.
- Nonpharmacologic measures should not be considered an "either/or" option with respect to pharmacologic therapy; often they allow pharmacologic therapy to be used more sparingly.[7]

Pharmacologic Choices (Table 2)

Alzheimer's Disease

Cholinesterase Inhibitors

The **cholinesterase inhibitors**, donepezil, rivastigmine and galantamine, are the mainstays of treatment for cognitive and functional symptoms, and may have a role with BPS, especially in mild-to-moderate dementia. Although they have distinct structures and modes of action, in the absence of blinded, controlled, head-to-head trials, they seem to be of equal efficacy. While clinically detectable, benefits are small to moderate on average,[8] and in many patients consist mainly of disease stabilization. Treatment effects and side effects can vary among individuals—patients who do not respond to one might respond to another. For each of the drugs, higher doses have better outcomes. The usual treatment response is that some symptoms improve, others stabilize and still others worsen. Reduction in repetitive questioning is a common treatment goal in patients with mild-to-moderate Alzheimer's disease and usually corresponds to a generally positive treatment effect.[9]

Target symptoms must be defined and monitored. Effectiveness is considered to be either improvement or no change in target symptoms. A strategy of setting individual goals for treatment and measuring their attainment at regular intervals has been shown to detect a range of beneficial treatment effects.[9,10] Follow-up to detect side effects is advised two weeks after initiating therapy or increasing dosage, then every three months to monitor treatment effects.

Most trials have had double-blind conditions for only 3 to 6 months, except for two 12-month[11,12] and one 24-month[13] placebo-controlled trial of **donepezil**. Donepezil was shown to be effective in 3- to 6-month trials in patients with *mild-to-moderate* Alzheimer's disease (MMSE scores 10 to 26).[14] It has also demonstrated efficacy in *moderate-to-severe* Alzheimer's disease,[14,15] although this indication has yet to be approved. The initial dose is 5 mg per day, often taken at night, but it can be taken in the morning if sleep disturbances occur. Generally, after 28 days try increasing the dose to 10 mg/day.

For **rivastigmine**, the initial dose is 1.5 mg po BID; after 30 days, the dose is doubled to 3 mg po BID, which is the minimum effective dose.[16] The maximum dose is 6 mg po BID, although a dose-response relationship has not been demonstrated consistently. For some patients, TID dosing is most effective, with the same maximum total daily dose of 12 mg.[17] Rivastigmine was effective in a double-blind trial in patients with Lewy body dementia,[18] and for patients with dementia associated with Parkinson's disease.[19]

Galantamine has been shown to be effective in several studies,[10,20] including one in patients with mixed Alzheimer's disease and vascular dementia.[21] A Canadian multicentre trial suggests that patients treated with galantamine were more likely to meet clinical treatment goals than those on placebo.[10] Galantamine is now available as an extended-release formulation administered once daily, not BID as the immediate-release formulation is administered. The recommended starting dose is 8 mg/day, increasing to 16 mg/day after 30 days. The dose can be increased to 24 mg/day if necessary.

N-methyl-D-aspartate (NMDA) Receptor Antagonists

The NMDA receptor antagonist **memantine** is also used to treat dementia. Its proposed mechanism of action is to block glutamate-induced neuronal excitotoxicity, which is implicated as a final common pathway in neuronal death. Meta-analyses suggest memantine has a small to moderately beneficial effect on cognition, ADL and behavior in moderate-to-severe Alzheimer's disease at 6 months.[22,23] The Cochrane review is more guarded.[24] A trial of memantine with donepezil suggested the combination added benefit in patients with moderate-to-severe Alzheimer's disease.[25] The generalizability of this remains unclear, and whether combination therapy has any role in mild disease is not yet known.

If memantine is used in patients in whom a greater response is sought than has been achieved with cholinesterase inhibitors, or when cholinesterase inhibitors are contraindicated or poorly tolerated (e.g., GI side effects), the approach of setting target symptoms and monitoring carefully remains the best standard for individualized clinical decision making. The initial dose of 5 mg daily should be increased by 5 mg daily at weekly intervals to a maximum of 10 mg BID. Reduce the dose to 5 mg BID in patients with mild-to-moderate renal failure. Dosage reduction may also be necessitated by other conditions (e.g., renal tubular acidosis, some urinary tract infections) or concomitant drug therapy (e.g., carbonic anhydrase inhibitors), in accordance with the manufacturer's product monograph.

Other Therapies

Despite many trials, clinically significant beneficial effects of **ergoloid mesylates** in Alzheimer's disease have not been demonstrated.

Vitamin E, in a dose of 2000 IU per day of alpha-tocopherol, appeared to slow the progression of dementia.[26] Few side effects were apparent beyond an increased incidence of falls. Given more recent data suggesting additional adverse effects or no benefit in a range of conditions, use of high-dose vitamin E is not recommended and any supplementation might be questionable.[27]

In the largest study of disease progression to date, **selegiline** proved more effective than placebo, but no more effective than Vitamin E alone in delaying death, institutionalization and progression to severe dementia.[26]

Vascular Dementia

With the aim of slowing disease progression, vascular risk factors should be modified, particularly to ensure good control of hypertension (< 140/80 mm Hg), and it seems reasonable to use lipid-lowering agents for dyslipidemias (see Chapter 32 and Chapter 31).

Dementia with Lewy Bodies and the Dementia of Parkinson's Disease

Patients with dementia with Lewy bodies often present with hallucinations and early parkinsonism, which can precede cognitive impairment. This psychosis can be worsened by antipsychotics.[28] Patients with dementia with Lewy bodies have severe antipsychotic sensitivity reactions which can precipitate irreversible parkinsonism, further impair consciousness and induce autonomic disturbances. These reactions occur in 40 to 50% of patients and increase mortality.

Clinical trial data for the use of **rivastigmine**[18] demonstrate that small doses can sometimes be dramatically effective, and leave the potential for subsequent dose titration over time. Prescribing considerations are similar to those for Alzheimer's disease. Similarly, a placebo-controlled trial in the treatment of patients with Parkinson's disease who had been diagnosed with dementia found statistically significant improvement in rivastigmine-treated patients for cognition, function and behaviour.[19] The size of the treatment effect appears to be comparable with that reported for cholinesterase inhibitors in Alzheimer's disease.

Prevention of Dementia

Cardiovascular risk factors increase the chance of all causes of late-life dementia, including Alzheimer's disease. Evidence from the Syst-Eur trial suggests that the incidence of dementia can be halved in elderly patients treated for systolic hypertension.[29] Despite the failure of some recent trials, there remains some evidence that long-term use of NSAIDs might be protective for Alzheimer's disease,[30] although their routine use is not recommended due to their associated adverse effects. There is not enough evidence to support the use of lipid-lowering agents, particularly statins, for prevention of dementia alone.[31] Prior enthusiasm for the use of estrogen, based on observational studies, has not been sustained by the experimental evidence, which on balance suggests net harm.

Behavioural and Psychological Symptoms (BPS)

Antidepressants

Many patients in the early stages of dementia suffer from depression. Occasionally, depression can manifest with prominent cognitive impairment. Previously known as pseudodementia, it is more commonly referred to as dementia of depression. A significant proportion of these patients will progress to dementia.

Most experienced psychiatrists agree that antidepressants are effective in the treatment of depression of demented patients.[32] However, there are few controlled studies specifically focused on the antidepressant treatment of these patients.

Citalopram and **sertraline**, both SSRIs, have been shown to be more effective than placebo in treating depression in patients with dementia in large, double-blind studies.[33,34,35] Generally, SSRIs are less likely than tricyclic antidepressants (TCAs) to cause anticholinergic side effects or to worsen orthostatic hypotension, which are common and problematic in this population. An increased risk of hyponatremia/SIADH, possibly potentiated by concurrent thiazide use, has been reported in elderly patients taking SSRIs.[36,37] Monitoring of electrolytes is recommended in this setting, because of the effect of hyponatremia on cognitive function. If using a TCA (because of lack of response or sensitivity to an SSRI) choose **desipramine** or **nortriptyline**. Older adults and those with dementia often require longer exposure to antidepressants; trials can be two to three months (see Chapter 5 for dosing information). Although trials should be longer, there are often early indications that the antidepressant is working—there may be improvement in vegetative symptoms such as sleep, appetite and energy before improvement of mood.

There is no evidence from randomized, controlled trials that antidepressants improve nondepression-related BPS in dementia,[35] although antidepressants are commonly used for anxiety (including compulsive behaviour), aggression and sexually inappropriate behaviour.

Antipsychotics

For BPS associated with dementia, especially if psychotic symptoms are evident, the second-generation antipsychotics are considered first-line. As the elderly demented brain is exquisitely sensitive to antipsychotics, initial doses should be small. **Risperidone** can be started at a daily dose of 0.25 mg with 1.0 mg being the optimal dose and 2 mg/day the upper limit.[38,39] **Olanzapine**, started at 2.5 mg and increased to 5 to 10 mg/day, was effective in a placebo-controlled trial in nursing home patients with Alzheimer's disease.[40] A recent review noted that there have been no published RCTs of **clozapine** or **quetiapine** in the treatment of BPS of dementia,[35] although individual considerations sometimes dictate the use of these medications, especially if risperidone or olanzapine have proved to be ineffective or have resulted in side effects. A Cochrane review of **haloperidol** for agitation in dementia recommended against its routine use.[41] Periodic reassessment of BPS is essential; even in the absence of therapy, the natural history is gradual diminution of these problems.

Extrapyramidal side effects are more commonly seen with the first-generation antipsychotics but can occur with the second-generation agents (especially with doses over 2 mg/day of risperidone). Tardive dyskinesia (TD), a potentially irreversible movement disorder, is also more common with first-generation antipsychotics. In patients over 60 years of age, TD occurs in 29% of patients after one year and in up to 63% after three years of use.[43] A shorter study found an incidence of TD of 2.6% with risperidone after nine months.[44] For patients with baseline movement disorders or those who develop EPS with other second-generation antipsychotics, **quetiapine** may be the best option.

The Clinical Antipsychotic Trials of Intervention Effectiveness (CATIE) study[45] found that people with dementia who received a placebo or any of the three atypical antipsychotics (risperidone, olanzapine, quetiapine) discontinued treatment at about the same rate. In general, patients were discontinued from placebo due to lack of effect, or from atypical antipsychotics due to adverse effects, after an average of eight weeks. The CATIE study reminds us to be cautious about using antipsychotics in people with dementia, and especially that they should not be used for a nonspecific complaint of agitation. A dilemma posed by the data is that psychotic symptoms will improve with antipsychotic therapy in some patients with dementia, but which patients will respond cannot be determined in advance. Consequently, a medication trial is needed for patients with psychotic symptoms.

The risk of serious adverse events with all antipsychotics is significant and indicates the need to reserve these drugs for patients with severe symptoms where alternative interventions have failed. An increased risk of stroke and death has been demonstrated with atypical antipsychotics compared to placebo, and observational comparisons suggest the risk may be higher when first-generation antipsychotics are used.[35,42,46]

Trazodone for Behavioural and Sleep Disturbances

Trazodone, a serotonin agonist, is often used successfully to manage agitated behaviour although this is not supported by randomized controlled trials.[35] Start with a low dose of 25 to 50 mg (initially given at night) and increase every few days until the desired effect is achieved (maximum dose of 400 mg/day in divided doses). Trazodone is also used to treat disrupted sleep/wake cycles and "sun downing" (worsening of behaviour as darkness falls).

Benzodiazepines

Data on the efficacy of benzodiazepines for BPS in dementia are conflicting. Although their use can result in oversedation, falls and worsening cognition, benzodiazepines are sometimes indicated for severe agitation, especially when other agents fail. Low doses of a short-acting agent without active metabolites (e.g., **lorazepam** 0.5 to 1 mg, **oxazepam** 5 to 10 mg, **temazepam** 15 mg) may be tried. In an acute situation, to manage severely agitated patients, **lorazepam** 0.5 to 1 mg can be mixed in the same syringe with **haloperidol** (0.5, 1 or 1.5 mg) and given im every eight hours for a maximum of three days. A recent review found only one placebo-controlled trial, in which intramuscular lorazepam was as effective as intramuscular olanzapine.[35]

Others

Beta-blockers (particularly **pindolol**), **carbamazepine, divalproex, lithium** and **buspirone** have been used successfully in case reports, but better evidence is lacking. These agents seem to work best when the problem behaviour mimics the psychiatric syndrome for which the drug is efficacious (e.g., lithium for cycling and manic features).

Therapeutic Tips

- Tips for *monitoring treatment effects* on target symptoms:
  - in certain provinces, drug reimbursement by the provincial formularies relies on monitoring of degrees of improvement or worsening of target symptoms. Symptoms should be described precisely, e.g., instead of "impaired function" state "cannot carry on a conversation; will call only one or two well-known numbers; cannot remember how often he has called." For many symptoms, it is important to quantify how often they occur, e.g., asks the same question up to 20 times per day
  - the most common target symptoms include repetitive questioning, decreased initiative (especially for social and leisure activities and for instrumental activities of daily living), irritability, impaired recent memory and disorientation. A web site

with the most common symptoms of dementia is available (www.dementiaguide.ca). Subscribers to the site can use a symptom tracking option to aid in communicating with their physicians about the effects of treatment.

- Tips for using **antidepressants** in dementia include:
  - start low
  - monitor for side effects
  - increase until the recommended dosage range is reached
  - once the lower end of the recommended dosage range has been reached, continue increasing the dose as side effects permit until the patient benefits, or the maximum dose has been reached; effective doses will be similar to those used to treat younger adults
  - maintain therapy for four to six weeks after the first indication of symptomatic improvement (e.g., improved mood, appetite, sleep or energy) *before* evaluating the success of treatment; symptoms like sleep, appetite and energy may improve earlier in treatment but it make take six to eight weeks for improvement in psychological symptoms such as depressed mood or anhedonia.
- Tips for using **antipsychotics** in dementia include:
  - start low, go slow; keep the dose as low as possible
  - treat to a designated endpoint, usually an improvement in symptoms, not their complete resolution
  - evaluate therapy at one, three and six months, then every six months. Symptoms may subside naturally and the antipsychotic can then be tapered
  - antipsychotic-induced akathisia (increased motor restlessness) may be misinterpreted as lack of drug effect. This can initiate a cycle of increased antipsychotic use and worsening akathisia; the escalating dose of antipsychotic can then result in extrapyramidal rigidity to the point of immobility. Beware the elderly patient with dementia who requires large or increasing doses of antipsychotics, especially if the patient seems even worse after their administration
  - beware of antipsychotic sensitivity, manifested as rigidity, autonomic dysregulation, cognitive deterioration (including delirium, and even coma). This can be a hallmark of Lewy body dementia, and antipsychotics are best avoided in these patients.

Figure 1: **Evaluation and Management of the Elderly Patient with Behavioural Problems**

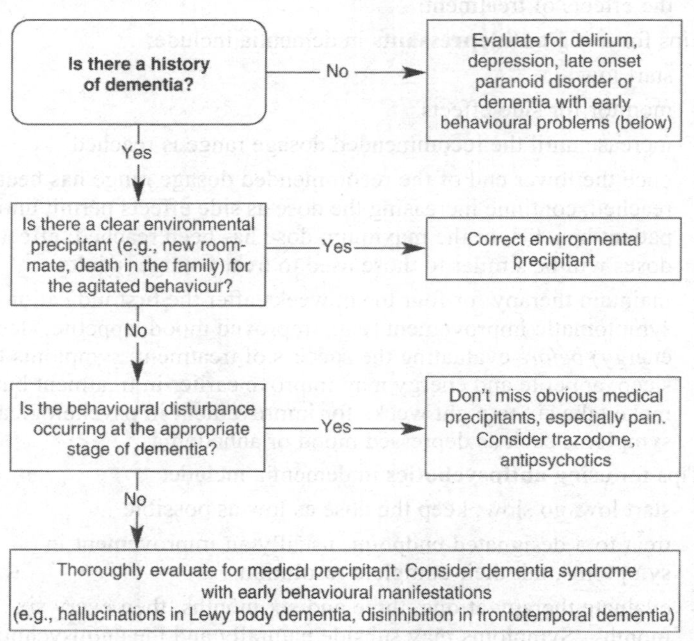

Table 2: **Drugs Used for the Treatment of Dementia**

Class	Drug	Dose	Adverse Effects	Drug Interactions	Cost[a]
Cholinesterase Inhibitors	*donepezil* Aricept, Aricept RDT	Initial: 5 mg/day Target: 10 mg/day Adjust dose after 4 wk	*Cholinesterase inhibitors*: Theoretically, these agents may lower seizure threshold, increase the risk of GI ulceration or bleeding or exacerbate COPD or asthma. *Donepezil*: > 10%: headache, nausea, diarrhea. < 10%: vomiting, anorexia, fatigue, sleep disturbance, syncope, muscle cramps, urinary frequency. Rare: bradycardia, heart block.	*Cholinesterase inhibitors*: Theoretical concern regarding antagonistic effect of combined therapy with cholinesterase inhibitors and drugs with anticholinergic activity, or additive bradycardic effects when combined with beta-blockers or calcium channel blockers; few reports of actual interactions. *Donepezil*: Toxicity may be ↑ by inhibitors of CYP2D6 or CYP3A4 (e.g., paroxetine, erythromycin, prednisone, grapefruit juice). Effectiveness may be ↓ by inducers of CYP2D6 or CYP3A4 (e.g., carbamazepine, phenytoin, rifampin).	$$$
	galantamine extended-release Reminyl ER	Initial: 8 mg daily Target: 16–24 mg daily Adjust dose at 4-wk intervals	See cholinesterase inhibitors. *Galantamine*: > 10%: nausea, vomiting, diarrhea. < 10%: bradycardia, syncope, dizziness, headache, sleep disturbance, fatigue, abdominal pain, weight loss, UTI, urinary incontinence, rhinitis. Rare: heart block, seizures, delirium.	See cholinesterase inhibitors. *Galantamine*: Toxicity may be ↑ by inhibitors of CYP2D6 or CYP3A4 (e.g., paroxetine, erythromycin, prednisone, grapefruit juice). Effectiveness may be ↓ by inducers of CYP2D6 or CYP3A4 (e.g., carbamazepine, phenytoin, rifampin).	$$$

(cont'd)

Table 2: **Drugs Used for the Treatment of Dementia** *(cont'd)*

Class	Drug	Dose	Adverse Effects	Drug Interactions	Cost[a]
	rivastigmine Exelon	Initial: 1.5 mg BID Target: 6–12 mg/day Adjust dose monthly; take with breakfast and dinner	See cholinesterase inhibitors. *Rivastigmine*: > 10%: headache, dizziness, nausea/vomiting, diarrhea, abdominal pain, anorexia. < 10%: fatigue, insomnia, syncope, dyspepsia, weight loss, UTI, rhinitis. Rare: heart block, delirium, seizures.	See cholinesterase inhibitors. *Rivastigmine*: None reported; not metabolized by cytochrome P450 system.	$$$
N-methyl-D-aspartate (NMDA) Receptor Antagonists	*memantine* Ebixa	Initial: 5 mg daily; increase by 5 mg daily, at weekly intervals, to 10 mg BID starting at wk 4	Generally well tolerated; dizziness (7%), headache (6%), confusion (6%), constipation (5%), nausea/vomiting (3%).	None reported. Not affected by cytochrome P450 system. Theoretically, urinary alkalizers (e.g., carbonic anhydrase inhibitors) may decrease the clearance of memantine.	$$$
Antipsychotics	*olanzapine* Zyprexa, Zypreda Zydis	Initial: 2.5 mg/day Target: 5–10 mg/day	Extrapyramidal symptoms, sedation, constipation, GI upset, weight gain, metabolic dysregulation (type 2 diabetes); ↑ risk of stroke and death	Toxicity may be ↑ by inhibitors of CYP3A4 (e.g., erythromycin, clarithromycin, grapefruit juice, prednisone). Effectiveness may be ↓ by inducers of CYP3A4 (e.g., carbamazepine, phenytoin, rifampin).	$$$-$$$$
	quetiapine Seroquel	Initial: 25 mg/day Up to: 150 mg/day	See olanzapine.	Toxicity may be ↑ by inhibitors of CYP2D6 (e.g., paroxetine, quinidine). Effectiveness may be ↓ by inducers of CYP2D6 (e.g., carbamazepine, phenytoin, rifampin).	$-$$

Class	Drug	Dose	Adverse Effects	Drug Interactions	Cost[a]
	risperidone (kidney symbol) Risperdal, Risperdal M-Tab, generics	Initial: 0.25 mg/day Target: 1 mg/day Max: 2 mg/day	See olanzapine.	Toxicity may be ↑ by inhibitors of CYP2D6 or CYP3A4 (e.g., paroxetine, erythromycin, prednisone, grapefruit juice). Effectiveness may be ↓ by inducers of CYP2D6 or CYP3A4 (e.g., carbamazepine, phenytoin, rifampin).	$
Serotonin Agonists	*trazodone* Desyrel, generics	Initial: 25–50 mg QHS Max: 400 mg/day in divided doses	Drowsiness, orthostatic hypotension, nausea, vomiting, headache, dry mouth, priapism (rare).	Toxicity may be ↑ by inhibitors of CYP2D6 or CYP3A4 (e.g., paroxetine, erythromycin, prednisone, grapefruit juice). Effectiveness may be ↓ by inducers of CYP2D6 or CYP3A4 (e.g., carbamazepine, phenytoin, rifampin).	$

[a] Cost of 30-day supply of target dose; includes drug cost only.

(kidney symbol) Dosage adjustment may be required in renal impairment; see Appendix I

Legend: $ < $50 $-$$ < $50–100 $$ $50–100 $$$ $100–150 $$$-$$$$ $100–250 $$$$ $150–250

Suggested Readings

Gauthier S, editor. *Clinical diagnosis and management of Alzheimer's disease.* 3rd ed. Boca Raton (FL): Taylor & Francis; 2006.

Patterson CJ, Gauthier S, Bergman H et al. The recognition, assessment and management of dementing disorders: conclusions from the Canadian Consensus Conference on Dementia. *CMAJ* 1999;160(12 Suppl):S1-S15.

Sink KM, Holden KF, Yaffe K. Pharmacological treatment of neuropsychiatric symptoms of dementia: a review of the evidence. *JAMA* 2005;293(5):596-608.

References

1. Reisberg B. Functional assessment staging (FAST). *Psychopharmacol Bull* 1988;24(4):653-9.
2. Folstein MF, Folstein SE, McHugh PR. "Mini-mental state". A practical method for grading the cognitive state of patients for the clinician. *J Psychiatr Res* 1975;12(3):189-98.
3. Gélinas I, Gauthier L, McIntyre M et al. Development of a functional measure for persons with Alzheimer's disease: the disability assessment for dementia. *Am J Occup Ther* 1999;53(5):471-81.
4. Clarfield AM. The decreasing prevalence of reversible dementias: an updated meta-analysis. *Arch Intern Med* 2003;163(18):2219-29.
5. Jelic V, Kivipelto M, Winblad B. Clinical trials in mild cognitive impairment: lessons for the future. *J Neurol Neurosurg Psychiatr* 2006;77(4):429-38.
6. Fick DM, Agostini JV, Inouye SK. Delirium superimposed on dementia: a systematic review. *J Am Geriatr Soc* 2002;50(10):1723-32.
7. Fossey J, Ballard C, Juszczak E et al. Effect of enhanced psychosocial care on antipsychotic use in nursing home residents with severe dementia: cluster randomised trial. *BMJ* 2006;332(7544):756-61.
8. Rockwood K. Size of the treatment effect on cognition of cholinesterase inhibition in Alzheimer's disease. *J Neurol Neurosurg Psychiatry*. 2004;75(5):677-85.
9. Rockwood K, Fay S, Jarrett P et al. Effect of galantamine on verbal repetition in AD: a secondary analysis of the VISTA trial. *Neurology* 2007;68(14):1116-21.
10. Rockwood K, Fay S, Song X et al. Attainment of treatment goals by people with Alzheimer's disease receiving galantamine: a randomized controlled trial. *CMAJ* 2006;174(8):1099-105.
11. Mohs RC, Doody RS, Morris JC et al. A 1-year, placebo-controlled preservation of function survival study of donepezil in AD patients. *Neurology* 2001;57(3):481-8.
12. Winblad B, Engedal K, Soininen H et al. A 1-year, randomized, placebo-controlled study of donepezil in patients with mild to moderate AD. *Neurology* 2001;57(3):489-95.
13. Courtney C, Farrell, Gray R et al. Long-term donepezil treatment in 565 patients with Alzheimer's disease (AD2000): randomised double-blind trial. *Lancet* 2004;363(9427):2105-15.
14. Birks J, Harvey RJ. Donepezil for dementia due to Alzheimer's disease. *Cochrane Database Syst Rev* 2006;(1):CD001190.
15. Winblad B, Kilander L, Eriksson S et al. Donepezil in patients with severe Alzheimer's disease: double-blind,parallel-group, placebo-controlled study. *Lancet* 2006;367(9516):1057-65.
16. Birks J. Cholinesterase inhibitors for Alzheimer's disease. *Cochrane Database Syst Rev* 2006;(1):CD005593.
17. Feldman HH, Lane R. Rivastigmine: a placebo-controlled trial of BID and TID regimens in patients with Alzheimer's disease. *J Neurol Neurosurg Psychiatry* 2007 Mar 12;[Epub ahead of print].
18. McKeith I, Del Ser T, Spano P et al. Efficacy of rivastigmine in dementia with Lewy bodies: a randomised, double-blind, placebo-controlled international study. *Lancet* 2000;356(9247):2031-6.
19. Emre M, Aarsland D, Albanese A et al. Rivastigmine for dementia associated with Parkinson's disease. *N Engl J Med* 2004;351(24):2509-18.
20. Loy C, Schneider L. Galantamine for Alzheimer's disease and mild cognitive impairment. *Cochrane Database Syst Rev* 2006;(1):CD001747.
21. Erkinjuntti T, Kurz A, Gauthier S et al. Efficacy of galantamine in probable vascular dementia and Alzheimer's disease combined with cerebrovascular disease: a randomised trial. *Lancet* 2002;359(9314):1283-90.
22. Smith M, Wells J, Borrie M. Treatment effect size of memantine therapy in Alzheimer disease and vascular dementia. *Alzheimer Dis Assoc Disord* 2006;20(3):133-7.
23. Winblad B, Jones RW, Wirth Y et al. Memantine in moderate to severe Alzheimer's disease: a meta-analysis of randomised clinical trials. *Dement Geriatr Cogn Disord* 2007;24(1):20-27.
24. McShane R, Areosa Sastre A, Minakaran N. Memantine for dementia. *Cochrane Database Syst Rev* 2006;(2):CD003154.

25. Tariot PN, Farlow MR, Grossberg GT et al. Memantine treatment in patients with moderate to severe Alzheimer disease already receiving donepezil: a randomized controlled trial. *JAMA* 2004;291(3):317-24.
26. Sano M, Ernesto C, Thomas RG et al. A controlled trial of selegiline, alpha-tocopherol, or both as treatment for Alzheimer's disease. The Alzheimer's Disease Cooperative Study. *N Engl J Med* 1997;336(17):1216-22.
27. Bjelakovic G , Nikolova D, Gluud LL et al. Mortality in randomized trials of antioxidant supplements for primary and secondary prevention: systematic review and meta-analysis. *JAMA* 2007;297(8):842-57.
28. McKeith IG , Galasko D, Kosaka K et al. Consensus guidelines for the clinical and pathologic diagnosis of dementia with Lewy bodies (DLB): report of the consortium on DLB international workshop. *Neurology* 1996;47(5):1113-24.
29. Forette F, Seux ML, Staessen JA et al. The prevention of dementia with antihypertensive treatment: new evidence from the Systolic Hypertension in Europe (Syst-Eur) study. *Arch Intern Med* 2002;162(18):2046-52.
30. Etminan M, Gill S, Samii A. Effect of non-steroidal anti-inflammatory drugs on risk of Alzheimer's disease: systematic review and meta-analysis of observational studies. *BMJ* 2003;327(7407):128.
31. Rockwood K. Epidemiological and clinical trials evidence about a preventive role for statins in Alzheimer's disease. *Acta Neurol Scand Suppl* 2006;185:71-7.
32. Swartz M, Barak Y, Mirecki I et al. Treating depression in Alzheimer's disease: integration of differing guidelines. *Int Psychogeriatr* 2000;12(3):353-8.
33. Nyth AL, Gottfries CG. The clinical efficacy of citalopram in treatment of emotional disturbances in dementia disorders. A Nordic multicentre study. *Br J Psychiatry* 1990;157:894-901.
34. Nyth AL, Gottfries CG, Lyby K. A controlled multicenter clinical study of citalopram and placebo in elderly depressed patients with and without concomitant dementia. *Acta Psychiatr Scand* 1992;86(2):138-45.
35. Sink KM, Holden KF, Yaffe K. Pharmacological treatment of neuropsychiatric symptoms of dementia: a review of the evidence. *JAMA* 2005;293(5):596-608.
36. Rosner MH. Severe hyponatremia associated with the combined use of thiazide diuretics and selective serotonin reuptake inhibitors. *Am J Med Sci* 2004;327(2):109-11.
37. Kirby D, Harrigan S, Ames D. Hyponatraemia in elderly psychiatric patients treated with Selective Serotonin Reuptake Inhibitors and venlafaxine: a retrospective controlled study in an inpatient unit. *Int J Geriatr Psychiatry* 2002;17(3):231-7.
38. Katz IR, Jeste DV, Mintzer JE et al. Comparison of risperidone and placebo for psychosis and behavioral disturbances associated with dementia: a randomized, double-blind trial. Risperidone Study Group. *J Clin Psychiatry* 1999;60(2):107-15.
39. De Deyn PP, Rabheru K, Rasmussen A et al. A randomized trial of risperidone, placebo, and haloperidol for behavioral symptoms of dementia. *Neurology* 1999;53(5):946-55.
40. Street JS, Clark WS, Gannon KS et al. Olanzapine treatment of psychotic and behavioral symptoms in patients with Alzheimer disease in nursing care facilities: a double-blind, randomized, placebo-controlled trial. The HGEU Study Group. *Arch Gen Psychiatry* 2000;57(10):968-76.
41. Lonergan E, Luxenberg J, Colford J. Haloperidol for agitation in dementia. *Cochrane Database Syst Rev* 2002(2):CD002852.
42. Gill SS, Rochon PA, Herrmann N et al. Atypical antipsychotic drugs and risk of ischaemic stroke: population based retrospective cohort study. *BMJ* 2005;330(7489):445.
43. Jeste DV. Tardive dyskinesia in older patients. *J Clin Psychiatry* 2000;61(Suppl 4):27-32.
44. Jeste DV, Lacro JP, Bailey A et al. Lower incidence of tardive dyskinesia with risperidone compared with haloperidol in older patients. *J Am Geriatr Soc* 1999;47(6):716-9.
45. Schneider LS, Tariot PN, Dagerman KS et al. Effectiveness of atypical antipsychotic drugs in patients with Alzheimer's disease. *N Engl J Med* 2006;355(15):1525-38.
46. Schneeweiss S, Setoguchi S, Brookhart A et al. Risk of death associated with the use of conventional versus atypical antipsychotic drugs among elderly patients. *CMAJ* 2007;176(5):627-32.

Pharmacoeconomic Considerations: Dementia

Nicole Mittmann, MSc, PhD

Epidemiology	
Country	**Prevalence (%)**
Canada (1991)[1]	8% of the population aged ≥ 65 years
Cost of Illness Data	
Country and Year of Estimate	**Direct Costs[a]**
Canada (1996)[2]	Cost per patient with Alzheimer's disease from a societal perspective: Mild disease: $9451 Mild-to-moderate disease: $16 054 Moderate disease: $25 724 Severe disease: $36 794

Commentary

Dementia has a significant impact on society from an economic perspective. Institutionalization is the largest cost component of direct and indirect care.[2] Unpaid caregiver time accounts for more than half of the overall costs in patients with mild and mild-to-moderate dementia.[2]

A number of cholinesterase inhibitors have been approved for the treatment of dementia. There appears to be no clear advantage of one agent over another.[3] The majority of economic evaluations have considered treatment of mild-to-moderate dementia and been conducted from a societal perspective.[4] Cholinesterase inhibitors are generally considered to be cost-effective compared with placebo in terms of delaying disease progression and the need for home care.[4] The economic benefits of treatment of mild-to-moderate dementia is relatively favourable for choices such as donepezil, rivastigmine and galantamine for improvements in meaningful outcomes such as delaying the progression of symptoms or improvement in cognitive impairment as rated by the Mini Mental State Exam.

Memantine is also considered to be cost-effective in patients with moderate-to-severe dementia, in whom it increases patient autonomy and time spent in an independent state.[5,6]

It should be noted, however, that the literature on the cost-effectiveness of cholinesterase inhibitors is dominated by noncomparative studies sponsored by pharmaceutical manufacturers.

[a] Direct costs include those associated with physician services, nursing care, diagnostic procedures, drugs and hospitalization.

References

1. Canadian Study of Health and Aging Working Group. Canadian Study of Health and Aging: study methods and prevalence of dementia. *CMAJ* 1994; 150(6):899-913.
2. Hux MJ, O'Brien BJ, Iskedjian, M et al. Relation between severity of Alzheimer's disease and costs of caring. *CMAJ* 1998;159(5):457-465.
3. Perras C, Shukla VK, Lessard C, et al. Cholinesterase inhibitors for Alzheimers disease: a systematic review of randomized controlled trials. [Technology report no 58] Ottawa: Canadian Coordinating Office for Health Technology Assessment; 2005.
4. Loveman E, Green C, Kirby J et al. The clinical and cost-effectiveness of donepezil, rivastigmine, galantamine and memantine for Alzheimer's disease. Health Technology Assessment 2006; 10(1): 1-183.
5. Francois C, Sintonen H, Sulkava R et al. Cost-effectiveness of memantine in moderately severe to severe Alzheimer's disease: a markov model in Finland. *Clin Drug Investig* 2004; 24(7): 373-384.
6. Feldman H, Gauthier S, Hecker J et al. Economic evaluation of donepezil in moderate to severe Alzheimer disease. *Neurology* 2004; 63(4): 644-650.

CHAPTER 5

Depression

Sidney H. Kennedy, MD, FRCPC
Sagar V. Parikh, MD, FRCPC and
Beata S. Eisfeld, Hons BSc

Depressive disorders (Table 1) include the specific illnesses of major depressive disorder (MDD), dysthymic disorder, and depressive disorder not otherwise specified (depressive episodes deviating from the precise criteria for MDD). Other illnesses producing depressive symptoms include: bipolar disorder, depressed phase (distinguished by a history of a previous manic, mixed or hypomanic episode); substance-induced mood disorder (caused by substances such as alcohol or medications); and mood disorder due to a general medical condition (when the depression is thought to be a direct physiological consequence of the medical disorder).[1,2]

Table 1: **Common Depressive Syndromes**

Syndrome	Essential Features[a]
Major Depressive Disorder (MDD)	Five (or more) of the following, at least one of which must be depressed mood or diminished interest/pleasure, on most days for at least two weeks: • Depressed mood • Diminished interest or pleasure • Significant weight loss or weight gain • Insomnia or hypersomnia • Psychomotor agitation or retardation • Fatigue or loss of energy • Feelings of worthlessness or excessive guilt • Diminished ability to think or concentrate, or indecisiveness • Recurrent thoughts of death/suicide or suicide attempt
Dysthymic Disorder	Depressed mood for most of the day, more days than not, for at least two years, plus at least two of the following: • Poor appetite or overeating • Insomnia or hypersomnia • Low energy or fatigue • Low self-esteem • Poor concentration or difficulty making decisions • Feelings of hopelessness

[a] Not due to medically or drug-induced conditions or normal bereavement.
Reprinted with permission from the *Diagnostic and Statistical Manual of Mental Disorders*, Fourth Edition, Text Revision. Copyright 2000 American Psychiatric Association.

Goals of Therapy

- Achieve remission of depressive symptoms
- Prevent suicide

- Restore optimal functioning
- Prevent recurrence

Investigations

The following screening questions/assessment tools are recommended for use by primary care physicians:

- "During the past month have you often been bothered by feeling down, depressed or hopeless?" and "During the past month have you often been bothered by little interest or pleasure in doing things?"[3]
- Patient Health Questionnaire (PHQ-9)[4] or seven-item Hamilton Depression Rating Scale (HAM-D-7)[5]
- Question patients about past manic or hypomanic episodes to rule out bipolar disorder, as many have difficulty recalling such episodes, and treatment differs significantly. The Mood Disorder Questionnaire (MDQ) is a useful screening instrument.[6]

Therapeutic Choices

The most impressive evidence for the success of antidepressant therapy and depression-specific psychotherapies, in terms of both clinical efficacy and restoration of occupational functioning, comes from controlled trials involving multifaceted health system interventions.[7,8] These interventions, often facilitated by a nonphysician health care provider, involve telephone contact to provide patient education about depression and to monitor progress during antidepressant treatment.[9,10] Multifaceted interventions add only modest costs but provide substantial long-term reductions in health care costs and increase the likelihood of returning to work.[11,12,13]

Nonpharmacologic Choices

Both *cognitive-behavioural* (CBT) and *interpersonal* (IPT) psychotherapy are as effective as antidepressants in mild to moderate depression;[14] antidepressants appear to be more effective in moderate to severe depression. For chronic depression, a modified form of CBT, the *Cognitive Behavioral Analysis System of Psychotherapy* (CBASP), is particularly effective in combination with pharmacotherapy.[15,16]

Psychoeducation improves adherence to treatment and enhances rates of response.[17] These simple messages significantly improve compliance:[18]

- Take medication daily
- Call this number for questions about side effects or other issues
- Antidepressants must be taken for two to four weeks for a noticeable effect
- Continue to take medication even if you are feeling better
- Do not stop taking the antidepressant without checking with the physician

Pharmacologic Choices (Table 2)

Although diagnostic criteria for MDD and dysthymic disorder differ (Table 1), there are no differences in recommendations for the use of antidepressants. The first step is to optimize dosing during the first four to six weeks. Consider switching within the same class during this time when a favourable response is overshadowed by intolerable side effects. Figure 1 provides a summary of current psychiatric practice in the absence of a remission of symptoms.

The safety of selective serotonin reuptake inhibitors (SSRIs) and dual action antidepressants is in question in relation to the risk of causing or worsening aggression and suicidality, especially in children and adolescents. This issue was addressed in a Canadian Psychiatric Association Position Statement[20] in which the authors reviewed recent reports and concluded that only fluoxetine is recommended as a first-line treatment for depression in children and adolescents. There is evidence that tricyclic antidepressants (TCAs) are no more effective than placebo in this population. Among published and unpublished randomized controlled trials of SSRIs and venlafaxine, a serotonin-norepinephrine reuptake inhibitor (SNRI), there is an increased rate of emergent suicidality (ranging from 2.6% to 7.7%) in the antidepressant groups compared to the placebo groups (0.6% to 3.8%).[21]

Selective Serotonin Reuptake Inhibitors (SSRIs)

Greater tolerability and *ease of dosing* are key reasons why SSRIs are first-choice antidepressants. Both time to onset (two to four weeks) and rate of response (60 to 70%) are comparable to tricyclic antidepressants (TCAs); side effects mainly affect sexual, gastrointestinal (GI) and/or central nervous system (CNS) function.[19] Unlike GI or CNS side effects, sexual dysfunction is more likely to persist during SSRI therapy and can involve impairment of desire, arousal and/or orgasm/ejaculation. When asked specifically about SSRI-induced sexual dysfunction, about 40% of depressed patients report onset or exacerbation of sexual dysfunction.[22] Consider the importance of sexual function to the patient when prescribing an antidepressant. Some non-SSRI antidepressants cause less sexual dysfunction (e.g., bupropion, mirtazapine, moclobemide) and may be used instead.[19] Some antidotes have been studied, including sildenafil, with modest benefits.[23] Easy-to-complete rating scales are available to monitor antidepressant-induced side effects.[24]

Six SSRIs are currently available in Canada (**citalopram**, **escitalopram**, **fluoxetine**, **fluvoxamine**, **paroxetine** and **sertraline**). Escitalopram, the stereoisomer of citalopram, has a similar side effect profile,[25] but preliminary evidence suggests superior efficacy relative to other SSRIs and potentially comparable efficacy to venlafaxine.[26] Among SSRIs, discontinuation effects are particularly prevalent with paroxetine.[27]

Dual Action Antidepressants

Bupropion is thought to exert antidepressant effects through norepinephrine and dopamine reuptake inhibition.[28] It is a first-line agent for major depression and is also indicated for smoking cessation.[29] Bupropion is contraindicated in patients with a history of anorexia or bulimia nervosa or a current seizure disorder and should be used with extreme caution in patients with a history of head trauma or prior seizure. It also has a favourable side effect profile and a low rate of sexual dysfunction.[22]

Trazodone is a potent postsynaptic serotonin ($5HT_2$) receptor antagonist with some serotonin reuptake inhibitory properties.[30] The use of trazodone as an antidepressant is limited by excessive sedation at therapeutic doses (300 to 400 mg daily); however, it is often prescribed at lower doses (50 to 100 mg) as a hypnotic in combination with other antidepressants. While the nonbenzodiazapines (zopiclone and zaleplon) are generally preferred as first-line hypnotics, trazodone is a favourable alternative in depressed patients, with potential advantages over benzodiazepines (lack of tolerance and potential antidepressant enhancement).

Mirtazapine acts directly on the noradrenergic system and indirectly on the serotonin system. It has a low rate of GI and sexual side effects but is associated with sedation and weight gain.[31]

Serotonin-norepinephrine Reuptake Inhibitors (SNRIs)

Venlafaxine has inhibitory effects on serotonin reuptake, and at doses of 150 mg daily and above, on norepinephrine reuptake as well. Higher rates of response[32] and remission[33] have been reported with venlafaxine compared to SSRIs, although these results have been questioned on the basis of differences among individual SSRIs.[34] Hypertension at doses of 225 mg and above is a rare side effect.

Duloxetine has been available in the United States and Europe since 2004. Since then, sporadic reports of hepatic injury have emerged.[35] Duloxetine is not yet available in Canada. Its actions on both serotonin and norepinephrine are approximately equal, and beneficial effects on pain and other physical symptoms have been reported.[36]

Tricyclic Antidepressants (TCAs)

Most clinicians reserve TCAs as second- or third-line agents when better-tolerated SSRIs or dual action agents have been ineffective.[32,37] For most cyclic antidepressants, it is best to *start low and go slow*. A usual starting dose for **amitriptyline** is 50 mg given at night, building to 100 mg after three to five days and increasing weekly, depending on tolerability and response. For many TCAs, the average dose can be approximated by calculating 3 mg/kg body weight. In elderly, cachexic or medically ill patients, lower starting doses (10 to 25 mg) are more appropriate and can be gradually increased to 1.5 mg/kg body weight.

TCAs are also used in some specific settings (e.g., **clomipramine** for obsessive-compulsive disorder, **nortriptyline** for elderly depressed patients and amitriptyline for patients with chronic pain). Unfavourable side effect profiles, lethality in overdose and poor adherence, especially during maintenance therapy, are limiting factors.[38]

Maprotiline, the only available tetracyclic antidepressant, is similar to TCAs in terms of its pharmacologic and toxicologic profile, although it has been associated with a higher risk of seizures than most other antidepressants.[39]

Monoamine Oxidase Inhibitors (MAOIs)

Moclobemide is the only *reversible* and selective inhibitor of MAO-A that is currently available. Dietary precautions are not required at standard doses. In the treatment of outpatient depression, clinical trials suggest comparable efficacy to TCAs and SSRIs and a lower rate of adverse effects.[40] Moclobemide is prescribed in divided doses (300 to 600 mg daily), although higher doses have been recommended to achieve remission of symptoms.[41] Nausea may be an early but brief adverse effect; insomnia may persist. Sexual dysfunction with moclobemide is rare.

Irreversible MAOIs, **phenelzine** and **tranylcypromine**, are reserved for the treatment of resistant depression in specialty clinics. Because of the irreversible enzyme inhibition, food and drug cautions must be followed during treatment and for two weeks after the last dose of the MAOI.[42,43]

Treatment-Resistant Depression

Antidepressants can be switched either within a medication class or to a different class. Most physicians switch out of class (e.g., from SSRI to SNRI or TCA) when there has been no response to the first drug. Switching within class should be considered in the presence of a favourable response but unfavourable side effects. Generally there is no need for a washout period, and a crossover technique can be applied (i.e., tapering one agent while titrating the other). Exceptions include: switching from an irreversible MAOI (phenelzine or tranylcypromine) to any other antidepressant, where a two-week washout is required; switching from moclobemide, where a five-day washout is recommended; and switching from fluoxetine to an irreversible MAOI, where a five-week washout is recommended. Similarly, due to its long half-life, caution should be exercised when starting other antidepressants after fluoxetine discontinuation.

Several *augmentation* and *combination* therapies have been evaluated in treatment-resistant depression and are best carried out in consultation with mood disorder specialists. While many agents have been evaluated as augmentation agents for various antidepressants, strong evidence exists only for the addition of **lithium** to TCAs.[44] The recommended dose of lithium is 600 mg to 900 mg daily. This is generally sufficient to achieve serum levels above 0.6 mmol/L; levels above 1.0 mmol/L are not recommended. Although evidence from randomized controlled trials is limited, **olanzapine**, **risperidone** and **quetiapine** are frequently used to augment antidepressant therapies, particularly where insomnia and anxiety symptoms persist.[45] These augmentations are not recommended for long-term use, and close monitoring of weight, cholesterol and glucose indices is indicated. The combination of bupropion with SSRIs is an alternative option.[46,47]

A combination of pharmacotherapy and psychotherapy (specifically IPT or CBT) is superior to either modality alone. In mild to moderate cases, combination therapy provides little synergy to either treatment alone, but does provide protection against early relapse compared to either treatment alone. Pharmacotherapy typically facilitates more rapid relief of symptoms, but does not prevent relapse if the medication is stopped; both IPT and CBT reduce relapse for up to three years after completion of a course of psychotherapy. For moderate to severe depression, or refractory depression, combination therapy should be strongly considered, particularly in individuals with a history of more than three previous depressions.[48]

Electroconvulsive therapy (ECT) is efficacious in 80 to 90% of depressed patients, a response rate that is superior to any single antidepressant drug, although relapse and recurrence rates are high in the absence of other prophylactic treatments.[49,50]

Duration of Antidepressant Treatment

Evidence supports the use of maintenance antidepressant therapies for a minimum period of one year, particularly when the intervals between depressive episodes become briefer and the disability associated with each depressive episode worsens. After one episode, treat for one year and after two or more episodes, treat for at least two years. CBT and IPT may also be effective in reducing the risk of relapse.[14]

In general, antidepressants should be tapered slowly to minimize the risk of discontinuation emergent symptoms. Among newer antidepressants, paroxetine and venlafaxine are most likely to produce discontinuation symptoms such as insomnia, dizziness, nausea and diarrhea.

Depression in Pregnancy

During pregnancy, symptoms of depression are common, and are highly predictive of subsequent postpartum depression. The decision to initiate or continue treatment during pregnancy should be based on a risk/benefit analysis. If treatment is necessary, there is most evidence to support IPT or fluoxetine;[51] however, a recent report suggests an association between SSRI use after the 20th week of gestation and persistent pulmonary hypertension of the newborn.[52] If antidepressants are prescribed, the dose should be reduced near term to decrease the risk of withdrawal symptoms in the infant, and a pediatrician should monitor the newborn.[51]

Postpartum Depression

Rates of postpartum depression vary according to the severity of the episode—postpartum "blues" affect up to 80%, major depression up to 15% and postpartum psychosis up to 0.1%. In the majority of cases, "the blues" are self-limited, requiring only monitoring and supportive care. Psychotherapy (particularly IPT) should be considered as the first option in the treatment of more persistent or severe postpartum depression unless it is inadequate or inappropriate for the patient's severity of illness, in which case antidepressant treatment should be initiated. For patients with postpartum depression who wish to breast-feed, citalopram, paroxetine and sertraline are considered first-line due to very low medication concentrations found in breast milk.[51]

Bipolar Disorder

Bipolar disorder is much less common (prevalence 1 to 2%) than MDD, but individuals with this disorder experience more depressive episodes than those with MDD.[53] Patients presenting with depression should be questioned about past manic or hypomanic episodes, as many have difficulty recalling such episodes, and treatment of bipolar disorder differs significantly. Pharmacotherapy for bipolar disorder, which includes a mood stabilizer and other medications as needed, is addressed in Chapter 6.

Therapeutic Tips

- Choose one or two agents from several antidepressant classes and use them consistently.
- Provide structured psychoeducation with the initial prescription.
- Reinforce the importance of maintenance therapy beyond the acute phase.
- Although serum drug concentrations are not useful with SSRIs, MAOIs and other new antidepressants, there is a role for such monitoring with some TCAs (e.g., desipramine, imipramine, amitriptyline and nortriptyline).
- Dietary restrictions for patients on irreversible MAOI therapy can be found at http://www.mayoclinic.com/health/maois/HQ01575, accessed May 2006.
- Review alcohol and drug abuse history in nonresponders.
- Refer for psychiatric consultation if the patient has psychotic symptoms or acute suicidal ideation, or after failure of three treatment trials.
- When initiating drug discontinuation, taper slowly over four to six weeks. This is particularly important for paroxetine and venlafaxine.
- For patient education, consider recommending web sites such as http://www.canmat.org or http://moodgym.anu.edu.au, or self-help books such as *Mind Over Mood*[54] or *Feeling Good*.[55]

Figure 1: **Pharmacologic Treatment of Depression**[19]

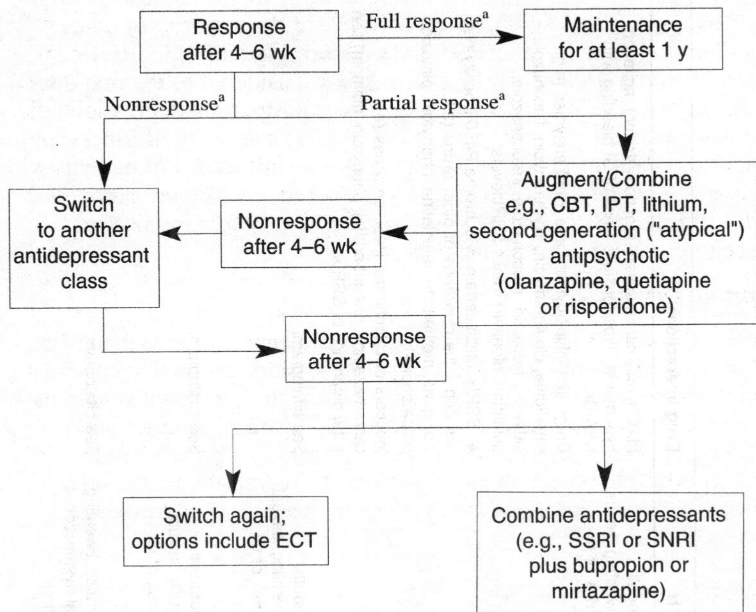

[a] Response definitions: Full = > 50% reduction; Partial = 25 to 50% reduction; Non = < 25% reduction.
Abbreviations: ECT = electroconvulsive therapy; SSRI = selective serotonin reuptake inhibitor; SNRI = serotonin and norepinephrine reuptake inhibitor; CBT = cognitive behavioural therapy; IPT = interpersonal psychotherapy

Table 2: Drug Therapy for Depression

Class	Drug	Dose	Adverse Effects	Drug Interactions	Cost[a]
SSRIs	*citalopram* Celexa, generics	Initial:[b] 10–20 mg/day Usual:[c] 20–40 mg/day High:[d] 60 mg/day	Nausea, dry mouth, somnolence, sweating, sexual dysfunction, ↑ risk of GI bleeding.	MAOIs may cause severe reaction—tremor, agitation, hypomania, hypertension; ↑ risk of GI bleeding with NSAIDs. Drugs that inhibit cytochrome P450 enzymes (e.g., cimetidine, clarithromycin, erythromycin, fluconazole, indinavir, isoniazid, itraconazole, ketoconazole, quinidine, ritonavir) may ↑ SSRI levels. All SSRIs inhibit certain cytochrome P450 isoenzymes and can ↓ the clearance of other drugs (e.g., clozapine, methadone, mexiletine, phenytoin, pimozide, propafenone). Inducers of cytochrome P450 enzymes (e.g., carbamazepine, phenobarbital, phenytoin, rifampin) can ↑ the clearance of SSRIs.	$$-$$$
	escitalopram Cipralex	Initial:[b] 10 mg/day Usual:[c] 10–20 mg/day High:[d] 20 mg/day	Nausea, dry mouth, somnolence, sweating, sexual dysfunction, ↑ risk of GI bleeding.	See citalopram.	$$$
	fluoxetine Prozac, generics	Initial:[b] 10–20 mg/day Usual:[c] 20–40 mg/day High:[d] 60–80 mg/day	Nausea, nervousness, anorexia, insomnia, sexual dysfunction, ↑ risk of GI bleeding.	See citalopram.	$$-$$$
	fluvoxamine Luvox, generics	Initial:[b] 50–100 mg/day Usual:[c] 150–200 mg/day High:[d] 400 mg/day	Nausea, drowsiness, sweating, anorexia, sexual dysfunction, ↑ risk of GI bleeding.	See citalopram.	$$$

Class	Drug	Dose	Adverse Effects	Drug Interactions	Cost[a]
	paroxetine, immediate-release Paxil, generics	Initial:[b] 10–20 mg/day Usual:[c] 20–40 mg/day High:[d] 60 mg/day	Nausea, drowsiness, fatigue, sweating, dizziness, sexual dysfunction, ↑ risk of GI bleeding.	See citalopram.	$$-$$$
	paroxetine, controlled-release Paxil CR	Initial:[b] 12.5–25 mg/day Usual:[c] 25–50 mg/day High:[d] 75 mg/day	Nausea, drowsiness, fatigue, sweating, dizziness, sexual dysfunction, ↑ risk of GI bleeding.	See citalopram.	$$$-$$$$$
	sertraline Zoloft, generics	Initial:[b] 25–50 mg/day Usual:[c] 50–100 mg/day High:[d] 150–200 mg/day	Nausea, tremors, diarrhea, dry mouth, sexual dysfunction, ↑ risk of GI bleeding.	See citalopram.	$$
Dual Action Antidepressants	*bupropion* Wellbutrin SR, Wellbutrin XL, generics	SR formulation: Initial:[b] 75 mg/day Usual: 150–300 mg/day High:[d] 375–450 mg/day XL formulation: Initial:[b] 150 mg/day Usual: 150–300 mg/day High:[d] 450 mg/day	Agitation, insomnia, anorexia; contraindicated in anorexia or bulimia nervosa and seizure disorders.	May ↑ levels of cyclophosphamide, ifosfamide and orphenadrine.	$-$$$$
	mirtazapine Novo-Mirtazapine, Remeron, Remeron RD, generics	Initial:[b] 15–30 mg/day Usual: 30–45 mg/day High:[d] 60 mg/day	Weight gain, sedation.	Sedative effects may be potentiated by alcohol or diazepam. Orally disintegrating tablets can be taken without water.	$$

(cont'd)

Table 2: **Drug Therapy for Depression** *(cont'd)*

Class	Drug	Dose	Adverse Effects	Drug Interactions	Cost[a]
	trazodone Desyrel, generics	Initial:[b] 150–200 mg/day Usual: 300–400 mg/day High:[d] 600 mg/day	Drowsiness, nausea, headache, dry mouth, priapism.	May potentiate effects of other CNS depressants and augment hypotensive effects of antihypertensives.	$$-$$$
SNRIs	*venlafaxine* Effexor XR, generic	Initial:[b] 37.5–75 mg/day Usual: 112.5–225 mg/day High:[d] 300–375 mg/day	Nausea, drowsiness, nervousness, dizziness, dry mouth, may ↑ BP if dose > 300 mg/day.	Drugs that inhibit cytochrome P450 may ↑ venlafaxine levels; may interact with MAOIs.	$$$$
TCAs	*amitriptyline* generics	Initial:[b] 25–50 mg/day Usual: 75–200 mg/day High:[d] 250–300 mg/day	Anticholinergic (dry mouth, blurred vision, constipation, urinary hesitancy, tachycardia, delirium), antihistaminergic (sedation, weight gain), orthostatic hypotension, lowered seizure threshold; sexual dysfunction.	Combination with MAOIs may result in mania, excitation, hyperpyrexia; barbiturates, carbamazepine and rifampin may ↓ effect; cimetidine and antipsychotics may ↑ effect and toxicity; possible interaction with antiarrhythmics (may lead to ↑ effect of either drug); may ↓ antihypertensive effect of clonidine; may augment hypotensive effect of thiazides.	$
	clomipramine Anafranil, generics	Initial:[b] 25–50 mg/day Usual: 75–200 mg/day High:[d] 250–300 mg/day	See amitriptyline.	See amitriptyline.	$$-$$$
	desipramine Norpramin, generics	Initial:[b] 25–50 mg/day Usual: 75–200 mg/day High:[d] 250–300 mg/day	See amitriptyline.	See amitriptyline.	$$-$$$
	doxepin Sinequan, generics	Initial:[b] 25–50 mg/day Usual: 75–200 mg/day High:[d] 250–300 mg/day	See amitriptyline.	See amitriptyline.	$-$$

Class	Drug	Dose	Adverse Effects	Drug Interactions	Cost[a]
	imipramine Tofranil, generics	Initial:[b] 25–50 mg/day Usual: 75–200 mg/day High:[d] 250–300 mg/day	See amitriptyline.	See amitriptyline.	$-$$
	nortriptyline Aventyl, generics	Initial:[b] 25–50 mg/day Usual: 75–150 mg/day High:[d] 200 mg/day	See amitriptyline.	See amitriptyline.	$$-$$$
	trimipramine Rhotrimine, generics	Initial:[b] 25–50 mg/day Usual: 75–200 mg/day High:[d] 250–300 mg/day	See amitriptyline.	See amitriptyline.	$-$$
Tetracyclic Antidepressants	*maprotiline* generics	Initial:[b] 75 mg/day Usual: 75–150 mg/day High:[d] 200 mg/day	See amitriptyline.	See amitriptyline.	$$-$$$
Reversible MAOIs	*moclobemide* Manerix, generics	Initial:[b] 200–300 mg/day Usual: 450–600 mg/day High:[d] 900 mg/day	Nausea, insomnia, dizziness.	Avoid sympathomimetics, meperidine. Caution with opioids, antihypertensives, antipsychotics, SSRIs, selegiline, excessive tyramine, alcohol. Reduce dose with cimetidine.	$$-$$$

(cont'd)

Table 2: **Drug Therapy for Depression** *(cont'd)*

Class	Drug	Dose	Adverse Effects	Drug Interactions	Cost[a]
Irreversible MAOIs	*phenelzine* Nardil	Initial:[b] 15–30 mg/day Usual: 30–75 mg/day High:[d] 90–120 mg/day	Edema, postural hypotension, insomnia, sexual dysfunction.	Sympathomimetics may ↑ BP; meperidine may cause agitation, hyperpyrexia, circulatory collapse; SSRIs, TCAs, levodopa may ↑ effects and side effects; tyramine-containing food may cause hypertensive crisis.	\$\$-\$\$\$
	tranylcypromine Parnate	Initial:[b] 10–20 mg/day Usual: 20–60 mg/day High:[d] 60–80 mg/day	See phenelzine.	See phenelzine.	\$\$-\$\$\$

[a] Cost of 30-day supply based on manufacturers' price lists, includes drug cost only; based on the upper and lower doses of the "usual" dose range.
[b] Lower starting dose indicated where previous side effect experience or polypharmacy; often applies to elderly patients.
[c] For SSRIs, upper starting dose may be usual dose, e.g., fluoxetine 20 mg or sertraline 50 mg; otherwise, increments every five to seven days.
[d] Higher doses often exceed upper doses in manufacturers' product monographs and usually result in more disabling side effects. These doses should be used with caution.
Dosage adjustment may be required in renal impairment; see Appendix I.
Legend: \$ < \$20 \$-\$\$ < \$20–40 \$\$ \$20–40 \$\$-\$\$\$ \$20–60 \$\$\$ \$40–60 \$\$\$\$ \$60–100 \$\$\$-\$\$\$\$\$ \$40– >100 \$\$\$\$\$ > \$100
Abbreviations: SSRIs = selective serotonin reuptake inhibitors; SNRIs = serotonin-norepinephrine reuptake inhibitors; TCAs = tricyclic antidepressants; MAOIs = monoamine oxidase inhibitors

Suggested Readings

Canadian Psychiatric Association; Canadian Network for Mood and Anxiety Treatments (CANMAT). Clinical guidelines for the treatment of depressive disorders. *Can J Psychiatry* 2001;46(Suppl 1):5S-90S.

Hollon SD, Jarrett RB, Nierenberg AA et al. Psychotherapy and medication in the treatment of adult and geriatric depression: which monotherapy or combined treatment? *J Clin Psychiatry* 2005;66(4):455-68.

Kennedy SH. Lam RW, Nutt DJ, Thase ME. *Treating depression effectively: applying clinical guidelines*. London (UK): Martin Dunitz; 2004.

Lam RW, Wan DD, Cohen NL, Kennedy SH. Combining antidepressants for treatment-resistant depression: a review. *J Clin Psychiatry* 2002;63(8):685-93.

Yatham LN, Kennedy SH, O'Donovan C et al. Canadian Network for Mood and Anxiety Treatments (CANMAT) guidelines for the management of patients with bipolar disorder: consensus and controversies. *Bipolar Disord* 2005;7(Suppl 3):5-69.

References

1. American Psychiatric Association. Task Force on DSM-IV. *Diagnostic and statistical manual of mental disorders: DSM-IV-TR*. Washington (DC): American Psychiatric Association; 2000.
2. Parikh SV, Lam RW; CANMAT Depression Work Group. Clinical guidelines for the treatment of depressive disorders, I. Definitions, prevalence, and health burden. *Can J Psychiatry* 2001;46(Suppl 1):13S-20S.
3. Arroll B, Khin N, Kerse N. Screening for depression in primary care with two verbally asked questions: cross sectional study. *BMJ* 2003;327(7424):1144-6.
4. Kroenke K, Spitzer RL, Williams JB. The PHQ-9: validity of a brief depression severity measure. *J Gen Intern Med* 2001;16(9):606-13.
5. McIntyre RS, Konarski JZ, Mancini DA et al. Measuring the severity of depression and remission in primary care: validation of the HAMD-7 scale. *CMAJ* 2005;173(11):1327-34.
6. Hirschfeld RM. The mood disorder questionnaire: a simple, patient-rated screening instrument for bipolar disorder. *Prim Care Companion J Clin Psychiatry* 2002;4(1):9-11.
7. Wells KB, Sherbourne C, Schoenbaum M et al. Impact of disseminating quality improvement programs for depression in managed primary care: a randomized controlled trial. *JAMA* 2000;283(2):212-20.
8. Von Korff M, Goldberg D. Improving outcomes in depression. *BMJ* 2001;323(7319):948-9.
9. Rost K, Nutting P, Smith JL et al. Managing depression as a chronic disease: a randomised trial of ongoing treatment in primary care. *BMJ* 2002;325(7370):934-7.
10. Katon W, Von Korff M, Lin E et al. Collaborative management to achieve depression treatment guidelines. *J Clin Psychiatry* 1997;58(Suppl 1):20-3.
11. Simon GE, Von Korff M, Ludman EJ et al. Cost-effectiveness of a program to prevent depression relapse in primary care. *Med Care* 2002;40(10):941-50.
12. Schoenbaum M, Unutzer J, McCaffrey D et al. The effects of primary care depression treatment on patients' clinical status and employment. *Health Serv Res* 2002;37(5):1145-58.
13. Lave JR, Frank RG, Schulberg HC et al. Cost-effectiveness of treatments for major depression in primary care practice. *Arch Gen Psychiatry* 1998;55(7):645-51.
14. Segal ZV, Whitney DK, Lam RW et al. Clinical guidelines for the treatment of depressive disorders. III. Psychotherapy. *Can J Psychiatry* 2001;46(Suppl 1):29S-37S.
15. Keller MB, McCullough JP, Klein DN et al. A comparison of nefazodone, the cognitive behavioral-analysis system of psychotherapy, and their combination for the treatment of chronic depression. *N Engl J Med* 2000;342(20):1462-70.
16. Klein DN, Santiago NJ, Vivian D et al. Cognitive-behavioral analysis system of psychotherapy as a maintenance treatment for chronic depression. *J Consult Clin Psychol* 2004;72(4):681-8.
17. Sperry L. *Psychopharmacology and psychotherapy*. New York (NY): Brunner/Mazel; 1995.
18. Lin EH, Von Korff M, Katon W et al. The role of the primary care physician in patients' adherence to antidepressant therapy. *Med Care* 1995;33(1):67-74.
19. Kennedy SH, Lam RW, Cohen NL et al. Clinical guidelines for the treatment of depressive disorders. IV. Medications and other biological treatments. *Can J Psychiatry* 2001;46(Suppl 1):38S-58S.

20. Lam RW, Kennedy SH. CPA Position Statement: Prescribing antidepressants for depression in 2005: recent concerns and recommendations. *Can J Psychiatry* 2004;49(12):1-6.
21. Whittington CJ, Kendall T, Fonagy P et al. Selective serotonin reuptake inhibitors in childhood depression: systematic review of published versus unpublished data. *Lancet* 2004;363(9418):1341-5.
22. Clayton AH, Pradko JF, Croft HA et al. Prevalence of sexual dysfunction among newer antidepressants. *J Clin Psychiatry* 2002;63(4):357-66.
23. Nurnberg HG, Hensley PL, Gelenberg AJ et al. Treatment of antidepressant-associated sexual dysfunction with sildenafil: a randomized controlled trial. *JAMA* 2003;289(1):56-64.
24. Vanderkooy JD, Kennedy SH, Bagby RM. Antidepressant side effects in depression patients treated in a naturalistic setting: a study of bupropion, moclobemide, paroxetine, sertraline, and venlafaxine. *Can J Psychiatry* 2002;47(2):174-80.
25. Wade A, Michael Lemming O, Bang Hedegaard K. Escitalopram 10 mg/day is effective and well tolerated in a placebo-controlled study in depression in primary care. *Int Clin Psychopharmacol* 2002;17(3):95-102.
26. Bielski RJ, Ventura D, Chang CC. A double-blind comparison of escitalopram and venlafaxine extended release in the treatment of major depressive disorder. *J Clin Psychiatry* 2004;65(9):1190-6.
27. Baldwin DS, Cooper JA, Huusom AK et al. A double-blind, randomized, parallel-group, flexible-dose study to evaluate the tolerability, efficacy and effects of treatment discontinuation with escitalopram and paroxetine in patients with major depressive disorder. *Int Clin Psychopharmacol* 2006;21(3):159-69.
28. Stahl SM. Basic psychopharmacology of antidepressants, part 1: Antidepressants have seven distinct mechanisms of action. *J Clin Psychiatry* 1998;59(Suppl 4):5-14.
29. Jorenby D. Clinical efficacy of bupropion in the management of smoking cessation. *Drugs* 2002;62(Suppl 2):25-35.
30. Kent JM. SNaRIs, NaSSAs, and NaRIs: new agents for the treatment of depression. *Lancet* 2000;355(9207):911-8.
31. Thase ME, Nierenberg AA, Keller MB et al. Efficacy of mirtazapine for prevention of depressive relapse: a placebo-controlled double-blind trial of recently remitted high-risk patients. *J Clin Psychiatry* 2001;62(10):782-8.
32. Stahl SM, Entsuah R, Rudolph RL. Comparative efficacy between venlafaxine and SSRIs: a pooled analysis of patients with depression. *Biol Psychiatry* 2002;52(12):1166-74.
33. Smith D, Dempster C, Glanville J. Efficacy and tolerability of venlafaxine compared with selective serotonin reuptake inhibitors and other antidepressants: a meta-analysis. *Br J Psychiatry* 2002;180:396-404.
34. Kennedy SH, Andersen HF, Lam RW. Efficacy of escitalopram in the treatment of major depressive disorder compared with conventional selective serotonin reuptake inhibitors and venlafaxine XR: a meta-analysis. *J Psychiatry Neurosci* 2006;31(2):122-31.
35. Malani AK, Ammar H. Medical management of depression. *N Engl J Med* 2006;354(6):646-8.
36. Detke MJ, Lu Y, Goldstein DJ et al. Duloxetine, 60 mg once daily, for major depressive disorder: a randomized double-blind placebo-controlled trial. *J Clin Psychiatry* 2002;63(4):308-15.
37. Anderson IM. Selective serotonin reuptake inhibitors versus tricyclic antidepressants: a meta-analysis of efficacy and tolerability. *J Affect Disord* 2000;58(1):19-36.
38. Montgomery SA, Kasper S. Comparison of compliance between serotonin reuptake inhibitors and tricyclic antidepressants: a meta-analysis. *Int Clin Psychopharmacol* 1995;9(Suppl 4):33-40.
39. Pisani F, Oteri G, Costa C et al. Effects of psychotropic drugs on seizure threshold. *Drug Saf* 2002;25(2):91-110.
40. Sogaard J, Lane R, Latimer P et al. A 12-week study comparing moclobemide and sertraline in the treatment of outpatients with atypical depression. *J Psychopharmacol* 1999;13(4):406-14.
41. Magder DM, Aleksic I, Kennedy SH. Tolerability and efficacy of high-dose moclobemide alone and in combination with lithium and trazodone. *J Clin Psychopharmacol* 2000;20(3):394-5.
42. Robinson DS. Monoamine oxidase inhibitors: a new generation. *Psychopharmacol Bull* 2002;36(3):124-38.
43. Gardner DM, Shulman KI, Walker SE et al. The making of a user friendly MAOI diet. *J Clin Psychiatry* 1996;57(3):99-104.
44. Lam RW, Wan DD, Cohen NL et al. Combining antidepressants for treatment-resistant depression: a review. *J Clin Psychiatry* 2002;63(8):685-93.
45. Kennedy SH, Lam RW. Enhancing outcomes in the management of treatment resistant depression: a focus on atypical antipsychotics. *Bipolar Disord* 2003;5(Suppl 2):36-47.
46. Kennedy SH, McCann SM, Masellis M et al. Combining bupropion SR with venlafaxine, paroxetine, or fluoxetine: a preliminary report on pharmacokinetic, therapeutic, and sexual dysfunction effects. *J Clin Psychiatry* 2002;63(3):181-6.
47. Zisook S, Rush AJ, Haight BR et al. Use of bupropion in combination with serotonin reuptake inhibitors. *Biol Psychiatry* 2006;59(3):203-10.
48. Hollon SD, Jarrett RB, Nierenberg AA et al. Psychotherapy and medication in the treatment of adult and geriatric depression: which monotherapy or combined treatment? *J Clin Psychiatry* 2005;66(4):455-68.

49. Sackeim HA, Haskett RF, Mulsant BH et al. Continuation pharmacotherapy in the prevention of relapse following electroconvulsive therapy: a randomized controlled trial. *JAMA* 2001;285(10):1299-307.
50. UK ECT Review Group. Efficacy and safety of electroconvulsive therapy in depressive disorders: a systematic review and meta-analysis. *Lancet* 2003;361(9360):799-808.
51. Moses-Kolko EL, Roth EK. Antepartum and postpartum depression: healthy mom, healthy baby. *J Am Med Womens Assoc* 2004;59(3):181-91.
52. Chambers CD, Hernandez-Diaz S, Van Marter LJ et al. Selective serotonin-reuptake inhibitors and risk of persistent pulmonary hypertension of the newborn. *N Engl J Med* 2006;354(6):579-87.
53. Kusumakar V. Antidepressants and antipsychotics in the long-term treatment of bipolar disorder. *J Clin Psychiatry* 2002;63(Suppl 10):23-8.
54. Greenberger D, Padesky CA. *Mind over mood: change how you feel by changing the way you think*. New York (NY): Guilford Press; 1996.
55. Burns DD. *Feeling good: the new mood therapy*. New York (NY): HarperCollins; 1999.

Pharmacoeconomic Considerations: Depression

Nicole Mittmann, MSc, PhD

Epidemiology

Country	Prevalence (%)
Canada (1995–96)[1]	33%

Cost of Illness Data

Country and Year of Estimate	Direct Costs[a]	Indirect Costs[b]
Canada (1998)[2]	$8 billion	$6 billion
United States (1990)[3]	US $20 billion	US $24 billion

Commentary

The economic burden associated with the treatment of depression is large. There are patient, health system and societal costs. Direct medical costs include hospital admissions, physician visits, emergency room visits and medications. Indirect costs include absenteeism, lost productivity and death.

The use of medications, in general, is 30% to 50% higher in patients who are depressed when compared with non-depressed individuals.[4,5]

From an indirect cost perspective, individuals who are depressed are more likely to be absent from work than those without depression.[6] Depressed patients are less productive than non-depressed patients.[7,8] Remission of depressive symptoms generally leads to fewer lost productivity days, use of fewer health care resources and improvement in quality of life.[9]

A number of new and more costly antidepressants have recently become available (e.g., citalopram, escitalopram, venlafaxine) to add to

(cont'd)

Commentary

the existing armamentarium of tricyclic antidepressants (TCAs) and selective serotonin reuptake inhibitors (SSRIs). These newer agents are as effective as older comparators, but have different adverse event profiles.[10,11,12] From an economic perspective, the different adverse event profiles of antidepressants can result in differential resource utilization (e.g., additional clinic visits, hospitalizations).

In general, the newer agents are reported to be more cost-effective than older or traditional agents. Use of escitalopram has been reported to have significantly lower direct costs (including hospitalization) than venlafaxine.[13,14]

It is important to note that the majority of economic analyses have been conducted by pharmaceutical manufacturers, and that studies sponsored by manufacturers generally produce results that favour the sponsor's product.[15] Despite the number of published economic evaluations, analyses often assume different perspectives, doses, costs and complications. This has prompted the authors of a recent review to argue that the quality of the pharmacoeconomic literature in this field needs to be improved.[16]

[a] Direct costs include those associated with physician services, nursing care, diagnostic procedures, drugs and hospitalization.

[b] Indirect costs are those associated with lost productivity and days off work due to morbidity or premature mortality.

References

1. Patten SB. Progress against major depression in Canada. *Can J Psychiatry* 2002;47(8):775-80.
2. Stephens T, Joubert N. The economic burden of mental health problems in Canada. *Chronic Dis Can* 2001;22(1):18-23.
3. Greenberg PE, Stiglin LE, Finkelstein SN et al. The economic burden of depression in 1990. *J Clin Psychiatry* 1993;54(11):405-18.
4. Unutzer J, Patrick DL. Simon G et al. Depressive symptoms and the cost of health services in HMO patients aged 65 years and older. A 4-yr prospective study. *JAMA* 1997;277(2):1618-23.
5. Simon G, Ormel J. VonKorff M et al. Health care costs associated with depressive and anxiety disorders in primary care. *Am J Psychiatry* 1995;152(3):352-7.
6. Kessler RC, Barber C, Birnbaum HG et al. Depression in the workplace: effect on short-term disability. *Health Aff (Millwood)* 1999;18(5):163-71.
7. Druss BG, Schlesinger M, Allen HM. Depressive symptoms, satisfaction with health cares, and 2-year work outcomes in an employed population. *Am J Psychiatry* 2001;158(5):731-4.
8. Wang PS, Beck AL, Berglund P et al. Effects of major depression on moment-in time work performance. *Am J Psychiatry* 2004;161(10):1885-91.
9. Sobocki P, Ekman M, Agren H et al. The mission is remission: health economic consequences of achieving full remission with antidepressant treatment for depression. *Int J Clin Pract* 2006;60(7):791-8.
10. Smith D, Dempster C, Glanville J et al. Efficacy and tolerability of venlafaxine compared with selective serotonin reuptake inhibitors and other antidepressants: a meta-analysis. *Br J Psychiatry* 2002;180:396-404.
11. Schatzberg AF. Efficacy and tolerability of duloxetine, a novel dual reuptake inhibitor, in the treatment of major depressive disorder. *J Clin Psychiatry* 2003;64(Suppl 13):30-7.
12. Einarson TR. Evidence based review of escitalopram in treating major depressive disorder in primary care. *Int Clin Psychopharmacol* 2004;19(5):305-10.
13. Fernandez JL, Montgomery S, Francois C. Evaluation of the cost effectiveness of escitalopram versus venlafaxine XR in major depressive disorder. *Pharmacoeconomics* 2005;23(2):155-67.
14. Francois C, Sintonen H, Toumi M. Introduction of escitalopram, a new SSRI in Finland: comparison of cost-effectiveness between the other SSRIs and SNRI for the treatment of depression and estimation of the budgetary impact. *J Med Econ* 2002;5:91-107.

15. Baker BC, Johnsrud MT, Crismon ML et al. Quantitative analysis of sponsorship bias in economic studies of antidepressants. *Br J Psychiatry* 2003;183:498-506.

16. Pirraglia PA, Rosen AB, Hermann RC et al. Cost-utility studies of depression management: a systematic review. *Am J Psychiatry* 2004;2005;161(12):2155-62.

CHAPTER 6
Bipolar Disorder

Sagar V. Parikh, MD, FRCPC

Bipolar disorder is a complex, recurrent mood disorder that affects 1–2% of the population.[1] It is defined as having either a manic, hypomanic or mixed episode (see Table 1),[2] and usually includes episodes of clinical depression.

Table 1: **Description of Bipolar Disorder Episodes[2]**

Type of Episode	Features
Mania	**Mood:** Abnormally and persistently elevated, expansive or irritable **Duration:** At least one week, causing significant distress/disability, or requiring hospital admission ***Plus:*** If mood is elevated or expansive, three or more of the following features must be present. If mood is predominantly irritable, four or more are required. • Grandiosity • More talkative • Excessive involvement in pleasurable activities • Less need for sleep • Flight of ideas • Distractability • More goal-directed activity
Hypomania	**Mood:** Same symptoms as for mania, but milder and not disabling; *no* psychotic symptoms **Duration**: four days or longer
Major Depressive Episode	**Mood:** Depressed most of the day OR markedly diminished interest or pleasure (anhedonia) **Duration:** At least two weeks, with significant change from previous functioning ***Plus:*** Four or more of the following: • Insomnia or hypersomnia • Significant weight loss/gain or change in appetite • Fatigue or loss of energy • Psychomotor retardation or agitation (observable) • Worthlessness or excessive guilt • Impaired thinking, concentrating or making decisions • Recurrent thoughts of death, suicidal ideation or attempt/plan
Mixed Episode	**Mood:** Criteria met *during same time period* for both a major depressive episode and a manic episode **Duration:** Nearly every day for at least one week or for any duration if hospitalized

Symptoms of mania include changes in mood, energy, sleep requirements and ability to concentrate, and in some cases psychotic symptoms.

Symptoms of depression include oversleeping or profound tiredness (the most common symptom of bipolar depression), pessimism, inability to socialize, decreased cognitive abilities and possibly suicidal or psychotic symptoms.

Bipolar disorder is formally divided into three categories: bipolar I disorder, bipolar II disorder and bipolar disorder not otherwise specified (Table 2).[2] Diagnosis of bipolar disorder is often difficult as the illness is perhaps the most complex psychiatric disorder. It has the most variable clinical presentation and is associated with the highest number of episodes, the highest degree of comorbidity and the highest mortality of the major psychiatric conditions. When bipolar disorder is severe and psychotic symptoms are present, it resembles schizophrenia. When accompanied by substance abuse, it mimics a pure substance abuse disorder. In a severe depression phase, it resembles unipolar major depression. When the symptoms are mild and changing rapidly, it resembles borderline personality disorder.

Table 2: **Classification of Bipolar Disorder[2]**

Disorder	Features
Bipolar I Disorder	Lifetime history of at least one clear-cut manic or mixed episode with or without episodes of depression
Bipolar II Disorder	History of hypomanic episodes and major depressive episodes, with no history of a full manic or a mixed episode
Bipolar Disorder Not Otherwise Specified	Bipolar disorder believed to be present but diagnostic criteria not strictly met
Bipolar Spectrum Disorder	Proposed category for mood conditions that appear to fall between traditional unipolar depression and bipolar disorder, e.g., major depression in person with first-degree relative with bipolar disorder
Cyclothymic Disorder	Recurrent episodes of hypomania and mild (subthreshold) depressive symptoms

Goals of Therapy

- Control symptoms of acute episode
- Prevent recurrences
- Provide ancillary care for comorbid psychiatric conditions such as anxiety or substance abuse or medical conditions such as endocrine/metabolic disorders

Investigations

- It is estimated that one-third of patients appearing in primary care settings with symptoms suggestive of unipolar major depression are actually experiencing depression in the context of bipolar illness.[3] Ask all depressed patients about possible hypomanic or manic symptoms in their past. While no screening test is ideal, the Mood

Disorder Questionnaire (MDQ) is a helpful, self-completed form that asks systematic yes/no questions about the symptoms of mania;[4] an adolescent version also has been developed.[5] Two or more "yes" answers on the MDQ should prompt a more thorough clinical review of symptoms, including questioning family/friends if possible.

- The diagnosis of bipolar disorder depends not just on the clinical presentation but, very importantly, on a reliable collateral history from a friend or family member who can corroborate episodes of elevated mood, inappropriate behaviour, decreased sleep with increased energy or grandiosity.
- It is critical to determine whether the patient has a *family history* of mood disorders, substance abuse or bipolar disorder itself.
- Laboratory investigations:
  - depend in part on the age and acute presentation of the patient
  - for all patients, basic blood tests include CBC, electrolytes, renal function, liver function and thyroid function
  - metabolic parameters including weight, lipid profile and fasting blood sugars at the time of initiation of any treatment
  - for patients with any unusual symptoms, neurologic signs or symptoms, or a first manic or hypomanic episode after age 50, include structural imaging of the brain such as CAT or MRI

Therapeutic Choices

Bipolar disorder is a complex illness that can only be partly managed by a sole physician; a team approach is ideal. At a minimum, it is helpful to have access to a nurse who will provide education and coping strategies as well as ongoing monitoring and support. The comprehensive treatment of bipolar disorder is reviewed in detail in the CANMAT treatment guidelines,[1,6] which are the basis for the recommendations that follow. Key additional resources such as treatment manuals and web sites are also listed in the CANMAT guidelines.

Nonpharmacologic Choices

- Psychoeducation consists of information about the illness as well as training in coping strategies and recognition of episodes early in their genesis. Structured group psychoeducational programs have been shown to substantially reduce the risk of relapse of manic, mixed and depressive episodes.[7] An excellent source of information on psychoeducation is a book called *Structured Group Psychotherapy for Bipolar Disorder* (see Suggested Readings), which is available in both English and French and provides explicit advice for effective psychoeducation over the course of six treatment sessions.
- To prevent an incipient manic or depressive episode from becoming a flagrant episode, conduct a "relapse drill," which trains patients to recognize their unique warning symptoms and respond in a specific treatment fashion which might include:

- changes in medication strategies
- rapid contact with the treating physician
- additional steps to regulate sleep and other behaviours

Pharmacologic Choices

Pharmacologic therapy varies according to the type and stage of the episode being treated. Since treatment for this condition is lifelong, engaging the patient in collaborative decision-making is critical. Except in situations where there is a severe episode or medical emergency, discuss the pros and cons of two or three pharmacologic options to inform and support the patient's decision.

Manic Episodes (Figure 1, Table 3, Table 6)

Moderate-to-severe mania is usually treated in hospital; mild mania, which by psychiatric definition is distinct from hypomania (see Table 1), may be treated on an outpatient basis. The first step in treating mania is to assess for risk of aggressive behaviour or violence to others, suicide, degree of insight and the ability to adhere to treatment (Figure 1).[6] If the patient is taking an antidepressant, it should be discontinued. Complicating issues such as other medical conditions, particularly substance abuse problems, will need attention.

Specific medication strategies for mania depend on whether the patient is already on maintenance therapy and is experiencing a breakthrough episode or whether the individual is unmedicated. If the patient is already taking a first-line agent (**lithium** or **divalproex** or an **atypical antipsychotic**), dosage adjustment may be sufficient after checking blood levels where appropriate. In moderate-to-severe manic episodes, addition of another medication is usually necessary.

In previously unmedicated patients, initiate treatment with a first-line agent (Table 3). When the episode is particularly severe, initiate treatment with a two-drug combination such as lithium or divalproex plus an atypical antipsychotic. Continue treatment on any particular regimen for two weeks at therapeutic doses before assessing whether a change is necessary. Various other treatment options are shown in Figure 1.

Depressive Episodes (Figure 2, Table 4, Table 7)

As with acute mania, first assess the patient for basic safety issues, including potential suicidality, comorbid medical problems or substance abuse (Figure 1). Next, the strategy depends on whether the patient is on medication and has had a breakthrough episode of major depression, or whether they are medication free (Table 4). In an unmedicated patient, therapy may begin with **lithium**, **lamotrigine** or **quetiapine**. If the depression is severe, therapy can be initiated with two agents, such as lithium plus quetiapine.

Table 3: **Treatment Regimens for Acute Mania in Bipolar Disorder**[a]

Place in Therapy	Drugs	Comments
First-line	lithium	Aim for blood levels near the high end of therapeutic range as tolerated, i.e., 1–1.2 mmol/L
	divalproex	Loading dose is possible; aim for blood levels high in therapeutic range
	olanzapine	May start with therapeutic dose of 15 mg; note peak sedation is 3–4 hours after ingestion, so may dose earlier in evening
	risperidone	Monitor regularly for orthostatic hypotension and extrapyramidal side effects, e.g., parkinsonism, akathisia
	quetiapine	Need to titrate dose rapidly; monitor for sedation, hypotension
	lithium or divalproex *plus* risperidone	Allows lower dosing of risperidone than in monotherapy; useful for more severe episodes; start risperidone first × 1–3 days
	lithium or divalproex *plus* quetiapine	Allows lower dosing of quetiapine than in monotherapy; useful for more severe episodes; start quetiapine first × 1–3 days
	lithium or divalproex *plus* olanzapine	Allows lower dosing of olanzapine than in monotherapy; useful for more severe episodes; start olanzapine first × 1–3 days
Second-line	carbamazepine oxcarbazepine ECT lithium *plus* divalproex	Try several first-line treatments first before going to second-line treatments
Third-line	haloperidol chlorpromazine lithium or divalproex *plus* haloperidol lithium *plus* carbamazepine clozapine	Haloperidol is well tolerated in severely medically ill patients, including iv formulation; clozapine is very useful in rapid-cycling patients
Not recommended	Monotherapy with gabapentin, topiramate, lamotrigine, verapamil, or combination therapy with risperidone and carbamazepine	Use of some of these agents as *adjuncts* may be appropriate, especially if initiated prior to mania for other symptoms (e.g., using gabapentin for anxiety, topiramate for alcohol craving)

[a] Treatment trials typically run two weeks at therapeutic doses. Adjunctive benzodiazepine use is common, e.g., clonazepam 1–2 mg BID. If patient is not on first-line agent, start first-line agent monotherapy; if more serious, consider dual therapy. If on maintenance therapy, optimize dosing prior to adding new medication.
Abbreviations: ECT = electroconvulsive therapy

Table 4: **Treatment Regimens for Acute Depression in Bipolar Disorder**[a]

Place in Therapy	Drugs	Comments
First-line	lithium	Aim for blood levels near the high end of therapeutic range as tolerated, i.e., 1–1.2 mmol/L. May be useful for those with high risk of suicide or self harm
	lamotrigine	Slow titration schedule in turn slows response but mitigates risk of adverse effects including rash; useful for milder episodes
	quetiapine	Monotherapy studies showed doses of 300 or 600 mg/day to be equally effective; lower dose preferred if patient is medication-naïve
	lithium or divalproex *plus* SSRI	Prefer shorter half-life SSRIs in case of switch to mania
	lithium or divalproex *plus* bupropion	As with all antidepressants, watch for switch into mania
	lithium *plus* divalproex	Aim for good blood levels of each mood stabilizer
	olanzapine *plus* fluoxetine	May have lower rates of switch into mania compared to mood stabilizer plus SSRI
Second-line	quetiapine *plus* SSRI lithium or divalproex *plus* lamotrigine	Try several first-line treatments before going to second-line options.
Third-line	carbamazepine olanzapine divalproex lithium *plus* carbamazepine lithium *plus* pramipexole lithium *plus* MAOI lithium or divalproex *plus* venlafaxine ECT lithium or divalproex *plus* atypical antipsychotic atypical antipsychotic *plus* TCA lithium or divalproex or carbamazepine *plus* SSRI lithium *plus* lamotrigine adjunctive eicosapentaenoic acid, riluzole or topiramate	Third-line choices best reserved for mood disorder specialists. ECT may be initial treatment in particularly severe depression or in medically ill patients
Not recommended	Monotherapy with gabapentin	

[a] Treatment trials typically run a minimum of four weeks at therapeutic doses. Response is often slower than in unipolar depression. Avoid antidepressants if possible, or shorten duration of antidepressant treatment to prevent switch into mania.

Abbreviations: SSRI = selective serotonin reuptake inhibitor; ECT = electroconvulsive therapy; MAOI = monoamine oxidase inhibitor; TCA = tricyclic antidepressant

Bipolar depression is difficult to treat; steps to follow if there is an inadequate response after two to four weeks of therapy are outlined in Figure 2. Two key emerging observations are that specific psychosocial strategies are potentially valuable for bipolar depression, and that combining two traditional mood stabilizers such as **lithium** plus **divalproex** may also be of some value. Although **antidepressants** can be considered in moderate-to-severe cases, there is some potential to destabilize and promote a more rapid-cycling course in susceptible individuals. Thus, the use (with caution) of short courses of antidepressants (e.g., ≤ 3 to 4 months), is prudent.

Maintenance Therapy for Bipolar Disorder (Table 5, Table 8)

When a patient recovers from an acute episode and remains well for at least two months, the patient is defined as being in the maintenance phase of the illness. Unmedicated, such individuals have an approximately 70% chance of experiencing another episode over the next year and an approximately 95% chance of having a recurrence within five years. To prevent relapse, interventions include psychosocial strategies such as psychoeducation, cognitive-behavioural therapy, family therapy, and interpersonal and social rhythm therapy. Key characteristics of effective psychosocial therapies that improve medication adherence include education about the disorder (including the likelihood of relapse), training in self-monitoring, education about how to manage side effects, development of strategies to manage stressors and attention to the patient's own belief system and attitude towards the illness.

Give patients the opportunity to discuss the impact of the illness on their life and their beliefs about potential effects of long-term medication use. To facilitate longer-term compliance, repeat a brief version of psychoeducation periodically, e.g., annually.

There is evidence of effective relapse prevention with **lithium**, **divalproex**, **olanzapine** and **lamotrigine** as maintenance therapy (Table 5). However, with the exception of lithium, evidence for long-term therapy is limited.

Table 5: **Maintenance Treatment Regimens for Bipolar Disorder[a]**

Place in Therapy	Drugs	Comments
First-line	lithium	Blood levels can be individualized — some patients have efficacy at lower end of normal therapeutic range; levels lower than for acute episode
	lamotrigine	Effective only for prophylaxis against depressive relapses

(cont'd)

Table 5: **Maintenance Treatment Regimens for Bipolar Disorder[a]** *(cont'd)*

Place in Therapy	Drugs	Comments
	olanzapine	Equal to lithium overall in relapse prevention, but better at preventing relapse to mixed episodes
	divalproex	RCT support is lacking but clinical observation suggests effective relapse prevention
Second-line	carbamazepine lithium *plus* divalproex lithium *plus* carbamazepine lithium or divalproex *plus* olanzapine risperidone quetiapine lithium *plus* risperidone or quetiapine lithium *plus* lamotrigine or SSRI or bupropion olanzapine *plus* fluoxetine	Try several first-line treatments before going to second-line treatments. These recommendations are based primarily on open-label studies. May be able to use antidepressants concurrently for a long time in some patients with clear histories of predominantly depressive relapses Aripiprazole and ziprasidone, not yet available in Canada, are also second-line options
Third-line	*adjunctive* therapy with: phenytoin clozapine ECT topiramate omega-3 fatty acids oxcarbazepine gabapentin	Third-line choices best reserved for mood disorder specialists
Not recommended	adjunctive flupenthixol; monotherapy with gabapentin, topiramate or antidepressants	Bipolar II patients may rarely benefit from monotherapy with antidepressants

[a] While the goal is ultimately complete relapse prevention, in individuals with severe illness reduction in the frequency, duration and intensity of relapse may be more realistic. Psychosocial interventions are critical to reduce relapse.

Abbreviations: RCT = randomized controlled trial; SSRI = selective serotonin reuptake inhibitor; ECT = electroconvulsive therapy

Bipolar Disorder in Children and Adolescents

Bipolar disorder typically emerges in adolescence, most often as depression.[8] An initial depressive episode is impossible to distinguish from unipolar depression. The existence of first-degree relatives with bipolar disorder in an adolescent presenting with an initial depression is suggestive of an eventual bipolar diagnosis, but treatment is usually initiated on the assumption that the teenager has unipolar depression. Other key predictors of an eventual shift to a bipolar diagnosis include the presence of particularly severe or psychotic symptoms in a teen who is unmistakably depressed (as opposed to someone who likely has schizophrenia). If the teen does have an initial presentation of hypomania or mania, the presentation is often one of a mixed state, where the mood is predominantly irritable and symptoms of both mania and depression are present in the same week (see Table 1).[9]

Both mania and depression have been documented in pre-teens, therefore bipolar disorder may be reliably diagnosed by a specialist at a very early age. ADHD presents a major differential challenge, with the key distinguishing feature remaining the episodic nature (weeks or months) of the bipolar disorder, while ADHD symptoms are present on a continuous daily basis. Bipolar treatment options are limited by a lack of drug studies in children and adolescents, but some evidence exists for the efficacy of the usual adult treatments such as **lithium**, **divalproex** and **quetiapine**.[10] Given the various diagnostic and medication controversies associated with children, refer to a child psychiatrist for treatment.

Bipolar Disorder in the Elderly

When bipolar disorder begins early in life, it is a lifelong illness that, if untreated, continues to manifest with more frequent episodes and shorter periods of recovery over the decades. The illness does *not* typically progress to an extremely rapid-cycling form of illness, and elderly bipolar patients usually will have major periods of euthymia. A small number of individuals experience a first onset of bipolar illness in their sixties or later; symptoms are typical of adult mania but irritability may be prominent.[11] Often these individuals have a history of comorbid neurologic problems and an elevated all-cause mortality rate. Clinical trials are relatively rare in the elderly, so most treatment parameters are extrapolated from the adult literature.[12] All atypical antipsychotics carry warnings about potential elevated stroke risk in the elderly, but the significant morbidity and mortality associated with bipolar disorder in this population compels consideration of these agents for treatment.

Bipolar Disorder in Pregnancy

Since bipolar disorder often starts early in life, many women will be living with the disorder at the time they are considering having children. Key management principles include careful risk assessment for each woman, namely the risk of pregnancy destabilizing the illness and the possibility of severe episodes resulting in the death of either the patient or child, or both. Untreated women with bipolar disorder are particularly susceptible to postpartum depression, including depression with psychotic features that may result in harm to the child. Despite such cautions, most women with bipolar disorder are able to manage pregnancy successfully. Collaborative management of the pregnancy by a psychiatrist, an obstetrician and a family physician is recommended, including consultation with an agency specializing in information on medications during and following pregnancy (e.g., Motherisk—www.motherisk.org).

Because most psychiatric medications pose some teratogenic risk, and many are excreted in breast milk, medication management during and following pregnancy requires extensive consideration and review with the patient.[13] If medication is to be discontinued prior to conception, it should be tapered with medical supervision.[14]

Creation of a "pregnancy contract" is recommended; in consultation with the doctor, a patient creates a one-page document that summarizes her typical symptoms in mania and in depression, and lists preferred treatment options for each phase of illness. That document is then shared among the treatment team and the patient's family, and serves as a nonbinding but helpful "advance directive" should a new episode of illness arise.

Therapeutic Tips

- A key feature of bipolar disorder is recurrent nonadherence to medication; including the patient in decision-making, together with psychoeducation, promotes a strong therapeutic alliance and enhances medication adherence.
- During acute manic episodes, patients may exhibit increased tolerance to lithium.
- Patients who experience diarrhea while taking slow-release lithium preparations may fare better with immediate-release formulations,[15] particularly the citrate salt.[16]
- Patients on lithium need to maintain their usual salt and caffeine intake and monitor fluid intake and output, making adjustments in the event of unexpected losses due to vomiting or diarrhea.

Figure 1: **Management of Acute Mania in Bipolar Disorder**

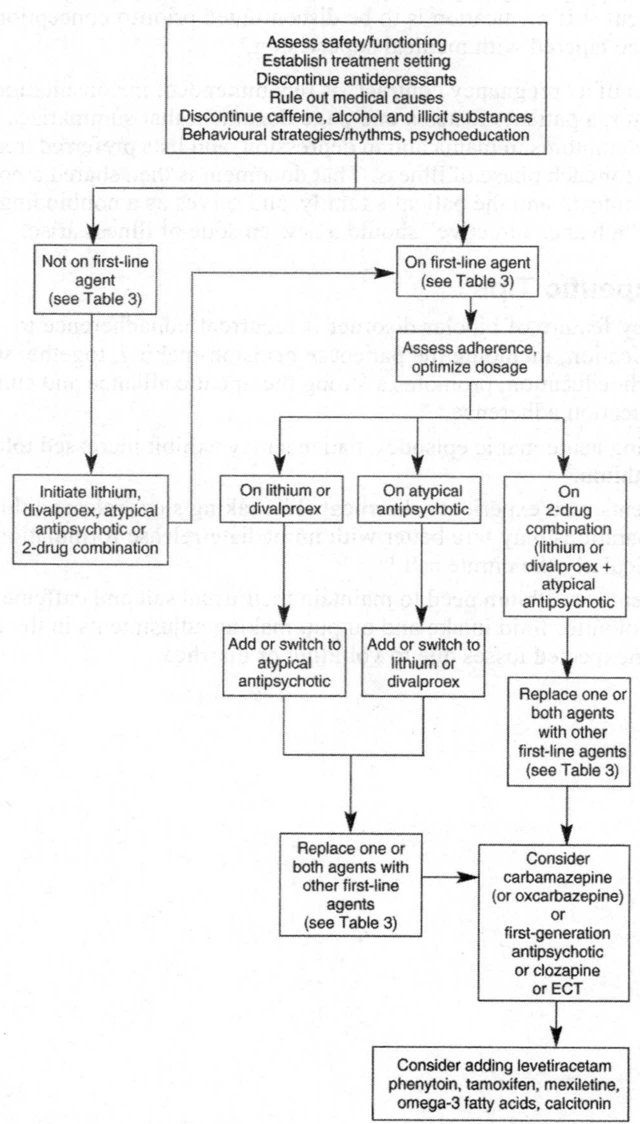

Abbreviations: ECT = electroconvulsive therapy
Adapted with permission from Yatham LN, Kennedy SH, O'Donovan C et al. Canadian Network for Mood and Anxiety Treatments (CANMAT) guidelines for the management of patients with bipolar disorder: update 2007. *Bipolar Disorder* 2006;8:721–739

Figure 2: **Management of Depressive Episodes in Bipolar Disorder**

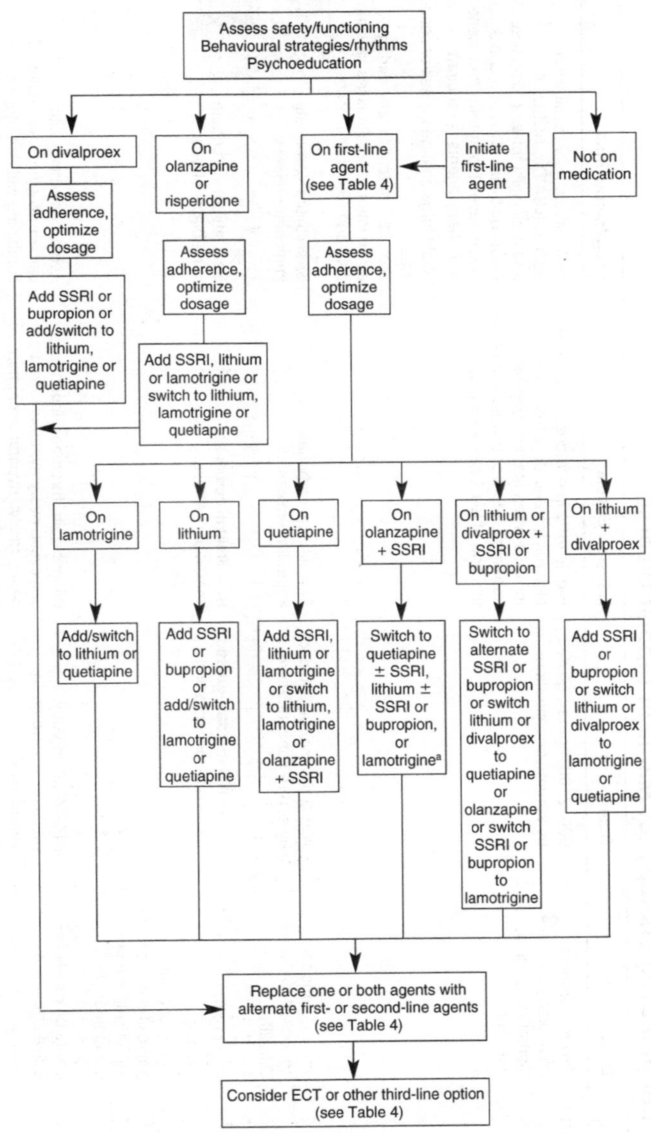

[a] Or switch SSRI to another SSRI.

Abbreviations: SSRI = selective serotonin reuptake inhibitor; ECT = electroconvulsive therapy

Adapted with permission from Yatham LN, Kennedy SH, O'Donovan C et al. Canadian Network for Mood and Anxiety Treatments (CANMAT) guidelines for the management of patients with bipolar disorder: update 2007. *Bipolar Disorder* 2006;8:721–739

Table 6: **First-line Drug Therapy for Mania in Bipolar Disorder**

Class	Drug	Dose	Adverse Effects	Drug Interactions	Cost[a]
Mood Stabilizers	*lithium carbonate immediate-release* Carbolith, Lithane, generics	900–2100 mg/day, guided by serum concentrations	Highly toxic in overdose. Measure electrolytes and do 24-hr urine for ClCr when starting long-term treatment. Monitor thyroid and renal function at least every six months.	Toxic levels may result when adding NSAIDs, ACEIs, ARBs and especially thiazide diuretics. Reduce lithium dose and check serum level if long-term treatment with these agents is required. Avoid large changes in salt or coffee intake. Stop lithium temporarily during acute intermittent illnesses causing fluid and electrolyte losses.	$
	lithium carbonate controlled-release Duralith	900–2100 mg/day, guided by serum concentrations	See lithium carbonate immediate-release.	See lithium carbonate immediate-release.	$$
	lithium citrate syrup generic (8 mmol/5 mL; approximately equivalent to 300 mg lithium carbonate/5 mL)	900–2100 mg/day, guided by serum concentrations	See lithium carbonate immediate-release.	See lithium carbonate immediate-release.	$
	divalproex sodium Epival, generics	750–2000 mg/day, adjusted according to serum levels	Weight gain, thrombocytopenia, polycystic ovary syndrome, teratogenic; rarely: hyperammonemia, hepatotoxicity.	Avoid combining with carbamazepine; use caution if combining with lamotrigine.	$$

Class	Drug	Dose	Adverse Effects	Drug Interactions	Cost[a]
	valproic acid Depakene, generics	750–2000 mg/day, adjusted according to serum levels	See divalproex sodium.	See divalproex sodium.	$$
Antipsychotics, Atypical	*risperidone* [renal] Risperdal, generics	3–6 mg/day	Weight gain, orthostasis, extrapyramidal symptoms, metabolic disturbances.	Avoid combining with carbamazepine.	$$$$
	olanzapine Zyprexa, Zyprexa Zydis	5–20 mg/day	Weight gain, metabolic disturbances, anticholinergic side effects in elderly, akathisia. Monitor periodically for movement disorders.	Fluvoxamine and ciprofloxacin raise olanzapine levels.	$$$$$
	quetiapine Seroquel	400–800 mg/day	Weight gain, sedation, orthostasis, metabolic disturbances. Monitor periodically for movement disorders.	Ketoconazole dramatically increases quetiapine levels. Watch for hypotension with antihypertensives.	$$$$$

[a] Cost of 30-day supply of mean dose; includes drug cost only.

[renal] Dosage adjustment may be required in renal impairment; see Appendix I.

Legend: $ < $25 $$ $25–50 $$$ $50–75 $$$$ $75–100 $$$$$ > $100

Table 7: **First-line Drug Therapy for Depression in Bipolar Disorder[a]**

Class	Drug	Dose	Adverse Effects	Drug Interactions	Cost[b]
Mood Stabilizers	*lithium carbonate immediate-release* Carbolith, Lithane, generics	600–1800 mg/day, adjusted according to serum levels	Highly toxic in overdose. Measure electrolytes and do 24-hr urine for ClCr when starting long-term treatment. Monitor thyroid and renal function at least every six months.	Toxic levels may result when adding NSAIDs, ACEIs, ARBs and especially thiazide diuretics. Reduce lithium dose and check serum level if long-term treatment with these agents is required. Avoid large changes in salt or coffee intake. Stop lithium temporarily during acute intermittent illnesses causing fluid and electrolyte losses.	$
	lithium carbonate controlled-release Duralith, generics	600–1800 mg/day, adjusted according to serum levels	See lithium carbonate immediate-release.	See lithium carbonate immediate-release.	$$
	lithium citrate syrup generic (8 mmol/5 mL; approximately equivalent to 300 mg lithium carbonate/5 mL)	600–1800 mg/day, adjusted according to serum levels	See lithium carbonate immediate-release.	See lithium carbonate immediate-release.	$
	divalproex sodium Epival, generics	750–2000 mg/day, adjusted according to serum levels	Weight gain, thrombocytopenia, polycystic ovary syndrome, teratogenic; rarely: hyperammonemia, hepatotoxicity.	Avoid combining with carbamazepine; use caution if combining with lamotrigine.	$$

Class	Drug	Dose	Adverse Effects	Drug Interactions	Cost[b]
	valproic acid Depakene, generics	750–2000 mg/day, adjusted according to serum levels	See divalproex.	See divalproex.	$$
	lamotrigine Lamictal, generics	100–300 mg/day	Rash common; severe rash rare.	Divalproex doubles blood level of lamotrigine; always initiate slowly.	$$
Antipsychotics, Atypical	*quetiapine* Seroquel	300–600 mg/day	Weight gain, sedation, orthostasis, metabolic disturbances.	Ketoconazole dramatically increases quetiapine levels. Monitor for hypotension with antihypertensives.	$$$$$

[a] Detailed information on antidepressants can be found in Chapter 5.
[b] Cost of 30-day supply for mean dose; includes drug cost only.
Dosage adjustment may be required in renal impairment; see Appendix I.
Legend: $ < $25 $$ $25–50 $$$ $50–75 $$$$ $75–100 $$$$$ > $100

Table 8: **First-line Maintenance Therapy for Bipolar Disorder**

Class	Drug	Dose	Adverse Effects	Drug Interactions	Cost[a]
Mood Stabilizers	*lithium carbonate immediate-release* Carbolith, Lithane, generics	600–1800 mg/day, adjusted according to serum levels	Highly toxic in overdose. Measure electrolytes and do 24-hr urine for ClCr when starting long-term treatment. Monitor thyroid and renal function at least every six months.	Toxic levels may result when adding NSAIDs, ACEIs, ARBs and especially thiazide diuretics. Reduce lithium dose and check serum level if long-term treatment with these agents is required. Avoid large changes in salt or coffee intake. Stop lithium temporarily during acute intermittent illnesses causing fluid and electrolyte losses.	$
	lithium carbonate controlled-release Duralith	600–1800 mg/day, adjusted according to serum levels	See lithium carbonate immediate-release.	See lithium carbonate immediate-release.	$$
	lithium citrate syrup generic (8 mmol/5 mL; approximately equivalent to 300 mg lithium carbonate/5 mL)	600–1800 mg/day, adjusted according to serum levels	See lithium carbonate immediate-release.	See lithium carbonate immediate-release.	$
	divalproex sodium Epival, generics	750–2000 mg/day, adjusted according to serum levels	Weight gain, thrombocytopenia, polycystic ovary syndrome, teratogenic; rarely: hyperammonemia, hepatotoxicity.	Avoid combining with carbamazepine; use caution if combining with lamotrigine.	$$

Class	Drug	Dose	Adverse Effects	Drug Interactions	Cost[a]
	valproic acid Depakene, generics	750–2000 mg/day, adjusted according to serum levels	See divalproex.	See divalproex.	$$
	lamotrigine Lamictal	100–300 mg/day	Rash common; severe rash rare.	Divalproex doubles blood level of lamotrigine; always initiate dosing slowly.	$$
Antipsychotics, Atypical	*olanzapine* Zyprexa, Zyprexa Zydis	5–20 mg/day	Weight gain, metabolic disturbances, anticholinergic side effects in elderly, akathisia. Monitor periodically for movement disorders.	Fluvoxamine and ciprofloxacin raise olanzapine levels.	$$$$$

[a] Cost of 30-day supply for mean dose; includes drug cost only.
Dosage adjustment may be required in renal impairment; see Appendix I.
Legend: $ < $25 $$ $25–50 $$$ $50–75 $$$$ $75–100 $$$$$ > $100

Suggested Readings

Bauer MS, McBride L. *Structured group psychotherapy for bipolar disorder: the Life Goals Program* (2nd Ed.), Springer, New York (NY) 2003.

Yatham LN, Kennedy SH, O'Donovan C et al. Canadian Network for Mood and Anxiety Treatments (CANMAT) guidelines for the management of patients with bipolar disorder: consensus and controversies. *Bipolar Disord* 2005;7(Suppl 3):5-69

Yatham LN, Kennedy SH, O'Donovan C et al. Canadian Network for Mood and Anxiety Treatments (CANMAT) guidelines for the management of patients with bipolar disorder: update 2007. *Bipolar Disord* 2006;8(6):721-39.

Yonkers KA, Wisner KL, Stowe Z et al. Management of bipolar disorder during pregnancy and the postpartum period. *Am J Psychiatry* 2004;161(4):608-20.

References

1. Yatham LN, Kennedy SH, O'Donovan C et al. Canadian Network for Mood and Anxiety Treatments (CANMAT) guidelines for the management of patients with bipolar disorder: consensus and controversies. *Bipolar Disord* 2005;7(Suppl 3):5-69.
2. American Psychiatric Association. *Diagnostic and statistical manual of mental disorders: DSM-IV-TR*. 4th edition. Washington (DC): American Psychiatric Association; 2000.
3. Berk M, Dodd S, Berk L. The management of bipolar disorder in primary care: a review of existing and emerging therapies. *Psychiatry Clin Neurosci* 2005;59(3):229-39.
4. Hirschfeld RM, Williams JB, Spitzer RL et al. Development and validation of a screening instrument for bipolar spectrum disorder: the Mood Disorder Questionnaire. *Am J Psychiatry* 2000;157(11):1873-5.
5. Wagner KD, Hirschfeld RM, Emslie GJ et al. Validation of the Mood Disorder Questionnaire for bipolar disorders in adolescents. *J Clin Psychiatry* 2006;67(5):827-30.
6. Yatham LN, Kennedy SH, O'Donovan C et al. Canadian Network for Mood and Anxiety Treatments (CANMAT) guidelines for the management of patients with bipolar disorder: update 2007. *Bipolar Disord* 2006;8(6):721-39.
7. Colom F, Vieta E, Martinez-Aran A et al. A randomized trial on the efficacy of group psychoeducation in the prophylaxis of recurrences in bipolar patients whose disease is in remission. *Arch Gen Psychiatry* 2003;60(4):402-7.
8. Schapiro NA. Bipolar disorders in children and adolescents. *J Pediatr Health Care* 2005;19(3):131-41.
9. Kowatch RA, Youngstrom EA, Danielyan A et al. Review and meta-analysis of the phenomenology and clinical characteristics of mania in children and adolescents. *Bipolar Disord* 2005;7(6):483-96.
10. Kowatch RA, DelBello MP. Pediatric bipolar disorder: emerging diagnostic and treatment approaches. *Child Adolesc Psychiatr Clin N Am* 2006;15(1):73-108.
11. Al Jurdi R, Pulakhandam S, Kunik ME et al. Late-life mania: assessment and treatment of late-life manic symptoms. *Geriatrics* 2005;60(10):18-20,22-3.
12. Aziz R, Lorberg B, Tampi RR. Treatments for late-life bipolar disorder. *Am J Geriatr Pharmacother* 2006:4(4):347-64.
13. Yonkers KA, Wisner KL, Stowe Z et al. Management of bipolar disorder during pregnancy and the postpartum period. *Am J Psychiatry* 2004;161(4):608-20.
14. Gentile S. Prophylactic treatment of bipolar disorder in pregnancy and breastfeeding: focus on emerging mood stabilizers. *Bipolar Disord* 2006;8(3):207-20.
15. Vismari L, Pires, MLN, Benedito-Silva AA et al. Bioavailability of immediate and controlled release formulations of lithium carbonate. *Rev Bras Psiquitr* 2002;24(2):74-9.
16. Bezchlibnyk-Butler KZ, Jeffries JJ, editors. *Clinical handbook of psychotropic drugs*. 15th ed. [Seattle]: Hogrefe & Huber Publishers; 2005.

CHAPTER 7
Psychoses

Heather Milliken, MDCM, FRCPC

Psychoses are brain disorders in which there is a distortion of or loss of contact with reality, affecting the ability to think, feel, perceive and act. Psychotic symptoms include delusions, hallucinations, disorganized thinking and bizarre or disorganized behaviour. Approximately 3% of people worldwide will experience at least one psychotic episode during their lifetime (Table 1).

The age of onset of schizophrenia spectrum psychotic disorders is usually late adolescence/early adulthood. There is increased emphasis on earlier detection and treatment of psychotic disorders[1,2,3] because the duration of untreated psychosis correlates with both short- and long-term outcomes.[4,5]

Table 1: **Differential Diagnosis of Psychotic Episodes**[6]

Disorder	Characteristics
Schizophrenia	Signs of illness for ≥ 6 mo; psychotic symptoms for ≥ 1 mo; social/occupational dysfunction
Schizophreniform psychosis	Similar to schizophrenia except duration of illness of < 6 mo
Schizoaffective disorder	Symptoms of schizophrenia and mood disorder occur concurrently and ≥ 2 wk of delusions or hallucinations in absence of prominent mood symptoms
Delusional disorder	Nonbizarre delusions for ≥ 1 mo and does not meet criteria for schizophrenia
Brief psychotic disorder	Psychotic symptoms for ≥ 1 day but < 1 mo; may or may not be related to marked stressor; eventual full return to premorbid level of functioning
Substance-induced psychotic disorder	Delusions or hallucinations develop during or within 1 mo of substance intoxication or withdrawal or are etiologically related to medication use and are not better accounted for by another psychotic disorder
Psychotic disorder due to a general medical condition	Delusions or hallucinations are direct physiological consequence of a medical condition and occur in absence of delirium
Psychotic disorder not otherwise specified	Psychotic symptoms present but criteria for specific disorder not met or there is insufficient or contradictory information
Major depression with psychotic features	Major depressive episode with concurrent mood-congruent (most common) or mood-incongruent psychotic symptoms
Bipolar disorder	Manic episode with concurrent mood-congruent (most common) or mood-incongruent psychotic symptoms.

Goals of Therapy

- Reduce psychotic agitation in acute episodes
- Achieve remission of specific psychotic symptoms such as delusions, hallucinations, disordered thinking and behaviour
- Facilitate recovery of functioning and healthy development
- Reduce risk of comorbidity, particularly suicide, depression and substance abuse
- Prevent recurrence of psychotic episodes

Investigations (Table 2)

- Family physicians are often the initial contact for a person experiencing a first psychotic episode. Have a high index of suspicion in any young individual who is experiencing persistent changes in behaviour, mood and functioning particularly in the presence of other risk factors such as substance abuse or a family history of psychosis
- Signs and symptoms of possible first-episode psychosis include:[1]
  - withdrawal from usual activities with friends and family
  - persistent decline in functioning in everyday activities, at school or at work
  - persistent dysphoria, anxiety or irritability, especially in the absence of identifiable stressors
  - rapid fluctuations in mood (emotional lability) or showing very little emotion or facial expression
  - unreasonable suspiciousness
  - insomnia; restlessness and pacing at night
  - unusual or bizarre behaviour
  - unusual perceptual experiences including hypersensitivity, illusions and/or brief intermittent hallucinations
  - difficulties in thinking such as organizing and/or expressing thoughts
  - problems with attention and concentration
- Substance use (particularly cannabis) is common in first-episode psychosis. Individuals may therefore be misdiagnosed with a substance-induced psychosis and not receive appropriate ongoing treatment. Even in the presence of substance use, have a high index of suspicion of a functional psychosis especially if:
  - symptoms precede the onset of substance use; if symptoms are bizarre or there is marked thought disorder
  - symptoms persist beyond the period of intoxication or withdrawal

  There is evidence that cannabis use can trigger the onset of a schizophrenia spectrum disorder in genetically vulnerable individuals[7]

- Individuals with a suspected first episode of psychosis require urgent services.[8] If available, refer to a psychiatrist, community mental health clinic or specialized early psychosis program[8]
- Appropriate investigations are based on both the phase of the psychotic disorder (see Table 2) and individual patient characteristics
- In an acute psychotic episode, assess the nature and extent of psychopathology:
  - thorough history of presenting problems with special attention to onset and course of prodromal symptoms
  - onset, characteristics and severity of psychotic symptoms
  - changes in behaviour and functioning
  - history of any suicidal ideation or behaviour and/or aggressive/violent ideation or behaviour
  - history of substance use/abuse in relation to onset and course of psychotic symptoms
- A thorough mental status examination is essential. Competency to consent to treatment needs to be assessed in all acutely psychotic individuals
- Obtain information from as many sources as possible since individuals with psychotic disorders are often poor historians
  - interview family members whenever possible with the consent of the individual
- A variety of clinical rating scales can be used at baseline and repeated periodically to monitor for symptomatic and functional recovery following an acute psychotic episode
  - the Clinical Global Impression Scales for Severity (CGI-S)[9] and for Change (CGI-C)[9] and Global Assessment of Functioning (GAF)[6] are easy to use for documenting changes over time.
  - the Brief Psychiatric Rating Scale (BPRS, available at www.priory.com/psych/bprs.htm) and the Positive and Negative Syndrome Scale (PANSS), require training to be used reliably. Use of the semistructured interview guide SCI-PANSS,[10] however, takes approximately 30–40 minutes to complete and can be helpful in eliciting signs and symptoms of psychopathology
- Patients with only partial symptomatic and/or functional recovery following an acute psychotic episode require diagnostic reassessment by a psychiatrist

Table 2: **Investigations and Monitoring of Psychoses**[8,11]

Parameter	Phase of Illness, Recommended Monitoring/Frequency
Psychopathology	**First episode**: baseline then weekly for first 4–8 wk; more often if clinically indicated **Recurrent acute episode**: baseline then weekly for first 4–8 wk; more often if clinically indicated **Stabilization phase**: monthly for first 6 mo following first or recurrent acute episode; more often if clinically indicated **Stable phase**: every 3 mo for individuals with good symptomatic and functional recovery and medication adherence; more often for individuals with poor medication adherence
Substance use	**First episode**: baseline **Recurrent acute episode**: baseline **Stabilization phase**: at every patient visit or as clinically indicated **Stable phase**: at every patient visit or as clinically indicated
Level of functioning (activities of daily living; social and occupational functioning)	**First episode**: premorbid level of functioning; baseline assessment of current functioning **Recurrent acute episode**: baseline assessment of current functioning **Stabilization phase**: monthly for first 6 mo following first or acute episode **Stable phase**: every 3 mo
Past psychiatric history	**First episode**: baseline **Recurrent acute episode**: baseline with focus on past antipsychotic treatment including type of medication, dose, side effects, response, duration of treatment and medication adherence. **Stabilization/Stable phase:** N/A
Family psychiatric history	**First episode**: baseline **Recurrent acute episode**: baseline **Stabilization/Stable phase:** N/A
Developmental history (mother's obstetrical history including pre- and perinatal complications); developmental milestones; history of learning disabilities	**First episode**: baseline **Recurrent acute episode**: N/A **Stabilization/Stable phase:** N/A
Medical history (past and current conditions including treatment)	**First episode**: baseline **Recurrent acute episode**: baseline **Stable phase**: yearly
Extrapyramidal signs and symptoms (parkinsonism, dystonia, akathisia, dyskinesia)	**First episode**: baseline; when dosage of antipsychotic is changed or new antipsychotic is started, then weekly for 2–4 wk. **Recurrent acute episode**: baseline; when dosage of antipsychotic is changed or new antipsychotic is started, then weekly for 2–4 wk. **Stabilization phase**: as clinically indicated **Stable phase**: every 6 mo or more often for individuals at higher risk

(cont'd)

Table 2: **Investigations and Monitoring of Psychoses**[8,11] *(cont'd)*

Parameter	Phase of Illness, Recommended Monitoring/Frequency
Cognitive functions (estimates of premorbid IQ, current IQ, attention and concentration, working memory, verbal and visual learning and memory, executive functions such as abstract thinking, reasoning, problem solving, judgment	**First episode**: referral to a psychologist is recommended for neurocognitive testing within 3 mo after psychotic symptoms have remitted **Recurrent acute episode**: N/A **Stabilization phase**: N/A **Stable phase**: referral to a psychologist for neurocognitive testing as clinically indicated (clinical evidence of ongoing cognitive impairment that affects functioning)
Functional enquiry and physical examination with focus on current complaints, endocrine and sexual function, vital signs, weight, body mass index (BMI)	**First episode**: baseline and then as clinically indicated; weight and BMI monthly for 6 mo; baseline waist circumference; blood pressure at baseline and 12 wk or more often if clinically indicated **Recurrent acute episode**: baseline and then as clinically indicated; weight and BMI monthly for 6 mo after initiation of a new antipsychotic; baseline waist circumference; blood pressure at baseline and 12 wk or more often if clinically indicated **Stabilization phase**: as clinically indicated **Stable phase**: as clinically indicated; weight and BMI every 3 mo when on stable antipsychotic dosage: waist circumference annually; blood pressure annually or more often if clinically indicated; functional enquiry (including endocrine and sexual function) and physical exam at least yearly
Laboratory investigations (including CBC and differential, electrolytes, kidney and liver function, fasting glucose and lipid profile, TSH, baseline prolactin, routine urinalysis, urine drug screen if clinically indicated, tests for STIs, HIV and hepatitis if clinically indicated	**First episode**: Baseline; fasting glucose at baseline and repeat at 12 wk or more often as clinically indicated; fasting lipid profile at baseline and 12 wk and repeat as clinically indicated **Recurrent acute episode**: baseline; fasting glucose at baseline and repeat at 12 wk after initiating a new antipsychotic or more often as clinically indicated; fasting lipid profile at baseline and 12 wk and repeat as clinically indicated **Stabilization phase**: as clinically indicated **Stable phase**: fasting glucose annually or more frequently if gaining weight or symptomatic; fasting lipid profile annually or every 6 mo if LDL or triglyceride levels above normal range; other tests as clinically indicated

Abbreviations: N/A = not applicable

Therapeutic Choices (Figure 1)

- Antipsychotic medications are the most effective treatment of schizophrenia and related psychotic disorders[12,13] but need to be integrated with psychosocial interventions to optimize outcome.[8]
- Both pharmacologic and psychosocial interventions should be tailored to the individual and to the phase of the illness.

Nonpharmacologic Choices

First Episode/Recurrent Acute Episode

- Determine appropriate treatment setting (least restrictive setting possible), ensure safety and reduce environmental stressors and stimuli.
- Acutely agitated patients and those at imminent risk of harm to self or others will require hospitalization, if necessary on an involuntary basis.
- See patient frequently (for outpatients at least weekly for first 4–6 weeks) in order to:
  - build rapport
  - provide support, practical advice and psychoeducation
  - promote medication adherence
  - monitor treatment response
- Foster a collaborative therapeutic relationship between the patient, family/caregivers and treatment team.

Stabilization/Stable Phases

- In schizophrenia and related psychotic disorders, recovery (stabilization phase) from an acute psychotic episode usually occurs over six months but may take longer and may be incomplete.
  - focus on medication adherence, stress management, assessment of signs and symptoms of postpsychotic depression and suicidality, assessment of substance use and education about early warning signs of relapse
- Psychosocial interventions such as individual and family psychoeducation, cognitive-behavioural therapies (CBT), social and vocational skills training and peer support groups have been shown to improve functional outcome and community reintegration, and help prevent relapse.[8]
- Maintain continuity of care with an individual clinician or multidisciplinary treatment team.
- Individuals with serious ongoing illness and functional disability or comorbid problems such as substance abuse may benefit from referral to an Assertive Community Treatment (ACT) team if available.[8]

Pharmacologic Choices (Table 4, Table 5)

Choice of Antipsychotic

Two major classes of antipsychotics are currently available in Canada:

- **First-generation** antipsychotics (FGAs), also known as "typical" or "conventional" antipsychotics, can be classified according to their chemical structure (e.g., phenothiazines such as **fluphenazine** or butyrophenones such as **haloperidol**) or potency (low, intermediate, high) as determined by dopamine D2-receptor binding affinity (see Table 5).

- **Second-generation** antipsychotics (SGAs) or "atypical" antipsychotics (**clozapine**, **olanzapine**, **quetiapine** and **risperidone**) have greater 5HT affinity relative to D2 affinity. The duration of binding to D2 receptors may account for clinical differences in dosing requirements and side effect profiles among SGAs (see Table 4).[14]
- Two newer antipsychotics, **ziprasidone** and **aripiprazole**, which have slightly different binding affinities, are not yet available in Canada.
- All FGAs and SGAs, with the exception of clozapine, have similar efficacy in treating the positive (psychotic) symptoms of schizophrenia and related disorders. SGAs may have advantages in first-episode psychosis,[15,16] in improving negative symptoms, mood and cognitive deficits[17,18] and in preventing relapse[19] and rehospitalization.[20] Clozapine is the only antipsychotic with proven efficacy in treatment-resistant schizophrenia,[12] in reducing hostility and aggression[21,22] and in reducing persistent suicidality.[23]
- SGAs are now considered first-line treatment.[17,18,24] The exception is clozapine which, because of the risk of agranulocytosis and the need for regular blood monitoring, is reserved for treatment-resistant schizophrenia. The major differences between the FGAs and SGAs are in side effect profiles, safety and tolerability (see Table 3).

Dosing and Duration of Treatment

Tailor treatment to the specific phase of the disorder.[8,24]

Acute Phase (see also Chapter 1)

- **Haloperidol** im has been the most widely used treatment for psychotic agitation. Haloperidol 5 mg im combined with **lorazepam** 2 mg im has been shown to be more effective than haloperidol alone.[25]
- **Olanzapine** im in doses of 2.5–10 mg is as effective as haloperidol and causes less EPS.[26,27] Do not combine with parenteral benzodiazepines because of reports of cardiac and respiratory problems including deaths.
- The rapid-dissolving oral formulations of olanzapine and risperidone are as effective as haloperidol im.[28]
- **Zuclopenthixol acetate** is an injectable FGA which, because of its pharmacokinetics (peak serum level in 24–48 hours declining to one-third of peak concentration in 72 hours), may reduce the number of injections required in severe acute agitation and/or aggression. It should not be used in antipsychotic-naïve patients.
- Patients with first-episode psychosis are more responsive to lower doses of antipsychotics,[29,30] have a greater rate of recovery[29] and are more prone to side effects.
  - begin with a low dose of an SGA and titrate gradually over one to two weeks up to the usual therapeutic range (see Table 4). Risperidone and olanzapine are usually administered once daily. Although twice-daily dosing is recommended for quetiapine, many patients can be maintained on one daily dose at bedtime.[31]

- if an FGA is used, consider an intermediate-potency agent such as loxapine, which has some "atypical" properties.
- benzodiazepines can be used to treat anxiety and agitation while titrating the dose of antipsychotic.

- Rapid titration and high doses of antipsychotics do not accelerate or enhance treatment response and are rarely indicated. Even in patients with a chronic course, doses in the range of 2–5 mg of haloperidol are as effective as 10–40 mg and are associated with fewer side effects and greater tolerability.[32] Only a very small subgroup of patients appear to benefit from high-dose therapy.[33] Doses exceeding the recommended daily maximum, (e.g., olanzapine > 20 mg/day or quetiapine > 800 mg/day) are sometimes required but should be used under the care of a psychiatrist.
- An adequate trial of antipsychotic therapy is four to eight weeks at a dose within the usual therapeutic range.[8,18,24] Patients who fail to demonstrate even minimal response by that time are unlikely to benefit from a longer trial; consider switching to a different antipsychotic and consulting a psychiatrist.
- There is no good evidence to guide switching from one antipsychotic medication to another. *Crossover medication strategies*, over two weeks to three months,[34] are preferred. It is important to complete the crossover; combination therapy with more than one antipsychotic medication is not supported by evidence and should be used only in exceptional circumstances under the care of a psychiatrist. Patients successfully stabilized on clozapine have not been shown to benefit from switching to any other antipsychotic medication.[8]

Stabilization/Stable Phases

- During the stabilization (recovery) phase patients are vulnerable to relapse; avoid changes in antipsychotic medication unless there are intolerable side effects or persistent residual symptoms that are distressing and/or disabling to the patient.
- *Maintenance* therapy is essential to prevent relapse. First-episode psychosis is associated with a 70 to 90% risk of relapse within five years.
  - patients who discontinue medication are five times more likely to relapse.[13] Recovery from recurrent acute psychotic episodes (relapse) may take longer with each subsequent episode and the degree of recovery may not be as great, resulting in persistent residual symptoms and functional disability.[13]
  - continue maintenance pharmacotherapy for at least one to two years for first-episode individuals who achieve symptom remission and functional recovery[8,24] Longer treatment (two to five years) may be required for individuals with a long duration of untreated psychosis, more severe illness, slower response, substance abuse and history of suicidal or aggressive behaviour.[8,24] For patients with two or more episodes, maintenance pharmacotherapy should continue for

at least five years, during which time the patient should be stable with no relapse.[8]

- many patients will require antipsychotic treatment indefinitely.
- in general, the lowest dose of antipsychotic that was effective in acute treatment should be used in maintenance treatment.[8,12]

- Consider long-acting intramuscular antipsychotics for individuals with poor treatment *adherence*.
- If *discontinuation* of medication is to be undertaken, gradually reduce the dose by not more than 20% at a time, every two to four weeks, over a period of 6 to 12 months (first episode) and 6 to 24 months (two or more episodes).[8,12] Monitor patients closely for early signs of relapse. If these occur, the patient should be re-stabilized as quickly as possible on the previously effective dose of antipsychotic.

Treatment of Comorbid Conditions

Depression and Suicidality

- Depressive symptoms are common in the prodromal phase preceding the onset of a first episode of psychosis. In the acute phase, particularly in multiple-episode patients, depressive symptoms usually remit along with the positive psychotic symptoms.
  - SGAs may be more effective than FGAs in treating depressive symptoms[35] in the acute phase; there is no evidence to support the use of an antidepressant in the acute phase.[8]
- Major depressive episodes occur as often in individuals diagnosed with schizophrenia as in those with either schizoaffective disorder or nonpsychotic major depression.[36]
  - patients with first-episode psychosis have a greater risk of depression compared to multiple-episode patients, particularly in the stabilization phase (postpsychotic depression),[37] and depressive symptoms tend to increase for the first three months following a first episode of psychosis.[38]
- It can be difficult to differentiate between depression and ongoing negative symptoms, and rating scales such as the HAM-D and Beck Depression Inventory have not been validated in individuals with schizophrenia. The Calgary Depression Scale for Schizophrenia[39] can be used to differentiate between negative symptoms and symptoms of major depression.
- Antidepressant medication may be useful in the treatment of major depression in the stabilization or stable phases.[38] Although there have been few studies, there is limited support for CBT.

Substance Abuse

- Higher rates of substance abuse/dependence disorders are found in individuals with schizophrenia (lifetime prevalence of 47–50%) compared to the general population. Persistent substance abuse is associated with significantly poorer outcomes.

- In individuals (particularly first-episode psychosis) who appear to have been using substances as a form of "self-medication," substance abuse may remit spontaneously with recovery from the acute episode.
- Refer individuals with persistent substance abuse to a mental health program that can provide a comprehensive, integrated approach.[40]

Antipsychotics in Pregnancy

Teratogenic effects have not been demonstrated with the use of antipsychotics during pregnancy. Their use is best avoided during the first trimester, but risks and benefits must be carefully weighed for each patient. The Motherisk program (www.motherisk.org) is a useful resource for information regarding antipsychotic use in pregnancy. Hypertonia in neonates has been noted following prepartum use of high-potency FGAs.

Side Effects of Antipsychotics

Neuroleptic Malignant Syndrome (NMS)

- Neuroleptic malignant syndrome is a rare but serious side effect, which can present as a medical emergency and has a high mortality rate. It is characterized by muscle rigidity, fever, autonomic disturbance, labile blood pressure, fluctuating levels of consciousness and elevated WBC and creatinine kinase.
- It has been reported with all antipsychotics and can occur at any dosage and at any time. Dehydration is also a risk factor.

Sedation and Cognitive Side Effects

- Sedation is a very common side effect, especially after initiating a new antipsychotic or after increasing the dose; it can be very disabling and distressing. It occurs most frequently with low-potency FGAs, clozapine, quetiapine and to a lesser extent olanzapine.[8] Risperidone may be associated with either mild sedation or insomnia.[41]
- FGAs can cause a subjective cognitive "dulling" effect and do not improve cognitive deficits, whereas SGAs have shown statistically significant improvement on a variety of cognitive measures.[42,43]
- Concomitant medications such as anticholinergics (used to treat EPS) and anticonvulsants (used as mood stabilizers) can worsen cognitive deficits.[44,45]
- Cognitive deficits have been shown to be correlated with functional outcomes such as social and occupational functioning and activities of daily living.[46]

Extrapyramidal Side Effects

- The major advantage of the SGAs is the significantly reduced risk of EPS (acute dystonia, parkinsonism, akathisia) and tardive dyskinesia (TD) compared to FGAs[12,17,18,47,48] However, higher doses of risperidone can cause EPS and akathisia and higher doses of olanzapine can cause akathisia.

- *Parkinsonism* can be associated with dysphoria, decreased concentration and slowing of cognition.
- *Akathisia* (subjective and objective restlessness) is often misidentified as psychotic agitation which can result in an increase in dose of the offending antipsychotic.
- *Tardive dyskinesia* consists of repetitive, involuntary choreoathetoid movements usually involving the buccal-oral-lingual musculature, face, trunk, extremities or respiratory muscles and can be permanent and disabling.
  - the incidence is 5% per year with FGAs and the cumulative risk is up to 50% even if low doses of FGAs are used. The incidence is significantly less with risperidone and olanzapine. Quetiapine and clozapine have rates of TD equivalent to placebo, and clozapine may improve existing TD.[8]
  - inform patients of the risk of TD when initiating treatment with any antipsychotic medication, especially if initiating treatment with an FGA.

Weight Gain, Diabetes and Dyslipidemia

- Antipsychotic-induced weight gain is a serious side effect given that individuals with schizophrenia and bipolar disorder are already at higher risk of obesity compared to the general population.
- For FGAs, the risk of weight gain is greatest with low-potency agents.
- The risk of weight gain with SGAs is higher compared to FGAs, although this varies. Clozapine and olanzapine are associated with the greatest weight gain followed by quetiapine and then risperidone.[49]
- Weight gain does not correlate with dosage in studies of one year or longer so reduction in dose is unlikely to result in weight loss. Weight gain may be rapid in some individuals, but usually plateaus over time, although it can continue for up to one year or longer. Weight gain is a common cause of nonadherence to treatment and of requests to discontinue or switch antipsychotic medication.
- Compared to FGAs, SGAs are associated with greater risk of glucose abnormalities including hyperglycemia, insulin resistance, new onset type 2 diabetes, exacerbation of type 1 diabetes and diabetic ketoacidosis.[50] This is a concern because type 2 diabetes is two to four times more prevalent in individuals with schizophrenia compared to the general population, and abnormal glucose tolerance and insulin resistance are also more common.[51]
- Differential risks among SGAs for glucose abnormalities (independent of risks associated with weight gain) have been reported, but further research is needed. In Canada, all SGAs carry a warning about potential glucose abnormalities.[52]
- Hyperlipidemia has been associated with clozapine and olanzapine. Increased triglycerides have been reported with quetiapine. Risperidone has not been associated with dyslipidemia.[53,54]

Cardiovascular Side Effects

- Orthostatic hypotension is the most common antipsychotic-induced cardiovascular side effect, particularly in patients with heart disease, diabetes or in the elderly. It is more common with low-potency first-generation antipsychotics and with clozapine, but can occur with quetiapine, risperidone or olanzapine.
- Prolongation of the QT_c interval is associated with the potentially lethal paroxysmal ventricular cardiac arrhythmia, torsades de pointes, which can cause recurrent syncope, ventricular fibrillation and sudden cardiac death. Clinically, a QT_c interval of > 450 msec is concerning.[55]
  - QT_c prolongation occurs with chlorpromazine, pimozide (particularly at doses > 8 mg/day) and haloperidol, although the incidence is low. The SGAs olanzapine, quetiapine and risperidone cause modest QT_c prolongation (mean < 30 msec).[56] Potentially clinically significant QT_c prolongation is infrequent with clozapine (1/100 to 1/1000 patients).[57]
- Clozapine is associated with an increased risk of myocarditis (especially in but not limited to the first month of therapy), pericarditis, pericardial effusion, cardiomyopathy, heart failure, myocardial infarction and mitral insufficiency. If signs and symptoms of any of these disorders appear, seek urgent assessment by a cardiologist.

Endocrine and Sexual Side Effects

- Hyperprolactinemia is a common side effect of FGAs (especially high-potency agents such as haloperidol) and risperidone (especially at higher doses). Transient hyperprolactinemia can occur with olanzapine. No differences in prolactin levels have been found with quetiapine or clozapine compared to placebo.[58,59]
  - hyperprolactinemia often causes no clinically significant effects but can be associated with menstrual irregularities and galactorrhea in women, galactorrhea and gynecomastia in men and sexual dysfunction in both men and women; sexual dysfunction, however, is associated with all antipsychotics independent of prolactin elevation.
  - the first approach to the management of clinically significant side effects due to hyperprolactinemia is to reduce the dose of antipsychotic.

Table 3: **Antipsychotic-induced Side Effects: Assessment, Monitoring and Management** [8,60]

Side Effect	Assessment, Monitoring and Management
Neuroleptic malignant syndrome	**Assessment**: physical exam with focus on level of consciousness; vital signs (fever, tachycardia, fluctuations in BP); look for evidence of muscle rigidity **Monitoring**: rare but can occur with any antipsychotic at any dose and at any time; risk factors include young age, male gender, neurologic disabilities, dehydration, agitation, exhaustion, rapid or parenteral administration of antipsychotic **Management**: medical emergency; discontinue antipsychotic and provide supportive care (hydration and cooling); other measures may include **dantrolene** 2–3 mg/kg TID to QID iv (max 10 mg/kg daily) and/or **bromocriptine** 2.5–5 mg TID po, increasing by 2.5 mg TID Q24H (max 60 mg daily)[34]
Sedation and cognitive effects	**Assessment**: ask patient about daytime drowsiness, excessive sleep, cognitive "dulling"; obtain collateral information from caregivers and family **Monitoring**: see outpatients at least weekly for first 4–6 wk after initiating new antipsychotic **Management**: use SGAs as first-line treatment to reduce risk of cognitive side effects; low initial dose and gradual titration based on degree of sedation (especially with clozapine and first-episode psychosis). Give entire daily dose at HS if possible to reduce daytime drowsiness; do not use anticholinergic antiparkinsonian agents prophylactically and avoid prolonged use when treating acute EPS
Extrapyramidal side effects (EPS; dystonia, parkinsonism, akathisia, tardive dyskinesia, tardive dystonia)	**Assessment**: rating scales such as Simpson Angus Scale, Barnes Akathisia Scale or Extrapyramidal Syndrome Rating Scale (ESRS)[61] are useful to assess EPS and the Abnormal Involuntary Movement Scale or the ESRS is used to assess tardive dyskinesia (TD) **Monitoring**: baseline assessment in antipsychotic-naïve first-episode patients, in multiple-episode patients when initiating a new antipsychotic and whenever dosage of antipsychotic is changed; repeat assessment weekly for 2–4 wk or until EPS resolves; in stable patients assess for TD every 6 mo or more often in patients at higher risk (on FGAs, erratic medication adherence or intermittent treatment, female, age > 55, diagnosis of an affective disorder, substance abuse, diabetes) **Management**: Prevention is key—use SGAs first-line; if EPS occurs, first reduce dose; consider switch to SGA if on FGA; anticholinergics such as benztropine, procyclidine and trihexyphenidyl should not be used prophylactically even with FGAs, and should usually only be used on a short-term basis to treat parkinsonism associated with FGAs; anticholinergics are generally not recommended with SGAs[62] For *akathisia*, if dose reduction is not effective, beta-blockers (e.g., **propranolol** 10–120 mg/day) are the treatment of choice with monitoring for hypotension; benzodiazepines also provide symptom relief; anticholinergics are ineffective IM **benztropine** or **diphenhydramine** can be used to treat *acute dystonia* (acute torticollis or oculogyric crisis), followed by reduction in dose or switch to SGA There is no evidence-based treatment for TD—some reports of limited benefit of vitamin E (D-isomer) 1600 IU daily;[63] prevention is key—use SGAs first-line; antiparkinsonian medications are not effective and may worsen symptoms; if TD occurs suggest consultation with a psychiatrist; consider switching to an SGA; clozapine trial should be considered with persistent, severe TD

(cont'd)

Table 3: **Antipsychotic-induced Side Effects: Assessment, Monitoring and Management** [8,60] *(cont'd)*

Side Effect	Assessment, Monitoring and Management
Weight gain	**Assessment**: baseline weight, body mass index (BMI) and waist circumference **Monitoring**: weight and BMI monthly for 6 mo after initiating new antipsychotic then every 3 mo when on a stable antipsychotic dosage; waist circumference annually **Management**: prevention is critical as weight reduction is difficult especially in individuals with mental illness; educate about risk of weight gain and provide dietary and exercise counselling; if weight increases > 7% over baseline implement behavioural weight reduction program; if unsuccessful assess risks/benefits of continuing current antipsychotic vs. switching; no consistent scientific evidence to date of efficacy of adjunctive weight loss pharmacotherapy
Glucose abnormalities	**Assessment**: baseline fasting plasma glucose; HbA1c as alternative if difficult to obtain fasting plasma glucose; oral glucose tolerance test (OGTT) if evidence of impaired glucose tolerance; obtain family history and medical history[60] **Monitoring**: enquire about signs and symptoms of emergent diabetes; fasting plasma glucose 12 wk after initiating new antipsychotic, then yearly; more frequent monitoring required in presence of significant weight gain or if symptomatic; OGTT if evidence of impaired glucose tolerance **Management**: educate about signs and symptoms of emergent diabetes; if diabetes is diagnosed, follow the Canadian Diabetes Association Guidelines (http://www.diabetes.ca/cpg2003/); consider switching to another antipsychotic
Dyslipidemias	**Assessment**: baseline fasting lipid profile (total cholesterol, LDL, HDL, triglycerides) **Monitoring**: fasting lipid profile annually; more frequent monitoring in presence of significant weight gain and every 6 mo if LDL and/or triglycerides above the normal range **Management**: change in diet; consider switching to a different antipsychotic although advantages still need to be confirmed; consult clinical guidelines for management of dyslipidemia at http://www.cmaj.ca and www.nhlbi.nih.gov/guidelines/cholesterol/index.htm
Cardiovascular side effects	**Assessment**: baseline vital signs; obtain family history and medical history; ECG as clinically indicated **Monitoring**: blood pressure at 12 wk then annually; vital signs and ECG as clinically indicated and with changes in medication; QT_c monitoring indicated when affected by multiple medications **Management**: educate about risks of orthostatic hypotension and strategies to avoid it; if symptoms persist, decrease dose of antipsychotic if possible or switch to another antipsychotic
Endocrine and sexual side effects	**Assessment**: baseline functional inquiry including menstrual history and libido in women and libido, erectile and ejaculatory function in men; baseline prolactin level when clinically indicated and before initiating antipsychotic associated with hyperprolactinemia **Monitoring**: monitor monthly for 3 mo after initiating a new antipsychotic, then yearly. **Management**: determine underlying cause of endocrine or sexual dysfunction and treat accordingly; consider drugs for erectile dysfunction For clinically significant hyperprolactinemia, first reduce dose of antipsychotic; if dose reduction not tolerated (emergence of or increase in psychotic symptoms) consider switching to an antipsychotic not associated with risk of hyperprolactinemia

Therapeutic Tips

- Initiate treatment before the development of a crisis such as self-harm, aggression or violence.[8,24]
- Provide treatment in the least restrictive setting, considering safety issues, availability of community resources (including both caregiver and mental health supports), the patient's insight and competency to consent to treatment and ability to cooperate with treatment.[8,24]
- Integrate psychosocial interventions such as patient and family psychoeducation, supportive therapy and stress management with the use of antipsychotic medications in order to promote adherence to treatment and optimize outcomes.[8,24]
- Conduct baseline and regular ongoing assessments of signs and symptoms, possible comorbid conditions, level of functioning, response to treatment, side effects and medication adherence during all phases of the disorder. A variety of standardized scales and semi-structured interviews facilitate these assessments.[8]
- To ensure continuity of care, longitudinal follow-up by the same clinician or multidisciplinary team is optimal.[8,24]

Figure 1: **Management of Acute Psychotic Episodes**

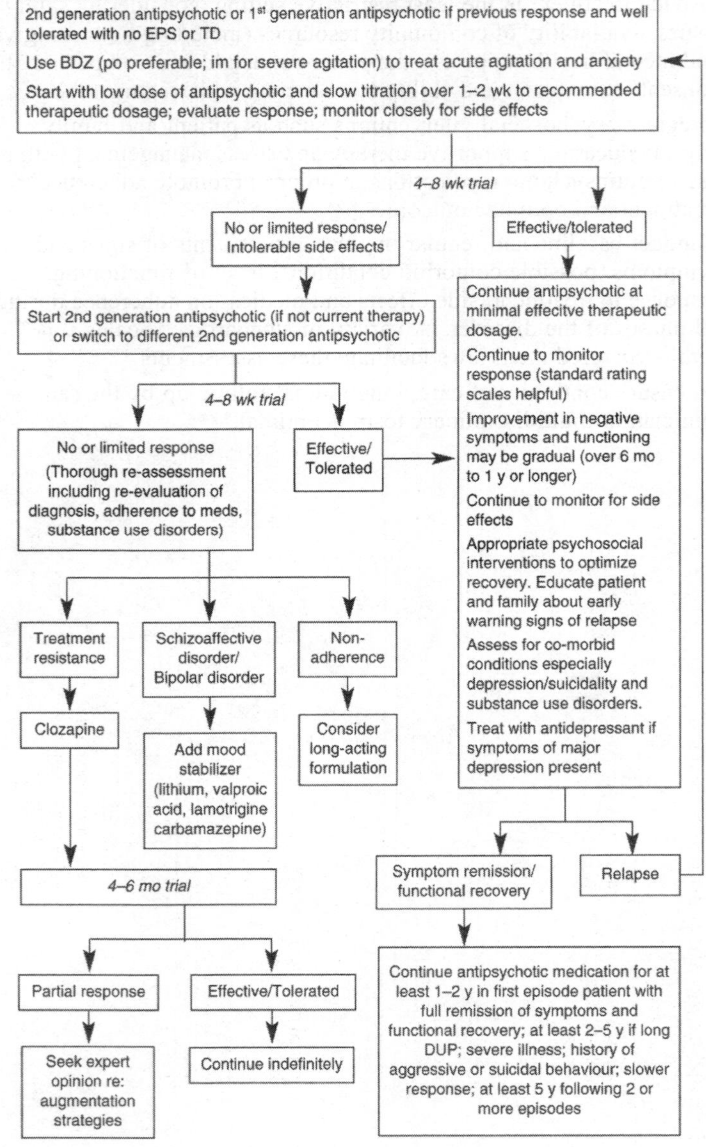

Abbreviations: BDZ = benzodiazepines; DUP = duration of untreated psychosis; EPS = extrapyramidal symptoms; TD = tardive dyskinesia

Table 4: **Second-generation Antipsychotics**

Class	Drug	Dose	Adverse Effects	Drug Interactions	Cost[a]
Second-generation Antipsychotics	*clozapine* Clozaril, Gen-Clozapine, generics	Initial: 12.5–25 mg/day po Titration: increase by 12.5–25 mg on second day and then by 25–50 mg po daily depending on tolerance Usual: 300–600 mg/day po Max: 900 mg/day Divided in 1–3 doses/day	Agranulocytosis (< 1%), seizures (5%; dose related), sedation, orthostatic hypotension, tachycardia, fever, nausea, weight gain, hypersalivation, urinary incontinence; ↑ risk of diabetes and hyperlipidemia; myocarditis and other cardiac effects (see Pharmacologic Choices).	Additive sedation with CNS depressants; may potentiate antihypertensive drug effects; inhibitors of CYP1A2 (e.g., diltiazem, fluvoxamine, propranolol) or CYP3A4 (e.g., clarithromycin, erythromycin, grapefruit juice, prednisone) may ↑ clozapine levels; inducers of CYP1A2 or CYP3A4 (e.g., carbamazepine, phenytoin, rifampin), may ↓ clozapine levels; respiratory depression with higher doses of benzodiazepines; avoid use with bone marrow suppressants and drugs that lower the seizure threshold.	$$$
	olanzapine, oral Zyprexa, Zyprexa Zydis (rapid-dissolving oral tablets)	Initial: 5–10 mg/day Titration: increase by 2.5–5 mg every 3–4 days Usual: 10–20 mg/day Max: 20 mg/day (product monograph). Doses of up to 40 mg/day are used in clinical practice under care of a psychiatrist Frequency: one dose/day; higher doses may be given in 2 divided doses	Weight gain, dizziness, sedation, anticholinergic effects, hepatic transaminase elevation, orthostatic hypotension, ↑ risk of diabetes and dyslipidemia, EPS (especially akathisia).	Sedation with CNS depressants; may potentiate antihypertensive drug effects; inhibitors of CYP1A2 or CYP2D6 (e.g., diltiazem, fluvoxamine, paroxetine) may ↑ olanzapine levels; inducers of CYP1A2 or CYP3A4 (e.g., barbiturates, carbamazepine, phenytoin, rifampin) may ↓ olanzapine levels.	$$$

(cont'd)

Table 4: **Second-generation Antipsychotics** *(cont'd)*

Class	Drug	Dose	Adverse Effects	Drug Interactions	Cost[a]
	olanzapine, intramuscular injection Zyprexa Intramuscular	Initial: 5–10 mg im Usual: 10 mg im. If necessary 2nd dose of 5–10 mg im may be given 2 h after first injection Max: 20 mg/day (oral and im) with no more than 3 injections in 24 h	See oral olanzapine.	See oral olanzapine. Should not be administered simultaneously with parenteral benzodiazepines due to reports of cardiac and respiratory problems including deaths.	$$$$
	quetiapine, oral Seroquel	Initial: 50–100 mg/day Titration: increase by 100 mg/day Usual: 600 mg/day Max: 800 mg/day (product monograph). Doses of up to 1200 mg/day used in clinical practice under care of a psychiatrist Divided in 1–3 doses/day	Sedation, dizziness, weight gain, orthostatic hypotension, hepatic transaminase elevation, headache, anticholinergic effects, ↑ risk of diabetes and dyslipidemia, possible ↑ risk of cataracts; may ↓ thyroid hormone levels.	Additive sedation with CNS depressants; may potentiate antihypertensive drug effects; inhibitors of CYP3A4 (e.g., clarithromycin, erythromycin, grapefruit juice, ketoconazole, prednisone) may ↑ quetiapine levels; inducers of CYP3A4 (e.g., carbamazepine, phenytoin, rifampin) may ↓ quetiapine levels.	$$ (depending on dose)
	risperidone, oral Risperdal, generics; Risperdal M Tabs (rapid-dissolving oral formulation)	Initial: 0.5–1 mg/day Titration: increase 0.5–1.0 mg every 3–4 days Usual: 2–6 mg/day Max: 8 mg/day Frequency: one dose/day, preferably HS	Insomnia, headaches, weight gain, orthostatic hypotension, rhinitis, anxiety, dose-related hyperprolactinemia and EPS.	Additive sedation with CNS depressants; may potentiate antihypertensive drug effects; inhibitors of CYP3A4 (e.g., clarithromycin, erythromycin, grapefruit juice, ketoconazole, prednisone) may ↑ risperidone levels; inducers of CYP3A4 (e.g., carbamazepine, phenytoin, rifampin) may ↓ risperidone levels.	$$

Class	Drug	Dose	Adverse Effects	Drug Interactions	Cost[a]
	risperidone long-acting intramuscular injection Risperdal Consta	Initial: 25 mg im every 2 wk (oral supplementation with current antipsychotic required for first 3 wk) Titration: depending on response, increase by 12.5 mg every 4–8 wk. Usual: 25–37.5 mg im every 2 wk. Max: 50 mg im every 2 wk	See oral risperidone, although potentially less severity due to decreased peak to trough serum fluctuations.	See oral risperidone.	$$$$ (depending on dose)

[a] Cost of 30-day supply of mean usual dose; includes drug cost only.
Dosage adjustment may be required in renal impairment; see Appendix I
Abbreviations: EPS = extrapyramidal symptoms
Legend: $ < $100 $$ $100–250 $$$ $250–400 $$$$ > $400

Table 5: **First-generation Antipsychotics**

Class	Drug	Dose	Adverse Effects	Drug Interactions	Cost[a]
Low Potency	*chlorpromazine* generics	Initial: 50–100 mg/day po Usual: 200–400 mg/day po Max: 1000–2000 mg/day po Divided in 1–3 doses/day	*First-generation antipsychotics:* sedation, cardiovascular effects, anticholinergic effects, weight gain, ↓ seizure threshold, photosensitivity (more common with low potency agents) ↑ prolactin, EPS, NMS, tardive movement disorders (more common with high-potency agents), liver function abnormalities.	*First-generation antipsychotics:* additive effects with other CNS depressants, anticholinergics, alpha-adrenergic antagonists; inhibitors of cytochrome P450 enzymes (e.g., TCAs, fluoxetine, fluvoxamine, paroxetine) may ↑ serum levels; inducers of cytochrome P450 enzymes (e.g., carbamazepine, phenytoin) may ↓ serum levels; effects of levodopa may be inhibited.	$$
	methotrimeprazine Nozinan, generics	Initial: 25–75 mg/day po Usual: 100–200 mg/day po Max: 1000 mg/day po Divided in 1–3 doses/day	See chlorpromazine.	See chlorpromazine.	$
Intermediate Potency	*loxapine* generics	Initial: 10–20 mg/day po Usual: 20–100 mg/day po Max: 250 mg/day po Divided in 2–3 doses/day	See chlorpromazine.	See chlorpromazine.	$
	perphenazine Trilafon, generics	Initial: 4–12 mg/day po Usual: 12–48 mg/day po Max: 48–64 mg/day po Divided in 2–3 doses/day	See chlorpromazine.	See chlorpromazine.	$

Class	Drug	Dose	Adverse Effects	Drug Interactions	Cost[a]
	zuclopenthixol Clopixol	Initial: 10–20 mg/day po Usual: 20–60 mg/day po Max: 100 mg/day po Divided in 1–3 doses/day	See chlorpromazine.	See chlorpromazine.	$$$
High Potency	*flupenthixol* Fluanxol	Initial: 3–6 mg/day po Usual: 9–24 mg/day po Max: 12–24 mg/day po Divided in 2 doses/day	See chlorpromazine.	See chlorpromazine.	$$$$
	fluphenazine generics	Initial: 2–5 mg/day po Usual: 2.5–10 mg/day po Max: 20 mg/day po Divided in 1–2 doses/day	See chlorpromazine.	See chlorpromazine.	$
	haloperidol generics	Initial: 1.5–3 mg/day Usual: 4–12 mg/day po Max: 20 mg/day po Divided in 1–3 doses/day	See chlorpromazine.	See chlorpromazine.	$
	pimozide Orap, generics	Initial: 2–4 mg/day po Usual: 2–12 mg/day Max: 12 mg/day po Divided in 1–2 doses/day	See chlorpromazine. Pimozide: QTc prolongation with doses > 8 mg/day.	See chlorpromazine. Pimozide: avoid use with sertraline due to ↑ risk of QTc prolongation.	$

(cont'd)

Table 5: **First-generation Antipsychotics** *(cont'd)*

Class	Drug	Dose	Adverse Effects	Drug Interactions	Cost[a]
	thiothixene Navane	Initial: 5–10 mg/day Usual: 15–30 mg/day po Max: 60 mg/day po Divided in 1–2 doses/day	See chlorpromazine.	See chlorpromazine.	$$
	trifluoperazine generics	Initial: 2–10 mg/day po Usual: 6–20 mg/day po Max: 40 mg/day po Divided in 1–2 doses/day	See chlorpromazine.	See chlorpromazine.	$

[a] Cost of 30-day supply of mean usual dose unless otherwise specified; includes drug cost only.
Legend: $ < $25 $$ $25–50 $$$ $50–75 $$$$ $75–100
Abbreviations: CV = cardiovascular; EPS = extrapyramidal symptoms; NMS = neuroleptic malignant syndrome; TCAs = tricyclic antidepressants; BDZs = benzodiazepines

Suggested Readings

Canadian Psychiatric Association. Clinical practice guidelines. Treatment of schizophrenia. *Can J Psychiatry* 2005;50(13 Suppl 1):7S-57S.

Faulkner G, Cohn TA. Pharmacologic and nonpharmacologic strategies for weight gain and metabolic disturbance in patients treated with antipsychotic medications. *Can J Psychiatry* 2006;51(8):502-11.

Gardner DM, Baldessarini RJ, Waraich P. Modern antipsychotic drugs: a critical overview. *CMAJ* 2005;172(13):1703-11.

Meltzer HY, Kostakoglu AE. Treatment-resistant schizophrenia. In: Lieberman JA, Murray RM, editors. *Comprehensive care of schizophrenia: a textbook of clinical management*. London (UK): Martin Dunitz; 2001. p. 181-203.

Newcomer JW, Haupt DW. The metabolic effects of antipsychotic medications. *Can J Psychiatry* 2006;51(8):480-91.

Remington G. Rational pharmacotherapy in early psychosis. *Br J Psychiatry Suppl* 2005;187(48):s77-84.

Siegfried SI, Fleischhacker W, Lieberman JA. Pharmacological treatment of schizophrenia. In: Lieberman JA, Murray RM, editors. *Comprehensive care of schizophrenia: a textbook of clinical management*. London (UK): Martin Dunitz; 2001. p. 59-94.

Tandon R, Fleischhacker WW. Comparative efficacy of antipsychotics in the treatment of schizophrenia: a critical assessment. *Schizophr Res* 2005;79(2-3):145-55.

References

1. Nova Scotia Early Psychosis Program, Capital Health Mental Health Program, Capital Health and the Department of Psychiatry, Dalhousie University. *The sooner the better: get help early for psychosis. Information guide*. Halifax (NS): Nova Scotia Early Psychosis Program; 2003. Available from: http://earlypsychosis.medicine.dal.ca/resources/FinalBooklet-Oct32005.pdf Accessed May 23, 2007.
2. Lieberman JA, Fenton WS. Delayed detection of psychosis: causes, consequences, and effect on public health. *Am J Psychiatry* 2000;157(11):1727-30.
3. Loebel AD, Lieberman JA, Alvir JM et al. Duration of psychosis and outcome in first-episode schizophrenia. *Am J Psychiatry* 1992;149(9):1183-8.
4. Craig TJ, Bromet EJ, Fennig S et al. Is there an association between duration of untreated psychosis and 24-month clinical outcome in a first-admission series? *Am J Psychiatry* 2000;157(1):60-6.
5. McGlashan TH. Duration of untreated psychosis in first-episode schizophrenia: marker or determinant of course? *Biol Psychiatry* 1999;46(7):899-907.
6. American Psychiatric Association; American Psychiatric Association. Task Force on DSM-IV. *Diagnostic and statistical manual of mental disorders: DSM-IV-TR*. 4th ed., text revision. Washington (DC): American Psychiatric Association; 2000.
7. Caspi A, Moffitt TE, Cannon M et al. Moderation of the effect of adolescent-onset cannabis use on adult psychosis by a functional polymorphism in the Catechol-O-Methyltransferase gene: longitudinal evidence of a gene x environment interaction. *Biol Psychiatry* 2005; 57:1117-27.
8. Canadian Psychiatric Association. Clinical practice guidelines. Treatment of schizophrenia. *Can J Psychiatry* 2005;50(13 Suppl 1):7S-57S.
9. Guy W; National Institute of Mental Health (U.S.). Psychopharmacology Research Branch; Early Clinical Drug Evaluation Program. *ECDEU assessment manual for psychopharmacology*. Rockville (MD): U. S. Dept. of Health, Education, and Welfare, Public Health Service, Alcohol, Drug Abuse, and Mental Health Administration, National Institute of Mental Health, Psychopharmacology Research Branch, Division of Extramural Research Programs; 1976. p. 217-22.
10. Kay SR, Fiszbein A, Opler LA. The positive and negative syndrome scale (PANSS) for schizophrenia. *Schizophr Bull* 1987;13(2):261-76.
11. American Diabetes Association; American Psychiatric Association; American Association of Clinical Endocrinologists et al. Consensus development conference on antipsychotic drugs and obesity and diabetes. *Diabetes Care* 2004;27(2):596-601

12. Siegfried SI, Fleischhacker W, Lieberman JA. Pharmacological treatment of schizophrenia. In: Lieberman JA, Murray RM, editors. *Comprehensive care of schizophrenia: a textbook of clinical management*. London (UK): Martin Dunitz; 2001. p. 59-94.
13. Zipursky RB. Optimal pharmacologic management of the first episode of schizophrenia. In: Zipursky RB, Schulz SC, editors. *The early stages of schizophrenia*. 1st ed. Washington (DC): American Psychiatric Pub; 2002.
14. Seeman P. Atypical antipsychotics: mechanism of action. *Can J Psychiatry* 2002;47(1):27-38.
15. Emsley RA. Risperidone in the treatment of first-episode psychotic patients: a double-blind multicenter study. Risperidone Working Group. *Schizophr Bull* 1999;25(4):721-9.
16. Sanger TM, Lieberman JA, Tohen M et al. Olanzapine versus haloperidol treatment in first-episode psychosis. *Am J Psychiatry* 1999;156(1):79-87.
17. Canadian Psychiatric Association. *Practical guide for schizophrenia management*. Ottawa (ON): Canadian Psychiatric Association; 2000.
18. Marder SR, Essock SM, Miller AL et al. The Mount Sinai conference on the pharmacotherapy of schizophrenia. *Schizophr Bull* 2002;28(1):5-16
19. Csernansky JG, Mahmoud R, Brenner R et al. A comparison of risperidone and haloperidol for the prevention of relapse in patients with schizophrenia. *N Engl J Med* 2002;346(1):16-22.
20. Conley RR, Love RC, Kelly DL et al. Rehospitalization rates of patients recently discharged on a regimen of risperidone or clozapine. *Am J Psychiatry* 1999;156(6):863-8.
21. Citrome L, Volavka J, Czobor P et al. Effects of clozapine, olanzapine, risperidone, and haloperidol on hostility among patients with schizophrenia. *Psychiatr Serv* 2001;52(11):1510-4.
22. Kane JM, Marder SR, Schooler NR et al. Clozapine and haloperidol in moderately refractory schizophrenia: a 6-month randomized and double-blind comparison. *Arch Gen Psychiatry* 2001;58(10):965-72.
23. Meltzer HY, Okayli G. Reduction of suicidality during clozapine treatment of neuroleptic-resistant schizophrenia: impact on risk-benefit assessment. *Am J Psychiatry* 1995;152(2):183-90.
24. International Early Psychosis Association. *Draft consensus statement - principles and practice in early psychosis*. Victoria (AU): IEPA; 2003. Available from: http://www.iepa.org.au/downloads/ics.pdf Accessed May 23, 2007.
25. Battaglia J, Moss S, Rush J et al. Haloperidol, lorazepam, or both for psychotic agitation? A multicenter, prospective, double-blind, emergency department study. *Am J Emerg Med* 1997;15(4):335-40.
26. Breier A, Meehan K, Birkett M et al. A double-blind, placebo-controlled dose-response comparison of intramuscular olanzapine and haloperidol in the treatment of acute agitation in schizophrenia. *Arch Gen Psychiatry* 2002;59(5):441-8.
27. Wright P, Birkett M, David SR et al. Double-blind, placebo-controlled comparison of intramuscular olanzapine and intramuscular haloperidol in the treatment of acute agitation in schizophrenia. *Am J Psychiatry* 2001;158(7):1149-51.
28. Currier GW, Chou JC, Feifel D et al. Acute treatment of psychotic agitation: a randomized comparison of oral treatment with risperidone and lorazepam versus intramuscular treatment with haloperidol and lorazepam. *J Clin Psychiatry* 2004;65(3):386-94.
29. Lieberman J, Jody D, Geisler S et al. Time course and biologic correlates of treatment response in first-episode schizophrenia. *Arch Gen Psychiatry* 1993;50(5):369-76.
30. Lieberman JA, Koreen AR, Chakos M et al. Factors influencing treatment response and outcome of first-episode schizophrenia: implications for understanding the pathophysiology of schizophrenia. *J Clin Psychiatry* 1996;57(Suppl 9):5-9.
31. Chengappa KN, Parepally H, Brar JS et al. A random-assignment, double-blind, clinical trial of once- vs twice-daily administration of quetiapine fumarate in patients with schizophrenia or schizoaffective disorder: a pilot study. *Can J Psychiatry* 2003;48(3):187-94.
32. Stone CK, Garve DL, Griffith J et al. Further evidence of a dose-response threshold for haloperidol in psychosis. *Am J Psychiatry* 1995;152(8):1210-2.
33. Thompson C. The use of high-dose antipsychotic medication. *Br J Psychiatry* 1994;164(4):448-58.
34. Weiden PJ et al. *Breakthroughs in antipsychotic medications : a guide for consumers, families, and clinicians*. New York (NY): Norton; 1999.
35. Davis JM, Chen N, Glick ID. A meta-analysis of the efficacy of second-generation antipsychotics. *Arch Gen Psychiatry* 2003;60(6):553-64.
36. Sands JR, Harrow M. Depression during the longitudinal course of schizophrenia. *Schizophr Bull* 1999;25(1):157-71.
37. Koreen AR, Siris SG, Chakos M et al. Depression in first-episode schizophrenia. *Am J Psychiatry* 1993;150(11):1643-8.
38. Addington D, Addington J, Patten S. Depression in people with first-episode schizophrenia. *Br J Psychiatry Suppl* 1998;172(33):90-2.
39. Addington D, Addington J, Schissel B. A depression rating scale for schizophrenics. *Schizophr Res* 1990; 3(4):247-51.
40. Drake RE, Mueser KT, Brunette MF et al. A review of treatments for people with severe mental illnesses and co-occurring substance use disorders. *Psychiatr Rehabil J* 2004;27(4):360-74.

41. Harvey PD, Meltzer H, Simpson GM et al. Improvement in cognitive function following a switch to ziprasidone from conventional antipsychotics, olanzapine, or risperidone in outpatients with schizophrenia. *Schizophr Res* 2004;66(2-3):101-13.
42. Bilder RM, Goldman RS, Volavka J et al. Neurocognitive effects of clozapine, olanzapine, risperidone, and haloperidol in patients with chronic schizophrenia or schizoaffective disorder. *Am J Psychiatry* 2002;159(6):1018-28.
43. Velligan DI, Miller AL. Cognitive dysfunction in schizophrenia and its importance to outcome: the place of atypical antipsychotics in treatment. *J Clin Psychiatry* 1999;60(Suppl 23):25-8.
44. Chakos M, Lieberman J, Hoffman E et al. Effectiveness of second-generation antipsychotics in patients with treatment-resistant schizophrenia: a review and meta-analysis of randomized trials. *Am J Psychiatry* 2001;158(4):518-26.
45. Raggi MA, Mandrioli R, Sabbioni C et al. Atypical antipsychotics: pharmacokinetics, therapeutic drug monitoring and pharmacological interactions. *Curr Med Chem* 2004;11(3):279-96.
46. Velligan DI, Mahurin RK, Diamond PL et al. The functional significance of symptomatology and cognitive function in schizophrenia. *Schizophr Res* 1997;25(1):21-31.
47. Casey DE. Tardive dyskinesia and atypical antipsychotic drugs. *Schizophr Res* 1999;35(Suppl):S61-6.
48. Leucht S, Pitschel-Walz G, Abraham D et al. Efficacy and extrapyramidal side-effects of the new antipsychotics olanzapine, quetiapine, risperidone, and sertindole compared to conventional antipsychotics and placebo. A meta-analysis of randomized controlled trials. *Schizophr Res* 1999;35(1):51-68.
49. Shriqui CL. Atypical antipsychotics. *Can J CME* 2002;65-80. Available from: http://www.stacommunications.com/journals/pdfs/cme/julycme/g.pdf Accessed May 23, 2007.
50. Sernyak MJ, Leslie DL, Alarcon RD et al. Association of diabetes mellitus with use of atypical neuroleptics in the treatment of schizophrenia. *Am J Psychiatry* 2002;159(4):561-6.
51. Buse JB. Metabolic side effects of antipsychotics: focus on hyperglycemia and diabetes. *J Clin Psychiatry* 2002;63(Suppl 4):37-41.
52. Canadian Pharmacists Association. *CPS: Compendium of pharmaceuticals and specialties*. Ottawa (ON): CPhA; 2006.
53. Casey DE. Dyslipidemia and atypical antipsychotic drugs. *J Clin Psychiatry* 2004; 65(Suppl 18):27-35.
54. Marder SR, Essock SM, Miller AL et al. Physical health monitoring of patients with schizophrenia. *Am J Psychiatry* 2004;161(8):1334-49.
55. Vieweg WV. Mechanisms and risks of electrocardiographic QT interval prolongation when using antipsychotic drugs. *J Clin Psychiatry* 2002;63(Suppl 9):18-24.
56. U.S. Food and Drug Administration. FDA Psychopharmacological Drugs Advisory Committee. *Briefing document for Zeldox capsules (Ziprasidone HCl)*. Rockville (MD): FDA; 2000. Available from: http://www.fda.gov/ohrms/dockets/ac/00/backgrd/3619b1a.pdf Accessed May 23, 2007.
57. Feinstein RE, Khawaja IS, Nurenberg JR et al. Cardiovascular effects of psychotropic drugs. *Curr Probl Cardiol* 2002; 27(5):190-240.
58. Atmaca M, Kuloglu M, Tezcan E et al. Quetiapine is not associated with increase in prolactin secretion in contrast to haloperidol. *Arch Med Res* 2002;33(6):562-5.
59. Knegtering H, van der Moolen AE, Castelein S et al. What are the effects of antipsychotics on sexual dysfunctions and endocrine functioning? *Psychoneuroendocrinology* 2003;28(Suppl 2):109-23.
60. Cohn TA, Sernyak MJ. Metabolic monitoring for patients treated with antipsychotic medications. *Can J Psychiatry* 2006;51(8):492-501.
61. De Deyn PP, Wirshing WC. Scales to assess efficacy and safety of pharmacologic agents in the treatment of behavioral and psychological symptoms of dementia. *J Clin Psychiatry* 2001;62(Suppl 21):19-22.
62. Serretti A, De Ronchi D, Lorenzi C et al. New antipsychotics and schizophrenia: a review on efficacy and side effects. *Curr Med Chem* 2004;11(3):343-58.
63. Jog M et al. *Movement disorders manual*. London (ON): Movement Disorders Program, London Health Sciences Centre; 2000.

Pharmacoeconomic Considerations: Psychoses

Nicole Mittmann, MSc, PhD

Epidemiology		
Country	**Prevalence (%)**	
Canada & Worldwide[1,2,3,4,5]	1%	
Cost of Illness Data		
Country and Year of Estimate	**Direct Costs[a]**	**Indirect Costs[b]**
Canada (2004)[5]	$2.02 billion	$4.83 billion

Commentary

Schizophrenia is associated with significant economic burden from a patient, health care and societal perspective.

Direct medical resources consumed in the care of patients with schizophrenia include physician visits, emergency department visits, acute and non-acute hospitalizations and residential care facilities. Nonmedical resources include social services and other government services, e.g., police, prisons. Lost work productivity is an important economic impact of schizophrenia. The average annual income of employed schizophrenics is relatively low, indicating underemployment.[5] A high proportion (30–70%) of individuals with schizophrenia are unemployed.[5]

Intangible costs (e.g., pain, suffering) associated with schizophrenia have not been well documented but may also have a significant impact on the overall societal costs of schizophrenia.

Newer atypical antipsychotic agents have higher acquisition costs compared with older antipsychotics. Atypical antipsychotics may reduce noncompliance relative to older antipsychotic agents.[6] In almost all published pharmacoeconomic analyses, atypical antipsychotic agents have been found to be cost-effective when compared with conventional antipsychotic agents, leading to reductions in hospitalization, use of other medical resources and improvements in quality of life.[6,7,8,9] Few economic evaluations have compared atypical antipsychotic agents with one another, although the majority of these analyses have been sponsored by pharmaceutical manufacturers.

[a] Direct costs include those associated with physician services, nursing care, diagnostic procedures, drugs and hospitalization.

[b] Indirect costs include those associated with lost productivity and days off work due to morbidity or premature mortality.

References

1. Goldner EM, Hsu L, Waraich P et al. Prevalence and incidence studies of schizophrenic disorders: a systematic review. *Can J Psychiatry* 2002;47(9):833-43.

2. World Health Organization. *Mental and neurological disorders*. Fact sheet no. 265. Geneva (CH): WHO; December 2001.
3. Bresnahan M, Menezes P, Varma V et al. Geographical variation in incidence, course and outcome in schizophrenia: a comparison of developing and developed countries. In: Murray R, Jones P, Susser E et al, editors. *Epidemiology of schizophrenia*. New York (NY): Cambridge University Press; 2003.
4. Saha S, Chant D, Welham J et al. A systematic review of the prevalence of schizophrenia. *PLoS Med* 2005;2(5):e141.
5. Goeree R, Farahati F, Burke N et al. The economic burden of schizophrenia in Canada in 2004. *Curr Med Res Opin* 2005;21(12):2017-28.
6. Dolder CR, Lacro JP, Dunn LB et al. Antipsychotic medication adherence: is there a difference between typical and atypical agents? *Am J Psychiatry* 2002;159(1):103-8.
7. Rosenheck R, Perlick D, Bingham S et al. Effectiveness and cost of olanzapine and haloperidol in the treatment of schizophrenia: a randomized controlled trial. *JAMA* 2003;290(20):2693-702.
8. Palmer CS, Revicki DA, Genduso LA et al. A cost-effectiveness clinical decision analysis model for schizophrenia. *Am J Manag Care* 1998;4(3):345-55.
9. Rosenheck R, Leslie DL, Sindelar J et al. Cost-effectiveness of second-generation antipsychotics and perphenazine in a randomized trial of treatment for chronic schizophrenia. *Am J Psychiatry* 2006;163(12) 2080-9.

CHAPTER 8
Insomnia

Jonathan A.E. Fleming, MB, FRCPC

Insomnia is a common symptom of a number of psychiatric, medical and sleep disorders. Primary insomnia[1] (chronic psychophysiological insomnia) is the focus of this chapter. Secondary insomnia (e.g., insomnia associated with a mood disorder or chronic pain)[2] usually responds to treatment of the underlying disorder.

Goals of Therapy

- Promote sound and restorative sleep when external (e.g., stress, noise, jet lag) or internal (e.g., pain, anxiety) factors disrupt natural sleep
- Reduce daytime impairment (e.g., dysphoria, fatigue, decreased alertness) associated with sleep loss
- Potentiate the effectiveness of behavioural interventions in managing patients with primary, chronic insomnia[3]

Investigations

- A complete sleep history (Table 1) is *essential:*
  - to quantify current sleep performance and daytime impairment
  - to determine the outcome of previous interventions
  - to rule out other sleep pathologies including those for which hypnotics are contraindicated and potentially lethal, e.g., obstructive sleep apnea[4]
- Completion of a sleep diary (Table 3) for one week, to quantify sleep performance and variability
- Psychiatric work-up to rule out associated mental disorders (especially mood and anxiety disorders, drug and alcohol use)
- Medical work-up to rule out associated medical disorders (especially those associated with nocturnal discomfort or pain such as arthritis, Parkinson's disease)
- Thorough drug history including prescription and nonprescription medications, herbal or other natural remedies, caffeine, nicotine, alcohol and recreational drugs
- Self-rating scales for depression (available at http://depression-webworld.com/zung_sdsndx.htm) and anxiety symptoms (available at http://depression-webworld.com/zung_anxietyndx.htm) are useful screening tools for identifying depressive or anxiety disorders causing insomnia (Note: insomnia can be both an early symptom and a cause of depression)

Therapeutic Choices (Figure 1)

Nonpharmacologic Choices

- Instruct patient in sleep hygiene (Table 2); monitor and encourage adherence throughout treatment and follow-up (important to success of *any* intervention).
- Suggest relaxation exercises (available as audio recordings for home use, e.g., http://www.calming.org/tapes.htm).
- Consider sleep restriction, stimulus control or other behavioural approaches,[5] alone or with pharmacologic interventions.
- Aerobic exercise, a useful modifier of stress and dysphoric moods, also promotes deeper and more restful sleep; encourage patients with insomnia to decrease daytime rest periods and increase exercise.

Table 1: **The Sleep History**

1. Time data (can also be collected as part of a sleep diary – Table 3)

Did you nap or lie down to rest today? If yes, when and for how long?
What time did you go to bed last night?
What time did you put out the lights?
How long did it take you to fall asleep?
How many times did you awaken last night?
How long was your longest awake period; when was it? What time did you finally awaken?
What time did you get out of bed?
How many hours sleep did you get last night?

2. Questions about the sleep period

Do physical symptoms, such as pain, prevent you from falling asleep?
Do mental or emotional symptoms (e.g., worry or anxiety) prevent you from falling asleep?
When you awaken during the night, what awakens you? (Snoring? Gasping for air? Dreams/nightmares? Noise?)
When you get up for the day, do you have any symptoms? (Headache? Confusion? Sleepiness?)

3. Questions for the patient's bed partner

Does your partner snore, gasp or make choking sounds during the night?
Does your partner stop breathing during the night?
Do your partner's legs twitch, jerk or kick during the night?
Has your partner's use of alcohol, nicotine, caffeine or other drugs changed recently?
Has your partner's mood or emotional state changed recently?
What do you think is the cause of your partner's sleep problem?

Pharmacologic Choices (Table 4)

Short courses (Figure 1) of hypnotics are useful combined with good sleep hygiene (Table 2). A comprehensive evaluation, education stressing the importance of sleep hygiene (especially preventing extended sleeping such as naps or nocturnal sleep periods of more than eight hours) and careful monitoring of progress are important. With these measures, the use of the preferred agents, the benzodiazepines or nonbenzodiazepines such as zaleplon and zopiclone, is usually straightforward in patients with primary insomnia.

Table 2: Sleep Hygiene Guidelines

1. Keep a regular sleep–wake schedule, 7 days per week.
2. Restrict the sleep period to the average sleep time you have obtained each night over the preceding week.
3. Avoid sleeping in, extensive periods of horizontal rest or daytime napping; these activities usually affect the subsequent night's sleep.
4. Get regular exercise every day: about 40 minutes of an activity with sufficient intensity to cause sweating. If evening exercise prevents sleep, schedule the exercise earlier in the day.
5. Avoid caffeine, nicotine, alcohol and other recreational drugs, all of which disturb sleep. If you must smoke do not do so after 7:00 p.m.
6. Plan a quiet period before lights out; a warm bath may be helpful.
7. Avoid large meals late in the evening; a light carbohydrate snack (e.g., crackers and warm milk) before bedtime can be helpful.
8. Turn the clock face away and always use the alarm. Looking at the clock time on awakening can cause emotional arousal (performance anxiety or anger) that prevents return to sleep.
9. As much as possible, keep the bedroom dark and soundproofed. If you live in a noisy area, consider ear plugs.
10. Use the bedroom only for sleep and intimacy; using the bed as a reading place, office or media centre conditions you to be alert in a place that should be associated with quiet and sleep. If you awaken during the night and are wide awake, get up, leave the bedroom and do something quiet until you feel drowsy-tired, then return to bed.

Note: Pharmacologic (or any) interventions will be less effective if these guidelines are not followed. In mild cases of insomnia, sleep hygiene guidelines, practised consistently and together, may be sufficient to reinstate a normal sleep pattern.

Benzodiazepines (BDZs)

All BDZs have sedative and hypnotic properties, but differ significantly in potency and pharmacokinetics. All may cause confusion and ataxia, especially in the elderly and the medically ill. For primary insomnia, BDZs that have been studied in sleep-disturbed patients are generally preferred over other BDZs. When insomnia is secondary to prominent anxiety symptoms, a long-acting BDZ (such as clonazepam) given at night may promote sleep and manage daytime anxiety. It is inappropriate to use one BDZ during the day to manage anxiety and a different BDZ as a hypnotic at night, in the same patient.

In Canada, four BDZs are officially indicated for insomnia: **flurazepam, nitrazepam, temazepam** and **triazolam**. Because of their longer half-lives, flurazepam and nitrazepam accumulate with repeated dosing and are associated with more hangover effects than shorter-acting BDZs. In the elderly, they cause higher cortical impairment resulting in confusion and falls. Flurazepam and nitrazepam are not recommended, particularly in the elderly.[6]

Temazepam is a good all-purpose hypnotic with a half-life sufficient to cover the sleep period without causing hangover effects. However, few hypnotics have proven tolerability in the elderly, and temazepam may be associated with falls in this population.[7] It causes less rebound insomnia than more potent BDZs such as lorazepam.

Triazolam has a fast onset and short duration of action, making it more suitable for managing *initial insomnia* (first third of the night) rather than *maintenance insomnia* (last third of the night). In addition to causing rebound insomnia, it has a unique adverse event profile (confusion, agitation, and amnesia) making it unsuitable for use in the elderly.[8] A shorter treatment course (five to seven days) is recommended for triazolam.

Although the number of comparative studies is relatively small, **oxazepam** is as effective as the BDZs that are officially indicated for insomnia.[9,10] In patients with *initial* insomnia, oxazepam should be given 60 to 90 minutes before bedtime because of its slow absorption. Conversely, patients who have no difficulty falling asleep but experience *maintenance* insomnia can take oxazepam when getting into bed.

There are few trials studying the effects of **lorazepam** on insomnia. Lorazepam may cause significant rebound effects such as anxiety and tension.[11]

Benzodiazepine–Receptor Agonists

Although not a BDZ, the cyclopyrrolone **zopiclone** acts at the BDZ receptor and so has similar therapeutic and side effects. Although psychomotor impairment associated with combined use of zopiclone and small amounts of alcohol has been shown to be minor, zopiclone can have residual or hangover effects that could impair morning driving, when used with or without alcohol.[12] Compared with BDZs, tolerance to zopiclone's hypnotic effect may be delayed and rebound insomnia may be reduced.[13] **Eszopiclone**, the active (S+) isomer of zopiclone, shares similar pharmacologic properties to the racemic compound but is more potent.[14] Several studies have demonstrated efficacy in transient and chronic insomnia with one demonstrating continued efficacy over 12 months of use with no evidence of tolerance or a withdrawal syndrome or rebound insomnia on discontinuation.[15] Eszopiclone in not available in Canada.

The pyrazolopyrimidine **zaleplon** was withdrawn voluntarily from the Canadian market in 2006. **Indiplon** is a short-acting pyrazolopyrimidine that binds to a specific site at the GABA-A receptor. Indiplon is not available in Canada; preliminary data from Phase III trials show good efficacy and safety.[16]

Other Hypnotics

The toxicity and drug interaction profile of **chloral hydrate** make it less safe than BDZs. Tolerance to its hypnotic effect typically develops within two weeks. Its use is not recommended.[17] **Barbiturates** are contraindicated in the management of insomnia due to their unacceptable safety profile.[18]

The Canadian supply of **L-tryptophan** has not been associated with the development of the eosinophilia–myalgia syndrome (a potentially lethal disorder) that has been described in the US. In high dosages (> 1 g), L-tryptophan has a hypnotic effect, but it is not as predictable as that seen with traditional hypnotics.[19] It may be useful when one wishes to avoid BDZs.

Use of **melatonin** (1 to 5 mg) in primary insomnia remains controversial.[20] More studies are required to determine if the slow-release form has a role in maintenance insomnia of middle and old age. **Ramelteon**, a novel compound with chronohypnotic properties (causing phase shifts in circadian rhythm) and high selectivity for MT1 and MT2 melatonin receptors, is available in the US but not in Canada. In various animal models, ramelteon has demonstrated hypnotic properties with no effect on learning, memory or motor coordination. Human studies in young adults[21] and elderly patients[22] show it is well tolerated, but further placebo-controlled studies are required to confirm its role as a sleep-promoting agent.[23]

Therapeutic Tips

- Always start hypnotics at the lowest dose and use them for the shortest possible time.
- Set realistic treatment goals with the patient, mainly to minimize daytime impairment; a chronic poor sleeper will not be turned into a good sleeper overnight.
- The degree of daytime impairment directs the intervention: if there is an acute change in daytime functioning, a short course of hypnotics may be indicated; if the daytime impairment is mild or chronic, try a behavioural intervention (e.g., sleep restriction) first.
- Sleep diaries (Table 3) are often helpful in delineating the initial complaint, monitoring progress and facilitating withdrawal.
- It is inappropriate to use the sedative side effect of another medication (e.g., diphenhydramine, antidepressants) to avoid using a BDZ or non-BDZ agonist when the latter agents are the treatment of choice. Self-medication with nonprescription agents is not recommended; patients should see their physician about distressing insomnia.
- Warn patients about combined effects when hypnotics are used with other CNS depressants, e.g., alcohol.
- If a short course of a hypnotic has been used, plan to withdraw it at a low-stress time, e.g., a weekend. Two nights before the planned withdrawal, the patient should shorten the sleep time (while staying on the medication) by 20 minutes. This modest degree of sleep deprivation will promote physiological sleepiness, which should counterbalance any sleep disruption associated with withdrawal. This shortened sleep period should be maintained for one week.
- Remain vigilant for the emergence of a mood disorder (which should always be treated with antidepressants rather than hypnotics alone)

as protracted insomnia may be the prodrome of an affective illness. Furthermore, one year of continued sleep disturbance increases the risk of a mood disorder in the subsequent year.[24]

Figure 1: **Management of Primary Insomnia**

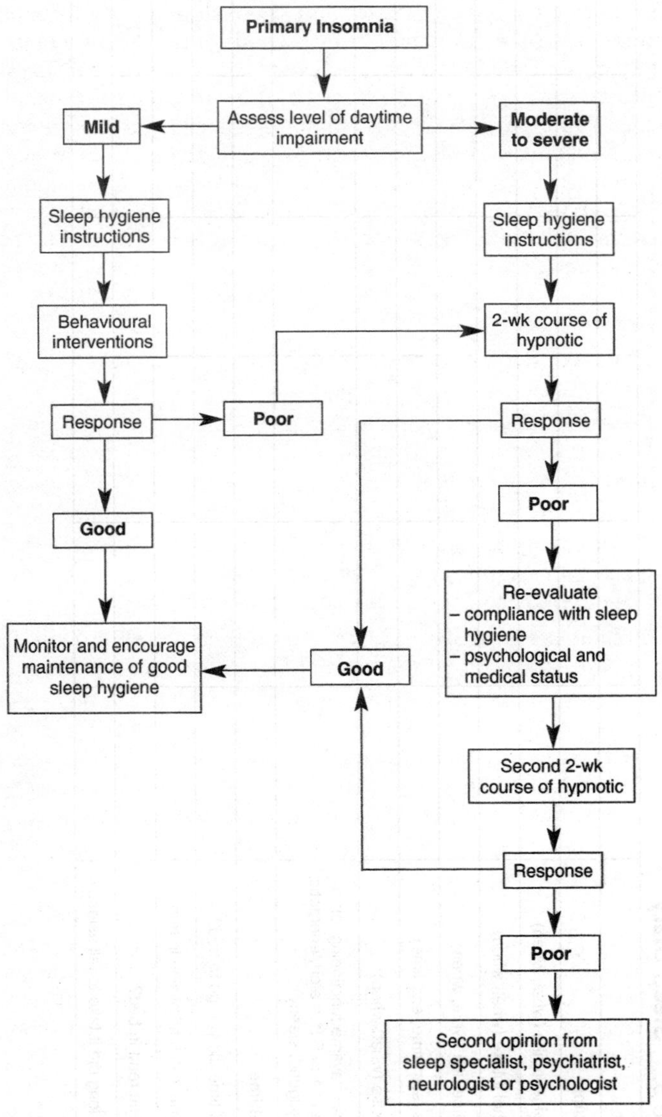

Table 3: Sleep Diary

Date							
Daytime							
Caffeine intake (what, when)							
Alcohol intake (what, when)							
Nicotine use (what, when)							
Naps (start time, end time)							
Exercise (what, when)							
Overall daytime functioning, on a scale of 1 to 5 (1 = alert, energetic; 5 = fatigued, sleepy)							
Nighttime							
What time did you go to bed?							
Did you watch television in bed?							
Did you read in bed?							
How long did it take to fall asleep?							

Date							
For each time you woke up during the night, record the following: 1. time you were awake (e.g., 1:10–2:30 a.m.) 2. what woke you up (e.g., snoring, gasping for air, bad dreams, pet, noise)?							
What time did you *wake up* for the day?							
What time did you *get out of bed* for the day?							
How many hours of sleep did you get?							
How did you feel when you woke up this morning, on a scale of 1 to 5 (1 = refreshed, alert; 5 = fatigued, sleepy)							

Table 4: **Drugs Used to Manage Primary Insomnia**

Class	Drug	Dose (nighttime)	Adverse Effects	Drug Interactions	Comments	Cost[a]
Benzodiazepines (BDZs)	*lorazepam* Ativan, generics	Initial: 0.5 mg Maximum: 1 mg	*Benzodiazepines*: dose-dependent ataxia, dizziness; dependence/withdrawal symptoms. *Lorazepam*: may cause more rebound insomnia on withdrawal than temazepam or oxazepam; may cause amnesia with higher dosages.	Additive sedation with CNS depressants such as alcohol.	Widely used as a hypnotic although not officially indicated.	$
	oxazepam generics	Initial: 15 mg Maximum: 30 mg	See benzodiazepines.	See lorazepam.	Slowly absorbed; onset of action is delayed; should be taken 60–90 min before retiring for *initial* insomnia; no hangover effects.	$
	temazepam Restoril, generics	Initial: 15 mg Maximum: 30 mg	See benzodiazepines.	Substrate of CYP3A4; metabolism could be increased by inducers (e.g., carbamazepine, smoking, phenytoin) or decreased by inhibitors (e.g., cimetidine, clarithromycin, efavirenz, erythromycin, grapefruit juice, itraconazole, ketoconazole, ritonavir) of the enzyme.	Good all-purpose hypnotic; does not accumulate.	$

Class	Drug	Dose (nighttime)	Adverse Effects	Drug Interactions	Comments	Cost[a]
	triazolam Halcion, generics	Initial: 0.125 mg Maximum: 0.25 mg	See benzodiazepines. *Triazolam*: anterograde amnesia (especially with higher dosages, concurrent use of alcohol) and other potency and dose-related side effects (rebound insomnia, daytime anxiety) have limited its use; useful for *initiating* sleep.	See temazepam.	Absence of hangover effects is an advantage (does not affect daytime alertness).	$
Cyclopyrrolones	*zopiclone* Imovane, Rhovane, generics	Initial: 3.75 mg (geriatric) Usual adult dose: 7.5 mg Maximum: 7.5 mg	Major adverse effect is bitter/metallic taste.	Minimal additive effects with low doses of alcohol.	Does not accumulate; minimal cognitive effects;[25] may cause less rebound on withdrawal.	$$$
Serotonin Precursors	*L-tryptophan* Tryptan, other generics	1–3 g 20 min before bedtime	May cause serotonin syndrome (shivering, diaphoresis, hypomanic behaviour and ataxia) alone or when combined with other serotonergic drugs.	Combined therapy with serotonergic drugs such as triptans, SSRIs, MAOIs and sibutramine can increase the risk of serotonin syndrome.	Alternative to BDZs and non-BDZ agonists; erratic response.	$$$$

[a] Cost of 14-day supply; includes drug cost only.
Legend: $ < $2 $$ $2–5 $$$ $5–10 $$$$ > $10

Suggested Readings

Benca RM. Diagnosis and treatment of chronic insomnia: a review. *Psychiatr Serv* 2005;56(3):332-43.

Sateia MJ, Nowell PD. Insomnia. *Lancet* 2004;364(9449):1959-73.

Silber MH. Clinical practice. Chronic insomnia. *N Engl J Med* 2005;353(8):803-10

References

1. American Psychiatric Association. *Diagnostic and statistical manual of mental disorders*. 4th ed. Text Revision. Washington (DC): American Psychiatric Association; 2000.
2. McCrae CS, Lichstein KL. Secondary insomnia: diagnostic challenges and intervention opportunities. *Sleep Med Rev* 2001;5(1):47-61.
3. Vallieres A, Morin CM, Guay B. Sequential combinations of drug and cognitive behavioral therapy for chronic insomnia: an exploratory study. *Behav Res Ther* 2005;43(12):1611-30.
4. Flemons WW. Clinical practice. Obstructive sleep apnea. *N Engl J Med* 2002;347(7):498-504.
5. Edinger JD, Means MK. Cognitive-behavioral therapy for primary insomnia. *Clin Psychol Rev* 2005;25(5):539-58.
6. Reynolds CF et al. Treatment of insomnia in the elderly. In: Salzman C, editor. *Clinical geriatric psychopharmacology*. 3rd ed. Baltimore (MD): Williams and Wilkins;1998.
7. Frels C, Williams P, Narayanan S et al. Iatrogenic causes of falls in hospitalised elderly patients: a case-control study. *Postgrad Med J* 2002;78(922):487-9.
8. Schneider DL. Insomnia. Safe and effective therapy for sleep problems in the older patient. *Geriatrics* 2002;57(5):24-6, 29, 32.
9. Bliwise D, Seidel W, Greenblatt DJ et al. Nighttime and daytime efficacy of flurazepam and oxazepam in chronic insomnia. *Am J Psychiatry* 1984;141(2):191-5.
10. Feldmeier C, Kapp W. Comparative clinical studies with midazolam, oxazepam and placebo. *Br J Clin Pharmacol* 1983;16(Suppl 1):151S-155S.
11. Kales A, Bixler EO, Soldatos CR et al. Lorazepam: effects on sleep and withdrawal phenomena. *Pharmacology* 1986;32(3):121-30.
12. Vermeeren A. Residual effects of hypnotics: epidemiology and clinical implications. *CNS Drugs* 2004;18(5):297-328.
13. Voderholzer U, Riemann D, Hornyak M et al. A double-blind, randomized and placebo-controlled study on the polysomnographic withdrawal effects of zopiclone, zolpidem and triazolam in healthy subjects. *Eur Arch Psychiatry Clin Neurosci* 2001;251(3):117-23.
14. Melton ST, Wood JM, Kirkwood CK. Eszopiclone for insomnia. *Ann Pharmacother* 2005;39(10):1659-66.
15. Roth T, Walsh JK, Krystal A et al. An evaluation of the efficacy and safety of eszopiclone over 12 months in patients with chronic primary insomnia. *Sleep Med* 2005;6(6):487-95.
16. Neubauer DN. Indiplon: the development of a new hypnotic. *Expert Opin Investig Drugs* 2005;14(10):1269-76.
17. Frankland A, Robinson MJ. Fatal chloral hydrate overdoses: unnecessary tragedies. *Can J Psychiatry* 2001;46(8):763-4.
18. Morgan WW. Abuse liability of barbiturates and other sedative-hypnotics. *Adv Alcohol Subst Abuse* 1990;9(1-2):67-82.
19. Schneider-Helmert D, Spinweber CL. Evaluation of L-tryptophan for treatment of insomnia: a review. *Psychopharmacology (Berl)* 1986;89(1):1-7.
20. Olde Rikkert MG, Rigaud AS. Melatonin in elderly patients with insomnia. A systematic review. *Z Gerontol Geriatr* 2001;34(6):491-7.
21. Erman M, Seiden D, Zammit G et al. An efficacy, safety, and dose-response study of Ramelteon in patients with chronic primary insomnia. *Sleep Med* 2006;7(1):17-24.
22. Roth T, Seiden D, Sainati S et al. Phase III outpatient trail of ramelteon for the treatment of chronic insomnia in the elderly [abstract]. *J Am Geriatr Soc* 2005;53(Suppl 4):S25.
23. Bellon A. Searching for new options for treating insomnia: are melatonin and ramelteon beneficial? *J Psychiatr Pract* 2006;12(4):229-43.
24. Ford DE, Kamerow DB. Epidemiologic study of sleep disturbances and psychiatric disorders. An opportunity for prevention? *JAMA* 1989;262(11):1479-84.
25. Silva A, Collao A, Orellana M et al. Zopiclone, but not brotizolam, impairs memory storage during sleep. *Neurosci Res* 2003;47(2):241-3.

CHAPTER 9

Drug Withdrawal Syndromes

James R. Kennedy, MD, FRCPC

Treatment of drug withdrawal syndromes requires attention to both the biological (medical) model and the behavioural (psychosocial) model. Alcohol and benzodiazepine withdrawal can result in medically important sequelae such as seizures and autonomic instability. Opioid withdrawal results in markedly unpleasant symptoms without important medical sequelae. Stimulant withdrawal is almost exclusively behavioural with the most important risks being suicidality and, less commonly, hallucinosis with amphetamines.

Withdrawal syndrome diagnosis requires:[1]

- The development of a substance-specific syndrome due to cessation or reduction of prolonged substance use
- Clinically significant distress or impairment of functioning
- The absence of a medical or other psychiatric disorder that can cause the syndrome

Table 1: **Diagnostic Criteria for Substance-specific Withdrawal Syndromes[1]**

Alcohol	Stimulants (Cocaine and Amphetamines)
Autonomic hyperactivity (e.g., sweating, pulse > 100 bpm)	Fatigue
Increased hand tremor	Vivid, unpleasant dreams
Insomnia	Insomnia or hypersomnia
Nausea/vomiting	Increased appetite
Transient visual, tactile or auditory hallucinations	Psychomotor retardation or agitation
Psychomotor agitation	Anxiety
Anxiety	Depression
Grand mal seizures	Craving for stimulant
Depression	Psychotic symptoms (amphetamines)
Opioids	**Benzodiazepines**
Dysphoric mood	Autonomic hyperactivity (e.g., sweating, pulse > 100 bpm)
Nausea/vomiting	Increased hand tremor
Muscle aches	Insomnia
Lacrimation, rhinorrhea	Nausea/vomiting
Pupillary dilation, piloerection, sweating	Transient visual, tactile or auditory hallucinations
Diarrhea	Psychomotor agitation
Yawning	Anxiety
Fever	Grand mal seizures (only after abrupt cessation of high doses)
Insomnia	

Goals of Therapy

- Relieve symptoms
- Anticipate, prevent and treat complications
- Assess for and treat comorbidities (medical and psychiatric)
- Facilitate definitive psychosocial/behavioural treatment
- Prevent relapse

Investigations

- Detailed history and physical examination to evaluate severity of abuse of the substance (amount, frequency, duration) and comorbid medical and psychiatric (axis II, depression or psychosis) conditions
- Specific assessment tools such as the Clinical Institute Withdrawal Assessment for Alcohol (CIWA-Ar)[2] or CIWA-Benzo[3]
- Laboratory tests and/or imaging to assess comorbidities/complications revealed in history and physical (complete blood count, renal/liver function, electrolytes, magnesium, phosphorus, chest x-ray, CT of head)
- Drug screening: blood alcohol or urine screen for benzodiazepines may be helpful in the trauma or emergency patient where history is inadequate

Therapeutic Choices (Figure 1)

Nonpharmacologic Choices

- Nonjudgmental approach to explain process, reassure and support.
- Psychosocial treatment program (cognitive behavioural therapy, motivational enhancement therapy, interpersonal therapy, 12-step, group and family therapies).[4]

Pharmacologic Choices

General principles:

- Monitor signs and symptoms.
- Treat specific symptoms of withdrawal and associated complications and comorbidities (medical and psychiatric).
- Substitute abused drug with one of same or similar class (a cross-tolerant agonist that is less likely to be abused, usually with longer half-life).
- Substitute abused drug with one that blocks its reinforcing effects (antagonist).

Alcohol Withdrawal Syndrome

Assessment (Table 1)

The severity of the alcohol withdrawal syndrome and its complications correlate directly but inconsistently with the intensity and duration of alcohol use. These complications can include undernutrition (e.g., thiamine deficiency), low potassium, magnesium and phosphorus, liver disease and bleeding diathesis (increased INR, impaired platelet function/thrombocytopenia), CNS disease (e.g., seizures, Wernicke encephalopathy, trauma), autonomic dysfunction (hypertension, dehydration, pyrexia), infections (pneumonia, aspiration, cellulitis), and psychosis (hallucinations, delusions). Mild withdrawal symptoms include tremor, irritability and insomnia, usually lasting 48–72 hours. Severe symptoms, with onset around 48 hours and lasting up to about five days, include autonomic instability, seizures, hallucinations, delusions and pyrexia. The CIWA-Ar is an effective assessment tool.[2]

Management (Table 3)

Approximately two-thirds of patients with mild-to-moderate withdrawal symptoms can be treated with support and monitoring, although comparison with pharmacotherapy is not described in the literature.[5] Blunting symptoms with low-dose, short-duration **benzodiazepine** therapy may be helpful and is of low risk.

Severe alcohol withdrawal syndrome always requires pharmacologic treatment, and guidelines usually recommend the same for moderate cases. Larger than usually recommended doses of **benzodiazepines** (> 50 mg diazepam iv in the first hour or > 200 mg in 3 hours) and/or addition of a different GABA-active drug like **phenobarbital** (130–1430 mg, mean dose 390 mg) may be required for resistant alcohol withdrawal (< 5% of cases), and these patients require monitoring in a critical care area (emergency room, intensive care unit or intermediate care unit).[6,7]

Although many emergency room physicians add an antipsychotic (usually **haloperidol** 5–10 mg) in resistant alcohol withdrawal, there is no good evidence to support their use, and there is risk of dystonia, akathisia and hypotension.

Patients admitted to hospital for surgical illness may have occult alcohol dependence, and appropriate prophylaxis and management of alcohol withdrawal syndromes with benzodiazepines can prevent complications.[8]

Rehabilitation

Cognitive therapy, group therapy and self-help groups like Alcoholics Anonymous form the mainstay of long-term rehabilitation, and there is conflicting evidence to support the use of pharmacotherapy (e.g., **naltrexone**) in this setting.[9] A Cochrane review reported a modest effect on reducing the quantity of alcohol intake.[10]

Stimulant (Cocaine and Amphetamine) Withdrawal Syndrome

Assessment (Table 1)

Symptoms of cocaine withdrawal include mostly psychosocial, subtle and medically unimportant symptoms and signs, except for the risk of acute severe depression and suicidality in a small percentage of patients. The toxic state is manifested by agitation, tachycardia and anorexia, and conversely the withdrawal state is characterized by somnolence and increased appetite. Depression, anxiety, anhedonia and sleep disturbance may also occur, resolving over several weeks. Suicidality is uncommon and requires direct assessment.

Amphetamine withdrawal shares most of the characteristics of cocaine withdrawal, but may include psychotic features or a more severe depressed mood and may last longer. Drug craving replaces the withdrawal syndrome and may last several months. After withdrawal from methamphetamine ("crystal meth"), a persistent psychosis may occur and become permanent (uncommon) or last several weeks, usually responding well to low-dose antipsychotics.[11] Medical complications of stimulant use should be surveyed, including cardiomyopathy, local or systemic abscess, endocarditis, HIV and hepatitis B and C.

Management

Evaluation of a variety of pharmacotherapy approaches both for treatment of the withdrawal syndrome and for relapse prevention yielded inconsistent results, reflecting ineffective treatment. Dopamine agonists, such as **amantadine**,[12] **bromocriptine**[13] and **pergolide**[14] have demonstrated no significant benefit. **Desipramine** and other antidepressants have little or no effectiveness for withdrawal or relapse prevention, but may have a role in comorbid depression or anxiety. Agonist replacement therapy with sustained-release **amphetamine** or **methylphenidate** has shown benefit in relapse prevention, but regulatory concerns may limit their use, unless underlying attention deficit disorder co-exists.[15] Making this diagnosis requires psychiatric expertise.

Rehabilitation

Although **buprenorphine** and **methadone** may offer benefit to patients with mixed opioid and stimulant dependence, no drug therapy is consistently effective for treating pure stimulant dependence. Intensive outpatient, abstinence-oriented psychosocial treatment, especially *cognitive behavioural therapy*, is the most effective treatment, in addition to addressing the psychiatric comorbidities.

Opioid Withdrawal Syndrome

Assessment (Table 1)

Symptoms of opioid withdrawal are not medically serious, with muscle aches, restlessness and insomnia predominating. The acute withdrawal syndrome usually lasts about one week, but is much longer in withdrawal from methadone, with drug craving often persisting for several months.

Management (Table 4)

Abstinence-based treatment may be desirable, but the most effective treatment by far continues to be replacement therapy with a long-acting agonist like **methadone** or the partial agonist **buprenorphine**, which is available through Health Canada's Special Access Programme. Methadone and buprenorphine can be initiated with the first withdrawal symptoms. Higher *maintenance* doses (methadone 60–100 mg or buprenorphine 8–32 mg/day) are more effective than lower doses. Because of methadone's long half-life of about 30 hours, the risk of narcosis in patients with an unknown degree of opioid tolerance is high in the first few days, and requires expertise and vigilance. Buprenorphine is a partial agonist with a long half-life (36 hours) and generally does not cause narcosis in overdose.[16]

Clonidine, an alpha-2 agonist that decreases the neuronal output of norepinephrine, can be used to blunt the symptoms of withdrawal, but muscle aches and craving usually persist. **Naltrexone**, a long-acting opioid antagonist, used to block opioid agonist effects like euphoria, is used to support long-term abstinence. However, both of these agents are ineffective in decreasing long-term opioid use, in spite of psychosocial supportive treatment.[17]

Rehabilitation

The best long-term results are obtained with replacement therapy (methadone or buprenorphine) combined with cognitive or group therapy, counselling and 12-step support. If methadone discontinuation is considered, the best outcomes occur with slow tapering over many weeks.[4]

Benzodiazepine Withdrawal Syndrome

Assessment (Table 1)

Assessing benzodiazepine withdrawal syndrome is associated with three challenges:

- distinguishing recurrence of anxiety, panic or insomnia from the onset of withdrawal symptoms
- assessing risk of seizures and autonomic hyperactivity
- selecting the best treatment for the underlying psychiatric condition.

The withdrawal syndrome begins within 1–2 days of abrupt discontinuation and can be severe, with hypertension, tachycardia and hyperreflexia progressing to seizures if there was long-term, high-dose use. In chronic anxiety and panic disorders, chronic dosing may be very high (even > 100 mg diazepam per day), and may be associated with alcohol overuse (i.e., sedative self-treatment). A number of factors correlate with severity of the benzodiazepine withdrawal syndrome: high daily dose, use of agents with short half-life, long duration of use, diagnosis of panic disorder, presence of severe Axis II disorders and concomitant alcohol or substance abuse.

Management

Replacement with a long half-life benzodiazepine and prolonged tapering of daily dose, combined with supportive and eventually cognitive therapy for the underlying condition, form the only effective treatment for high-dose, prolonged benzodiazepine dependence. Most Canadian experts use diazepam or clonazepam for replacement therapy (Table 2). Initial tapering of the daily dose to 50% of the starting dose can usually occur over a 2–4 week period; the last 50% frequently takes many weeks, sometimes with periods of weeks with no dosage change.[18]

Since patients with personality disorders tolerate distress poorly, they often drop out early, and an intensive supportive and cognitive program should coincide with benzodiazepine tapering and may include periods of maintenance. Patients can be managed in an intensive outpatient program. Few patients (those with associated cardiovascular disease, severe alcoholism or previous seizures) require a short hospitalization.

Table 2: **Dose Equivalents of Benzodiazepines**

Benzodiazepine	Elimination Half-life[a]	Approximate Oral Dosage Equivalent[19] (mg)
Clorazepate	Long	10
Chlordiazepoxide	Long	25
Diazepam	Long	5
Flurazepam	Long	15
Alprazolam	Intermediate	0.5
Bromazepam	Intermediate	3
Clonazepam	Intermediate	0.25
Lorazepam	Intermediate	1
Nitrazepam	Intermediate	2.5
Oxazepam	Intermediate	15
Temazepam	Intermediate	10
Triazolam	Short	0.25

[a] Short = ≤ 5 h; Intermediate = 5–60 h; Long = ≥ 100 h.

Rehabilitation

The best treatment for the underlying condition (e.g., insomnia, generalized anxiety, panic disorder, mood disorder) is *cognitive behavioural therapy*.[4, 20] Pharmacotherapy should be directed to the specific underlying condition and should have a low risk for dependence;

options include low-dose, low-potency antipsychotics. Insomnia can be treated with these agents or with **trazodone** (25-100 mg at bedtime). **Buspirone** can be effective treatment for generalized anxiety and has low abuse potential and reasonable but not dramatic efficacy.

Figure 1: **Management of Drug Withdrawal Syndromes**

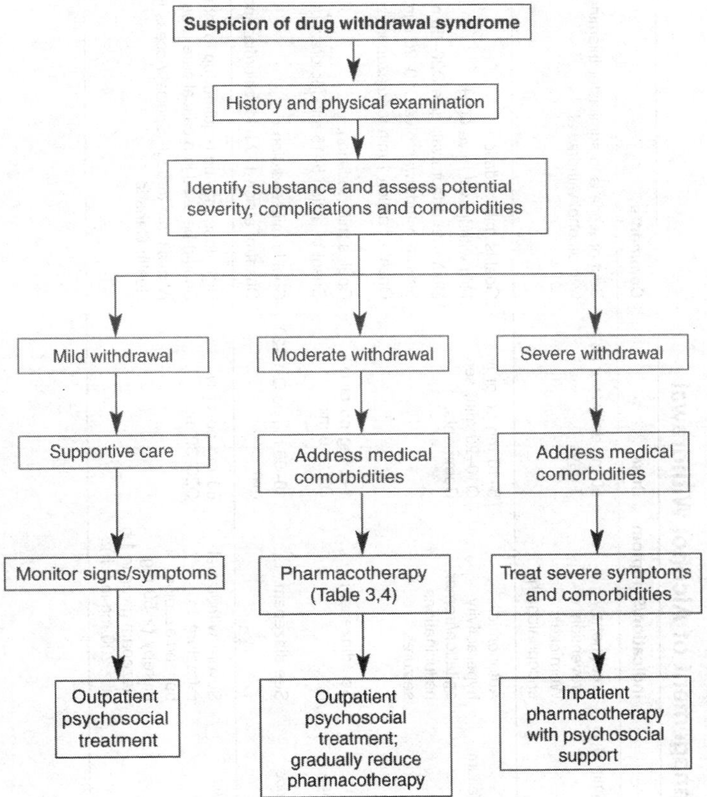

Table 3: Pharmacologic Management of Alcohol Withdrawal

Class	Drug	Indication/Symptom	Dose	Comments	Cost[a]
Vitamins	*thiamine* (vitamin B_1) Betaxin, generics	Treatment/ prevention of Wernicke's encephalopathy	50 mg daily iv or po × 3 days	Best practice is to administer thiamine to all patients with alcohol withdrawal.	$$
Benzodiazepines	*diazepam* Diazemuls, Valium, generics	Autonomic hyperactivity, agitation/tremor, hallucinations, seizures	5–10 mg po or iv Q10–20 min; see Comments.	Goal is mild sedation. Mild withdrawal: give Q1H. Moderate withdrawal: give Q20–60 min. Severe withdrawal: give Q10–20 min. Onset of action 1 min for diazepam iv.	$$
	lorazepam Ativan, generics	See diazepam.	1–2 mg po or iv Q20–60 min	Goal is mild sedation. Onset of action 5–15 min for lorazepam iv.	$$
	chlordiazepoxide generics	See diazepam.	10–50 mg po Q10–20 min	Goal is mild sedation. Onset of action 1–2 h for chlordiazepoxide po.	$
Barbiturates	*phenobarbital*[6,7] generics	Severe withdrawal refractory to benzodiazepine therapy (> 50 mg diazepam given in 1 h or > 200 mg in 3 h)	60 mg po or iv Q20–30 min	High dose may be required (up to total of 1000 mg). Should be used in a critical care area. IV available through Special Access Programme, Health Canada.	$

Class	Drug	Indication/Symptom	Dose	Comments	Cost[a]
Antipsychotics	*haloperidol* generics	Psychosis refractory to benzodiazepines	0.5–5 mg im or po Q2H Max: 20 mg in 24 h	May lower blood pressure or cause acute dystonia. Continue appropriate benzodiazepine dosing.	po:$ im:$$
Antiepileptic Drugs	*phenytoin* Dilantin Capsules, Dilantin Infatabs, generics	Seizures only if previous seizure history or cause of seizure unrelated to alcohol	Loading dose: 300–400 mg po Q2H up to 1 g in total, or 1 g iv. If phenytoin already on board, half or no loading dose required. Maintenance: 100 mg po or iv Q8H or 300 mg once daily po or iv.	Measure trough level in 3–5 days.	po:$ iv: $$$

[a] Cost of a single administration; includes drug cost only.
Legend: $ < $1 $$ $1–5 $$$ > $5

Table 4: **Pharmacologic Management of Opioid Withdrawal**

Class	Treatment Drug	Dose	Comments	Cost[a]
Opioid Agonists	*methadone*[16] generics	Acute withdrawal symptoms in new patients: 10–20 mg po Q2–4H until stable (usually 20–60 mg). If not to be continued as maintenance, taper by 5 mg/day over 1–2 wk Maintenance: 40–100 mg/day po	High relapse rate without maintenance therapy. Long half-life (24–36 h). Higher maintenance doses (60–100 mg) associated with better outcomes.	$$$-$$$$
Partial Opioid Agonists	*buprenorphine* Subutex	Long-term maintenance: 8–32 mg sl daily	Start with first signs of withdrawal. Available through Special Access Programme, Health Canada.	c
Opioid Antagonists	*naltrexone* ReVia	50 mg daily or 100 mg 3 times weekly	Administer a naloxone 0.8 mg im test dose to detect occult opioid dependence. If withdrawal symptoms occur, do not start naltrexone. Clinical trials fail to show efficacy.	$$$$
Alpha$_2$-adrenergic Agonists	*clonidine* Catapres, Dixarit, generics	0.1–0.5 mg/day Q8H po for 7 days, then taper over 3–5 days	Blunts some withdrawal symptoms. Use only for acute detoxification and when patient prefers over methadone. Maintain fluid intake and monitor for hypotensive effects.	$-$$

[a] Cost of 7-day supply; includes drug cost only.
[b] Duration of study, not necessarily the recommended clinical treatment regimen.
[c] Available through Special Access Programme, Health Canada.
Legend: $ < $5 $-$$ < $5–15 $$ $5–15 $$$ $15–30 $$$-$$$$ $15–45 $$$$ $30–45

Suggested Readings

Practice guideline for the treatment of patients with substance use disorders. 2nd ed. American Psychiatric Association. *Am J Psychiatry* 2007;164(4 Suppl):1-124.

Spies CD, Rommelspacher H. Alcohol withdrawal in the surgical patients: prevention and treatment. *Anesth Analg* 1999;88(4):946-54.

Voshaar RC, Couvee JE, van Balkom AJ et al. Strategies for discontinuing long-term benzodiazepine use: meta-analysis. *Br J Psychiatry* 2006;189:213-20.

References

1. American Psychiatric Association. Task Force on DSM-IV. *Diagnostic and statistical manual of mental disorders: DSM-IV-TR*. Washington (DC): American Psychiatric Association; 2000.
2. Sullivan JT, Sykora K, Schneiderman J et al. Assessment of alcohol withdrawal: the revised clinical institute withdrawal assessment for alcohol scale (CIWA-Ar). *Br J Addict* 1989;84(11):1353-7.
3. Busto UE, Sykora K, Sellers EM. A clinical scale to assess benzodiazepine withdrawal. *J Clin Psychopharmacol* 1989;9(6):412-6.
4. Practice guideline for the treatment of patients with substance use disorders. 2nd ed. American Psychiatric Association. *Am J Psychiatry* 2007;164(4 Suppl):1-124.
5. Naranjo CA, Sellers EM, Chater K et al. Nonparmacologic intervention in acute alcohol withdrawal. *Clin Pharmacol Ther* 1983;34(2):214-9.
6. Hack JB, Hoffman RS, Nelson LS. Resistant alcohol withdrawal: does an unexpectedly large sedative requirement identify these patient early? *J Med Toxicol* 2006;2(2):55-60.
7. Gold JA, Rimal B, Nolan A et al. A strategy of escalating doses of benzodiazepines and phenobarbital administration reduce the need for mechanical ventilation in delirium tremens. *Crit Care Med* 2007;35(3):724-30.
8. Spies CD, Dubisz N, Funk W et al. Prophylaxis of alcohol withdrawal syndrome in alcohol dependent patients admitted to the intensive care unit following tumour resection. *Br J Anaesth* 1995;75(6):734-9.
9. Krystal JH, Cramer JA, Krol WF et al. Naltrexone in the treatment of alcohol dependence. *N Engl J Med* 2001;345(24):1734-9.
10. Srisurapanont M, Jarusuraisin N. Opioid antagonists for alcohol dependence. *Cochrane Database Syst Rev* 2005;(1):CD001867.
11. Curran C, Byrappa N, McBride A. Stimulant psychosis: systematic review. *Br J Psychiatry* 2004;185:196-204.
12. Weddington WW, Brown BS, Haertzen CA et al. Changes in mood, craving, and sleep during short-term abstinence reported by male cocaine addicts: a controlled, residential study. *Arch Gen Psychiatry* 1990;47(9):861-8.
13. Moscovitz H, Brookoff D, Nelson L. A randomized trial of bromocriptine for cocaine users presenting to the emergency department. *J Gen Intern Med* 1993;8(1):1-4.
14. Malcolm R, Kajdasz DK, Herron J et al.. A double-blind, placebo-controlled outpatient trial of pergolide for cocaine dependence. *Drug Alcohol Depend* 2000;60:161-8.
15. Grabowski J, Shearer J, Merril J et al. Agonist-like, replacement pharmacotherapy for stimulant abuse and dependence. *Addict Behav* 2004;29(7):1439-64.
16. Petry NM, Bickel WK, Badger GJ. A comparison of four buprenorphine dosing regimens in the treatment of opioid dependence. *Clin Pharmacol Ther* 1999;66(3):306-14.
17. Kirchmayer U, Davoli M, Verster A. Naltrexone maintenance treatment for opioid dependence. *Cochrane Database Syst Rev* 2003;(2):CD001333.
18. Rickels K, DeMartinis N, Rynn M et al. Pharmacologic strategies for discontinuing benzodiazepine treatment. *J Clin Psychopharmacol* 1999:19(6 Suppl 2):12S-16S.
19. Bezchlibnyk-Butler KZ, Jeffries JJ, editors. *Clinical handbook of psychotropic drugs*. 15th ed. Ashland (OH): Hogrefe & Huber Publishers; 2005.
20. Spiegel DA. Psychological strategies for discontinuation in benzodiazepine treatment. *J Clin Psychopharmacol*1999:19(6 Suppl 2):17S-22S.

CHAPTER 10
Smoking Cessation

Peter Selby, MBBS, CCFP

Tobacco use kills approximately 48 000 Canadians annually, primarily from cardiac disease, lung cancer and respiratory diseases such as COPD.[1] The toxicity of cigarette smoke is due to the inhalation of about 4000 chemicals including 50 to 60 carcinogens.[2] Cigarettes are highly addictive because of the rapid delivery of nicotine to the mesolimbic reward pathways in the brain and development of tolerance. The short half-life of nicotine (60 to 90 minutes) forces repeated administration to maintain nicotine levels.[3] Other psychoactive compounds in smoke include MAOA and MAOB inhibitors.[4] The polyaromatic hydrocarbons (PAHs) are inducers of CYP1A1, 1A2 and 2E1 enzymes that have clinical implications when smokers quit.[5]

Goals of Therapy[8]

- The ultimate goal is to help smokers achieve complete and sustained remission from tobacco use and nicotine dependence
- An intermediate goal is to help them achieve complete and sustained remission from cigarette smoking and/or other forms of tobacco products such as chewing tobacco
- To help smokers understand that:
  - smoking cessation is a process not a singular event; helping smokers stay engaged in the process of behaviour change is a major objective of therapy
  - the best odds of quitting are when behavioural and pharmacologic interventions complement each other
  - reduction in smoking by 50% in those unable or unwilling to quit is controversial because there is no long-term health benefit.[9] However, reduction is associated with subsequent successful quitting[10]

Investigations (Figure 1)

- Figure 1 provides a general assessment questionnaire for patients who have not previously stopped smoking for more than 24 hours
- Measures of physical dependence include the Fagerström Test of Nicotine Dependence[11]. A shorter version is the Heaviness of Smoking Index, which asks about the time to first cigarette of the day and the number of cigarettes smoked per day[12]
- Motivation can be assessed by asking the following two questions:[3]
  - "Given everything going on in your life right now, on a scale of 1 to 10, where 10 is the most important thing to do right now, how important is it for you to quit smoking altogether?"

– "Given everything going on in your life right now, on a scale of 1 to 10, where 10 is the most confident you have felt about anything, how confident do you feel you will be able to quit smoking altogether?"

Therapeutic Choices (Figure 2, Table 2)

This chapter will focus on smokers who want to quit in the next 30 days.

Nonpharmacologic Choices

Most smokers try to quit on several occasions though success rates over the long term are generally low. Many methods for quitting smoking have been advocated; however, few have been demonstrated to be effective. This type of evidence generally requires randomized controlled trials with a minimum follow-up assessment of self-reported quit rates at six months along with supportive objective evidence, e.g., measurement of exhaled carbon monoxide or cotinine levels in urine, saliva or serum.[8] Though widely promoted, there is no evidence for the efficacy of hypnosis or acupuncture.

The five evidence-based steps required to successfully quit include the following[8]

- setting a target quit date
- getting professional help
- enlisting social support
- using medication to quit smoking
- using problem-solving methods of counselling to quit and remain smoke free.

There is a dose-response relationship between counselling and quit success.[8] Estimated abstinence rates increase from 13.4% with minimal counselling contact time (< 3 minutes) to an average of 22% with contact time > 10 minutes. Optimal total contact time is 91–300 minutes, yielding abstinence rates of approximately 28%.[8] Smokers who are attempting to quit should be counselled at least once prior to their quit date, the week following their quit date and weekly thereafter as necessary to optimize therapy and to identify and manage early relapse.[8] Formats that have been shown to be effective include face-to-face (individual or group) counselling as well as contact by telephone, Internet and mail.

Pharmacologic Choices

The addition of pharmacotherapy increases the odds of quitting (see Table 1) and should be offered to all patients who smoke 10 or more cigarettes per day and are attempting to quit. Pharmacotherapy can be divided into first-line and second-line medications.[8] First-line medications include all forms of **nicotine replacement therapy** and **bupropion**. Second-line pharmacotherapies have evidence of efficacy but are not officially indicated for smoking cessation. These include **nortriptyline** and **clonidine**.[14,15,16,17] **Varenicline**, an $alpha_4beta_2$-nicotinic receptor partial agonist, with quit rates higher than previously existing therapies, recently became available.[18,19,20] In two comparative trials, varenicline increased the odds of successfully quitting over bupropion and placebo at 12 weeks (varenicline 44%, bupropion 29.5% and placebo 17.7%).[21,22] However, differences at 6 months (i.e., 3 months after treatment was stopped) were smaller (varenicline 22%, bupropion 16%, placebo 8.4%).

Table 1: **Estimated Abstinence Rates with Pharmacotherapy**

Drug	Estimated 6-month Abstinence Rate (%)	
	Drug	**Placebo**
Nicotine replacement therapy[23]	17[a]	10
Varenicline[21,22]	22	8.4
Bupropion[21,22]	16	8.4
Nortriptyline[8]	30	11.7
Clonidine[8]	25	13.9

[a] Pooled data from any form of nicotine replacement therapy

Nortriptyline can be used in otherwise healthy individuals with minimal risk for overdose or cardiac disease when first-line therapies are either unaffordable or have not worked. Clonidine may be used in those with coexisting hypertension. However, postural hypotension can be problematic and the drug must be tapered to prevent rebound hypertension.

Choice of medication should depend on patient preference and absence of contraindications.

Monotherapy is the norm. There is evidence that combination therapy such as the nicotine patch combined with either nicotine gum[24], nicotine inhaler,[25] nicotine spray[25] or bupropion[26] is better in the short term than monotherapy. However, cost is a limiting factor and combination therapy should be reserved for those in whom quitting immediately is essential. Varenicline has not been studied in combination with other medications and is contraindicated in combination with nicotine replacement therapy. The nicotine lozenge, nasal spray and sublingual tablet are not available in Canada. Rimonabant, a cannabinoid receptor 1 antagonist approved in Europe for weight loss, has shown mixed results in two smoking cessation trials.[27,28] It is not approved for smoking cessation in either Europe or the United States and is not available in Canada.

Therapeutic Tips

- Encourage smokers who have slips while on medication to continue medication for at least four weeks and use behavioural interventions to help them to stop smoking.[29]

- If smokers using the patch complain of unmanageable cravings and smoke cigarettes, add nicotine gum or inhaler as a breakthrough medication.[8]
- It is important to monitor for low mood and emergence of depression in smokers who quit.[30]
- Potential weight gain following smoking cessation should be addressed before quitting and practical advice should be offered to help the smoker avoid gaining weight, i.e., healthy diet and exercise and avoidance of high-sugar products which the patient craves when quitting smoking.[31,32]
- Create a therapeutic relationship in which the patient can report back at the first signs of a relapse to abort it as soon as possible.

Figure 1: Tobacco-smoking History Questionnaire

1. Tobacco use history

a. Current (past year):

i. Quantity: number of cigarettes smoked per day ______

ii. Frequency/pattern:

a. weekday ____

b. weekend ______

iii. Time to first cigarette after waking up (in minutes): ______

iv. Type(s):
cigarettes: ❑yes ❑no;
cigars: ❑yes ❑no;
cigarellos: ❑yes ❑no;
others (❑bidis, ❑kretek)

b. Past history:

i. Age of onset of smoking (years) ______

ii. Maximum smoked per day (lifetime) ______

iii. Number of past quit attempts (24 hours or more of intentional cessation) ______

iv. Past methods used to quit:
____

v. Utility of method used to quit:
____

vi. What led to a relapse? (check all that apply)
withdrawal: ❑yes ❑no
negative mood: ❑yes ❑no
habit: ❑yes ❑no
being with other smokers: ❑yes ❑no
stress: ❑yes ❑no
other______________________

2. Other drug use

a. Caffeine: ❑no
❑yes: cups per day ______

b. Alcohol: ❑no
❑yes: drinks per day ______

c. Marijuana: (especially if smoked)
❑no ❑yes: joints per day ______

3. Concurrent mental health problems

a. Depression: ❑yes ❑no
b. Anxiety: ❑yes ❑no
c. Eating disorders: ❑yes ❑no
d. Bipolar disease: ❑yes ❑no
e. Schizophrenia: ❑yes ❑no

4. Environmental assessment

a. Living with smokers: ❑yes ❑no
b. Workplace smoking: ❑yes ❑no

5. Consequences of smoking

a. Health — cardiac: ❑yes ❑no
respiratory: ❑yes ❑no
cancer: ❑yes ❑no
others: ❑yes ❑no

b. Social/Family — feeling ostracized, advice to stop from friends/family

c. Financial: costs of cigarettes ______ per pack of 20 (small pack)

6. Concurrent medications

a. Benzodiazepines: ❑yes ❑no
b. Antipsychotics: ❑yes ❑no
c. Antidepressants: ❑yes ❑no
d. Others:______________________

7. Allergies and intolerances especially to smoking cessation medications

❑yes ❑no

8. A rapid assessment of motivation

a. High importance and confidence, ready to quit in the next 30 days
b. High importance low confidence, wants to quit but needs help
c. Low importance, low confidence, doesn't want to quit
d. Low importance, high confidence, discounts the importance of quitting but has high self efficacy

9. Physical examination

a. Blood pressure ______ mm Hg
b. Height ______ metres
c. Weight ______ kg
c. Waist circumference ______ cm

Treatment plan for those who want to quit within 30 days:

10. Quit date

a. ❑yes________________; If yes offer self-help material and follow up

b. ❑no: If no, within 6 months? Advise to quit and follow up as needed

11. Counselling

a. In person: ❑yes ❑no
b. Telephone: ❑yes ❑no
c. Internet: ❑yes ❑no

12. Pharmacotherapy

Drug	Start date
NRT	
a. Patch: ❑ 21 mg ❑ 14 mg ❑ 7 mg	
b. Gum: ❑ 2 mg ❑ 4 mg	
c. Inhaler: ❑ 4 mg	
Bupropion: dose ______	
Varenicline: dose ______	
Nortriptyline: dose ______	
Clonidine: dose ______	

Signature______________________ Date__________

Figure 2: **Management of Smoking Cessation**

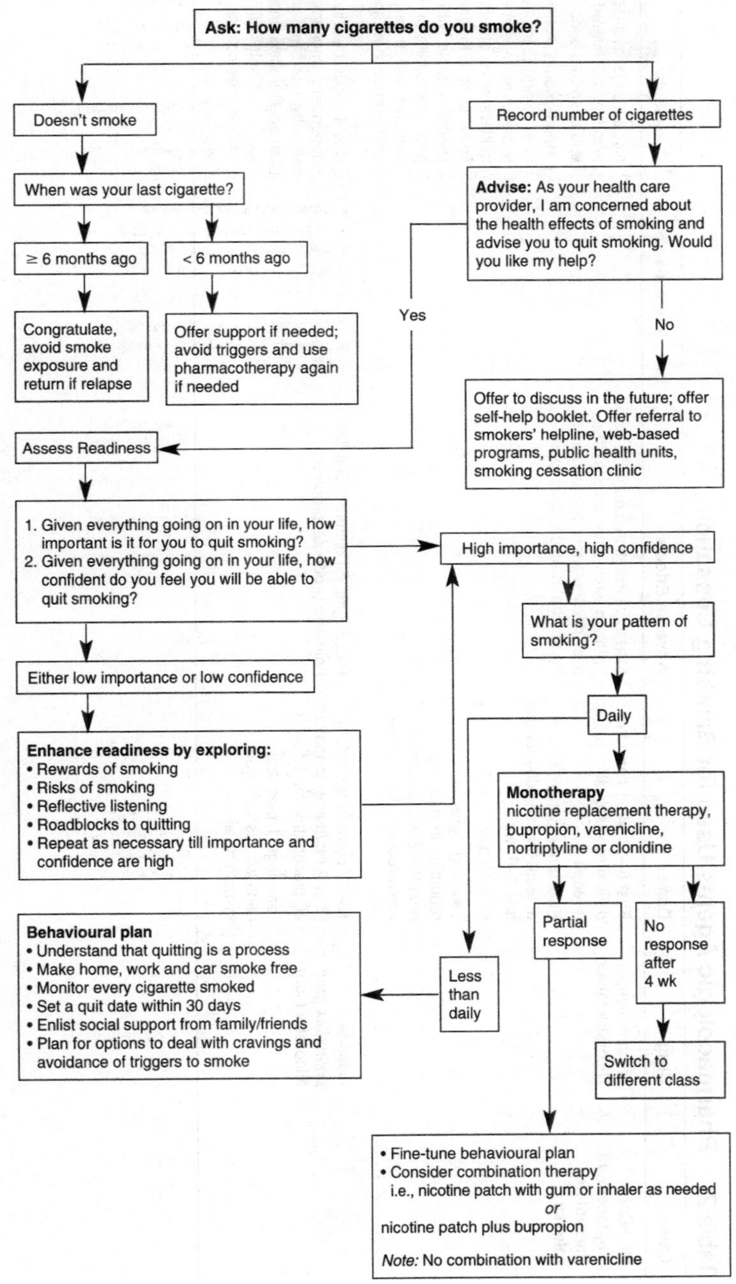

Table 2: **Pharmacologic Agents Used for Smoking Cessation**

Class	Drug	Dose	Adverse Effects	Drug Interactions[a]	Comments	Cost[b]
Nicotine Replacement, immediate-release	*nicotine inhaler* Nicorette Inhaler	First 6–12 wk: 1 cartridge delivering 4 mg nicotine, as needed Encourage patient to use at least 6 doses/day for the first 3–6 wk Max 12/day Tapering: gradual reduction in use over next 6–12 wk, stopping when reduced to 1–2/day	Mild local irritation (cough, throat irritation, stomatitis, rhinitis) that may decline with continued use; headache, nausea, dyspepsia.		Not a true inhaler—the nicotine is delivered and absorbed buccally. "Hand–mouth" activity from using the inhaler is preferred by some quitters while others find it to be a trigger. Useful in those with poor oral health or dentures and in those who cannot chew gum.	$$
	nicotine polacrilex gum Nicorette Gum	10–12 pieces/day initially (2 or 4 mg/piece) to max of 20 pieces/day, for 12 wk Tapering: 1 piece/day each wk, as withdrawal symptoms allow	Hiccoughs, GI disturbances, jaw pain and orodental problems.		Use 4 mg in heavily dependent smokers. May be used for temporary abstinence, e.g., to comply with smoking restrictions on airplanes.	$$

Class	Drug	Dose	Adverse Effects	Drug Interactions[a]	Comments	Cost[b]
Nicotine Replacement, sustained-release	*nicotine transdermal patch* Habitrol, Nicoderm, generics	**Habitrol:** > 20 cigarettes/day: 1 patch (21 mg/24 h) daily × 3–4 wk ≤ 20 cigarettes/day: 1 patch (14 mg/24 h) daily × 3–4 wk Tapering: reduce strength of patch (i.e., from 21 to 14 to 7 mg/24 h) every 3–4 wk **Nicoderm:** 21 mg/24 h × 6 wk then 14 mg/24 h × 2 wk then 7 mg/24 h × 2 wk If patient has cardiovascular disease, weighs less than 45 kg or smokes < ½ pack/day begin with 14 mg/24 h × 6 wk then ↓ to 7 mg/24 h × 2 wk	Skin sensitivity and irritation (most common); abnormal dreams; insomnia; nausea, dyspepsia.		Start patch on the quit date. Advise not to smoke cigarettes while using the patch, though this is generally safe and does not indicate treatment failure. Educate users on the signs and symptoms of nicotine toxicity. **Habitrol:** Takes longer to reach peak levels than Nicoderm; should not use while exercising; major supplier of the generic/store brands. **Nicoderm:** More rapid onset and shorter time to peak effects; may be worn while exercising; although not recommended by the manufacturer, can be cut without damaging the delivery device.	$$$$

(cont'd)

Table 2: **Pharmacologic Agents Used for Smoking Cessation** *(cont'd)*

Class	Drug	Dose	Adverse Effects	Drug Interactions[a]	Comments	Cost[b]
Nicotine Receptor Partial Agonists	*varenicline* Champix	0.5 mg daily for 3 days then BID for 3 days then 1 mg po BID for 12 wk. Patient should quit smoking 1–2 wk after starting the medication. Reassess if patient is still smoking 4 wk after starting medication; can be continued for an additional 12 wk if patient has benefited. No tapering necessary	Nausea (30%); can be mitigated by increasing water intake or dosage reduction.	Should not be combined with nicotine replacement therapy due to increased risk of adverse effects.	Does not induce cytochrome P450 enzymes; excreted renally unchanged.	$$$$$
Antidepressants	*bupropion* Zyban, generics	150 mg daily × 3 days then 150 mg BID × 7–12 wk. Begin 1–2 wk before the selected quit date	Usual: insomnia, dry mouth, dizziness, restlessness, difficulty concentrating. Unusual: hypersensitivity reactions, ↑ risk of seizures at higher dosages.	Clearance of bupropion may be ↓ by inhibitors (e.g., ticlopidine) or ↑ by inducers (e.g., phenobarbital, phenytoin, primidone) of CYP2B6. May ↓ clearance of other substrates of CYP2B6 (e.g., cyclophosphamide, ketamine, promethazine, propofol, selegiline). MAOIs, levodopa, amantadine may ↑ toxicity. May be safely combined with NRT (monitor for	Not recommended in patients with conditions predisposing to seizures, history of seizures, current eating disorder or severe hepatic impairment. Least expensive of oral medications officially indicated for smoking cessation.	$$$

Class	Drug	Dose	Adverse Effects	Drug Interactions[a]	Comments	Cost[b]
				treatment-emergent hypertension).		
	nortriptyline generics	25 mg/day titrated to 75–100 mg/day. Quit day is usually set between 1 and 4 wk; medication is continued for 12 wk	Common: dry mouth, blurred vision, constipation, dizziness, sedation. Less common: confusion, arrhythmias, urinary retention.	Avoid with MAOIs—may cause mania, excitation, hyperpyrexia. Inducers of CYP2D6 or CYP3A4 (e.g., carbamazepine, phenytoin, rifampin) may ↓ effect. Inhibitors of CYP2D6 or CYP3A4 (e.g., clarithromycin, erythromycin, grapefruit juice, fluoxetine, paroxetine) may ↑ effect and toxicity.	Caution in patients with cardiovascular disease or arrhythmias. Consider measuring serum levels to reach therapeutic dose.	$$
Alpha$_2$-adrenergic Receptor Agonists	*clonidine* Catapres, Dixarit, generics	0.1 mg po BID starting up to 3 days before or on the quit date. Increase by 0.1 mg/day once per wk if needed. Duration of therapy ranges from 3–10 wk	Common: sedation, dizziness, hypotension, dry mouth. Less common: anxiety, irritability, memory problems, rebound hypertension.	Avoid concurrent use with tricyclic antidepressants. Additive effects with other CNS depressants such as ethanol.	Monitor blood pressure and heart rate during treatment initiation. Taper off gradually to avoid rebound hypertension when stopping treatment.	$

[a] Smoking is associated with increased CYP1A1/ 1A2 and 2E1 activity. Upon smoking cessation, reduced clearance of substrates of these enzymes (e.g., theophylline, clozapine, caffeine, fluvoxamine, haloperidol, olanzapine, lorazepam, alprazolam and diazepam) may necessitate dose adjustments.

[b] Cost of 105 pieces of gum, 42 inhalations, 28 patches or 30-day supply of tablets; includes drug cost only.

Dosage adjustment may be required in renal impairment; see Appendix I.

Abbreviations: CVS = cardiovascular; NRT = nicotine replacement therapy

Legend: $ < $25 $$ $25–50 $$$ $50–75 $$$$ $75–100 $$$$$ $100–120

Suggested Readings

Foulds J, Steinberg MB, Williams JM et al. Developments in pharmacotherapy for tobacco dependence: past, present and future. *Drug Alcohol Rev* 2006;25(1):59-71.

George TP, editor. *Medication treatments for nicotine dependence*. Boca Raton (FL): CRC/Taylor & Francis; 2007.

McEwen A, Hajek P, McRobbie H et al. *Manual of smoking cessation: a guide for counsellors and practitioners*. Malden (MA): Addiction Press, Blackwell; 2006.

West R. Bupropion SR for smoking cessation. *Expert Opin Pharmacother* 2003;4(4):533-40.

www.treatobacco.net. Database & educational resource for treatment of tobacco dependence. Available from: www.treatobacco.net Accessed June 1, 2007.

References

1. Makomaski Illing EM, Kaiserman MJ. Mortality attributable to tobacco use in Canada and its regions, 1998. *Can J Public Health* 2004;95(1):38-44.
2. Hoffmann D, Djordjevic MV, Hoffmann I. The changing cigarette. *Prev Med* 1997;26(4):427-34.
3. Le Houezec J. Role of nicotine pharmacokinetics in nicotine addiction and nicotine replacement therapy: a review. *Int J Tuberc Lung Dis* 2003;7(9):811-9.
4. Fowler JS, Logan J, Wang GJ et al. Monoamine oxidase and cigarette smoking. *Neurotoxicology* 2003;24(1):75-82.
5. Desai HD, Seabolt J, Jann MW. Smoking in patients receiving psychotropic medications: a pharmacokinetic perspective. *CNS Drugs* 2001;15(6):469-94.
6. Song F, Raftery J, Aveyard P et al. Cost-effectiveness of pharmacological interventions for smoking cessation: a literature review and a decision analytic analysis. *Med Decis Making* 2002;22(5 Suppl):S26-37.
7. Parrott S, Godfrey C. Economics of smoking cessation. *BMJ* 2004;328(7445):947-9.
8. Fiore MC, Bailey WC, Cohen SJ et al. *Clinical practice guideline. Treating tobacco use and dependence.* Washington (DC): Public Health Service, US Department of Health and Human Services; 2000. Available from: http://www.surgeongeneral.gov/tobacco/treating_tobacco_use.pdf Accessed June 1, 2007.
9. Tverdal A, Bjartveit K. Health consequences of reduced daily cigarette consumption. *Tob Control* 2006;15(6):472-80.
10. Hyland A, Levy DT, Rezaishiraz H et al. Reduction in amount smoked predicts future cessation. *Psychol Addict Behav* 2005;19(2):221-5.
11. Heatherton TF, Kozlowski LT, Frecker RC et al. The Fagerstrom Test for Nicotine Dependence: a revision of the Fagerstrom Tolerance Questionnaire. *Br J Addict* 1991;86(9):1119-27.
12. Kozlowski LT, Porter CQ, Orleans CT et al. Predicting smoking cessation with self-reported measures of nicotine dependence: FTQ, FTND, and HSI. *Drug Alcohol Depend* 1994;34(3):211-6.
13. Rollnick S, Mason P, Butler C. *Health behavior change: a guide for practitioners*. New York (NY): Churchill Livingstone; 1999.
14. Hughes JR, Stead LF, Lancaster T. Antidepressants for smoking cessation. *Cochrane Database Syst Rev* 2007;1:CD000031.
15. Frishman WH, Mitta W, Kupersmith A et al. Nicotine and non-nicotine smoking cessation pharmacotherapies. *Cardiol Rev* 2006;14(2):57-73.
16. Gourlay S, Forbes A, Marriner T et al. A placebo-controlled study of three clonidine doses for smoking cessation. *Clin Pharmacol Ther* 1994;55(1):64-9.
17. Glassman AH, Stetner F, Walsh BT et al. Heavy smokers, smoking cessation, and clonidine. Results of a double-blind, randomized trial. *JAMA* 1988;259(19):2863-6.
18. Keating GM, Siddiqui MA. Varenicline: a review of its use as an aid to smoking cessation therapy. *CNS Drugs* 2006;20(11):945-60.
19. Oncken C, Gonzales D, Nides M et al. Efficacy and safety of the novel selective nicotinic acetylcholine receptor partial agonist, varenicline, for smoking cessation. *Arch Intern Med* 2006;166(15):1571-7.
20. Tonstad S, Tonnesen P, Hajek P et al. Effect of maintenance therapy with varenicline on smoking cessation: a randomized controlled trial. *JAMA* 2006;296(1):64-71.
21. Jorenby DE, Hays JT, Rigotti NA et al. Efficacy of varenicline, an alpha4beta2 nicotinic acetylcholine receptor partial agonist, vs placebo or sustained-release bupropion for smoking cessation: a randomized controlled trial. *JAMA* 2006;296(1):56-63.

22. Gonzales D, Rennard SI, Nides M et al. Varenicline, an alpha4beta2 nicotinic acetylcholine receptor partial agonist, vs sustained-release bupropion and placebo for smoking cessation: a randomized controlled trial. *JAMA* 2006;296(1):47-55.
23. Silagy C, Lancaster T, Stead L, et al. Nicotine replacement therapy for smoking cessation. *Cochrane Database Syst Rev*, 2004;(3):CD000146
24. Haustein KO, Krause J, Haustein H et al. Comparison of the effects of combined nicotine replacement therapy vs. cigarette smoking in males. *Nicotine Tob Res* 2003;5(2):195-203.
25. Sweeney CT, Fant RV, Fagerstrom KO et al. Combination nicotine replacement therapy for smoking cessation: rationale, efficacy and tolerability. *CNS Drugs* 2001;15(6):453-67.
26. Jorenby DE, Leischow SJ, Nides MA et al. A controlled trial of sustained-release bupropion, a nicotine patch, or both for smoking cessation. *N Engl J Med* 1999;340(9):685-91.
27. Foulds J, Steinberg MB, Williams JM et al. Developments in pharmacotherapy for tobacco dependence: past, present and future. *Drug Alcohol Rev* 2006;25(1):59-71.
28. Henningfield JE, Fant RV, Buchhalter AR et al. Pharmacotherapy for nicotine dependence. *CA Cancer J Clin* 2005;55(5):281-99.
29. Mallin R. Smoking cessation: integration of behavioral and drug therapies. *Am Fam Physician* 2002;65(6):1107-14.
30. Smith SS, Jorenby DE, Leischow SJ et al. Targeting smokers at increased risk for relapse: treating women and those with a history of depression. *Nicotine Tob Res* 2003;5(1):99-109.
31. O'Hara P, Connett JE, Lee WW et al. Early and late weight gain following smoking cessation in the Lung Health Study. *Am J Epidemiol* 1998;148(9):821-30.
32. Fagerstrom K, Balfour DJ. Neuropharmacology and potential efficacy of new treatments for tobacco dependence. *Expert Opin Investig Drugs* 2006;15(2):107-16.

CHAPTER 11
Eating Disorders

C. Laird Birmingham, MD, MHSc, FRCPC

A disturbance in the perception of body image and weight is an essential feature of both anorexia nervosa and bulimia nervosa.

Anorexia nervosa is characterized by a deliberate loss of weight (to ≤ 85% of expected weight), refusal to maintain a normal body weight, fear of weight gain and amenorrhea. The two subtypes, *restricting* and *binge-eating/purging*, indicate the presence or absence of regular binge-eating or purging.

Bulimia nervosa is characterized by repeated episodes of binge-eating followed by inappropriate compensatory behaviours such as self-induced vomiting, misuse of laxatives, diuretics, emetics or other medications, fasting or excessive exercise. The two subtypes of bulimia nervosa are *purging* and *nonpurging* (uses inappropriate compensatory behaviours, e.g., fasting or excessive exercise but does not regularly engage in self-induced vomiting, misuse of laxatives).

Goals of Therapy

- Assess and treat coexistent nutritional deficiencies
- Assess and treat the effects of malnutrition, e.g., osteoporosis, hypoglycemia, dehydration
- Improve cognitive and emotional function
- Identify and treat psychiatric comorbidity, e.g., anxiety, depression, family dysfunction, self-injurious behaviour, suicidal ideation
- Treat binge and purge behaviour
- Develop healthy eating habits
- For anorexia nervosa, achieve and maintain a healthy weight/body mass index (BMI)

Investigations

- A thorough history with special attention to:
  - weight, eating habits, binge and purge behaviour, menstruation (in females), body image, use of vomiting, laxatives (oral formulations or rectal suppositories), diuretics, ipecac, fasting and excessive exercising
  - developmental and psychological history
  - depression, anxiety, suicidal ideation, family dysfunction and sexual abuse

- symptoms of malnutrition including chest wall pain, palpitations, loss of consciousness, hematemesis, seizures, abdominal pain, muscle weakness or cramping, episodes of confusion
- dietary history

- Physical examination for parotid hypertrophy, jugular venous pressure, edema, abnormal dentition, Russell's sign (scarring over the knuckles caused by using the hand to induce vomiting); for anorexia nervosa, look also for postural hypotension, tachycardia, lanugo hair, hypercarotenemia, height, weight, measurements of body fat, proximal myopathy, neuromuscular hyperirritability (Chvostek's and Trousseau's signs)[1]
- Laboratory tests:
  - sodium, potassium, chloride, bicarbonate, creatinine, magnesium, calcium, phosphorus, zinc, B_{12}, ferritin; for anorexia nervosa, add ECG, hemoglobin, WBC count, urinalysis, RBC, folate and blood glucose (fasting and two hours after eating)
- For anorexia nervosa, a psychiatric and nutritional assessment if symptoms continue and weight does not normalize after weekly follow-up and counselling[2]

Anorexia Nervosa

Therapeutic Choices (Figure 1)

Nonpharmacologic Choices

- Develop and maintain a rapport and therapeutic alliance.
- Consider the need for and role of family intervention and treatment (especially for children and adolescents).
- Set step-wise nutritional goals.
- Use nutritional supplements (e.g., Ensure, Boost) to achieve weight gain if not possible through food. Supportive nursing care at mealtime may improve success;[3] tube feeding may be necessary if oral feeding fails.
- Exercise should be limited. However, a supervised graded exercise plan (such as non-exercise yoga) can reduce anxiety while not interfering with the rate of weight gain.[4]
- Warming, by means of a warm room or warming vest, may reduce anxiety, hasten recovery and improve the chances of long-term recovery.[5]
- Monitor binge and purge behaviour and set goals for normalization, e.g., a gradual tapering of laxatives.

Pharmacologic Choices[6] (Table 1)

Prokinetic Agents

Domperidone and **metoclopramide** usually help to reduce the feeling of fullness caused by decreased intestinal motility during the early stages of feeding.[7] Of the prokinetic agents, only cisapride has been compared to placebo in this patient group, but it was withdrawn from the market because of its association with an increased rate of dysrhythmia and death.

Unless the antinauseant effect of metoclopramide is needed, domperidone is preferred because it has a lower incidence of extrapyramidal side effects. Rarely, if the feeling of fullness is limiting treatment and domperidone or metoclopramide is ineffective, the addition of **erythromycin** may help.[8,9]

The potential for these drugs to cause QT prolongation should be considered, especially in patients with other risk factors such as hypokalemia or hypoglycemia.

Other Therapies

Zinc gluconate supplementation (100 mg daily for two months) increases the rate of weight gain irrespective of the serum zinc measurement.[10] Zinc causes nausea in about 2% of patients when taken orally, but it can be taken with food to reduce this adverse effect.

Olanzapine decreases anorexic rumination resulting in improved motivation and may thereby promote weight gain, even in chronic anorexia nervosa.[11,12] A randomized controlled trial supports these findings and demonstrates that the rate of weight gain is not increased in patients with anorexia nervosa (beyond the weight gain olanzapine would be expected to cause in a person without anorexia).[13] This is important in anorexia nervosa sufferers because they would not use the medication if weight gain were rapid. Doses of 2.5 to 5 mg/day have been effective, with a maximum dose of 20 mg/day. Because of extrapyramidal side effects it should not be used long term unless the benefits outweigh the risks of developing a movement disorder. Usually, the appropriate duration of therapy is until it is no longer needed for weight gain (around 3 months) and to a maximum BMI of 17 kg/m^2. Beyond that, a rapid increase in appetite and weight gain may occur if olanzapine is continued. Diabetes due to reduced insulin sensitivity is a commonly observed adverse effect of olanzapine, but not in this patient group to date.

Cyproheptadine 4 to 16 mg at bedtime may be useful, particularly in chronic anorexia nervosa. It may cause a modest weight gain and can be used as a hypnotic.[14,15]

Benzodiazepines (e.g., **clonazepam**) can be used to treat severe anxiety. Take care to avoid dependence. Begin with clonazepam at 0.25 to 0.5 mg BID and cautiously titrate upward if necessary, no more often than every three days. The atypical antipsychotic **quetiapine** is often used instead of a benzodiazepine to manage anxiety in this setting, because it is more effective and not addictive.[16,17]

Selective serotonin reuptake inhibitor (SSRI) antidepressants should be used only for coexistent depression or purge behaviour, and if cardiac status is stable (e.g., QTc less than 450 milliseconds; see Bulimia Nervosa, Antidepressants.)[18]

Give **thiamine** in a dose of 100 mg/day for five days at the beginning of feeding to prevent the development of Wernicke-Korsakoff syndrome (encephalopathy).

Ondansetron is not effective in controlling the nausea or vomiting associated with eating disorders.[19]

Therapeutic Tips

- Hypoglycemia can occur after eating because liver glycogen is depleted. Blood glucose should be measured two hours after meals for the first day or two of feeding and if confusion occurs.[20]
- Chronic laxative abuse can be treated by slowly tapering laxatives over months to years.[21]
- Normalizing body fat is necessary for psychological treatment to be effective and for cure.
- Women with anorexia nervosa can become pregnant when amenorrheic.[22]
- Treatment refusal is common. A careful reassessment of the treatment plan is necessary.[23] Family therapy is particularly important for the treatment of children and adolescents.
- Suicidality, worsening depression and/or an inability to gain weight are indications for referral to an eating disorders specialist. Outpatient, residential or inpatient eating disorder treatment may be required.[24]

Bulimia Nervosa

Therapeutic Choices (Figure 2)

Nonpharmacologic Choices

- Cognitive behavioural therapy and interpersonal therapy are helpful in addressing cognitive and emotional issues and reinforcing normal eating behaviour. Follow progress.[2]
- Assess patients for suicidal ideation and depression; treat if present.
- Psychoeducational groups addressing nutritional and psychological issues can enhance individual therapy.[25,26]

Pharmacologic Choices (Table 2)

Antidepressants

Two-thirds of patients taking an antidepressant experience a ≥ 50% reduction in binge episodes. There is no correlation between the presence of comorbid depression and antibulimic effects of the antidepressant, nor is there any evidence that one antidepressant is more effective than another.[27] However, because of toxicity and poor compliance, do not prescribe tricyclic antidepressants, MAOIs, or bupropion (which has been associated with an increased likelihood of seizures in patients with eating disorders). **SSRIs**, **venlafaxine** or **trazodone** can be used; **fluoxetine** is supported by the most evidence.[28,29,30] Trazodone can be particularly useful in patients with insomnia associated with bulimia nervosa.

Maintain therapy for at least six months, preferably one year. If symptoms persist after a trial of counselling and an antidepressant, treatment by a multidisciplinary team may be necessary.

Therapeutic Tips

- If effective, continue antidepressants for 6 to 12 months. Individual response to medication varies, so a series of antidepressants may have to be tried until an effective one is found.
- Treatment with more than one antidepressant at the same time has no proven advantages and has the potential to increase adverse effects and cost.
- Often during psychological treatment (e.g., when a long-suppressed traumatic event such as sexual abuse is uncovered and addressed) or with significant life stress, a temporary worsening of binge and purge behaviour occurs. This does not indicate a worsening in the patient's overall condition.
- Treatment of psychiatric comorbidity is necessary for long-term cure.

Figure 1: Management of Anorexia Nervosa

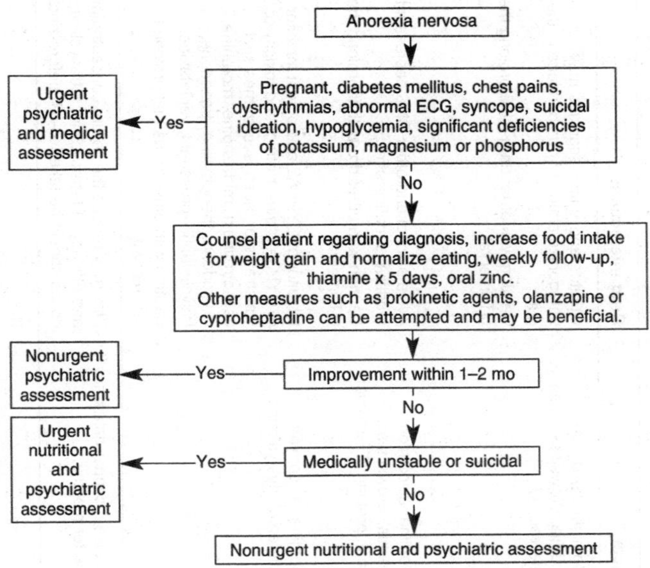

Figure 2: Management of Bulimia Nervosa

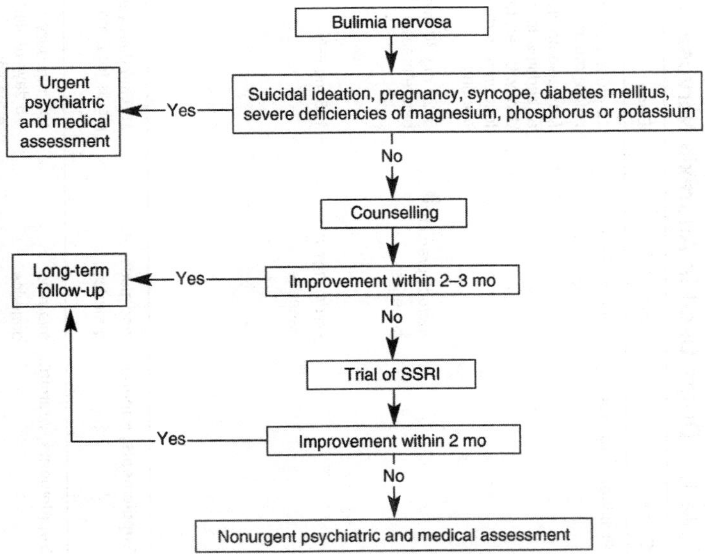

Table 1: **Drugs Used in Anorexia Nervosa**

Class	Drug	Dose	Adverse Effects	Drug Interactions	Cost[a]
Prokinetic Agents	*domperidone* generics	10–20 mg 30 min before meals May also be given at bedtime to deal with residual food ingested in evening.	Diarrhea, abdominal discomfort, hyperprolactinemia, drowsiness; can prolong QT interval.	Opiates and antimuscarinics may antagonize action of domperidone in the gut. Caution with other drugs that prolong the QT interval.	$
	metoclopramide generics	5–20 mg 30 min before meals	Diarrhea, abdominal discomfort, hyperprolactinemia, drowsiness, restlessness; can prolong QT interval.	Avoid alcohol and other CNS depressants (additive sedative effects). Caution with other drugs that prolong the QT interval.	$
	erythromycin generics	125 mg BID	Diarrhea, abdominal discomfort, prolonged QT interval, dysrythmias.	Inhibitor of CYP1A2 and potent inhibitor of CYP3A4; may ↑ effect and toxicity of substrates of these isoenzymes such as isotretinoin, mirtazapine, morphine, oxycodone, theophylline, trazodone, tricyclic antidepressants, venlafaxine. Caution with other drugs that prolong the QT interval.	$
Supplements, mineral	*zinc gluconate* generics	100 mg daily with meals for 2 mo	Nausea; can cause a copper deficiency if taken in excess for months.	Zinc may reduce the serum concentration and efficacy of tetracycline; tetracycline doses should be taken 2–3 h before zinc.	$
Supplements, vitamin	*thiamine* generics	100 mg daily × 5 days at start of re-feeding	N/A	N/A	$

Class	Drug	Dose	Adverse Effects	Drug Interactions	Cost[a]
Benzodiazepines	*clonazepam* Rivotril, generics	Initial: 0.25–0.5 mg BID May titrate up cautiously at 3-day intervals if needed Usual maximum: 2–5 mg/day	Sedation, ataxia, weakness, dependence.	Potentiates effects of other CNS depressants, including alcohol.	$
Antipsychotics, second-generation	*olanzapine* Zyprexa	2.5–20 mg/day	Drowsiness, akathisia.	Fluvoxamine may ↑ olanzapine serum concentrations; other SSRIs are less likely to exhibit this interaction.	$$$
	quetiapine Seroquel	12.5–50 mg before meals and at bedtime Used to manage severe anxiety in this setting	Drowsiness, extrapyramidal side effects, QT prolongation.	↑ hypotension with antihypertensives; additive sedation with CNS depressants, including alcohol; inhibitors of CYP3A4 such as erythromycin, clarithromycin, fluoxetine or ketoconazole can increase the effects and toxicity of quetiapine.	$-$$

[a] Cost of 30-day supply; includes drug cost only.

Dosage adjustment may be required in renal impairment; see Appendix I.

Legend: $ < $15 $-$$ < $15–30 $$ $15–30 $$$ > $30

Table 2: **Drugs Used in Bulimia Nervosa**

Class	Drug	Dose	Adverse Effects	Drug Interactions	Cost[a]
Selective Serotonin Reuptake Inhibitors[b]	*fluoxetine* Prozac, generics	20–60 mg daily	Anxiety, GI discomfort (common), sexual dysfunction, ↑ risk of GI bleeding.	Avoid use with MAOIs, L-tryptophan (serotonin syndrome); inhibits cytochrome P450 enzymes, especially CYP2D6—may ↑ effects and toxicity of many drugs including atomoxetine, methamphetamine, mirtazapine, TCAs, tramadol; ↑ risk of GI bleeding with NSAIDs.	$$–$$$$
Serotonin-norepinephrine Reuptake Inhibitors	*venlafaxine* (renal symbol) Effexor XR, generic	75–150 mg daily	Nausea, drowsiness, nervousness, dizziness, dry mouth, hypertension at doses > 300 mg.	Inhibitors of CYP2D6 or CYP3A4 (e.g., erythromycin, clarithromycin, fluphenazine, ketoconazole) can ↑ effects and toxicity of venlafaxine; do not use with MAOIs.	$$
Serotonin Agonists	*trazodone* Desyrel, generics	100–500 mg daily in single or divided doses	Sedation (common), anticholinergic adverse effects less common than with other TCAs.	Avoid use with MAOIs; inhibitors of CYP3A4 such as erythromycin, clarithromycin or ketoconazole can ↑ effects and toxicity of trazodone.	$–$$$

[a] Cost of 30-day supply; includes drug cost only.
[b] For other SSRIs see Chapter 5.
(renal symbol) Dosage adjustment may be required in renal impairment; see Appendix I.
Abbreviations: TCA = tricyclic antidepressant; XR = extended-release
Legend: $ < $25 $–$$$ < $25–75 $$ $25–50 $$–$$$$ $25–100 $$$ $50–75 $$$$ $75–100

Suggested Readings

American Dietetic Association. Position of the American Dietetic Association: nutrition intervention in the treatment of anorexia nervosa, bulimia nervosa, and other eating disorders. *J Am Diet Assoc* 2006;106(12):2073-82.

American Psychiatric Association. Treatment of patients with eating disorders, third edition. *Am J Psychiatry* 2006;163(7 Suppl):4-54.

Bacaltchuk J, Hay P. Antidepressants versus placebo for people with bulimia nervosa. *Cochrane Database Syst Rev* 2003;(4):CD003391.

Beumont P, Hay P, Beumont D et al. Australian and New Zealand clinical practice guidelines for the treatment of anorexia nervosa. *Aust N Z J Psychiatry* 2004;38(9):659-70.

National Collaborating Centre for Mental Health; National Institute of Clinical Excellence. Eating disorders: core interventions in the treatment and management of anorexia nervosa, bulimia nervosa and related eating disorders. London (UK): National Institute for Clinical Excellence; 2004. Available from www.nice.org.uk/CG009NICEguideline Accessed May 14, 2007.

References

1. Tyler I, Birmingham CL. The interrater reliability of physical signs in patients with eating disorders. *Int J Eat Disord* 2001;30(3):343-5.
2. American Dietetic Association. Position of the American Dietetic Association: nutrition intervention in the treatment of anorexia nervosa, bulimia nervosa, and other eating disorders. *J Am Diet Assoc* 2006;106(12):2073-82.
3. Leichner P, Hall D, Calderon R. Meal support training for friends and families of patients with eating disorders. *Eat Disord* 2005;13(4):407-11.
4. Thien V, Thomas A, Markin D et al. Pilot study of a graded exercise program for the treatment of anorexia nervosa. *Int J Eat Disord* 2000;28(1):101-6.
5. Bergh C, Brodin U, Lindberg G et al. Randomized controlled trial of a treatment for anorexia and bulimia nervosa. *Proc Natl Acad Sci U S A* 2002;99(14):9486-91.
6. Zhu AJ, Walsh BT. Pharmacologic treatment of eating disorders. *Can J Psychiatry* 2002;47(3):227-34.
7. Leung M, Birmingham CL. Food fight. *Pharmacy Practice* 1997;13(10):62-72.
8. Stacher G, Peeters TL, Bergmann H et al. Erythromycin effects on gastric emptying, antral motility and plasma motilin and pancreatic polypeptide concentrations in anorexia nervosa. *Gut* 1993;34(2):166-72.
9. Ray WA, Murray KT, Meredith S, et al. Oral erythromycin and the risk of sudden death from cardiac causes. *N Engl J Med* 2004;351(11):1089-96.
10. Su JC, Birmingham CL. Zinc supplementation in the treatment of anorexia nervosa. *Eat Weight Disord* 2002;7(1):20-2.
11. La Via MC, Gray N, Kaye WH. Case reports of olanzapine treatment of anorexia nervosa. *Int J Eat Disord* 2000;27(3):363-6.
12. Mehler C, Wewetzer C, Schulze U et al. Olanzapine in children and adolescents with chronic anorexia nervosa. A study of five cases. *Eur Child Adolesc Psychiatry* 2001;10(2):151-7.
13. Mondraty NK et al. A randomized controlled trial of olanzapine versus chlorpromazine in anorexia nervosa. *Int J Eat Disord.* In press 2003.
14. Halmi KA, Eckert E, LaDu TJ et al. Anorexia nervosa. Treatment efficacy of cyproheptadine and amitriptyline. *Arch Gen Psychiatry* 1986;43(2):177-81.
15. Halmi KA, Eckert E, Falk JR. Cyproheptadine for anorexia nervosa. *Lancet* 1982;1(8285):1357-8.
16. Powers PS, Bannon Y, Eubanks R et al. Quetiapine in anorexia nervosa patients: an open label outpatient pilot study. *Int J Eat Disord* 2007;40(1):21-6.
17. Sattar SP, Bhatia SC, Petty F. Potential benefits of quetiapine in the treatment of substance dependence disorders. *J Psychiatry Neurosci* 2004;29(6):452-7
18. Walsh BT, Kaplan AS, Attia E et al. Fluoxetine after weight restoration in anorexia nervosa: a randomized controlled trial. *JAMA* 2006;295(22):2605-12.
19. Fung SM, Ferrill MJ. Treatment of bulimia nervosa with ondansetron. *Ann Pharmacother* 2001;35(10):1270-3.
20. Puddicombe DM, Birmingham CL. Using the glucagon test to predict hypoglycemia in anorexia nervosa. *Eat Weight Disord* 2006;11(2):e72-4.

21. Harper J, Leung M, Birmingham CL. A blinded laxative taper for patients with eating disorders. *Eat Weight Disord* 2004;9(2):147-50.
22. Mehler PS. Diagnosis and care of patients with anorexia nervosa in primary care settings. *Ann Intern Med* 2001;134(11):1048-59.
23. Geller J, Cockell SJ, Drab DL. Assessing readiness for change in the eating disorders: the psychometric properties of the readiness and motivation interview. *Psychol Assess* 2001;13(2):189-98.
24. Kaplan AS. Psychological treatments for anorexia nervosa: a review of published studies and promising new directions. *Can J Psychiatry* 2002;47(3):235-42.
25. Davis R, McVey G, Heinmaa M et al. Sequencing of cognitive-behavioral treatments for bulimia nervosa. *Int J Eat Disord* 1999;25(4):361-74.
26. Hay PJ, Bacaltchuk J, Stefano S. Psychotherapy for bulimia nervosa and binging. *Cochrane Database Syst Rev* 2004;(3):CD000562.
27. Bacaltchuk J, Hay P. Antidepressants versus placebo for people with bulimia nervosa. *Cochrane Database Syst Rev* 2003;(4):CD003391.
28. Goldstein DJ, Wilson MG, Thompson VL et al. Long-term fluoxetine treatment of bulimia nervosa: Fluoxetine Bulimia Nervosa Research Group. *Br J Psychiatry* 1995;166(5):660-6.
29. Romano SJ, Halmi KA, Sarkar NP et al. A placebo-controlled study of fluoxetine in continued treatment of bulimia nervosa after successful acute fluoxetine treatment. *Am J Psychiatry* 2002;159(1):96-102.
30. [No authors listed]. Fluoxetine in the treatment of bulimia nervosa. A multicenter, placebo-controlled, double-blind trial. Fluoxetine Bulimia Nervosa Collaborative Study Group. *Arch Gen Psychiatry* 1992;49(2):139-47.

CHAPTER 12
Headache in Adults

R. Allan Purdy, MD, FRCPC

Goals of Therapy

- Relieve or abolish pain and associated symptoms such as nausea/vomiting
- Prevent recurrent symptoms in primary headache disorders, e.g., migraine, tension-type and cluster
- Diagnose and manage serious causes of headache, e.g., tumor, arteritis, infection, hemorrhage
- Prevent complications of medication usage

Investigations (Figure 1)

- A thorough history and physical examination are most important for a correct diagnosis.[1] Note characteristics of the headache:
  - onset: sudden versus gradual
  - temporal profile: progressive versus self-limited
  - frequency/pattern of recurrence: e.g., during menses (menstrual migraine), strictly unilateral and occurring in clusters separated by months or years, always on the same side (episodic cluster headache)
  - associated symptoms: nausea, vomiting, sensitivity to light, noise or odours, systemic or other neurologic signs or symptoms
  - degree of interference with activities of daily life caused by migraine
- The physical examination should be normal; if any abnormalities are found (especially visual, motor, reflex, sensory, speech or cognitive), investigation is warranted
- CT/MR scans are not routine but must be done if any organic etiology is suspected (see Table 1)
- Lumbar puncture if subarachnoid hemorrhage, encephalitis, high- or low-pressure headache syndromes or meningitis is suspected
- Laboratory tests (on an individual basis)
  - ESR for suspected temporal arteritis
  - endocrine, biochemical, infection work-up
  - search for malignancy if indicated
- Facial pain may need a thorough assessment by a dental specialist familiar with headaches and facial pain and/or an ENT specialist if sinus or other ENT disorders are suspected

Table 1: **Red Flags for Serious Headache**

	Red Flags
Age of onset	Middle-aged to elderly patient
Type of onset	Severe and abrupt
Temporal sequence	Progressive severity or increased frequency
Pattern	Significant change in headache pattern
Neurologic signs	Stiff neck, focal signs, reduced consciousness
Systemic signs	Fever, appears sick, abnormal examination
Caution: If headache does not fit typical pattern, a serious diagnosis can be missed	

Therapeutic Choices

If serious structural CNS causes for headache and facial pain have been ruled out, the primary headache disorders can be managed as follows.[2,3]

Nonpharmacologic Choices

- The management of headache is as much art as science; the science is improving, but the art remains important:
  - after serious causes are excluded, the interaction with the patient is the first and most important therapeutic choice
  - communicate with patients to let them know their headache is real, and that they have a specific diagnosis
  - determine patients' expectations and explain management options
- Advise patients to:
  - avoid triggers, especially in migraine, e.g., too much or too little sleep, irregular meals, lack of regular exercise, extremes of stress or relaxation, known dietary triggers
  - apply ice; sleep or rest in a dark, noise-free room
- Try informal psychotherapy (family physician); refer to psychiatrist if psychiatric comorbidity present
- Try biofeedback, relaxation therapy, cognitive-behavioural therapy, psychotherapy, acupuncture and/or nerve blocks, individualized to each patient[3]
- Refer to neurologist and/or specialized headache or pain management unit if problems too complex or require multidisciplinary approach

Pharmacologic Choices (Table 2)

Evidence-based guidelines for symptomatic and prophylactic therapies have been published.[4,5]

Symptomatic Treatment

Analgesics

Ibuprofen, naproxen, and **ASA** or **acetaminophen** with or without **codeine** and/or **butalbital,** are used with some success for mild to moderate headache pain. Medication-overuse headache can result from overuse of analgesics, which limits their long-term potential. To avoid medication-overuse headache, nonopioid analgesics should be used less than 15 days per month; opioids and combination analgesics should be used less than 10 days per month. Butalbital compounds and opioids have limited use in benign headache disorders because of the potential for dependency.

Ergot Derivatives

Ergotamine acts on serotonin receptors and is classically used for migraine and cluster headaches but use is limited by side effects. Ergotamine is available in many formulations and routes of administration. Ergot derivatives may produce rebound headaches if used 10 days per month or more.

Dihydroergotamine mesylate (DHE) has similar actions to the triptans but also interacts centrally with dopamine and adrenergic receptors, accounting for some of its side effects. It can be used to treat acute intractable headache or withdrawal from analgesics. DHE produces no dependence.

Triptans

The triptans currently available to abort migraine include **almotriptan, eletriptan, naratriptan, rizatriptan, sumatriptan** and **zolmitriptan**. All act on serotonin (5-HT) subclass 1B and 1D receptors, on extracerebral blood vessels and neurons respectively. The supposed mechanism of action is prevention of neurogenically sterile inflammatory responses around vessels and vasoconstriction. The newer agents may alter pain transmission centrally at the level of the trigeminal nucleus of the medulla, an action that may or may not have clinical benefits.

Subcutaneous sumatriptan has the fastest onset of action and remains the most efficacious triptan for a severe migraine attack. It is also useful in an acute cluster headache. Naratriptan has the slowest onset of action with maximal efficacy at four hours, less headache recurrence than the other agents and near placebo rates of side effects. Naratriptan may be best for moderately severe migraine attacks and for individuals who have low tolerance for side effects or high pain recurrence rates.

Overall, there is now good evidence that the available triptans are efficacious, generally well tolerated and safe.[6] Meta-analyses reveal that differences among the triptans are relatively small, but may be clinically relevant to patients.[7,8] However, the benefits in individual patients may vary, as may patient preference for specific formulations (i.e., injection, nasal spray, tablets or fast-melt tablets).[9] All triptans are contraindicated in patients with cardiac disorders, sustained hypertension, basilar and hemiplegic migraine.

To avoid medication-overuse headache, triptans should be used less than 10 days per month.

Others

Corticosteroids can be useful in many headache disorders, including status migraine, cluster headache and cerebral neoplasms with edema (especially metastatic lesions). Corticosteroids in temporal arteritis relieve headache and may prevent blindness.

Phenothiazines (e.g., **prochlorperazine** or **chlorpromazine**) have been used in the emergency room for treatment of migraine and other intractable headaches.

If no success is obtained with the above treatments for acute migraine, **ketorolac** im may be effective. **Meperidine**, administered iv or im, should be regarded as a treatment of last resort. **Indomethacin** has been found useful in chronic paroxysmal hemicrania and related disorders.

Antinauseants (e.g., **dimenhydrinate** 50 to 100 mg po PRN) and antiemetic/prokinetic agents (e.g., **metoclopramide** 10 mg po or iv and **domperidone** 10 to 20 mg po) are useful as adjunctive or primary (i.e., metoclopramide iv) therapy in headache disorders associated with nausea and vomiting, or to facilitate absorption of medications in some patients.

Prophylactic Therapy (Table 3)

Prophylaxis is indicated if the migraine attacks are severe enough to interfere with the patient's quality of life, or if the patient has three or more severe attacks per month that fail to respond adequately to symptomatic therapy.

Beta-blockers

Beta-blockers are commonly used and efficacious in migraine prophylaxis; their mechanism of action is uncertain. Effective agents lack partial agonist activity, but CNS penetration, membrane stabilization and cardioselectivity do not influence efficacy. **Metoprolol** has the best evidence to support its use but there is more experience with **propranolol**. Because they may cross the blood-brain barrier less than other beta-blockers, **nadolol** and **atenolol** may have fewer CNS side effects.

Calcium Channel Blockers

These drugs may work by modulating neurotransmitter function rather than producing vasodilation or protecting against hypoxia. **Verapamil** is useful in migraine and cluster headache prophylaxis. **Flunarizine** is a selective calcium entry blocker and has good efficacy in migraine.

Tricyclic Analgesics

Amitriptyline, nortriptyline and **doxepin** are effective for migraine and tension-type headache, acting as analgesics at doses lower than those required for affective disorders. They do not produce dependence and are relatively safe medications in this setting.

Antiepileptic Drugs

Valproic acid and **divalproex sodium** are effective in migraine prophylaxis and may work by modulating gamma aminobutyric acid (GABA) receptors in the peripheral trigeminovascular system. Guidelines for use have been published.[10] Teratogenicity (neural tube defects) occurs.

Topiramate can be helpful in the management of some patients in doses up to 100 mg or occasionally higher. Randomized trial data support its use.[11] It should be avoided in patients with renal stones and can cause increased intraocular pressure that responds to drug discontinuation; one side effect that can be beneficial in some patients is weight loss. Start topiramate at a very low dose of 25 mg and increase very slowly to avoid cognitive side effects.[12]

Gabapentin shows promise in the prophylactic management of migraine. It is generally well tolerated and has few side effects or drug interactions.[13]

Serotonin Antagonists

Methysergide is a potent prophylactic medication for migraine and cluster headaches. It has potentially serious long-term side effects which can be avoided by limiting duration of treatment. Although less potent than methysergide, **pizotifen** (pizotyline) is helpful in migraine if tolerated at maximal dosage.

Others

Oral **riboflavin** (400 mg/day)[14] has shown some efficacy in migraine prophylaxis but more trials are needed.

Lithium 300 mg TID is useful in the prophylactic management of chronic cluster headache.[15]

The role of **botulinum toxin** in the management of migraine is under investigation.

Chronic Daily Headache and Medication-overuse Headache

Chronic headache occurs daily or almost daily for 15 days per month, for six months or longer. The most common causes of these headaches are *transformed migraine* and *chronic tension-type headache*. In the former there is history of migraine attacks and over several years the migraine attacks become more frequent. Soon the migraine characteristics give way to chronic daily headache with a daily or near-daily background headache that often resembles a typical "tension-type headache." People with chronic tension-type headache may have no history of distinct migraine.

Patients with these disorders frequently use excessive amounts of abortive agents, including ergots, acetaminophen, ASA and opioid analgesics. They can have *rebound headaches* as a result of *medication-overuse headache,* while some may have symptoms of depression or other psychological comorbidities. Rebound headaches can also occur with the overuse of triptans.[16] Most will improve in days or a few weeks with the discontinuation of these medications, especially mixed analgesics.

Generally, simple analgesics should be used less than 15 days per month in primary headache disorders such as migraine or tension-type headache or they will lead to the development of medication-overuse headache and chronic daily headache. [17] Further, if chronic daily headache develops, other useful abortive and prophylactic medications usually have less efficacy.

Management includes recognition of these disorders, tapering and stopping the offending agent(s), and starting a prophylactic medication such as **amitriptyline** or another agent listed in Table 3. During withdrawal, particularly in patients with transformed migraine, use abortive agents such as **DHE** or a **triptan** for treatment of the migraine headaches that emerge. Short-term admission to hospital may be required to use the Raskin protocol (using DHE)[18,19] and give support. If psychological comorbidities, including depression, are present they must be managed and treated. Consider referral to a multidisciplinary pain management clinic for cases failing to respond to therapy.

Therapeutic Tips

- Give abortive treatment, without exceeding recommended dosages, as soon as possible.
- Use simple analgesics less than 15 days per month, and ergots, triptans, opioids or analgesic combinations less than 10 days per month.
- A calendar or diary of headaches is useful in follow-up assessment.
- A record of medications (usefulness, dosage and side effects) should be kept.
- If migraine that does not respond adequately to symptomatic therapy occurs more than three to four times per month, try prophylactic medications for several months and then discontinue if possible, to assess ongoing need.[2]
- Different medications may need to be tried, including different members of the same class, such as triptans.
- Follow-up is most important in managing chronic headache.
- Reassurance and explanation are most important to the patient in the long term.
- Always offer hope to patients with chronic headache even if no cure is available; most primary headaches can be controlled.

Figure 1: Diagnosis and Initial Assessment of Headache

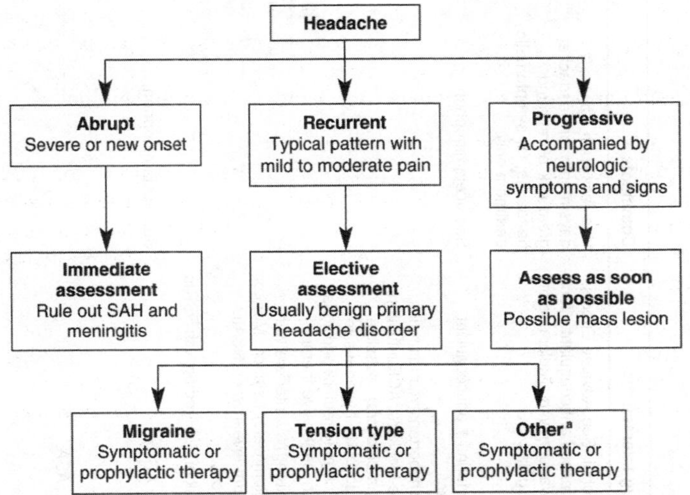

[a] Any headache not recognized as migraine, tension headache or known cause is in the "other" group. Investigate if no response to usual treatments.

Abbreviations: SAH = subarachnoid hemorrhage.

Table 2: **Medications for Symptomatic Treatment of Headache**

Class	Drug	Dose (per attack)	Adverse Effects	Drug Interactions	Comments	Cost[a]
Analgesics	*acetaminophen* Tylenol, generics	650–1300 mg Q4H X 2 doses	Potential hepatoxicity with chronic use of high doses (particularly in heavy drinkers) or in acute overdose.	Alcohol: See Adverse Effects; enhanced anticoagulant effect of warfarin with regular use of > 2 g/day.	Use less than 15 days/month for headache; great risk of rebound headache; for symptomatic treatment only.	$
	ASA Coated Aspirin, Bufferin, Aspirin, generics	650–1300 mg Q4H X 2 doses	GI upset.	Warfarin: ↑ anticoagulant effect. Antihypertensives (diuretics, beta-blockers, ACE inhibitors, alpha-blockers): possible reduction in hypertensive effect; may require additional antihypertensive therapy. Lithium may interfere with sodium/water balance. Monitor lithium levels when NSAID added. ↑ risk of GI bleeding with SSRIs	See acetaminophen.	$
	ibuprofen Advil, Motrin, generics	400–800 mg Q6H X 2 doses	GI upset.	See ASA.	See acetaminophen.	$
	ketorolac Toradol IM	30–60 mg im; max. 120 mg/24h		See ASA.		$

Class	Drug	Dose (per attack)	Adverse Effects	Drug Interactions	Comments	Cost[a]
	naproxen Naprosyn, generics	250–500 mg Q2–6H; max. 1000 mg per day	GI upset.	See ASA.	Use less than 15 days/month for symptomatic treatment of headache.	$
	naproxen sodium Anaprox, generics	275–550 mg Q2–6H; max. 1100 mg per day	GI upset.	See ASA.	See naproxen. Useful in preventing premenstrual migraine attacks when taken BID perimenstrually for 2 weeks, starting 7 days before menses.[20]	$
Analgesics, Combination	*butalbital (with ASA, caffeine ± codeine)* Fiorinal, Fiorinal C ¼, C ½	50–100 mg Q4H X 2 doses	Dependence, tolerance.	Additive sedation with other CNS depressants (e.g., alcohol).	Use less than 10 days/month to avoid medication-overuse headache.	$
	codeine (with ASA or acetaminophen ± caffeine) 222s, Tylenol No 1, 2 or 3, generics	15–60 mg Q4H X 2 doses	Dependence, tolerance.	Additive sedation with other CNS depressants (e.g., alcohol); inhibitors of CYP2D6 (e.g., amiodarone, cimetidine, fluoxetine, moclobemide, paroxetine, quinidine) may antagonize codeine's analgesic effect.	See butalbital.	$

(cont'd)

Table 2: **Medications for Symptomatic Treatment of Headache** *(cont'd)*

Class	Drug	Dose (per attack)	Adverse Effects	Drug Interactions	Comments	Cost[a]
Ergot Derivatives	*ergotamine* *(± belladonna alkaloids ± caffeine ± dimenhydrinate ± phenobarbital)* Bellergal Spacetabs, Cafergot, Gravergol	Oral: 2 mg at onset then 1 mg Q1H PRN X 3 doses Rectal: 1 mg at onset; max. 3 mg in 24 h	Chest pain, tingling, nausea, vomiting, paresthesias, cramps, vasoconstriction; ergot dependence producing ergotism.	See Comments.	Use less than 10 days/month to avoid medication-overuse headache; contraindicated in pregnancy, cardiac disorders, hypertension, sepsis, PVD, PUD, renal or liver disease or in patients taking potent inhibitors of CYP3A4 (e.g., cimetidine, clarithromycin, efavirenz, erythromycin, itraconazole, ketoconazole and ritonavir); caution in elderly.	$
	dihydroergotamine (DHE) Migranal	Parenteral: 0.5–1 mg sc, im or iv; may repeat at 1 h; max. 4 doses/24 h (Administration of DHE is preceded by metoclopramide 10 mg iv or prochlorperazine 5 mg iv)[18,19] Deliver iv meds *slowly.* Nasal: 1 spray (0.5 mg) in each nostril; may repeat in 15 min if no effect; max. 2 mg/day	Same as for ergotamine but less frequent and less prolonged; watch for hypotension (rare). Nasal formulation: rhinitis, nausea, taste disturbance.	See ergotamine, Comments.	Not as potent a vasoconstrictor as ergotamine; mainly venoconstrictor; same contraindications as ergotamines; no dependence; good for attacks beginning in emergency room and in treating medication-overuse headaches. Nasal spray: convenient, bypasses GI tract.	Parenteral: $ Nasal: $

Class	Drug	Dose (per attack)	Adverse Effects	Drug Interactions	Comments	Cost[a]
Triptans	*almotriptan* Axert	Oral: 6.25–12.5 mg; may repeat in 2 h; max. 2 doses/24 h	*All triptans:* chest discomfort, fatigue, dizziness, paresthesias, drowsiness, nausea, throat symptoms.	See Comments. *Almotriptan:* inhibitors of CYP3A4 (e.g., cimetidine, clarithromycin, efavirenz, erythromycin, grapefruit juice, itraconazole, ketoconazole and ritonavir) may increase bioavailability of almotriptan.	*All triptans:* do not use if *any* cardiac-like symptoms; contraindicated in ischemic heart disease, sustained hypertension, pregnancy, basilar or hemiplegic migraine, ergotamine-containing products or with MAOIs (except eletriptan and naratriptan); caution with SSRIs; do not use a triptan within 24 h after another triptan; use less than 10 days/month to avoid medication-overuse headache.	$$$
	eletriptan Relpax	Oral: 20–40 mg; if 20 mg taken initially, may take an additional 20 mg-dose in 2 h; max. 40 mg/24 h	See almotriptan.	See almotriptan, Comments. *Eletriptan*: contraindicated within 72 hours of the following inhibitors of CYP3A4: clarithromycin, itraconazole, ketoconazole, nelfinavir and ritonavir, or any potent inhibitor of CYP3A4.	See almotriptan.	$$$
	naratriptan ❸ Amerge	Oral: 1–2.5 mg; may repeat in 4 h; max. 5 mg/24 h	See almotriptan. Naratriptan may be associated with fewer side effects than the other triptans.	See almotriptan, Comments.	See almotriptan.	$$$

(cont'd)

Table 2: **Medications for Symptomatic Treatment of Headache** *(cont'd)*

Class	Drug	Dose (per attack)	Adverse Effects	Drug Interactions	Comments	Cost[a]
	rizatriptan Maxalt, Maxalt RPD	Oral: 5–10 mg; may repeat in 2 h; max. 20 mg/24 h	See almotriptan.	See almotriptan, Comments. *Rizatriptan:* use with caution in patients taking propranolol (↑ bioavailability of rizatriptan).	See almotriptan. *Rizatriptan:* fastmelt wafers can be taken without water.	$$$
	sumatriptan Imitrex, Imitrex DF	Oral: 25–100 mg; may repeat in 2 h; max. 200 mg/24 h Injectable: 6 mg sc; may repeat in 1 h; max. 2 injections/24 h Nasal spray: 5–20 mg intranasally; may repeat in 2 h; max. 40 mg/24 h	See almotriptan. Nasal spray: taste disturbance, nausea.	See almotriptan, Comments.	See almotriptan. *Sumatriptan nasal spray:* faster onset than with oral formulations.	Oral: $$$ SC: $$$$$ Nasal: $$$
	zolmitriptan Zomig, Zomig Rapimelt, Zomig Nasal Spray	Oral: 2.5–5 mg; may repeat in 2 h;max. 10 mg/24 h Nasal Spray: 2.5 or 5 mg; may repeat in 2 h; max. 10 mg/24 h	See almotriptan.	See almotriptan, Comments. Maximum dose of zolmitriptan 5 mg/24 h if also on fluvoxamine or cimetidine.	See almotriptan. *Zolmitriptan:* orally dispersible tablets can be taken without water; nasal spray available as 2.5 or 5 mg per dose.	$$$

[a] Cost per dose; includes drug cost only.

Dosage adjustment may be required in renal impairment; see Appendix I.

Abbreviations: PVD = peripheral vascular disease; PUD = peptic ulcer disease

Legend: $ < $5 $$ $5–10 $$$ $10–20 $$$$ $20–30 $$$$$ > $30

Table 3: **Medications for Prophylactic Treatment of Headache**

Class	Drug	Dose	Adverse Effects	Drug Interactions	Comments	Cost[a]
Beta$_1$-adrenergic Antagonists	*atenolol* Tenormin, generics	50–150 mg per day	Fatigue, impotence, bradycardia and hypotension, GI symptoms, bronchospasm, CHF, depression.	Possible bradycardia with dipyridamole; antacids may decrease absorption.	Contraindicated in asthma, insulin-dependent diabetes, heart block or pregnancy; avoid abrupt withdrawal; consider long-acting formulations. Atenolol and nadolol may have fewer CNS side effects.	$–$$
	metoprolol Lopresor, Betaloc, generics	100–200 mg per day	See atenolol.	See atenolol.	See atenolol.	$
	nadolol generics	20–160 mg per day	See atenolol.	See atenolol.	See atenolol. Nadolol and atenolol may have fewer CNS side effects.	$
	*propranolol*generics	40–240 mg per day	See atenolol.	See atenolol.	See atenolol.	$
Calcium Channel Blockers	*flunarizine* Sibelium, generics	5–10 mg QHS	Weight gain, extrapyramidal effects, drowsiness, depression.		Long latency to onset; many patients have side effects; contraindicated in hypotension, heart failure and arrhythmia; avoid if severe constipation. Do not use flunarizine in depressed patients or those with extrapyramidal disorders.	$–$$

(cont'd)

Table 3: **Medications for Prophylactic Treatment of Headache** *(cont'd)*

Class	Drug	Dose	Adverse Effects	Drug Interactions	Comments	Cost[a]
	verapamil Isoptin SR, generics	240–320 mg per day	Bradycardia, hypotension, constipation.	Inhibits CYP3A4 and may decrease the clearance of CYP3A4 substrates (e.g., lovastatin, sildenafil).	See flunarizine.	$$
Antiepileptic Drugs	*topiramate* Topamax	Start with 25 mg daily, titrate slowly to minimum effective dose (usual maintenance range 50 to 100 mg daily in 2 divided doses)	CNS effects (e.g., dizziness, ataxia, tremor, sedation, cognitive impairment), GI symptoms (e.g., nausea, dyspepsia, constipation), weight loss (can be beneficial in some patients).	Additive depressant effects with other CNS depressants. May ↓ effectiveness of low dose oral contraceptives; use at least 30 µg estrogen. Inhibitors of CYP2C19 may ↑ topiramate levels (e.g., SSRIs, isoniazid, omeprazole, moclobemide). Phenytoin and carbamazepine can ↓ topiramate levels.	May increase risk of nephrolithiasis; maintain adequate hydration during therapy; avoid in patients with renal stones. May cause acute myopia, with consequent angle closure glaucoma that responds to drug discontinuation; advise patients to consult an ophthalmologist or emergency room*immediately* if they have acute painful/red eyes or decreased/blurred vision. Warn patients about CNS depressant effects; possible risk associated with driving, other hazardous activities.	$$
	valproic acid, (valproate) Depakene, generics	500–1500 mg per day	Nausea, alopecia, tremor, weight gain, ↑ hepatic enzymes; neural tube defects can occur if used during pregnancy.	Inhibits CYP2C9 and may ↓ the clearance of substrates (e.g., fluoxetine, fluvastatin, sertraline, verapamil, warfarin); avoid ASA or warfarin; carbamazepine, phenytoin and phenobarbital can significantly ↑ clearance; may ↑ depressant effect of alcohol.	Start with low dosage (250–500 mg/day); do liver function tests prior to initiation of therapy and periodically, especially in the 1st 6 mo of therapy and if symptoms of hepatic dysfunction occur.	$–$$$
	divalproex sodium Epival, generics	500–1500 mg per day	See valproic acid.	See valproic acid.	See valproic acid.	$–$$$

Class	Drug	Dose	Adverse Effects	Drug Interactions	Comments	Cost[a]
Tricyclic Analgesics (TCAs)	*amitriptyline* generics	10–150 mg QHS	All TCAs: weight gain, drowsiness, anticholinergic symptoms (e.g., dry mouth, constipation), lower seizure threshold, confusion.	All TCAs: ↑ sedation with other CNS depressants (e.g., alcohol). *Amitriptyline*: metabolized by many cytochrome P450 enzymes — clearance may be affected by inhibitors (e.g., cimetidine, ciprofloxacin, clarithromycin, diltiazem, erythromycin, fluoxetine, fluvoxamine, isoniazid, itraconazole, ketoconazole, paroxetine, valproic acid), inducers (e.g., phenobarbital, carbamazepine, phenytoin, rifampin, smoking) or other substrates of these enzymes.	All TCAs: dose can be cumulative, adjustments needed; contraindicated if significant cardiac disease, glaucoma, prostate disease or hypotension; start with low dosage in elderly or in patients sensitive to these agents.	$
	doxepin Sinequan, generics	25–100 mg QHS	See amitriptyline.	All TCAs: ↑ sedation with other CNS depressants (e.g., alcohol). *Doxepin*: metabolized by CYP2D6; clearance may be altered by inducers (e.g., carbamazepine, phenobarbital, phenytoin, rifampin), inhibitors (e.g., celecoxib, fluoxetine, imatinib, paroxetine, quinidine) or other substrates of the enzyme.	See amitriptyline.	$
	nortriptyline Aventyl, generics	10–150 mg QHS	See amitriptyline.	All TCAs: ↑ sedation with other CNS depressants (e.g., alcohol). *Nortriptyline*: metabolized by CYP1A2 and CYP2D6. Clearance may be affected by inducers (e.g., carbamazepine, phenobarbital, primidone, phenytoin, rifampin, smoking), inhibitors (e.g., celecoxib, cimetidine, ciprofloxacin, clarithromycin, diltiazem, erythromycin, ethinyl estradiol, fluvoxamine, isoniazid,	See amitriptyline.	$

(cont'd)

Table 3: **Medications for Prophylactic Treatment of Headache** *(cont'd)*

Class	Drug	Dose	Adverse Effects	Drug Interactions	Comments	Cost[a]
				ketoconazole, fluoxetine, imatinib, paroxetine, quinidine) or other substrates of either enzyme.		
Serotonin Antagonists	*pizotifen (pizotyline)* Sandomigran, Sandomigran DS	Start with 0.5 mg QHS, gradually ↑ to TID; if necessary to 3 or 6 mg/day (usual dose: 1–6 mg)	Drowsiness, weight gain.	Additive sedation with other CNS depressants (e.g., alcohol).	Consider QHS dosing at increasingly higher doses.	$–$$$$
	methysergide Sansert	Start with 2 mg QHS, gradually ↑ to TID; if necessary ↑ to 8 mg/day (usual dose: 4–8 mg)	Weight gain; retroperitoneal, cardiac and pulmonary fibrosis associated with long-term use.	Concurrent use with inhibitors of CYP3A4 (e.g., macrolide antibiotics, protease or reverse transcriptase inhibitors, azole antifungals) and vasoconstrictors (e.g., ergot derivatives, triptans) is contraindicated according to the manufacturer's product monograph, although published evidence of clinical interactions is lacking.	*Never* use methysergide for more than 6 mo without a 1 mo drug holiday, and ↓ dosage gradually before discontinuation; methysergide is not a first-line medication; many contraindications to use; review every time medication prescribed.	$–$$$$
Others	*lithium* Carbolith, Lithane, Duralith, generics	300 mg TID	GI upset, tremor, polyuria, hypothyroidism.	ACE inhibitors and angiotensin II receptor blockers ↓ lithium clearance; NSAIDs and thiazide diuretics ↑ lithium serum levels; a potential effect on lithium levels should be considered whenever other drugs are started or discontinued.	Used in chronic cluster headache; contraindicated in renal dysfunction, dehydration, CHF.	$

[a] Cost of 30-day supply; includes drug cost only.

Dosage adjustment may be required in renal impairment; see Appendix I.

Legend: $ < $20 $-$$ < $20–40 $$ $20–40 $-$$$ < $20–60 $$$ $40–60 $-$$$$ < $20– > 60 $$$$ > $60

Suggested Readings

Pryse-Phillips WE, Dodick DW, Edmeads JG et al. Guidelines for the diagnosis and management of migraine in clinical practice. Canadian Headache Society. *CMAJ* 1997;156(9):1273-87.

Pryse-Phillips WE, Dodick DW, Edmeads JG et al. Guidelines for the nonpharmacologic management of migraine in clinical practice. Canadian Headache Society. *CMAJ* 1998;159(1):47-54.

References

1. Purdy RA. Clinical evaluation of a patient presenting with headache. *Med Clin North Am* 2001;85(4):847-63.
2. Pryse-Phillips WE, Dodick DW, Edmeads JG et al. Guidelines for the diagnosis and management of migraine in clinical practice. Canadian Headache Society. *CMAJ* 1997;156(9):1273-87.
3. Pryse-Phillips WE, Dodick DW, Edmeads JG et al. Guidelines for the nonpharmacologic management of migraine in clinical practice. Canadian Headache Society. *CMAJ* 1998;159(1):47-54.
4. Silberstein SD. Practice parameter: evidence-based guidelines for migraine headache (an evidence-based review): report of the Quality Standards Subcommittee of the American Academy of Neurology. *Neurology* 2000;55(6):754-62.
5. Snow V, Weiss K, Wall EM et al. Pharmacologic management of acute attacks of migraine and prevention of migraine headache. *Ann Intern Med* 2002;137(10):840-9.
6. Dodick D, Lipton RB, Martin V et al. Consensus statement: cardiovascular safety profile of triptans (5-HT agonists) in the acute treatment of migraine. *Headache* 2004;44(5):414-25.
7. Ferrari MD, Goadsby PJ, Roon KI et al. Triptans (serotonin, 5-HT1B/1D agonists) in migraine: detailed results and methods of a meta-analysis of 53 trials. *Cephalalgia* 2002;22(8):633-58.
8. Ferrari MD, Roon KI, Lipton RB et al. Oral triptans (serotonin 5-HT(1B/1D) agonists) in acute migraine treatment: a meta-analysis of 53 trials. *Lancet* 2001;358(9294):1668-75.
9. Dodick DW, Silberstein S, Dahlof CG. Is there a preferred triptan? *Headache* 2002;42(1):1-7.
10. Silberstein SD. Divalproex sodium in headache: literature review and clinical guidelines. *Headache* 1996;36(9):547-55.
11. Brandes JL, Saper JR, Diamond M et al. Topiramate for migraine prevention: a randomized controlled trial. *JAMA* 2004;291(8):965-73.
12. Young WB, Hopkins MM, Shechter AL et al. Topiramate: a case series study in migraine prophylaxis. *Cephalalgia* 2002;22(8):659-63.
13. Silberstein SD, Goadsby PJ. Migraine: preventive treatment. *Cephalalgia* 2002;22(7):491-512.
14. Schoenen J, Jacquy J, Lenaerts M. Effectiveness of high-dose riboflavin in migraine prophylaxis. A randomized controlled trial. *Neurology* 1998;50(2):466-70.
15. Bussone G, Leone M, Peccarisi G et al. Double blind comparison of lithium and verapamil in cluster headache prophylaxis. *Headache* 1990;30(7):411-7.
16. Limmroth V, Katsarava Z, Fritsche G et al. Features of medication overuse headache following overuse of different acute headache drugs. *Neurology* 2002;59(7):1011-4.
17. Silberstein SD, Welch KM. Painkiller headache. *Neurology* 2002;59(7):972-4.
18. Raskin NH. Repetitive intravenous dihydroergotamine as therapy for intractable migraine. *Neurology* 1986;36(7):995-7.
19. Raskin NH. Modern pharmacotherapy of migraine. *Neurol Clin* 1990;8(4):857-65.
20. Sances G, Martignoni E, Fioroni L et al. Naproxen sodium in menstrual migraine prophylaxis: a double-blind placebo controlled study. *Headache* 1990;30(11):705-9.

CHAPTER 13
Headache in Children

Sharon Whiting, MBBS, FRCPC

Headaches occur commonly in children and adolescents. They may occur as a primary disorder such as migraine, or accompany systemic disorders or infectious diseases. In Canada, more than 25% of 12- to 13-year-olds experience headache at least weekly.[1] The prevalence of migraine shows an increase with age, i.e., 2.4% in 12- to 14-year-olds and 5% in 15- to 19-year-olds.[2]

Migraine in children is usually associated with at least one of the following: vomiting, photophobia, family history of migraine.

Goals of Therapy

- Make an accurate diagnosis of headache
- Relieve or abort pain and associated symptoms
- Prevent further headaches

Investigations (Figure 1)

- The history is the key to the diagnosis of headache and should be obtained from both parent and child with attention to:
  - specific questions such as where pain began, progress, duration, frequency, relieving and aggravating factors (especially sleep loss, excitement, certain foods, relief with activity) and associated symptoms such as vomiting and photophobia
  - specific neurologic symptoms such as seizures, visual disturbances, difficulty with balance, personality change, weakness
  - analgesic use
  - degree of interference with school and social life, e.g., pedMIDAS questionnaire[3]
  - symptoms suggestive of renal, cardiac, dental or infectious disease
  - mother's pregnancy/labour/delivery, with respect to the child in question
  - child's growth and development, behaviour, academic function

Note: During the interview, observe interaction between parent and child.

- Physical examination:
  - blood pressure, vital signs, palpation of sinuses, examination of teeth, neck stiffness, examination of optic fundi
  - height, weight, head circumference
  - a thorough neurologic examination including cranial nerves, muscle tone, power and reflexes and coordination tests

- Investigations:
  - sinus x-rays if sinusitis suspected
  - CT followed by lumbar puncture with measurement of opening pressure if pseudotumor cerebri suspected based on history of raised intracranial pressure with a negative CT
  - lumbar puncture if infectious process suspected
  - CT and/or MRI if abnormal neurologic examination, decreased visual acuity, recent behaviour change, increasing severity and frequency of headaches, or if headache does not fit a known pattern
- The routine use of any diagnostic study is not indicated when the clinical history has no associated risk factors and the child's examination is normal[4]

Tension-type Headache

Therapeutic Choices

Nonpharmacologic Choices

- Psychological evaluation
- Relaxation therapy
- Biofeedback

Pharmacologic Choices

- Simple analgesics (**acetaminophen**, **ASA**) and **NSAIDs** are effective (Table 1).[5]
- **Amitriptyline** (Table 2) is effective in patients with a component of depression.[6]

Medication-overuse Headache

The occurrence of headache induced by chronic use of analgesics such as acetaminophen and NSAIDs is now recognized in pediatric patients. Treatment involves education and gradual withdrawal of analgesic drugs. Consider use of a prophylactic agent (Table 2).[7]

Migraine

Therapeutic Choices

Nonpharmacologic Choices

After exclusion of mass lesion or other causes:

- Reassure and explain.
- Discuss triggers of migraine, e.g., lack of sleep, too much sleep, excitement, foods, stress, menstruation.

- Encourage sleep at the time of headache and medication early in the course of the headache.
- Biofeedback and relaxation therapy are effective.

Pharmacologic Choices

These can be divided into medication given at the time of the headache (symptomatic) and medication to prevent headache (prophylactic).

Symptomatic Treatments (Table 1)

Analgesics

Intermittent oral analgesics, given as early in the course of the headache as feasible, are the mainstay of pharmacologic management of childhood migraine. **Acetaminophen**, **ibuprofen** and **ASA** are effective at appropriate doses.[8] Two evaluations of the evidence for treatment of migraine in children concluded that ibuprofen and acetaminophen are effective.[9,10]

Combination products, such as ASA, caffeine and butalbital ± codeine (e.g., Fiorinal), play secondary roles should the initial agents fail. These sedating drugs have abuse potential and should be reserved for adolescents (12 to 18 years) for brief periods only. Take care to avoid unnecessary opioids.

Antiemetics

Nausea and vomiting occur in up to 90% of young migraine sufferers and besides being disabling, inhibit oral administration of analgesics. Antiemetics alone (e.g., **chlorpromazine**, **prochlorperazine**, **metoclopramide**) are surprisingly effective in relieving all symptoms including the headache.[11] Chlorpromazine combined with **chloral hydrate** to induce sleep is an effective regimen in childhood migraine.

Ergot Derivatives

Ergotamine compounds have very limited use in pediatrics for the following reasons:

- Auras are uncommon and inconsistent; therefore, warning indicators that trigger the time to treat with ergot are often unreliable.
- Ergots can exacerbate gastrointestinal upset.
- Ergots are contraindicated in complicated migraine syndromes because of the risk of increasing vasospasm.

Oral dihydroergotamine showed no significant difference in headache improvement in a study comparing it with placebo.[12] In severe intractable headache, dihydroergotamine can be used iv in combination with an antiemetic in the emergency department.[13]

Triptans

Of the six agents available in Canada (**almotriptan**, **eletriptan**, **naratriptan**, **rizatriptan**, **sumatriptan** and **zolmitriptan**), none are specifically approved for use in children, though several studies have demonstrated an excellent safety profile in children age 12 to 18 years.[14] Consider triptans for use in adolescents with moderate to severe headaches unresponsive to conventional analgesics.[15] Nasal sumatriptan is effective and should be considered for acute treatment in adolescents 12 years and older.[9,10,14] Unpleasant taste is a common side effect.

Prophylactic Agents (Table 2)

In a practice parameter on the pharmacologic treatment of childhood migraine, the evidence for efficacy was examined for several medications.[9] Although many are in current use and may be effective, only **flunarizine** was deemed probably effective based on evidence. Flunarizine has been shown to significantly reduce headache frequency and severity in children.[16,17]

Although evidence of its efficacy is lacking, **pizotifen** (pizotyline) may be helpful and is less potent than **methysergide**, which is *not* used in pediatric headache because of potentially serious long-term side effects.

Evidence for **propranolol** is conflicting, although it is commonly used and is effective in some cases.[18] Propranolol is contraindicated in reactive airway disease, diabetes mellitus and bradyarrhythmias. Symptoms of depression are an under-reported but common side effect in adolescents.

Despite a lack of evidence of efficacy, **cyproheptadine,** an antihistamine with antiserotonergic and calcium channel blocking properties, is widely used as a prophylactic agent. Its use in older children and adolescents is limited by sedative properties and increased appetite/weight gain.

Amitriptyline has shown efficacy in adults; studies in children are limited.[19]

NSAIDs reduce headache frequency and severity in adults, presumably through prostaglandin inhibition. Although evidence of efficacy in children is lacking, **naproxen sodium** can be tried in adolescents as prophylaxis (see Therapeutic Tips).

Valproic acid has been studied in children;[20] however, there is insufficient evidence to recommend its use.[9] Phenobarbital and phenytoin are no longer used.

Therapeutic Tips

- There are very few controlled trials of pharmacologic management of childhood migraine; hence, anecdotal experience prevails. Most young patients with migraine do not require daily medication but need access to reliable analgesia at home and at school.

- Children are debilitated by nausea and vomiting and benefit greatly from antiemetics. Rest and sleep are usually very helpful.
- Consider prophylactic agents for children who cycle through periods of time when they experience such frequency of headache that their lifestyle is disrupted, or when isolated or infrequent events are severe and complex.
- Calendars/diaries are helpful in identifying triggers, headache patterns, frequency and severity and are invaluable for management and evaluation of response to therapy.
- For *prophylaxis*, consider medications with the fewest side effects first. Cyproheptadine is usually used in younger children. For adolescents, consider using propranolol, amitriptyline, naproxen sodium or flunarizine.
- The prognosis for children with migraine is favourable with 50% of patients reporting improvement within six months after medical intervention, regardless of treatment methods used.
- Most children respond to reassurance, general advice and simple remedies for attacks when they occur.

Figure 1: **Investigations Based on Headache Profile**

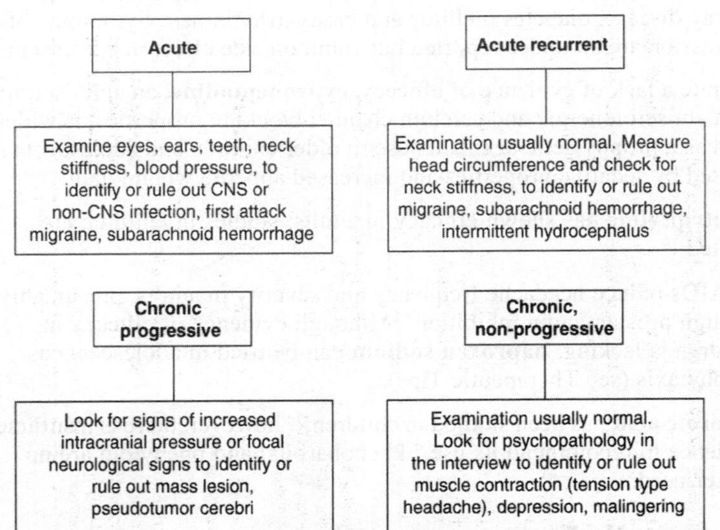

Table 1: **Treatment of Headache in Children**

Class	Drug	Dose[a]	Adverse Effects	Drug Interactions	Comments	Cost[b]
Analgesics	*acetaminophen* Atasol Preparations, Tempra, Tylenol, generics	10–15 mg/kg/dose Q4H	GI upset; liver toxicity in overdose.	Enhanced anticoagulant effect of warfarin with regular use of > 2 g/day; heavy alcohol use can increase risk of liver toxicity.	Analgesics are the most commonly used medications at time of headache.	$
	ASA Aspirin, Bufferin, Coated Aspirin, generics	Age ≥ 12 y: single dose of 500–650 mg per headache	GI upset.	Warfarin: ↑ anticoagulant effect.	Because of the concern of Reye's syndrome, ASA should *not* be used in the context of fever or a viral illness; should not be used more frequently than Q4–6H.	$
	ibuprofen Advil, Motrin Children's, Motrin IB, generics	5–10 mg/kg/dose, up to 4 times daily	GI upset.	See ASA.		$
	naproxen sodium Anaprox, generics	Age > 2 y: 5–7 mg/kg/dose Q8–12H	GI upset.	See ASA.		$
Analgesics, combination	*butalbital + ASA + caffeine ± codeine* Fiorinal, Fiorinal C1/4, C1/2 , generics	1–2 tablets 4 times daily	GI upset; dependence and tolerance to barbiturates and opioids.	Possible additive sedation with other CNS depressants, e.g., alcohol.	Reserved for adolescents; no more than 2 days/wk; risk of tolerance, addiction and misuse.	$

(cont'd)

Table 1: **Treatment of Headache in Children** *(cont'd)*

Class	Drug	Dose[a]	Adverse Effects	Drug Interactions	Comments	Cost[b]
Antiemetics	*chlorpromazine* generics	Oral/IM: 1 mg/kg to a maximum of 25 mg Q8H IV: 0.1 mg/kg Q10–15 min to a max of 30 mg	Hypotension.	Possible additive sedation with other CNS depressants, e.g., alcohol.	Can be used with chloral hydrate 25–50 mg/kg po Q8H. Can cause hypotension when given iv; use in the emergency department.	$
	prochlorperazine Stemetil, generics	Oral: 2.5–5 mg twice daily IV: 10 mg	Extrapyramidal dysfunction.	Possible additive sedation with other CNS depressants, e.g., alcohol.	Use iv in adolescents in the emergency department.	$
	metoclopramide generics	Oral: 0.1– 0.2 mg/kg (≤ 10 mg) IV: 10 mg	Extrapyramidal dysfunction.	Possible enhanced sedative effect of alcohol.	Use iv in adolescents in the emergency department.	$
Ergot Derivatives	*dihydroergotamine (DHE)* Migranal	Parenteral: 0.1–0.25 mg/dose iv. May be repeated Q20 min × 3. Give metoclopramide 0.2 mg/kg/dose (max 20 mg) 30 min prior to iv DHE. Nasal spray: 1 spray into each nostril. May repeat in 15 min	Parenteral: Flushed feeling, tingling in extremities, nausea and vomiting. Nasal Spray: Nausea, taste disturbance, rhinitis.	Do not use with potent inhibitors of CYP3A4 such as cimetidine, clarithromycin, efavirenz, erythromycin, itraconazole, ketoconazole and ritonavir.	Parenteral: useful in patients with severe and prolonged migraine headache; protocol to take place in hospital; contraindicated in complicated migraine, coronary heart disease, abnormal blood pressure, abnormal ECG.	$
Triptans	*almotriptan* Axert	Oral: 6.25 mg at start of headache; if headache returns, dose may be repeated after 2 h; no more	Chest discomfort, fatigue, dizziness, paresthesias, drowsiness,	Do not use with ergotamine-containing products. Caution with SSRIs. Do not use a triptan within 24 h after another triptan. Do not use with MAOIs.	Consider for adolescents 12–18 years unresponsive to conventional analgesics; do not use if *any* cardiac-like symptoms; contraindicated in	$$$$

Class	Drug	Dose[a]	Adverse Effects	Drug Interactions	Comments	Cost[b]
		than 2 doses in a 24-h period	nausea, throat symptoms.	Inhibitors of CYP3A4 (e.g., cimetidine, clarithromycin, efavirenz, erythromycin, grapefruit juice, itraconazole, ketoconazole and ritonavir) may increase bioavailability of almotriptan.	ischemic heart disease, sustained hypertension, pregnancy, basilar or hemiplegic migraine; use less than 10 days/month to avoid medication-overuse headache.	
	eletriptan Relpax	Oral: 20–40 mg as soon after headache onset as possible; if initial dose is 20 mg and headache returns after ≥ 2 hours, may repeat 20 mg dose; max 40 mg in a 24-h period	See almotriptan.	Do not use with ergotamine-containing products. Caution with SSRIs. Do not use a triptan within 24 h after another triptan. Contraindicated within 72 hours of the following inhibitors of CYP3A4: clarithromycin, itraconazole, ketoconazole, nelfinavir and ritonavir, or any potent inhibitor of CYP3A4.	See almotriptan.	$$$$
	naratriptan Amerge	Oral: 1 mg at start of headache; if partial response or headache returns, dose may be repeated once after 4 hours; max dose of 5 mg in a 24-h period	See almotriptan. Naratriptan may be associated with fewer side effects than the other triptans.	Do not use with ergotamine-containing products. Caution with SSRIs. Do not use a triptan within 24 h after another triptan.	See almotriptan.	$$$$
	rizatriptan Maxalt, Maxalt RPD	Oral: 5–10 mg (tablet or wafer) at start of headache. Do not repeat if no relief from 1st dose; if headache returns 2 h	See almotriptan.	Do not use with ergotamine-containing products. Caution with SSRIs. Do not use a triptan within 24 h after another triptan. Do not use with MAOIs. Use with caution	See almotriptan. Fastmelt wafers can be taken without water.	$$$$

(cont'd)

Table 1: **Treatment of Headache in Children** *(cont'd)*

Class	Drug	Dose[a]	Adverse Effects	Drug Interactions	Comments	Cost[b]
		or more after partial or complete relief from an initial 5 mg dose, may repeat 5 mg dose (daily max 10 mg)		in patients taking propranolol (↑ bioavailability of rizatriptan).		
	sumatriptan Imitrex Nasal Spray, Imitrex DF, generics	25 mg tablet or 20 mg nasal spray at start of headache. Do not repeat if no relief from 1st dose; if headache returns 2 h or more after 1st dose, may repeat dose (daily max 2 doses)	See almotriptan. Nasal spray may cause taste disturbance.	Do not use with ergotamine-containing products. Caution with SSRIs. Do not use a triptan within 24 h after another triptan. Do not use with MAOIs.	See almotriptan. Faster onset with nasal spray than with oral formulations.	$$$
	zolmitriptan Zomig, Zomig Rapimelt, Zomig Nasal Spray	2.5–5 mg (tablet, orally dispersible tablet or nasal spray) at start of headache. Do not repeat if no relief from 1st dose; if headache returns 2 h or more after 1st dose, may repeat dose (daily max 2 doses)	See almotriptan. Nasal spray may cause taste disturbance.	Do not use with ergotamine-containing products. Caution with SSRIs. Do not use a triptan within 24 h after another triptan. Do not use with MAOIs. Maximum dose of 5 mg/24 h if also taking fluvoxamine or cimetidine.	See almotriptan. Zolmitriptan orally dispersible tablets can be taken without water.	$$$$

[a] Not to exceed maximum adult dose.
[b] Cost per dose, based on 20 kg body weight; includes drug cost only.
Dosage adjustment may be required in renal impairment; see Appendix I.
Legend: $ < $1 $$ $1–5 $$$ $5–10 $$$$ > $10

Table 2: **Prophylaxis of Headache in Children**

Class	Drug[a]	Dose	Adverse Effects	Drug Interactions	Comments	Cost[b]
$Beta_1$-adrenergic Antagonists	*propranolol* generics	Oral: 0.6–1.5 mg/kg/day in divided doses	Fatigue, bradycardia, hypotension, depression.	Antacids may decrease absorption.	Contraindicated in asthma, diabetes, heart block, bradyarrhythmias, pregnancy; avoid abrupt withdrawal.	$
Calcium Channel Blockers	*flunarizine* Sibelium, generics	Oral: 5 mg/day	Bradycardia, hypotension, depression, drowsiness.	Additive sedation with other CNS depressants.	May take several weeks to be effective; do not use in depressed patients or those with extrapyramidal disorders.	$
Antihistamines	*cyproheptadine* generics	Age 2–6 y: 2 mg Q8–12H (max. 12 mg/day) Age 7–14 y: 4 mg Q8–12H (max 16 mg/day)	Drowsiness, weight gain.	Possible additive sedation with other CNS depressants, e.g., alcohol.		$-$$
NSAIDs	*naproxen sodium* Anaprox, generics	275–550 mg twice daily	GI upset.	Warfarin: ↑ anticoagulant effect. Antihypertensives (diuretics, beta-blockers, ACE inhibitors, alpha-blockers): possible reduction in hypertensive effect; may require additional antihypertensive therapy. Lithium may interfere with sodium/water balance. Monitor lithium levels when NSAID added.	Use in adolescents.	$$

(cont'd)

Table 2: **Prophylaxis of Headache in Children** *(cont'd)*

Class	Drug[a]	Dose	Adverse Effects	Drug Interactions	Comments	Cost[b]
Tricyclic Analgesics (TCAs)	*amitriptyline* generics	10–150 mg/day	Weight gain, drowsiness; anticholinergic symptoms such as dry mouth and constipation.	Possible additive sedation with other CNS depressants, e.g., alcohol; metabolized by cytochrome P450 enzyme system—clearance may be affected by inhibitors (e.g., erythromycin, fluoxetine, fluvoxamine, isoniazid, itraconazole, ketoconazole, paroxetine, valproic acid), inducers (e.g., phenobarbital, carbamazepine, phenytoin, rifampin) or other substrates of these enzymes.	Contraindicated in significant cardiac disease or hypotension.	$
Serotonin Antagonists	*pizotifen* Sandomigran	Oral: 0.5–1.5 mg/day in divided doses	Sedation and weight gain.	Possible additive sedation with other CNS depressants including alcohol.	Start medication slowly and increase over 1–3 wk.	$-$$

[a] Not to exceed maximum adult dose.
[b] Cost of 30-day supply based on 20 kg body weight; includes drug cost only.
Dosage adjustment may be required in renal impairment; see Appendix I.
Legend: $ < $20 $-$$ < $20–40 $$ $20–40

Suggested Readings

Friedman G. Advances in paediatric migraine. *Paediatr Child Health* 2002;7(4):239-43.

Guidetti V, Galli F. Recent development in paediatric headache. *Curr Opin Neurol* 2001;14(3):335-40.

Lewis DW. Headaches in children and adolescents. *Am Fam Physician* 2002;65(4):625-32.

Lewis DW. Toward the definition of childhood migraine. *Curr Opin Pediatr* 2004;16(6):628-36.

References

1. Dooley JM, Gordon KE, Wood EP. Frequent headaches in Canadian adolescents: prevalence and associated features. *Eur J Pediatr Neurol* 2003;7:357-8.
2. Gordon KE, Dooley JM, Wood EP. Prevalence of reported migraine headaches in Canadian adolescents. *Can J Neurol Sci* 2004;31(3):324-7.
3. Hershey AD, Powers SW, Vockell AL et al. PedMIDAS: development of a questionnaire to assess disability of migraines in children. *Neurology* 2001;57(11):2034-9.
4. Lewis DW, Ashwal S, Dahl G et al. Practice parameter: evaluation of children and adolescents with recurrent headaches: report of the Quality Standards Subcommittee of the American Academy of Neurology and the Practice Committee of the Child Neurology Society. *Neurology* 2002;59(4):490-8.
5. Steiner TJ, Lange R, Voelker M. Aspirin in episodic tension-type headache: placebo-controlled dose-ranging comparison with paracetamol. *Cephalalgia* 2003;23(1):59-66.
6. Hershey AD, Powers SW, Bentti AL et al. Effectiveness of amitriptyline in the prophylactic management of childhood headaches. *Headache* 2000;40(7):539-49.
7. Mathew NT, Kurman R, Perez F. Drug induced refractory headache--clinical features and management. *Headache* 1990;30(10):634-8.
8. Hamalainen ML, Hoppu K, Valkeila E et al. Ibuprofen or acetaminophen for the acute treatment of migraine in children: a double-blind, randomized, placebo-controlled, crossover study. *Neurology* 1997;48(1):103-7.
9. Lewis D, Ashwal S, Hershey A et al. Practice parameter: pharmacological treatment of migraine headache in children and adolescents: report of the American Academy of Neurology Quality Standards Subcommittee and the Practice Committee of the Child Neurology Society. *Neurology* 2004;63(12):2215-24.
10. Damen L, Bruijn JK, Verhagen AP et al. Symptomatic treatment of migraine in children: a systematic review of medication trials. *Pediatrics* 2005;116(2):e295-302.
11. Iserson KV. Parenteral chlorpromazine treatment of migraine. *Ann Emerg Med* 1983;12(12):756-8.
12. Hamalainen ML, Hoppu K, Santavuori PR. Oral dihydroergotamine for therapy-resistant migraine attacks in children. *Pediatr Neurol* 1997;16(2):114-7.
13. Linder SL. Treatment of childhood headache with dihydroergotamine mesylate. *Headache* 1994;34(10):578-80.
14. Ahonen K, Hamalainen ML, Rantala H. Nasal sumatriptan is effective in treatment of migraine attacks in children: a randomized trial. *Neurology* 2004;62(6):883-7.
15. Friedman G. Advances in paediatric migraine. *Paediatr Child Health* 2002;7(4):239-43.
16. Sorge F, De Simone R, Marano E et al. Flunarizine in prophylaxis of childhood migraine. A double-blind, placebo-controlled, crossover study. *Cephalalgia* 1988;8(1):1-6.
17. Martinez-Lage JM. Flunarizine (Sibelium) in the prophylaxis of migraine. An open, long-term, multicenter trial. *Cephalalgia* 1988;8(Suppl 8):15-20.
18. Ludvigsson J. Propranolol used in prophylaxis of migraine in children. *Acta Neurol Scand* 1974;50(1):109-15.
19. Hershey AD, Powers SW, Bentti AL et al. Effectiveness of amitriptyline in the prophylactic management of childhood headaches. *Headache* 2000;40(7):539-49.
20. Caruso JM, Brown WD, Exil G et al. The efficacy of divalproex sodium in the prophylactic treatment of children with migraine. *Headache* 2000;40(8):672-6.

CHAPTER 14
Acute Pain

Benoit Bailey, MD, MSc, FRCPC

Pain is one of the commonest symptoms. It needs to be recognized, assessed for cause and treated appropriately as soon as possible. The absence of treatment can lead to physiological and psychological adverse effects. Treatment should be tailored to the level of pain; an analgesic that is effective in one patient may not necessarily be helpful in another with the same type of pain. The absence of a diagnosis should not delay measures to relieve pain.

Goals of Therapy

- Recognize that the patient is experiencing pain
- Relieve the pain until the cause is treated
- Identify and treat the cause of pain

Investigations

- Observe the patient for behavioural signs of pain, e.g., agitation, anxiety, crying, gritting of teeth, withdrawal from activities
- Solicit self-reports of the pain
- Inquire about the medical history and perform a physical examination to determine the cause and severity of the pain
- Inquire about medication self-treatment history and possible allergy or adverse reactions to analgesics
- Use laboratory investigations as appropriate to determine the cause of the pain
- Use a *pain scale* to measure and assess pain

Note: The use of a pain scale is increasingly encouraged; this can help reduce oligoanalgesia (undertreatment of pain).[1] The results of this assessment should be recorded as for a vital sign. The visual analog scale (a 100 mm horizontal line anchored by "no pain" at 0 mm and "worst pain imaginable" at 100 mm) is the pain scale used most. It is validated in adults and in children ≥ 5–6 years. Other pain scales such as the standardized colour analog scale or the Wong-Baker Faces Pain Rating Scale can be used in children as young as 4–5 years or 3–6 years, respectively.[2,3]

Therapeutic Choices (Figure 1)
Nonpharmacologic Choices

Patients presenting with acute pain should be quickly and calmly assessed with empathy and reassurance. Encourage patients to verbalize their pain at all stages of treatment. Initiate measures to decrease pain immediately (e.g., immobilize a fracture, apply dressings to burns, employ cold or heat or other techniques such as relaxation, imagery and distraction) until pharmacologic treatment is started. Do not wait until a full assessment is made to start pharmacologic treatment.

Pharmacologic Choices (Table 2)

Oral Analgesics

For mild to moderate pain, the first step should be the use of a nonopioid analgesic alone or in combination with a weak opioid. If the pain is still present or worsening, use a weak opioid alone or in combination with a nonopioid analgesic. Alternatively, an NSAID can be tried. If necessary, the next step is to use a stronger opioid alone or with a nonopioid analgesic. For severe pain, starting with a strong opioid is usually more appropriate (Figure 1).

Nonopioid Analgesics

Acetaminophen can be used for mild to moderate pain. Its advantages include having analgesic and antipyretic onset and efficacy equal to ASA and fewer adverse reactions and drug interactions than NSAIDs.[4] However, it has no anti-inflammatory action. It can be used with opioids for additive analgesic effect.[5,6]

Nonsteroidal anti-inflammatory drugs (NSAIDs) are a heterogeneous group of medications with analgesic, antipyretic and anti-inflammatory action that can be used for mild to moderate pain. Nonselective NSAIDs are divided into five classes: salicylates, fenamates, propionic acid derivatives, oxicams and acetic acid derivatives (see Chapter 71). COX-2 selective NSAIDs should not be used at this time for treatment of acute pain until their adverse effects in the acute pain setting, although unlikely, are well defined.

Adverse effects associated with single (or few) doses of nonselective NSAIDs are limited and are qualitatively similar to those of ASA. Chronic use is associated with GI effects (ulceration, bleeding and perforation) and renal failure. ASA, unlike other NSAIDs, irreversibly inhibits platelet function for the lifetime of the platelet (8 to 10 days) even after a single therapeutic dose. In contrast, platelet function returns to normal when other NSAIDs have been eliminated from the body (approximately 24 hours for most NSAIDs). NSAIDs can precipitate asthma in ASA-sensitive patients.

Avoid NSAIDs in patients with a history of peptic ulcer disease, renal failure, congestive heart failure or asthma.

Choosing an NSAID is difficult. Some patients respond well to a certain class but not to others. Also, it appears that full single doses of most NSAIDs are more effective analgesics than full doses of ASA or acetaminophen.[4,6,7] Cost can be an important factor.

ASA can be given with opioids for additive analgesic effect.[7] It should be avoided in children, particularly those less than 16 years of age with chickenpox or flu-like symptoms, because of possible association with Reye's syndrome. It can also precipitate asthma in ASA-sensitive patients.

Ibuprofen 200 mg is equivalent to 650 mg ASA or acetaminophen in terms of analgesia; a dose of 400 mg is superior and longer acting, and provides comparable analgesia to the combination of acetaminophen/codeine.[4,6] A 10 mg/kg dose of ibuprofen is as safe as a 15 mg/kg dose of acetaminophen, although GI bleeding has been reported with ibuprofen.[8]

Naproxen 250 mg is equivalent to a dose of 650 mg of ASA; a dose of 500 mg is superior. At either dose, naproxen has a longer duration of action than ASA.[4]

Opioids

Opioids can be used orally for the treatment of moderate to severe pain. However, for severe pain the parenteral route is preferred because of its faster onset of action. Opioids may be substituted using equipotent doses. However, the adverse effects of codeine and meperidine can limit this process. Caution should always be used when switching among opioids, to minimize any adverse events, particularly when substituting to the highly potent hydromorphone. Adverse effects include constipation (codeine may be the worst offender), nausea, sedation, respiratory depression and (if used for long period of time) tolerance, dependence and withdrawal symptoms.

Codeine is frequently given concomitantly with acetaminophen or ASA for additive analgesic effect without increasing the adverse effects.[4,5] Approximately 6 to 10% of the general population does not possess sufficient CYP2D6 to transform codeine to morphine, and experiences no analgesic response to codeine. Increasing the dose is not effective. Drugs that inhibit CYP2D6 can also decrease the analgesic effect of codeine. The use of codeine, particularly in the elderly, should be accompanied by stool softeners and/or bulk-forming laxatives.

Morphine is available in several immediate-release dosage forms and in sustained-release preparations. However, sustained-release preparations should rarely be given for the treatment of acute pain. Because of fewer adverse effects compared to codeine, morphine can be titrated to achieve pain-free status.

Tramadol is a unique analgesic structurally related to morphine and codeine that acts through opioid and nonopioid mechanisms.[9] Although it appears to have less abuse potential and minimal effect on respiratory function, tramadol causes more nausea compared to other opioids and may not be as effective unless combined with another analgesic such as acetaminophen.[9,10] Tramadol should not be used as a first-line analgesic.

Parenteral Analgesics

The intravenous route of administration is preferred to subcutaneous and intramuscular use because it is pain free and onset of action is predictable.

NSAIDs

Ketorolac is an NSAID that can be given im or iv for the treatment of moderate to severe pain. A dose of 30 mg is comparable to approximately 12 mg of morphine.[4] Ketorolac has the same adverse effect profile as the oral nonselective NSAIDs. The pharmacologic effect cannot be titrated but the drug can be used when opioids are contraindicated. Ketorolac is effective for the treatment of pain associated with renal colic.

Opioids

Morphine is the standard to which other opioids are compared. Its advantages over meperidine include longer duration of action, and metabolism not affected by liver and renal disease. It can be administered as continuous infusion or as patient-controlled analgesia (PCA), a pump programmed to deliver a preset amount of drug by continuous infusion or repeated boluses, as well as smaller bolus doses for breakthrough pain.

Avoid using **meperidine** in patients with renal failure because an active metabolite (normeperidine) will accumulate and cause seizures in some patients. This same metabolite causes the adverse CNS effects of meperidine (tremors, hyperreflexia, hallucinations). Meperidine should also be avoided in patients with liver disease and those who have received MAOIs in the past 14 days. Usually, meperidine should not be given for pain that is expected to last more than three hours, where morphine is a better choice. In some hospitals, meperidine has been removed from the formulary because of all these concerns.

Fentanyl is a synthetic opioid which has a duration of action of only 30 to 60 minutes, making it an ideal analgesic for brief procedures but limiting its usefulness for managing acute pain. This can be overcome by giving fentanyl by infusion, but this offers no advantage over morphine and is much more costly. Fentanyl has almost no hemodynamic effects and does not induce histamine release, unlike morphine and meperidine. Rapid iv administration can lead to chest wall rigidity that could interfere with ventilation.

Topical and Local Anesthesia

Infiltrative techniques using **lidocaine** are the most frequently used for minor procedures. A dose of 3 to 5 mg/kg (maximum 300 mg) can be used for direct infiltration or regional nerve block. Coadministration of **epinephrine** allows an increase of lidocaine dose to 5 to 7 mg/kg, unless epinephrine is contraindicated (e.g., if tissue vascularity is poor or if distal vasculature is involved). If allergy to amide type local anesthetics (e.g., lidocaine, bupivacaine) is suspected, an ester (e.g., procaine, tetracaine, benzocaine) can be used because of the absence of cross-reactivity.

For small facial lacerations, a mixture of **tetracaine** 0.5 to 1%, **epinephrine** (adrenaline) 0.25 to 0.5% and **cocaine** 1 to 4% (**TAC**) can be applied topically (3 mL—maximum cocaine 6 mg/kg). The restricted status of cocaine limits its usefulness. A mixture of lidocaine 0.4%, epinephrine 0.1% and tetracaine 0.05% (**LET**), in a dose of 2 mL topically, is as effective as TAC.

Topical anesthetics such as eutectic mixture of local anesthetics (**EMLA**), **amethocaine** (tetracaine; Ametop) or **liposomal lidocaine** (Maxilene) can be used to reduce pain associated with minor procedures such as needle insertion on intact skin. EMLA, containing **prilocaine** and **lidocaine**, causes vasoconstriction potentially making cannulation difficult. To be effective, a large amount should be applied for at least 45–60 minutes with an occlusive dressing.

Amethocaine is superior to EMLA in preventing pain associated with needle insertion in children.[11] It requires a shorter application time than EMLA (30 minutes). Amethocaine causes vasodilation and may induce hypersensitivity with repeated use. Liposomal lidocaine is as effective as EMLA in decreasing pain associated with venipuncture or intravenous cannulation. It has minimal vasoactive properties and requires an application time of 30 minutes. An occlusive dressing is not required but it is recommended in young children.

Inhalation Pain Management

Nitrous oxide (N_20) at a concentration of 30 to 50% can be used as an analgesic. Advantages include rapid onset and short duration of action. Contraindications include altered level of consciousness, severe maxillofacial injuries, chronic obstructive pulmonary disease, acute pulmonary edema, pneumothorax, shock, decompression sickness, bowel obstruction and major chest injury. It can produce lightheadedness, drowsiness, nausea, vomiting and excitement.

Therapeutic Tips

- Choose the medication and route of administration according to the severity of the pain, the desired onset and duration of action.
- Consider sedatives as well, particularly for procedures, but their use should not replace analgesics.
- For the elderly, choose the right analgesic, considering hepatic and renal function as well as concurrent medications.
- Always wait the appropriate amount of time, according to the onset of action of the analgesic, to perform a procedure or to assess whether an analgesic was effective.
- Monitor the level of consciousness and presence of adverse effects after administration of an analgesic.
- Reassess the need for analgesics frequently, using a pain scale.

- Avoid the use of opioids on an as-needed basis. A regular schedule of administration is more effective.
- Consult specialized acute pain services as needed.
- In case overdosage occurs, keep **naloxone** (Table 1) on hand when administering opioids parenterally. Overdosage will not occur as long as the patient has pain.

Table 1: **Treatment of Opioid-induced Respiratory Depression**

Class	Drug	Dose
Opioid Antagonist	*naloxone* Naloxone Hydrochloride Injection USP	Adults and children > 5 y or > 20 kg weight: 0.4 to 2 mg iv Q2–3 min, depending on response Children birth–5 y or 20 kg weight: 0.1 mg/kg Q2–3 min, depending on response Maximum dose: 10 mg. **Note:** May need to repeat in 1 to 2 h, depending on half-life of opioid. Continuous infusion may be used for overdoses of long-acting opiates. Starting dose is 2/3 of the initial dose that was effective for the patient, administered per hour by infusion *or* 0.4–0.8 mg/h in adults and 0.05–0.15 mg/kg/h in children. Titrate to effect.

Figure 1: Management of Acute Pain

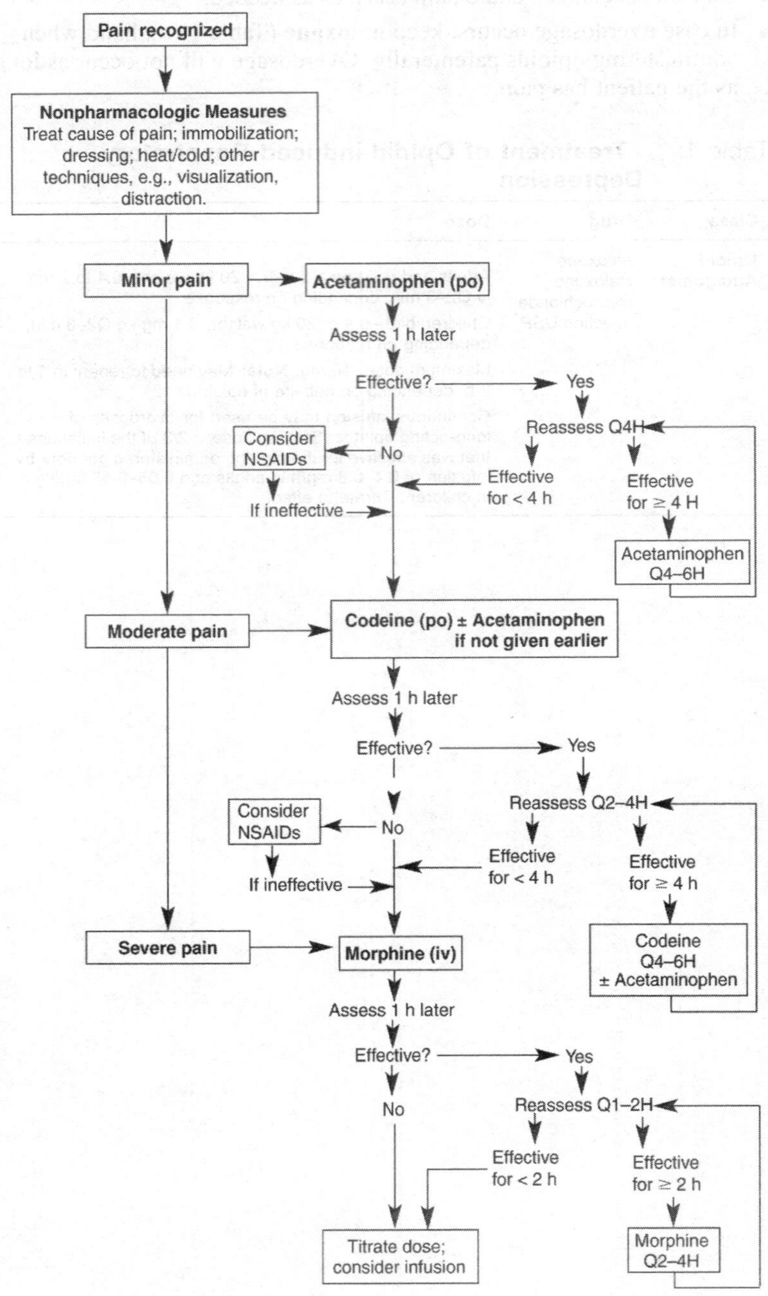

Table 2: **Analgesics for the Treatment of Acute Pain**

Class	Drug	Dose	Adverse Effects	Drug Interactions	Cost[a]
Analgesics, nonopioid	*acetaminophen* Atasol Preparations, Tempra, Tylenol, generics	Children: 10–15 mg/kg/dose po Q4H; oral suspension available 15–20 mg/kg/dose pr Q4H Max: 5 doses/day Adults: 325–650 mg po or pr Q4H Max: 4 g/day	Hepatotoxicity in overdose or supratherapeutic dosing.	Enhanced anticoagulant effect of warfarin with regular use of > 2 g/day of acetaminophen.	$–$$
	ASA Aspirin, Bufferin, Coated Aspirin, generics	Children: 10–15 mg/kg/dose po Q4H Max: 5 doses/day Adults: 325–650 mg po Q4H Max: 4 g/day	GI upset.	Warfarin: ↑ anticoagulant effect. Antihypertensives (diuretics, beta-blockers, ACE inhibitors, alpha-blockers): possible reduction in hypertensive effect; may require additional antihypertensive therapy. Lithium may interfere with sodium/water balance. Monitor lithium levels when NSAID added. ↑ risk of GI bleeding with SSRIs.	$
	ibuprofen Advil, Motrin IB, Motrin (Children's), generics	Children: 10 mg/kg/dose po Q6–8H; oral suspension available Max: 40 mg/kg/day, not to exceed adult dose Adults: 200–400 mg po Q6–8H Max: 1.2 g/day	GI upset.	See ASA.	$

(cont'd)

Table 2: **Analgesics for the Treatment of Acute Pain** *(cont'd)*

Class	Drug	Dose	Adverse Effects	Drug Interactions	Cost[a]
	ketorolac Toradol, generics	Children: 0.2–1 mg/kg/dose im or iv Q4–6H Max: 30 mg/dose Adults: 10–30 mg im or iv Q4–6H Max: 120 mg/day	GI upset.	See ASA.	$$$-$$$$
	naproxen Naprosyn, generics	Children: 5–7 mg/kg/dose po Q8–12H; oral suspension available Max: 1000 mg/day Adults: 500 mg initially, then 250 mg po Q6–8H Max: 1250 mg/day	GI upset.	See ASA.	$
Analgesics, opioid	*morphine* M.O.S., MS-IR, generics	Titrate to effect. **Immediate-release oral:** Children: 0.2–0.5 mg/kg/dose po Q4–6H Adults: 10–30 mg po Q4–6H **Intravenous:** Children: Intermittent: 0.1–0.2 mg/kg/dose Q2–4H Continuous infusion: 0.01–0.05 mg/kg/h Breakthrough pain during infusion: 0.01–0.05 mg/kg/dose Adults: Intermittent: 2.5–10 mg iv Q2–4H Continuous infusion: 1–10 mg/h Breakthrough pain during infusion: 2.5–5 mg/dose	*All opioids:* sedation, constipation.	*All opioids:* additive sedation with other CNS depressants, e.g., alcohol; potential enhancement of opioid effects with lidocaine.	$–$$

Class	Drug	Dose	Adverse Effects	Drug Interactions	Cost[a]
	codeine generics	Children: 0.5–1 mg/kg/dose po Q4–6H; oral liquid formulation available Max: 60 mg/dose Adults: 15–60 mg po Q4–6H Max: 60 mg/dose	See morphine.	See morphine. *Codeine:* ↓ analgesic effect with somatostatin, rifampin. Inhibitors of CYP2D6 (e.g., celecoxib, cimetidine, desipramine, fluoxetine, imatinib, paroxetine, quinidine) may antagonize codeine's analgesic effect.	$
	meperidine (pethidine) Demerol Injectable, generics	Children: 1–1.5 mg/kg/dose iv Q3–4H Max: 100 mg/dose Adults: 50–100 mg iv Q3–4H Max: 100 mg/dose	See morphine. Seizures can occur when used in renal failure. May cause tremors, hyperreflexia, hallucinations. Avoid in liver disease and those who have received MAOIs within the last 14 days.	See morphine. *Meperidine:* potentially life-threatening serotonin syndrome with nonselective MAOIs.	$-$$
	fentanyl generics	Children: 0.5–3 μg/kg/dose iv Q1–2H Adults: 50–100 μg iv Q1–2H Titrate to effect	See morphine.	See morphine. *Fentanyl*: inhibitors of CYP3A4 (e.g., cimetidine, efavirenz, erythromycin, itraconazole, ketoconazole, ritonavir) may potentiate fentanyl's opioid effects.	$$-$$$

[a] Cost per dose (based on body weights of 20 kg for children and 70 kg for adults); includes drug cost only.

Dosage adjustment may be required in renal impairment; see Appendix I.

Legend: $ < $0.50 $–$$ < $0.50–1.00 $$ $0.50–1.00 $$-$$$ $0.50–2.00 $$$ $1.00–2.00 $$$-$$$$ $1.00–4.00 $$$$ $2.00–4.00

Suggested Readings

Berde CB, Sethna NF. Analgesics for the treatment of pain in children. *N Engl J Med* 2002;347(14):1094-103.

Collège des médecins du Québec. *L'analgésie à l'urgence.* Lignes directrices du Collège des Médecins du Québec. Montreal (QC): Collège des médecins du Québec, 2006. Available from http://www.cmq.org/DocumentLibrary/UploadedContents/CmsDocuments/Lignes-analgesie-urgence-complet-2006.pdf Assessed May 7, 2007.

Falanga IJ, Lafrenaye S, Meyer SK et al. Management of acute pain in children: safety and efficacy of a nurse-controlled algorithm for pain relief. *Acute Pain* 2006;8:45-54.

[No authors listed]. Drugs for pain. *Treat Guidel Med Lett* 2004;2(23):47-54.

Ranji SR, Goldman LE, Simel DL et al. Do opiates affect the clinical evaluation of patients with acute abdominal pain? *JAMA* 2006;296(14):1764-74.

Sachs CJ. Oral analgesics for acute nonspecific pain. *Am Fam Physician* 2005;71(5):913-8.

References

1. Drendel AL, Brousseau DC, Gorelick MH. Pain assessment for pediatric patients in the emergency department. *Pediatrics* 2006;117(5):1511-8.
2. O'Rourke D. The measurement of pain in infants, children, and adolescents: from policy to practice. *Phys Ther* 2004;84(6):560-70.
3. Hain RD. Pain scales in children: a review. *Palliat Med* 1997;11(5):341-50.
4. [No authors listed]. Drugs for pain. *Treat Guidel Med Lett* 2004;2(23):47-54.
5. Moore A, Collins S, Carroll D et al. Single dose paracetamol (acetaminophen), with and without codeine, for postoperative pain. *Cochrane Database Syst Rev* 2000;(2):CD001547.
6. McQuay HJ, Moore RA. *An evidence-based resource for pain.* Oxford (UK): Oxford University Press; 1998.
7. McQuay H, Moore A, Justins D. Treating acute pain in hospital. *BMJ* 1997;314(7093):1531-5.
8. Lesko SM, Mitchell AA. An assessment of the safety of pediatric ibuprofen. A practitioner-based randomized clinical trial. *JAMA* 1995;273(12):929-33.
9. Grond S, Sablotzki A. Clinical pharmacology of tramadol. *Clin Pharmacokinet* 2004;43(13):879-923.
10. Sachs CJ. Oral analgesics for acute nonspecific pain. *Am Fam Physician* 2005;71(5):913-8.
11. Lander JA, Weltman BJ, So SS. EMLA and amethocaine for reduction of children's pain associated with needle insertion. *Cochrane Database Syst Rev* 2006;(3):CD004236.

Concurrently with instituting an antiviral agent, it is important to relieve the acute pain. This may be accomplished with **opioids** if necessary, *nerve blocks* and early treatment with **amitriptyline** and/or **gabapentin**.

A **vaccine** to prevent herpes zoster and postherpetic neuralgia[3] is expected to be available soon in Canada and is available now in the United States.

Recurrent Neuralgia—Trigeminal Neuralgia (TN)

TN (also known as tic douloureux) is confined to the face and shows a predilection for the second or third trigeminal divisions. Almost always unilateral, it generally afflicts persons over the age of 50, and often follows a remitting course. TN usually responds very well to therapy with **carbamazepine**.[1] The sustained-release form (given every 8–12 hours) may improve compliance, lessen untoward effects and provide a more sustained effect. Measuring serum levels may help in assessing adherence and titrating dose. **Oxcarbazepine** is a new antiepileptic drug related to carbamazepine. Advantages include twice daily dosing and fewer side effects and drug interactions, but it appears to have a higher propensity to cause hyponatremia, particularly in the young. Randomized controlled trials are lacking.

Clinical experience has shown that other pharmacologic approaches are inferior to carbamazepine. Therefore, if some relief is achieved with carbamazepine but side effects are unacceptable, a good strategy is to try oxcarbazepine or reduce the dose to tolerability and add **baclofen**. Should this fail, add **phenytoin** or replace baclofen with phenytoin. **Gabapentin**, **pregabalin**, **clonazepam** and **valproic acid** may be tried if other strategies fail.

Should medical therapy fail, a variety of *neurosurgical options* have a high success rate in experienced hands; procedures include potentially curative microvascular decompression, ablative procedures such as glycerol instillation or balloon compression of the gasserian ganglion, and more recently, the gamma knife. MRI can help identify candidates for microvascular decompression by ruling out other causes of nerve compression. There is a risk of recurrence with all ablative surgeries and a < 10 percent risk of anesthesia dolorosa (nerve injury pain caused by surgery) with all procedures.

Chronic Neuralgia

Nerve Root Compression: Cervical and Lumbar Radiculopathy

Disc material may be extruded through the ligamentum flavum. This sequestrum may cause nerve root compression (cervical and lumbar radiculopathies). In the acute phase, **NSAIDs** or **acetaminophen/codeine** may be effective. Where necessary, additional pain relief can be achieved with strong **opioids**, an appropriate regimen of rest and avoidance of further aggravation.

This pain often settles with conservative management. Consider surgical treatment if medical treatment fails over 6 to 12 weeks and if neuroimaging with CT or MR shows a surgically treatable lesion, if acute pain is excruciating and intractable or if a neurologic deficit and a correctable lesion are present. Signs of a progressive neurologic deficit such as weakness or muscle wasting should prompt surgical consultation as early as possible. Investigate if pain does not resolve within a reasonable time frame, or if this is the first episode in an elderly person (because of possible malignancy or other serious illness).

Complex Regional Pain Syndrome Type I (CRPS I)[4]

CRPS I, formerly known as reflex sympathetic dystrophy or sympathetically maintained pain, may cause neuropathic pain and neurovascular and dystrophic changes. It may result from penetrating or crush injuries to nerve but sometimes occurs after stroke or myocardial infarction. Characteristics include burning pain, hyperalgesia, hyperpathia and allodynia, sweating, rubor and coldness of the limb.

If symptoms persist, after a few months one may see widening of the painful area, cool cyanotic skin, a glossy appearance to the skin, altered hair growth and progressive loss of function. Some will progress to dystrophic changes, osteoporosis, nail changes, subcutaneous thinning with pointed digits and further loss of function with contractures or frozen shoulder and continued severe pain.

While CRPS I was thought to be due to sympathetic overactivity, evidence now points to a disorder involving upregulation of adrenergic receptors. Although sympathetic blocks often provide temporary relief, sympathectomy does not necessarily result in permanent resolution. Bier blocks using guanethidine are ineffective. Physical therapy, corticosteroids, sympathectomies and repeated sympathetic blocks have limited success. At follow-up, two-thirds are likely to have continued pain, and only about one-quarter return to fully normal activity. Treat these patients as for other neuropathic pain; some may require chronic opioid therapy.

Chronic Peripheral Neuropathic Pain[1]

This category of neuropathic pain conditions includes *postherpetic neuralgia*, *diabetic* and other *neuropathy*, *causalgia* (CRPS II), *phantom limb pain* and others. **Tricyclic antidepressants** (TCAs), antiepileptic drugs such as **gabapentin** and **pregabalin** and **opioids** such as morphine, oxycodone and tramadol are proven therapies for PHN and diabetic neuropathy. The standard therapy has been **amitriptyline** but gabapentin and pregabalin are alternative first-line agents. **Nortriptyline** and **desipramine** may be tried in sequence as some patients may respond better to one of these agents. **Bupropion** and serotonin-norepinephrine reuptake inhibitor (SNRI) antidepressants such as duloxetine (not yet available in Canada) and **venlafaxine** have recently been shown to relieve neuropathic pain, but seem less effective than TCAs.[1] A stool softener and mouth spray of artificial saliva might pre-empt the common side effects of constipation and dry mouth. Randomized controlled trials in painful diabetic neuropathy indicate relief of pain in some patients with the serotonergic antidepressants **paroxetine** and **citalopram**.

If pain is severe and refractory to antidepressants and antiepileptic drugs, **opioid** therapy may be prescribed. Psychological dependence, tolerance and physical dependence are not major problems when opioids are used for chronic, severe, nonmalignant pain. Guidelines are suggested in Table 2. A variety of opioids may be tried such as **morphine**, **oxycodone**, **hydromorphone**, **tramadol**, transdermal **fentanyl** and **methadone**, which requires special knowledge and prescribing authorization. **Codeine** alone or combined with **acetaminophen** is a poor choice for severe pain of any kind.

Table 2: **Guidelines for Opioids in Chronic Nonmalignant Pain**

- Consider after other reasonable therapies have failed.
- Perform a complete pain and psychosocial history and physical examination. A history of substance abuse, tension-type headaches and pain that appears to be largely determined by psychologic factors is a relative contraindication to the use of opioid therapy.
- A single physician/prescriber/pharmacy is optimal. The prescriber may choose to set up a contract with the patient. The agreement should specify the drug regimen, possible side effects, the functional restoration program and that violations may result in termination of opioid therapy.
- The opioid analgesic of choice should be administered around the clock and may include a provision of "rescue doses" for breakthrough pain. Controlled-release preparations include morphine, oxycodone, hydromorphone, tramadol and transdermal fentanyl. Drug administration should include a titration phase to minimize side effects. If a graded analgesic response to incremental doses is not observed, the patient may not be opioid-responsive and opioid treatment should probably be terminated.
- The patient should be seen monthly for the first few months and every two to three months thereafter. At each visit assess pain relief (0–10 scale), mood, side effects, quality of life, adherence to functional goals and presence of drug-related behaviour. Optimally, affix a copy of the prescription and drug therapy flow sheet to the medical record.
- The goal of opioid therapy is to make the pain tolerable. For some patients with nonmalignant pain (e.g., postherpetic neuralgia), the administration of an opioid analgesic can mean the difference between bearable and unbearable pain.

Lidocaine 5% topical gel and transdermal patch have been shown to relieve PHN;[5] the patch is available in the United States but not yet in Canada.

Other treatments, such as topical **ASA**, **menthol** and **capsaicin**, are unproven or of modest efficacy, but may be helpful in refractory patients for psychological support or a potential analgesic response, placebo benefit or antidepressant effect, while awaiting the possibility of spontaneous pain resolution.

Although the evidence for these therapeutic approaches is mainly from studies of patients with PHN and diabetic neuropathy, they can be tried in patients with phantom limb pain or other chronic peripheral neuropathic pain. Surgical treatment has no role in PHN and other types of neuropathic pain in the majority of patients.

Therapeutic Tips

- While patients frequently say they have used amitriptyline or carbamazepine or other agents, these drugs have often been used in too high or too low a dose and for too short a period of time. It is useful to re-institute these drugs to evaluate their effectiveness when used appropriately: start low, go slow, increase dose until relief of symptoms or side effects occur and treat side effects when possible.
- Be sure the patient understands the goals of therapy: reduction in pain from moderate or severe to mild, at the price of some side effects that may be tolerable or treatable.
- Use a pain assessment tool, such as a scale of 0–10 where 0 is no pain and 10 the worst pain imaginable, to evaluate pain relief.
- Prescribe an **artificial saliva mouth spray** with TCAs and a **stool softener** for TCAs and opioids as a matter of course.
- Use controlled-release formulations of carbamazepine and opioids (see Table 2).
- Try different drugs within a class (e.g., TCAs), drugs of different classes and combination therapy (polypharmacy) for possible additive or synergistic effect.
- After a period of relief of one to three months it may be possible to reduce or stop the drugs. Gradual reduction is important to avoid withdrawal symptoms.
- If opioids are used, guidelines (see Table 2) are important and should be worked through with the patient.
- A trial and error approach of scientifically unproven treatments is reasonable if standard therapy fails.
- Repeated visits can provide important psychological support and hope for desperate patients as trial and error approaches are utilized.
- If chronic neuropathic pain is being managed in general practice, semi-annual or annual visits to a pain specialist, where available, help provide support to the family practitioner for contentious approaches such as opioids, and offer the chance of a novel therapy for the patient.

Figure 1: **Pharmacologic Management of Neuropathic Pain**[a]

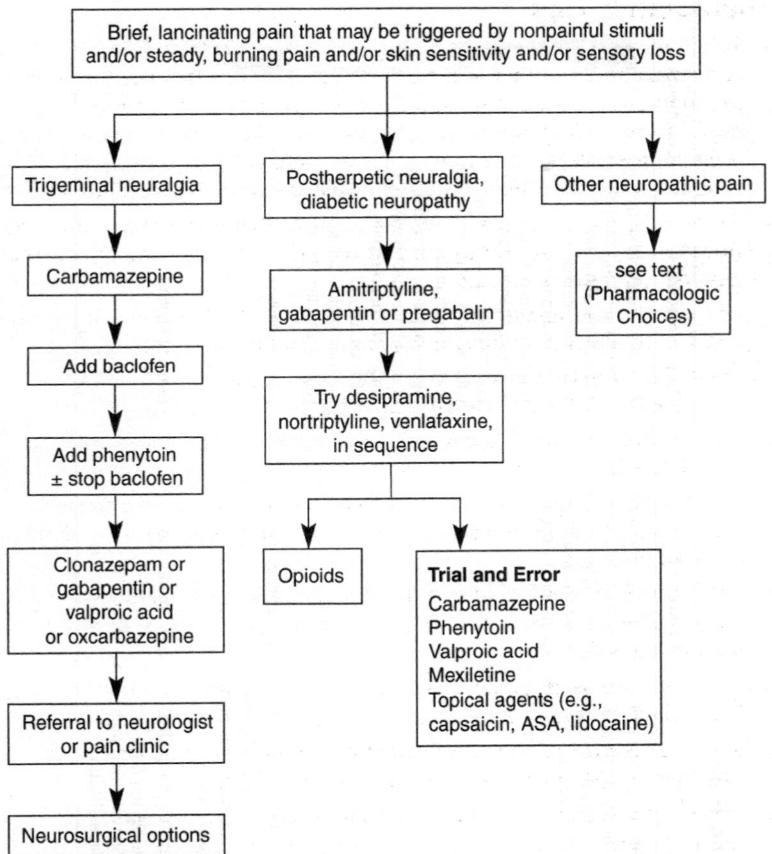

[a] Two to three months constitutes a reasonable trial of medication for neuropathic pain.

Table 3: Drugs Used in Neuropathic Pain

Class	Drug	Dose	Adverse Effects	Drug Interactions	Comments	Cost[a]
Tricyclic Antidepressants (TCAs)	*amitriptyline* generics	Begin with 10–25 mg QHS Increase by 10 to 25 mg daily at weekly intervals, until pain relief or side effects	All TCAs: dry mouth, constipation, drowsiness, blurred vision, urinary retention, weight gain, confusion, tachycardia.	All TCAs: metabolized by cytochrome P450; potential interactions with other substrates, inhibitors (e.g., erythromycin, fluoxetine, fluvoxamine, isoniazid, itraconazole, ketoconazole, paroxetine, valproic acid), or inducers (e.g., phenobarbital, carbamazepine, phenytoin, rifampin); ↑ sedation with other CNS depressants such as alcohol; ↑ anticholinergic effects with other anticholinergics.		$
	desipramine Norpramin, generics	Begin with 10–25 mg QHS Increase by 10 to 25 mg daily at weekly intervals, until pain relief or side effects	See amitripyline.	See amitripyline.		$
	nortriptyline Aventyl, generics	Begin with 10–25 mg QHS ↑ by 10 to 25 mg daily at weekly intervals, until pain relief or side effects	See amitripyline.	See amitripyline.		$

Class	Drug	Dose	Adverse Effects	Drug Interactions	Comments	Cost[a]
Serotonin-norepinephrine Reuptake Inhibitors	*venlafaxine* Effexor XR, generic	Initial: 37.5 mg daily Increase weekly by 37.5 mg/day Usual effective dose: 150–225 mg/day Max: 375 mg/day	Hypertension, ataxia, sedation, insomnia, nausea, hyperhidrosis, dry mouth, constipation, anxiety, anorexia.	Clearance may be ↓ by inhibitors of CYP2D6 such as cannabidiol, fluoxetine, paroxetine or quinidine, or by inhibitors of CYP3A4 such as erythromycin, itraconazole, ketoconazole or grapefruit juice. Contraindicated with MAOIs.		$$$-$$$$
Muscle Relaxants	*baclofen* Lioresal Oral, generics	Initial: 10 mg BID Max: 20 mg TID	Sedation, muscle weakness, nausea, dizziness.	Potential additive CNS depression with TCAs, opioids, benzodiazepines and antihypertensives.	Gradual withdrawal is important.	$$
Antiepileptic Drugs	*carbamazepine immediate-release* Tegretol, generics	Initial: 100 mg BID to QID Increase by 100 mg daily at weekly intervals to 400–1200 mg/day or more, in 2–4 divided doses, until good pain control or intolerable side effects	Drowsiness, ataxia, dizziness, nausea, hyponatremia; allergic reactions, e.g., rash.	Induces several cytochrome P450 isoenzymes, potentially ↑ the clearance of many drugs, such as OCs, warfarin, risperidone or TCAs; clearance may be ↓ by CYP3A4 inhibitors such as erythromycin, grapefruit juice, itraconazole or ketoconazole.	Serum levels may help assess adherence and guide dosage.	$$
	carbamazepine controlled-release Tegretol CR, generics	Initial: 200 mg once daily Increase at weekly intervals as needed to 400–1200 mg daily in 2 divided doses	See carbamazepine immediate-release.	See carbamazepine immediate-release.	See carbamazepine immediate-release.	$$

(cont'd)

Table 3: **Drugs Used in Neuropathic Pain** *(cont'd)*

Class	Drug	Dose	Adverse Effects	Drug Interactions	Comments	Cost[a]
	oxcarbazepine Trileptal	Initial: 75–150 mg BID Max: 1200 mg/day	See carbamazepine immediate-release. Hyponatremia may be more common than with carbamazepine, especially in younger patients.	May have lower propensity for drug interactions than carbamazepine, but comparative trials are lacking.	May be alternative to carbamazepine in terms of efficacy; generally fewer side effects.	$$$-$$$$
	clonazepam Rivotril, generics	Initial: 1.5 mg/day Max: 20 mg/day	Sedation.	Additive sedation with CNS depressants such as alcohol; serum levels potentially ↑ by CYP3A4 inhibitors, such as cimetidine, clarithromycin, erythromycin, grapefruit juice, ketoconazole, lamotrigine, ritonavir or verapamil, or ↓ by inducers of CYP3A4, such as carbamazepine, phenytoin or rifampin.	Important to withdraw gradually.	$–$$
	gabapentin Neurontin, generics	Initial: 300–400 mg/day May increase at weekly intervals to BID then TID Max: 3600 mg/day	Sedation, ataxia, tremor; less commonly, GI upset, peripheral edema, vision changes.	Administration with aluminum/magnesium-containing antacids may ↓ bioavailability.		$$$–$$$$

Class	Drug	Dose	Adverse Effects	Drug Interactions	Comments	Cost[a]
	pregabalin Lyrica	Initial: 50–150 mg daily in 2 divided doses Increase dose weekly by 50–150 mg/day Usual effective dose: 300-600 mg/day Max: 600 mg/day	Sedation, ataxia, edema, diplopia, weight gain, dry mouth.	No known significant drug interactions.	BID dosing is an advantage. Pain relief similar to gabapentin (about 30% have moderate relief or better over placebo).	$$$-$$$$
	phenytoin Dilantin Capsules, Dilantin Infatabs, generics	100–300 mg QHS, depending on age	Ataxia, drowsiness, nausea; gingival hyperplasia; skin rash 5–10%, rarely very serious; ↑ liver enzymes; blood dyscrasias; dose-related encephalopathy; coarse facial features with long-term use.	Induces several cytochrome P450 isoenzymes, potentially increasing the clearance of many drugs, such as OCs, warfarin, risperidone and TCAs.	Dosage increments should be small and gradual because of saturation kinetics. Serum levels may help assess adherence and guide dosage.	$
	valproic acid Depakene, generics	Initial: 15 mg/kg/day in divided doses Max: 60 mg/kg/day in divided doses	Nausea, alopecia, tremor, weight gain, ↑ hepatic enzymes; neural tube defects can occur if used during pregnancy; do liver function tests prior to initiation of therapy and periodically, especially in 1st 6 mo of therapy and if symptoms of hepatic dysfunction occur.	Inhibits CYP2C9 and may ↓ clearance of its substrates, such as fluoxetine, fluvastatin, sertraline, verapamil or warfarin; avoid with ASA or warfarin; carbamazepine, phenytoin and phenobarbital can significantly ↑ clearance of valproic acid; may ↑ depressant effect of alcohol.	Serum levels may help assess adherence and guide dosage.	$$–$$$$[b]

(cont'd)

Table 3: **Drugs Used in Neuropathic Pain** *(cont'd)*

Class	Drug	Dose	Adverse Effects	Drug Interactions	Comments	Cost[a]
	divalproex sodium Epival, generics	Initial: 15 mg/kg/day in divided doses Max: 60 mg/kg/day in divided doses	See valproic acid.	See valproic acid.	See valproic acid.	$$-$$$$ [b]
Opioids	*oxycodone immediate-release* Oxy-IR, Supeudol, generics	5–10 mg Q4–6H Start low and go slow; increase to relief or unacceptable side effects	All opioids: nausea, constipation, drowsiness; allergic reactions, e.g., rash.	All opioids: additive sedation with other CNS depressants such as alcohol; potential enhancement of opioid effects with lidocaine.		$$–$$$
	oxycodone controlled-release OxyContin	20–40 mg/day Start low and go slow; increase to relief or unacceptable side effects	See oxycodone immediate-release.	See oxycodone immediate-release.		$$-$$$
	morphine immediate-release Statex, generics	Initial: 5–15 mg Q4–6H PRN Start low and go slow; increase until relief of symptoms or unacceptable side effects	See oxycodone immediate-release.	See oxycodone immediate-release. ↓ analgesic effect with somatostatin, rifampin.	After 1–2 weeks, convert to equivalent daily dose of controlled-release formulation.	$$
	morphine controlled-release Kadian, M-Eslon, MS Contin, generics	20–30 mg/day Titrate slowly as needed until relief of symptoms or unacceptable side effects	See oxycodone immediate-release.	See oxycodone immediate-release. ↓ analgesic effect with somatostatin, rifampin.		$$

Class	Drug	Dose	Adverse Effects	Drug Interactions	Comments	Cost[a]
	hydromorphone immediate-release Dilaudid, Hydromorph IR, generics	Initial: 1–2 mg Q4H PRN Start low and go slow; increase until relief of symptoms or unacceptable side effects	See oxycodone immediate-release.	See oxycodone immediate-release.		$$
	hydromorphone controlled-release Hydromorph Contin	Initial: 3 mg Q8–12H Start low and go slow; increase until relief of symptoms or unacceptable side effects	See oxycodone immediate-release.	See oxycodone immediate-release.		$$$-$$$$
	fentanyl transdermal Duragesic, generics	Initial: One 2.5 mg patch, delivering 25 μg/h, Q3 days Start low and go slow; increase until relief of symptoms or unacceptable side effects	See oxycodone immediate-release.	See oxycodone immediate-release. Inhibitors of CYP3A4, such as cimetidine, efavirenz, erythromycin, itraconazole, ketoconazole or ritonavir, may potentiate fentanyl's pharmacologic effects.		$$$$
	tramadol controlled-release Zytram XL	Initial: 150 mg daily May increase at weekly intervals to 200-400 mg/day	Respiratory depression, sedation, ataxia, constipation, seizures, nausea, orthostatic hypotension.	Do not use if MAOIs taken within past 14 days. Caution with drugs that ↓ seizure threshold, e.g., SSRIs, TCAs, bupropion. ↑ sedation with other CNS depressants. Carbamazepine may ↓ analgesic effect of tramadol. Clearance may be ↓ by inhibitors of CYP2D6 such as		$$$

(cont'd)

Table 3: **Drugs Used in Neuropathic Pain** *(cont'd)*

Class	Drug	Dose	Adverse Effects	Drug Interactions	Comments	Cost[a]
				fluoxetine, paroxetine or quinidine or by inhibitors of CYP3A4 such as erythromycin, itraconazole or ketoconazole.		

[a] Cost of 30-day supply of usual dose; includes drug cost only.
[b] Cost based on 70 kg body weight.
Dosage adjustment may be required in renal impairment; see Appendix I.
Abbreviations: TCAs = tricyclic antidepressants; OCs = oral contraceptives
Legend: $ < $10 $–$$ < $10–50 $$ $10–50 $$–$$$ $10–100 $$–$$$$ $10– > 100 $$$ $50–100 $$$–$$$$ $50– > 100 $$$$ > $100

Suggested Readings

Gilron I, Watson CP, Cahill CM et al. Neuropathic pain: a practical guideline for the clinician. *CMAJ* 2006;175(3):265-75.

Harden RN, Baron R, Janig W, editors. *Complex regional pain syndrome.* Seattle (WA): IASP Press; 2001.

Oxman MN, Levin MJ, Johnson GR et al. A vaccine to prevent herpes zoster and postherpetic neuralgia in older adults. *N Eng J Med* 2005;352(22):2271-84.

Watson CPN, Gershon AA, editors. *Herpes zoster and postherpetic neuralgia.* 2nd ed. New York (NY): Elsevier; 2001.

References

1. Gilron I, Watson CP, Cahill CM et al. Neuropathic pain: a practical guideline for the clinician. *CMAJ* 2006;175(3):265-75.
2. Watson CPN, Gershon AA, editors. *Herpes zoster and postherpetic neuralgia.* 2nd ed. New York (NY): Elsevier; 2001.
3. Oxman MN, Levin MJ, Johnson GR et al. A vaccine to prevent herpes zoster and postherpetic neuralgia in older adults. *N Eng J Med* 2005;352(22):2271-84.
4. Harden RN, Baron R, Janig W, editors. *Complex regional pain syndrome.* Seattle (WA): IASP Press; 2001.
5. Hansson PT et al., editors. *Neuropathic pain: pathophysiology and treatment.* Seattle (WA): IASP Press; 2001.

CHAPTER 16
Bell's Palsy

William Pryse-Phillips, MD, FRCP, FRCPC

Bell's palsy is a lower motor neuron paralysis of the facial nerve, often due to herpes simplex virus-1 infection, causing inflammation and edema.[1] It affects about 20 per 100 000 per year without gender predominance.[2] The incidence increases until age 40 and then remains static until late adult life when it again increases. Bell's palsy occurs more frequently in pregnant women and in patients with diabetes or hypertension.

Up to 85% of patients achieve spontaneous complete recovery without treatment; those who will not recover cannot be identified clinically,[3] although incomplete paralysis carries a better prognosis. In < 10% of cases the palsy recurs on either side.

Goals of Therapy

- Promote complete recovery of function through prevention of denervation
- Protect the eye from corneal abrasion
- Alleviate pain

Investigations

The classic presentation of Bell's palsy includes abrupt onset of facial weakness affecting the upper and lower face, ear pain and altered taste. Involvement of other cranial nerves, remote CNS signs and systemic features would indicate further inquiry for the conditions listed in Table 1.

Table 1: **Differential Diagnosis of Unilateral Bell's Palsy**

- Ramsay Hunt syndrome (herpes zoster infection; vesicles in the ear or throat)
- Facial nerve tumors (usually painless; examine for neurofibromatosis)
- Cerebellopontine angle tumors (added neurologic signs)
- Parotid tumors (clinical examination)
- Mastoiditis (clinical examination; deafness, discharge)
- Lyme disease (skin and joint signs)
- Neurosarcoidosis (chest x-ray)
- Brainstem lesions such as multiple sclerosis (other neurologic signs)

Bilateral facial palsy is a feature of Guillain-Barré syndrome, Lyme disease, sarcoid and Wegener's granulomatosis, and of even more rare conditions.

Investigations are seldom needed after a complete history and physical examination have excluded other causes of peripheral facial palsy.

- EMG and facial nerve conduction studies may help with prognosis but only after 8 to 10 days

- Computed tomography (CT) scan is appropriate if trauma is a likely cause
- Magnetic resonance imaging (MRI) is indicated in the presence of atypical features such as slow progression or associated neurologic signs
- No laboratory tests are useful

Therapeutic Choices (Figure 1)

Pharmacologic Choices (Table 2)

Eye Care

- To prevent corneal abrasions in any eye that cannot be closed voluntarily:
  - lubricate with ophthalmic drops or ointment
  - tape the eyelid closed at night and protect with glasses during the day

Analgesics

- **Ibuprofen** or **acetaminophen** with or without **codeine** is occasionally required for the first day or two.
- More potent opioids such as meperidine or morphine are rarely needed.

Corticosteroids

Theoretically, the anti-inflammatory action of corticosteroids minimizes nerve damage and thus improves outcomes. Steroids have been used empirically for many years for treatment of Bell's palsy, but the evidence for their use is not compelling after meta-analysis.[4] However, data from pooled Class I and II studies do suggest that steroids are "probably effective."[5] In addition, there is good anecdotal evidence for a reduction in pain with early steroid therapy, and clinical experience suggests that steroid-treated patients achieve better recovery and are less likely to develop denervation. Therefore, the following basic regimen is reasonable: **prednisone** 1 mg/kg po daily for five days, then taper over another five days (See Figure 1 and Table 2).

In the case of *complete* facial paralysis, corticosteroid treatment showed clinically and statistically significant improvement in recovery of function,[6] a report not cited in the American Academy of Neurology (AAN) Practice Parameter.[5] A systematic review of the use of steroids in children with Bell's palsy concluded that in cases of complete facial paralysis, corticosteroid therapy is not advisable.[7]

Antivirals

Acyclovir is seldom given without prednisone. The doses used in the few reported studies (none a Class I trial) range from 5 to 24 g over 5 to 10 days. A Cochrane review [8] concluded that before a definitive recommendation can be made regarding the effect of acyclovir or valacyclovir on Bell's palsy, data are needed from a large, multicentre, randomized controlled and blinded study with at least 12 months' follow-up. The AAN concluded that the benefit of acyclovir is not definitively established.[5] However, in Ramsay Hunt syndrome (herpes zoster infection of the VII cranial nerve), acyclovir therapy seems appropriate.

Reports of decompressive surgery have also been scrutinized[5] but the quality of evidence is insufficient to allow a recommendation.

Therapeutic Tips

- No treatment is needed for mild weakness that is no longer evolving.
- Use prednisone as soon as possible in all other cases of Bell's palsy unless there is a potential contraindication to steroid use, such as diabetes or peptic ulcer disease.
- There is no good evidence for benefit from prednisone if it is started more than seven days after the onset of symptoms.
- No evidence supports the use of acyclovir alone.
- The combination of acyclovir and prednisone is not proven to be superior to prednisone alone, although at least one retrospective study concluded that it was.[9] The optimal dose of acyclovir is not established and its risk-benefit ratio makes it inappropriate for routine use.[5]

Figure 1: **Management of Bell's Palsy**

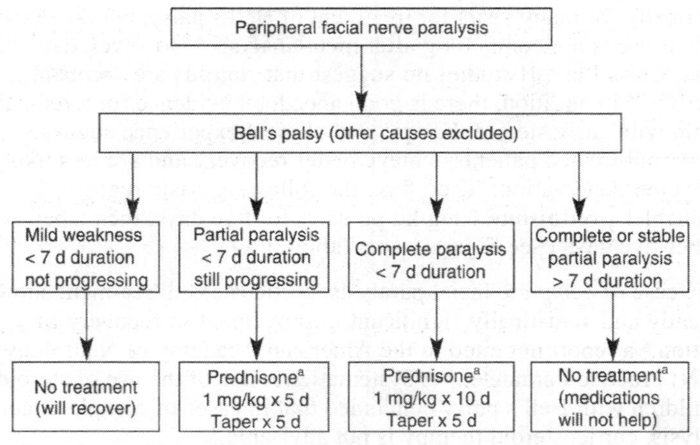

[a] The addition of acyclovir is an option but is not routinely warranted based on current evidence.

Table 2: **Drugs Used for the Treatment of Bell's Palsy**

Class	Drug	Dose	Adverse Effects	Cost[a]
Corticosteroids	*prednisone* Winpred, generics	1 mg/kg daily × 5 days,[b] then taper over another 5 days	GI upset, hyperglycemia, sodium and fluid retention, hypokalemia, hypocalcemia.	$
Antivirals	*acyclovir* ➔ Zovirax Oral, generics	400 mg 5 × daily × 10 days	Headache, GI upset. Avoid concurrent use with probenecid.	$$$

[a] Cost of one course of treatment, based on 70 kg weight; includes drug cost only.
[b] In cases of complete facial paralysis, treat for 10 days then taper over another 5 days.
➔ Dosage adjustment may be required in renal impairment; see Appendix I.
Abbreviation: GI = gastrointestinal
Legend: $ < $5 $$ $5–85 $$$ $85–90

Suggested Readings

Baringer JR. Herpes simplex virus and Bell palsy. *Ann Intern Med* 1996;124(1 Pt 1):63-5.

Roob G, Fazekas F, Hartung HP. Peripheral facial palsy: etiology, diagnosis and treatment. *Eur Neurol* 1999;41(1):3-9.

Salinas RA, Alvarez G, Ferreira J. Corticosteroids for Bell's palsy (idiopathic facial paralysis). *Cochrane Database Syst Rev* 2004;(4):CD001942.

References

1. Morrow MJ. Bell's palsy and herpes zoster oticus. *Curr Treat Options Neurol* 2000;2(5):407-16.
2. Rowlands S, Hooper R, Hughes R et al. The epidemiology and treatment of Bell's palsy in the UK. *Eur J Neurol* 2002;9(1):63-7.
3. Jabor MA, Gianoli G. Management of Bell's palsy. *J La State Med Soc* 1996;148(7):279-83.
4. Salinas RA, Alvarez G, Ferreira J. Corticosteroids for Bell's palsy (idiopathic facial paralysis). *Cochrane Database Syst Rev* 2004;(4):CD001942.
5. Grogan PM, Gronseth GS. Practice parameter: Steroids, acyclovir, and surgery for Bell's palsy (an evidence-based review): report of the Quality Standards Subcommittee of the American Academy of Neurology. *Neurology* 2001;56(7):830-6.
6. Ramsey MJ, DerSimonian R, Holtel MR et al. Corticosteroid treatment for idiopathic facial nerve paralysis: a meta-analysis. *Laryngoscope* 2000;110(3 Pt 1):335-41.
7. Salman MS, MacGregor DL. Should children with Bell's palsy be treated with corticosteroids? A systematic review. *J Child Neurol* 2001;16(8):565-8.
8. Allen D, Dunn L. Aciclovir or valaciclovir for Bell's palsy (idiopathic facial paralysis). *Cochrane Database Syst Rev* 2004;(3):CD001869.
9. Hato N, Matsumoto S, Kisaki H et al. Efficacy of early treatment of Bell's palsy with oral acyclovir and prednisolone. *Otol Neurotol* 2003;24(6):948-51.

CHAPTER 17
Chronic Spasticity

Virginia Devonshire, MD, FRCPC

Spasticity is an involuntary velocity-dependent increase in muscle tone resulting from injury to the motor pathways in the brain or spinal cord. It is common in spinal cord injury, multiple sclerosis, stroke and cerebral palsy. Spasticity usually occurs as part of the upper motor neuron (UMN) complex which consists of weakness, hyper-reflexia, Babinski's sign and slow coordination.

Spasticity can impair feeding, dressing, bowel/bladder function, hygiene and gait. It can also reduce range-of-movement of joints, cause contractures (shortening of muscles, which can cause joint dysfunction) and result in significant pain and skin breakdown. However, spasticity is not always impairing and can facilitate some movements by providing posture and tone in what would otherwise be a flaccid limb. It can allow weight bearing in a plegic limb by essentially "bracing" that limb. Further, treatment of spasticity can sometimes worsen ambulation by unmasking limb weakness. Thus, spasticity should only be treated when it interferes with function and care, or results in pain.

Goals of Therapy

- Improve functional movements and gait
- Improve range of movement and limit contracture formation
- Reduce pain and spasms
- Improve seating and positioning, and reduce skin breakdown
- Improve care, e.g., perineal care and catheterization

Investigations

- No investigations needed if seen as part of a UMN complex already diagnosed.
- Spasticity in isolation needs investigation for the underlying pathology.

Therapeutic Choices (Figure 1)

Nonpharmacologic Choices

Search for aggravating factors if spasticity has increased in a stable patient. This can include pressure areas, infections (bladder, toenail, etc.), bladder stones, constipation and DVTs.

Physical measures should always be undertaken and include daily stretching and range-of-movement exercises. Braces may be used to maintain a spastic limb in a reflex-inhibiting posture and prevent contractures.

Surgical treatment of spasticity tends to be reserved for the most refractory cases. Many destructive procedures such as myelotomy and cordotomy have significant complications and are rarely performed. Selective dorsal rhizotomy can be effective in limited patients but can affect trunk tone and sensation. Orthopedic procedures, such as lengthening, releasing or transferring a tendon, are helpful in optimizing function and preventing contractures but do not treat the underlying spasticity.

Pharmacologic Choices (Table 1)

Oral medications remain important in the treatment of spasticity. A number of randomized clinical trials have demonstrated efficacy of antispasticity medications, although recent reviews found the studies were limited.[1,2] Although level I evidence is lacking, clinical experience has shown that efficacy is better in spasticity of spinal origin (multiple sclerosis, spinal cord injury) than cerebral origin (brain injury and stroke). With the exception of dantrolene, which acts directly on the muscle, these drugs have a central mode of action.

Baclofen is the standard initial medication for spasticity. It must be gradually titrated and the typical effective dose is 30 to 80 mg/day. Abrupt discontinuation can result in confusion, seizures and hallucinations.

Tizanidine is also a good first-line treatment,[3] or it can be combined with baclofen as they have different sites of action. Side effects of dry mouth and drowsiness can limit its use. It is best to start with a low dose of 2 mg at night and increase gradually.

Dantrolene is effective in the management of spasticity, although it is used less frequently because of an association with liver toxicity and muscle weakness. Liver function tests should be carried out before the start of treatment and every 3 to 6 months thereafter.

Benzodiazipines such as **diazepam** and **clonazepam** can be useful for treating spasms especially if these are problematic at night. The sedating effects of these drugs otherwise limit their use.

Gabapentin may be a useful alternative or addition in spasticity management especially if there is concurrent neuropathic pain.[4]

Cannabinoids (e.g., **dronabinol, nabilone, Sativex**) may emerge as another option for managing spasticity. Several trials have shown mixed results.[5,6] Their efficacy compared with other medications requires evaluation.

Focal treatment of spastic muscles may have advantages over the global approach to spasticity control through oral medications. Focal treatments are useful in spasticity of cerebral origin where current drug therapies are less successful. They also reduce spasticity selectively, leaving some muscle groups with tone that is functional. **Phenol** injections are used to block nerves going to specific spastic muscle groups. Injections can be uncomfortable and need to be repeated in six months; adverse effects can include pain, dysesthesias and infection. **Botulinum toxin A** injections can also be used and may be better tolerated than phenol.[7] The toxin blocks the release of acetylcholine at the neuromuscular junction, causing weakness (reduced tone) in that muscle. The effect lasts three months, after which collateral sprouting occurs. It is a relatively safe medication with few serious side effects.

Intrathecal delivery of medication is usually indicated when oral medications fail to control spasticity or side effects are intolerable. The medication is delivered via a programmable pump that is usually implanted in the anterior abdominal wall. It delivers small continuous or bolus amounts of drug (usually **baclofen**) into the spinal fluid. Because the drug is acting locally at the level of the spinal cord, there are minimal cognitive side effects. The effect on spasticity can be profound, although it is more effective for lower limb tone as there is a concentration gradient from lumbar to cervical levels.[8]

Therapeutic Tips

- Treat the patient, not the spasticity. The goal is improved comfort or function.
- Titrate medications slowly and to a maximum tolerated dose before switching/adding.
- Consider earlier referral to a neurologist/physiatrist for focal treatment if the spasticity is limited to a focal area and/or is of cerebral origin (therefore less likely to respond to oral agents).
- Muscle spasms occurring during the night can interrupt sleep. Diazepam or clonazepam can be very helpful in reducing these nocturnal spasms.

Figure 1: **Management of Chronic Spasticity**

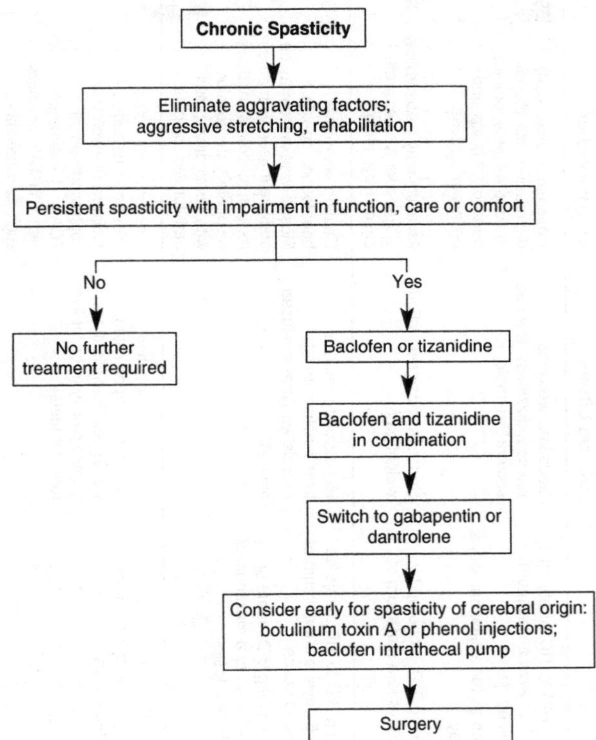

Table 1: Drug Therapy for Chronic Spasticity

Class	Drug	Dose	Adverse Effects	Drug Interactions	Cost[a]
Gamma Aminobutyric Acid Derivatives	*baclofen* Lioresal, generics	Adults: Start with 5 mg BID to TID; titrate up by 5–15 mg per day Q3–5 days to a maximum of 120 mg/day in 3–4 divided doses Children: Same titration as for adults, but with a maximum of 60 mg/day	Sedation, weakness, nausea, dizziness, lowered seizure threshold.	Potential additive CNS depression with tricyclic antidepressants, opioids, benzodiazepines and antihypertensives.	$$$
	gabapentin Neurontin, generics	Adults: Start with 100 mg TID; titrate up by 100 mg per dose Q3 days to a maximum of 800 mg QID	Sedation, dizziness, fatigue, weight gain.	Antacids may ↓ absorption of gabapentin; separate doses by at least 2 h.	$$$$
Skeletal Muscle Relaxants, Direct-acting	*dantrolene* Dantrium	Adults: Start with 25 mg BID to TID; titrate up by 25 mg per day Q3–5 days to a maximum of 400 mg/day in 3–4 divided doses Children: Start with 0.5 mg/kg BID; titrate up by 0.5 mg/kg per day Q3–7 days to a maximum of 400 mg daily in 3–4 divided doses	Hepatoxicity (monitor liver function tests), muscle weakness, nausea, sedation.	Caution with other hepatotoxic agents. Muscle weakness may be additive if used with other muscle relaxants. Additive respiratory depression with benzodiazepines, barbiturates, opioids.	$$$
Alpha$_2$-Adrenergic Agonists	*tizanidine* Zanaflex, generics	Adults: Start with 2 mg QHS; titrate up by 2 mg per day Q3–5 days to a maximum of 36 mg/day in 3–4 divided doses	Dry mouth, sedation, dizziness, hypotension, weakness, hallucinations, hepatotoxicity (monitor liver function tests).	↑ hypotensive effect with antihypertensives. ↓ clearance with oral contraceptives or TCAs. ↓ clearance with CYP1A2 inhibitors such as cimetidine, ciprofloxacin, fluvoxamine, ketoconazole. May ↑ phenytoin levels.	$$$$

Class	Drug	Dose	Adverse Effects	Drug Interactions	Cost[a]
Benzodiazepines	*diazepam* Valium, generics	Adults: Start with 2.5 mg QHS; titrate up by 2.5 mg Q3–7 days to a maximum of 60 mg/day in 3–4 divided doses For nocturnal spasms: 5–10 mg QHS Children: 0.1–0.8 mg/kg/day in 2–3 divided doses	Sedation, ataxia, weakness, dependence.	Potentiates effects of other CNS depressants including alcohol.	$
	clonazepam Rivotril, generics	Adults: 0.5–2 mg QHS	See diazepam.	See diazepam.	$

[a] Cost of 30-day supply at the maximum dose; includes drug cost only.
Dosage adjustment may be required in renal impairment; see Appendix I.
Legend: $ < $25 $$ $25–75 $$$ $75–125 $$$$ $125–175

Suggested Readings

Gracies J, Elovic E, McGuire J, Simpson D. Traditional pharmacologic treatments for spasticity. Part II. General and regional treatments. *Muscle Nerve Suppl* 1997;6:S92-120.

Katz RT, Campagnolo DE. Pharmacologic management of spasticity. In: Katz RT, editor. *Spasticity: state of the art review.* Vol. 8. Philadelphia (PA): Hanley & Belfus;1994. p. 473-80.

References

1. Shakespeare DT, Boggild M, Young C. Anti-spasticity agents for multiple sclerosis. *Cochrane Database Syst Rev* 2003;(4):CD001332.
2. Taricco M, Pagliacci MC, Telaro E et al. Pharmacological interventions for spasticity following spinal cord injury: results of a Cochrane systematic review. *Eura Medicophys* 2006;42(1):5-15.
3. Nance PW, Bugaresti J, Shellenberger K et al. Efficacy and safety of tizanidine in the treatment of spasticity in patients with spinal cord injury. North American Tizanidine Study Group. *Neurology* 1994;44(11 Suppl 9):S44-51
4. Cutter NC, Scott DD, Johnson JC et al. Gabapentin effect on spasticity in multiple sclerosis: a placebo-controlled, randomized trial. *Arch Phys Med Rehabil* 2000;81(2):164-9.
5. Zajicek J, Fox P, Sanders H et al. Cannabinoids for treatment of spasticity and other symptoms related to multiple sclerosis (CAMS study): multicentre randomised placebo-controlled trial. *Lancet* 2003;362(9395):1517-26.
6. Petro DJ, Ellenberg C. Treatment of human spasticity with delta 9-tetrahydrocannabinol. *J Clin Pharmacol* 1981;21(8-9 Suppl):413S-416S.
7. Simpson DM. Clinical trials of botulinum toxin in the treatment of spasticity. *Muscle Nerve Suppl* 1997;6:S169-75.
8. Coffey JR, Cahill D, Steers W et al. Intrathecal baclofen for intractable spasticity of spinal origin: results of a long-term multicenter study. *J Neurosurg* 1993;78(2):226-32.

CHAPTER 18
Muscle Cramps

Virginia Devonshire, MD, FRCPC

Muscle cramps are sudden, involuntary contractions of one or more muscle groups. They are caused by hyperexcitability of the anterior horn cells or peripheral nerves that subserve them. Cramps are common and increase in frequency with age. They can last up to a quarter of an hour and are typically painful. They often recur multiple times and can leave residual pain. Common cramps typically occur at rest (usually at night, involving the calf or foot) or after overuse. Cramps are usually idiopathic but can be associated with acute extracellular volume depletion (diarrhea, vomiting, excessive sweating; "heat cramps"), medications, metabolic disorders including hormonal changes (pregnancy, hypothyroidism, uremia, liver disease), hereditary disorders and rarely, autoimmune conditions (antibodies against voltage-gated potassium channels).

Goals of Therapy

- Prevent and relieve cramps

Investigations

- Check for contributing factors such as excessive muscle use, acute volume depletion.
- Perform laboratory tests for BUN, creatinine, sodium, potassium, magnesium, calcium, thyroid, glucose and CK.
- Check for iatrogenic causes: diuretics, angiotensin receptor blockers, lithium, cyclosporine, nifedipine, cholesterol-lowering agents, salbutamol, donepezil, phenothiazines and alcohol.
- Consider underlying pathology if cramps occur in unusual muscle groups or during activities, or if they occur in the setting of weakness, muscular atrophy/fasciculations or sensory symptoms, though some may still be benign, i.e., cramp-fasciculation syndrome.
  - electromyography to rule out motor neuron disease or peripheral neuropathy
- Differentiate from spasms, spasticity, dystonia (co-contraction of agonist/antagonist muscles during a movement or posture), restless legs, tetany, myalgias and contractures (originate from muscle; associated with exercise and metabolic myopathies).

Therapeutic Choices

Nonpharmacologic Choices

Patients should be reassured of the benign nature of cramps, and nonpharmacologic treatments should be the mainstay. Most cramps can be relieved by stretching the affected muscle. For calf cramps, the patient stands two feet from a wall and leans into the wall, stretching the Achilles tendon. Fluid imbalances can be corrected, and regular stretching may be of benefit in preventing cramps.

Pharmacologic Choices

Quinine sulfate has been used for decades to manage nocturnal leg cramps; its proposed mechanism of action involves decreasing the responsiveness of the motor endpoint to nerve stimulation by increasing the muscle refractory period.

Clinical trials have not conclusively demonstrated its effectiveness. A meta-analysis did show a reduction in frequency of cramps but not in severity or duration.[1] It is reasonable to give a patient a four- to six-week trial of quinine at a dose of 200 to 300 mg at bedtime. Higher doses of quinine are associated with dizziness, visual impairment, tinnitus, gait disturbance, headache and hypersensitivity reactions. Fatal thrombocytopenia has also been reported. At the lower doses used for nocturnal cramps, usually only tinnitus is commonly reported. However, patients need to be counselled about the more serious side effects. Treatment should be interrupted every three months to assess further need.[2]

There is minimal evidence for other therapies for leg cramps. A crossover trial of vitamin E failed to show any benefit.[3] Results for magnesium supplementation (300 to 900 mg per day) have been mixed.[4,5] Small, randomized, double-blind or cross-over studies have shown potential benefit of diltiazem 30 mg daily,[6] vitamin B complex[7] and orphenadrine citrate.[8] Open-labelled trials of gabapentin[9] and verapamil[10] showed some potential benefit. These studies are of insufficient sample size to allow for recommendation of the respective therapies; therefore, risk-benefit analysis must guide therapy for individual patients.

Therapeutic Tips

- Check patient's medication history carefully before treating cramps.
- Use quinine cautiously, only if cramps are frequent and severe and nonpharmacologic measures have failed.
- Regularly reassess use of quinine, as cramps can resolve spontaneously or after a short duration of therapy.
- Cramps rarely need referral unless associated with other neurologic complaints or signs.

Table 1: Management of Nocturnal Leg Cramps

Class	Drug	Dose	Adverse Effects	Drug Interactions	Comments	Cost[a]
Cinchona Alkaloids	*quinine sulfate* generics	200–300 mg QHS	Tinnitus; higher doses have been associated with dizziness, gait disturbances, visual impairment, headache, potentially fatal thrombocytopenia.	May potentiate the effect of warfarin — monitor INR; may ↓ digoxin clearance — monitor serum concentration; ketoconazole may reduce quinine clearance and ↑ toxicity; rifampin may ↑ quinine clearance and reduce effectiveness.	Withdraw therapy every 3 months to reassess need.	$

[a] Cost of 30-day supply; includes drug cost only.
Legend: $ $5–15

Suggested Readings

Butler JV, Mulkerrin EC, O'Keeffe ST. Nocturnal leg cramps in older people. *Postgrad Med J* 2002;78(924):596-8.

MedicineNet.com. *Muscle cramps (of skeletal muscles).* San Clemente (CA): MedicineNet; 2005. Available from: http://www.medicinenet.com/script/main/art.asp?articlekey=2024&pf=3&page=3 Accessed January 30, 2007.

References

1. Man-Son-Hing M, Wells G, Lau A. Quinine for nocturnal leg cramps: a meta-analysis including unpublished data. *J Gen Intern Med* 1998;13(9):600-6.
2. Coppin RJ, Wicke DM, Little PS. Managing nocturnal leg cramps–calf-stretching exercises and cessation of quinine treatment: a factorial randomized controlled trial. *Br J Gen Pract* 2005;55(512):186-91.
3. Connolly PS, Shirley EA, Wasson JH et al. Treatment of nocturnal leg cramps. A crossover trial of quinine vs vitamin E. *Arch Intern Med* 1992;152(9):1877-80.
4. Frusso R, Zarate M, Augustovski F et al. Magnesium for the treatment of nocturnal leg cramps: a crossover randomized trial. *J Fam Pract* 1999;48(11):868-71.
5. Roffe C, Sills S, Crome P et al. Randomised, cross-over, placebo controlled trial of magnesium citrate in the treatment of chronic persistent leg cramps. *Med Sci Monit* 2002;8(5):CR326-30.
6. Voon WC, Sheu SH. Diltiazem for nocturnal leg cramps. *Age Ageing* 2001;30(1):91-2.
7. Chan P, Huang TY, Chen YJ et al. Randomized, double-blind, placebo-controlled study of the safety and efficacy of vitamin B complex in the treatment of nocturnal leg cramps in elderly patients with hypertension. *J Clin Pharmacol* 1998;38(12):1151-4.
8. Latta D. An alternative to quinine in nocturnal leg cramps. *Current Therapeutic Research* 1989;45(5):833-7.
9. Serrao M, Rossi P, Cardinali P et al. Gabapentin treatment for muscle cramps: an open-label trial. *Clin Neuropharmacol* 2000;23(1):45-9.
10. Baltodano N, Gallo BV, Weidler DJ. Verapamil vs quinine in recumbent nocturnal leg cramps in the elderly. *Arch Intern Med* 1988;148(9):1969-70.

CHAPTER 19
Restless Legs Syndrome

Anne-Louise Lafontaine, MD

Restless legs syndrome (RLS) is a neurologic disorder characterized by an unpleasant sensation in the legs accompanied by an urge to move the legs, especially at bedtime.[1] In severe cases, symptoms may extend to the arms and trunk. The prevalence of RLS in the general population is estimated to be 5-15%;[1,2] prevalence is higher in women and increases with age. Patients often use the following terms to describe the symptoms of RLS: a "creepy-crawly," "burning," "nagging," "aching," "painful," "itching-bones" or "electric-current" sensation.

Diagnostic criteria have recently been established:[3]

- An urge to move the legs, usually accompanied or caused by unpleasant sensations in the legs.
- Symptoms begin or worsen during periods of rest or inactivity such as lying or sitting.
- Symptoms are partially or totally relieved by movement, such as walking or stretching, for at least as long as the activity continues.
- Symptoms are worse in the evening or at night than during the day, or occur only in the evening or at night.

Supportive clinical features include a positive family history, response to dopaminergic therapy and periodic limb movements during wakefulness (PLM) or during sleep (PLMS).[3]

Intermittent RLS is defined as symptoms that are troublesome enough to require treatment but not frequent enough to require daily therapy. *Daily* RLS involves symptoms that are frequent and bothersome enough to require daily therapy. Patients with *refractory* RLS are those who experience inadequate response and/or intolerable side effects and/or "augmentation" (see Goals of Therapy) not responding to more frequent dosing, while receiving dopamine agonist therapy for daily symptoms.

Goals of Therapy

- Improve the symptoms of motor restlessness and discomfort
- Improve sleep
- Reduce the PLMS, if disruptive
- Reduce the potential for "rebound" or "augmentation"
  - "rebound" is the recurrence of symptoms during the night or early morning coinciding with the end-of-dose wearing off of effectiveness[4]
  - "augmentation" is the occurrence of symptoms earlier in the day than they occurred prior to treatment, a shorter latency time to

symptom onset when at rest, an increase in the severity of symptoms with shorter treatment effect, and/or spread of symptoms to involve the upper extremities and trunk.[5]

Investigations

- History from patient and partner regarding sleep and PLMS
- CBC, electrolytes, BUN, creatinine, fasting glucose, serum iron, ferritin and iron saturation
- Nerve conduction studies can be performed if peripheral neuropathy is suspected
- Polysomnography should be performed if there is a clinical suspicion of sleep apnea or concurrent sleep disorder

Therapeutic Choices

Nonpharmacologic Choices

- Mental alertness activities (playing cards or video games or doing crossword puzzles) to reduce symptoms during times of boredom.[6]
- Abstinence from alcohol, caffeine and nicotine.[6]
- Hot baths, stretching and moderate exercise.[7]
- Discontinuing medications that may be contributing to symptoms, e.g., antidepressants, antipsychotics, dopamine-blocking antiemetics and sedating antihistamines.[6]

Pharmacologic Choices

Iron deficiency states are a known cause of secondary RLS; **iron replacement therapy** is indicated in the presence of low serum ferritin level or iron deficiency.

Dopamine agonists are considered the drugs of choice for most patients with daily RLS because of their long elimination half-life. Efficacy has been established in controlled clinical studies for **bromocriptine,**[8] **pergolide,**[9,10] **pramipexole**[11] and **ropinirole.**[12] These drugs improve sleep efficiency and decrease frequency of PLMS. Pergolide and bromocriptine are ergoline derivatives and are more frequently associated with adverse effects. Pergolide has been associated with restrictive valvular heart disease in patients being treated for Parkinson's disease.[13] Ropinirole and pramipexole are nonergoline derivatives and have a more favourable side effect profile overall, although they have been associated with a higher incidence of sudden sleep attacks in patients treated with higher doses for Parkinson's disease. The starting dose of pramipexole for RLS is 0.125 mg, taken two hours before the onset of symptoms, and can be increased every two to three days to effectiveness. The average effective dose is 0.5 mg but doses of up to 2 mg may be required. The starting dose of ropinirole is 0.25 mg. The average effective dose lies between 1 and 4 mg. Some patients may require a second dose in late afternoon if symptoms arise earlier in the day. Side effects of dopamine agonists include nausea, sedation and lightheadedness.

Levodopa/carbidopa has been shown in many clinical trials to be effective for the treatment of RLS.[14] The main limitation of levodopa/carbidopa is its short half-life, which increases the potential for rebound and augmentation. While levodopa/carbidopa may be appropriate for the treatment of *intermittent* RLS, dopamine agonists are the treatment of choice in *daily* RLS.

Gabapentin may be an alternative to dopamine agonists in the event of intolerability or augmentation (see Goals of Therapy). Effectiveness of gabapentin has been demonstrated in open[15] and randomized controlled trials.[16] It can be considered the drug of choice in the presence of a particularly *painful* RLS. Major side effects include drowsiness and unsteady gait, especially in the elderly.

Opioids have been used since the earliest descriptions of the treatment of RLS. Clinical effectiveness has been demonstrated in a few controlled as well as open clinical trials.[17] Opioids may be effective by virtue of their strong sedating properties rather than their effect on leg movements. Because of the potential for dependence, low-potency opioids such as **propoxyphene** and **codeine** are reserved for intermittent or daily RLS, and more potent agents such as **oxycodone** or **methadone** for refractory RLS.

Benzodiazepines have been demonstrated in clinical trials to significantly improve objective sleep efficiency and subjective sleep quality in both RLS and PLMS.[18] The main limitation of this class of drugs is the potential for dependence. Benzodiazepines are appropriate for the treatment of intermittent RLS or in refractory RLS where they can be added to first-line therapy. Given the long half-life of **clonazepam** and its potential to cause morning sedation and dizziness, consideration should be given to agents with short or intermediate duration of action in elderly patients.

Therapeutic Tips

- Always consider nonpharmacologic management.
- Start with a single dose of dopamine agonist 1–2 hours prior to bedtime. Titrate to effectiveness.
- In the event of symptoms beginning earlier in the day, a second dose of dopamine agonist can be prescribed in the afternoon, and if needed in the morning.
- Rebound can be avoided by prescribing dopamine agonists rather than levodopa.
- Augmentation has been reported less frequently with dopamine agonists than with levodopa. This can also be managed by alternating medications, i.e., switching between medication classes every few months as needed.

Figure 1: Management of Restless Legs Syndrome

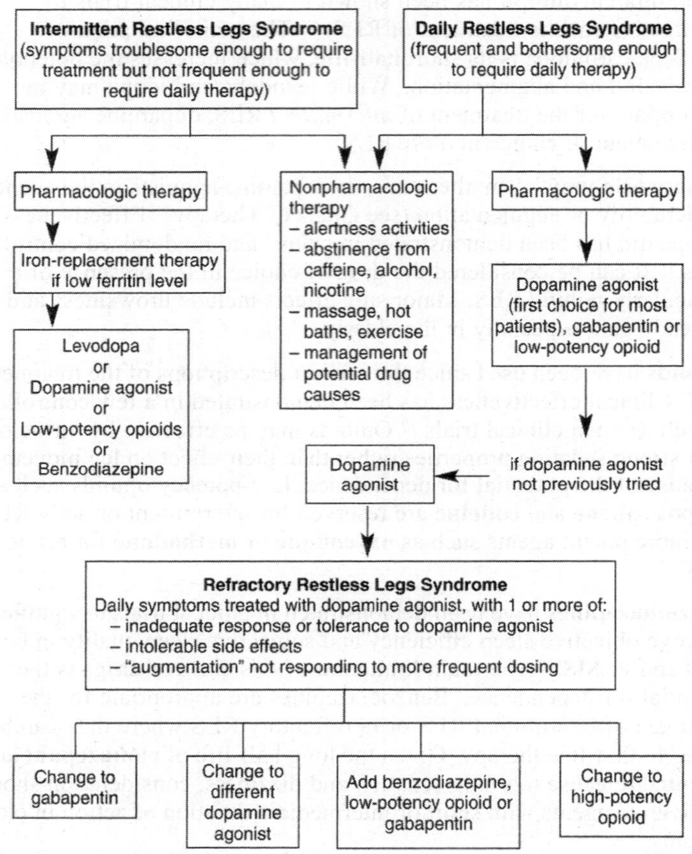

Adapted with permission from Silber MH, Ehrenberg BL, Allen RP et al. An algorithm for the management of restless legs syndrome. *Mayo Clin Proc* 2004;79(7):916-22.

Table 1: Drug Therapy for Restless Legs Syndrome

Class	Drug	Dose	Adverse Effects	Drug Interactions	Cost[a]
Dopamine Agonists	*bromocriptine* Parlodel, generics	7.5 mg HS	Nausea, vomiting, lightheadedness; hallucinations, psychosis, erythromelalgia (burning pain, warmth and redness of the extremities), pleural fibrosis.	First-generation antipsychotics ↓ effect of dopamine agonists.	$$
	pergolide Permax	0.025–0.5 mg per day in 2–3 divided doses if needed	See bromocriptine. Reports of cardiac valve regurgitation.	See bromocriptine.	$
	pramipexole Mirapex, generics	0.125–2 mg per day in 2–3 divided doses if needed	Lightheadedness, confusion, hallucinations, nausea, vomiting, sedation.	See bromocriptine.	$$$
	ropinirole ReQuip	0.25–4 mg per day in 2–3 divided doses if needed	See pramipexole.	See bromocriptine.	$$
Levodopa Preparations	*levodopa/ carbidopa* Sinemet, Sinemet CR, generics	50/12.5–200/50 mg HS	Nausea, vomiting, lightheadedness, dry mouth, "rebound" and "augmentation."	First-generation antipsychotics ↓ effect of levodopa. Antihypertensives, diuretics, tricyclic antidepressants may ↑ hypotensive action. Decreased absorption with high-protein meals.	$
Antiepileptics	*gabapentin* Neurontin, generics	300–3600 mg daily in 2–3 divided doses if needed	Sedation, dizziness, ataxia, tremor, vision changes, weight gain.	No known significant interactions.	$$$$

(cont'd)

Table 1: **Drug Therapy for Restless Legs Syndrome** *(cont'd)*

Class	Drug	Dose	Adverse Effects	Drug Interactions	Cost[a]
Opioids	*propoxyphene napsylate* Darvon-N, generics	100–600 mg per day in 2–3 divided doses if needed	Sedation, constipation, dependence.	Additive sedation with other CNS depressants such as alcohol.	$$
	codeine immediate-release, generics	30–180 mg per day in 2–3 divided doses if needed	See propoxyphene.	See propoxyphene.	$
	codeine sustained-release Codeine Contin	30–180 mg daily divided Q12H	See propoxyphene.	See propoxyphene.	$$
	oxycodone immediate-release Oxy-IR	5–30 mg daily in 2–3 divided doses if needed	See propoxyphene.	See propoxyphene.	$
	oxycodone sustained-release Oxycontin	10–20 mg at bedtime	See propoxyphene.	See propoxyphene.	$
	methadone generics	2.5–20 mg in 2 divided doses if needed	See propoxyphene.	See propoxyphene.	$
Benzodiazepines	*clonazepam* Rivotril, generics	0.25–2 mg HS	Sedation, dizziness, dependence.	Additive sedation with other CNS depressants such as alcohol.	$
	triazolam Halcion, generics	0.125–0.25 mg HS	See clonazepam.	See clonazepam.	$
	temazepam Restoril, generics	15–30 mg HS	See clonazepam.	See clonazepam.	$

Class	Drug	Dose	Adverse Effects	Drug Interactions	Cost[a]
Nonbenzodi-azepine Agonists	*zopiclone* Imovane, generics	3.75–7.5 mg HS	Bitter metallic taste.	Minimal additive effects with low doses of alcohol.	$

[a] Cost of 30-day supply of mean dose; includes drug cost only.
Legend: $ < $25 $$ $25–50 $$$ $50–75 $$$$ > $75

Suggested Readings

Comella CL. Restless legs syndrome: treatment with dopaminergic agents. *Neurology* 2002;58(4 Suppl 1):S87-S92.

Earley CJ. Clinical practice. Restless legs syndrome. *N Engl J Med* 2003;348(21):2103-9.

Silber MH, Ehrenberg BL, Allen RP et al. An algorithm for the management of restless legs syndrome. *Mayo Clin Proc* 2004;79(7):916-22.

References

1. Ekbom KA. Restless legs syndrome. *Neurology* 1960;10:868-73.
2. Lavigne GJ, Montplaisir JY. Restless legs syndrome and sleep bruxism: prevalence and associations among Canadians. *Sleep* 1994;17(8):739-43.
3. Allen RP, Picchietti D, Hening WA et al. Restless legs syndrome: diagnostic criteria, special considerations, and epidemiology. A report from the restless legs syndrome diagnosis and epidemiology workshop at the National Institutes of Health. *Sleep Med* 2003;4(2);101-19.
4. Guilleminault C, Cetel M, Philip P. Dopaminergic treatment of restless legs and rebound phenomenon. *Neurology* 1993;43(2):445.
5. Allen RP, Earley CJ. Augmentation of the restless legs syndrome with carbidopa/levodopa. *Sleep* 1996;19(3):205-13.
6. Silber MH, Ehrenberg BL, Allen RP et al. An algorithm for the management of restless legs syndrome. *Mayo Clin Proc* 2004;79(7):916-22.
7. Ryan M, Slevin JT. Restless legs syndrome. *Am J Health Syst Pharm* 2006;63(17):1599-612.
8. Walters AS, Hening WA, Kavey N et al. A double-blind randomized crossover trial of bromocriptine and placebo in restless legs syndrome. *Ann Neurol* 1988;24(3):455-8.
9. Wetter TC, Stiasny K, Winkelmann J et al. A randomized controlled study of pergolide in patients with restless legs syndrome. *Neurology* 1999;52(5):944-50.
10. Trenkwalder C, Hundemer HP, Lledo A et al. Efficacy of pergolide in treatment of restless legs syndrome: the PEARLS Study. *Neurology* 2004;62(8):1391-7.
11. Montplaisir J, Nicolas A, Denesle R et al. Restless legs syndrome improved by pramipexole: a double-blind randomized trial. *Neurology* 1999;52(5):938-43.
12. Adler CH, Hauser RA, Sethi K et al. Ropinirole for restless legs syndrome: a placebo-controlled crossover trial. *Neurology* 2004;62:1405-7.
13. Van Camp G, Flamez A, Cosyns B et al. Treatment of Parkinson's disease with pergolide and relation to restrictive valvular heart disease. *Lancet* 2004;363(9416):1179-83.
14. Montplaisir J, Lapierre O, Warnes H et al. The treatment of the restless legs syndrome with or without periodic leg movements in sleep. *Sleep* 1992;15(5):391-5.
15. Happe S, Klosch G, Saletu B et al. Treatment of idiopathic restless legs syndrome (RLS) with gabapentin. *Neurology* 2001;57(9):1717-19.
16. Garcia-Borreguero D, Larrosa O, de la Llave Y et al. Treatment of restless legs syndrome with gabapentin: a double-blind, cross-over study. *Neurology* 2002;59(10):1573-9.
17. Ondo WG. Methadone for refractory restless legs syndrome. *Mov Disord* 2005;20(3):345-8.
18. Saletu M, Anderer P, Saletu-Zyhlarz G, Prause W, Semler B, Zoghlami A et al. Restless legs syndrome (RLS) and periodic limb movement disorder (PLMD): acute placebo-controlled sleep laboratory studies with clonazepam. *Eur Neuropsychopharmacol* 2001;11(2):153-61.

CHAPTER 20
Parkinson's Disease

D.A. Grimes, MD, FRCPC

Parkinson's disease (PD) is a chronic, progressive, neurodegenerative disease whose cardinal features are tremor, bradykinesia and rigidity. Currently available treatments significantly decrease morbidity and mortality; however, no treatment to date has been shown to impact the underlying disease process.[1] Medications providing the most benefit are directed at replenishing dopamine within the brain.

Goals of Therapy

- Improve functioning and quality of life
- Minimize acute and long-term side effects of medications
- Instil a positive outlook, despite the chronic, progressive nature of PD

Investigations

- The clinical diagnosis of PD can be made with confidence if the classic features of a unilateral or asymmetric resting tremor plus bradykinesia and rigidity are present. The patient's earliest complaints may include fatigue, general slowness, poor handwriting and a tremulous feeling in one arm, without obvious tremor.
- Postural instability, autonomic dysfunction, dementia, impaired eye movements, rapid progression and poor response to dopaminergic therapy are not features of early PD, and if present suggest a different diagnosis.
- Perform imaging studies in young patients or those with atypical features. Exclude Wilson's disease in young patients by performing a serum ceruloplasmin, a slit-lamp examination and a 24-hour urine for copper.
- Exclude drug-induced parkinsonism. The most common drug causes include first- and second-generation antipsychotics and central dopamine-blocking antiemetics, e.g., metoclopramide and prochlorperazine.

Therapeutic Choices

Nonpharmacologic Choices

- Patient education via books, websites and local and national Parkinson societies (all available through the Parkinson Society of Canada, www.parkinson.ca).
- Stress importance of staying active and having a regular exercise routine.
- Encourage awareness of the important roles of allied health professionals such as speech, physical and occupational therapists.

Pharmacologic Choices (Figure 1)

Levodopa

Levodopa is converted to dopamine within presynaptic dopaminergic neurons. Although used alone when first discovered, today it is combined with a dopamine decarboxylase inhibitor, **carbidopa** or **benserazide**, to minimize acute side effects.

There has been concern that levodopa could be toxic to already damaged dopaminergic neurons through a mechanism involving excess oxidative stress.[2] There is little evidence for this in recent in vitro studies and no good evidence from in vivo animal models or human studies.[3]

Over time, many PD patients develop symptoms such as dysarthria, gait disorders, postural instability and cognitive dysfunction that are poorly responsive to levodopa therapy. The cause is mainly disease-related degeneration of nondopaminergic neuronal systems, and not that levodopa has become ineffective for the initial symptoms for which it was started.[2,3]

Though initially effective, levodopa therapy is eventually complicated by motor fluctuations and dyskinesia; these complications develop in up to 50% of patients after five years.[4,5] In the early stages of PD, patients enjoy a long-lasting response following a single dose of levodopa. With disease progression and longer-term treatment, patients begin to experience motor fluctuations, such as end-of-dose "wearing-off" of effectiveness or periods of fluctuating response known as "on-off" phenomena, and a variety of patterns of dyskinesia such as peak-dose dyskinesia (occurring during the peak effect of the dose), diphasic dyskinesia (occurring at the beginning and/or end of a dosing interval) and off-period dystonia (painful spasms, usually of the feet, occurring upon morning rising or when a dose is wearing off). The pathophysiology of these motor complications is not completely understood, but the leading theory suggests they are related to pulsatile stimulation of dopamine receptors resulting from intermittent dosing and levodopa's short plasma half-life.[5]

Factors shown to increase the risk of levodopa-induced dyskinesia include higher doses of levodopa, longer duration of treatment, severity of the underlying nigral degeneration and a younger age of disease onset.[5] Delaying the use of levodopa, especially in young-onset patients, has become the standard of practice in many movement disorder centres. Slow-release preparations of levodopa benefit patients having difficulty with "wearing-off," although good randomized trials are lacking;[6] there is no evidence that initiating treatment with controlled-release levodopa provides an advantage over immediate-release formulations.[7] A variety of strategies can be used to help treat patients who have developed "wearing-off" or dyskinesia (Figure 2).

Dopamine Agonists

Bromocriptine, pergolide, pramipexole and **ropinirole** are effective as monotherapy in the early stages of the disease, and as adjunctive therapy with levodopa for more advanced patients with motor complications.[6,7] A transdermal patch containing **rotigotine** is expected to become available. Compared to levodopa, dopamine agonists are associated with fewer motor complications in the first five years of the disease, but it is unknown if this translates into long-term benefit for patients.[6,7] Although all clinical trials demonstrate a lower efficacy compared to levodopa, this difference does not seem to affect quality-of-life scores in early disease.[7,8] Because of the lower incidence of motor complications, dopamine agonists are typically used as initial therapy in younger patients, then levodopa is added in the case of poor tolerance or inadequate benefit, or later because of waning efficacy of the dopamine agonist.

Because pergolide has recently been associated with a high rate of cardiac valve fibrosis and bromocriptine can cause pulmonary fibrosis, the newer, non-ergot dopamine agonists (pramipexole and ropinirole) are better choices.[9,10] Daytime sleepiness or sudden irresistible attacks of sleep can occur with all of the dopamine replacement medications, including levodopa. Sudden attacks of sleep seem to occur more frequently with the newer dopamine agonists.[11] Personality changes such as hypersexual behaviour and pathologic gambling have also been associated with these medications; discuss these rare but important side effects with your patient.[12] Additional difficulties with dopamine agonists, compared to levodopa, include more GI upset, orthostatic hypotension and psychiatric reactions (hallucinations and confusion); in addition, supplementary levodopa is almost always required for supervening disability after varying periods of time. For these reasons, dopamine agonists tend to be used less frequently in older individuals.

MAO-B Inhibitors

Early clinical evaluations of **selegiline**, an irreversible inhibitor of monoamine oxidase B (MAO-B), suggested that it might slow the progression of PD. The weight of evidence now indicates that it does not have a substantial neuroprotective effect, and most of the apparent benefit during the first year of treatment is likely due to its very mild effects on symptoms.[7] In addition, it does not delay the development of dyskinesia or fluctuations associated with chronic levodopa therapy. A second, more potent, MAO-B inhibitor **rasagiline** is now available as initial treatment to improve motor symptoms and for patients with more advanced disease to help with "wearing-off." Initial studies suggested it may slow disease progression but further evidence is needed.[13]

Amantadine

Amantadine provides mild-to-modest improvement in about two-thirds of early PD patients and improves levodopa-induced dyskinesia in the later stages of the disease.[6] Its exact mechanism of action is unclear but it may act by releasing dopamine from the presynaptic terminals or by blocking its reuptake. Amantadine is an N-methyl-D-aspartate (NMDA) antagonist, which may account for some of its antiparkinsonian efficacy. NMDA receptor blockade confers a neuroprotective effect in some animal models of parkinsonism, and it has been suggested that amantadine improves survival in PD patients; however, this is far from proven. It is easy to use and usually well tolerated, with leg edema, erythema and livedo reticularis (a reversible condition characterized by bluish, mottled appearance of the skin, mainly of the lower extremities) being the most common adverse events. In patients with cognitive deficits, amantadine can increase confusion and should not be used.

Anticholinergics

Anticholinergic drugs such as **benztropine**, **biperiden**, **ethopropazine**, **procyclidine** and **trihexyphenidyl** have been used in the treatment of PD for decades, since before the availability of levodopa. Their major putative effect is on tremor, with little or no effect on bradykinesia; however, this has not been well studied.[2] They can be used as monotherapy or as adjuncts to dopaminergic therapy. Their many side effects (e.g., dry mouth, urinary retention, constipation) limit their use, especially in the elderly.

COMT Inhibitors

COMT (catechol-O-methyl transferase), an enzyme that helps metabolize levodopa, is found in both the brain and in the peripheral nervous system. COMT inhibitors such as **entacapone** and **tolcapone** help prevent peripheral metabolism of levodopa, which increases its availability to the brain. They have no effect if not used in conjunction with levodopa. Despite some studies showing additional improvement in activities of daily living, in non-fluctuating patients their use should be limited to patients with wearing-off.[6] Most of their side effects relate to increased dopaminergic activity in the brain (e.g., dyskinesia and, less often, confusion/hallucinations). Because of this, levodopa dosage may have to be reduced by up to 30% when a COMT inhibitor is initiated. Tolcapone was the first COMT inhibitor to be approved, but because of associated hepatotoxicity it is now available only through the Special Access Programme, Health Canada, for use in exceptional cases. Entacapone is not associated with liver toxicity, but two other potential side effects are diarrhea (often weeks to months after initiation) and a harmless discolouration of the urine that patients need to be warned about.

Surgery

Recognition that there is a limit to the medical management of PD brought about a resurgence of surgical treatments. Two main surgical procedures have been shown to be effective — lesioning procedures and deep brain stimulation. Surgical treatment of PD mainly targets the thalamus (improves tremor), globus pallidum (improves dyskinesia) and the subthalamic nucleus (improves bradykinesia, tremor and dyskinesia). These are performed only in patients with advanced disease in whom medications can no longer control symptoms. It is important for patients to understand that these surgeries are not a cure and will only improve function to the level of their best "on" times.

Complications — Depression, Psychosis, Dementia

Depression is common in PD, but keep in mind that a lack of facial expression in a patient with PD does not necessarily indicate sadness or depression. Selective serotonin reuptake inhibitors (SSRIs) and tricyclic antidepressants (TCAs) have been the mainstay of therapy for depression in patients with PD, yet there is a surprising lack of evidence to guide the choice of antidepressant.[14] TCAs should be used cautiously because their anticholinergic effects are more likely to induce delirium, especially in memory-impaired patients; they may also aggravate orthostatic hypotension, which can increase the risk of falls.

Psychosis and *dementia* are also very common in PD, typically in patients with more advanced disease. All medications used to treat the motor symptoms can contribute to psychosis in a dose-related fashion. As the disease progresses, PD medications often need to be withdrawn because of worsening of the patient's cognitive status. Usually, anticholinergics are withdrawn first, then selegiline, rasagiline, amantadine and dopamine agonists, until only levodopa remains. Review other (non-PD) medications carefully to ensure they are not also contributing to the psychosis. The atypical antipsychotics **clozapine** and **quetiapine** can be used for patients in whom an optimum balance cannot be found by adjusting the PD medication.[14] Avoid olanzapine as it has not been shown to be effective and is poorly tolerated.[14]

Cholinesterase inhibitors (e.g., **donepezil** and **rivastigmine**) have a modest impact on improving dementia, but careful observation for deterioration in motor function is required.[14]

Therapeutic Tips

- In the early stage of PD when symptoms are noticed but not troublesome, symptomatic treatment is not necessary, remembering that all drugs have potential side effects.
- To minimize the acute side effects of medications it is important to start at low doses and titrate slowly, especially in the elderly.
- To minimize gastric upset or orthostatic hypotension, **domperidone** (10 to 20 mg ½ hr prior to each dose) can be very helpful when starting levodopa or a dopamine agonist.
- Individualize patient management based on the severity of disease, level of disability, cost, patient preference and patient's age.
- Nonmotor difficulties (e.g., dysarthria, sleep disturbance, depression, dementia and postural instability) are common, especially as the disease progresses. Managing these effectively with the assistance of allied health professionals is important for maximizing a patient's quality of life.

Figure 1: **Initial Pharmacologic Management of Parkinson's Disease**

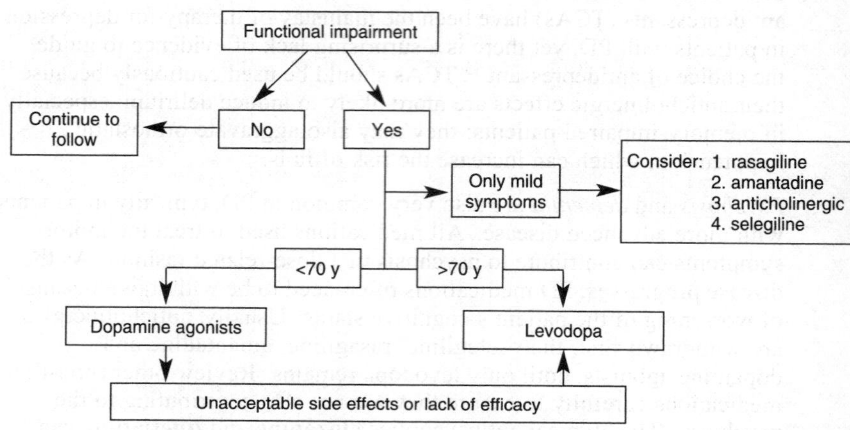

Figure 2: **Management of Levodopa-associated Motor Complications**

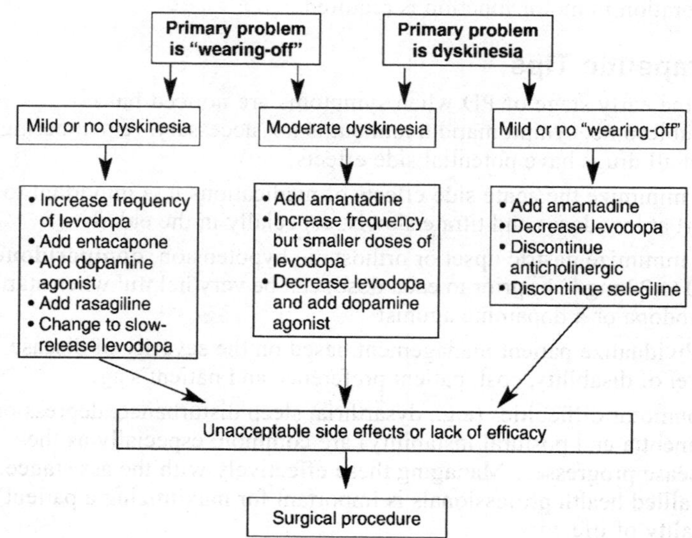

Table 1: **Drugs Used in the Treatment of Parkinson's Disease**

Class	Drug	Dose	Adverse Effects	Drug Interactions	Cost[a]
Levodopa Preparations	*levodopa/carbidopa, immediate-release* Sinemet, generics	Initial: 50/12.5 mg BID Usual: 100/25 mg – 150/37.5 mg TID–QID	Nausea, vomiting, orthostatic hypotension, dyskinesias, hallucinations, confusion.	First-generation antipsychotics ↓ effect of dopaminergic drugs. Antihypertensives, diuretics, tricyclic antidepressants may ↑ hypotensive action.	$
	levodopa/carbidopa, controlled-release Sinemet CR, generics	Initial:[b] 100/25 mg BID Usual:[b] 200/50 mg QID	See levodopa/carbidopa, immediate-release. ↓ "kick" compared to Sinemet immediate-release; patterns of dyskinesia may be more complex.	See levodopa/carbidopa, immediate-release.	$$
	levodopa/benserazide Prolopa	Initial: 50/12.5 mg BID Usual: 100/25 mg – 150/37.5 mg TID–QID	See levodopa/carbidopa, immediate-release.	See levodopa/carbidopa, immediate-release.	$
Dopamine Agonists	*bromocriptine* Parlodel, generics	Initial: 1.25 mg BID Usual: 5–10 mg TID	Nausea, vomiting, orthostatic hypotension, hallucinations, psychosis, erythromelalgia (burning pain, warmth and redness of the extremities), pleural fibrosis (do a baseline chest x-ray before initiating therapy).	See levodopa/carbidopa, immediate-release.	$$-$$$

(cont'd)

Table 1: Drugs Used in the Treatment of Parkinson's Disease *(cont'd)*

Class	Drug	Dose	Adverse Effects	Drug Interactions	Cost[a]
	pergolide Permax	Initial: 0.05 mg daily Usual: 0.5–1.5 mg TID	See bromocriptine. Reports of cardiac valve regurgitation.	See levodopa/carbidopa, immediate-release.	\$\$\$\$-\$\$\$\$\$
	pramipexole Mirapex	Initial: 0.125 mg TID Usual: 0.5–1 mg TID	Orthostatic hypotension, somnolence, confusion, hallucinations, nausea, vomiting, sudden sleep attacks; caution patients about driving or operating dangerous machinery.	See levodopa/carbidopa, immediate-release.	\$\$\$\$
	ropinirole ReQuip	Initial: 0.25 mg TID Usual: 3–6 mg TID	See pramipexole.	See levodopa/carbidopa, immediate-release. Ciprofloxacin ↑ levels of ropinirole.	\$\$\$\$-\$\$\$\$\$
MAO-B Inhibitors	*rasagiline* Azilect	Monotherapy: 1 mg daily Adjunctive therapy: 0.5–1 mg daily	Insomnia, confusion, hallucinations, ↑ dyskinesia, autonomic dysfunction. Use lower dose of 0.5 mg in patients with mild hepatic impairment and avoid in patients with severe impairment.	Avoid use with antidepressants such as TCAs, MAO-A inhibitors, SNRIs, SSRIs. Use lower dose of 0.5 mg daily in patients taking ciprofloxacin or other CYP1A2 inhibitors.	\$\$\$\$\$

Class	Drug	Dose	Adverse Effects	Drug Interactions	Cost[a]
	selegiline (deprenyl) generics	2.5 mg daily – 5 mg BID Give before 1 p.m.	See rasagiline.	Avoid use with pseudoephedrine, meperidine, dextromethorphan, TCAs, MAO-A inhibitors, SSRIs, atomoxetine, bupropion, dextroamphetamine. May need to reduce dose in women taking oral contraceptives.	$-$$
COMT Inhibitors	*entacapone* Comtan	200 mg with each dose of levodopa; max 8 × daily	Dyskinesia, nausea, sleep disorder, anorexia, diarrhea, hallucinations; urine discolouration.	Potentiates levodopa; increased dyskinesia, psychosis. Avoid nonselective MAOIs, isoproterenol, epinephrine, dopamine, dobutamine.	$$$-$$$$
Anticholinergic Agents	*benztropine* Cogentin, generics	1 mg BID – 2 mg BID	Dry mouth, blurred vision, constipation, urinary retention, aggravation of glaucoma, confusion, memory impairment. Avoid in elderly.	Amantadine may ↑ anticholinergic effects.	$
	ethopropazine Parsitan	25 mg BID – 50 mg TID	See benztropine.	See benztropine.	$
	procyclidine generics	5 mg TID	See benztropine.	See benztropine.	$

(cont'd)

Table 1: **Drugs Used in the Treatment of Parkinson's Disease** *(cont'd)*

Class	Drug	Dose	Adverse Effects	Drug Interactions	Cost[a]
	trihexyphenidyl generics	Initial: 1 mg BID Usual: 2 mg TID	See benztropine.	See benztropine.	$
N-methyl-D-aspartate (NMDA) Receptor Antagonists	*amantadine* ❥ Symmetrel (Antiparkinson), generics	Usual: 100 mg BID	Nausea, constipation, dry mouth, insomnia, anxiety, impaired concentration, livedo reticularis, orthostatic hypotension, ankle edema. Use with caution in elderly; avoid in patients with cognitive deficits.	Anticholinergic agents may ↑ effects.	$

[a] Cost of 30-day supply of usual dose; includes drug cost only.
[b] Compared to Sinemet immediate-release formulation, bioavailability of Sinemet CR is 25–30% lower and duration of action 25–30% longer.
❥ Dosage adjustment is required in renal impairment; see Appendix I.
Abbreviations: MAOIs = monoamine oxidase inhibitors; SNRIs = serotonin-norepinephrine reuptake inhibitors; SSRIs = selective serotonin reuptake inhibitors; TCAs = tricyclic antidepressants
Legend: $ < $50 $-$$ < $50–100 $$ $50–100 $$-$$$ $50–150 $$$ $100–150 $$$-$$$$ $100–200 $$$$ $150–200 $$$$-$$$$$ $150– >200 $$$$$ > $200

Suggested Readings

Lang AE, Lozano AM. Parkinson's disease. Second of two parts. *N Engl J Med* 1998;339(16):1130-43.

Miyasaki JM, Martin W, Suchowersky O et al. Practice Parameter: initiation of treatment for Parkinson's disease: an evidence-based review: report of the Quality Standards Subcommittee of the American Academy of Neurology. *Neurology* 2002;58(1):11-7.

Pahwa R, Factor SA, Lyons KE et al. Practice Parameter: treatment of Parkinson disease with motor fluctuations and dyskinesia (an evidence-based review): report of the Quality Standards Subcommittee of the American Academy of Neurology. *Neurology* 2006;66(7):983-95.

Suchowersky O, Gronseth G, Perlmutter J et al. Practice Parameter: neuroprotective strategies and alternative therapies for Parkinson disease (an evidence-based review): report of the Quality Standards Subcommittee of the American Academy of Neurology. *Neurology* 2006;66(7):976-82.

References

1. Suchowersky O, Gronseth G, Perlmutter J et al. Practice Parameter: neuroprotective strategies and alternative therapies for Parkinson disease (an evidence-based review): report of the Quality Standards Subcommittee of the American Academy of Neurology. *Neurology* 2006;66(7):976-82.
2. Grimes DA, Lang AE. Treatment of early Parkinson's disease. *Can J Neurol Sci* 1999;26(Suppl 2):S39-44.
3. Fahn S. Does levodopa slow or hasten the rate of progression of Parkinson's disease? *J Neurol* 2005;252(Suppl 4):IV37-IV42.
4. Lang AE, Lozano AM. Parkinson's disease. Second of two parts. *N Engl J Med* 1998;339(16):1130-43.
5. Olanow CW, Agid Y, Mizuno Y et al. Levodopa in the treatment of Parkinson's disease: current controversies. *Mov Disord* 2004;19(9):997-1005.
6. Pahwa R, Factor SA, Lyons KE et al. Practice Parameter: treatment of Parkinson disease with motor fluctuations and dyskinesia (an evidence-based review): report of the Quality Standards Subcommittee of the American Academy of Neurology. *Neurology* 2006;66(7):983-95.
7. Miyasaki JM, Martin W, Suchowersky O et al. Practice Parameter: initiation of treatment for Parkinson's disease: an evidence-based review: report of the Quality Standards Subcommittee of the American Academy of Neurology. *Neurology* 2002;58(1):11-7.
8. Holloway RG, Shoulson I, Fahn S et al. Pramipexole vs levodopa as initial treatment for Parkinson disease: a 4-year randomized controlled trial. *Arch Neurol* 2004;61(7):1044-53.
9. Baseman DG, O'Suilleabhain PE, Reimold SC et al. Pergolide use in Parkinson disease is associated with cardiac valve regurgitation. *Neurology* 2004;63(2):301-4.
10. Van Camp G, Flamez A, Cosyns B et al. Treatment of Parkinson's disease with pergolide and relation to restrictive valvular heart disease. *Lancet* 2004;363(9416):1179-83.
11. Hobson DE, Lang AE, Martin WR et al. Excessive daytime sleepiness and sudden-onset sleep in Parkinson disease: a survey by the Canadian Movement Disorders Group. *JAMA* 2002;287(4):455-63.
12. Dodd ML, Klos KJ, Bower JH et al. Pathological gambling caused by drugs used to treat Parkinson disease. *Arch Neurol* 2005;62(9):1377-81.
13. Parkinson Study Group. A controlled, randomized, delayed-start study of rasagiline in early Parkinson disease. *Arch Neurol* 2004;61(4):561-6.
14. Miyasaki JM, Shannon K, Voon V et al. Practice Parameter: evaluation and treatment of depression, psychosis, and dementia in Parkinson disease (an evidence-based review): report of the Quality Standards Subcommittee of the American Academy of Neurology. *Neurology* 2006;66(7):996-1002.

CHAPTER 21
Seizures and Epilepsy

R. Mark Sadler, MD, FRCPC

Goals of Therapy

- Decide whether treatment with antiepileptic drugs (AEDs) is indicated for the patient presenting with the first seizure
- Prevent seizure recurrence in patients with an established diagnosis of epilepsy, i.e., patients with recurrent seizures
- Prevent or minimize adverse effects of AEDs
- Optimize quality of life, e.g., employment, psychosocial interactions, driving

Investigations (Figure 1)

History

- Most important factor in making a diagnosis is a detailed history of the patient's "spells" obtained from both the patient and a witness (see Clinical Features).
- Is there an aura? An aura signifies the onset of the seizure, and its features provide valuable clues to the anatomic site of the seizure onset. Lack of an aura indicates partial seizures that spread very rapidly or that the seizures are of the primary generalized variety.
- Inquire about history of intracranial sepsis, head trauma, stroke, any systemic disorders that may affect the central nervous system (e.g., malignancies, fluid and electrolyte disorders), drugs (prescribed or recreational), sleep deprivation, symptoms of raised intracranial pressure and family history of seizures or other neurologic diseases.

Clinical Features[1,2]

- Simple partial seizures:
  - motor or sensory features
  - no impairment of consciousness
  - usually brief (< 60 seconds)
- Complex partial seizures:
  - focally originating seizures characterized by impaired awareness and a blank stare
  - duration of one to two minutes
  - frequently accompanied by motor automatisms, e.g., lip smacking and chewing movements
  - brief postictal confusion is common
  - begin with simple partial features or impaired consciousness, and are commonly misdiagnosed as absence seizures

- Absence ("petit mal"):
  - primary generalized seizure type
  - last only seconds, usually 5–10
  - recur daily (often in clusters) in the untreated patient
  - no warning signs or postictal confusion
  - onset in childhood or adolescence (almost never *begin* in adulthood)
- Primary or secondarily generalized tonic-clonic ("grand mal"):
  - fairly uniform sequence of motor features (tonic and clonic phases)
  - impaired consciousness
  - duration of one to two minutes
  - postictal stupor, confusion and headache
  - a careful history may reveal a partial seizure (e.g., simple partial or complex partial) that secondarily evolves to a generalized tonic-clonic seizure
- Atonic seizures:
  - abrupt loss of consciousness and muscle tone
  - no other motor features
  - return to awareness in seconds
  - occur as part of a clinical scenario in patients with childhood onset epilepsy, significant intellectual handicaps and other seizure types
  - virtually never occur in otherwise intellectually and physically intact adults
- Myoclonic seizures:
  - a generalized seizure type consisting of brief, bilateral "shock-like" jerks
  - multifocal asynchronous myoclonic jerks most commonly occur in the setting of a metabolic encephalopathy
- Consider whether the clinical features suggest one of the entities (e.g., syncope or psychogenic nonepileptic seizures) commonly mistaken for epileptic seizures

Physical Examination

- Look for evidence of any systemic disorder that can affect the central nervous system, e.g., a malignancy
- Look for focal or lateralizing findings in the neurologic examination (hemianopia, motor weakness, hemisensory disturbance, reflex asymmetry)
- Assess potential injuries sustained during a generalized tonic-clonic seizure, such as tongue laceration, shoulder dislocation or vertebral compression fracture

Laboratory Investigations

- For the patient presenting with the *first seizure,* consider:

- CBC, glucose, electrolytes, calcium, renal and hepatic function
- chest x-ray if metastatic disease is a consideration
- electroencephalogram (EEG) to support the clinical impression of seizures and to determine if the seizure is partial (focally originating) or primary generalized. The interictal EEG may show focal spikes in patients with partial seizures or generalized spike-waves in the primary generalized epilepsies
- computed tomography (CT) head scan. Adults should have a CT scan unless the patient is otherwise well and their EEG demonstrates generalized spike-and-wave discharges (which indicates one of the primary generalized seizure syndromes that are not accompanied by gross structural brain abnormalities). Patients should have a CT scan before a lumbar puncture
- lumbar puncture if the presenting clinical features suggest intracranial infection (meningitis, encephalitis) or a CT-negative subarachnoid hemorrhage
- magnetic resonance imaging (MRI) scan if the patient has partial seizures of unknown etiology and negative CT scan

- For the patient with *known epilepsy treated with AEDs* and presenting with a *seizure recurrence*, assess:
  - factors that may precipitate loss of seizure control (medication noncompliance, intercurrent illness with fever and vomiting, sleep deprivation, alcohol and other nonprescription drug use)
  - the addition (or sudden withdrawal) of a drug that may promote seizures or may cause a drug interaction with AEDs
- Measure AED serum levels (phenytoin, phenobarbital, primidone, carbamazepine, valproic acid). Serum levels for other AEDs are not available or are of limited clinical value

Therapeutic Choices

Nonpharmacologic Choices

- Avoid sleep deprivation.
- Keep alcohol consumption to a minimum. Cocaine and amphetamines must be forbidden because of their proconvulsant properties. The evidence for marijuana as a "pro-" or "anti-" seizure drug is inconclusive.

Pharmacologic Choices[3,4,5]

The choice of an AED depends on the seizure type (Table 1), potential for drug interactions and side effects (Table 3), cost (Table 3) and physician familiarity with the drug. Current evidence does not allow an evidence-based recommendation for initial AED monotherapy.[5]

Basic principles are:

- Select a single AED.

- Start the AED at a fraction of the initial target dose to minimize the risk of dose-dependent adverse effects (exceptions are phenytoin and phenobarbital).
- Inform patient of potential risks of treatment (especially hypersensitivity reactions).
- Evaluate the patient after the initial target dose has been achieved. Make a small dose reduction if dose-related adverse effects are problematic. Slowly increase the dose if seizures have recurred.
- Add a second AED if the maximum tolerated dose of the first AED has failed to achieve satisfactory seizure control. Gradually withdraw the first AED after the maintenance dose of the second drug has been achieved. Polytherapy is usually reserved until monotherapy with two to three drugs has failed.

Table 1: **Suggested Therapeutic Choices for Antiepileptic Drugs (AEDs)[a]**

Seizure Type	First Choice Monotherapy[a]	Alternate Monotherapy or Add-on[a]
Generalized Tonic-clonic	carbamazepine lamotrigine phenytoin valproic acid	clobazam levetiracetam topiramate
Absence	ethosuximide valproic acid	clobazam lamotrigine levetiracetam topiramate
Myoclonic and Atonic	valproic acid	clobazam lamotrigine levetiracetam topiramate
Partial (simple or complex) with or without 2° Generalization	carbamazepine lamotrigine phenytoin	clobazam gabapentin levetiracetam oxcarbazepine phenobarbital primidone topiramate valproic acid vigabatrin

[a] AEDs are listed alphabetically; the order does not reflect a preference ranking.

The First Seizure[6,7]

- The decision of whether or not to treat with AEDs after the first seizure can be difficult for the patient and physician and must be individualized.

- Most patients come to medical attention with a primary or secondarily generalized tonic-clonic seizure. At least one-third of these patients have experienced prior unrecognized nocturnal tonic-clonic seizures and/or nonconvulsive seizures. It is important to determine if the event was *truly* the first seizure. Patients with unequivocal prior seizures should generally be treated, as the risk for seizure recurrence is high.
- Not all patients with a single convulsion will have a recurrence. The overall risk of recurrence after a single unprovoked seizure is 40% within two years, but the degree of risk can be stratified based on other factors. For example, the recurrence risk over two years after a single idiopathic seizure with a normal EEG is 24%. In this situation most would not advocate treatment.
- The risks of treatment must be weighed against the likelihood of seizure recurrence. An increased risk of recurrence is suggested if one or more of the following features are present:
  - clear, known remote cause of seizure
  - focally originating seizure
  - abnormal neurologic examination
  - abnormal EEG (particularly if the EEG demonstrates epileptiform discharges)

Women with Epilepsy[8,9,10]

- There is an increased risk of oral contraceptive (OC) failure in women taking enzyme-inducing AEDs. (The OC should contain > 35 micrograms of estradiol.)
- Discuss pregnancy plans *prior* to conception:
  - is AED treatment still required?
  - withdraw least helpful AEDs if the patient is treated with AED polytherapy (determined by the history of which drug seemed to be more or less helpful when added).
  - over 90% of women with epilepsy treated with AEDs have successful pregnancies and outcomes. AEDs confer an increased risk of congenital malformations and other adverse effects. Current evidence does not allow selection of an AED that is "best" for this patient population, but recent data suggest that valproic acid is associated with the highest risk of adverse outcomes among the commonly used AEDs.
  - women of childbearing potential who take AEDs should receive continuous **folic acid** supplementation (5 mg/day) to potentially reduce the risk of teratogenic effects associated with AEDs.
- During pregnancy:
  - follow AED levels as they may drop significantly.
  - obtain expert obstetrical advice on timing and type of ultrasound to detect fetal malformations.
  - start oral **vitamin K** (10 mg/day) in last four weeks of pregnancy.

- Postpartum:
  - breastfeeding is generally acceptable. Babies whose mothers are taking barbiturates may be sedated; babies exposed to barbiturates prepartum and not breastfeeding may have barbiturate withdrawal symptoms in the first week after delivery.
  - follow AED levels as they may rise precipitously in the first weeks post-delivery.

Status Epilepticus (SE)[11,12]

- "Convulsive" SE was traditionally defined as recurrent primary or secondarily generalized tonic-clonic seizures lasting > 30 minutes, or intermittent seizures lasting > 30 minutes, from which the patient does not return to consciousness.

  Note: Almost all "isolated" tonic-clonic seizures last < 2 minutes. A tonic-clonic seizure lasting > 5 minutes is therefore "different" and has been defined as "impending SE." Impending SE should be treated aggressively in the first 30 minutes.[12]
- Any seizure type can evolve to "nonconvulsive" status epilepticus (absence, partial complex, simple partial).
- Psychogenic nonepileptic seizures (psychiatrically based behaviours that are not associated with abnormal EEG rhythms) can be confused with convulsive SE because of some superficial similarities. Conversely, absence or partial complex SE is often misdiagnosed as a psychiatric condition.
- Convulsive SE is associated with high morbidity and mortality, related to underlying cause and effects on the brain caused by the seizures. Brain injury begins at 30 to 45 minutes of SE; aggressive treatment of seizures is important to optimize outcome. Table 2 outlines a suggested treatment protocol.

Table 2: **Initial Management of Convulsive Status Epilepticus**

Time	Management
0–5 min	History, physical examination. Oral airway, oxygen. Consider intubation. Venous blood (glucose, blood counts, electrolytes, calcium, renal and liver function, AED blood levels, consider drug screen). Arterial blood gases. Monitor ECG, pulse oximetry, blood pressure.
5–10 min	Start 2 large-bore iv saline infusions. 50 mL dextrose 50% iv. Thiamine 50–100 mg im. Lorazepam 2 mg/min iv, to max dose of 0.1 mg/kg ***or*** diazepam 5 mg/min iv, to max dose of 0.25–0.4 mg/kg.

(cont'd)

Table 2: **Initial Management of Convulsive Status Epilepticus** *(cont'd)*

Time	Management
10–30 min	Phenytoin 20 mg/kg iv (maximum rate = 50 mg/min) ***or*** phenobarbital[a] 20 mg/kg iv (50–75 mg/min) ***or*** midazolam 10 mg iv bolus, then 0.05–0.4 mg/kg/h ***or*** propofol 2–5 mg/kg iv bolus followed by infusion at 2–10 mg/kg/h.
30–60 min	Obtain neuroimaging (CT, MRI) if etiology of SE not known; consider lumbar puncture if a possibility of meningitis-encephalitis. Admit to critical care unit, obtain expert advice, arrange EEG.

[a] Phenobarbital injection is available through Health Canada's Special Access Programme.
Abbreviations: AED = antiepileptic drug; EEG = electroencephalogram; ECG = electrocardiogram

Other General Measures

- To reduce the risk of burns during seizures:
  - discourage smoking
  - encourage patients to use microwave ovens and place pots and pans on the rear burners of stoves
- Showers are preferable to tub baths because of the risk of drowning.
- Assess recreational activities, current and planned employment.
- Patients with active epilepsy who are caregivers for young children should not bathe them without assistance and should not use change tables for clothing or diaper changes.
- Assess driving status. Physicians should be aware of their legal obligations to local departments of transportation (mandatory vs. discretional reporting).
- Some patients may benefit from the activities of epilepsy support groups.

Therapeutic Tips

- Obtain a baseline CBC and serum liver transaminases (and repeat in four to six weeks) if treating with an AED that may cause a hypersensitivity syndrome involving blood or liver. Mild elevations (< 2–3 times normal) of liver enzymes and/or modest reductions in blood counts (e.g., neutropenia with carbamazepine; thrombocytopenia with valproic acid) are relatively common. Neither requires discontinuation of treatment but the abnormality should be followed with serial studies.
- Do not rely on serum AED levels alone to guide therapy as their validity is not established. Some patients will have satisfactory seizure control at low AED levels, while others have dose-related toxicity below the upper end of the quoted "therapeutic" range. A useful adage is "treat the patient, not the serum level."
- With many AEDs, drug interactions are potential problems. Drugs with hepatic enzyme-inducing properties (carbamazepine, phenytoin,

phenobarbital, primidone) may reduce the levels of concomitant medications. The presence (or absence) of other medications should be considered when selecting an AED.

- Consider epilepsy surgery for patients with medically refractory partial seizures. Refer these patients to tertiary-care epilepsy programs for evaluation.

Figure 1: **Management of Seizures and Epilepsy**

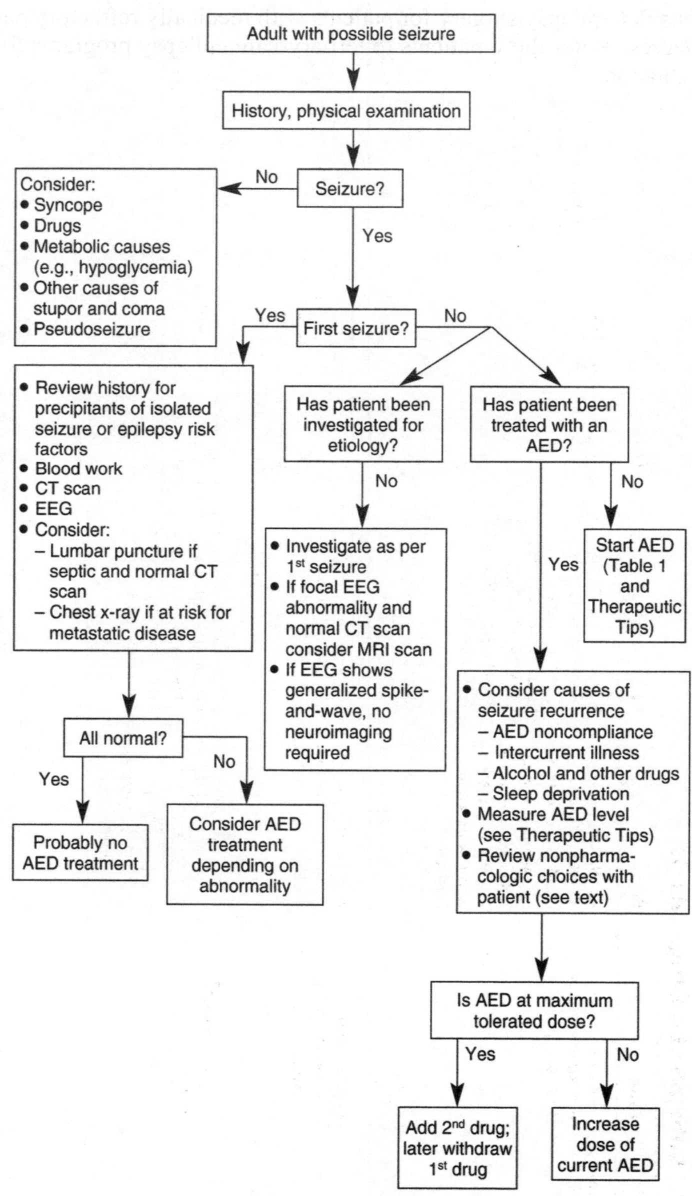

Abbreviations: CT=computed tomography; MRI=magnetic resonance imaging; EEG=electroencephalogram; AED=anti-epileptic drugs

Table 3: **Antiepileptic Drugs (AEDs)**

Class	Drug	Dose	Adverse Effects[a]	Advantages	Disadvantages	Cost[b]
Iminostilbene Derivatives	*carbamazepine immediate-release* Tegretol, generics	Initial: 100 mg BID; increase by 200 mg/day Q3–4 days Usual maintenance: 800–1200 mg/day in 2–4 divided doses, with meals when possible	Rash 5–10%; rarely, can be very serious. ↑ liver enzymes; transient neutropenia (common); aplastic anemia (extremely rare); hyponatremia.	Linear pharmacokinetics.	Substrate of CYP3A4 and inducer of CYP1A2, 3A4, 2C9, 2C19, 2D6, 3A4 and 2C8, therefore many potential drug interactions; may ↓ effectiveness of oral contraceptives; available only as oral formulations; may worsen absence seizures; may produce or exacerbate myoclonus.	$
	carbamazepine controlled-release Tegretol CR, generics	800–1200 mg/day in 2 divided doses with meals	See carbamazepine immediate-release.	BID dosing; linear pharmacokinetics; CR preparation may be better tolerated and improve compliance.	See carbamazepine immediate-release.	$
	oxcarbazepine Trileptal	Initial: 300 mg BID; ↑ by ≤ 600 mg/day at weekly intervals Usual maintenance: 1200–2400 mg/day in 2 divided doses	Similar to carbamazepine but slightly higher risk of hyponatremia; skin rash cross-reaction with carbamazepine.	BID dosing; efficacy may be similar to carbamazepine but better tolerated; no autoinduction of liver enzymes.	↓ efficacy of oral contraceptives; available only as oral formulation.	$$$$$

(cont'd)

Table 3: **Antiepileptic Drugs (AEDs)** *(cont'd)*

Class	Drug	Dose	Adverse Effects[a]	Advantages	Disadvantages	Cost[b]
Benzodi-azepines	*clobazam* Frisium, generics	Initial: 5–15 mg/day, preferably at HS Usual maintenance: 20–40 mg/day in 1 or 2 divided doses	Irritability, depression.	Very safe; daily or BID dosing; broad spectrum; rapid onset; few drug interactions; can be useful as "add-on" for patients "nearly" seizure free.	Tolerance (initial good response followed by loss of seizure control).	$
Succinimide Derivatives	*ethosuximide* Zarontin	Initial: 500 mg/day in 1 or 2 divided doses; ↑ by 250 mg/day Q4–7 days Usual maintenance: 750–1000 mg/day	GI upset.	Few drug interactions.	For absence seizures only; confers no protection for generalized tonic-clonic seizures.	$
Gamma Aminobutyric Acid (GABA) Derivatives	*gabapentin* Neurontin, generics	Initial: 300 mg TID Usual maintenance: 200–3600 mg/day divided Q6–8H	Tremor; vision changes.	No known significant drug interactions; well tolerated; safe; not metabolized; can use in liver failure.	TID dosing; not for 1° generalized seizures; expensive at high doses; best used as "add on" drug.	$$–$$$$
	vigabatrin Sabril	Initial: 1000 mg/day in 1–2 divided doses Usual maintenance: 2000–4000 mg/day in 1–2 divided doses	Low incidence of psychosis, depression; irreversible visual field problems.	BID dosing; well tolerated; few drug interactions; easy to use; linear pharmacokinetics; does not exhibit dermatologic, hepatic or hematologic adverse effects.	May worsen absence seizures, myoclonus; expensive at high doses; reports of visual field defects have severely limited use of this drug.	$$$–$$$$$

Class	Drug	Dose	Adverse Effects[a]	Advantages	Disadvantages	Cost[b]
Barbiturates	*phenobarbital* generics	90–120 mg/day at HS	Sedation prominent; skin rash 5%; depression; diminished libido.	Long $t_{1/2}$; daily dosing; inexpensive.	Potent inducer of cytochrome P450, therefore many potential drug interactions; metabolism inhibited by valproic acid; declining use because of adverse effect profile.	$
	primidone generics	Initial: 125 mg HS × 3 days, 125 mg BID × 3 days, 125 mg TID × 3 days Usual maintenance: 500–1000 mg/day in 3–4 divided doses	See phenobarbital. Some patients intolerant of low-dose primidone.	Primidone metabolized to phenobarbital but parent compound has significant antiseizure properties.	Potent inducer of cytochrome P450, therefore many potential drug interactions; metabolism inhibited by valproic acid; declining use because of adverse effect profile; QID dosing (to maintain high primidone/phenobarb ratio); slow dose titration.	$
Hydantoin Derivatives	*phenytoin* Dilantin, generics	300–400 mg/day If used, loading doses should be administered carefully	Gingival hyperplasia. Skin rash 5–10%; rarely can be very serious. ↑ liver enzymes. Blood dyscrasias. Dose-related encephalopathy. Coarse facial features with long-term use.	Daily or BID dosing; parenteral form available; inexpensive.	Inducer of cytochrome P450, therefore many potential drug interactions; long-term cosmetic adverse effects; dosing complicated by saturation kinetics.	$

(cont'd)

Table 3: **Antiepileptic Drugs (AEDs)** *(cont'd)*

Class	Drug	Dose	Adverse Effects[a]	Advantages	Disadvantages	Cost[b]
Carboxylic Acid Derivatives	*valproic acid* Depakene, generics	750–1000 mg/day in 2–4 divided doses	Nausea; weight gain; tremor; hair loss; blood dyscrasias; hepatotoxicity rarely; edema rarely; menstrual irregularities; teratogenicity.	Often may use BID dosing; broad spectrum; no hepatic enzyme induction; very low incidence of rash; cognitive effects generally less than with other older AEDs; drug of first choice for patients with mixed 1° generalized seizures (generalized tonic-clonic, myoclonus, absence).	Inhibits hepatic enzymes, therefore many potential drug interactions (but does not reduce oral contraceptive efficacy).	$
	divalproex sodium Epival, generics	750–1000 mg/day in 2 divided doses	See valproic acid.	Often may use BID dosing; broad spectrum; no hepatic enzyme induction; very low incidence of rash; cognitive effects generally less than other older AEDs; drug of first choice for patients with mixed 1° generalized seizures (generalized tonic-clonic, myoclonus, absence); GI tolerability may be better than with valproic acid.	Inhibits hepatic enzymes, therefore many potential drug interactions (but does not reduce oral contraceptive efficacy).	$

Class	Drug	Dose	Adverse Effects[a]	Advantages	Disadvantages	Cost[b]
Other Antiepileptic Drugs	*lamotrigine* Lamictal, generics	Initial: 25 mg Q2 days to 50 mg/day, depending on concurrent AED therapy; after 2 wk give same dose BID × 2 wk, then ↑ by 100 mg/day at 1- to 2-wk intervals Usual maintenance: 300–400 mg/day in 2 divided doses	Rash 5–10%, which rarely can be very serious; insomnia.	BID dosing; broad spectrum; no enzyme induction (few interactions); some patients more "alert;" increasing evidence for monotherapy; increasing use for 1° generalized seizures.	Very slow dose titration; metabolism markedly inhibited by valproic acid/divalproex sodium and increased by enzyme-inducing AEDs (carbamazepine, phenytoin, primidone, phenobarbital); available only as oral formulation; expensive at high doses.	$$
	levetiracetam[renal] Keppra, generics	Initial: 1000 mg/day in 2 divided doses; ↑ by 1000 mg/day at weekly intervals Usual maintenance: 1000–3000 mg/day in 2 divided doses	Sleepiness, ↓ energy, headache, irritability, depression.	BID dosing; broad spectrum; no drug interactions; rapid titration.	Expensive.	$$$–$$$$$
	topiramate[renal] Topamax, generics	Initial: 100 mg/day in 2 divided doses Usual maintenance: 200–400 mg/day	Cognitive problems common; kidney stones; weight loss; headache; fingers/toes paresthesias.	BID dosing; broad spectrum; safe; few drug interactions; potent AED with broad spectrum of activity.	Slow titration; ↓ efficacy of oral contraceptives; expensive; cognitive effects commonly limit use.	$$–$$$

[a] Virtually all AEDs can produce sedation, fatigue, cognitive impairment, dizziness and ataxia in a dose-dependent fashion.
[b] Cost of 30-day supply for usual maintenance dose; includes drug cost only.
[renal] Dosage adjustment may be required in renal impairment; see Appendix I.
Abbreviations: AED = antiepileptic drug; CR = controlled-release; GI = gastrointestinal
Legend: $ < $50 $$ $50–100 $$-$$$ $50–150 $$$ $100–150 $$–$$$$ $50–200 $$$$ $150–200 $$$–$$$$$ $100– > 200 $$$$–$$$$$ $150– > 200 $$$$$ > $200

Suggested Readings

Browne TR, Holmes GL. Epilepsy. *N Engl J Med* 2001;344(15):1145-51.

Chen JW, Wasterlain CG. Status epilepticus: pathophysiology and management in adults. *Lancet Neurol* 2006;5(3):246-56.

Glauser T, Ben-Menachem E, Bourgeois B et al. ILAE treatment guidelines: evidence-based analysis of antiepileptic drug efficacy and effectiveness as initial monotherapy for epileptic seizures and syndromes. *Epilepsia* 2006;47(7):1094-120.

Pohlman-Eden B, Behgi E, Camfield C et al. The first seizure and its management in adults and children. *BMJ* 2006;332(7537):339-42.

References

1. Mosewich RK, So EL. A clinical approach to the classification of seizures and epileptic syndromes. *Mayo Clin Proc* 1996;71(4):405-14.
2. Browne TR, Holmes GL. Epilepsy. *N Engl J Med* 2001;344(15):1145-51.
3. Brodie MJ, Dichter MA. Antiepileptic drugs. *N Engl J Med* 1996;334(3):168-75.
4. Dichter MA, Brodie MJ. New antiepileptic drugs. *N Engl J Med* 1996;334(24):1583-90.
5. Glauser T, Ben-Menachem E, Bourgeois B et al. ILAE treatment guidelines: evidence-based analysis of antiepileptic drug efficacy and effectiveness as initial monotherapy for epileptic seizures and syndromes. *Epilepsia* 2006;47(7):1094-120.
6. Wiebe S. An evidence based approach to the first unprovoked seizure. *Can J Neurol Sci* 2002;29(2):120-4.
7. Pohlman-Eden B, Behgi E, Camfield C et al. The first seizure and its management in adults and children. *BMJ* 2006;332(7537):339-42.
8. [No authors listed]. Practice parameter: management issues for women with epilepsy (summary statement). Report of the Quality Standards Subcommittee of the American Academy of Neurology. *Neurology* 1998;51(4):944-8.
9. Tettenborn B. Management of epilepsy in women of childbearing age: practical recommendations. *CNS Drugs* 2006;20(5):373-87.
10. Tatum WO. Use of antiepileptic drugs in pregnancy. *Expert Rev Neurother* 2006;6(7):1077-86.
11. Lawn ND, Wijdicks EF. Progress in clinical neurosciences: Status epilepticus: a critical review of management options. *Can J Neurol Sci* 2002;29(3):206-15.
12. Chen JW, Wasterlain CG. Status epilepticus: pathophysiology and management in adults. *Lancet Neurol* 2006;5(3):246-56.

CHAPTER 22
Cataract Surgery Postoperative Care

Stan P. George, MD, FRCSC

It is understandably difficult for a primary care practitioner to manage and diagnose the complications of a postoperative cataract patient without the benefit of a slit lamp, indirect ophthalmoscope, and frequently without even a Snellen acuity chart. The goal of this chapter is to review symptoms and signs that would allow a primary care practitioner to identify cases that should be urgently referred to the ophthalmologist.

Goals of Therapy

- Control inflammation
- Prevent infection
- Maintain eye comfort
- Promote early visual rehabilitation

The goals of the *postoperative assessment* are to:

- Detect intraocular infection in its early stages
- Detect postoperative uveitis or intraocular pressure (IOP) elevation
- Detect other abnormalities in the postoperative course such as a retinal detachment, iris prolapse, wound leak, flat anterior chamber or intraocular hemorrhage

Investigations

- Pain:
  - the postoperative eye should be comfortable; at worst, patient may have a mild foreign-body sensation
  - more intense pain suggests increased IOP, increased inflammation and/or infection
- History of recent trauma:
  - any trauma to the eye in the early postoperative phase requires thorough reassessment with a slit lamp
- Change in vision (worsening, darkening, loss of detail or peripheral visual loss):
  - any significant change could indicate infection, hemorrhage, retinal detachment or other acute intraocular pathology requiring immediate attention
- Visual phenomena (flashing lights, dark shadows or floaters):
  - requires thorough reassessment to rule out infection, retinal tear or detachment or uveitis

  - using a pinhole to test visual acuity will eliminate the effect of refractive error if the patient has apparent reduced acuity
- Itching of the eye (as predominant symptom):
  - suggests allergy to medications
- Examination of eye:
  - swelling of lids and/or conjunctiva suggests drug allergy or infection
  - pupil(s) should react normally to light unless a mydriatic agent has been used. Photophobia (glare sensitivity and pain from light exposure) can indicate anterior uveitis or corneal haze (from infection, inflammation or increased IOP)
  - the cornea should be clear of any clouding or infiltrates (to rule out corneal or anterior segment infection, inflammation or intraocular pressure elevation); the cornea should reflect a clear, well-demarcated image when the direct ophthalmoscope or pupil light is shined on it
  - use the ophthalmoscope to see if the disc is clearly viewed and a red reflex is present (to rule out vitreous clouding, inflammation or infection)
- Review of ocular medications:
  - reinforce proper use
  - clarify any confusion
  - discuss with family member
- Verify follow-up visits with surgeon

Therapeutic Choices (Figure 1)

Postoperative ophthalmic medications may include:

- **Antibacterials (Table 1)**
  - a broad-spectrum antibacterial is used perioperatively to reduce the risk of endophthalmitis. Although there is some evidence that prophylactic antibacterials are beneficial,[1] the evidence is weak.[2] Nonetheless, not using perioperative topical antibacterials could be problematic from a medical-legal point of view.
  - one study demonstrated the efficacy of preoperative topical **povidone iodine** in reducing the rate of endophthalmitis.[3] The use of perioperative fourth-generation topical fluoroquinolones (**gatifloxacin, moxifloxacin**)[4,5] is gaining widespread acceptance; however, many surgeons still prefer an agent that combines the antibacterial with a corticosteroid in the same bottle, e.g., ciprofloxacin/dexamethasone (Ciprodex).
- **Dilators** and **cycloplegics (Table 2)**
  - used to keep iris away from implant during early healing period and to improve comfort by decreasing ciliary muscle spasm.

- **Anti-inflammatory agents (Table 3)**
  - used during the first few weeks to reduce postoperative inflammation.
- **Glaucoma medications (Table 4)**
  - used to lower the intraocular pressure after eye surgery; in patients with pre-existing glaucoma, medication regimen may be modified in postoperative period to protect against early postoperative intraocular pressure rise.
- A mild analgesic may be required (e.g., **acetaminophen** 500 mg every four to six hours).
- Sedation is rarely needed.
- Other systemic medications should be continued.

Therapeutic Tips

- No changes to postoperative ophthalmic medications should be made without discussion with the treating ophthalmologist.
- Advise patients not to administer different eye drops at the same time, and to separate their administration by a period of 15 minutes.
- Worsening vision, floaters and increasing eye redness, especially in the first postoperative week, should be considered an endophthalmitis until proven otherwise, and necessitates an urgent assessment by an ophthalmologist.
- Because treatment with many medications in this setting is for a limited course, any remaining ophthalmic medication should be disposed of properly.

Figure 1: **Evaluation of the Postoperative Cataract Patient by the Primary Care Practitioner**

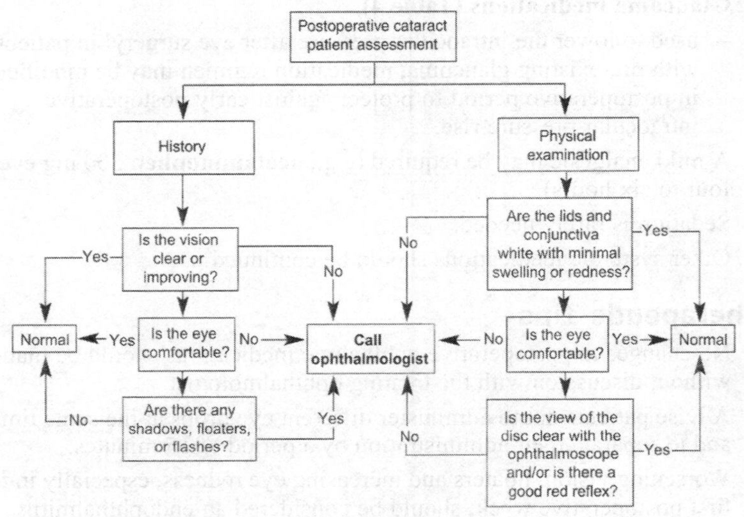

Table 1: **Antibacterials for Cataract Surgery Postoperative Care**

Class	Drug	Duration of Use	Adverse Effects	Comments	Cost[a]
Miscellaneous Antibacterials	*bacitracin ± polymyxin B ± gramicidin* Polysporin, generics	7–10 days	Allergic/hypersensitivity reactions.	Good broad-spectrum coverage but hypersensitivity reactions in some patients, especially with longer use.	$
	chloramphenicol Chloroptic, Pentamycetin, generics	7–10 days	Very small risk of idiosyncratic aplastic anemia.	Bacteriostatic; well tolerated.	$
Aminoglycosides	*gentamicin* Garamycin Ophthalmic, generics	7–10 days	Extended use may cause conjunctivitis or epitheliopathy reactions to the eye.	High concentrations on and in the eye lead to broader bacterial coverage than traditional in vitro testing suggests.	$
	neomycin combinations Neosporin, generics	7–10 days	See gentamicin.	See gentamicin.	$
	tobramycin Tobrex, generics	7–10 days	See gentamicin.	See gentamicin.	$

(cont'd)

Table 1: Antibacterials for Cataract Surgery Postoperative Care *(cont'd)*

Class	Drug	Duration of Use	Adverse Effects	Comments	Cost[a]
Fluoroquinolones	*ciprofloxacin, ophthalmic* Ciloxan	7–10 days	Formation of white crystalline precipitate after administration.	Excellent broad-spectrum profile and minimal ocular surface toxicity; very commonly used; may be used orally if lens capsule ruptured during cataract surgery.	$$
	ciprofloxacin, oral (renal) Cipro, generics	500 mg po Q12H × 7–10 days	Abdominal pain, headache, dizziness, photosensitivity, hepatitis, pseudomembranous colitis, cartilage toxicity.	Used orally if lens capsule ruptured during cataract surgery.	$$$
	gatifloxacin Zymar	7–10 days	See ciprofloxacin, ophthalmic.	4th generation fluoroquinolone; improved broad-spectrum activity, especially against gram-positive organisms.	$$
	moxifloxacin Vigamox	7–10 days	See ciprofloxacin, ophthalmic.	See gatifloxacin.	$$
	ofloxacin, ophthalmic Ocuflox, generics	7–10 days	See ciprofloxacin, ophthalmic.	See ciprofloxacin, ophthalmic.	$
	ofloxacin, oral (renal) Floxin, generics	400 mg po Q12H× 7–10 days	See ciprofloxacin, oral.	Used orally if lens capsule ruptured during cataract surgery.	$$$

[a] Cost of smallest available pack size or 10-day supply for oral treatment; includes drug cost only.

(renal) Dosage adjustment may be required in renal impairment; see Appendix I.

Legend: $ < $10 $$ $10–20 $$$ $20–30

Table 2: **Dilators and Cycloplegics for Cataract Surgery Postoperative Care**

Class	Drug	Duration of Use	Adverse Effects	Comments	Cost[a]
Dilators and Cycloplegics	*cyclopentolate* Cyclogyl, generics	First few weeks after surgery.	Uncommonly, systemic anticholinergic side effects (e.g., flushing, tachycardia, urinary retention).	Less commonly used with modern cataract surgery in light of smaller incisions and less postoperative inflammation.	$$
	phenylephrine Mydfrin, generics	First few weeks after surgery.	Rarely, tachycardia and hypertension.	See cyclopentolate.	$
	tropicamide Mydriacil, generics	First few weeks after surgery.		See cyclopentolate.	$$

[a] Cost of smallest available pack size; includes drug cost only.
Legend: $ < $10 $$ $10–20

Table 3: Anti-inflammatories for Cataract Surgery Postoperative Care

Class	Drug	Duration of Use	Adverse Effects	Comments	Cost[a]
Corticosteroids	*dexamethasone* Maxidex, generics	3–4 wk; longer if evidence of cystoid macular edema.	Elevated intraocular pressure; anti-inflammatory effects can mask signs of infection.	Commonly used after all types of eye surgery.	$
	fluorometholone Flarex, FML, generics	3–4 wk; longer if evidence of cystoid macular edema.	See dexamethasone.	See dexamethasone.	$$
	prednisolone Pred Mild, Pred Forte, generics	3–4 wk; longer if evidence of cystoid macular edema.	See dexamethasone.	See dexamethasone.	$$
	rimexolone Vexol	3–4 wk; longer if evidence of cystoid macular edema.	See dexamethasone.	See dexamethasone.	$$
NSAIDs	*diclofenac* Voltaren Ophtha	3–4 wk; longer if evidence of cystoid macular edema.	Mild to moderate burning on instillation; epitheliopathy with prolonged and frequent use.	Used as a substitute for steroids to ↓ inflammation without the risk of elevating intraocular pressure; should not be used in asthmatics or patients with allergies to ASA or NSAIDs.	$
	flurbiprofen Ocufen	3–4 wk; longer if evidence of cystoid macular edema.	See diclofenac.	See diclofenac.	$$$
	ketorolac Acular, generics	3–4 wk; longer if evidence of cystoid macular edema.	See diclofenac.	See diclofenac.	$$

[a] Cost of smallest available pack size; includes drug cost only.
Legend: $ < $10 $$ $10–20 $$$ $20–30

Table 4: **Glaucoma Medications for Cataract Surgery Postoperative Care**

Class	Drug	Duration of Use	Adverse Effects	Comments	Cost[a]
Beta$_1$-adrenergic Antagonists	*timolol* Timoptic, generics	Used as long as intraocular pressure is elevated, or permanently in patients with pre-existing glaucoma.	Symptoms of systemic beta blockade can be precipitated or aggravated with beta-blocking eye drops (e.g., bradycardia, arrhythmia, hypotension, bronchospasm); potentially serious systemic effects in asthmatics or patients with obstructive lung disease or borderline cardiac function.	Efficacious and cost effective with minimal ocular toxicity; avoid in asthmatics or patients with obstructive lung disease or borderline cardiac function.	$
	timolol gel-forming solution Timoptic XE	Used as long as intraocular pressure is elevated, or permanently in patients with pre-existing glaucoma.	See timolol.	See timolol.	$
	betaxolol Betoptic S, generics	Used as long as intraocular pressure is elevated, or permanently in patients with pre-existing glaucoma.	See timolol.	See timolol.	$
	levobunolol Betagan, generics	Used as long as intraocular pressure is elevated, or permanently in patients with pre-existing glaucoma.	See timolol.	See timolol.	$

(cont'd)

Table 4: **Glaucoma Medications for Cataract Surgery Postoperative Care** *(cont'd)*

Class	Drug	Duration of Use	Adverse Effects	Comments	Cost[a]
Alpha$_2$-adrenergic Agonists	*apraclonidine* Iopidine	Used as long as intraocular pressure is elevated, or permanently in patients with pre-existing glaucoma.	Common ocular reactions include hyperemia and a burning sensation.	Potent in controlling postoperative pressure spikes; avoid in patients with severe cardiovascular disease in light of alpha-adrenergic effects; use with caution in patients taking tricyclic antidepressants.	$$$
	brimonidine 0.2% Alphagan, generics	Used as long as intraocular pressure is elevated, or permanently in patients with pre-existing glaucoma.	See apraclonidine.	See apraclonidine.	$$
	brimonidine 0.15% Alphagan P	Used as long as intraocular pressure is elevated, or permanently in patients with pre-existing glaucoma.	See apraclonidine.	See apraclonidine. Contains purite as preservative rather than benzalkonium chloride; may have slightly lower incidence of ocular allergy than brimonidine 0.2%.	$$
Prostaglandins	*bimatoprost* Lumigan	Used as long as intraocular pressure is elevated, or permanently in patients with pre-existing glaucoma.	Brown pigmentation of the iris or darkening or thickening of eye lashes may develop.	Very potent pressure-lowering agents with once-daily application.	$$$
	latanoprost Xalatan	Used as long as intraocular pressure is elevated, or permanently in patients with pre-existing glaucoma.	See bimatoprost.	See bimatoprost.	$$$

Class	Drug	Duration of Use	Adverse Effects	Comments	Cost[a]
	travoprost Travatan	Used as long as intraocular pressure is elevated, or permanently in patients with pre-existing glaucoma.	See bimatoprost.	See bimatoprost.	$$$
Carbonic Anhydrase Inhibitors	*acetazolamide*, oral (renal) Acetazolam, generics	250 mg up to QID; used for very high intraocular pressure on a short-term basis.	Should not be used in patients with sulfonamide allergy; conjunctivitis and blepharitis are not uncommon side effects; systemic hypersensitivity reactions may develop.	Carbonic anhydrase inhibitors more commonly used *topically* as adjunctive agents to reduce intraocular pressure.	$
	methazolamide, oral generics	50–100 mg BID–TID; used for very high intraocular pressure on a short-term basis.	See acetazolamide.	See acetazolamide.	$$$$
	brinzolamide Azopt	Topical use may be long term.	See acetazolamide.	See acetazolamide.	$$
	dorzolamide Trusopt	Topical use may be long term.	See acetazolamide.	See acetazolamide.	$$

[a] Cost of smallest available pack size or 30-day supply of oral therapy; includes drug cost only.
(renal) Dosage adjustment may be required in renal impairment; see Appendix I.
Legend: $ < $10 $$ $10–20 $$$ $20–30 $$$$ > $30

Suggested Readings

American Academy of Ophthalmology. Cataract and Anterior Segment Panel. *Cataract in the adult eye, preferred practice pattern.* San Francisco (CA): The Academy; 2006. Available from: http://www.aao.org/education/library/ppp/upload/Cataract_in_the_Adult_Eye.pdf Accessed April 17, 2007

Bradford CA, editor. *Basic ophthalmology for medical students and primary care residents.* 7th ed. San Francisco (CA): American Academy of Ophthalmology; 2004.

Kunimoto DY, Kanitkar KD, Makar MS, editors. *The Wills eye manual: office and emergency room diagnosis and treatment of eye disease.* 4th ed. Philadelphia (PA): Lippincott Williams & Wilkins; 2004.

Tasman W, Jaeger EA, editors. *Duane's ophthalmology.* Philadelphia (PA): Lippincott Williams & Wilkins; 2006.

References

1. Allen HF, Mangiaracine AB. Bacterial endophthalmitis after cataract extraction. II. Incidence in 36,000 consecutive operations with special reference to preoperative topical antibiotics. *Arch Ophthalmol* 1974;91(1):3-7.
2. Ciulla TA, Starr MB, Masket S. Bacterial endophthalmitis prophylaxis for cataract surgery: an evidence-based update. *Ophthalmology* 2002;109(1):13-24.
3. Speaker MG, Menikoff JA. Prophylaxis of endophthalmitis with topical povidone-iodine. *Ophthalmology* 1991;98(12):1769-75.
4. Callegan MC, Ramirez R, Kane ST et al. Antibacterial activity of the fourth generation flouroquinolones gatifloxacin and moxifloxacin against ocular pathogens. *Adv Ther* 2003;20(5):246-52.
5. Deramo VA, Lai JC, Fastenberg DM et al. Acute endophthalmitis in eyes treated prophylactically with gatifloxacin and moxifloxacin. *Am J Ophthmol* 2006;142(5):721-5.

CHAPTER 23
Glaucoma

Mark R. Lesk, MSc, MD, FRCSC and
Paul Rafuse, MD, PhD, FRCSC

Glaucoma is a group of ocular diseases that have in common an optic neuropathy that causes visual loss. Characteristically, the optic disc is cupped, and peripheral field loss precedes deterioration of visual acuity. Elevated intraocular pressure (IOP) is the most important, and only modifiable, risk factor for glaucoma.[1] Other risk factors (see Table 1) are likely important in the pathogenesis of this neurodegenerative condition.[2]

Goals of Therapy

- Prevent, halt or slow progressive visual loss
- Preserve the structure and function of the optic nerve
- Eliminate pain and improve vision in acute forms

Investigations

- Thorough history with special attention to:
  - nature of any ocular disturbances, e.g., loss of peripheral vision, halos around lights, decreased visual acuity
  - quality of any pain, e.g., deep orbital, brow or headache
  - associated systemic symptoms, e.g., abdominal pain, nausea and vomiting

  Note: The most common varieties of glaucoma are chronic. Generally, symptoms are associated only with *acute* types of glaucoma, which warrant urgent referral to an ophthalmologist or emergency room. Most patients with chronic glaucoma are asymptomatic until they reach the advanced stages of the disease.
- Careful assessment of risk factors (Table 1)
- History of drug use that can cause or worsen glaucoma
  - corticosteroids (common)
  - drugs with antimuscarinic activity (rare), e.g., antihistamines, decongestants, antidepressants, antispasmodics
  - the anticonvulsant topiramate has been associated with acute angle-closure glaucoma[3]
- Physical examination
  - positive findings include constricted visual field, optic disc cupping and elevated IOP

  Note: Screening for elevated IOP *alone* lacks adequate sensitivity and specificity for the detection of glaucoma, as up to 50% of people with glaucoma have IOP in the normal range (< 21 mm Hg).[4] Further, about

90% of people with elevated IOP do *not* have glaucoma, although they are at increased risk of developing it.[5]

- Comprehensive eye examination by an ophthalmologist or optometrist
- Laboratory tests:
  - automated perimetry
  - optic disc photography

Table 1: **Risk Factors for the Development of Glaucoma**

Type of Glaucoma	Open-angle Glaucoma	Angle-closure Glaucoma: Acute	Angle-closure Glaucoma: Chronic
Acquired, Primary	Elevated IOP Advanced age[6] Black ethnicity[7] Positive family history Myopia[8] Vascular diseases such as migraine,[9] hypertension[10] or nocturnal hypotension[11]	Female gender Advanced age[6] Positive family history Hyperopia White ethnicity	Advanced age[6] Black ethnicity[7] Positive family history Hyperopia
Acquired, Secondary	Blunt or penetrating trauma Previous intraocular surgery Previous intraocular inflammation Corticosteroid use (ophthalmic, systemic, nasal or inhaled)	Proliferative diabetic retinopathy and central retinal vein occlusion (neovascular angle-closure glaucoma)	
Congenital	Positive family history		

Therapeutic Choices (Figure 1)

The therapeutic goals (see Goals of Therapy) are achieved by lowering the IOP, even in patients with glaucoma whose pressures are in the normal range, through the use of medications, laser and/or surgery.

Nonpharmacologic Choices

- There are no lifestyle modifications proven to alter the outcome of the disease. Aerobic exercise can lower IOP modestly in some patients with glaucoma.[12]
- Laser or surgical procedures are options if drug therapy is unsuccessful (Figure 1, Table 2).

Table 2: **Laser and Surgical Treatment of Glaucoma**

Procedure	Indication	Description
Laser Treatment		
Laser trabeculoplasty (argon or selective laser)	Open-angle glaucoma	Laser applications to trabecular meshwork (drainage system). Effect is short term, e.g., 2 y; most suitable for elderly patients.
Laser iridotomy	Angle-closure glaucoma	A neodymium: yttrium-aluminum-garnet (Nd:YAG) laser cuts holes in iris to permit flow of aqueous humor directly from posterior to anterior chamber; can be done without incising eyeball. Simple office procedure.
Laser ciliary body ablation	Advanced refractory glaucomas	Used where other options are limited.
Surgical Treatment		
Filtration procedures (e.g., trabeculectomy, nonpenetrating deep sclerotomy, viscocanalostomy)	Open-angle glaucoma, in cases refractory to medical or laser treatment	A channel is created, allowing aqueous flow from anterior chamber to a subconjunctival space. Healing and surgical success improved with topical use of antiproliferative agents, such as mitomycin C or 5-fluorouracil, during or following procedure.
Iridectomy	Angle-closure glaucoma	Used in affected eye and prophylactically in other eye. Reserved for rare cases refractory to Nd:YAG laser iridotomy.
Drainage tube insertion	Any form of glaucoma, where other surgical procedures have not succeeded	Small tube, inserted into anterior chamber, drains aqueous to a plate that is implanted on the sclera, beneath the conjunctiva.

Pharmacologic Choices (Table 3)

- Treat reversible causes of *secondary* and *angle-closure* glaucoma.

  Note: The definitive treatment for *acute angle-closure* glaucoma is a surgical or laser iridectomy. Aggressive medical treatment is required to ameliorate the damaging effects of extreme IOP elevation until the iridectomy is performed.
- Treat excessive IOP, the only modifiable risk factor in chronic primary *open-angle* glaucoma (the most prevalent form); all treatment measures in Figure 1 are believed to exert their therapeutic effect by lowering IOP.
- Selected patients with risk factors in addition to elevated IOP may require treatment even in the absence of glaucomatous optic disc and visual field damage.[5]
- Patients with open-angle glaucoma at normal pressures will benefit from further lowering of their IOP.[13]

- Target IOPs for a specific patient are set on the basis of:
  - the extent of glaucomatous damage
  - the IOP range believed to have been associated with that damage
  - the burden of therapy to achieve the desired IOP.
- Target pressure is adjusted downward if progressive damage to the optic disc or visual field occurs at the target IOP.[14]
- In some cases, clinicians may want to consider the potential neuroprotective effects or improvement in ocular blood flow afforded by some of the existing ocular hypotensive agents.[15]

Open-angle Glaucoma

Beta-blockers

Topical **timolol, levobunolol** and **betaxolol** are effective ocular hypotensive agents that lack significant ocular side effects.[16] They decrease IOP by inhibiting the formation of aqueous humor. Beta-blockers are contraindicated when certain pulmonary and cardiac diseases are present (Table 3). Betaxolol hydrochloride is relatively specific for beta$_1$-receptor blockade and may be used with caution in selected patients with mild obstructive pulmonary disease.[17]

Topical Carbonic Anhydrase Inhibitors

Dorzolamide and **brinzolamide** are the two available agents in this class. Like oral carbonic anhydrase inhibitors, they decrease IOP by inhibiting an enzyme involved in the formation of aqueous humor. Both have limited systemic effects when compared to oral formulations, but they do not lower IOP to the same extent.[18] Brinzolamide appears to be as efficacious as dorzolamide and may be more comfortable on instillation.[19] These drugs can be considered for adjunctive therapy, or for primary treatment in patients with cardiopulmonary contraindications to beta-blockers.

Prostaglandin Analogues

Latanoprost and **travoprost** are prostaglandin $F_{2\alpha}$ analogues that lower IOP by increasing outflow through the uveoscleral pathway.[20] **Bimatoprost**, a prostamide analogue, may act by increasing both uveoscleral and trabecular outflow.[21] These agents are slightly more efficacious than nonselective beta-blockers. Clinical experience with this class has not revealed any significant systemic adverse effects, but a few ocular effects have been noted, including darkening of some brown-coloured irides, lengthening of the eyelashes and mild conjunctival hyperemia.[22] Any of these agents may be considered first-line therapy because of their potencies and excellent safety profiles.

Alpha$_2$-Adrenergic Agonists

Topical epinephrine, the prototype in this class, has not been available in Canada for some time, because of unacceptable adverse ocular effects. The epinephrine prodrug dipivefrin has also been discontinued. **Apraclonidine** was the first alpha$_2$-specific agonist introduced, but local allergic reactions have limited its use to the management of acute IOP spikes.[23] Also with a significant incidence of allergy, **brimonidine** has a higher specificity for the alpha$_2$-receptor and is associated with a less severe conjunctival hyperemia.[24] A new formulation of brimonidine (0.15%, preserved with purite rather than benzalkonium chloride) may have a slightly lower rate of ocular allergy than brimonidine 0.2%. Like apraclonidine, brimonidine supresses the formation of aqueous humor and can be used for a variety of open-angle and angle-closure glaucomas.[25] Brimonidine may also increase uveoscleral outflow.

Cholinergic Agonists

The topical cholinergic agonists **pilocarpine** and **carbachol** directly stimulate muscarinic receptors to contract the ciliary muscle and increase trabecular outflow.[26] These drugs are characterized by ocular side effects, including miosis (with reduced night vision), accommodative spasm (including myopia) and brow ache, and rarely, in predisposed patients, retinal detachment. Rarely is sufficient drug absorbed systemically to cause abdominal cramping or diarrhea. These drugs are poorly tolerated in children and young adults.

Fixed-combination Preparations

There are currently four fixed-combination topical glaucoma therapies, each containing timolol, available in Canada. **Dorzolamide/timolol,**[27] **brimonidine/timolol,**[28] **latanoprost/timolol**[29] and **travoprost/timolol**[30] are all more effective than the individual agents, and they have similar ocular hypotensive effects. Dorzolamide/timolol has by far the longest track record. The combined agents are thought to have advantages with respect to adherence to therapy.

Oral Carbonic Anhydrase Inhibitors

Acetazolamide and **methazolamide** lower IOP by decreasing the production of aqueous humor. Their use is normally reserved for emergencies because of significant side effects. Approximately 50% of patients are unable to use these agents long term because of GI or CNS difficulties, paresthesias or renal lithiasis.[31] Oral and topical carbonic anhydrase inhibitors can show cross-reactivity in patients allergic to sulfonamides.

Therapeutic Tips

- Topical glaucoma medications are highly concentrated to allow adequate intraocular penetration. Systemic absorption occurs through the nasal mucosa. This can be reduced through digital occlusion of the nasolacrimal drainage system for several minutes following instillation of the drops,[32] or through eyelid closure for three to five minutes.
- Nonprescription antihistamine products (which carry a caution against use in glaucoma patients due to anticholinergic side effects) and anticholinergic drugs will rarely cause a problem in open-angle glaucoma with intermittent use. The caution is included primarily to

warn that, rarely, drugs with anticholinergic activity can precipitate angle-closure glaucoma in predisposed individuals[33] (e.g., elderly white or Asian females who are significantly hyperopic, have a positive family history and have not yet had a therapeutic or prophylactic iridectomy — see Table 1).

Figure 1: **Management of Open-angle Glaucoma**

Treatment is stepped up if optic disc cupping progresses, the visual field deteriorates or intraocular pressure control is inadequate.

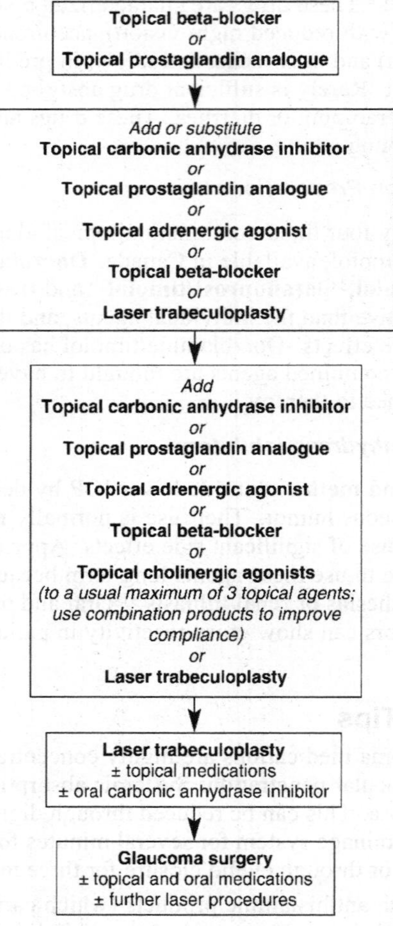

Table 3: **Drugs Used in Glaucoma**

Class	Drug	Dose	Adverse Effects	Comments	Cost[a]
$Beta_1$-adrenergic Antagonists, ophthalmic	*timolol 0.25%, 0.5%* Timoptic, generics	Q12H	Local adverse effects usually minimal — stinging, dry eyes, rarely conjunctivitis; systemic effects can include bronchospasm, exacerbation of CHF, bradycardia, syncope, depression, impotence, altered response to hypoglycemia, reduction of high-density lipoproteins.	Avoid in patients with bronchial asthma; caution in patients with a history of syncope or bradycardia.	$
	timolol gel-forming solution 0.25%, 0.5% Timoptic-XE	Once daily	See timolol.	See timolol.	$$
	betaxolol 0.25% Betoptic S	Q12H	See timolol.	See timolol.	$$
	levobunolol 0.25%, 0.5% Betagan, generics	Q12H	See timolol.	See timolol.	$
Carbonic Anhydrase Inhibitors, ophthalmic	*dorzolamide 2%* Trusopt	Q8–12H	Bitter, sour or unusual taste, stinging, local allergic reaction.	Cross-reactivity in patients allergic to sulfonamides.	$$
	dorzolamide 2% preservative-free Trusopt	Q8–12H	Bitter, sour or unusual taste, stinging, local allergic reaction.	Advantageous for patients with allergies to benzalkonium chloride. Cross-reactivity in patients allergic to sulfonamides.	$$

(cont'd)

Table 3: **Drugs Used in Glaucoma** *(cont'd)*

Class	Drug	Dose	Adverse Effects	Comments	Cost[a]
	brinzolamide 1% Azopt	Q12H	See dorzolamide.	Cross-reactivity in patients allergic to sulfonamides; dose can be increased to Q8H after 4 wk if inadequate response.	$$
Prostaglandin Analogues, ophthalmic	*latanoprost 0.005%* Xalatan	Once daily	Foreign body sensation, burning, stinging, itching, increased iris pigmentation, increased eyelash length.	Once-daily dosing should not be exceeded; more frequent administration may reduce effectiveness.	$$$
	travoprost 0.004% Travatan	Once daily	Conjunctival hyperemia, foreign body sensation, burning, stinging, itching, increased iris pigmentation, increased eyelash length.	See latanoprost.	$$$
	bimatoprost 0.03% Lumigan	Once daily	See travoprost.	See latanoprost.	$$$
Alpha$_2$-Adrenergic Agonists, ophthalmic	*apraclonidine 0.5%, 1%* Iopidine	Q8H	Local allergic reaction, tachycardia, hypotension, headache, tremor.	Contraindicated with MAO inhibitors. Can rarely be used chronically due to more than 40% incidence of marked blepharoconjunctivitis.	$$-$$$
	brimonidine 0.2% Alphagan, generics	Q12H	Local allergic reaction, tachycardia, hypotension, headache, tremor.	Contraindicated with MAO inhibitors; not recommended in pediatric patients. Lower incidence of allergy than apraclonidine when used chronically.	$$

Class	Drug	Dose	Adverse Effects	Comments	Cost[a]
	brimonidine 0.15% Alphagan P	Q12H	See brimonidine 0.2%.	See brimonidine 0.2%. Contains purite as preservative rather than benzalkonium chloride; may have slightly lower incidence of ocular allergy than brimonidine 0.2%.	$$
Cholinergic Agonists, ophthalmic	*pilocarpine 1%, 2%, 4%, 6%* Isopto Carpine drops, others;Pilopine HS gel	Drops: QID Gel: QHS	Reduced vision in patients with cataracts, blurred vision due to refractive shift, brow ache, GI upset (rare).	Poorly tolerated in children and younger adults.	Drops: $ Gel: $$
	carbachol Isopto Carbachol	Q8H	See pilocarpine.	See pilocarpine.	$
Carbonic Anhydrase Inhibitor/Beta-blocker Combinations, ophthalmic	*dorzolamide 2%/timolol 0.5%* Cosopt	Q12H	See dorzolamide. See timolol.	Cross-reactivity in patients allergic to sulfonamides.	$$$
	dorzolamide 2%/ timolol 0.5%, preservative-free Preservative-free Cosopt	Q12H	See dorzolamide. See timolol.	Advantageous for patients with allergies to benzalkonium chloride. Cross-reactivity in patients allergic to sulfonamides.	$$$
Prostaglandin/Beta-blocker Combinations, ophthalmic	*latanoprost 0.005%/ timolol 0.5%* Xalacom	Once daily	See latanoprost. See timolol.	See latanoprost. See timolol.	$$$$
	travoprost 0.004%/ timolol 0.5% DuoTrav	Once daily	See travoprost. See timolol.	See travoprost. See timolol.	$$$$

(cont'd)

Table 3: **Drugs Used in Glaucoma** *(cont'd)*

Class	Drug	Dose	Adverse Effects	Comments	Cost[a]
Alpha$_2$-adrenergic Agonist/ Beta-blocker Combinations, ophthalmic	*brimonidine 0.2%/timolol 0.5%* Combigan	Q12H	See brimonidine 0.2%. See timolol.	See brimonidine. 0.2%. See timolol.	$$
Carbonic Anhydrase Inhibitors, oral	*acetazolamide* ◗ Diamox Sequels, generics	250 mg up to QID Diamox Sequels: 500 mg Q12H	Paresthesias of the extremities, metabolic acidosis, hypokalemia, GI upset, urolithiasis, lethargy and depression, aplastic anemia (rare), Stevens-Johnson syndrome (rare).	Cross-reactivity in patients allergic to sulfonamides.	$
	methazolamide generics	50–100 mg BID-TID	See acetazolamide. Side effects are less severe than with acetazolamide.	See acetazolamide.	$$-$$$$

[a] Cost of smallest available pack size or 30–day supply for oral medications; includes drug cost only.

◗ Dosage adjustment may be required in renal impairment; see Appendix I.

Legend: $ < $10 $$ $10–20 $$-$$$ $10–30 $$$ $20–30 $$-$$$$ $10– >30 $$$$ > $30

Suggested Readings

American Academy of Ophthalmology. Glaucoma Panel. *Primary angle closure: preferred practice pattern.* San Francisco (CA): AAO; 2005. Available from: http://www.aao.org/education/library/ppp/upload/Primary_Angle_Closure-3.pdf Accessed December 18, 2006.

American Academy of Ophthalmology. Glaucoma Panel. *Primary open-angle glaucoma: preferred practice pattern.* San Francisco (CA): AAO; 2005. Available from: http://www.aao.org/education/library/ppp/upload/Primary_Open_Angle_Glaucoma-2.pdf Accessed December 18, 2006.

American Academy of Ophthalmology. Glaucoma Panel. *Primary open-angle glaucoma suspect: preferred practice pattern.* San Francisco (CA): AAO; 2005. Available from: http://www.aao.org/education/library/ppp/upload/Primary_Open_Angle_Glaucoma_Suspect-2.pdf Accessed December 18, 2006.

Morrison JC, Pollack IP, editors. *Glaucoma: science and practice.* New York (NY): Thieme; 2003.

Rafuse PE. Screening those at risk for glaucoma. *Can J Diagn* 1999;16:105-12.

References

1. Sommer A, Tielsch JM, Katz J et al. Relationship between intraocular pressure and primary open angle glaucoma among white and black Americans. The Baltimore Eye Survey. *Arch Ophthalmol* 1991;109(8):1090-5.
2. Drance SM. Bowman Lecture. Glaucoma--changing concepts. *Eye* 1992;6(Pt 4):337-45.
3. Fraunfelder FW, Fraunfelder FT, Keates, EU. Topiramate-associated acute, bilateral, secondary angle-closure glaucoma. *Ophthalmology* 2004;111(1):109-11.
4. Grodum K Heijl A, Bengtsson B. A comparison of glaucoma patients identified through mass screening and in routine clinical practice. *Acta Ophthalmol Scand* 2002;80(6):627-31.
5. Kass MA, Heuer DK, Higginbotham EJ et al. The Ocular Hypertension Treatment Study: a randomized trial determines that topical ocular hypotensive medication delays or prevents the onset of primary open-angle glaucoma. *Arch Ophthalmol* 2002;120(6):701-13.
6. Quigley, HA, Vitale S. Models of open-angle glaucoma prevalence and incidence in the United States. *Invest Ophthalmol Vis Sci* 1997;38(1):83-91.
7. Tielsch JM, Sommer A, Katz J et al. Racial variations in the prevalence of primary open angle glaucoma. The Baltimore Eye Survey. *JAMA* 1991;266(3):369-74.
8. Hitchings R. Normal-tension glaucoma. In: Yanoff M, Duker JS, editors. *Ophthalmology.* London (UK): Mosby; 1999. p.1-4.
9. Phelps CD Corbett JJ. Migraine and low-tension glaucoma. A case-control study. *Invest Ophthalmol Vis Sci* 1985;26(8):1105-8.
10. Tielsch JM Katz J, Sommer A et al. Hypertension, perfusion pressure, and primary open-angle glaucoma. A population-based assessment. *Arch Ophthalmol* 1995;113(2):216-21.
11. Graham SL Drance SM, Wijsman K et al. Ambulatory blood pressure monitoring in glaucoma. The nocturnal dip. *Ophthalmology* 1995;102(1):61-9.
12. Passo MS, Goldberg L, Elliot DL et al. Exercise training reduces intraocular pressure among subjects suspected of having glaucoma. *Arch Ophthalmol* 1991;109(8):1096-8.
13. [No authors listed]. Comparison of glaucomatous progression between untreated patients with normal-tension glaucoma and patients with therapeutically reduced intraocular pressures. Collaborative Normal-Tension Glaucoma Study Group. *Am J Ophthalmol* 1998;126(4):487-97.
14. Damji KF, Behki R, Wang L et al. Canadian perspectives in glaucoma management: setting target intraocular pressure range. *Can J Ophthalmol* 2003;38(3):189-97.
15. Lesk MR, Lachaine J. Medical therapy of glaucoma: focus on newer agents. *Ophthalmic Practice* 2003;21(2):46-52.
16. Rafuse PE. Adrenergic antagonists. In: Morrison JC, Pollack IP, editors. *Glaucoma: science and practice.* New York (NY): Thieme; 2003.
17. Berry DP, Van Buskirk EM, Shields MB. Betaxolol and timolol. A comparison of efficacy and side effects. *Arch Ophthalmol* 1984;102(1):42-5.
18. Goldberg I. Carbonic anhydrase inhibitors. In: Morrison JC, Pollack IP, editors. *Glaucoma: science and practice.* New York (NY): Thieme; 2003.

19. Stewart R. *Invest Ophthalmol Vis Sci* 1997;38(Suppl):559.
20. Lawlor D et al. Prostaglandin analogs. In: Morrison JC, Pollack IP, editors. *Glaucoma: science and practice*. New York (NY): Thieme; 2003.
21. Brubaker RF, Schoff EO, Nau CB et al. Effects of AGN 192024, a new ocular hypotensive agent, on aqueous dynamics. *Am J Ophthalmol* 2001;131(1):19-24.
22. Johnstone MA. Hypertrichosis and increased pigmentation of eyelashes and adjacent hair in the region of the ipsilateral eyelids of patients treated with unilateral topical latanoprost. *Am J Ophthalmol* 1997;124(4):544-7.
23. Butler P, Mannschreck M, Lin S et al. Clinical experience with the long-term use of 1% apraclonidine. Incidence of allergic reactions. *Arch Ophthalmol* 1995;113(3):293-6.
24. Blondeau P, Rousseau JA. Allergic reactions to brimonidine in patients treated for glaucoma *Can J Ophthalmol* 2002;37(1):21-6.
25. Serle JB et al. Adrenergic agonists. In: Morrison JC, Pollack IP, editors. *Glaucoma: science and practice*. New York (NY): Thieme; 2003.
26. Derick RJ. Cholinergic agonists. In: Morrison JC, Pollack IP, editors. *Glaucoma: science and practice*. New York (NY): Thieme; 2003.
27. Strohmaier K, Snyder E, DuBiner H et al. The efficacy and safety of the dorzolamide-timolol combination versus the concomitant administration of its components. Dorzolamide-Timolol Study Group. *Ophthalmology* 1998;105(10):1936-44.
28. Craven ER, Walters TR, Williams R et al. Brimonidine and timolol fixed-combination therapy versus monotherapy: a 3-month randomized trial in patients with glaucoma or ocular hypertension. *J Ocul Pharmacol Ther* 2005;21(4):337-48.
29. Higginbotham EJ, Feldman R, Stiles M et al. Latanoprost and timolol combination therapy vs monotherapy: one-year randomized trial. *Arch Ophthalmol* 2002;120(7):915-22.
30. Schuman JS, Katz GJ, Lewis RA et al. Efficacy and safety of a fixed combination of travoprost 0.004%/timolol 0.5% ophthalmic solution once daily for open-angle glaucoma or ocular hypertension. *Am J Ophthalmol* 2005;140(2):242-50.
31. Stamper RL et al. Carbonic anhydrase inhibitors. In: *Becker-Shaffer's diagnosis and therapy of the glaucomas*. 7th ed. St. Louis (MO): Mosby; 1999.
32. Zimmerman TJ, Kooner KS, Kandarakis AS et al. Improving the therapeutic index of topically applied ocular drugs. *Arch Ophthalmol* 1984;102(4):551-3.
33. Abelson MB et al. Antiallergic therapies. In: Zimmerman TJ et al., editors. *Textbook of ocular pharmacology*. Philadelphia (PA): Lippincott-Raven; 1997.

CHAPTER 24
Red Eye

Sueda Akkor, MD, FRCSC

Red eye is common in a wide variety of ocular conditions, some of which have serious consequences and require immediate referral to an ophthalmologist.

Goals of Therapy

- Preserve eyesight
- Control infection
- Control inflammation
- Provide symptomatic relief

Investigations (Figure 1)

The first step is to differentiate the major/serious causes from the minor causes (Table 1). The presence of one or more warning signs requires referral to an ophthalmologist (Table 2).

Table 1: **Etiology of Red Eye**

Cause	Examples
Infection	Conjunctivitis/keratitis (bacterial, viral, other), lacrimal system infection
Allergy	
Dry eyes (keratoconjunctivitis sicca)	Sjögren's syndrome, vitamin A deficiency, other
Blepharitis and secondary conjunctivitis/keratitis	
Toxic/chemical/other irritants	Topical drugs, contact lens solutions, acids/alkalis, smoke, wind, UV light (e.g., tanning bed, welder's arc)
Traumatic injury	Corneal abrasions, foreign bodies, hyphema (bleeding into the anterior chamber), heat exposure, other
Ocular inflammation	Iritis, episcleritis, scleritis
Glaucoma	Acute angle-closure glaucoma
Other	Pterygium, subconjunctival hemorrhage

Table 2: **Warning Signs for Ophthalmologist Referral**

- Limbal/ciliary injection (redness dominant at the corneoscleral junction)
- Pain *not* relieved by test dose of topical anesthetic drop (proparacaine, tetracaine)
- Pupil abnormalities (miotic or mid-dilated and fixed)
- Signs and symptoms of acute angle-closure glaucoma such as red painful eye with raised intraocular pressure, blurred vision, headache, vomiting or coloured halos around lights
- History of iritis/angle-closure glaucoma
- Recent trauma to eye

Therapeutic Choices (Figure 1)

Nonpharmacologic Choices

Instruct patient to:

- Stop wearing contact lenses until the problem is resolved
- Avoid makeup, smoke, wind and other irritants
- Apply cold wet compresses for allergic or viral conjunctivitis
- Apply hot wet compresses for blepharitis/styes
- Practise lid hygiene for blepharitis:
  - warm water compresses applied to closed eyelids for 5 to 10 minutes, followed by gentle scrubbing of lid margins with warm water, a commercial eyelid scrub or a few drops of baby shampoo in a small amount of warm water
  - repeat daily at bedtime

Pharmacologic Choices

Choice depends on underlying cause (see Table 3). Once the major/serious conditions are ruled out, treatment can be initiated. In general, if no improvement is seen after one week, refer.

For symptomatic relief (decreased redness, edema) of allergic or viral conjunctivitis or minor eye irritation, ophthalmic vasoconstrictors should be reserved for occasional and short-term use. Overuse may cause rebound hyperemia.

Therapeutic Tips

- Most topically administered eye drops used in therapy are themselves capable of causing irritation or toxicity.
- Corticosteroids or antibiotic/corticosteroid combinations may worsen herpetic/fungal keratitis and should not be used indiscriminately.
- Long-term use of topical corticosteroids may cause glaucoma and/or cataracts.
- Topical decongestants/vasoconstrictors may provoke angle-closure glaucoma in those predisposed (see Chapter 23).

- Some patients may react to preservatives in artificial tears. In those who use drops more than four to five times daily and who experience irritation, nonpreserved lubricants may be preferable.

Figure 1: **Management of Red Eye**

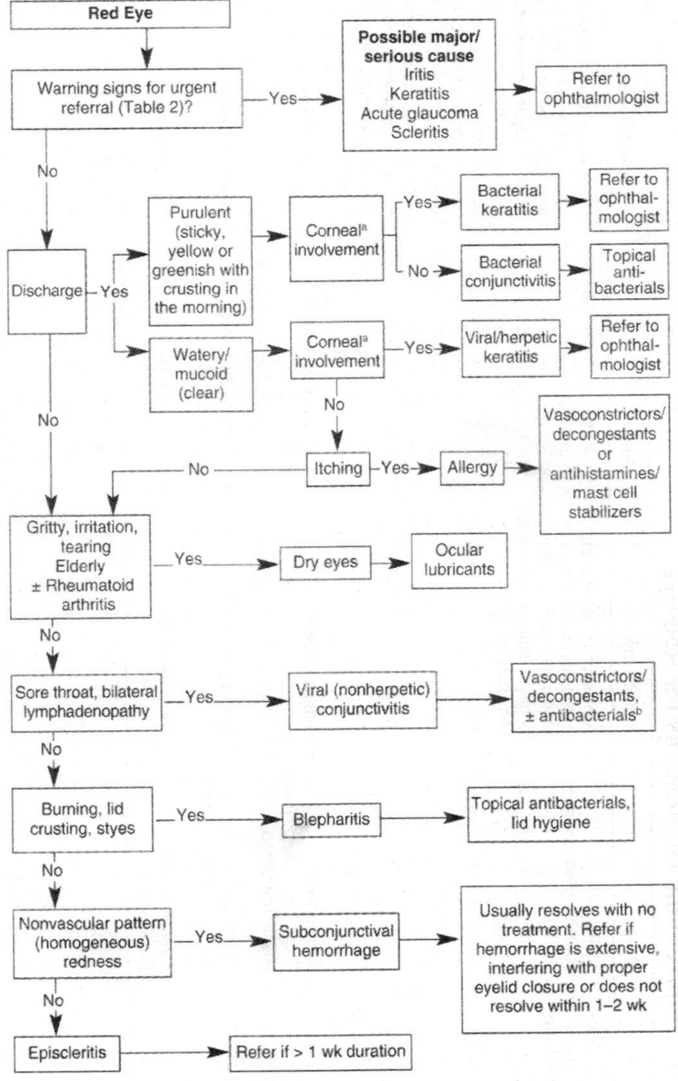

[a] Corneal staining with fluorescein strip indicates corneal involvement.
[b] Used rarely to prevent secondary bacterial infection.

Table 3: **Ophthalmic Medications for Red Eye**

Class	Drug	Indications	Dose	Adverse Effects	Cost[a]
Vasoconstrictors/ Decongestants, ophthalmic	*naphazoline* Naphcon Forte, others	Alleviation of redness and/or eyelid edema in allergic or viral conjunctivitis, minor irritation (smoke, dust, wind, chlorinated pool).	1–2 drops Q3–4H PRN × 3–4 days	Minor stinging on instillation; pupillary dilation and angle-closure glaucoma in predisposed persons, e.g., elderly white or Asian females who are significantly hyperopic, have a positive family history and have not had a therapeutic or prophylactic iridectomy. Ophthalmic vasoconstrictors are meant for occasional and short-term use. Overuse may cause rebound hyperemia.	$
	oxymetazoline Claritin Eye Allergy Relief, Visine Workplace	See naphazoline.	1–2 drops Q6H PRN × 3–4 days	See naphazoline.	$
	phenylephrine Mydfrin, Prefrin, generics	See naphazoline.	1–2 drops QID PRN × ≤ 3 days	See naphazoline.	$
	tetrahydrozoline Visine, others	See naphazoline.	1–2 drops BID-QID	See naphazoline.	$

Class	Drug	Indications	Dose	Adverse Effects	Cost[a]
Antibacterials, ophthalmic	*chloramphenicol* Pentamycetin, generics	Bacterial conjunctivitis/keratitis; blepharitis/styes; prophylactically in corneal epithelial disorders such as dry eyes, exposure, lid malpositions; choose broad-spectrum agent first, guided by patient allergies.	1 drop, or 1 cm ointment Q3H × 48 h, then frequency may decrease.	*Antibacterials*: Chronic use may cause corneal epithelial toxicity; allergy. *Chloramphenicol*: Controversial/theoretical risk of blood dyscrasias with ophthalmic use of chloramphenicol; in patients at increased risk, consider using other broad-spectrum ophthalmic antibacterials such as fusidic acid or framycetin.	$
	ciprofloxacin Ciloxan	See chloramphenicol. Fluoroquinolones should be reserved for serious infections such as Pseudomonas.	Drops: 1–2 drops Q2H while awake × 2 days then 2 drops Q4H while awake × 5 days Ointment: 1.25 cm TID × 2 days then BID × 5 days	See chloramphenicol.	$$
	erythromycin Diomycin, generics	See chloramphenicol.	Ointment: 1.25 cm 2–6 times/day	See chloramphenicol.	$
	framycetin Soframycin	See chloramphenicol.	Drops: 1–2 drops Q1–2H × 2–3 days then 1–2 drops TID-QID Ointment: 1.25 cm BID-TID, or at bedtime if drops used during the day	See chloramphenicol.	Drops: $ Ointment: $$
	fusidic acid Fucithalmic	See chloramphenicol. Due to its broad spectrum and BID dosing, fusidic acid is especially useful in children and elderly patients.	1 drop Q12H × 7 days	See chloramphenicol.	$

(cont'd)

Table 3: **Ophthalmic Medications for Red Eye** *(cont'd)*

Class	Drug	Indications	Dose	Adverse Effects	Cost[a]
	gatifloxacin Zymar	See chloramphenicol. Fluoroquinolones should be reserved for serious infections such as Pseudomonas.	First 2 days: 1 drop in affected eye(s) Q2H while awake, up to 8 times daily. Days 3 to 7: 1 drop QID	See chloramphenicol.	$$
	gentamicin Alcomicin, Garamycin Ophthalmic Drops/ Ointment, generics	See chloramphenicol.	Drops: 1–2 drops Q2–4H Ointment: 1.2 cm BID-TID, or up to Q3–4H	See chloramphenicol.	Drops: $ Ointment: $$
	moxifloxacin Vigamox	See chloramphenicol.	1 drop TID × 7 days	See chloramphenicol.	$$
	ofloxacin Ocuflox, generics	See chloramphenicol. Fluoroquinolones should be reserved for serious infections such as Pseudomonas.	1–2 drops Q2–4H x 2 days then QID × 5 days	See chloramphenicol.	$
	polymyxin B/trimethoprim Polytrim	See chloramphenicol.	Initially 1–3 drops Q1H, gradually decreasing to 1–2 drops 4–6 times daily	See chloramphenicol.	$$$
	polymyxin B ± bacitracin ± gramicidin ± neomycin Neosporin Eye and Ear Solution, Polysporin Eye/Ear Drops, Polysporin Ophthalmic Ointment, generics	See chloramphenicol.	Drops: initially 1–3 drops Q1H, gradually decreasing to 1–2 drops 4–6 times daily Ointment: apply 2–5 times daily	See chloramphenicol.	$

Class	Drug	Indications	Dose	Adverse Effects	Cost[a]
	sulfacetamide Cetamide, generics	See chloramphenicol.	Ointment: 1.5 cm at bedtime	See chloramphenicol.	$
	tobramycin Tobrex, generics	See chloramphenicol.	Drops: 1–2 drops Q4H Ointment: 1.25 cm BID-TID	See chloramphenicol.	$
Antivirals, ophthalmic	*trifluridine* Viroptic, generics	Herpes simplex; *not* for herpes zoster infections.	1 drop Q2H while awake, maximum 9 drops per day, until lesion re-epithelialized, then 1 drop Q4H, maximum 5 drops per day, × 7 days	Chronic use may cause corneal epithelial toxicity.	$$$
Antivirals, systemic	*acyclovir* Zovirax Oral, generics	Herpes zoster, herpes simplex.	Herpes zoster: 800 mg po 5 times/day × 7 days Herpes simplex: 200 mg po QID × 2 wk	GI upset (uncommon); well tolerated.	$$$$
	famciclovir Famvir, generics	Herpes zoster, herpes simplex.	Herpes zoster: 500 mg po TID × 7 days	GI upset (uncommon); well tolerated.	$$$$
	valacyclovir Valtrex	Herpes zoster, herpes simplex.	Herpes zoster: 1 g po TID × 7 days	GI upset (uncommon); well tolerated.	$$$$

(cont'd)

Table 3: **Ophthalmic Medications for Red Eye** *(cont'd)*

Class	Drug	Indications	Dose	Adverse Effects	Cost[a]
Antihis-tamines/Mast Cell Stabilizers, ophthalmic	*sodium cromoglycate* Opticrom, generics	Ocular allergies; contact lens wear-related giant papillary conjunctivitis (a hypersensitivity disorder seen in patients with contact lenses or artificial eyes; family practitioners may suspect it in patients complaining of itch and ropy whitish discharge, but diagnosis requires slit lamp exam by an ophthalmologist).	1–2 drops 4–6 times/day	Minor stinging on instillation.	$
	emedastine Emadine	Ocular allergies.	1 drop up to QID	Minor stinging on instillation.	$$
	ketotifen fumarate Zaditor	Ocular allergies.	1 drop Q8–12H	Minor stinging on instillation.	$$$
	lodoxamide Alomide	Ocular allergies.	1–2 drops QID	Minor stinging on instillation.	$$
	levocabastine Livostin	Ocular allergies.	1 drop QID for up to 2 wk	Minor stinging on instillation.	$$$
	nedocromil Alocril	Ocular allergies.	1–2 drops BID	Minor stinging on instillation.	$$$
	olopatadine Patanol	Ocular allergies.	1–2 drops Q6–8H	Minor stinging on instillation.	$$$

Class	Drug	Indications	Dose	Adverse Effects	Cost[a]
	antazoline/naphazoline Albalon-A Liquifilm	Ocular allergies.	1–2 drops Q3–4H	Minor stinging on instillation.	$
	pheniramine/naphazoline Diopticon A, Naphcon-A, Opcon-A	Ocular allergies.	1–2 drops up to QID	Minor stinging on instillation.	$
Ocular Lubricants	*carboxymethylcellulose* Celluvisc, Refresh Liquigel, Refresh Plus, Refresh Tears	Dry eyes, exposure, lid malpositions, blepharitis, minor irritations.	1–2 drops TID-QID	Preservative toxicity, filmy vision.	$
	dextran 70 /hypromellose (hydroxypropyl methylcellulose) Bion Tears, Tears Naturale, Tears Naturale Free, Tears Naturale II	See carboxymethylcellulose.	1–2 drops TID-QID	See carboxymethylcellulose.	$
	hypromellose (hydroxypropyl methylcellulose) Genteal, Isopto Tears	See carboxymethylcellulose.	1–2 drops TID-QID	See carboxymethylcellulose.	$
	polysorbate Dioptears, Tears Encore	See carboxymethylcellulose.	1–2 drops TID-QID	See carboxymethylcellulose.	$
	polyvinyl alcohol Hypotears Ophthalmic Solution, Liquifilm Tears, Refresh, generics	See carboxymethylcellulose.	1–2 drops TID-QID	See carboxymethylcellulose.	$

(cont'd)

Table 3: **Ophthalmic Medications for Red Eye** *(cont'd)*

Class	Drug	Indications	Dose	Adverse Effects	Cost[a]
	mineral oil/petrolatum Duolube, Hypotears Eye Ointment, Lacri-Lube S.O.P., generics	See carboxymethylcellulose.	Ointment: 0.6 cm to inside of lower lid as needed	See carboxymethylcellulose.	$
	propylene glycol/polyethylene glycol-400 Systane	See carboxymethylcellulose.	1–2 drops as needed	See carboxymethylcellulose.	
	sodium hyaluronate Eyestil	See carboxymethylcellulose.	With preservative: 1 drop up to QID; preservative-free drops can be used more frequently as needed	See carboxymethylcellulose.	$
Corticosteroids, ophthalmic	*dexamethasone* Maxidex, generics	Episcleritis, iritis, scleritis, some keratitis, ocular allergy.	Drops: 2 drops Q1H during the day and Q2H during the night; gradually ↓ to Q3–4H then to TID-QID Ointment: small amount to conjunctival sac TID-QID	Minor stinging on instillation; may worsen herpetic/fungal keratitis; long-term use may cause glaucoma, cataracts.	$
	fluorometholone FML, FML Forte, Flarex, generics	See dexamethasone.	1–2 drops BID-QID; may be used more frequently during initial 48 h if needed	See dexamethasone.	$
	prednisolone Pred Mild/Forte, generics	See dexamethasone.	1–2 drops Q1H during the day and Q2H at night until favourable response, then 1 drop Q4H	See dexamethasone.	$$

Class	Drug	Indications	Dose	Adverse Effects	Cost[a]
	rimexolone Vexol	Inflammation following ocular surgery; anterior uveitis.	Postoperative inflammation: 1–2 drops QID × 2 wk, beginning 24 h post-op Uveitis: 1–2 drops Q1H while awake × 1 wk, then Q2H while awake × 1 wk, then QID × 1 wk, then TID × 4 days, then BID × 3 days	See dexamethasone.	$$
NSAIDs, ophthalmic	*diclofenac* Voltaren Ophtha	Episcleritis, minor corneal abrasions; as an adjunct to topical corticosteroids in scleritis, iritis.	1 drop 4–5 times daily	Minor stinging on instillation.	$$
	flurbiprofen Ocufen	Episcleritis, minor corneal abrasions; as an adjunct to topical corticosteroids in scleritis, iritis.	1 drop QID	See diclofenac.	$$
	ketorolac Acular, generics	Episcleritis, minor corneal abrasions; as an adjunct to topical corticosteroids in scleritis, iritis.	1 drop QID	See diclofenac.	$

[a] Cost of smallest available pack size or 7-day supply of oral medications; includes drug cost only.

Dosage adjustment may be required in renal impairment; see Appendix I.

Legend: $ < $10 $$ $10–20 $$$ $20–30 $$$$ > $30

Suggested Readings

Abnormal eye appearances. In: Frith P. *The eye in clinical practice*. 2nd ed. Oxford (UK): Blackwell Science; 2001. p. 57-84.

Canadian Ophthalmological Society. Self-directed learning modules. *Assessment of the red eye*. Available from: http://www.eyesite.ca/7modules/Module2/html/Mod2_TOC.html Accessed Jan 16, 2007.

Chern, Kenneth C, editor. *Emergency ophthalmology : a rapid treatment guide*. New York (NY): McGraw-Hill; 2002. p. 85-128.

Maclean, Hunter. *The eye in primary care : a symptom-based approach*. Oxford (UK): Butterworth-Heinemann; 2002. p. 96-114.

Trobe, Jonathan D; American Academy of Family Physicians. *The physician's guide to eye care*. 2nd ed. San Francisco (CA): American Academy of Ophthalmology; 2001. p. 41-67.

CHAPTER 25

Age-related Macular Degeneration

Michael J. Potter, MD, FRCSC

Age-related macular degeneration (AMD) is classified as *dry* or *wet* (*exudative*) AMD. The dry form is characterized by drusen (white to yellow spots in the central retina) and may or may not be associated with gradual deterioration in central vision. Wet AMD is responsible for the vast majority of severe vision loss, and always occurs in the setting of pre-existing dry AMD. The wet form is caused by the presence of a choroidal neovascular membrane (CNV). There are a number of similar conditions causing central visual loss, the most common of which is pathologic myopia.

In the Western world, almost a third of people over the age of 75 develop the dry form of AMD.[1] About 90% of severe vision loss, however, is seen in the 5% of these individuals who go on to develop the wet form of the disease.

Up to 30% of the risk of vision loss in AMD is attributable to smoking.[2] Hypertension[2,3,4] and family history[2] of AMD are also risk factors. Vision loss from wet AMD in one eye is associated with a 50% risk[5,6,7] of vision loss in the unaffected eye over five years. Whether nutrition (aside from eating a balanced diet) or wearing sunglasses makes a significant impact is currently unclear.

Goals of Therapy

- Minimize loss of vision
- Improve vision if possible
- Minimize enlargement of central scotomas
- Optimize function and quality of life

Investigations

- Thorough history with attention to:
  - vision loss
    - recent changes
    - central visual changes such as a central scotoma (blank spot in centre of visual field)
    - metamorphopsia (distortion such that straight lines appear curved or crooked)
  - AMD in patient or first-degree relatives
- Physical examination with attention to:
  - visual acuity

- Amsler grid (available at www.stlukeseye.com/eyeq/AmslerPrint.htm)
- funduscopy (dilated fundus exam with slit-lamp biomicroscopy; performed by ophthalmologist)

Note: The retinal exam alone may be inadequate to exclude the presence of a treatable lesion in wet AMD.

- Fluorescein angiography
  - available only at large centres and interpreted by retinal specialists
  - involves intravenous injection of fluorescein sodium, followed by photography of the ocular fundus
  - considered the gold standard for investigating AMD

Note: Some patients have allergic reactions to fluorescein sodium, which is chemically unrelated to x-ray contrast and contains no iodine. Severe reactions are quite rare.

- Optical coherence tomography
  - widely available
  - uses infrared light to generate a cross-sectional view of the macula in false colours
  - considered the gold standard for treatment decisions using vascular endothelial growth factor inhibitors

Therapeutic Choices (Figure 1)

Nonpharmacologic Choices

The *Amsler grid* is useful for self-monitoring by patients. A central blur or distortion in either eye can indicate the onset of the wet form of AMD. The test must be performed with one eye closed, then repeated with the other eye. Reading glasses must be used for the test, if the patient customarily requires them.

Aids such as magnifiers, high-power glasses and reading machines can enable many visually handicapped persons to read enough to perform common household tasks. Low vision clinics sponsored by the Canadian National Institute for the Blind (CNIB) are widely available in Canada.

Pharmacologic Choices

Photodynamic Therapy (PDT)

In patients with a suitable CNV lesion from wet AMD or related conditions, photodynamic therapy [8,9,10,11] with **verteporfin** may be indicated. Verteporfin is a porphyrin derivative that, when activated by light in the presence of oxygen, generates free radicals that damage the neovascular endothelium and occlude the vessels. Verteporfin is contraindicated in patients with porphyria; severe liver disease is a relative contraindication.

PDT has been shown to significantly reduce vision loss compared to placebo.[9,10,11] Patients usually do not recover lost vision, and indeed often lose further vision after the initiation of therapy before plateauing at levels higher than untreated patients. Individual patient response may vary from the averages in the large studies.

Treatment decisions require the interpretation of fluorescein angiograms together with clinical evaluation by a retinal specialist. PDT involves administration of intravenous verteporfin followed by a low-level (nonthermal) laser light that is aimed at the CNV lesion through a magnifying contact lens using a slit-lamp. The 10-minute infusion is followed by a 5-minute waiting period. The laser light is then applied for 83 seconds.

Patients must be in semi-darkness for the treatment, and remain so for 48 hours afterward. Skin is photosensitive during this time, and a severe burn may result if sunlight or bright lights strike the patient anywhere on the body. This warning includes tanning salons, halogen examination lights used in emergency wards, surgical lights and lighting used for dental procedures. Ultraviolet sunscreens provide no protection from this photosensitivity reaction.

Inadvertent subcutaneous extravasation of verteporfin can cause pain and prolonged photosensitivity of the overlying skin until the drug has been metabolized.

Severe back pain during verteporfin infusion, occurring in 2.2% of patients, is an idiosyncratic reaction that improves immediately upon discontinuing the infusion. Uncommonly (less than 5%), patients may experience a severe decrease in vision following therapy, and some may recover this loss with time. It is important to note that the likelihood of severe decrease in vision associated with verteporfin therapy is lower than in untreated patients. Patients are monitored every three months for choroidal neovascular leakage; treatment may need to be repeated at these intervals.

A course of photodynamic therapy can cost over $10,000. Most provincial health plans cover some of these treatments.

Vascular Endothelial Growth Factor (VEGF) Inhibitors

Recent studies have proven the efficacy of inhibitors of vascular endothelial growth factor in decreasing vision loss in wet AMD.[12,13,14,15] These drugs decrease VEGF levels in the extracellular space, which inhibits growth and causes regression of new blood vessels in CNV membranes. They also stabilize the blood-retinal barrier and thereby reduce macular edema, restoring normal anatomy.

Two VEGF inhibitors, **pegaptanib** (Macugen) and **bevacizumab** (Avastin) are available in Canada. Large multicentre randomized controlled clinical trials have been performed with pegaptanib; it was shown to reduce vision loss at a rate similar to that of PDT.[12,13]

Bevacizumab is in widespread use worldwide since it was approved in 2005 for the treatment of colon cancer. It is frequently used off-label for several retinal diseases, including wet AMD. Large-scale studies currently underway are evaluating the efficacy of bevacizumab in AMD, but preclinical and small-scale clinical reports support its safety and clinical effectiveness.[16,17,18,19]

A third agent, **ranibizumab**, is derived from a fragment of bevacizumab but has a higher binding affinity for VEGF. Ninety percent of patients receiving ranibizumab lost less than three lines on a specialized vision chart and 40% showed improvement at two years.[14] There is excellent evidence supporting the use of ranibizumab, and approval for the use of this drug in Canada may be granted in 2007.[14,15]

VEGF inhibitors are injected into the vitreous cavity of the eye (intravitreal injection) every one to two months. The endpoints of treatment have yet to be established, but six injections or more are often required. Optical coherence tomography studies are performed at each visit to determine whether further treatment is needed.

Combination therapy including PDT and VEGF inhibitors is sometimes used.[20] Studies are currently underway to determine optimal treatment guidelines.

Side effects of these drugs are uncommon; the most worrisome is bacterial endophthalmitis from the injection procedure, which occurs at a frequency of 2 in 1000 procedures or less.[21] Severe loss of vision is the hallmark of endophthalmitis. Pain and redness of the eye may also be present. Because irreversible blindness may occur, endophthalmitis is considered a medical emergency that requires immediate treatment by an ophthalmologist; management includes biopsy for bacterial culture followed by intravitreal injection of antibiotics. Often surgery is necessary, and outcomes vary widely depending on the duration and etiology of the infection. Patients receiving intravitreal VEGF inhibitors are warned to come to medical attention immediately if they develop symptoms of endophthalmitis. Many patients will have mild pain from the drug injection procedure, which does not necessarily indicate a problem. Subconjunctival hemorrhage is also common and generally resolves within two weeks.

Costs of the VEGF inhibitors vary from $300 to $2000 per injection depending on the medication and the province.

Prevention

A combination of **beta-carotene** 25 000 IU, **vitamin C** 500 mg, **vitamin E** 400 IU, **zinc** 80 mg and **copper** 2 mg per day reduced AMD-associated vision loss in suitable patients by 25% over seven years in the Age-Related Eye Disease Study (AREDS), a large multicentre trial.[22] Copper was included to reduce the likelihood of anemia in patients taking large amounts of zinc. A commercial preparation of the above vitamins and supplements is available (Table 1). The ingredients and strengths of such products should be carefully checked to ensure they reflect the evidenced-based combination.

Smokers who take supplemental beta-carotene have an increased risk of lung cancer, and should *not* take such preparations.[23,24] Patients who have smoked within the last five to ten years may also be advised not to take supplemental beta-carotene; this duration has not been firmly established. Contraindications to beta-carotene also include severe liver disease, renal insufficiency, renal dialysis and pregnancy. While beta-carotene appears to be less teratogenic than vitamin A, no definitive data on risk are available. Women of child-bearing potential are below the age for which vitamins have been proven effective. High-dose vitamin C and E supplementation is contraindicated in renal disease, and vitamin C has been noted to cause oxalosis in such patients. High-dose zinc may cause gastric disturbances as well as severe anemia. Fish liver oils may contain high doses of vitamins A and E, and toxicity could result from taking multiple supplements with overlapping constituents.

Lutein and **zeaxanthin** are carotenoids similar in structure and function to beta-carotene. They occur naturally in foods and are concentrated in the macula. There is some evidence that they may play a role in normal macular function, and that supplementation may be helpful. Studies are currently underway to determine the efficacy of these compounds, and the same cautions apply as to beta-carotene. Effective and safe doses of lutein and zeaxanthin have not been established.

Omega-3 and -6 fatty acids may also play a role in macular function. Their role in prevention of vision loss is the subject of current investigations.

Figure 1: **Management of Age-related Macular Degeneration**

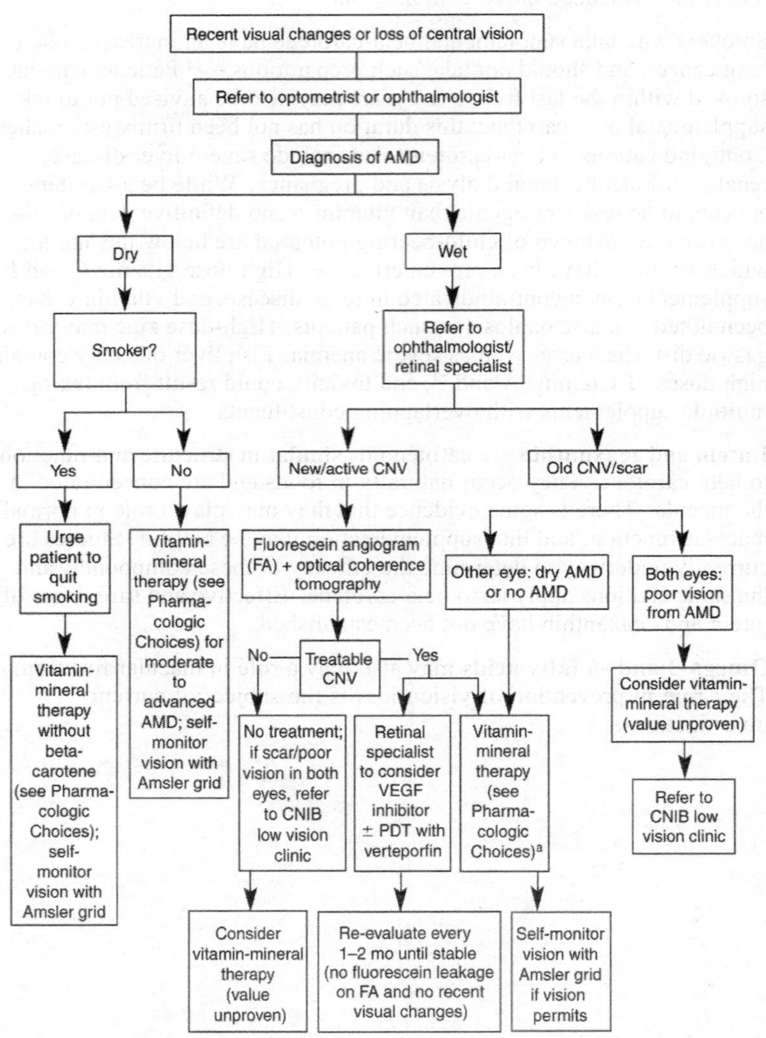

[a] If smoker, vitamin-mineral therapy without beta-carotene and counsel to quit smoking

Abbreviations: AMD = age-related macular degeneration; CNV = choroidal neovascular membrane; CNIB = Canadian National Institute for the Blind; PDT = photodynamic therapy; VEGF = vascular endothelial growth factor

Table 1: Vitamin-mineral Supplements for Wet AMD

Class	Drug	Dose	Comments	Cost[a]
Combination Vitamin/Mineral Supplements, for nonsmokers	*beta-carotene 12 500 IU + vitamin C 250 mg + vitamin E 200 IU + copper 1 mg + zinc 40 mg* Vitalux	1 tablet twice daily	Formulated to match the doses in the AREDS trial.[22] Do not use this formula containing beta-carotene in smokers, due to increased risk of lung cancer. Contraindicated in renal failure, pregnancy. Caution with other vitamin-mineral supplements containing overlapping ingredients.	$$
Combination Vitamin/Mineral Supplements, for smokers	*vitamin C 250 mg + vitamin E 200 IU + copper 1 mg + zinc 40 mg* Vitalux-S	1 tablet twice daily	Alternative formulation for smokers and those who have smoked within the last 5–10 y (duration uncertain) – no beta-carotene. Caution with other vitamin-mineral supplements containing overlapping ingredients.	$$

[a] Cost of 30-day supply; includes drug cost only.
Legend: $ < $10 $$ $10–15

Suggested Readings

Age-Related Eye Disease Study Research Group. A randomized, placebo-controlled, clinical trial of high-dose supplementation with vitamins C and E, beta carotene, and zinc for age-related macular degeneration and vision loss: AREDS report no. 8. *Arch Ophthalmol* 2001;119(10):1417-36.

Bressler NM; Treatment of Age-Related Macular Degeneration with Photodynamic Therapy (TAP) Study Group. Photodynamic therapy of subfoveal choroidal neovascularization in age-related macular degeneration with verteporfin: two-year results of 2 randomized clinical trials-TAP Report 2. *Arch Ophthalmol* 2001;119(2):198-207.

de Jong PT. Age-related macular degeneration. *N Engl J Med* 2006;355(14):1474-85.

Klein R, Klein BE, Tomany SC et al. Ten-year incidence and progression of age-related maculopathy: the Beaver Dam eye study. *Ophthalmology* 2002;109(10):1767-79.

Verteporfin In Photodynamic Therapy Study Group. Verteporfin therapy of subfoveal choroidal neovascularization in age-related macular degeneration: two-year results of a randomized clinical trial including lesions with occult with no classic choroidal neovascularization—Verteporfin in Photodynamic Therapy Report 2. *Am J Ophthalmol* 2001;131(5):541-60.

Verteporfin Roundtable 2000 and 2001 Participants; Treatment of age-related macular degeneration with photodynamic therapy (TAP) study group principal investigators; Verteporfin in photodynamic therapy (VIP) study group principal investigators. Guidelines for using verteporfin (Visudyne) in photodynamic therapy to treat choroidal neovascularization due to age-related macular degeneration and other causes. *Retina* 2002;22(1):6-18.

References

1. Leibowitz HM, Krueger DE, Maunder LR et al. The Framingham Eye Study monograph: an ophthalmological and epidemiological study of cataract, glaucoma, diabetic retinopathy, macular degeneration, and visual acuity in a general population of 2631 adults, 1973-1975. *Surv Ophthalmol* 1980;24(Suppl):335-610.
2. Hyman LG, Lilienfeld AM, Ferris FL et al. Senile macular degeneration: a case-control study. *Am J Epidemiol* 1983;118(2):213-27.
3. Kahn HA, Leibowitz HM, Ganley JP et al. The Framingham Eye Study. II. Association of ophthalmic pathology with single variables previously measured in the Framingham Heart Study. *Am J Epidemiol* 1977;106(1):33-41.
4. Klein BE, Klein R. Cataracts and macular degeneration in older Americans. *Arch Ophthalmol* 1982;100(4):571-3.
5. Bressler SB, Bressler NM, Fine SL et al. Natural course of choroidal neovascular membranes within the foveal avascular zone in senile macular degeneration. *Am J Ophthalmol* 1982;93(2):157-63.
6. Chandra SR, Gragoudas ES, Friedman E et al. Natural history of disciform degeneration of the macula. *Am J Ophthalmol* 1974;78(4):579-82.
7. Gass JD. Drusen and disciform macular detachment and degeneration. *Arch Ophthalmol* 1973;90(3):206-17.
8. Verteporfin Roundtable Participants. Guidelines for using verteporfin (Visudyne) in photodynamic therapy for choroidal neovascularization due to age-related macular degeneration and other causes: update. *Retina* 2005;25(2)119-34.
9. Verteporfin Roundtable 2000 and 2001 Participants; Treatment of age-related macular degeneration with photodynamic therapy (TAP) study group principal investigators; Verteporfin in photodynamic therapy (VIP) study group principal investigators. Guidelines for using verteporfin (Visudyne) in

photodynamic therapy to treat choroidal neovascularization due to age-related macular degeneration and other causes. *Retina* 2002(1);6-18.

10. Verteporfin In Photodynamic Therapy Study Group. Verteporfin therapy of subfoveal choroidal neovascularization in age-related macular degeneration: two-year results of a randomized clinical trial including lesions with occult with no classic choroidal neovascularization—Verteporfin in Photodynamic Therapy Report 2. *Am J Ophthalmol* 2001;131(5)541-60.
11. Bressler NM; Treatment of Age-Related Macular Degeneration with Photodynamic Therapy (TAP) Study Group. Photodynamic therapy of subfoveal choroidal neovascularization in age-related macular degeneration with verteporfin: two-year results of 2 randomized clinical trials-TAP Report 2. *Arch Ophthalmol* 2001;119(2):198-207.
12. Gragoudas ES, Adamis AP, Cunningham ET et al. Pegaptanib for neovascular age-related macular degeneration. *N Engl J Med* 2004;351(27):2805-16.
13. VEGF Inhibition Study in Ocular Neovascularization (V.I.S.I.O.N.) Clinical Trial Group; Chakravarthy U, Adamis AP et al. Year 2 efficacy results of 2 randomized controlled clinical trials of pegaptanib for neovascular age-related macular degeneration. *Ophthalmology* 2006;113(9):1508.e1-25.
14. Rosenfeld PJ, Brown DM, Heier JS et al. Ranibizumab for neovascular age-related macular degeneration. *N Engl J Med* 2006;355(14):1419-31.
15. Brown DM, Kaiser PK, Michels M et al. Ranibizumab versus verteporfin for neovascular age-related macular degeneration. *N Engl J Med* 2006;355(14):1432-44.
16. Avery RL, Pieramici DJ, Rabena MD et al. Intravitreal bevacizumab (Avastin) for neovascular age-related macular degeneration. *Ophthalmology* 2006;113(3):363-372.e5.
17. Lazic R, Gabric N. Intravitreally administered bevacizumab (Avastin) in minimally classic and occult choroidal neovascularization secondary to age-related macular degeneration. *Graefes Arch Clin Exp Ophthalmol* 2007;245(1):68-73.
18. Rich RM, Rosenfeld PJ, Puliafito CA, et al. Short-term safety and efficacy of intravitreal bevacizumab (Avastin) for neovascular age-related macular degeneration. *Retina* 2006;26(5):495-511.
19. Yoganathan P, Deramo VA, Lai JC et al. Visual improvement following intravitreal bevacizumab (Avastin) in exudative age-related macular degeneration. *Retina* 2006;26(9):994-8.
20. Heier JS, Boyer DS, Ciulla TA et al. Ranibizumab combined with verteporfin photodynamic therapy in neovascular age-related macular degeneration: year 1 results of the FOCUS Study. *Arch Ophthalmol* 2006;124(11):1532-42.
21. Chakravarthy U, Soubrane G, Bandello F et al. Evolving European guidance on the medical management of neovascular age related macular degeneration. *Br J Ophthalmol* 2006;90(9):1188-96.
22. Age-Related Eye Disease Study Research Group. A randomized, placebo-controlled, clinical trial of high-dose supplementation with vitamins C and E, beta carotene, and zinc for age-related macular degeneration and vision loss: AREDS report no. 8. *Arch Ophthalmol* 2001;119(10):1417-36.
23. Albanes D, Heinonen OP, Huttunen JK et al. Effects of alpha-tocopherol and beta-carotene supplements on cancer incidence in the Alpha-Tocopherol Beta-Carotene Cancer Prevention Study. *Am J Clin Nutr* 1995;62(6 Suppl):1427S-1430S.
24. Omenn GS, Goodman GE, Thornquist MD et al. Risk factors for lung cancer and for intervention effects in CARET, the Beta-Carotene and Retinol Efficacy Trial. *J Natl Cancer Inst* 1996;88(21):1550-9

CHAPTER 26
Thyroid Disorders

Heather Lochnan, MD, FRCPC

Thyroid disease is extremely common, with women more frequently affected than men. The symptoms associated with thyroid disease are often nonspecific. A high index of suspicion coupled with a low threshold for screening for thyroid disease will capture most affected patients.

Goals of Therapy

- Achieve a euthyroid state in patients with hyperthyroidism or hypothyroidism
- Recognize which patients with goitre or thyroid nodules require treatment
- Manage patients with thyroid disease during all stages of life, including pregnancy

Hypothyroidism

Hypothyroidism is a clinical syndrome that usually results from a deficiency of thyroid hormone (Table 1). Rarely, it can be due to resistance to thyroid hormone. A thyroid-stimulating hormone (TSH) measurement is a very sensitive indicator of hypothyroidism but may be low or normal in pituitary or hypothalamic disease. *Subclinical hypothyroidism* is defined by an elevated TSH with normal thyroid hormone levels.[1] If subclinical hypothyroidism is confirmed, consider treatment, especially in patients with TSH > 10 mU/L (normally 0.3 to 6.0 mU/L, depending on the laboratory), an abnormal lipid profile, symptoms of hypothyroidism and in patients who are antithyroid peroxidase (anti-TPO) positive or who are planning a pregnancy.[2]

Investigations

- Thorough history with attention to:
  - symptoms such as fatigue, weight gain, impaired memory, constipation and cold intolerance
- Physical examination with attention to:
  - appearance, e.g., coarse features, dry skin and hair
  - hypertension, bradycardia
  - delayed relaxation phase of reflexes
  - extreme cases may present with myxedema coma (hypotension, coma, hypothermia)
- Laboratory investigations:
  - TSH

- free triiodothyronine (fT_3)
- free thyroxine (fT_4)
- antithyroid peroxidase (anti-TPO or antimicrosomal antibodies)

Table 1: Causes of Hypothyroidism

Cause	Comments
Hashimoto's thyroiditis	Most common cause; anti-TPO levels very high
Iatrogenic	Surgical removal of thyroid; ^{131}I therapy; drugs such as lithium, amiodarone, sulfonylureas, iodinated contrast agents
Hypothyroid phase of subacute thyroiditis	Usually transient
Congenital	Aplasia of thyroid; dyshormonogenesis
Iodine deficiency	Rare in North America
Recovering phase of nonthyroidal illness	Transiently elevated TSH
Pituitary disorder	*Secondary* hypothyroidism; TSH low or normal; fT_4 usually low
Hypothalamic disorder	*Tertiary* hypothyroidism; TSH low or normal; fT_4 usually low
Resistance to thyroid hormone	High TSH, fT_3 and fT_4

Abbreviations: fT_3 = free triiodothyronine; fT_4 = free thyroxine

Therapeutic Choices

Pharmacologic Choices (Table 4)

Levothyroxine (L-T_4)

The goal of L-T_4 replacement therapy is to normalize the TSH level. Replacement dosages average 1.6 µg/kg/day in adults and 10 to 16 µg/kg/day in newborns. Dosage adjustment is made every four to six weeks as needed. Generally, it takes six weeks to attain a new steady state after dosage adjustments. In the elderly, or in patients with coronary artery disease, start with a dose as low as 12.5 µg/day as tolerated, and titrate every four weeks.

Liothyronine (Triiodothyronine, T_3)

T_3 is used for short-term management of patients with thyroid cancer undergoing withdrawal of L-T_4. The combination of L-T_4 and T_3 is occasionally used for replacement therapy, though recent studies have shown little or no benefit of combination therapy and there is concern of causing adverse effects with T_3.[3]

Therapeutic Tips

- Because thyroid binding globulins increase during *pregnancy*, requirements for L-T_4 replacement may increase by up to 50% during pregnancy to maintain TSH at around 1 to 3 mU/mL.[5]
- Numerous drugs can interfere with the absorption and metabolism of L-T_4 (Table 4). Iron supplementation frequently decreases L-T_4 absorption.
- *Myxedema coma* is treated with L-T_4 300 to 500 µg iv initially, followed by 100 µg iv daily. These patients are concomitantly treated with corticosteroids, such as hydrocortisone 100 mg iv Q8H. Supportive therapy and passive rewarming are indicated as required.

Hyperthyroidism

Hyperthyroidism (thyrotoxicosis) is defined as the syndrome of excessive thyroid hormone production and its effects (Table 2). *Subclinical hyperthyroidism* is common and can be a risk factor for atrial fibrillation.[6,7] In subclinical hyperthyroidism, TSH is suppressed while thyroid hormone levels are normal. Treatment is indicated if the patient is frail and/or elderly, has other risk factors for atrial fibrillation or has symptoms of hyperthyroidism.

Thyroid storm is a life-threatening medical emergency characterized by severe thyrotoxicosis as well as other signs and symptoms. It can be precipitated by many causes including radioactive iodine, infection, trauma, surgery or withdrawal from antithyroid drugs.

Investigations

- A thorough history with attention to:
  - symptoms such as weight loss, palpitations, diarrhea, heat intolerance and anxiety
- Physical examination with attention to:
  - signs such as eyelid lag, stare and the ophthalmopathy associated with Graves' disease; tachycardia; hyperreflexia; warm, moist skin; goitre or nodules
- Laboratory tests, nuclear medicine and imaging:
  - TSH, fT_3, fT_4
  - thyroid scan
  - radioactive iodine uptake (RAIU)

Note: Suppression of TSH can be seen in nonthyroidal illness, depression or treatment with corticosteroids and some centrally acting medications (e.g., domperidone, metoclopramide, dopamine).

Table 2: **Causes of Hyperthyroidism**

Cause	Comments
Graves' disease	Due to thyroid-stimulating immunoglobulins activating the TSH receptor; most common cause of hyperthyroidism; patients frequently have eye disease and possibly pretibial myxedema;[8] RAIU is elevated and thyroid scan with pertechnetate or ^{123}I shows a diffuse pattern
Subacute thyroiditis	Scan poorly defines the gland; RAIU is very low
Postpartum thyroiditis	Scan poorly defines the gland; RAIU is very low (not usually done if patient is lactating)
Toxic nodule	Thyroid scan shows hot area
Toxic multinodular goitre	Scan shows multiple hot areas; RAIU is slightly elevated
Iodine excess	Usually in setting of multinodular goitre; RAIU is low
Iatrogenic	Due to overtreatment with thyroid hormones; scan shows no thyroid; 0% RAIU
Struma ovarii	Very rare; thyroid hormone production in ectopic sites; RAIU is 0%; body scan will show thyroid tissue in ovary
Metastatic thyroid cancer	With large tumor burden
TSH–producing pituitary adenoma	TSH elevated
Stimulation of TSH receptor by excessive human chorionic gonadotropin	Examples are hydatidiform mole, hyperemesis gravidarum, other tumors

Abbreviations: RAIU = radioactive iodine uptake; TSH = thyroid-stimulating hormone

Therapeutic Choices

Nonpharmacologic Choices

Consider thyroid surgery in patients with thyroid nodules, large goitre, and occasionally in patients with Graves' disease. Surgery is part of the management of thyroid cancer and ectopic production of thyroid hormone. Medical therapy is frequently initiated prior to surgery to make the patient euthyroid if possible.

Pharmacologic Choices (Table 5)

Use **radioactive iodine (^{131}I)** to ablate thyroid tissue in patients with Graves' disease, toxic autonomous nodules and toxic multinodular goitres. Inducing hypothyroidism is the main risk associated with its use. It is contraindicated in pregnancy. Use with caution, or concomitantly with **corticosteroids**, in patients with significant ophthalmopathy.[9]

Methimazole (MMI) and **propylthiouracil (PTU)** decrease the production of thyroid hormones; PTU can also block the conversion of T_4 to T_3. PTU is the drug of choice for the treatment of hyperthyroidism in pregnant women. Both drugs must be stopped about five days prior to a thyroid scan, RAIU or treatment with ^{131}I. PTU may make the thyroid more resistant to ^{131}I.[10] Side effects of these agents include allergy, rash, agranulocytosis and, rarely, hepatotoxicity and nephrotoxicity.

Beta-adrenergic blockers ameliorate the symptoms of adrenergic excess and are usually used adjunctively in the management of Graves' disease or toxic nodules. Nonselective agents such as propranolol can decrease the conversion of T_4 to T_3. Avoid beta-blockers in patients with asthma.

Iodine, in the form of oral **Lugol's solution** (6.3 mg iodide per drop) or iv **sodium iodide**, blocks thyroid hormone production. Iodine can be used in the acute management of severe hyperthyroidism.

Consider **corticosteroids** as adjuvant therapy in treatment-resistant cases.

The management of *thyroid storm* involves supportive therapy in conjunction with aggressive treatment with antithyroid medications, beta-blockers and corticosteroids. Use acetaminophen for hyperthermia, and avoid ASA and other NSAIDs.[11] Plasmapheresis can be considered in unresponsive cases.

Therapeutic Tips

- Patients with Graves' disease may have prolonged suppression of TSH, despite normalization or decreased levels of thyroid hormones. Follow TSH, fT_4 and fT_3 levels.
- Patients on propylthiouracil or methimazole can develop a gradual neutropenia which may be detected by regular measurement of white blood cell counts with a differential. In many cases it occurs suddenly, and patients should be advised to contact their physician immediately if symptoms of infection occur.
- Warn patients who decline treatment of the risks of untreated hyperthyroidism, which include myopathy, cardiac arrhythmias, cardiomyopathy and osteoporosis.

Thyroid Nodules and Goitre

Individuals with *goitre* may be at higher risk for disorders of thyroid function and should be screened with a TSH level. Goitres in euthyroid patients can be problematic if growing or causing compressive symptoms. The usual treatment is surgery. Thyroid suppression with L-T_4 may help prevent further growth and occasionally shrink the gland.

Thyroid *nodules* are very common. They may be identified incidentally by ultrasound, CT or MRI of the neck.[12] Solitary nodules are concerning, but large or growing nodules within a multinodular goitre should be investigated similarly to a solitary nodule. Thyroid suppression therapy for nodules is no longer routinely used.[13] Table 3 lists risk factors for thyroid cancer.

Table 3: **Risk Factors for Thyroid Cancer**[14]

< 20 or > 60 years of age
Prior radiation exposure
Male gender
Family history of thyroid cancer
Previous malignancy
Nodule > 4 cm in size or rapidly growing
Nodule fixed to soft tissue
Vocal cord paralysis
Lymphadenopathy

Therapeutic Choices (Figure 1)

Nonpharmacologic Choices

Surgery is the definitive therapy. Surgical pathology will confirm or exclude malignancy and reduce compressive symptoms. The risks associated with surgery include hypothyroidism, hypoparathyroidism and vocal cord paralysis. Consider surgery if two or more risk factors for malignancy are present.

Pharmacologic Choices (Table 4)

Radioactive iodine therapy can be used to treat a multinodular goitre or a *hot* nodule, with an associated risk of hypothyroidism.

Levothyroxine can be considered to prevent further growth of a *benign* nodule.[15] The goal is to keep TSH below 1.0 mU/L, and above the lower limit of the normal range. In this setting, the risk of inducing hyperthyroidism is minimal.

Therapeutic Tips

- Ultrasound can be helpful to document the size of a goitre or nodule and whether it is changing in size. Some features on ultrasound may raise suspicion of malignancy.
- A thyroid scan is rarely needed if the TSH is normal.
- Repeat fine needle aspiration biopsy (FNAB) if a nodule is growing.

Figure 1: **Management of Thyroid Nodules**

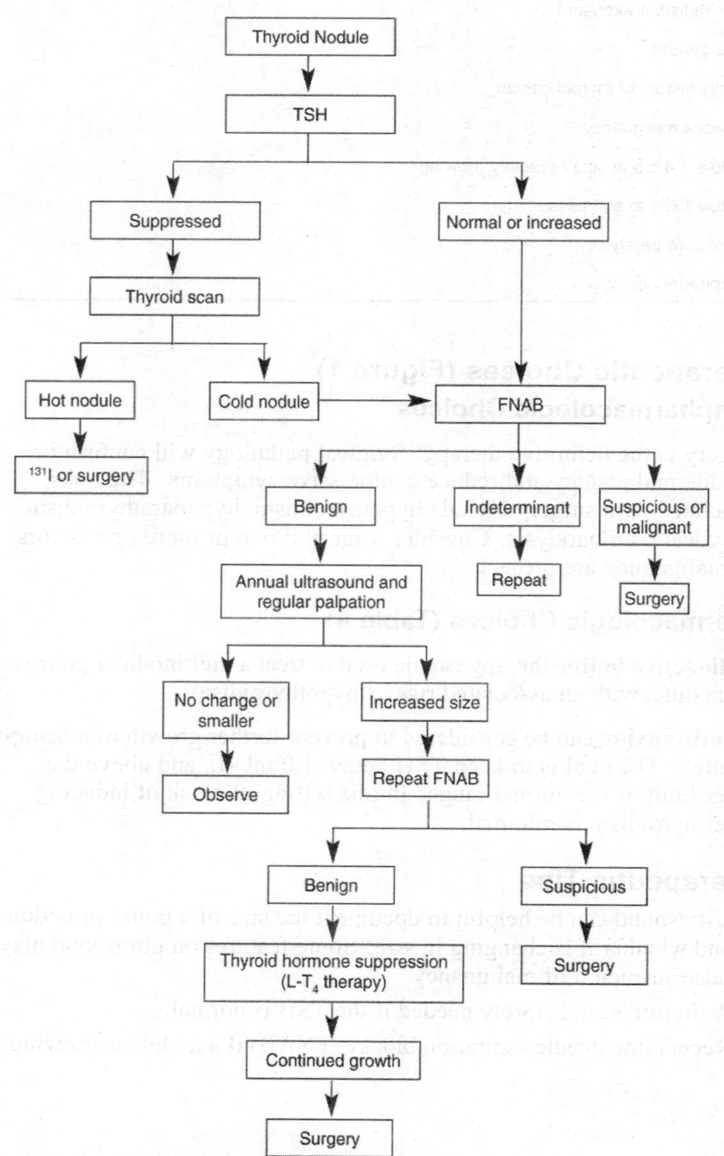

Abbreviations: TSH = thyroid-stimulating hormone; FNAB = fine needle aspiration biopsy.

Table 4: **Drugs Used in the Management of Hypothyroidism**

Class	Drug	Dose	Adverse Effects	Drug Interactions	Comments	Cost[a]
Thyroid Hormones	*levothyroxine* Eltroxin, Euthyrox, Synthroid, generics	Average adult replacement: 1.6 µg/kg/day; elderly patients may need less Start with 12.5–25 µg/day in those at risk of angina	Symptoms of hyperthyroidism if over-treated; possible exacerbation of angina.	Absorption may be ↓ by iron salts, calcium salts, cholestyramine (separate administration by 6 hours), colestipol and sucralfate. Response to warfarin may vary. Glycemic control may decline with initiation of levothyroxine, potentially necessitating dosage adjustment of antihyperglycemic agents.	Monitor TSH levels to adjust initial dosage after 6–8 wk, then as required or annually; adrenal insufficiency may be uncovered; dosage may have to be increased during pregnancy to maintain TSH in desired range; check TSH each trimester and 4–6 wk after any dosage adjustment.	$
	liothyronine (triiodothyronine) Cytomel	Up to 25 µg BID for short-term management of thyroid cancer patients off L-T_4	See levothyroxine.			$$$

[a] Cost of 30-day supply; includes drug cost only.
Legend: $ < $5 $$ $5–30 $$$ $30–35

Table 5: **Drugs Used in the Management of Hyperthyroidism**

Class	Drug	Dose	Adverse Effects	Drug Interactions	Comments	Cost[a]
Antithyroid Agents	*methimazole* (MMI) Tapazole, generic	10–30 mg daily in 2–3 divided doses; higher doses are sometimes necessary *Thyroid storm*: up to 40 mg BID may be required	Risk of skin rash, allergic reaction, agranulocytosis, rarely hepatotoxicity, nephrotoxicity.	May potentiate the action of warfarin.	Warn patient to stop medication if rash, fever, sore throat, or jaundice develop.	$$–$$$
	propylthiouracil (PTU) Propyl-Thyracil	Initially 50–100 mg TID in most cases; reduce dose in renal failure *Thyroid storm*: up to 1200 mg daily in divided doses	Risk of skin rash; allergic reaction; agranulocytosis; rarely, hepatotoxicity.	See methimazole.	See methimazole. Preferred drug during pregnancy and lactation; in pregnancy, use the lowest dose necessary to maintain thyroid hormone in the upper normal range.	$$
Iodine	*iodine*	*Thyroid storm*: sodium iodide 0.5–1 g iv Q12H for several days, or Lugol's solution, 3–5 drops Q6H po, 1 h after antithyroid drug *Prior to thyroidectomy*: if hyperthyroidism reasonably controlled, use Lugol's solution 2–6 drops TID po × 7 d preceding operation	Allergy, hypersensitivity.		Administer 1 h after PTU or MMI; blocks radioactive iodine uptake.	$

Class	Drug	Dose	Adverse Effects	Drug Interactions	Comments	Cost[a]
Beta$_1$-adrenergic Antagonists, nonselective	*propranolol* generics	*Hyperthyroidism*: 10–40 mg QID *Thyroid storm*: 40–120 mg Q6H po or 0.5–2 mg iv slowly Q4–6H, if no evidence of cardiac decompensation	Fatigue, bradycardia.		Avoid in patients with asthma or conditions associated with bradycardia; taper once thyrotoxicosis improved. Controls tachycardia.	$–$$
Beta$_1$-adrenergic Antagonists, selective	*atenolol* Tenormin, generics	Initial dose: 25–50 mg daily, may ↑ to 200 mg daily	See propranolol.		See propranolol. May have faster onset of action compared to propranolol. Controls tachycardia.	$$
	metoprolol Betaloc, Lopresor, generics	50 mg QID, may ↑ to 100 mg QID	See propranolol.		See propranolol. May have faster onset of action compared to propranolol. Controls tachycardia.	$$–$$$
Corticosteroids, oral	*dexamethasone* generics	*Thyroid storm*: 2 mg Q6H po or iv; continue until free T_3 level controlled	Numerous effects especially if prolonged use; acutely: elevated blood glucose, risk of avascular necrosis, altered mood.	Effects can be diminished with concomitant medications such as phenytoin.	Reserved for emergency adjunctive management of hyperthyroidism or myxedema coma, in conjunction with specific management of thyroid disorder.	$ (3 days' oral therapy)

(cont'd)

Table 5: **Drugs Used in the Management of Hyperthyroidism** *(cont'd)*

Class	Drug	Dose	Adverse Effects	Drug Interactions	Comments	Cost[a]
	hydrocortisone sodium succinate Solu-Cortef, generics	*Myxedema coma*: 100 mg iv Q8H; taper when stable	See dexamethasone.	See dexamethasone.	See dexamethasone.	$$$$ (3 days' iv therapy)
Iodine, radioactive	*sodium iodide* *^{131}I* Iodotope	*Graves' disease*: ~ 370 MBq (10 mCi); more might be used for a toxic nodule or nodular goitre, or less if uptake is very high	High risk of hypothyroidism; possible worsening of Graves' ophthalmopathy; risk of radiation thyroiditis.		Given as single oral dose; usually only one dose required.	$$$$ (per dose)

[a] Cost of 30-day supply unless otherwise specified; includes drug cost only.

Dosage adjustment may be required in renal impairment; see Appendix I

Abbreviations: TSH = thyroid-stimulating hormone; T_3 = triiodothyronine; MBq = megabecquerels; mCi = megacurie; MMI = methimazole; PTU = propylthiouracil

Legend: $ < $10 $–$$ < $10–20 $$ $10–20 $$–$$$ $10–30 $$$ $20–30 $$$$ > $30

Suggested Readings

AACE/AME Task Force on Thyroid Nodules. American Association of Clinical Endocrinologists and Associazione Medici Endocrinologi medical guidelines for clinical practice for the diagnosis and management of thyroid nodules. *Endocr Pract* 2006;12(1):63-102. Available from: http://www.aace.com/pub/pdf/guidelines/thyroid_nodules.pdf Accessed May 29, 2007.

American Association of Clinical Endocrinologists. American Association of Clinical Endocrinologists medical guidelines for clinical practice for the evaluation and treatment of hypothyroidism and hyperthyroidism. *Endocr Pract* 2002;8(6):457-69. Available from: http://www.aace.com/pub/pdf/guidelines/hypo_hyper.pdf Accessed May 29, 2007.

Cooper DS. Antithyroid Drugs. *N Engl J Med* 2005;352(9):905-917.

Klein I, Ojamaa K. Thyroid hormone and the cardiovascular system. *N Engl J Med* 2001;344(7):501-9.

Thyroid disease manager. South Dartmouth (MA): Endocrine Education. Available from: http://www.thyroidmanager.org/ Accessed May 29, 2007.

References

1. Cooper DS. Clinical practice. Subclinical hypothyroidism. *N Engl J Med* 2001;345(4):260-5.
2. Surks MI, Ortiz E, Daniels GH et al. Subclinical thyroid disease: scientific review and guidelines for diagnosis and management. *JAMA* 2004;291(2):228-38.
3. Escobar-Morreale HF, Botella-Carretero JI, Escobar del Rey F et al. Review: Treatment of hypothyroidism with combinations of levothyroxine plus liothyronine. *J Clin Endocrinol Metab* 2005;90(8):4946-54.
4. Bunevicius R, Kazanavicius G, Zalinkevicius R et al. Effects of thyroxine as compared with thyroxine plus triiodothyronine in patients with hypothyroidism. *N Engl J Med* 1999;340(6):424-9.
5. Alexander EK, Marqusee E, Lawrence J et al. Timing and magnitude of increases in levothyroxine requirements during pregnancy in women with hypothyroidism. *N Engl J Med* 2004;351(3):241-9.
6. Weetman AP. Graves' disease. *N Engl J Med* 2000;343(17):1236-48.
7. Toft AD. Clinical practice. Subclinical hyperthyroidism. *N Engl J Med* 2001;345(7):512-6.
8. Sawin CT, Geller A, Wolf PA et al. Low serum thyrotropin concentrations as a risk factor for atrial fibrillation in older persons. *N Engl J Med* 1994;331(19):1249-52.
9. Bartalena L, Marcocci C, Bogazzi F et al. Relation between therapy for hyperthyroidism and the course of Graves' ophthalmopathy. *N Engl J Med* 1998;338(2):73-8.
10. Imseis RE, Vanmiddlesworth L, Massie JD et al. Pretreatment with propylthiouracil but not methimazole reduces the therapeutic efficacy of iodine-131 in hyperthyroidism. *J Clin Endocrinol Metab* 1998;83(2):685-7.
11. Larsen PR. Salicylate-induced increases in free triiodothyronine in human serum: Evidence of inhibition of triiodothyronine binding to thyroxine-binding globulin and thyroxine-binding prealbumin. *J Clin Invest* 1972;51:1125-1134.
12. Tan GH, Gharib H. Thyroid incidentalomas: management approaches to nonpalpable nodules discovered incidentally on thyroid imaging. *Ann Intern Med* 1997;126(3):226-31.
13. Gharib H, Mazzaferri EL. Thyroxine suppressive therapy in patients with nodular thyroid disease. *Ann Intern Med* 1998;128(5):386-94.
14. Mazzaferri EL, Kloos RT. Clinical review 128: current approaches to primary therapy for papillary and follicular thyroid cancer. *J Clin Endocrinol Metab* 2001;86(4):1447-63.
15. Ridgway EC. Medical treatment of benign thyroid nodules: have we defined a benefit? *Ann Intern Med* 1998;128(5):403-5.

CHAPTER 27
Diabetes Mellitus

M.A. Boctor, MD, DMSc, FRCPC

Diabetes mellitus is a chronic metabolic disturbance characterized by fasting or postprandial hyperglycemia. Rather than a single disease entity, diabetes mellitus is a heterogeneous syndrome that is caused by an absolute or relative lack of insulin, resistance to the action of insulin, or both. When severe, it affects carbohydrate, lipid and protein metabolism.

Severe long-term diabetes mellitus may lead to complications involving small blood vessels (microangiopathy), large blood vessels (macroangiopathy) and nerve damage (neuropathy), affecting multiple organs and systems.

Dysglycemia describes abnormal blood glucose levels without definite threshold. The term reflects current evidence that even minor degrees of blood glucose abnormalities increase cardiovascular risk, but that optimal blood glucose levels have not yet been identified.

Classification

Type 1 diabetes mellitus is due to beta cell destruction, usually leading to absolute insulin deficiency. It is most often immune mediated, but occasionally is idiopathic. Type 1 diabetes usually presents as acute metabolic symptoms of relatively short duration in a child, adolescent or young adult. If untreated, ketoacidosis may supervene. Onset is unusual after 30 years of age; the presentation may be more gradual in older individuals. In North America, type 1 accounts for 5 to 10% of all patients with diabetes.

Type 2 diabetes mellitus ranges from predominant insulin resistance with relative insulin deficiency, to a predominant insulin secretory defect with insulin resistance. This entity is commonly discovered incidentally, or is diagnosed in an adult who is most often obese and has nonspecific symptoms. Presentation with chronic complications is becoming increasingly frequent. The incidence and prevalence of type 2 diabetes is rising rapidly in certain ethnic groups, notably aboriginal populations around the world. It is also being diagnosed more frequently in obese children and adolescents.

Gestational diabetes is defined as onset or recognition of glucose intolerance in pregnancy.

Other specific causes of diabetes mellitus include genetic syndromes such as maturity-onset diabetes of the young, pancreatic diseases, infectious agents, other diseases leading to carbohydrate intolerance or drug-induced carbohydrate intolerance. Drugs that can perturb blood glucose levels and interfere with glycemic control in patients with diabetes are presented in Table 1.

Table 1: **Drugs That Can Cause Dysglycemia**

- Atypical antipsychotic agents, e.g., clozapine, olanzapine, risperidone, quetiapine, ziprasidone
- Beta-adrenergic agonists, e.g. atenolol, metoprolol, propranolol
- Diazoxide
- Glucocorticoids, e.g., prednisone
- Interferon alfa
- Nicotinic acid
- Pentamidine
- Phenytoin
- Protease inhibitors (amprenavir, atazanavir, fosamprenavir, darunavir, indinavir, lopinavir, nelfinavir, ritonavir, saquinavir, tipranavir)
- Thiazide diuretics, e.g., hydrochlorothiazide

Goals of Therapy

- Control symptoms
- Establish and maintain optimum metabolic control, while avoiding hypoglycemia
- Prevent or minimize the risk of complications
- Achieve optimal control of comorbidities such as hypertension and dyslipidemia

Investigations (Figure 1)

- Diabetes mellitus may present in a variety of settings:
  - asymptomatic; incidental discovery through screening
  - nonspecific signs and symptoms such as fatigue, lassitude, weight changes
  - presence of diabetic complications such as macrovascular or microvascular changes, neuropathy, kidney disease, erectile dysfunction
  - acute metabolic symptoms such as polyuria, polydipsia, weight loss
  - diabetic ketoacidosis
- The diagnosis of diabetes is established by:[1]
  - a casual (random) plasma glucose ≥ 11.1 mmol/L in the presence of classic symptoms of diabetes (polyuria, polydipsia and unexplained weight loss)

    or
  - a fasting plasma glucose (FBG) ≥ 7.0 mmol/L confirmed by a second test done on a subsequent day (fasting is defined as no caloric intake for ≥ 8 hours)

    or

  - a plasma glucose level ≥ 11.1 mmol/L two hours after a 75 g oral glucose load

Screening

All individuals should be evaluated annually for diabetes risk. A fasting plasma glucose level should be measured every three years in individuals over 40 years of age. Consider earlier and more frequent testing in individuals at a higher risk (Table 2).[2]

Fasting plasma glucose (FPG) levels are less sensitive screening tests than postprandial glucose levels or those measured by oral glucose tolerance testing.[3] They also are not as good at predicting cardiovascular risk in patients with diabetes or states of carbohydrate intolerance.[4] However, measurement of FPG is the recommended screening test because it is less expensive, more reproducible and easier to standardize than other alternatives.

Table 2: **Risk Factors for Diabetes Mellitus**[2]

- 1st degree relative with diabetes mellitus
- History of impaired glucose tolerance or impaired fasting glucose
- Vascular disease
- Hypertension
- Overweight
- Polycystic ovary syndrome
- Schizophrenia

Type 1 and Type 2 Diabetes Mellitus

Therapeutic Choices

Therapy for type 2 diabetes should be aimed at achieving glycemic targets as close to normal as possible as early as possible. Aim to achieve target glycosylated hemoglobin (HbA_{1c}) within 6–12 months.[5] If nonpharmacologic therapy fails to establish euglycemia, institute drug therapy promptly. In patients with marked hyperglycemia (HbA_{1c} ≥ 9%) at the time of diagnosis, institute drug therapy in conjunction with nonpharmacologic therapy.

Nonpharmacologic Choices

Nonpharmacologic therapy plays a pivotal role in the treatment of both type 1 and type 2 diabetes. Those with type 1 diabetes must be initiated on insulin therapy at the time of diagnosis, along with nonpharmacologic therapy.

- *Education* is vital in making the patient a full participant in the diabetes health care delivery team and ensuring that they can effectively and safely manage the disease. A well-structured educational program teaches the patient:

- a basic understanding of diabetes
- the role of diet, exercise and medications
- how and when to self-monitor blood glucose and why it is necessary
- management of sick days
- recognition and treatment of hypoglycemia
- knowledge of the major side effects of medications and how to adjust drugs in response to changes in diet and activity
- care of the feet

- *Nutritional management* should be individualized. Provide counselling by a registered dietitian and include instruction on nutrients from all the basic food groups. Total caloric consumption in patients with type 2 diabetes should be reduced to decrease weight and improve metabolic control. For patients on insulin, tailor the distribution of food intake into meals and snacks according to the individual's preference, lifestyle and medications taken. In patients with type 1 diabetes, the amount and type of carbohydrate have the most immediate impact on blood glucose levels. Advise patients to fix carbohydrate consumption or count the amount of carbohydrate ingested and adjust the insulin dose accordingly.
- *Self-monitoring of blood glucose levels* usually results in improved control of blood glucose, allows appropriate recognition of low blood glucose levels and provides immediate feedback about the effects of therapy. Monitoring blood sugar levels before each meal and before bedtime is an absolute minimum in individuals on intensive therapy, and postprandial testing (2 hours after meals) is recommended. Self-monitoring is an integral component of therapeutic plans for patients treated with insulin and oral antihyperglycemic agents. It is also useful in those treated with diet alone.[4]
- *Physical activity* and *exercise* improve cardiovascular function, enhance insulin sensitivity, lower blood pressure and lipid levels and improve glycemic control in type 2 diabetes. Educate patients treated with insulin about the effect of exercise on blood glucose and how to adjust the insulin dosage. Teach patients how to time their meals and/or regulate food consumption to ensure the safety of the prescribed exercise regimen.[5]
- *Periodic reassessments* including directed histories and physical examinations are intended to detect comorbidities and complications; assessments should include:
  - blood pressure measurements
  - foot examinations
  - tests of long-term control (HbA_{1c}). Individualize the frequency of testing—every 3–4 months for patients on insulin; at least every 6

months for those on nutritional therapy or oral antihyperglycemic agents
- assuring the accuracy of blood glucose measurements made by the patient
- reinforcing skills learned in education and dietary counselling
- urinary albumin excretion rate, using the albumin-creatinine ratio, at least annually
- fasting lipid profile, at the time of diagnosis and every 1–3 years if initially normal
- eye examination using dilated fundoscopy or wide-angle stereoscopic retinal photography at the time of diagnosis in patients with type 2 diabetes, and 5 years after diagnosis or at puberty in patients with type 1 diabetes; repeat at least every 2 years if initially normal
- annual influenza immunization and one-time pneumococcal immunization

Pharmacologic Choices

Type 1 Diabetes

Insulin may be administered by syringe, pen or continuous subcutaneous insulin infusion (CSII). Inhaled insulin has a rapid onset and a short duration of action suitable for use at mealtimes. It is available in the US and Europe but has not yet been approved in Canada. Either human insulin preparations or insulin analogues may be used (Table 6). Pure pork insulin preparations are still available, but beef/pork preparations are no longer produced in North America. The long-acting insulin analogues (insulin glargine and insulin detemir) produce more predictable effects than other intermediate- or long-acting insulin preparations, allowing for better control of FPG levels with fewer hypoglycemic episodes, especially nocturnal.[6,7,8]

Insulin Regimens (Table 3)

The Diabetes Control and Complications Trial (DCCT) showed that intensive treatment regimens control blood glucose more effectively than conventional regimens and reduce the risk of long-term diabetic microangiographic complications (retinopathy, nephropathy, neuropathy).[9] Follow-up data from the trial demonstrate a long-term benefit of intensive therapy on the risk of cardiovascular events.[10] Newly diagnosed patients and those with poor glycemic control on conventional regimens should be offered the option of an intensive diabetes management regimen.

Most patients require approximately 0.5 U of insulin per kg of lean body mass. To avoid hypoglycemia, initiate therapy with a lower dose and adjust the dose according to blood glucose response. Regular home monitoring allows patients to adjust the dose of insulin to correct abnormal blood glucose levels, to adjust the dose more accurately for diet and exercise and to readjust the insulin dose based on blood glucose patterns. For optimal control, regular insulin should be administered 20 to 30 minutes before meals. Alternatively, a very rapid acting insulin analogue may be more conveniently administered shortly before eating.

The use of CSII or regimens involving multiple doses of rapid-acting insulin improves the stability of postprandial glucose levels and may also diminish the frequency and severity of hypoglycemia, especially early nocturnal hypoglycemia. CSII using insulin pumps can achieve a tighter and more reproducible degree of glycemic control, but at a significantly increased cost to the patient.

Table 3: **Insulin Regimens in Type 1 Diabetes Mellitus**

	Rapid- or Short-acting	Intermediate- or Long-acting	Comments
Intensive: Multiple Dose Insulin Regimens	R, insulin aspart, glulisine or lispro before each meal	N, insulin glargine, insulin detemir at supper *or* bedtime	Flexible Usually good BG control
	R, insulin aspart, glulisine or lispro before each meal	N, twice daily at breakfast and supper *or* bedtime	Better for people with varying schedules
Intensive: Continuous Subcutaneous Insulin Infusion	R, insulin aspart, glulisine or lispro basal and boluses as per program	None	Most flexible and expensive May have advantages over multiple dose regimens DKA may occur quickly after discontinuation
Conventional	None	N or long acting analogue once daily before breakfast	Unlikely to control BG
	None	N at breakfast *and* supper	Improved a.m. BG levels
	R, insulin aspart, glulisine or lispro at breakfast and supper	N at breakfast *and* supper	Most widely used regimen; better meal control
	R, insulin aspart, glulisine or lispro at breakfast and supper	N at breakfast *and* bedtime	More likely to be effective until morning

Abbreviations: BG = blood glucose; DKA = diabetic ketoacidosis; N = NPH insulin; R = Regular insulin

Adverse Effects of Insulin Therapy

- *Hypoglycemia* is the most common side effect of insulin therapy and occurs more frequently in patients on tight diabetic control.
  - the only way to completely avoid hypoglycemia is through unacceptably loose glycemic control. Hypoglycemia is most

commonly the result of either a missed meal or an unusual amount of exercise. Frequent hypoglycemic events may lead to hypoglycemia unawareness. Teach patients to account for diet and physical activity when planning insulin treatment regimens.

- *mild* hypoglycemia is manifested by adrenergic symptoms: sweating, tremors, tachycardia, hunger and a general sensation of weakness. It can easily be treated by the patient with an oral source of sugar. A small glass of unsweetened juice will usually raise the blood glucose approximately 2 mmol/L.
- *severe* hypoglycemia requires assistance in its recognition and/or treatment. Neuroglycopenic symptoms, confusion, altered behaviour and disorientation can progress to seizures and coma and prevent the patient from appropriately treating the hypoglycemic episode. If the patient is conscious, an **oral glucose** preparation should be used. Unsweetened juice, Lifesavers or sugar cubes may be useful. Oral glucose and dextrose do not require digestion before absorption.
- in *unconscious* patients, 1 mg of **glucagon** im or sc temporarily increases blood glucose, allowing for the intake of oral carbohydrate. Glucagon is *not* effective in malnourished patients or in alcohol-induced hypoglycemia. Intravenous administration of 50 mL of 50% dextrose in water is the treatment of choice under these circumstances.

- *Localized fat hypertrophy* is most often the result of frequent use of the same injection site.
- *Allergic reactions*, such as urticaria, angioedema, rashes and local erythema, are rare with human insulin.
- Immune-mediated *insulin resistance*, due to the production of anti-insulin antibodies, is rare with human insulin. Patients who have developed immune-mediated resistance to animal insulins should be switched to human insulin. Reduce the dose substantially at the initiation of the switch. Concentrated regular insulin, 500 U/mL, may be useful in the treatment of patients requiring very large doses of insulin.

Type 2 Diabetes Mellitus (Figure 2)

Pharmacologic therapy for type 2 diabetes is indicated if blood glucose control is not achieved within 2 to 3 months after initiating nonpharmacologic therapy. Drug treatment is warranted initially (i.e., without delay) in the presence of severe hyperglycemia ($HbA_{1c} \geq 9\%$) or diabetic symptoms.[5]

The choice of therapeutic agent should be tailored to the patient's needs, the desired therapeutic effect and the presence of contraindications. Patients are usually started on one oral drug; however, if the clinical condition warrants it, or if it is unreasonable to expect excellent control with oral monotherapy, then treatment may be initiated with a combination of oral agents and/or insulin. In patients with $HbA_{1c} \geq 9\%$ at presentation, combination therapy with two antihyperglycemic agents from different classes or insulin is recommended.[5,11] If adequate control is not achieved with monotherapy within 2 to 3 months, the addition of a second oral agent from a different therapeutic class should not be delayed. If blood glucose is not controlled by a combination of oral agents, insulin therapy may be instituted.

Oral agents (Table 7) can be divided into several broad categories: insulin secretagogues (sulfonylureas and meglitinides); drugs that decrease hepatic glucose production (the biguanide metformin); drugs that increase tissue sensitivity to insulin (thiazolidinediones and metformin); and drugs that delay or prevent the digestion of complex carbohydrates (the alpha-glucosidase inhibitor acarbose) or lipids (the intestinal lipase inhibitor orlistat). The mean decrease in HbA_{1c} achieved with metformin, sulfonylureas, repaglinide and the thiazolidinediones has generally ranged from 1% to 1.5% in clinical trials. In contrast, the mean decrease in HbA_{1c} achieved with acarbose, nateglinide and orlistat has been lower ($\leq 1\%$).[11]

When used as initial monotherapy, rosiglitazone, metformin and glyburide were associated with therapeutic failure rates, defined as a confirmed FPG > 10 mmol/L, of 15%, 21% and 34% after five years of follow-up in the ADOPT trial ($p < 0.001$ for rosiglitazone vs. either comparator).[12] Consistent with the primary outcome, 40%, 36% and 26% of patients treated with rosiglitazone, metformin and glyburide, respectively, had HbA_{1c} levels < 7% after 4 years of treatment. Patients eligible for the randomized double-blind trial had been diagnosed with diabetes mellitus within the previous 3 years, had previously been treated with diet and exercise alone, and had a baseline FPG between 7 and 10 mmol/L.

The adverse event profile of the three therapies differed markedly in ADOPT. Rosiglitazone was associated with the highest rates of weight gain (6.9% of patients) and edema (14.1%); metformin was associated with the highest overall rate of gastrointestinal events (38.3%), the most common of which was diarrhea (23.7%); and glyburide was associated with the highest rate of hypoglycemia (38.7%).[13] Among the three therapies, glyburide was associated with the lowest risk of cardiovascular events. The risk of heart failure was similar in patients treated with rosiglitazone (1.5%) and metformin (1.3%), but was lowest in those treated with glyburide (0.6%).[13]

The ADOPT trial did not address the merits of early use of combination therapy. The results of smaller trials with shorter durations of follow-up suggest that the combination of a thiazolidinedione and metformin is associated with overall lower glucose and HbA_{1c} levels and a higher probability of reaching control targets as compared with monotherapy with either agent alone.[14,15]

The results of the UK Prospective Diabetes Study suggest that *obese* patients with good blood sugar control on metformin therapy have better outcomes than those treated with insulin or sulfonylureas.[16] In general, consider metformin the initial drug of choice for obese patients unless contraindicated.

The addition of metformin or a thiazolidinedione to the regimen of patients not well controlled on insulin may improve control in some patients and lower insulin requirements. The combination of a thiazolidinedione plus insulin has not been approved by Health Canada.

Insulin Secretagogues, Sulfonylureas

Sulfonylureas (**gliclazide, glimepiride, glyburide, chlorpropamide** and **tolbutamide**) stimulate basal insulin secretion and increase meal-stimulated insulin release. They do not correct the impaired early-phase insulin response. Sulfonylureas can cause hypoglycemia and weight gain to varying degrees.[16,17,18,19] They differ from each other in the dose, rate of absorption, duration of action, route of elimination and site of attachment to the receptor on pancreatic beta cells. Some agents, notably gliclazide, produce an earlier insulin release than others.

Insulin Secretagogues, Meglitinides

Repaglinide and **nateglinide** induce an early insulin response to meals, thereby lowering postprandial glucose levels. Both are short acting, and should be taken only with meals. Repaglinide produces a dose-related increase in insulin release.[11] FPG usually drops after about one month of regular use.[20] Nateglinide results in a metabolically sensitive insulin response that is modulated by blood glucose level.[21]

Biguanides

Metformin decreases hepatic glucose production and may lower glucose absorption and enhance insulin-mediated glucose uptake. Metformin is the only oral antihyperglycemic agent not associated with weight gain. When used alone, metformin does not cause hypoglycemia, but it can potentiate the hypoglycemic effects of insulin and sulfonylureas. Metformin should not be used in patients at high risk of lactic acidosis, such as those with renal disease, hepatic disease, congestive heart failure or hypoxemic states.

Thiazolidinediones (TZDs)

Rosiglitazone and **pioglitazone** are agonists at nuclear PPARγ receptors that enhance insulin sensitivity and lower both blood glucose and circulating insulin levels.[22] These drugs increase peripheral glucose uptake, enhance fat cell sensitivity to insulin and lower hepatic glucose output. They do not produce hypoglycemia, although they may enhance the hypoglycemic effects of insulin and sulfonylureas. Individual TZDs may differ in their effects on serum lipids. TZDs are associated with weight gain due to increased subcutaneous fat deposition, fluid retention and edema, and also with an increased incidence of heart failure.[22,23] They have also been associated with worsening macular edema.[24]

The cardiovascular safety of rosiglitazone is under scrutiny. A meta-analysis of data from 42 clinical trials concluded that patients treated with rosiglitazone have a small but significant increase in the incidence of myocardial infarction (MI) as compared with placebo or other antihyperglycemic agents.[25] These findings are yet to be confirmed. In contrast, interim analysis of a randomized trial designed to examine the cardiovascular safety of rosiglitazone suggested that there is no evidence of an increased incidence of death from cardiovascular or other causes as compared with metformin plus sulfonylurea, but confirmed the increased risk of heart failure with TZDs.[26]

Alpha-glucosidase Inhibitors

Acarbose and **miglitol** (not available in Canada) inhibit intestinal alpha-glucosidases, which delay the digestion of starches and disaccharides, thereby reducing postprandial glucose levels. They do not significantly inhibit intestinal lactase. Acarbose does not cause hypoglycemia but can increase the risk of hypoglycemia when combined with insulin or insulin secretagogues. Because the digestion of sucrose is impaired by acarbose, hypoglycemia in patients taking acarbose should be treated with glucose rather than sucrose.

Intestinal Lipase Inhibitors

Orlistat is an intestinal lipase inhibitor used initially as an anti-obesity agent, which can produce modest improvements in glycemic control in patients with type 2 diabetes.[27] The hypoglycemic effect is small and in proportion to the degree of weight loss. Orlistat should not be used as monotherapy for glycemic control.

Insulin Regimens for Type 2 Diabetes Mellitus

In patients with type 2 diabetes, insulin may be used singly or in combination with oral agents in a nighttime insulin/daytime pill regimen.[28] Because of their underlying resistance to insulin, many patients require high doses of insulin. There are several commonly used insulin regimens:

- Single bedtime injection of insulin added to an ongoing oral antihyperglycemic regimen. Start with a dose of 0.1–0.2 units/kg of insulin NPH or long-acting analogue and adjust the dose to achieve morning euglycemia. The dose of oral agents may need to be reduced once control is achieved. Reduce the dose of sulfonylurea if necessary.
- Twice daily injections of a premixed insulin with two-thirds of the daily dose administered in the morning before breakfast and the remaining one-third of the daily dose administered before the evening meal (e.g., usually 30/70 in the a.m. and 50/50 or 30/70 in the p.m., 0.5 units/kg). These regimens provide convenience at the expense of flexibility and the ability to correct for abnormal results. The dose and type of mixture may have to be adjusted to achieve glycemic targets.
- Intensive insulin therapy may be started with 40% of the total daily dose (0.5 units/kg) administered as a basal insulin (NPH or long-acting analogue) and 20% of the daily dose administered before meals three

times daily (Regular or very rapid acting analogues). The dose is then adjusted to achieve glycemic targets.

Targets for Control

Control of *blood glucose* (Table 4) reduces the risk of long-term complications in type 1 and type 2 diabetes. Euglycemia is difficult to attain and maintain. The main risk of tight control of blood glucose levels is the increased risk of hypoglycemic episodes.[9] Frequent hypoglycemia may lead to hypoglycemia unawareness.[29]

Table 4: **Recommended Targets for Blood Glucose Control**[38]

	HbA_{1c} (%)	FPG/ preprandial glucose (mmol/L)	2-hour PPG (mmol/L)
Target for most patients	≤ 7.0	4.0–7.0	5.0–10.0
Normal range (for those in whom it can be achieved safely)	≤ 6.0	4.0–6.0	5.0–8.0

Abbreviations: HbA_{1C} = glycosylated hemoglobin; FPG = fasting plasma glucose; PPG = postprandial plasma glucose

Vascular protection is a priority in patients with diabetes. Vascular protection encompasses comprehensive reduction of cardiovascular risk. In addition to glycemic control, achieve blood pressure (see Chapter 32) and serum lipid targets (see Chapter 31), encourage smoking cessation (see Chapter 10) and prescribe antiplatelet therapy as indicated.[30]

- **Antiplatelet therapy** is recommended for both primary and secondary prevention of cardiovascular events in adults with type 1 and type 2 diabetes.[30,31] Several analyses support the use of aspirin for primary prevention in this population,[32,33,34] although one has provided discordant results.[35,36] No large randomized trials have addressed this question exclusively in this population.
- Control of *serum lipids* reduces the risk of cardiovascular events, which are the main cause of morbidity and mortality in diabetes. Patients aged > 30 years are at very high risk for coronary artery disease. Therapy includes **statins** for elevated LDL-C and **fibrates** for elevated triglycerides and/or low HDL-C. **Niacin** can increase blood glucose levels; thus antihyperglycemic therapy will require adjustment if this agent is used to manage dyslipidemia.
- Control of *blood pressure* (< 130/80 mm Hg) is an additional goal of therapy. Diabetes, particularly type 2, is frequently associated with hypertension. Monitor blood pressure regularly and control hypertension if it occurs, especially in the elderly.
- A targeted, intensified, multifactorial intervention involving behaviour modification, pharmacologic therapy targeting hyperglycemia, hypertension, dyslipidemia and microalbuminuria, and *secondary*

prevention of cardiovascular disease with low-dose ASA and ACE-inhibitor therapy, improves HbA_{1c} levels, blood pressure and serum lipid control, and reduces albumin excretion and the incidence of cardiovascular endpoints, nephropathy, retinopathy and autonomic neuropathy.[37]

Therapeutic Tips

- Assess all patients every 3 to 6 months. Study their home monitoring records and note the occurrence and frequency of hypoglycemia. Monitor control of blood sugar and blood pressure levels, body weight and the presence of complications. Foot examination is an integral part of such monitoring.
- Inadequate control is frequently related to inadequate dietary compliance or poor adherence to medications.
- The use of snacks is important in patients on conventional insulin therapy and may be important in those treated with a sulfonylurea. Those treated with acarbose, metformin, thiazolidinedione, meglitinide or a multidose rapid-acting insulin regimen may not require snacks.
- Encourage all patients to wear a Medic Alert bracelet or the equivalent.

Diabetes Mellitus in Pregnancy

Carbohydrate intolerance during pregnancy can occur in patients with diabetes prior to pregnancy and in those who become diabetic during pregnancy.

Pre-existing Diabetes

Poor diabetic control at the time of conception increases the risk of spontaneous abortion, prenatal mortality and morbidity and congenital malformations. Both retinal and renal disease may worsen significantly in the mother during pregnancy. Pregnancy should therefore be planned carefully. Patients should be followed by specialized diabetes health care teams with experience in the management of diabetic pregnancy.

Optimize diabetic control prior to pregnancy and screen for microvascular complications. Women with pre-existing diabetes are at risk of progressive retinopathy if glycemic control is suboptimal during pregnancy. Microalbuminuria is associated with increased risk of maternal and fetal complications.

Discontinue oral antihyperglycemic agents, and certain teratogenic antihypertensive agents (ACE inhibitors[39] and angiotensin II receptor antagonists) prior to conception. Optimize glycemic control with diet or, if necessary, diet and insulin. Prescribe folic acid at a dose of 1 to 4 mg/day before conception until 13 weeks of gestation. If conception occurs in a patient treated with oral antihyperglycemics, stop these drugs as soon as pregnancy is diagnosed and switch the patient to insulin.

Gestational Diabetes (Figure 3)

Gestational diabetes mellitus is carbohydrate intolerance of varying severity that is detected, or first recognized, during pregnancy. It is associated with increased risk of macrosomia (high birth weight), neonatal hypoglycemia, hyperbilirubinemia, hypocalcemia and polycythemia. It may be associated with an increased risk of childhood obesity and diabetes in the offspring and an increased risk for future diabetes in the mother. Gestational diabetes is usually detected towards the end of the second trimester based on an abnormal response to a 75 g oral glucose tolerance test.

Women who have had gestational diabetes should have a 2-hour oral glucose tolerance test 6 weeks to 6 months postpartum, to rule out the presence of ongoing glucose intolerance.

Therapeutic Choices

Nonpharmacologic Choices

- *Dietary counselling* by a registered dietitian is essential. The diet is divided into meals and snacks, and should provide for the nutritional needs of the pregnant woman and the fetus while avoiding starvation and ketosis.
- *Self-monitoring* of pre- and postprandial blood glucose levels is important. Targets for control are an FPG < 5.3 mmol/L, and 1- and 2-hour PPG < 7.8 mmol/L and < 6.7 mmol/L, respectively. Elevated PPG is more predictive of macrosomia than is FPG.
- *Aerobic exercise*, particularly use of the upper body, should be encouraged.

Pharmacologic Choices

Insulin is the only approved pharmacologic therapy for hyperglycemia in pregnant women. Tailor its use to achieve the targets outlined above. Tight control frequently necessitates multidose insulin regimens. Rapid-acting insulin analogues, although not specifically approved for this purpose, are now widely used to better control postprandial glucose levels. Limited data are available regarding the use of insulin glargine during pregnancy.[40,41,42,43]

The results of one small study suggest that glyburide may be safe and effective when used in the later stages of pregnancy, although glycemic control was relatively loose and the data are yet to be independently confirmed.[44]

Preventing Type II Diabetes Mellitus

Individuals with blood glucose elevations below the diabetic thresholds may be described as having *prediabetes* or *dysglycemia*. The term includes both *impaired fasting glucose* (FPG 6.1 to 7.0 mmol/L) and *impaired glucose tolerance* (plasma glucose of 7.8 to 11.0 mmol/L two hours after a 75 g oral glucose load).

Metabolic syndrome is a common, multifeatured constellation of central obesity, hypertension, dyslipidemia, insulin resistance and glucose abnormalities. It carries a significant risk of diabetes and cardiovascular disease.[45,46]

Several large studies have examined nonpharmacologic and pharmacologic strategies aimed at preventing the onset of type 2 diabetes mellitus in high-risk individuals.

The Finnish Diabetes Prevention Study (DPS)[47] and the Diabetes Prevention Program (DPP)[48] showed that calorie restriction and reduced fat intake combined with supervised, moderately intense physical activity of about 150 minutes/week significantly reduced the relative risk of progression from prediabetes to diabetes by 58% at four years. In the DPS the incidence of diabetes was 11% in those randomized to the life-style intervention versus 23% in the control group; in the DPP the incidence of diabetes was 4.8%, 7.8% and 11% in those randomized to the life-style intervention, metformin and placebo, respectively. The weight loss associated with life-style interventions was about 5 to 6% of initial body weight in these studies.

The benefits of the life-style changes were maintained after the discontinuation of the active intervention in the DPS. The relative risk of diabetes remained 36% lower in those originally randomized to the life-style intervention compared with the control group after a further 3 years of follow-up (4.3% vs 7.4%).[49]

Metformin 850 mg twice daily reduced the relative risk of progression from prediabetes to diabetes by 31% versus placebo in the DPP. After a 1- to 2-week washout period, the risk of progression to diabetes remained 25% lower in those treated with metformin than placebo.[50]

Acarbose has also been evaluated in prevention trials.[51] In STOP-NIDDM, acarbose 100 mg TID resulted in a 30% reduction of progression to diabetes at 14 months (32% vs. 42% with placebo).[52]

TZDs also reduce the risk of progression from prediabetes to diabetes.[54,56,57]

The DREAM study evaluated the effects of rosiglitazone and ramipril on progression from prediabetes to type 2 diabetes.[53,54,55] **Rosiglitazone** significantly reduced the risk of progression to diabetes or death by 60% over three years compared with placebo (11.6% versus 26%) in patients with prediabetes and no other cardiovascular risk factors. The benefit of rosiglitazone in preventing progression to diabetes was offset to some extent by a significantly higher incidence of heart failure relative to placebo (0.5% vs. 0.1%).[54] In contrast to the demonstrated benefit of rosiglitazone, ramipril did not prevent the progression from prediabetes to diabetes in the DREAM trial.[55] The use of ramipril was, however, associated with higher rates of normalization of glucose tolerance and lower overall blood glucose levels.

The results of DREAM are consistent with 2 large prospective studies (TRIPOD[56] and the DPP[57]) that showed that troglitazone, a TZD that is no longer available, delayed progression from prediabetes to diabetes.

There are no known safe and effective measures to prevent *type 1* diabetes.

Diabetic Ketoacidosis

Diabetic ketoacidosis is a potentially fatal complication that results from severe insulin deficiency and is characterized by severe hyperglycemia, volume depletion, acidosis, depressed levels of consciousness and marked ketonemia.[58] Patients are depleted in sodium, potassium, chloride and water. Despite potassium depletion, serum potassium is frequently elevated at the time of presentation. Prerenal azotemia may be present. Hyperglycemia, as well as high triglycerides and free fatty acids, may result in pseudohyponatremia. Diabetic ketoacidosis may be seen at first presentation in patients with type 1 diabetes and may also occur when insulin is discontinued. It often occurs in patients with established diabetes who have a severe stressful illness (e.g., severe infection), surgery, trauma or MI. Patients with diabetic ketoacidosis should be hospitalized (Table 5).

Table 5: Management of Diabetic Ketoacidosis

Fluids: Patients are always volume depleted (average 7 L). Give iv NS (0.9% NaCl) 2 L in the first 2 h, then individualize. Good urinary output is reassuring. May use 0.45% NaCl (½ NS) initially if the blood glucose is > 50 mmol/L. Change to 5% D5W when blood glucose drops to ≤ 14 mmol/L.

Insulin: Give 10 units of insulin R iv bolus, then infuse at 0.1 U/kg/hr (5–10 U/h). Mix 50 U in 500 mL NS and piggyback into a main iv. Continue iv insulin until the anion gap resolves.

Potassium: Potassium chloride is the preparation of choice. If serum K^+ is < 3.5 mmol/L, add 40 mmol/L of fluid; if 3.5–5.5 mmol/L, add 20 mmol/L; if > 5.5 mmol/L, do not add K^+, especially if anuric.

Bicarbonate: Give sodium bicarbonate if acidosis is severe (e.g., pH < 7.0) but only for partial correction (e.g., 10 mL 8.4% $NaHCO_3$), then reassess.

Laboratory tests: Initial CBC, glucose, electrolytes, urea, creatinine and ABG. Cultures as indicated. Radiology as indicated. Repeat electrolyte and glucose hourly, ABG only if severe acidosis persists.

Supportive care: Keep the patient warm and rested. Insert an NG tube if vomiting, and a urinary catheter if anuric (urinary retention may be significant).

Pitfalls:

- Acetone smell may be absent, undetected or unrecognized by some.
- Temperature may be low initially — absence of fever does not rule out infection.
- Leukocytosis is usually present and does not necessarily mean infection.
- Low serum sodium may be due to pseudohyponatremia.
- High serum potassium is caused by acidosis and may be seen in spite of severe total body potassium depletion.
- Ketostix detects aceto-acetate but not hydroxybutyrate.
- Dehydration may mask a respiratory infection; reassess after rehydration and stabilization.
- Severe abdominal pain or signs of an acute abdomen need to be reassessed after stabilization — they often disappear.
- A premature switch to sc insulin and/or discharge results in high recurrence and readmission rates.

Abbreviations: R = regular; NS = normal saline

Figure 1: **Diagnosis of Diabetes Mellitus**

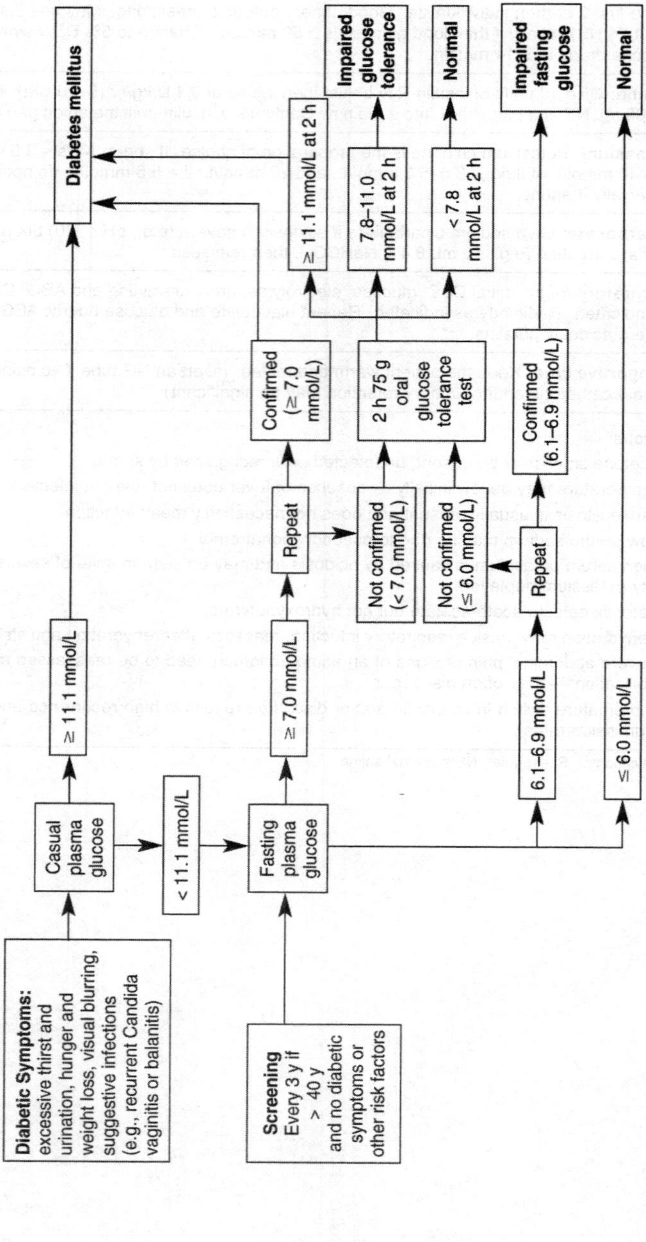

Diabetic Symptoms: excessive thirst and urination, hunger and weight loss, visual blurring, suggestive infections (e.g., recurrent Candida vaginitis or balanitis)

Casual plasma glucose

≥ 11.1 mmol/L

< 11.1 mmol/L

Screening Every 3 y if > 40 y and no diabetic symptoms or other risk factors

Fasting plasma glucose

≥ 7.0 mmol/L

Repeat

Confirmed (≥ 7.0 mmol/L)

Not confirmed (< 7.0 mmol/L)

Not confirmed (≤ 6.0 mmol/L)

2 h 75 g oral glucose tolerance test

≥ 11.1 mmol/L at 2 h

7.8–11.0 mmol/L at 2 h

< 7.8 mmol/L at 2 h

Diabetes mellitus

Impaired glucose tolerance

Normal

6.1–6.9 mmol/L

Repeat

Confirmed (6.1–6.9 mmol/L)

Impaired fasting glucose

≤ 6.0 mmol/L

Normal

Figure 2: **Stepwise Approach to Type 2 Diabetes**

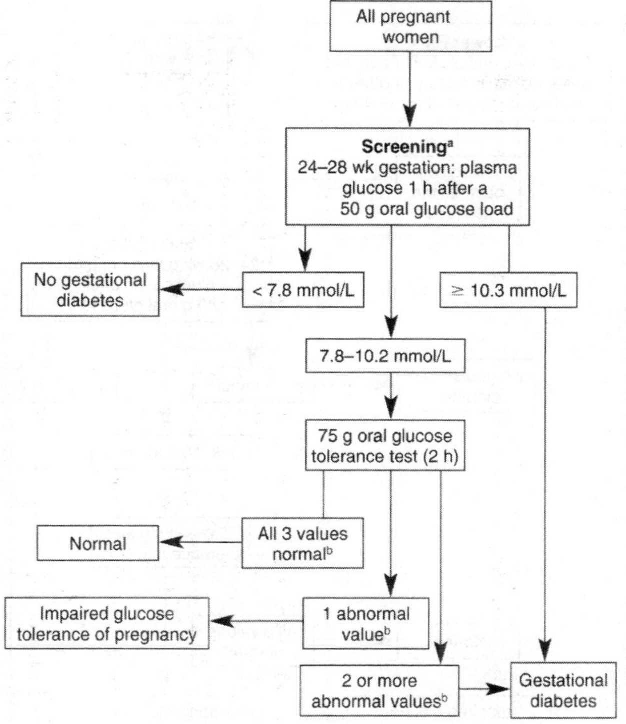

[a] *Screening may be done earlier if very high risk or previous gestational diabetes mellitus.*

[b] *Abnormal values: fasting blood glucose > 5.3 mmol/L*
blood glucose > 10.6 mmol/L 1 h post glucose load
blood glucose > 8.9 mmol/L 2 h post glucose load

Figure 3: **Diagnosis of Gestational Diabetes**

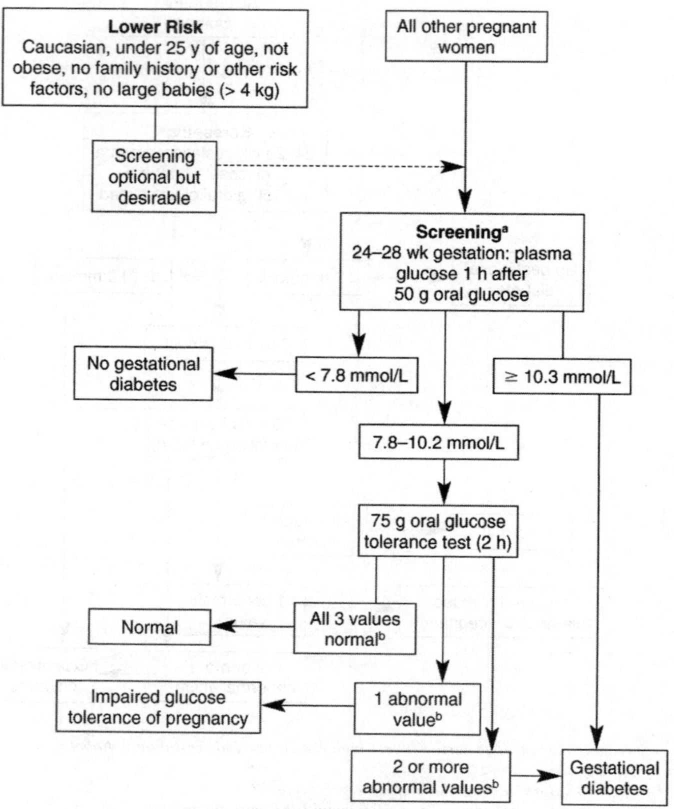

[a] Screening may be done earlier if very high risk or previous gestational diabetes mellitus.

[b] Abnormal values: fasting blood glucose > 5.3 mmol/L; blood glucose > 10.6 mmol/L 1 h post glucose load; blood glucose > 8.9 mmol/L 2 h post glucose load

Table 6: **Human Insulin and Analogues**

Class	Drug	Onset	Peak	Duration	Comments	Cost[a]
Very Rapid-acting Insulin Analogues	*insulin aspart* NovoRapid	10–15 min	60–90 min	4–5 h	Appearance: clear.	$$$$
	insulin glulisine Apidra[b]	10–15 min	60–90 min	4–5 h	Appearance: clear.	
	insulin lispro Humalog	10–15 min	60–90 min	4–5 h	Appearance: clear.	$$$$$
Rapid-acting Human Insulin	*insulin regular* Humulin R, Novolin ge Toronto	30–60 min	2–4 h	5–8 h	Appearance: clear.	$$$
Intermediate-acting Human Insulin	*insulin NPH* Humulin N, Novolin ge NPH	1–2 h	5–8 h	14–18 h	Appearance: cloudy.	$$$
Long-acting Insulin Analogues	*insulin detemir* Levemir	1.5 h	Flat, no discernible peak.	24 h	Appearance: clear. Do not mix with other insulins. Contains a C14 fatty acid chain and is highly bound (98%) to serum albumin.	$$$$$

(cont'd)

Table 6: **Human Insulin and Analogues** *(cont'd)*

Class	Drug	Onset	Peak	Duration	Comments	Cost[a]
	insulin glargine Lantus	1.5 h	Flat, no discernible peak.	24 h	Appearance: clear. Do not mix with other insulins. An acidic solution (pH 4). After injection the solution is neutralized, and microprecipitates form, from which the drug is slowly released. Do not inject im or iv.	$58/ 10 mL vial
Mixed (regular/NPH) Human Insulin	*insulin regular/insulin NPH* Humulin 20/80, 30/70, Novolin ge 10/90, 20/80, 30/70, 40/60, 50/50				Appearance: cloudy.	$$$
Mixed Insulin Analogues	*insulin lispro/lispro protamine* Humalog Mix25				Appearance: cloudy	$$$$

[a] Cost of 5 × 3 mL cartridges unless otherwise specified; drug cost only.
[b] Approved by Health Canada but not yet marketed.
Legend: $ < $15 $$ $15–30 $$$ $30–45 $$$$ $45–60 $$$$$ > $60

Table 7: **Oral Antihyperglycemic Agents**

Class	Drug[a]	Dose	Adverse Effects	Drug Interactions	Comments	Cost[b]
Insulin Secretagogues, Sulfonylureas	*chlorpropamide* generics	100–500 mg daily in one dose	Sulfonylureas: prolonged hypoglycemia; weight gain. Chlorpropamide: alcohol-associated flushing; hyponatremia.	Hypoglycemic effect potentiated by salicylates, sulfonamides and monoamine oxidase inhibitors; beta-blockers may mask hypoglycemic symptoms.	Contraindicated in type 1 diabetes, pregnancy.	$
	gliclazide Diamicron, generics	40–320 mg/day; give in 2 divided doses if daily dose ≥ 160 mg	Prolonged hypoglycemia; weight gain. Antiplatelet effect.	See chlorpropamide.	See chlorpropamide.	$
	gliclazide, long-acting Diamicron MR	30–120 mg once daily	Prolonged hypoglycemia; weight gain. Antiplatelet effect.	See chlorpropamide.	See chlorpropamide.	$-$$$
	glimepiride Amaryl, generics	1–4 mg once daily	Prolonged hypoglycemia; weight gain.	See chlorpropamide.	See chlorpropamide.	$$
	glyburide Diabeta, generics	2.5–20 mg/day; give in 2 divided doses if daily dose > 10 mg	Prolonged hypoglycemia; weight gain.	See chlorpropamide.	See chlorpropamide.	$

(cont'd)

Table 7: **Oral Antihyperglycemic Agents** *(cont'd)*

Class	Drug[a]	Dose	Adverse Effects	Drug Interactions	Comments	Cost[b]
	tolbutamide generics	500 mg BID–TID Max. 3 g/day	Prolonged hypoglycemia; weight gain. GI upset, skin rash, hemolytic anemia, jaundice.	See chlorpropamide. Alcohol and rifampin may accelerate clearance.	See chlorpropamide.	$
Insulin Secretagogues, Meglitinides	*nateglinide* Starlix	60–180 mg 0–3 min before meals	Hypoglycemia, esp. if meal not taken.	Clearance of meglitinides is reduced by strong CYP3A4 inhibitors, e.g., imidazole antifungals, macrolides, protease inhibitors. Clearance of meglitinides is enhanced by strong CYP3A4 inducers, e.g., rifampin, carbamazepine.	Contraindicated in type 1 diabetes, pregnancy.	$$$
	repaglinide GlucoNorm	0.5–4 mg 0–3 min before meals	Hypoglycemia, esp. if meal not taken; weight gain.	See nateglinide. Strong inhibitors of CYP2C8 have the potential to ↓ metabolism of repaglinide, e.g., atazanavir, ritonavir, gemfibrozil. Enhanced and prolonged hypoglycemia occurs when taken with gemfibrozil (avoid combined use). Cyclosporine ↑ plasma concentrations of repaglinide.	Contraindicated in type 1 diabetes, pregnancy.	$$$

Class	Drug[a]	Dose	Adverse Effects	Drug Interactions	Comments	Cost[b]
Biguanides	*metformin* Glucophage, generics	500–2500 mg/day divided BID or TID; start low and go slow to minimize GI side effects; little additional benefit above 1500 mg/day	Nausea, diarrhea, abdominal discomfort, anorexia, metallic taste, lactic acidosis if hepatic or renal disease.	Potentiates other oral antihyperglycemic agents; alcohol potentiates hypoglycemic effect.	No weight gain; contraindicated in hepatic impairment, renal impairment, previous lactic acidosis.	$–$$
Alpha-glucosidase Inhibitors	*acarbose* Glucobay	50–100 mg TID with each meal; start low and go slow	Flatulence, diarrhea, abdominal pain, cramps, nausea.	Potentiates other antihyperglycemic agents; may ↓ metformin bioavailability.	No weight gain; not absorbed; contraindicated in irritable bowel syndrome or inflammatory bowel disease.	$$
Thiazolidinediones (TZDs)	*pioglitazone* Actos	15–45 mg once daily	Weight gain, fluid retention and hemodilution; worsening heart failure; macular degeneration. Increased incidence of distal limb fractures in women treated with pioglitazone.	Potentiates the effect of other antihyperglycemic agents. Gemfibrozil inhibits metabolism and ↑ plasma levels.	Avoid in patients with heart failure. TZDs have variable effects on lipids; (pioglitazone ↑ HDL, ↓ TG; rosiglitazone↑ HDL,↑ LDL), Ovulation resumes in previously anovulatory women, e.g., polycystic ovarian syndrome; ↑ risk of pregnancy if adequate contraception not used.	$$$$–$$$$$
	rosiglitazone Avandia	4–8 mg daily in 1–2 doses	See pioglitazone.	See pioglitazone.	See pioglitazone.	$$$$

(cont'd)

Table 7: **Oral Antihyperglycemic Agents** *(cont'd)*

Class	Drug[a]	Dose	Adverse Effects	Drug Interactions	Comments	Cost[b]
Intestinal Lipase Inhibitors	*orlistat* Xenical	120 mg TID with meals	Diarrhea, steatorrhea, abdominal discomfort, oily leakage.	May impair absorption of fat-soluble vitamins (A, D, E, K).		$$$$
Combination Products	*rosiglitazone/glimepiride* Avandaryl	Initial: 4 mg/1 mg or 4 mg/2 mg once daily. Maximum: 4 mg/4 mg once daily	See pioglitazone. See chlorpropamide.	See pioglitazone. See chlorpropamide.	See pioglitazone. See chlorpropamide.	$$$$
	rosiglitazone/metformin Avandamet	If on metformin monotherapy: start with rosiglitazone 2 mg BID. If on rosiglitazone monotherapy start with metformin 500 mg BID. Maximum: 8 mg/1000 mg BID	See pioglitazone. See metformin.	See pioglitazone. See metformin.	See pioglitazone. See metformin.	$$$$–$$$$$

[a] Combination therapy: always use agents from different classes; combinations can be used as initial therapy if hyperglycemia is not expected to be controlled by a single agent.
[b] Cost of 30-day supply; includes drug cost only.
Dosage adjustment may be required in renal impairment; see Appendix I.
Legend: $ < $10 $–$$ < $10–25 $$ $10–25 $–$$$ <$10– 50 $$$ $25–50 $$$$ $50–100 $$$$–$$$$$ $50– >100 $$$$$ > $100

Suggested Readings

Canadian Diabetes Association. 2003 Clinical practice guidelines for the prevention and management of diabetes in Canada. *Canadian Journal of Diabetes* 2003;27(Suppl 2): S1-152.

Cheng AY, Fantus IG. Oral antihyperglycemic therapy for type 2 diabetes mellitus. *CMAJ* 2005;172(2):213-26.

Daneman D. Type 1 diabetes. *Lancet* 2006;367(9513):847-58.

Drucker DJ, Nauck MA. The incretin system: glucagon-like peptide-1 receptor agonists and dipeptidyl peptidase-4 inhibitors in type 2 diabetes. *Lancet* 2006;368(9548):1696-705.

Heine RJ, Diamant M, Mbanya JC et al. Management of hyperglycaemia in type 2 diabetes: the end of recurrent failure? *BMJ* 2006;333(7580):1200-4.

[No authors listed]. The effect of intensive treatment of diabetes on the development and progression of long-term complications in insulin-dependent diabetes mellitus. The Diabetes Control and Complications Trial Research Group. *N Engl J Med* 1993;329(14):977-86.

Stumvoll M, Goldstein BJ, van Haeften TW. Type 2 diabetes: principles of pathogenesis and therapy. *Lancet* 2005;365(9467):1333-46.

References

1. Canadian Diabetes Association Clinical Practice Guidelines Expert Committee. Definition, classification and diagnosis of diabetes and other dysglycemic categories. *Canadian Journal of Diabetes* 2003;27(Suppl 2):S7-9.
2. Charles MA, Fontbonne A, Thibult N et al. Risk factors for NIDDM in white population. Paris prospective study. *Diabetes* 1991;40(7):796-9.
3. American Diabetes Association. Screening for type 2 diabetes. *Diabetes Care* 2003;26(Suppl 1):S21-4.
4. [No authors listed]. Is fasting glucose sufficient to define diabetes? Epidemiological data from 20 European studies. The DECODE-study group. European Diabetes Epidemiology Group. Diabetes Epidemiology: Collaborative analysis of Diagnostic Criteria in Europe. *Diabetologia* 1999;42(6):647-54.
5. Canadian Diabetes Association Clinical Practice Guidelines Expert Committee. Pharmacologic management of type 2 diabetes. *Canadian Journal of Diabetes* 2003;27(Suppl 2):S37-42.
6. Ratner RE, Hirsch IB, Neifing JL et al. Less hypoglycemia with insulin glargine in intensive insulin therapy for type 1 diabetes. U.S. Study Group of Insulin Glargine in Type 1 Diabetes. *Diabetes Care* 2000;23(5):639-43.
7. Home P, Bartley P, Russell-Jones D et al. Insulin detemir offers improved glycemic control compared with NPH insulin in people with type 1 diabetes: a randomized clinical trial. *Diabetes Care* 2004;27(5):1081-87.
8. Vague P, Selam JL, Skeie S et al. Insulin detemir is associated with more predictable glycemic control and reduced risk of hypoglycemia than NPH insulin in patients with type 1 diabetes on a basal-bolus regimen with premeal insulin aspart. *Diabetes Care* 2003;26(3):590-6.
9. [No authors listed]. The effect of intensive treatment of diabetes on the development and progression of long-term complications in insulin-dependent diabetes mellitus. The Diabetes Control and Complications Trial Research Group. *N Engl J Med* 1993;329(14):977-86.
10. Nathan DM, Cleary PA, Backlund JY et al. Intensive diabetes treatment and cardiovascular disease in patients with type 1 diabetes. *N Engl J Med* 2005;353(25):2643-53.
11. Cheng AY, Fantus IG. Oral antihyperglycemic therapy for type 2 diabetes mellitus. *CMAJ* 2005;172(2):213-26.
12. Kahn SE, Haffner SM, Heise MA et al. Glycemic durability of rosiglitazone, metformin, or glyburide monotherapy. *N Engl J Med* 2006;355(23):2427-43.
13. Viberti G, Kahn SE, Greene DA et al. A diabetes outcome progression trial (ADOPT): an international multicenter study of the comparative efficacy of rosiglitazone, glyburide, and metformin in recently diagnosed type 2 diabetes. *Diabetes Care* 2002;25(10):1737-43.
14. Rosenstock J, Rood J, Cobitz A et al. Improvement in glycaemic control with rosiglitazone/metformin fixed-dose combination therapy in patients with type 2 diabetes with very poor glycaemic control. *Diabetes Obes Metab* 2006;8(6):643-9.

15. Rosenstock J, Rood J, Cobitz A et al. Initial treatment with rosiglitazone/metformin fixed-dose combination therapy compared with monotherapy with either rosiglitazone or metformin in patients with uncontrolled type 2 diabetes. *Diabetes Obes Metab* 2006;8(6):650-60.
16. [No authors listed]. Effect of intensive blood-glucose control with metformin on complications in overweight patients with type 2 diabetes (UKPDS 34). UK Prospective Diabetes Study (UKPDS) Group. *Lancet* 1998;352(9131):854-65.
17. Dills DG, Schneider J. Clinical evaluation of glimepiride versus glyburide in NIDDM in a double-blind comparative study. Glimepiride/Glyburide Research Group. *Horm Metab Res* 1996;28(9):426-9.
18. Jennings AM, Wilson RM, Ward JD. Symptomatic hypoglycemia in NIDDM patients treated with oral hypoglycemic agents. *Diabetes Care* 1989;12(3):203-8.
19. Lebovitz HE. Oral therapies for diabetic hyperglycemia. *Endocrinol Metab Clin North Am* 2001;30(4):909-33.
20. Jovanovic L, Dailey G, Huang WC et al. Repaglinide in type 2 diabetes: a 24-week, fixed-dose efficacy and safety study. *J Clin Pharmacol* 2000;40(1):49-57.
21. Keilson L, Mather S, Walter YH et al. Synergistic effects of nateglinide and meal administration on insulin secretion in patients with type 2 diabetes mellitus. *J Clin Endocrinol Metab* 2000;85(3):1081-6.
22. Yki-Jarvinen H. Thiazolidinediones. *N Engl J Med* 2004;351(11):1106-18.
23. Dormandy JA, Charbonnel B, Eckland DJ et al. Secondary prevention of macrovascular events in patients with type 2 diabetes in the PROactive Study (PROspective pioglitAzone Clinical Trial In macroVascular Events): a randomised controlled trial. *Lancet* 2005;366(9493):1279-89.
24. Ryan EH, Han DP, Ramsay RC et al. Diabetic macular edema associated with glitazone use. *Retina* 2006;26(5):562-70.
25. Nissen SE, Wolski K. Effect of rosiglitazone on the risk of myocardial infarction and death from cardiovascular causes. *N Engl J Med* 2007 May 21; [Epub ahead of print].
26. Home PD, Pocock SJ, Beck-Nielsen H et al. Rosiglitazone evaluated for cardiovascular outcomes – an interim analysis. *N Engl J Med* 2007 Jun 5; [Epub ahead of print].
27. Hollander PA, Elbein SC, Hirsch IB et al. Role of orlistat in the treatment of obese patients with type 2 diabetes. A 1-year randomized double-blind study. *Diabetes Care* 1998;21(8):1288-94.
28. Yki-Jarvinen H, Ryysy L, Nikkila K et al. Comparison of bedtime insulin regimens in patients with type 2 diabetes mellitus. A randomized, controlled trial. *Ann Intern Med* 1999;130(5):389-96.
29. Ovalle F, Fanelli CG, Paramore DS et al. Brief twice-weekly episodes of hypoglycemia reduce detection of clinical hypoglycemia in type 1 diabetes mellitus. *Diabetes* 1998;47(9):1472-9.
30. Canadian Diabetes Association Clinical Practice Guidelines Expert Committee. Macrovascular complications, dyslipidemia and hypertension. *Canadian Journal of Diabetes* 2003;27(Suppl 2):S58-65.
31. Colwell JA, American Diabetes Association. Aspirin therapy in diabetes. *Diabetes Care* 2004;27(Suppl 1)S72-3.
32. [No authors listed]. Final report on the aspirin component of the ongoing Physicians' Health Study. Steering Committee of the Physicians' Health Study Research Group. *N Engl J Med* 1989;321(3):129-35.
33. [No authors listed]. Aspirin effects on mortality and morbidity in patients with diabetes mellitus. Early Treatment Diabetic Retinopathy Study report 14. ETDRS Investigators. *JAMA* 1992;268(10):1292-300.
34. Hansson L, Zanchetti A, Carruthers SG et al. Effects of intensive blood-pressure lowering and low-dose aspirin in patients with hypertension: principal results of the Hypertension Optimal Treatment (HOT) randomised trial. HOT Study Group. *Lancet* 1998;351(9118):1755-62.
35. Sacco M, Pellegrini F, Roncaglioni MC et al. Primary prevention of cardiovascular events with low-dose aspirin and vitamin E in type 2 diabetic patients: results of the Primary Prevention Project (PPP) trial. *Diabetes Care* 2003;26(12):3264-72.
36. Colwell JA. Aspirin for primary prevention of cardiovascular events in diabetes. *Diabetes Care* 2003;26(12):3349-50.
37. Gaede P, Vedel P, Larsen N et al. Multifactorial intervention and cardiovascular disease in patients with type 2 diabetes. *N Engl J Med* 2003;348(5):383-93.
38. Canadian Diabetes Association Clinical Practice Guidelines Expert Committee. Targets for glycemic control. *Canadian Journal of Diabetes* 2003;27(Suppl 2):S18-20.
39. Cooper WO, Hernandez-Diaz S, Arbogast PG et al. Major congenital malformations after first-trimester exposure to ACE inhibitors. *N Engl J Med* 2006;354(23):2443-51.
40. Di Cianni G, Volpe L, Lencioni C et al. Use of insulin glargine during the first weeks of pregnancy in five type 1 diabetic women. *Diabetes Care* 2005;28(4):982-3.
41. Graves DE, White JC, Kirk JK. The use of insulin glargine with gestational diabetes mellitus. *Diabetes Care* 2006;29(2):471-2.
42. Holstein A, Plaschke A, Egberts EH. Use of insulin glargine during embryogenesis in a pregnant woman with Type 1 diabetes. *Diabet Med* 2003;20(9):779-780.

43. Wolderink JM, van Loon AJ, Storms F et al. Use of insulin glargine during pregnancy in seven type 1 diabetic women. *Diabetes Care* 2005;28(10):2594-5.
44. Langer O, Conway DL, Berkus MD et al. A comparison of glyburide and insulin in women with gestational diabetes mellitus. *N Engl J Med* 2000;343(16):1134-8.
45. Expert Panel on Detection, Evaluation, and Treatment of High Blood Cholesterol in Adults. Executive Summary of The Third Report of The National Cholesterol Education Program (NCEP) Expert Panel on Detection, Evaluation, And Treatment of High Blood Cholesterol In Adults (Adult Treatment Panel III). *JAMA* 2001;285(19):2486-97.
46. Alberti KG, Zimmet PZ. Definition, diagnosis and classification of diabetes mellitus and its complications. Part 1: diagnosis and classification of diabetes mellitus provisional report of a WHO consultation. *Diabet Med* 1998;15(7):539-53.
47. Tuomilehto J, Lindstrom J, Eriksson JG et al. Prevention of type 2 diabetes mellitus by changes in lifestyle among subjects with impaired glucose tolerance. *N Engl J Med* 2001;344(18):1343-50.
48. Knowler WC, Barrett-Connor E, Fowler SE et al. Reduction in the incidence of type 2 diabetes with lifestyle intervention or metformin. *N Engl J Med* 2002;346(6):393-403.
49. Lindstrom J, Ilanne-Parikka P, Peltonen M et al. Sustained reduction in the incidence of type 2 diabetes by lifestyle intervention: follow-up of the Finnish Diabetes Prevention Study. *Lancet* 2006;368(9548):1673-9.
50. Diabetes Prevention Program Research Group. Effects of withdrawal from metformin on the development of diabetes in the diabetes prevention program. *Diabetes Care* 2003;26(4):977-80.
51. Van de Laar FA, Lucassen PL, Akkermans RP et al. Alpha-glucosidase inhibitors for people with impaired glucose tolerance or impaired fasting blood glucose. *Cochrane Database Syst Rev* 2006;(4):CD005061
52. Chiasson JL, Josse RG, Gomis R et al. Acarbose for prevention of type 2 diabetes mellitus: the STOP-NIDDM randomised trial. *Lancet* 2002;359(9323):2072-7.
53. Gerstein HC, Yusuf S, Holman R et al. Rationale, design and recruitment characteristics of a large, simple international trial of diabetes prevention: the DREAM trial. *Diabetologia* 2004;47(9):1519-27.
54. Gerstein HC, Yusuf S, Bosch J et al. Effect of rosiglitazone on the frequency of diabetes in patients with impaired glucose tolerance or impaired fasting glucose: a randomised controlled trial. *Lancet* 2006;368(9541):1096-105.
55. Bosch J, Yusuf S, Gerstein HC et al. Effect of ramipril on the incidence of diabetes. *N Engl J Med* 2006;355(15):1551-62.
56. Buchanan TA, Xiang AH, Peters RK et al. Preservation of pancreatic beta-cell function and prevention of type 2 diabetes by pharmacological treatment of insulin resistance in high-risk hispanic women. *Diabetes* 2002;51(9):2796-803.
57. Knowler WC, Hamman RF, Edelstein SL et al. Prevention of type 2 diabetes with troglitazone in the Diabetes Prevention Program. *Diabetes* 2005;54(4):1150-6.
58. Kitabchi AE, Umpierrez GE, Murphy MB et al. Hyperglycemic crises in adult patients with diabetes: a consensus statement from the American Diabetes Association. *Diabetes Care* 2006;29(12):2739-48.

Pharmacoeconomic Considerations: Diabetes Mellitus

Blair Jarvis, MSc, BSP

Epidemiology	
Country (Year)	**Prevalence (%)**
Canada (1995)[1]	Adults (self-reported): 5.1%
Canada (1997)[2]	Adults with type 2 diabetes in Sandy Lake First Nation (age-standardized): 26.1%

(cont'd)

Country (Year)	Prevalence (%)	
Canada (2001):[3]	Primary care patients aged ≥ 40 years: • 16.4% with known diabetes • 2.2% with undiagnosed diabetes	
Cost of Illness Data		
Country and Year of Estimate	**Total Costs[a]**	**Indirect Costs[b]**
Canada (1998)[4]	US $3.7 billion	
Canada (1998)[4]		Before considering complications: US $573 million
Canada (1998)[4]		Related to cardiovascular complications: US $637 million
Commentary		

The prevalence of diabetes mellitus and associated complications is rising in step with the increasing incidence of obesity in Canada. It is estimated that the prevalence of this disease will increase by 35% between 1995 and 2025.[5]

The medical costs associated with diabetes are substantial and incorporate not only those associated with screening patients and controlling blood sugar levels (i.e., test supplies and drugs), but also considerable costs associated with the microvascular and macrovascular complications of the disease. For example, total health care expenditures for people with diabetes in Saskatchewan in 1996 were estimated to be $134.3 million, which amounted to approximately 15% of all expenditures for hospitalizations, physician's services and prescription drugs.[6] In this analysis more than one-third (36.4%) of medical costs were associated with the management of the major comorbid conditions associated with diabetes. Because type 2 diabetes is much more prevalent than type 1 diabetes in the population, the total direct costs to health care systems are driven almost entirely by the cost of type 2 diabetes.[7]

Tight control of blood glucose levels as practised in the Diabetes Control and Complications Trial is cost-effective. This approach greatly reduces the incidence of blindness, end-stage renal disease and amputation at an estimated cost of US $28 661 (1996) per QALY in patients with type 1 diabetes.[8]

There is little evidence that any one antihyperglycemic agent is better than others at lowering blood glucose levels in patients with type 2 diabetes. Use of the older agents is appealing from an economic

(cont'd)

Commentary

perspective and is necessary because combinations of drugs from two or more classes are often required to achieve blood glucose targets in patients with type 2 diabetes. A number of new drugs for diabetes have recently been introduced (i.e., thiazolidinediones,[9] insulin analogues) or are poised to enter the Canadian market (e.g., inhaled insulin, exenatide, sitagliptin). Thus, in addition to the increasing prevalence of diabetes, higher drug costs will likely contribute to the economic burden of diabetes.

Prevention of type 2 diabetes through lifestyle intervention and antihyperglycemic drug therapy is a topic of great interest with huge cost implications for the health care system. A cost-effectiveness analysis based on data from the Diabetes Prevention Program showed that, from a societal perspective the cost per additional QALY gained from intensive lifestyle intervention (US $8800, 2005) was considerably lower than that for metformin ($29 900).[10]

[a] Total costs include direct costs and mortality costs.
[b] Direct costs include those associated with physician services, nursing care, diagnostic procedures, drugs and hospitalization.

DM = diabetes mellitus; IGT = impaired glucose tolerance as measured by a 75 g oral glucose tolerance test; QALY = quality-adjusted life-year.

References

1. Tan MH, MacLean DR. Epidemiology of diabetes mellitus in Canada. *Clin Invest Med* 1995;18(4):240-6.
2. Harris SB, Gittelsohn J, Hanley A et al. The prevalence of NIDDM and associated risk factors in native Canadians. *Diabetes Care* 1997;20(2):185-7.
3. Leiter LA, Barr A, Belanger A et al. Diabetes Screening in Canada (DIASCAN) Study: prevalence of undiagnosed diabetes and glucose intolerance in family physician offices. *Diabetes Care* 2001;24(6):1038-43.
4. Dawson KG, Gomes D, Gerstein H et al. The economic cost of diabetes in Canada, 1998. *Diabetes Care* 2002;25(8):1303-7.
5. King H, Aubert RE, Herman WH. Global burden of diabetes, 1995-2025: prevalence, numerical estimates, and projections. *Diabetes Care* 1998;21(9):1414-31.
6. Simpson SH, Corabian P, Jacobs P et al. The cost of major comorbidity in people with diabetes mellitus. *CMAJ* 2003;168(13):1661-7.
7. Johnson JA, Pohar SL, Majumdar SR. Health care use and costs in the decade after identification of type 1 and type 2 diabetes: a population-based study. *Diabetes Care* 2006;29(11):2403-8.
8. [No authors listed]. Lifetime benefits and costs of intensive therapy as practiced in the diabetes control and complications trial. The Diabetes Control and Complications Trial Research Group. *JAMA* 1996;276(17):1409-15.
9. Boucher M, McAuley L, Brown A et al. *Comparative clinical and budget evaluations of rosiglitazone and pioglitazone with other anti-diabetic agents.* Ottawa (ON): Canadian Coordinating Office for Health Technology Assessment; 2003. Technology overview no. 9. Available from: http://www.cadth.ca/media/pdf/143_diones_ov_e.pdf Accessed June 13, 2007.
10. Herman WH, Hoerger TJ, Brandle M et al. The cost-effectiveness of lifestyle modification or metformin in preventing type 2 diabetes in adults with impaired glucose tolerance. *Ann Intern Med* 2005;142(5):323-32.

CHAPTER 28

Obesity

Arya M. Sharma, MD

Obesity is a complex heterogeneous disorder that places individuals at increased risk for adverse mental and/or physical health consequences from excess body fat. The current definition of obesity is based on body mass index (BMI = weight/height^2 [kg/m^2]; Table 1). In 2004, 23.1% of Canadians aged 18 or older—an estimated 5.5 million adults—had a body mass index (BMI) of 30 kg/m^2 or more; the prevalence of class II and III obesity was 5.1% and 2.7%, respectively.[1] Childhood obesity is likewise on the rise, currently affecting more than 500 000 children in Canada.[1]

These figures likely underestimate the impact of excess body weight on health, as weight distribution (central versus peripheral) and ectopic adiposity (hepatic steatosis, increased intramyocellular fat) may increase health risks, even at BMI levels well below the conventional BMI cut-offs.[2] Thus, measures of abdominal obesity, such as waist circumference values exceeding 102 cm (40 inches) in men and 88 cm (35 inches) in women, have been suggested as markers of increased cardiometabolic risk. Limitations to the BMI and waist circumference classification system exist with respect to young adults who have not yet reached full growth, lean or muscular adults, adults over age 65, and some racial and ethnic groups such as Asian, Black and Canadian First Nations, including Inuit.

Table 1: WHO Classification of Overweight and Obesity in Adults According to Body Mass Index

Classification	BMI[a]	Risk of Comorbidities[b]
Underweight	< 18.5	Mildly increased
Normal	18.5–24.9	Average
Overweight	25.0–29.9	Mildly increased
Obese	≥ 30.0	
Class I	30–34.9	Moderate
Class II	35–39.9	Severe
Class III	≥ 40.0	Very severe

[a] Values are age and gender independent.
[b] Both BMI and a measure of fat distribution (e.g., waist circumference) are important in estimating the risk of comorbidities (type 2 diabetes, hypertension, dyslipidemia).

Adapted with permission from the National Heart, Lung and Blood Institute. Preventing and Managing the Global Epidemic of Obesity. *Report of the World Health Organization Consultation of Obesity.* Geneva (SZ): WHO, June 1997.

Goals of Therapy

- The overall aim is to reduce excess body fat for health and not for cosmetic reasons; reducing weight by 5 to 10% can result in important health benefits
- Minimum goal: stabilize and prevent further weight gain
- Prevent weight regain
- Prevent and treat obesity-related comorbidities and complications

Strategies for Obesity Treatment

As obesity is a heterogeneous condition, no single management strategy works for every patient. Psychosocial, emotional or physical barriers may make it difficult for patients to adhere to management strategies. There is currently no "cure" for obesity, implying that any strategy has to be a long-term "coping" strategy that allows the patient to reduce their body weight and prevent weight regain. Typically, treatment is characterized by intermittent periods of "remission" and "relapse," commonly referred to as "weight cycling." The health risks of weight cycling versus maintaining a long-term stable weight remain controversial.

Treatment strategies should acknowledge two distinct phases in obesity management:[3]

Phase 1: Induction of weight loss

Weight loss requires caloric restriction. A negative energy balance of about 500 kcal/day results in weight loss of about 1 to 2 kg (2 to 4 lb) per month. A kilogram of fat is equivalent to 7780 kcal (3500 kcal/lb). A challenge in this phase is to prevent the concomitant loss of lean body mass, which can be minimized by ensuring the intake of high-quality protein and participation in resistance training. This phase lasts until the patient achieves the weight-loss plateau (usually three to six months into the weight-loss phase), at which time the focus of treatment changes to phase 2.

Phase 2: Prevention of weight regain

The induction of weight loss results in complex hormonal and neurobehavioural changes that seek to restore body weight to its original level. There is no evidence that these responses diminish over time. The patient will thus have to continue restricting energy intake indefinitely to the same level as was consumed at the time of the weight-loss plateau. Any increase in energy intake will result in weight regain. Deep-rooted lifestyle changes, intense physical activity, medication and surgery can significantly reduce the likelihood of weight regain.

Setting Treatment Goals

- **Treatment goals should focus on improving health status and/or quality of life rather than on just reducing numbers on the scale.**

- Significant health benefits can be achieved with a 5-10% weight loss; further weight loss in class I and II obesity may be difficult to achieve and maintain.
- In phase 2 of treatment, the principal goal is to prevent weight regain.
- Increased physical activity in phase 2 can help maintain weight loss and result in further improvements in health and quality of life.

Investigations

- Thorough history including:
  - weight history, including previous attempts at weight loss, precipitating events (e.g., pregnancy, injury) and contributing factors (e.g., steroids, antihyperglycemic, anticonvulsant or antipsychotic medications)
  - lifestyle (diet and activity), readiness for change, psychosocial, emotional and physical barriers to lifestyle change, smoking, alcohol, substance abuse
  - reasons for willingness to change and possible health and quality-of-life goals
  - family history of obesity and comorbidities
  - support system and insurance coverage for obesity treatment
  - assess as indicated for depression (see Chapter 5), anxiety (see Chapter 2), attention deficit (see Chapter 3), insomnia (see Chapter 8) and eating disorders (see Chapter 11)
- Physical examination:
  - weight, height, waist circumference, visual impression of weight distribution; calculate BMI
  - vital signs
  - target organ damage, including hepatomegaly, abdominal wall hernias, acanthosis nigricans, intertrigo
  - identify genetic and associated conditions
  - assess for osteoarthritis (see Chapter 71) and low back pain (see Chapter 75) as indicated
  - assess for fibromyalgia (see Chapter 67) and chronic fatigue syndrome (see Chapter 68) as indicated
- Laboratory and diagnostic procedures:
  - screen for hypertension (see Chapter 32), diabetes mellitus (see Chapter 27), dyslipidemia (see Chapter 31) and gout (see Chapter 70)
  - liver function tests—liver ultrasound where indicated
  - discourage routine TSH testing
  - pulmonary functions and sleep studies where indicated
  - ECG, exercise test and echocardiography where indicated

- assess for gastroesophageal reflux and gallbladder disease where indicated

Therapeutic Choices (Figure 1)

Nonpharmacologic Choices

Nutrition Planning and Diet Composition

- Regular eating (three meals, three snacks) is an important measure for weight control. Discourage prolonged fasting and skipping of meals — people who eat breakfast are less likely to be obese than people who do not.
- Weight-management strategies include grocery shopping after meals, using smaller dishes and glasses and avoiding energy-dense foods, empty calories in soda pop and snacking in front of the TV.
- All weight-loss diets must be nutritionally adequate to ensure optimal health and well balanced with respect to macronutrient composition. Discourage extreme diets.
- Ensure an adequate carbohydrate intake of ≥ 100 g/day (400 kcal/day) to avoid protein breakdown and muscle wasting, and to avoid large shifts in fluid balance. Complex carbohydrates that are high in fibre (e.g., kidney beans) and have a low glycemic index require more time to eat and digest and are associated with greater satiety.
- Ensure a protein intake of ≥1 g/kg/day of high quality mixed proteins to maintain lean body mass and other essential body functions. When energy intake falls below that needed to maintain energy balance, protein requirements increase by 1.75 g for every 100 kcal deficit.
- Fat intake should not exceed 30 to 35% of total calories consumed, with ≤ 10% from trans and saturated fat. Low-fat diets are not more effective in weight loss than other hypocaloric diets, but they do reduce cardiovascular risk.
- Use of commercial meal replacements can provide a simple and sustainable adjunct to weight management. A comparison of adult nutrition products, including meal replacement products, is available in the current edition of *Compendium of Self-Care Products* published by the Canadian Pharmacists Association.
- All popular diets result in weight loss, but weight maintenance is generally disappointing. The long-term efficacy and safety of various diets have not been established in randomized controlled trials.

Physical Activity

Increased physical activity and fitness are clearly associated with a reduction in cardiometabolic risk.[4] Regular physical activity also enhances the patient's sense of well-being, promotes weight maintenance, improves insulin resistance and reduces the loss of bone mineral density that is associated with weight loss.[5] However, exercise alone is not an effective strategy for weight loss.

Individual patients should be assessed to determine the level of fitness before starting an exercise program. A treadmill stress test should be considered for individuals with elevated cardiovascular risk.

- Exercise coupled with a judicious caloric-deficit meal plan accelerates fat loss while maintaining lean body mass, and helps sustain weight loss over the long term.
- Encourage all patients to spend ≥30 minutes doing continuous or intermittent (minimum of 10-minute bouts accumulated throughout the day) physical activity at least five days each week. Initially, physical activity could begin with 5 to 10 minute bouts, with increasing frequency, duration and intensity over time.
- The initial goal is to increase energy expenditure by 700 to 1000 kcal/week or about 100 to 130 kcal daily (Table 2).
- Walking 10 000 steps a day (measured by a pedometer) is associated with increased weight maintenance.
- Promote a daily energy expenditure of about 300 kcal. Recommend a variety of activities that are enjoyable and can be continued for life.
- Resistance training to build lean body mass sustains weight loss in the long term.

Table 2: **Average Energy Consumption Per Hour of Low-intensity Forms of Physical Activity**

Activity	Average Energy Cost[a] Kilocalories	Kilojoules
Shopping	150	630
Light housework (cleaning, vacuuming)	220	920
Dancing	250	1050
Walking		
4 km/h or 2.5 mph	200	840
6 km/h or 4 mph	300	1260

[a] 1 kilocalorie is approximately 4.2 kilojoules. The calories consumed per hour depend on the intensity of the activity, and can range from 150 calories for shopping to just over 300 calories for brisk walking at 6 km/h. An example of low-intensity endurance exercise activity is walking at a brisk pace (6 km/h) for 60 minutes daily (about 50% of maximal oxygen consumption, VO_{2max}).

Pharmacologic Choices

- The combination of lifestyle modification and anti-obesity drug therapy is superior to lifestyle modification alone in achieving a target weight loss of 5 to 10% over the long term, and may improve health status.
- Discontinuation of anti-obesity medication generally results in weight regain and should therefore be continued as long as there is benefit; however, long-term studies are only available for sibutramine and orlistat.

- No anti-obesity drugs have shown an effect on mortality; long-term cardiovascular risk reduction and safety studies are ongoing.
- There is no indication that currently available anti-obesity medications are associated with pulmonary hypertension, valvular dysfunction or other cardiovascular abnormalities associated with earlier anti-obesity medications.

Appetite Suppressants

Diethylpropion and **bupropion** are sympathomimetic drugs that have a mild appetite-suppressant effect and can be used for short-term induction of weight loss.

Satiety Enhancers

Sibutramine, a serotonin and norepinephrine reuptake inhibitor (SNRI), primarily acts by increasing the sense of satiety after meals, thereby allowing patients to reduce portion size and avoid snacking between meals.[6] The average weight loss at one year was 4.9% greater with sibutramine than placebo. The adverse effect profile of sibutramine is similar to that of venlafaxine, an SNRI that is used for depression.

Lipase Inhibitors

Orlistat is a pancreatic and gastric lipase inhibitor that reduces dietary fat absorption by 30%, resulting in an effective reduction in caloric intake of around 180 kcal/day on a diet containing 60 g of fat.[7] A high fat intake is poorly tolerated during orlistat therapy because of an increased incidence of gastrointestinal adverse effects, including bloating, steatorrhea and oily discharge. Orlistat is less effective in patients on low-fat diets and is difficult to take for individuals with irregular eating patterns. In randomized, double-blind long-term trials, patients lost on average 2.9% more weight over one year than those on placebo. Orlistat is approved for use in obese patients with type 2 diabetes mellitus, in whom it improves glycemic and metabolic control.

Cannabinoid Type 1 Receptor Antagonists

Rimonabant is the prototype of a new class of anti-obesity drugs that block the central and peripheral effects of the endocannabinoid system mediated by cannabinoid (CB)-1 receptors.[8] This system is activated in obese individuals, and clinical trials have shown sustained 5 to 10% weight loss over two years during treatment in obese patients with or without comorbidities, including dyslipidemia and diabetes. Rimonabant was well tolerated in clinical trials; the principal side effects were depression, anxiety, dizziness, nausea and vomiting. It has been licensed for obesity treatment in Europe but has not yet been approved in the US or Canada.

Bariatric Surgery

There is good evidence that bariatric surgery provides significant psychosocial and health benefits in patients with morbid obesity.[9] The best outcomes are achieved by interdisciplinary teams working in high-volume centres and are largely dependent on appropriate patient selection and follow-up. Patients must be counseled on the need for lifelong nutritional changes to avoid nutritional complications. Patients with underlying psychiatric or emotional issues should be carefully evaluated.

Therapeutic Tips

- Obesity is a chronic disease—focus on long-term strategies rather than short-term interventions.
- Identify psychosocial, emotional and physical barriers—addressing these may be required before obesity treatment is initiated.
- Focus on improvements in health and quality of life, not on changes in body weight.
- Correct disordered eating; encourage three meals and three snacks. Avoid hunger, which leads to binging.
- Meal replacements are an easy, efficient and inexpensive way to facilitate portion control. Recommend meal replacements that do not contain trans fats, have a low glycemic load and are high in fibre.
- Exercise is not the best way to lose weight, but can reduce visceral fat, increase cardiovascular fitness and help with weight maintenance.
- Prepare the patient for the weight-loss plateau; managing expectations is an important part of obesity management.

Figure 1: **Management of Obesity**

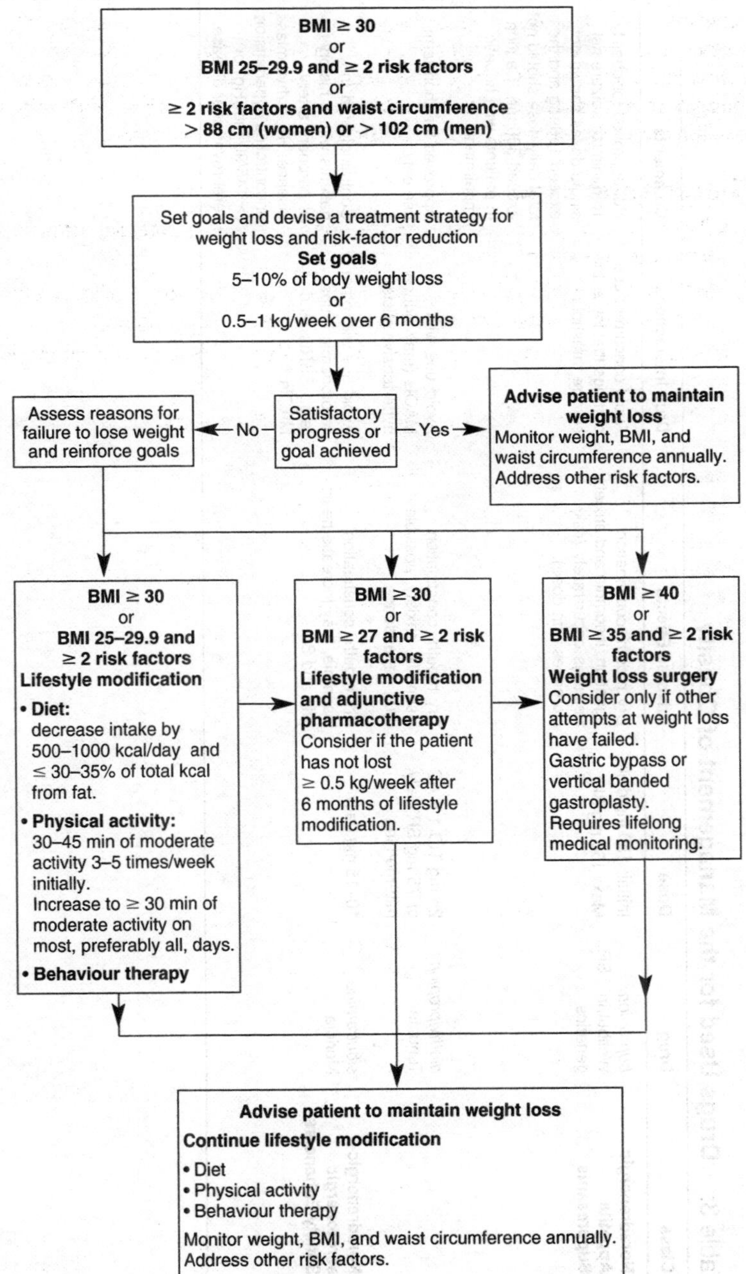

Table 3: Drugs Used for the Management of Obesity

Class	Drug	Dose	Adverse Effects	Drug Interactions	Comments	Cost[a]
Noradrenergic Appetite Suppresants	*bupropion* Wellbutrin SR, generics	Initial: 150 mg daily Max: 150 mg BID	Dry mouth, constipation, agitation, insomnia and anxiety. Seizures occur rarely (risk increases with dose).	Avoid concurrent use of drugs that lower the seizure threshold.	Not approved for obesity. To minimize seizure risk, single doses should not exceed 150 mg and the total daily dose should not exceed 300 mg. Caution in patients with hepatic impairment.	$
	diethylpropion Tenuate	25 mg TID 1 h AC or 75 mg SR daily, mid-morning	Dry mouth, constipation, insomnia, anxiety, possible drug dependence.	Avoid use with MAOIs (may induce hypertensive crisis).	Approved for short-term use only.	$
Noradrenergic–serotonergic Satiety Enhancers	*sibutramine* Meridia	10–15 mg daily	Dry mouth, constipation, insomnia, may increase heart rate and BP.	Avoid use with other serotonergic drugs (e.g., SSRIs) and MAOIs.	Contraindicated in patients with a history of coronary artery disease, HF, arrhythmias, uncontrolled hypertension (> 145/90 mm Hg) or cerebrovascular disease.	$$

Class	Drug	Dose	Adverse Effects	Drug Interactions	Comments	Cost[a]
Lipase Inhibitors	*orlistat* Xenical	120 mg daily to TID with each meal containing fat	Oily spotting, flatus with discharge, fecal urgency.	Decreased absorption of soluble vitamins. Administer cyclosporine at least 2 h apart from orlistat.	Contraindicated in patients with chronic malabsorption syndrome or cholestasis. Minimal systemic absorption. Advise patients to take a multivitamin daily ≥ 2 h before or after orlistat or at bedtime.	$$

[a] Cost of 30-day supply; includes drug cost only.
Abbreviations: HF = heart failure; MAOI = monoamine oxidase inhibitor; SSRI = selective serotonin reuptake inhibitor
Legend: $ < $50 $$ $100–150

Suggested Readings

Dietz WH, Robinson TN. Clinical practice. Overweight children and adolescents. *N Engl J Med* 2005;352(20):2100-9.

Haslam DW, James WP. Obesity. *Lancet* 2005;366(9492):1197-209.

Lau DC, Douketis JD, Morrison KM et al. 2006 Canadian clinical practice guidelines on the management and prevention of obesity in adults and children [summary]. *CMAJ* 2007;176(8):S1-13.

Strychar I. Diet in the management of weight loss. *CMAJ* 2006;174(1):56-63.

References

1. Tjepkema M. *Measured obesity. Adult obesity in Canada: measured height and weight.* Nutrition: Findings from the Canadian Community Health Survey 2004;(1). Available from: http://www.statcan.ca/english/research/82-620-MIE/2005001/pdf/aobesity.pdf Accessed December 21, 2006.
2. Franzosi MG. Should we continue to use BMI as a cardiovascular risk factor? *Lancet* 2006;368(9536):624-5.
3. Merchant A, Yusuf S, Sharma AM. A cardiologist's guide to waist management. *Heart* 2006;92(7):865-6.
4. Shaw K, Gennat H, O'Rourke P et al. Exercise for overweight or obesity. *Cochrane Database Syst Rev* 2006;(4):CD003817.
5. Villareal DT, Fontana L, Weiss EP et al. Bone mineral density response to caloric restriction-induced weight loss or exercise-induced weight loss: a randomized controlled trial. *Arch Intern Med* 2006;166(22):2502-10.
6. Arterburn DE, Crane PK,Veenstra DL. The efficacy and safety of sibutramine for weight loss: a systematic review. *Arch Intern Med* 2004;164(9):994-1003.
7. Hutton B, Fergusson D. Changes in body weight and serum lipid profile in obese patients treated with orlistat in addition to a hypocaloric diet: a systematic review of randomized clinical trials. *Am J Clin Nutr* 2004;80(6):1461-8.
8. Curioni C, Andre C. Rimonabant for overweight or obesity. *Cochrane Database Syst Rev* 2006;(4):CD006162.
9. Buchwald H, Avidor Y, Braunwald E et al. Bariatric surgery: a systematic review and meta-analysis. *JAMA* 2004;292(14):1724-37.

CHAPTER 29
Nutritional Supplements for Adults

L. John Hoffer, MD, CM, PhD, FRCPC

Goals of Therapy

- Prevent or treat nutritional deficiency disease
- Prevent or treat nondeficiency diseases whose progression may be mitigated by increased intake of certain nutrients

Therapeutic Choices
Preventive Supplements

Table 1: Indications For Preventive Supplements[a]

Clinical evidence of deficient intake:[b]
Voluntary or involuntary weight loss (< 1500 kcal/d)
History of inadequate intake of certain nutrient groups:
dairy products and fluid milk (calcium, vitamin D)
deeply coloured vegetables and fruits (folic acid, carotenoids, vitamin C)
whole grains (folic acid, vitamin B_6, vitamin E)
Patient populations at risk of deficient intake or malabsorption:
Prolonged hospital admission
Institutionalization
Poverty, social isolation
GI tract symptoms (nausea, pain, diarrhea, anorexia)
GI disease known to cause malabsorption or maldigestion
Reduced functional and activity status
Multiple comorbidities, especially organ failure
Swallowing, chewing or dental problems
Psychiatric or neurologic disease
Chronic substance abuse, especially alcoholism
Increased vitamin/mineral needs
Hemo- or peritoneal dialysis
Pregnancy
Drug-nutrient interactions

[a] This table identifies situations in which the risk of overt deficiency is sufficiently great that preventive therapy is indicated. Large segments of the normal population consume inadequate amounts of calcium, zinc, certain B vitamins and vitamin D, and for this reason some authorities now advise *all* adults to use a daily preventive supplement.[1,2,3,4]

[b] Formal dietetic assessment advised

Preventive supplements are vitamin or vitamin/mineral supplements formulated to compensate for inadequacies in the diet of normal persons. They are also useful for patients with excellent diets but increased requirements, mild malabsorption or increased nutrient losses (Table 1).

Traditionally, preventive supplements contained 50 to 150% of the recommended dietary allowance (RDA) for some or many vitamins, but products currently on the market vary considerably, especially with regard to folic acid, vitamin B_{12}, vitamin C, vitamin A, iron and zinc. Some common vitamin/mineral deficiencies and recommendations are listed in Table 2. See Table 3 for preventive supplementation in special populations.

Prevention of Deficiencies (Table 2, Table 3)

Table 2: **Common Vitamin/Mineral Deficiencies**

Preventive Supplement	Recommendations
Calcium	Children age 9 to 18 require 1300 mg/day, adults age 19 to 50 require 1000 mg/day and persons over 50 require 1200 mg/day. Most people need supplements to accomplish this. In order to maximize absorption, calcium carbonate (1200 mg provides 500 mg elemental calcium) should generally be taken with food in individual divided doses not exceeding 500 mg of calcium. In addition to preventing osteoporosis-associated bone fractures, calcium and vitamin D supplements may delay tooth loss in the elderly.[5]
Folic acid	All women of child-bearing potential should consume a supplement providing 0.4 mg/day of folic acid prior to conception to reduce the risk of congenital birth defects. Women with a history of neural tube defect pregnancy require 5 mg/day. Better folic acid status is associated with lower plasma homocysteine levels, which in turn are predictive, in epidemiologic studies, of a reduced risk of vascular disease,[6,7] stroke, Alzheimer's disease,[7,8] osteoporosis[9] and colon cancer.[10] Prospective clinical trials using very high-dose folic acid and pyridoxine to reduce plasma homocysteine levels in non-folate deficient patients with cardiovascular disease have, so far, been disappointing.[11] The Canadian and American food supply has been fortified with synthetic folic acid since 1999 to prevent congenital birth defects.
Iron	Because it is potentially toxic, iron supplementation at or above the recommended intake should be used only on a case-by-case basis for at-risk persons (e.g., adolescents and women with heavy menstrual losses) or people clearly not meeting the recommended intake, until the dietary inadequacy is corrected. Dietary iron deficiency occurs in the elderly but there is a comparable risk of iron storage disease from excessive intake.
Multivitamin	Select a preventive multiple vitamin/mineral containing the daily iron recommendation for persons who require supplementation or whose diet lacks iron, and a product specific to patients over age 50 containing less iron (~4 mg) for more general use. A multivitamin should be taken with food containing some fat. It should provide approximately 800 retinol activity equivalents (RAE) equivalent to ~2500 IU retinol, but preferably partly as beta-carotene; 0.4 to 1 mg folic acid; at least 2 µg vitamin B_{12}; other B vitamins; 400 IUvitamin D_3; and 10 to 15 mg zinc.
Vitamin A and beta-carotene	The recommended daily vitamin A intake of ~800 RAE can be achieved by 2500 IU of retinol or 10 mg (equivalent to 1600 IU) of its plant-derived precursor, beta-carotene. Multivitamins typically contain a mixture of the two forms.

(cont'd)

Table 2: **Common Vitamin/Mineral Deficiencies** *(cont'd)*

Preventive Supplement	Recommendations
Vitamin B_{12}	All persons over age 50 are advised to consume approximately 2 μg of synthetic vitamin B_{12} daily in enriched foods (e.g., some cold breakfast cereals) or as a supplement since achlorhydria is common and impairs the absorption of food-bound vitamin B_{12}.[12] Doses range from 50 μg/day orally for mild deficiency to 1 to 2 mg orally daily or 1 mg monthly im or sc in pernicious anemia.[13] Patients lacking their stomach or terminal ileum require parenteral vitamin B_{12}.
Vitamin D	Canadians consuming less than 1 litre of fluid milk/day (which provides 400 IU vitamin D_3) are dependent on endogenous skin photosynthesis for this vitamin, but this is lessened in fall and winter, prevented by sun block and decreases with age. Biochemical vitamin D deficiency is highly prevalent in Canada, and the amount of dietary vitamin D and sunlight exposure required for optimum vitamin D nutrition is controversial.[2,14,15] Institutionalized persons and those who shield themselves from sunlight are extremely likely to be vitamin D deficient if not provided with supplements.[16] Persons with or at high risk of osteoporosis, including those being treated with bisphosphonates, should consume 800 to 1200 IU vitamin D_3/day (as well as calcium). Vitamin D_2 (ergocalciferol) is less active than vitamin D_3. Some patients with fat malabsorption will benefit from the better water solubility of calcitriol (1,25-dihydroxycholecalciferol), but must be monitored for toxicity (hypercalciuria, hypercalcemia).

Table 3: **Preventive Supplementation in Special Populations**

Special Population	Recommendations
Pregnancy	All pregnant women should have taken folic acid prior to conception, and continue it during pregnancy with a standard supplement containing **folic acid** and a moderate increase in **iron** during the second and third trimesters. Adequate **vitamin A** nutrition is very important, but do not exceed ~3300 IU of supplemental vitamin A in the form of retinol.
Vegetarian diet	Vegans require a **vitamin D_3** supplement unless direct skin sunlight exposure is guaranteed and, unless a dietetic evaluation demonstrates otherwise, also require **calcium** supplements. Both vegans and lacto-ovo-vegetarians should use a **vitamin B_{12}** supplement providing 2 μg/day. Vegetarians are not especially iron deficient and do not routinely require iron supplements.

Therapeutic Supplementation

Therapeutic supplements contain 5 to 50-times more than the RDA of specific vitamins for therapeutic or pharmacologic purposes. Some indications for the use of therapeutic supplements are listed in Table 4. Examples of common therapeutic supplements and recommendations are listed in Table 5.

Table 4: Indications for Therapeutic Supplements

Overt deficiency disease[a]

Compensation for maldigestion or malabsorption:[a]
- extensive gastric resection (calcium, folic acid, vitamin B_{12} and iron)
- absent or diseased terminal ileum (vitamin B_{12})
- decreased absorptive surface area (most micronutrients)
- fat maldigestion (vitamins A, D, E, calcium, magnesium and essential fatty acids)

Certain inborn errors of metabolism

Nutrient-responsive nondeficiency diseases

[a] Formal dietetic assessment advised

Table 5: Therapeutic Supplements

Therapeutic Supplement	Recommendations
Antioxidant vitamin therapy	Despite epidemiologic, biologic and metabolic clinical data indicating that combination antioxidant vitamin therapy could prevent atherosclerotic events, several hard endpoint clinical trials have failed to confirm this. Clinical trials have employed greatly varying doses of vitamin E, ignored its very poor bioavailability when not consumed with fat, and/or included high-dose beta-carotene, which may specifically increase cardiovascular and cancer risk.[17] Nevertheless, current evidence does not justify the use of vitamin E or other antioxidant vitamins to prevent cardiovascular disease, with the possible exception of hemodialysis patients.[18] In sufficiently high doses (1200 mg/day of the natural form), vitamin E may arrest neuroleptic-induced tardive dyskinesias.[19]
Combination supplementation for age-related macular degeneration	A nutritional supplement providing vitamin C 500 mg, synthetic vitamin E 400 IU, beta-carotene 15 mg, zinc 80 mg (as zinc oxide) and copper 2 mg reduced the risk of progression to advanced disease by ~25% from baseline in patients with intermediate macular degeneration, from a baseline risk of roughly 20 to 30%. However, the trial was not sufficiently powered to detect a treatment effect on the low rate of progression in persons with only mild disease.[20,21]
Omega-3 fatty acids	Consumption of the marine oil–derived polyunsaturated omega-3 fatty acids, docosahexaenoic acid (DHA) and eicosapentaenoic acid (EPA) substantially reduces the risk of cardiac arrhythmias and cardiac death.[22,23] Persons with cardiovascular disease and especially those at risk of arrhythmias should eat certain fatty fish (e.g., salmon) two to three times/week to achieve an average daily intake of ~1 g DHA plus EPA/day, or use supplements.[24] The quality of fish oil capsules on the market is not standardized. Flaxseed oil contains the 18-carbon omega-3 fatty acid, alpha-linolenic acid, which, although not significantly converted to EPA and DHA by humans, could theoretically benefit by reducing formation of the potential antagonist omega-6 fatty acid, arachidonic acid.[22]
Thiamine	Wernicke's encephalopathy is under-diagnosed in malnourished persons because it frequently presents nonspecifically as confusion or decreased consciousness. All patients at risk (chronic alcoholism, hyperemesis gravidarum and AIDS) should receive oral thiamine, and those with altered mental status should be treated presumptively with 50 to 100 mg parenterally for three days.

(cont'd)

Table 5: **Therapeutic Supplements** *(cont'd)*

Therapeutic Supplement	Recommendations
Zinc	Zinc intake is marginal in adults consuming diets low in meat, fish or fowl. Zinc deficiency impairs immunity and wound healing, and may impair taste sensation; skin rash and diarrhea occur in severe cases. Deficiency should be suspected and treated in patients with poor diet, malabsorption, inflammatory diarrhea or severe sickle cell disease.[25] Zinc lozenges or nasal gels may shorten the duration of the common cold through a direct antiviral action, but the product must actually release zinc; effective products may be identified by an astringent feeling in the mouth.[26]

Micronutrient Toxicity

Although often considered innocuous, micronutrients can cause toxicities and be involved in drug–nutrient interactions. Table 6 lists some vitamin/mineral toxicities and Table 7 provides examples of some drug–nutrient interactions.

Table 6: **Vitamin/Mineral Toxicities**

Supplement	Toxicity
Folic Acid	In doses greater than 1 mg/day, folic acid may mask the hematologic picture of concurrent vitamin B_{12} deficiency, delaying the diagnosis and allowing the neurologic lesion to progress.
Iron	Therapy with iron should be monitored (e.g., to normalize serum ferritin) and/or time limited to avoid iron storage disease. There is also theoretical concern that increased tissue iron may catalyze free radical production even in persons without classical iron storage disease. In the absence of an obvious explanation, the diagnosis of iron deficiency should prompt investigation (e.g., GI blood loss, occult celiac disease).
Vitamin A and beta-carotene	Except in malabsorption/maldigestion and the treatment of retinitis pigmentosa, there is no indication for intakes of vitamin A (as retinol) in excess of the recommended intake of 2500 IU. Patients with renal failure accumulate retinol and hence are not normally prescribed supplements containing it. Heavy cigarette smokers who used a specially formulated 30 mg beta-carotene product had an increased death rate from lung cancer and cardiac causes. It is possible that high dose beta-carotene could mitigate the beneficial effects of other antioxidants.[27] No increased risk (or benefit) was seen in smokers or nonsmokers in a large clinical trial that combined vitamins E and C and high-dose beta-carotene.[28] Despite having depleted liver retinol, patients with chronic liver disease and alcohol abusers are prone to hepatotoxicity from retinol and high-dose beta-carotene.[29] Retinol consumption of 10 000 IU or more from fish has been associated with lower bone density and a higher hip fracture rate.[10,30] Pregnant women require adequate vitamin A, but should not exceed a daily supplement of 3300 IU.

(cont'd)

Table 6: Vitamin/Mineral Toxicities *(cont'd)*

Supplement	Toxicity
Vitamin C	There is no good evidence of toxicity especially below ~2 g/day.[31] High-dose vitamin C is an osmotic laxative with predictable effects. Although it is metabolized to oxalate, the risk of urolithiasis is not increased by high-dose vitamin C consumption, at least in persons lacking a prior history of oxalate stone formation. Vitamin C can theoretically increase iron absorption and interact with iron to promote oxidative damage, so large doses should be avoided in persons with iron storage disease. It should also be avoided by persons with advanced renal disease, whose renal oxalate clearance is reduced. "Chewable" vitamin C is somewhat acidic and if used as a lozenge could promote tooth enamel loss.
Vitamin D	The upper safe daily intake of 2000 IU/day[16] is a conservative estimate, and toxicity due to vitamin D has not been well described except as a result of errors by food producers.[14] At potential risk, either from vitamin D ingestion or sunlight exposure, are some patients with granulomatous diseases (lymphoma, sarcoidosis, tuberculosis), in which cholecalciferol may be converted in an uncontrolled fashion to the active vitamin, 1,25-dihydroxycholecalciferol. Early toxicity manifests as hypercalciuria, progressing to hypercalcemia.
Vitamin E	Daily intake of 1600 mg of natural vitamin E appears to be safe.[31] A meta-analysis suggested that long-term intake of 400 mg/day or the equivalent dose of the synthetic form marginally increased all-cause mortality,[32] but may have been biased by including studies in which high-dose beta-carotene was co-administered.[33] High-dose vitamin E has a mild antiplatelet effect, potentially increasing the risk of hemorrhage; it should, like aspirin, be avoided in persons with a bleeding diathesis or uncontrolled hypertension. There is a theoretical risk that high-dose vitamin E can increase prothrombin time although a systematic study failed to show this.[34]
Zinc	The RDA for zinc is approximately 15 mg/day. Long-term high-dose zinc intake (e.g., 50 mg/day) may block iron and copper absorption.

Table 7: Drug–Nutrient Interactions

Drug	Interaction
Anticonvulsants	Anticonvulsant drugs induce **folic acid** and **vitamin D** deficiency. Preventive folic acid and vitamin D supplements are indicated.
Antidepressants	Depression may not respond optimally to antidepressant therapy when folic acid status is marginal or deficient.[35,36] Assess nutritional status of depressed patients and prescribe a multiple vitamin providing the RDA for **thiamine, folic acid** and synthetic **vitamin B_{12}**.
Glucocorticoids	The adverse bone effects of systemic glucocorticoids are magnified when **calcium** or **vitamin D** intake are inadequate. Routine supplementation with calcium and vitamin D is recommended.
Isoniazid	Isoniazid increases **pyridoxine (vitamin B_6)** needs and can induce peripheral neuropathy. Patients who require this drug should be prescribed a preventive supplement. Clinically malnourished patients should receive 10 to 50 mg pyridoxine every day.

(cont'd)

Table 7: **Drug–Nutrient Interactions** *(cont'd)*

Drug	Interaction
Loop diuretics	Especially when used in high doses or in combination with other diuretics, loop diuretics increase urinary loss of calcium, magnesium, potassium, thiamine and zinc. Supplementation may be indicated.
Metformin	Metformin use may cause malabsorption of dietary vitamin B_{12}. Hematologic testing for vitamin B_{12} levels should be considered.
Methotrexate	Patients receiving low-dose methotrexate therapy (as used to treat rheumatoid arthritis) should receive **folic acid** (1 to 5 mg/day) to reduce the risk of GI and liver toxicity.
Orlistat	Orlistat induces fat malabsorption; suggest a preventive multivitamin containing the **fat-soluble vitamins** and **beta-carotene**.

Suggested Readings

Institute of Medicine (US). Panel on Dietary Antioxidants and Related Compounds. *Dietary reference intakes for vitamin C, vitamin E, selenium and carotenoids.* Washington (DC): National Academy Press; 2000.

Institute of Medicine (US). Panel on Dietary Antioxidants and Related Compounds. *Dietary reference intakes for calcium, phosphorus, magnesium, vitamin D and fluoride.* Washington (DC): National Academy Press; 1997.

Institute of Medicine (US). Panel on Dietary Antioxidants and Related Compounds. *Dietary reference intakes for thiamin, riboflavin, niacin, vitamin B_6, folate, vitamin B_{12}, pantothenic acid, biotin and choline.* Washington (DC): National Academy Press; 1998.

Fletcher RH, Fairfield KM. Vitamins for chronic disease prevention in adults: clinical applications. *JAMA* 2002; 287(23):3127-9.

References

1. Dollahite J, Franklin D, McNew R. Problems encountered in meeting the Recommended Dietary Allowances for menus designed according to the Dietary Guidelines for Americans. *J Am Diet Assoc* 1995; 95(3):341-4.
2. Willett WC, Stampfer MJ. Clinical practice. What vitamins should I be taking, doctor? *N Engl J Med* 2001;345(25):1819-24.
3. Fletcher RH, Fairfield KM. Vitamins for chronic disease prevention in adults: clinical applications. *JAMA* 2002;287(23):3127-9.
4. Centers for Disease Control and Prevention (CDC). Use of vitamins containing folic acid among women of childbearing age--United States, 2004. *MMWR Morb Mortal Wkly Rep* 2004;53(36):847-50.
5. Krall EA, Wehler C, Garcia RI et al. Calcium and vitamin D supplements reduce tooth loss in the elderly. *Am J Med* 2001;111(6):452-6.
6. Malinow MR, Bostom AG, Krauss RM. Homocyst(e)ine, diet, and cardiovascular diseases: a statement for healthcare professionals from the Nutrition Committee, American Heart Association. *Circulation* 1999;99(1):178-82.
7. Goldstein LB, Adams R, Becker K et al. Primary prevention of ischemic stroke: a statement for healthcare professionals from the Stroke Council of the American Heart Association. *Circulation* 2001;103(1):163-82.
8. Seshadri S, Beiser A, Selhub J et al. Plasma homocysteine as a risk factor for dementia and Alzheimer's disease. *N Engl J Med* 2002;346(7):476-83.
9. Raisz LG. Homocysteine and osteoporotic fractures--culprit or bystander? *N Engl J Med* 2004;350(20):2089-90.

10. Fairfield KM, Fletcher RH. Vitamins for chronic disease prevention in adults: scientific review. *JAMA* 2002;287(23):3116-26.
11. Loscalzo J. Homocysteine trials--clear outcomes for complex reasons. *N Engl J Med* 2006;354(15):1629-32.
12. Baik HW, Russell RM. Vitamin B12 deficiency in the elderly. *Annu Rev Nutr* 1999;19:357-77.
13. Seal EC, Metz J, Flicker L, Melny J. A randomized, double-blind, placebo-controlled study of oral vitamin B12 supplementation in older patients with subnormal or borderline serum vitamin B12 concentrations. *J Am Geriatr Soc* 2002;50(1):146-51.
14. Vieth R. Vitamin D supplementation, 25-hydroxyvitamin D concentrations, and safety. *Am J Clin Nutr* 1999;69(5):842-56.
15. Vieth R, Fraser D. Vitamin D insufficiency: no recommended dietary allowance exists for this nutrient. *CMAJ* 2002;166(12):1541-2.
16. Institute of Medicine (US). Panel on Dietary Antioxidants and Related Compounds. *Dietary reference intakes for calcium, phosphorus, magnesium, vitamin D and fluoride.* Washington (DC): National Academy Press; 1997.
17. Omenn GS, Goodman GE, Thornquist MD et al. Effects of a combination of beta carotene and vitamin A on lung cancer and cardiovascular disease. *N Engl J Med* 1996;334(18):1150-5.
18. Boaz M, Smetana S, Weinstein T et al. Secondary prevention with antioxidants of cardiovascular disease in endstage renal disease (SPACE): randomised placebo-controlled trial. *Lancet* 2000;356(9237):1213-8.
19. Soares KV, McGrath JJ. Vitamin E for neuroleptic-induced tardive dyskinesia. *Cochrane Database Syst Rev* 2001;(4):CD000209.
20. Age-related Eye Disease Study Group. A randomized, placebo-controlled, clinical trial of high-dose supplementation with vitamins C and E, beta carotene, and zinc for age-related macular degeneration and vision loss: AREDS report no. 8. *Arch Ophthalmol* 2001;119(10):1417-36.
21. Jampol LM. Antioxidants and zinc to prevent progression of age-related macular degeneration. *JAMA* 2001;286(19):2466-8.
22. De Lorgeril M, Salen P. Fish and N-3 fatty acids for the prevention and treatment of coronary heart disease: nutrition is not pharmacology. *Am J Med* 2002;112(4):316-9.
23. Kris-Etherton PM, Harris WS, Appel LJ et al. Fish consumption, fish oil, omega-3 fatty acids, and cardiovascular disease. *Circulation* 2002;106(21):2747-57.
24. Holub BJ. Clinical nutrition: 4. Omega-3 fatty acids in cardiovascular care. *CMAJ* 2002;166(5):608-15.
25. Prasad AS, Beck FW, Kaplan J et al. Effect of zinc supplementation on incidence of infections and hospital admissions in sickle cell disease (SCD). *Am J Hematol* 1999;61(3):194-202.
26. Eby GA. Elimination of efficacy by additives in zinc acetate lozenges for common colds. *Clin Infect Dis* 2000;32(10):1520.
27. Baron JA, Cole BF, Mott L et al. Neoplastic and antineoplastic effects of beta-carotene on colorectal adenoma recurrence: results of a randomized trial. *J Natl Cancer Inst* 2003;95(10):717-22.
28. Heart Protection Study Collaborative Group. MRC/BHF Heart Protection Study of antioxidant vitamin supplementation in 20,536 high-risk individuals: a randomised placebo-controlled trial. *Lancet* 2002;360(9326):23-33.
29. Leo MA, Lieber CS. Alcohol, vitamin A, and beta-carotene: adverse interactions, including hepatotoxicity and carcinogenicity. *Am J Clin Nutr* 1999;69(6):1071-85.
30. Feskanich D, Singh V, Willett WC, Colditz GA. Vitamin A intake and hip fractures among postmenopausal women. *JAMA* 2002;287(1):47-54.
31. Hathcock JN, Azzi A, Blumberg J et al. Vitamins E and C are safe across a broad range of intakes. *Am J Clin Nutr* 2005;81(4):736-45.
32. Miller ER, Pastor-Barriuso R, Dalal D et al. Meta-analysis: high-dosage vitamin E supplementation may increase all-cause mortality. *Ann Intern Med* 2005;142(1):37-46.
33. Greenberg ER. Vitamin E supplements: good in theory, but is the theory good? *Ann Intern Med* 2005;142(1):75-6.
34. Kim JM, White RH. Effect of vitamin E on the anticoagulant response to warfarin. *Am J Cardiol* 1996;77(1):545-6.
35. Alpert JE, Fava M. Nutrition and depression: the role of folate. *Nutr Rev* 1997;55(5):145-9.
36. Coppen A, Bailey J. Enhancement of the antidepressant action of fluoxetine by folic acid: a randomised, placebo controlled trial. *J Affect Disord* 2000;60(2):121-30.

CHAPTER 30
Primary Prevention of Vascular Disease

Tania Mysak, BSP, PharmD

Vascular disease remains a top contributor to morbidity and mortality in Canada. It is well recognized that many modifiable risk factors are undertreated, leaving a care gap with costly consequences for our health care system.[1,2]

Prevention of morbidity and mortality from vascular disease requires early recognition and management of modifiable risk factors such as poor diet, sedentary lifestyle, obesity, elevated blood pressure, elevated cholesterol, diabetes mellitus and smoking.

Primary prevention of vascular disease involves management of risk factors before the patient suffers a vascular event such as myocardial infarction or stroke.[3] While the data supporting pharmacologic therapies in secondary prevention of vascular disease (i.e., management of risk factors after the patient has suffered a vascular event) are fairly robust, evidence supporting primary prevention strategies is relatively sparse in comparison.

Goals of Therapy

- Prevent vascular events, including myocardial infarction, stroke or amputation
- Prevent vascular mortality
- Minimize adverse effects from drug therapy
- Preserve quality of life

Investigations

- At all appropriate visits determine:
  - blood pressure using standardized techniques[4]
  - smoking status[3]
  - patient weight. Calculate hip-to-waist ratio and body mass index (BMI)[3]
- All men ≥ 40 years, all women who are postmenopausal or ≥ 50 years, and any adult with vascular risk factors including diabetes mellitus, cigarette smoking, hypertension, obesity and/or a family history of premature coronary artery disease should:
  - have a lipid profile done every one to three years. The more frequent screening is for patients with abnormal values or those requiring treatment.[5]

  - be screened for peripheral arterial disease (PAD) on the basis of symptoms and measurement of the ankle-brachial index (ABI).[5,6,7] This recommendation is controversial. The ABI is the ratio of systolic blood pressure in the dorsalis pedis or posterior tibial artery to the systolic blood pressure in the brachial artery and is performed using a blood pressure cuff assisted by an ultrasound Doppler device instead of a stethoscope. An ABI < 0.9 is indicative of PAD.
- All individuals ≥ 40 years of age should be screened for diabetes by measuring fasting plasma glucose every three years. More frequent and/or earlier testing should be considered in people with first-degree relatives with diabetes, members of high-risk populations (e.g., Aboriginal, Hispanic, Asian, South Asian or African) and those with hypertension, dyslipidemia, obesity or schizophrenia[8]
- Calculate the patient's cardiovascular risk (see back cover). Management of the patient depends on their risk score. Most patients with type 1 or 2 diabetes mellitus are considered "high risk"[5]
- Rule out secondary causes of hypertension, dyslipidemia and elevated blood glucose

Therapeutic Choices

Nonpharmacologic Choices

- Lifestyle modification including weight loss, increased physical activity, reduced sodium intake and adherence to the DASH (Dietary Approaches to Stop Hypertension) diet can improve control of risk factors and, potentially, reduce vascular risk.[9,10]
- Based primarily on observational studies, current guidelines recommend a diet that emphasizes fruits, vegetables, fish and low-fat dairy products, and limits intake of saturated and trans fatty acids, simple sugars and refined carbohydrates.[4,5,6,10,11]
- Encourage regular physical activity to maintain physical fitness, vascular health, optimal body weight and sustain weight loss. Most guidelines suggest 30–60 minutes of moderate intensity exercise (walking, jogging, cycling or swimming) four to seven days of the week.[12]
- Encourage patients to achieve and maintain a healthy body weight (BMI of 18.5–24.9 kg/m^2).[3,4,5] Bariatric surgery may be required for the morbidly obese.[13]
- Counsel patients to stop using tobacco and minimize exposure to second-hand smoke.[14] Nonpharmacologic therapies may include psychological counselling.
- Patients should limit alcohol intake to a maximum of two standard drinks per day for men and one standard drink per day for women.[3]

Pharmacologic Choices

Absolute risk reductions (ARR) for primary preventive strategies are small compared with secondary preventive strategies. Refer to Table 1 for the ARR and number needed to treat (NNT) to prevent vascular events with the pharmacologic therapies discussed below.

Hypertension

Lowering blood pressure (BP) with antihypertensive therapy reduces the relative risk of a first major vascular event by ~20–40% when compared with placebo.[15,16] Larger reductions in BP produce larger reductions in risk.[15] ARR are small (Table 1); however, the higher the BP, the greater the potential benefits.[17] In the absence of other vascular risk factors (e.g., age > 55, male gender, positive family history, abdominal obesity) or macrovascular target organ damage, antihypertensive treatment should be initiated if the average BP is ≥ 160/100 mm Hg. In the presence of target organ damage or other vascular risk factors, treatment should be initiated if the average BP is ≥ 140/90 mm Hg. The target BP is <140/90 mm Hg for most patients. In patients with diabetes mellitus or chronic kidney disease, the target BP is < 130/80 mm Hg.[4] The choice of antihypertensive agent is less important than achieving target BP. See Chapter 32 for current recommendations on the choice of antihypertensive agents.

Dyslipidemia

Cholesterol-lowering therapy with **HMG Co-A reductase inhibitors (statins)** reduces the relative risk of a first major vascular event by ~15–30% (Table 1) when compared with placebo.[18] The primary target of therapy is LDL-C with the specific target number based on individual patient risk (as per Framingham Risk Score; see Figure 2, Chapter 31). While controversial, current guidelines recommend patients at low risk should target LDL-C < 5.0 mmol/L; those at medium risk, < 3.5 mmol/L; and those at high risk, < 2.0 mmol/L.[5] The lower LDL target for high-risk individuals is based on secondary prevention trials, and the routine use of statins in medium-risk individuals is controversial.[5,18] Data for aggressive LDL reduction in primary prevention are limited. The majority of primary prevention trials involving statins included primarily younger (< 65 years) men, therefore robust evidence for primary prevention in women and older adults is lacking.[19,20]

Most patients are able to achieve target levels of LDL-C on statin monotherapy, however some patients may require combination therapy to achieve targets. Evidence is lacking for the use of agents aside from statins in primary prevention. See Chapter 31 for current recommendations on the choice of antihyperlipidemic agents.

Diabetes Mellitus

The target hemoglobin A_{1c} for most patients with type 1 or type 2 diabetes is ≤ 7% and ≤ 6% for those in whom it can be safely achieved.[8] Such tight control of blood glucose reduces the risk of microvascular complications (e.g., retinopathy), but evidence linking tight glycemic control to prevention of macrovascular complications is less robust.[21,22] The Canadian Diabetes Association Guidelines provide an algorithm to assist in evidence-based choices for drug therapy.[8] See Chapter 27 for current recommendations on the choice of antihyperglycemic agents.

Antithrombotics

The role of antiplatelet therapy in primary prevention of vascular disease is controversial. A meta-analysis of data from five major primary prevention trials suggests that treating 143 patients for five years with **ASA** prevents one nonfatal MI (30% RRR) and treating 270 patients for five years prevents one "important vascular event" (15% RRR). This benefit is offset by a 1% increase in the annual risk of a GI bleed. The risk of stroke was not significantly reduced by ASA.[23,24] Guidelines recommend ASA 75–162 mg/day for patients at "moderate risk" (defined as 10-year CV risk > 10% according to FRS).[3]

The data on which this recommendation is based were obtained from studies that enrolled predominantly men. The Women's Health Study (WHS) found that ASA 100 mg every other day reduces the relative risk of stroke in women aged 45 years or older by 17% (ARR 0.3%, NNT 333), but not the risk of MI or vascular death.[25] A subsequent meta-analysis of this and other studies of ASA concluded that there are differences between men and women.[26] However, older women in the WHS (those aged 65 years and older) experienced a vascular benefit from ASA in the form of a 26% relative reduction in the risk of major vascular events (ARR 2.2%, NNT 46), a 34% relative reduction in the risk of MI (ARR 1%, NNT 100), but no reduction in the risk of stroke.[25] Epidemiologic data from the Nurses' Health Study also suggests a possible age-related vascular benefit from ASA.[27] At this time a standard recommendation for use of ASA that applies to all persons cannot be made.

Patients with atrial fibrillation are at high risk for cardioembolic stroke and may be candidates for **warfarin** therapy to prevent a first stroke or transient ischemic attack (TIA). $CHADS_2$ is a risk assessment tool that can be used to stratify patients by their risk of stroke on the basis of risk factors including congestive heart failure ("C"), hypertension ("H"), age > 75 years ("A"), diabetes mellitus ("D") and history of stroke or TIA ("S").[23] ASA 325 mg daily is an alternative to warfarin for low-risk patients.[28,29] A complete description of $CHADS_2$ is provided in Chapter 39.

Smoking Cessation

Observational studies suggest that the elevated vascular risk induced by cigarette smoking can be decreased by quitting and reversed after five years of abstinence.[30] Successful smoking cessation can be enhanced by **nicotine replacement therapy** (NRT) (gum, patch, inhalers), **bupropion** and **varenicline**. Bupropion and NRT are roughly equivalent in terms of efficacy, and either varenicline or the combination of bupropion and NRT may provide higher success rates.[31,32,33]

Nonpharmacologic interventions, in combination with pharmacologic therapies, are effective in optimizing success rates, and may be superior to pharmacologic therapies alone.[32] See Chapter 10 for current recommendations on the choice of nonpharmacologic and pharmacologic therapies.

Obesity

Current drugs approved for obesity include **orlistat** and **sibutramine** (**rimonabant** is approved in the US and elsewhere, but not in Canada). Each drug produces a 5–10% weight loss that is maintained over two years in ~60% of patients; however, the impact of drug-induced weight loss of this magnitude on vascular morbidity and mortality is unknown.[34] Discontinuation of therapy generally leads to weight regain, therefore, effective management must focus on lifestyle changes. Drug therapy should be regarded as a therapeutic trial and stopped if significant weight loss is not achieved after several months.[35] See Chapter 28 for current recommendations on the choice of nonpharmacologic and pharmacologic therapies.

Nutritional Supplements

There is no conclusive evidence that omega-3 supplementation reduces vascular risk, although dietary recommendations suggest including these foods in a balanced diet.[36] Interpretation of data regarding **omega-3 fatty acids** (found in oily fish and plants) is hindered by poor study design. Reduction of risk by vitamin therapy (e.g., folic acid, vitamin E) in patients with established vascular disease has largely been shown to be ineffective, and current data do not support supplementation in primary prevention.[37,38,39,40]

Hormone Therapy (HT)

Women should not be encouraged to continue HT if the sole reason is vascular protection. While observational data suggested a vascular risk reduction benefit of hormone therapy in postmenopausal women, experimental data have refuted that claim.[41]

Therapeutic Tips

- View every patient encounter as an opportunity to identify risk factors, discuss risk factor modification and encourage patient progress.
- Consider nonpharmacologic management to be an essential component of risk reduction strategies. Drugs can have adverse effects. Patients suitable for primary prevention have not yet experienced symptoms of disease and may not wish to be "medicalized."
- Individualize patient goals based on the risk of having an event. The comparatively small absolute benefits of many drug therapies for

primary prevention warrant discussion with patients regarding their personal health goals and willingness to undertake drug therapy.

- Patients must make the link between risk factors and potential consequences (i.e., major vascular events). Stress the importance of risk factor reduction in these terms, not simply to reduce surrogate markers (e.g., cholesterol, blood pressure).
- Pharmacologic choices should include consideration of significant cost differences between therapies that are equally effective.

Table 1: Primary Prevention of Coronary Events and Stroke

Outcome Prevented	Intervention	Comparator	ARR (%)	NNT	Potential Risks
Coronary event[42]	Antihypertensive therapy	Placebo	0.7[a]	143 over 4–5 years	Symptoms of hypotension Side effects of drug therapy
Coronary event[18]	Statin	Placebo	1.4	73 over 4–5 years	Rhabdomyolysis 0.2% per year[43]
Coronary event[26]					
• Men	ASA	Placebo	0.85	118 over 5 years	GI bleed 1% per year[24]
• Women	ASA	Placebo	NS	NS	GI bleed 1% per year[24]
Stroke[42]	Antihypertensive therapy	Placebo	1.3	77 over 4–5 years	Symptoms of hypotension Side effects of drug therapy
Stroke[18]	Statin	Placebo	0.4	280 over 5 years	Rhabdomyolysis 0.2% per year[43]
Stroke[26]					
• Men	ASA	Placebo	NS	NS	GI bleed 1% per year[24]
• Women	ASA	Placebo	0.24	417 over 10 years	GI bleed 1% per year[24]

[a] Absolute benefits are correlated with baseline risk.[17]

Abbreviations: ARR = absolute risk reduction; NNT = number needed to treat to prevent one outcome; NS = not significant

Suggested Readings

Abramson BL, Huckell V, Anand S et al. Canadian Cardiovascular Society Consensus Conference: peripheral arterial disease—executive summary. *Can J Cardiol* 2005;21(12):997-1006.

Canadian Diabetes Association Clinical Practice Guidelines Expert Committee. Canadian Diabetes Association 2003 clinical practice guidelines for the prevention and management of diabetes in Canada. *Can J Diabetes* 2003:27(Suppl 2):S1-152. Available from: http://www.diabetes.ca/cpg2003/ Accessed March 20, 2007.

Canadian Hypertension Education Program. *CHEP 2007 recommendations*. Available from: http://www.hypertension.ca/chep/en/Recommendations.asp Accessed March 20, 2007.

Lau DC, Douketis JD, Morrison KM, et al. 2006 Canadian clinical practice guidelines on the management and prevention of obesity in adults and children [summary]. *CMAJ* 2007;176(8):S1-13.

McPherson R, Frohlich, J, Fodor G et al. Canadian Cardiovascular Society position statement—recommendations for the diagnosis and treatment of dyslipidemia and prevention of cardiovascular disease. *Can J Cardiol* 2006;22(11):913-27.

References

1. Joffres MR, Ghadirian P, Fodor JG et al. Awareness, treatment, and control of hypertension in Canada. *Am J Hypertens* 1997;10(10 Pt 1):1097-102.
2. McLean DL, Simpson SH, McAlister FA et al. Treatment and blood pressure control in 47,964 people with diabetes and hypertension: a systematic review of observational studies. *Can J Cardiol* 2006;22(10):855-60.
3. Pearson TA, Blair SN, Daniels SR et al. AHA Guidelines for Primary Prevention of Cardiovascular Disease and Stroke: 2002 Update: Consensus Panel Guide to Comprehensive Risk Reduction for Adult Patients Without Coronary or Other Atherosclerotic Vascular Diseases. American Heart Association Science Advisory and Coordinating Committee. *Circulation* 2002;106(3):388-91.
4. Canadian Hypertension Education Program. *CHEP 2007 recommendations*. Available from: http://www.hypertension.ca/chep/en/Recommendations.asp Accessed March 20, 2007.
5. McPherson R, Frohlich, J, Fodor G et al. Canadian Cardiovascular Society position statement—recommendations for the diagnosis and treatment of dyslipidemia and prevention of cardiovascular disease. *Can J Cardiol* 2006;22(11):913-27.
6. Abramson BL, Huckell V, Anand S et al. Canadian Cardiovascular Society Consensus Conference: peripheral arterial disease-executive summary. *Can J Cardiol* 2005;21(12):997-1006.
7. Beckman JA, Jaff MR, Creager MA. The United States preventive services task force recommendation statement on screening for peripheral arterial disease: more harm than benefit? *Circulation* 2006;114(8):861-6.
8. Canadian Diabetes Association Clinical Practice Guidelines Expert Committee. Canadian Diabetes Association 2003 clinical practice guidelines for the prevention and management of diabetes in Canada. *Can J Diabetes* 2003:27(Suppl 2):S1-152. Available from: http://www.diabetes.ca/cpg2003/ Accessed March 20, 2007.
9. Elmer PJ, Obarzanek E, Vollmer WM et al. Effects of comprehensive lifestyle modification on diet, weight, physical fitness and blood pressure control: 18-month results of a randomized trial. *Ann Intern Med* 2006;144(7):485-95.
10. Appel LJ, Moore TJ, Obarzanek E et al. A clinical trial of the effects of dietary patterns on blood pressure. DASH Collaborative Research Group. *N Engl J Med* 1997;336(16):1117-24.
11. Health Canada. *Eating well with Canada's food guide*. Ottawa (ON): Health Canada; 2007. Available from: http://www.hc-sc.gc.ca/fn-an/food-guide-aliment/order-commander/index_e.html Accessed March 20, 2007.
12. American Heart Association Nutrition Committee; Lichtenstein AH, Appel LJ, Brands M et al. Diet and lifestyle recommendations revision 2006: a scientific statement from the American Heart Association Nutrition Committee. *Circulation* 2006;114(1):82-96.
13. Kral JG. ABC of obesity. Management part III–surgery. *BMJ* 2006;333(7574):900-3.
14. [No authors listed]. A clinical practice guideline for treating tobacco use and dependence: A US Public Health Service report. The Tobacco Use and Dependence Clinical Practice Guideline Panel, Staff, and Consortium Representatives. *JAMA* 2000;283(24):3244-54.

15. Neal B, MacMahon S, Chapman N et al. Effects of ACE inhibitors, calcium antagonists, and other blood-pressure-lowering drugs: results of prospectively designed overviews of randomised trials. Blood Pressure Lowering Treatment Trialists' Collaboration. *Lancet* 2000;355(9246):1955-64.
16. Turnbull F; Blood Pressure Lowering Treatment Trialists' Collaboration. Effects of different blood-pressure-lowering regimens on major cardiovascular events: results of prospectively designed overviews of randomized trials. *Lancet* 2003;632(9395):1527-35.
17. Ogden L, He J, Lydick E et al. Long-term absolute benefit of lowering blood pressure in hypertensive patients according to JNC VI risk stratification. *Hypertension* 2000;35(2):539-43.
18. Thavendiranathan P, Bagai A, Brookhart MA et al. Primary prevention of cardiovascular diseases with statin therapy: a meta-analysis of randomized controlled trials. *Arch Intern Med* 2006;166(21):2307-13.
19. Walsh JM, Pignone M. Drug treatment of hyperlipidemia in women. *JAMA* 2004;291(18):2243-52.
20. Shepherd J, Blauw GJ, Murphy MB et al. Pravastatin in elderly individuals at risk of vascular disease (PROSPER): a randomized controlled trial. *Lancet* 2002;360(9346):1623-30.
21. [No authors listed]. Intensive blood-glucose control with sulphonylureas or insulin compared with conventional treatment and risk of complications in patients with type 2 diabetes (UKPDS 33). UK Prospective Diabetes Study (UKPDS) Group. *Lancet* 1998;352(9131):837-53.
22. Nathan DM, Cleary PA, Blacklund JY et al. Intensive diabetes treatment and cardiovascular disease in patients with type 1 diabetes. *N Eng J Med* 2005;353(25):2643-53.
23. Eidelman RS, Hebert PR, Weisman SM et al. An update on aspirin in the primary prevention of cardiovascular disease. *Arch Intern Med* 2003;163(17):2006-10.
24. Derry S, Loke YK. Risk of gastrointestinal hemorrhage with long term use of aspirin: meta-analysis. *BMJ* 2000;321(7270):1183-7.
25. Ridker PM, Cook NR, Lee IM et al. A randomized trial of low-dose aspirin in the primary prevention of cardiovascular disease in women. *N Engl J Med* 2005;352(13):1293-304.
26. Berger JS, Roncaglioni MC, Avanzini F et al. Aspirin for the primary prevention of cardiovascular events in women and men; a sex specific meta-analysis of randomized controlled trials. *JAMA* 2006;295(3):306-13.
27. Chan AT, Manson JE, Feskanich D et al. Long-term aspirin use and mortality in women. *Arch Intern Med* 2007;167(6):562-72.
28. Goldstein LB, Adams R, Alberts MJ et al. Primary prevention of ischemic stroke: a guideline from the American Heart Association/American Stroke Association Stroke Council: cosponsored by the Atherosclerotic Peripheral Vascular Disease Interdisciplinary Working Group; Cardiovascular Nursing Council; Clinical Cardiology Council; Nutrition, Physical Activity, and Metabolism Council; and the Quality of Care and Outcomes Research Interdisciplinary Working Group: the American Academy of Neurology affirms the value of this guideline. *Stroke* 2006;37(6):1583-633.
29. Singer DE, Albers GW, Dalen JE et al. Antithrombotic therapy in atrial fibrillation: the Seventh ACCP Conference on Antithrombotic and Thrombolytic Therapy. *Chest* 2004;(Suppl 3):429S-56S.
30. Wolf PA, D'Agostino RB, Kannel WB et al. Cigarette smoking as a risk factor for stroke. The Framingham Study. *JAMA* 1988;259(7):1025-9.
31. Okuyemi KS, Nollen NL, Ahluwalia JS. Interventions to facilitate smoking cessation. *Am Fam Physician* 2006;74(2):262-71.
32. Ranney L, Melvin C, Lux L et al. Systematic review: smoking cessation intervention strategies for adults and adults in special populations. *Ann Intern Med* 2006;145(11):845-56.
33. Wu P, Wilson K, Dimoulas P et al. Effectiveness of smoking cessation therapies: a systematic review and meta-analysis. *BMC Public Health* 2006;6:300.
34. Padwal RS, Majumdar SR. Drug treatments for obesity: orlistat, sibutramine, and rimonabant. *Lancet* 2007;369(9555):71-7.
35. Lean M, Finer N. ABC of obesity. Management: part II—drugs. *BMJ* 2006;333(7572):794-7.
36. Hooper L, Thompson RL, Harrison RA et al. Omega 3 fatty acids for prevention and treatment of cardiovascular disease. *Cochrane Database Syst Rev* 2004;(4):CD003177.
37. Toole JF, Malinow MR, Chambless LE et al. Lowering homocysteine in patients with ischemic stroke to prevent recurrent stroke, myocardial infarction, and death: the Vitamin Intervention for Stroke Prevention (VISP) randomized controlled trial. *JAMA* 2004;291(5):565-75.
38. Bonaa KH, Njolstad I, Ueland PM et al. Homocysteine lowering and cardiovascular events after acute myocardial infarction. *N Engl J Med* 2006;354(15):1578-88.
39. Lonn E, Yusuf S, Arnold MJ et al. Homocysteine lowering with folic acid and B vitamins in vascular disease. *N Engl J Med* 2006;354(15):1567-77.
40. Lonn E, Bosch J, Yusuf S et al. Effects of long-term vitamin E supplementation on cardiovascular events and cancer: a randomized controlled trial. *JAMA* 2005;293(11):1338-47.
41. Gabriel SR, Carmona L, Roque M et al. Hormone replacement therapy for preventing cardiovascular disease in post-menopausal women. *Cochrane Database Syst Rev* 2005;(2):CD002229.
42. Herbert PR, Moser M, Mayer J et al. Recent evidence on drug therapy of mild to moderate hypertension and decreased risk of coronary heart disease. *Arch Intern Med* 1993;153(5):578-81.
43. Kashani A, Phillips CO, Foody JM et al. Risks associated with statin therapy: a systematic overview of randomized clinical trials. *Circulation* 2006;114(25):2788-97.

CHAPTER 31
Dyslipidemias

Ghislaine O. Roederer, MD, PhD

Goals of Therapy

- Reduce risk of cardiovascular disease (CVD) and renal disease
- Prevent pancreatitis from severe hypertriglyceridemia

Investigations

- Medical history with attention to CVD (past or present), possible causes of secondary dyslipidemia (Table 1) and major cardiovascular risk factors (Figure 1, Figure 2)
- Family history:
  – premature CVD (before age 55 in males, age 65 in females) in first degree relatives
  – dyslipidemia
- Physical examination:
  – BMI (weight (kg)/height (m)^2)
  – waist circumference
  – bilateral brachial blood pressure
  – arcus corneae (especially in the young patient)
  – funduscopy (lipemia retinalis, retinopathies)
  – peripheral pulses
  – cardiac auscultation
  – arterial bruits
  – hepatosplenomegaly
  – lipid deposits (xanthomas, xanthelasmas)
- Laboratory tests: lipid and lipoprotein levels[1]

  Note that the Friedewald equation, LDL-C=Total-C - (HDL-C+TG/2.2) cannot be used if triglyceride levels are > 4.52 mmol/L, if type III dysbetalipoproteinemia or if chylomicrons are present.

  – use the same laboratory for repeated measurements
  – a 12-hour fast is required for triglyceride levels
  – obtain two or three measurements at four- to six-week intervals to establish a baseline before initial diagnosis of a dyslipidemic phenotype. At least one measurement should include a lipoprotein profile, i.e., high-density lipoprotein cholesterol (HDL-C), low-density lipoprotein cholesterol (LDL-C)
  – other lab investigations to rule out frequent causes of secondary dyslipidemias (Table 1)

Classification of Dyslipidemias

Primary (genetic) versus secondary dyslipidemias: The WHO classification of dyslipidemia is based on lipoprotein phenotyping. Phenotypes, either primary or secondary, can result from interaction between environmental and genetic factors often polygenic and therefore rather ill-defined. Nevertheless, the genetic component is clear for monogenic familial hypercholesterolemia, type III dysbetalipoproteinemia and hyperchylomicronemia. Seek possible causes for secondary dyslipidemia and address them if present. If secondary dyslipidemia persists despite proper management of the underlying disease and constitutes an additional risk factor for the condition, lipid-lowering treatment then becomes necessary, e.g., diabetic dyslipidemia.

Table 1: **Common Causes of Secondary Hyperlipidemia**

Conditions	Medications
Hypothyroidism	Thiazide diuretics
Pregnancy	Beta-blockers without intrinsic sympathomimetic or alpha-blocking activity
Excess weight	Oral contraceptives
Alcohol excess	Highly active antiretroviral therapy (HAART)
Obstructive liver disease	Hormone replacement therapy (HRT)
Nephrotic syndrome	Corticosteroids
Chronic renal failure	
Diabetes/Metabolic syndrome	

Criteria for Intervention

Global cardiovascular risk assessment described in the recommendations from the Canadian Working Group on Hypercholesterolemia and Other Dyslipidemias[1] includes clinical status (primary, i.e., patients with no previous CVD versus secondary prevention, i.e., patients with prior CVD/atherosclerotic disease and/or at very high risk), risk factors and both *LDL-C* and *Total-C:HDL-C ratio* (Figure 1). Also consider additional CV risk imparted by a positive family history (less than 55 years old for men and 65 years old for women), the presence of at least three risk factors for metabolic syndrome and/or other biochemical markers. Modifiable risk factors for CV include smoking, poor glycemic control, hypertension and abdominal obesity. Nonmodifiable risk factors include a positive family history, male sex and age.

Metabolic syndrome is characterized by abdominal obesity, atherogenic dyslipidemia (high triglycerides, small LDL particles, low HDL cholesterol), hypertension, insulin resistance and prothrombotic and proinflammatory states (Table 2).[2] Management includes weight reduction, increased physical activity and treatment of lipid and nonlipid risk factors.

Table 2: **Clinical Identification of the Metabolic Syndrome**[a]

Risk Factor	Defining Level
Abdominal obesity	
Men	Waist circumference > 102 cm
Women	Waist circumference > 88 cm
Triglyceride level	≥ 1.7 mmol/L
HDL-C level	
Men	< 1.0 mmol/L
Women	< 1.3 mmol/L
Blood pressure	≥ 130/85 mm Hg
Fasting glucose level	5.7–7.0 mmol/L

[a] Criteria: three or more risk factors.
Abbreviations: HDL-C = high density lipoprotein cholesterol
Reprinted from *Can J Cardiol* September 2006; 22(11), Pages 913-927 by permission of the publisher (c) 2006 Pulsus Group Inc.

Diabetics, end-stage renal disease and renal transplant patients are considered very high risk. High triglyceride levels (2.3 to 11.3 mmol/L) are an additional CV risk factor when associated with atherogenic dyslipidemias, e.g., familial combined hyperlipidemia, insulin resistance, diabetes, renal failure. Very high triglyceride levels (> 10 mmol/L) are a risk factor for pancreatitis.

Therapeutic Choices

Nonpharmacologic Choices

- *Diet*, aimed at reducing blood lipid levels and weight (if needed), should always be part of the treatment. For secondary prevention and very high risk individuals, medication is introduced simultaneously. For primary prevention, a six-month dietary trial (Table 3) is recommended before considering medication; during this time, take two (ideally three) lipid and lipoprotein measurements.
- Encourage other lifestyle changes to further modify lipoprotein profile and reduce the risk of CVD, e.g., weight loss, physical activity and smoking cessation. Smoking cessation can help raise HDL-C.

Table 3: **Dietary Interventions**

Step I **Primary Prevention** **(patients with no previous CVD)**	**Step II** **Secondary Prevention[a]** **(patients with prior CVD/atherosclerotic disease and/or at very high risk)**
↓ dietary cholesterol intake to < 300 mg/day Restrict fat intake to 30% of calories Increase proportion of mono- and polyunsaturated fats in diet Restrict saturated and trans-fatty acids in diet Favour fruit and vegetable intake Increase omega-3 fatty acids from fish and plant sources Favour high-fibre intake Limit simple sugars to 8% of total calories Limit alcohol consumption to 5% of total calories	Same as Step I, but further ↓ dietary cholesterol intake to < 200 mg/day Restrict fat intake to 20% of calories and less than 7% of daily calories as saturated fat and trans-fatty acids

[a] A dietitian's help is usually required to reach and maintain these goals.

Pharmacologic Choices (Table 6)

Table 4 summarizes the effects of lipid-lowering drugs on lipoproteins.

Resins

The bile acid-sequestering resins **cholestyramine** and **colestipol** reduce plasma LDL and can slightly increase HDL levels. They have a strong safety record. Resins are the only lipid-lowering agents appropriate for use in children (> 2 years) or in pregnant or lactating women.

Table 4: **Lipid-lowering Agents—Effect on Lipoproteins**

	LDL	**HDL**	**TG**
Resins	↓↓	↑	↑
HMG CoA reductase inhibitors	↓↓↓	↑	↓↔↓↓[a]
Niacin	↓↓	↑↑	↓↓
Fibrates	↓↔↓	↑↑	↓↓↓
Ezetimibe	↓↓	↑↔	↓

[a] Atorvastatin and rosuvastatin have the greatest TG-lowering effect.

HMG CoA Reductase Inhibitors (Statins)

HMG CoA reductase inhibitors, the most potent LDL-lowering agents, interfere with the atherosclerotic disease process. Significant reductions in CVD morbidity, CVD mortality and total deaths in both primary and secondary prevention have been associated with their use.[3,4] Initiating a statin for primary prevention depends on the individual's global cardiovascular risk (Figure 2). For patients at high risk of coronary artery disease, statins should be initiated at the recommended starting doses and titrated to reach targets (Figure 1). However, different statins have different degrees of lipid-lowering potential [5] (Table 4). Atorvastatin is indicated for the reduction of stroke and heart attack in individuals with type 2 diabetes without evidence of heart disease but with other risk factors and also to reduce the risk of stroke in individuals without evidence of heart disease but with multiple risk factors other than diabetes.[6]

Effect on HDL is modest. Statins differ in their structure, pharmacokinetics, in vitro properties and efficacy; no dose-to-dose equivalence can be drawn among them. Increasing the dose may result in further decrease in LDL and global cardiovascular risk.[7] Statin- and patient-related factors influencing potential myotoxic effects must be considered to avoid this complication[8] (Table 5).

Table 5: **Patient- and Statin-related Factors That May Influence Myotoxic Effects**

Patient Characteristics	Concomitant Medications	Statin Properties
Advanced age (> 80 y) Women are more affected than men Frailty, small body frame Chronic renal insufficiency Hepatic dysfunction Untreated hypothyroidism Polypharmacy Perioperative periods Alcohol abuse Grapefruit juice intake	Fibrates (particularly gemfibrozil) Nicotinic acid (rarely) Cyclosporine Azole antifungals: (itraconazole, ketoconazole) Macrolide antibiotics (erythromycin, clarithromycin) HIV protease inhibitors Nondihydropyridine calcium channel blockers Amiodarone	High systemic exposure Lipophilicity High bioavailability Limited protein binding Potential for drug–drug interactions metabolized by cytochrome P450 pathways, especially 3A4 and 2C9 (Table 6)

Nicotinic Acid (Niacin)

Niacin is a B vitamin that, at high doses, lowers triglycerides and LDL and raises HDL more than any other lipid-lowering agent. It lowers lipoprotein(a), although the clinical significance of this effect is not yet known. The unpleasant side effects of niacin make patient compliance difficult, limiting its usefulness. Slow-release formulations appear to be more hepatotoxic than standard-release products.[4] A “no-flush” formulation combining inositol and niacin purports to reduce this adverse effect. A “once a day at night” dosage of an extended-release formulation of niacin recently marketed in Canada appears promising in terms of tolerability[9]. Further, it seems to have a lower rate of hepatotoxicity than other formulations. More clinical experience with these formulations are nevertheless required. Glucose intolerance is not an absolute contraindication to the use of niacin. Antihyperglycemic agents can be pre-emptively adjusted to maintain glycemic control.

Fibrates

Gemfibrozil, fenofibrate and **bezafibrate** lower triglyceride levels and raise HDL and may benefit patients with diabetic dyslipidemias. The effect of fibrates on LDL is variable; bezafibrate and fenofibrate lower LDL more consistently. Except for gemfibrozil, combining a fibrate with a statin can be safe. Fenofibrate was shown to significantly reduce total CVD events, particularly due to reductions in nonfatal MI and coronary revascularization, without reducing fatal events in patients with type 2 diabetes.[10]

Cholesterol Absorption Inhibitors

Ezetimibe, an intestinal cholesterol absorption inhibitor, is useful as monotherapy or in combination with statins. It is better tolerated than resins, has low potential for drug interactions with cytochrome P450 substrates and does not affect the absorption of fat-soluble vitamins.[11]

Combination Therapy

Agents from different classes can be combined to reach maximal efficacy with an acceptable level of safety, especially if a single drug fails to achieve targets. However, since some combination therapies (such as fibrates and statins) carry an increased risk of drug toxicity, consider referral for such patients.[12]

Therapeutic Tips

- Lipid-lowering drugs must always be an adjunct to, not a substitution for, diet therapy.
- Except for resins, avoid lipid-lowering drugs in children and pregnant or lactating women.
- Maintain therapy at the lowest dosage required to reach the target levels.
- Try different agents within the same class in cases of intolerance or insufficient efficacy.
- Long-term clinical and laboratory follow-up is essential to monitor lipid-lowering efficacy and safety of therapy.
- Allow three months for a stabilized and representative plasma lipid profile after a major medical event. Acute coronary syndromes require immediate statin therapy regardless of the lipid profile.
- Doubling the dose of a statin will further reduce the LDL-C level by only 6% (Figure 1, Figure 2).
- It appears safe to lower target LDL-C levels to 1.8 mmol/L (< 70 mg/dL) in individuals with overt coronary heart disease and multiple risk factors.

Figure 1: **Management of Dyslipidemia**[1]

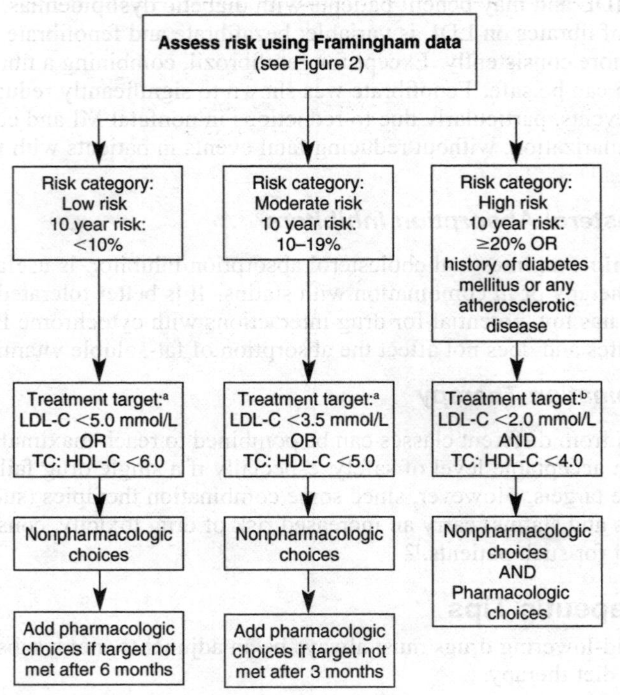

[a] In patients with low to moderate risk who are candidates for statin therapy, treatment to lower LDL-C by at least 40% is generally appropriate.

[b] In patients with established atherosclerosis, treatment to lower LDL-C by at least 50% is generally appropriate.

Abbreviations: HDL-C = high density lipoprotein cholesterol; LDL-C = low density lipoprotein cholesterol; TG = triglyceride

Figure 2: **Model for Estimating the 10-year Risk of Coronary Artery Disease in a Patient Without Diabetes Mellitus or Clinically Evident Cardiovascular Disease**[a]

MEN

Risk Factor	Risk Points
Age group, yr	
20–34	-9
35–39	-4
40–44	0
45–49	3
50–54	6
55–59	8
60–64	10
65–69	11
70–74	12
75–79	13

Total cholesterol Level, mmol/L	Age Group, yr 20–39	40–49	50–59	60–69	70–79
<4.14	0	0	0	0	0
4.15–5.19	4	3	2	1	0
5.20–6.19	7	5	3	1	0
6.20–7.20	9	6	4	2	1
≥7.21	11	8	5	3	1

Smoker	Age Group, yr 20–39	40–49	50–59	60–69	70–79
No	0	0	0	0	0
Yes	8	5	3	1	1

HDL-C Level, mmol/L	
≥1.55	-1
1.30–1.54	0
1.04–1.29	1
<1.04	2

Systolic Blood Pressure, mm Hg	Untreated	Treated
<120	0	0
120–129	0	1
130–139	1	2
140–159	1	2
≥160	2	3

Total Risk Points	10-year Risk, %
<0	<1
0–4	1
5–6	2
7	3
8	4
9	5
10	6
11	8
12	10
13	12
14	16
15	20
16	25
≥17	≥30

10-year Risk: ______ %

WOMEN

Risk Factor	Risk Points
Age group, yr	
20–34	-7
35–39	-3
40–44	0
45–49	3
50–54	6
55–59	8
60–64	10
65–69	12
70–74	14
75–79	16

Total cholesterol Level, mmol/L	Age Group, yr 20–39	40–49	50–59	60–69	70–79
<4.14	0	0	0	0	0
4.15–5.19	4	3	2	1	1
5.20–6.19	8	6	4	2	1
6.20–7.20	11	8	5	3	2
≥7.21	13	10	7	4	2

Smoker	Age Group, yr 20–39	40–49	50–59	60–69	70–79
No	0	0	0	0	0
Yes	9	7	4	2	1

HDL-C Level, mmol/L	
≥1.55	-1
1.30–1.54	0
1.04–1.29	1
<1.04	2

Systolic Blood Pressure, mm Hg	Untreated	Treated
<120	0	0
120–129	1	3
130–139	2	4
140–159	3	5
≥160	4	6

Total Risk Points	10-year Risk, %
<9	<1
9–12	1
13–14	2
15	3
16	4
17	5
18	6
19	8
20	11
21	14
22	17
23	22
24	27
≥25	≥30

10-year Risk: ______ %

[a] using Data from the Framingham Heart Study

Recommendations for the management of dyslipidemia and the prevention of cardiovascular disease: summary of the 2003 update

Reprinted from CMAJ 28-Oct-03; 169(9), Page(s) 921-924 by permission of the publisher © 2003 CMA Media Inc.

Table 6: Lipid-lowering Agents

Class	Drug	Dose	Adverse Effects	Drug Interactions	Comments	Cost[a]
Resins	*cholestyramine* generics	Adult: 4 g BID–TID AC Max: 24 g/day and 3 doses/day Children: 240 mg/kg/day divided in 3 doses	Common: Constipation (>10%), bloating, abdominal fullness, flatulence, ↑ triglycerides, ↑ transaminases (reversible). Rare: hyperchloremic acidosis, cholecystitis, cholelithiasis, pancreatitis, malabsorption syndrome, GI bleeding, peptic ulceration.	Administer 1 h before or 4–6 h after concurrent medications due to possible adsorption of other drugs in the GI tract.	Recommend high-fibre diet and high water intake to minimize constipation. Monitor serum electrolytes periodically. Long-term and high-dose use can prevent the absorption of fat-soluble vitamins and folic acid. Monitor liver function and triglycerides. May be mixed with juice, soups and applesauce. Can be used to lower cholesterol and LDL in pregnancy and in children. In general, can use in children ≥10 y. Add granules to at least 90 mL of fluid. Contraindications: biliary obstruction, dysbetalipoproteinemia, TG > 4.6 mmol/L; phenylketonurics.	$$$
	colestipol Colestid	Granules: 5 g BID–TID AC Max: 30 g/day Tablets: 2 g once daily–BID. Max: 16 g/day.	See cholestyramine.	See cholestyramine.	See cholestyramine.	$$$

Class	Drug	Dose	Adverse Effects	Drug Interactions	Comments	Cost[a]
Cholesterol Absorption Inhibitor	*ezetimibe* Ezetrol	10 mg once daily at any time	Well tolerated. Common: back pain, arthralgia, diarrhea, abdominal pain, fatigue, dizziness, headache. Rare: myopathy, rhabdomyolysis, hepatitis, acute pancreatitis, thrombocytopenia.	Low potential for drug interactions. Potential pharmacokinetic interaction with cyclosporine. Exercise caution when initiating ezetimibe in patients receiving cyclosporine, especially if severe renal insufficiency.	Monitor liver function and CK. In general, can use in children ≥ 12 y. Not recommended in moderate to severe hepatic impairment.	$$$
HMG CoA Reductase Inhibitors	*atorvastatin* Lipitor	10–80 mg at any time	Common: ↑ CPK, ↑ transaminases (reversible), mild upper GI disturbances, myalgias (with and without CPK elevation), sleep disturbances, headache, rash. Rare: myopathy, rhabdomyolysis, peripheral neuropathy, lupus-like symptoms, impotence.	Avoid with CYP3A4 inhibitors: macrolide antibiotics, gemfibrozil, grapefruit juice, azoles, protease inhibitors, amiodarone, cyclosporine, nondihydropyridine calcium channel blockers, e.g., verapamil.	Start with low doses and titrate up to reach targets while monitoring biochemical markers. Monitor liver function and CK at 3, 6 and 12 mo, then yearly. If LFTs (AST, ALT) > 3 × normal, discontinue statin. LFT elevations are dose dependent. Excellent safety profile. Use caution in patients with moderate to severe renal impairment (< 60 mL/min). Contraindications: active liver disease, high alcohol consumption, pregnancy.	$$–$$$

(cont'd)

Table 6: **Lipid-lowering Agents** *(cont'd)*

Class	Drug	Dose	Adverse Effects	Drug Interactions	Comments	Cost[a]
	fluvastatin Lescol	20–80 mg with evening meal	See atorvastatin.	Monitor INR with concomitant warfarin use. Avoid with CYP P450 2C9 inhibitors: amiodarone, fluconazole, fluoxetine, fluvoxamine.	See atorvastatin.	$$
	lovastatin Mevacor, generics	20–80 mg with evening meal; max. 40 mg BID	See atorvastatin.	See atorvastatin.	See atorvastatin.	$$–$$$$$
	pravastatin Pravachol, generics	10–40 mg QHS	See atorvastatin.	Not metabolized through CYP P450 pathway, thus low potential for drug interactions.	See atorvastatin.	$$–$$$
	rosuvastatin Crestor	10–40 mg at any time Initial dose 10 mg/day except in Asian patients and those receiving cyclosporine. (Initial dose 5 mg/day)	See atorvastatin.	See fluvastatin. ↓ levels with concomitant use of magnesium/aluminum hydroxide-containing antacids.	See atorvastatin. Administer antacids 2 h after rosuvastatin.	$$$
	simvastatin Zocor, generics	10–80 mg with evening meal	See atorvastatin.	See atorvastatin.	See atorvastatin.	$$

Class	Drug	Dose	Adverse Effects	Drug Interactions	Comments	Cost[a]
Niacin (Nicotinic Acid) derivatives	*niacin, immediate release* Niacin, generics	Start with 50 mg TID; double dose Q5 days to 1.5–2 g/day. If tolerated, maximum is 4 g/day after meals Usual dose: 1.5–4 g/day divided TID, PC Reassure and instruct the patient (see comments)	Common: hot flushes and pruritus, dry skin, acanthosis nigricans (reversible), reactivation of peptic ulcer, GI disturbances, ↑ blood glucose, glucose intolerance, uric acid and transaminases. Rare: torsades de pointes, severe hepatotoxicity (more frequent with slow-release formulation), ↑ blood glucose, uric acid, transaminases.	Use caution if using with statins because of potential hepatotoxicity and myopathy.	Greatest HDL-raising effect. Monitor blood glucose, uric acid, transaminases at 3, 6 and 12 months, then yearly. Contraindications: severe peptic ulcer disease, uncontrolled hyperglycemia, severe gout, hepatic disease. Flushing abates with time. Avoid hot drinks, hot showers, spicy food, alcohol for 1–2 h after a dose; uncoated ASA 325 mg daily in the first few weeks of treatment or when increasing the dose may be helpful. Tolerance develops within several weeks. Avoid missing a dose.	$$–$$$
	niacin, slow release (SR), generics	0.5–2 g/day divided BID after meals	Same as niacin immediate release, although less flushing. See niacin, immediate release. Severe hepatotoxicity more frequent with slow-release formulation, thus not recommended.	See niacin, immediate release.	Similar to niacin immediate release, although fewer measures required. See niacin, immediate release.	$$–$$$

(cont'd)

Table 6: Lipid-lowering Agents *(cont'd)*

Class	Drug	Dose	Adverse Effects	Drug Interactions	Comments	Cost[a]
	niacin, extended release (ER) Niaspan	Titrate the dose: 0.5 g HS after a low-fat snack × 1 month, 1 g HS for 1 mo, then 1.5 g HS. May ↑ to 2 g HS if required	Similar adverse effects to niacin immediate release, although less severe. See niacin, immediate release.	See niacin, immediate release.	Less flushing because taken at bedtime. Less hepatotoxic effects relative to SR formulations.	$$–$$$
Fibrates	*bezafibrate* Bezalip, generics	200 mg BID–TID SR: 400 mg/day with evening meal	Upper GI disturbances (nausea, abdominal pain, flatulence), myalgias ↑ bile lithogenicity, ↑ CK, ↑ creatinine (not representative of renal function deterioration).	Caution when combining with statins. Monitor INR with concomitant warfarin use. ↑ ezetimibe levels. Monitor for signs of cholelithiasis.	Monitor CK, liver and renal function at 3, 6 and 12 mo, then yearly. Useful in diabetic dyslipidemias. Contraindications: hepatic impairment, renal dysfunction, pre-existing gallbladder disease.	$$$
	fenofibrate generics	100 mg BID–QID with meals	See bezafibrate.	See bezafibrate. Monitor renal function with concomitant cyclosporine use.	See bezafibrate.	$$–$$$
	fenofibrate microcoated Lipidil Supra	160 mg/day, once daily with largest meal	See bezafibrate.	See bezafibrate. Monitor renal function with concomitant cyclosporine use.	See bezafibrate.	$$
	fenofibrate micronized Lipidil Micro, generics	200 mg/day, once daily with largest meal	See bezafibrate.	See bezafibrate. Monitor renal function with concomitant cyclosporine use.	See bezafibrate.	$$

Class	Drug	Dose	Adverse Effects	Drug Interactions	Comments	Cost[a]
	fenofibrate nanocrystals Lipidil EZ	145 mg/day, once daily with or without food Recommended starting dose for patients with renal impairment and in the elderly is 48 mg daily	See bezafibrate.	See bezafibrate. Monitor renal function with concomitant cyclosporine use.	See bezafibrate.	$$–$$$
	gemfibrozil Lopid, generics	300–1200 mg/day divided BID 30 min prior to meals	See bezafibrate.	Not to be used in combination with statins. May increase repaglinide and rosiglitazone levels; metabolized by CYP2C8. Monitor INR with concomitant warfarin use.	See bezafibrate.	$–$$
Combination products	*niacin, extended release / lovastatin* Advicor	Dose is individualized. 500 mg/20 mg or 1000 mg/20 mg: 1 tab HS with low-fat snack	Niacin: Similar adverse effects to niacin immediate release, although less severe. See niacin, immediate release Lovastatin:See atorvastatin	Niacin:See niacin, immediate release Lovastatin:See atorvastatin	Not recommended as initial therapy. May switch to combination therapy when on stable doses of lovastatin and niacin, extended release. See niacin, extended release See atorvastatin	$$–$$$

[a] Cost of 30-day supply; includes drug cost only.
Dosage adjustment may be required in renal impairment; see Appendix I.
Legend: $ < $20 $-$$ < $20–40 $$ $20–40 $$-$$$ $20–60 $$$ $40–80 $$$$ $60–80 $$-$$$$$ $20– > 80 $$$$$ > $80

Suggested Readings

Armitage J. The safety of statins in clinical practice. *Lancet* 2007 Jun 6; [Epub ahead of print].

Gotto AM, Pownall HJ. *Manual of lipid disorders: reducing the risk for coronary heart disease.* 3rd ed. Philadelphia (PA): Lippincott Williams & Wilkins; 2003.

Grundy SM, Cleeman JI, Merz CN et al. Implications of recent clinical trials for the National Cholesterol Education Program Adult Treatment Panel III guidelines. *Circulation* 2004;110(2):227-39.

Jialal I. A practical approach to the laboratory diagnosis of dyslipidemia. *Am J Clin Pathol* 1996;106(1):128-38.

LaRosa JC, Gotto AM. Past, present, and future standards for management of dyslipidemia. *Am J Med* 2004;116(Suppl 6A):3S-8S.

References

1. McPherson R, Frolich J, Fodor G et al. Canadian Cardiovascular Society position statement--recommendations for the diagnosis and treatment of dyslipidemia and prevention of cardiovascular disease. *Can J Cardiol* 2006;22(11):913-27.
2. Ford ES. The metabolic syndrome and mortality from cardiovascular disease and all-causes: findings from the National Health and Nutrition Examination Survey II Mortality Study. *Atherosclerosis* 2004;173(2):309-14.
3. Evans M, Roberts A, Davies S, Rees A. Medical lipid-regulating therapy: current evidence, ongoing trials and future developments. *Drugs* 2004;64(11):1181-96.
4. Vrecer M, Turk S, Drinovec J, Mrhar A. Use of statins in primary and secondary prevention of coronary heart disease and ischemic stroke. Meta-analysis of randomized trials. *Int J Clin Pharmacol Ther* 2003;41(12):567-77.
5. Grundy SM, Cleeman JI, Merz CN et al. Implications of recent clinical trials for the National Cholesterol Education Program Adult Treatment Panel III guidelines. *Circulation* 2004;110(2):227-39.
6. Colhoun HM, Betteridge DJ, Durrington PN et al. Primary prevention of cardiovascular disease with atorvastatin in type 2 diabetes in the Collaborative Atorvastatin Diabetes Study (CARDS): multicentre randomized placebo-controlled trial. *Lancet* 2004;364(9435):685-96.
7. LaRosa JC, Grundy SM, Waters DD et al. Intensive lipid lowering with atorvastatin in patients with stable coronary disease. *N Engl J Med* 2005;352(14):1425-35.
8. Rosenson RS. Current overview of statin-induced myopathy. *Am J Med* 2004;116(6):408-16.
9. Carlson LA. Niaspan, the prolonged release preparation of nicotinic acid (niacin), the broad-spectrum lipid drug. *Int J Clin Pract* 2004;58(7):706-13.
10. Keech A, Simes RJ, Barter P et al. Effects of long-term fenofibrate therapy on cardiovascular events in 9795 people with type 2 diabetes mellitus (the FIELD study): randomised controlled trial. *Lancet* 2005;366(9500):1849-61.
11. Jialal I, Kappagoda T. Therapy and clinical trials: ezetimibe.*Curr Opin Lipidol* 2003 Dec;14(6):643-6.
12. Thompson PD, Clarkson P, Karas RH. Statin-associated myopathy. *JAMA* 2003;289(13):1681-90.

Pharmacoeconomic Considerations: Dyslipidemias

Blair Jarvis, MSc, BSP

Epidemiology	
Country (Year)	**Prevalence**
Canada (2006[a])[1]	~2.3 million adults aged 40–74 years require lipid treatment based on 2003 guidelines

(cont'd)

Cost of Illness Data		
Type of Costs and Year	**Direct Costs[b]**	**Indirect Costs[c]**
Canada (1998)[2]	Cardiovascular disease: $6.8 billion	Cardiovascular disease: $11.7 billion
Canada (2004)[1]	Expenditures on lipid lowering drugs: $1.39 billion	Not applicable

Commentary

Lowering low-density lipoprotein (LDL) cholesterol levels with statins reduces overall mortality and the rate of MI, stroke and revascularization in patients at risk. The benefits are not dependent on the baseline LDL cholesterol level and are in proportion to the extent of the reduction achieved.[3] This suggests that any reduction in LDL levels is beneficial in patients at increased risk. Lipid-lowering trials have generally enrolled approximately 75% to 85% male participants; therefore, the evidence of benefit in women is less convincing than in men, particularly in the setting of primary prevention.

The 2006 Canadian Cardiovascular Society guidelines recommend estimating a patient's risk of cardiovascular events, which is then used to determine the target LDL level.[4] In patients at low to intermediate 10-year risk of a cardiovascular event, reduction of LDL levels by at least 40% is considered appropriate rather than treating to an exclusive fixed target. High-risk patients (10-year risk ≥ 20%) should be treated with the goal of achieving an LDL level of < 2.0 mmol/L. Most patients can achieve these targets with statin monotherapy, but a significant minority will require combination regimens. However, data are lacking as to the impact on clinical outcomes and the cost-effectiveness of combination regimens.[4]

Most available cost-effectiveness analyses have been based on data from early intervention trials and do not reflect all currently available therapies or current treatment targets. Newer, more potent statins may be required to achieve target lipid levels in some patients, although older, generic statins remain useful, particularly for those with financial constraints.

The Heart Protection Study showed that achievement of a mean reduction in LDL of 1 mmol/L produced significant reductions in mortality over five years in moderate to high risk patients, 75% of whom were men.[5] A lifetime cost-effectiveness analysis based on this study concluded that treatment with a generic statin (simvastatin 40 mg/day) would produce gains in life expectancy for patients aged between 35 and 85 years, and that treatment would be cost saving

(cont'd)

Commentary

or would cost < £2500 per-life-year-gained in those with a five-year cardiovascular risk > 5%.[6]

On the basis of Canadian data it has been estimated that 20-person-years of dyslipidemia treatment will result in one year of life saved.[1] This estimate assumes that patients will achieve target lipid levels, which is not always the case in the "real world." In fact, it has been reported that patients with the lowest risk are more likely to receive treatment than those with the highest risk.[7] The causes of this "treatment-risk paradox" are complex. A large prospective study in Alberta found that high-risk patients were more likely than low-risk patients to be taking a statin one month after an angiogram. The key driver of this phenomenon was reduced functional status and an increased burden of depressive symptoms in the high-risk patients. These findings suggest that, in addition to calculating baseline cardiovascular risk to identify patients who will benefit from treatment, primary caregivers must identify and address barriers to adherence if the full benefit of lipid-lowering therapy is to be realized.

[a] Extrapolated from Canadian Heart Health Survey data collected between 1986 and 1992.

[b] Direct costs include those associated with physician services, nursing care, diagnostic procedures, drugs and hospitalization.

[c] Indirect costs include those associated with lost productivity and days off work due to morbidity or premature mortality.

References

1. Grover SA, Coupal L, Kaouache et al. Preventing cardiovascular disease among Canadians: What are the potential benefits of treating hypertension or dyslipidemia? *Can J Cardiol* 2007;23(6):467–473.
2. Health Canada. Economic burden of illness in Canada, 1998. Health Canada Publications, 2002. Available at www.phac-aspc.gc.ca/publicat/ebic-femc98/pdf/ebic1998.pdf
3. Baigent C, Keech A, Kearney PM et al. Efficacy and safety of cholesterol-lowering treatment: prospective meta-analysis of data from 90,056 participants in 14 randomised trials of statins. *Lancet* 2005;366(9493):1267-78.
4. McPherson R, Frohlich J, Fodor G et al. Canadian Cardiovascular Society position statement—recommendations for the diagnosis and treatment of dyslipidemia and prevention of cardiovascular disease. *Can J Cardiol* 2006;22(11):913-27.
5. Heart Protection Study Collaborative Group. MRC/BHF Heart Protection Study of cholesterol lowering with simvastatin in 20,536 high-risk individuals: a randomised placebo-controlled trial. *Lancet* 2002;360(9326):7-22.
6. Heart Protection Study Collaborative; Mihaylova B, Briggs A et al. Lifetime cost effectiveness of simvastatin in a range of risk groups and age groups derived from a randomised trial of 20,536 people. *BMJ* 2006;333(7579):1145.
7. McAlister FA, Oreopoulos A, Norris CM et al. Exploring the treatment-risk paradox in coronary disease. *Arch Intern Med* 2007;167(10):1019-25.

CHAPTER 32
Hypertension

Norm R.C. Campbell, MD, FRCPC

Goals of Therapy

- Reduce the risk of cardiac, cerebrovascular and renal morbidity and mortality
- Targets for blood pressure control in treated patients are shown in Table 1

Table 1: **Blood Pressure Targets in Treated Patients**[1]

In general	< 140/90 mm Hg
Isolated systolic hypertension	SBP < 140 mm Hg
Diabetes mellitus	< 130/80 mm Hg
Chronic kidney disease	< 130/80 mm Hg

Reproduced with permission from Canadian Hypertension Education Program. 2007 Hypertension Recommendations, available from http://www.hypertension.ca.
Abbreviations: SBP = systolic blood pressure

Investigations

- History:
  - duration of hypertension, usual level of blood pressure and any sudden change in severity of hypertension
  - history of antihypertensive drug use, reason for changing therapy, effectiveness, side effects and intolerance
  - drugs that may cause hypertension (Table 2)
  - family history of hypertension, cardiovascular risk factors and premature cardiovascular disease
  - personal history of cigarette and alcohol use, usual physical activity, usual diet, current weight and recent weight change, diabetes and dyslipidemia
  - cerebrovascular, cardiac and peripheral vascular symptoms to assess for target organ damage
  - symptoms of secondary hypertension, which include, for example, pheochromocytoma (hyperadrenergic symptoms), hyper- and hypothyroidism, Cushing's syndrome, renal/urinary symptoms or a past history of renal disease

Table 2: **Drugs and Other Exogenous Factors That Can Induce or Aggravate Hypertension**

Drugs	NSAIDs including coxibs
	Corticosteroids and anabolic steroids
	Oral contraceptive and sex hormones
	Vasoconstricting, sympathomimetic decongestants
	Calcineurin inhibitors, e.g., cyclosporine, tacrolimus
	Erythropoietin and analogues
	Monoamine oxidase inhibitors
	Midodrine
Other factors	Licorice root
	Stimulants, including cocaine
	Salt
	Excessive alcohol use
	Sleep apnea

Reproduced with permission from Canadian Hypertension Education Program. 2006 Hypertension Recommendations, available from http://www.hypertension.ca.

- Diagnosis:[1]
  - the diagnosis of hypertension is immediate in the case of hypertensive emergencies and urgencies. This includes patients with hypertension that is compromising vital organ function (encephalopathy, cardiac, or rapidly decreasing renal function), hypertension and a major artery dissection, or those with DBP ≥ 130 mm Hg
  - hypertension may be diagnosed in two office visits if the blood pressure is ≥ 180/110, or ≥ 140/90 mm Hg in the presence of diabetes, renal disease, atherosclerotic cardiovascular disease or cerebrovascular disease
  - the diagnosis may be arrived at after two visits if self–blood pressure measurement or ambulatory blood pressure measurement is used
  - the diagnosis may require three visits if the blood pressure is ≥ 160/100 mm Hg. However, up to five visits may be required to establish the diagnosis if the initial blood pressure is < 160/100 mm Hg and there is no target organ dysfunction. Attention to the details of measuring blood pressure is essential to making a correct diagnosis[1]
- Physical exam:
  - fundi for hypertensive retinopathy
  - bruits and peripheral pulses for vascular disease and renovascular hypertension

- edema and lung fields for signs of heart failure
- heart sounds and apex for left ventricular hypertrophy
- abdominal mass for polycystic kidneys and aortic aneurysm
- neurologic exam for cerebrovascular disease

- Initial laboratory testing:
  - serum potassium, sodium and creatinine
  - urinalysis
  - fasting glucose, total cholesterol, HDL-C, LDL-C, triglycerides
  - standard 12-lead ECG
  - select patients should have additional testing (Table 3)

Table 3: **Hypertensive Patients Requiring Additional Laboratory Testing[1]**

If these characteristics are present:			
Two or more of: • Sudden onset or worsening of hypertension in patients aged > 55 or < 30 y • Abdominal bruit • Uncontrolled hypertension despite use of ≥ 3 drugs • Decreased renal function associated with use of an ACE inhibitor or ARB • Overt atherosclerotic vascular disease • Recurrent episodes of hypertension and flash pulmonary edema	• Paroxysmal and/or severe sustained hypertension refractory to usual antihypertensive therapy • Hypertension and symptoms suggestive of catecholamine excess (two or more of headaches, palpitations, sweating, etc.) • Hypertension triggered by beta-blockers, monoamine oxidase inhibitors, micturition, or changes in abdominal pressure • Incidentally discovered adrenal adenoma • MEN 2A or 2B; von Recklinghausen's neurofibromatosis, or von Hippel-Lindau disease	• Spontaneous hypokalemia • Profound diuretic-induced hypokalemia (K^+ < 3.0 mmol/L) • Hypertension refractory to treatment with ≥ 3 drugs • Incidental adrenal adenoma	High SCr (high normal in the elderly)
Check for:			
Renovascular disease	Pheochromocytoma	Hyperaldosteronism	Renal disease

Abbreviations: ARB = angiotensin receptor blocker; MEN = multiple endocrine neoplasia

Therapeutic Choices

Nonpharmacologic Choices

All individuals should be advised about a healthy lifestyle to prevent or control hypertension and cardiovascular disease (Table 4).

- Weight loss of 4 kg or more if overweight (target body mass index: 18.5 to 24.9 kg/m²; waist circumference <102 cm in men and < 88 cm in women).
- Healthy diet (high in fresh fruits, vegetables, soluble fibre and low-fat dairy products; low in saturated fats and salt).
- Regular, moderate intensity cardiorespiratory physical activity for 30–60 minutes on most days.
- Low risk alcohol consumption (0 to 2 drinks/day, < 9 drinks/week for women and < 14 drinks/week for men).
- Smoke-free environment.

Table 4: **Effect of Lifestyle Changes on Blood Pressure in Adults with Hypertension**

Intervention	Target	Change in BP (systolic/diastolic) mm Hg
Sodium reduction	100 mmol/day	−5.8/−2.5
Weight loss	4.5 kg	−7.2/−5.9
Alcohol reduction	2.7 drinks/day	−4.6/−2.3
Exercise	3 times/week	−10.3/−7.5
Dietary recommendations	DASH diet	−11.4/−5.5

Reproduced with permission from Campbell N. Canadian Hypertension Education Program: brief overview of 2004 recommendations. *Can Fam Physician* 2004;50:1411-2.

Pharmacologic Choices[1] (Table 6)

If the average SBP/DBP is 140–159/90–99 mm Hg, treatment is recommended in the presence of either:

- hypertensive target organ damage or
- other independent risk factors for cardiovascular disease, e.g., cigarette smoking, dyslipidemia, strong family history of premature cardiovascular disease, truncal obesity, sedentary lifestyle, males older than 55 years, females older than 60 years. It is unusual to have hypertension in the absence of other cardiovascular risk factors.[2]

If the average SBP/DBP is 140–159/90–99 mm Hg and the individual does not have additional risk factors, the short-term benefits of pharmacotherapy are small; discuss the risks and benefits of therapy with the patient. Monitor blood pressure and other risk factors regardless of whether such a patient chooses to begin drug therapy.

Consider **ASA** in patients over age 50 once blood pressure is controlled. Consider **lipid-lowering therapy** in patients with three cardiovascular risk factors in addition to hypertension.

In general, the reduction in cardiovascular risk depends more on the extent of the reduction in blood pressure than on the specific blood pressure medication. Pharmacologic therapy should usually be started with a low dose of the initial drug. Consider concurrent risk factors and disease states when selecting initial therapy (Table 5). Dose titration to achieve goal blood pressure should be done every four to eight weeks for all but those with severe hypertension or target organ damage or high cardiovascular risk, for whom closer follow-up and more frequent dosage titration is required.

Diuretics

Diuretics are first-line therapy for uncomplicated hypertension. They are inexpensive and well tolerated, and extensive data support their efficacy. Therefore, low-dose thiazide or related diuretics (e.g., indapamide) should generally be selected first, unless there are specific indications for other drugs. Diuretics have proven antihypertensive effectiveness in patients with isolated systolic hypertension, the elderly and black patients.

Diuretics can cause hypokalemia that may be associated with adverse cardiovascular outcomes. Consider alternative first-line agents in those with or strongly predisposed to a serious arrhythmia, for example, prolonged QT syndrome. Consider using a combination product to minimize the risk of hypokalemia (i.e., hydrochlorothiazide plus a potassium-sparing diuretic—spironolactone, amiloride or triamterene). Reserve the use of high doses (e.g., > 25 mg/day of hydrochlorothiazide) for patients with resistant hypertension unresponsive to treatment with multiple drugs or secondary to renal impairment. Consider using a loop diuretic in patients with renal impairment. Diuretics can also cause diabetes, although cardiovascular outcomes in patients with diabetes who are treated with diuretics are similar to those treated with ACE inhibitors.[3]

Beta-blockers

Beta-blockers are first-line therapy in patients who are younger than 60 years of age, or who have stable angina, heart failure or a history of myocardial infarction. Beta-blockers are also useful in patients who have migraine headaches, tachycardia or essential tremor. However, beta-blockers are not as effective as angiotensin II receptor blockers (ARBs), calcium channel blockers (CCBs) or diuretics as initial therapy for primary prevention of cardiovascular events in patients over the age of 60 years. In addition, they may be ineffective in preventing cardiovascular events in people who smoke.[4]

Angiotensin Converting Enzyme Inhibitors

Angiotensin converting enzyme (ACE) inhibitors are first-line agents for patients with uncomplicated hypertension and for patients with diabetes, recent myocardial infarction, heart failure or chronic kidney disease. ACE inhibitors are contraindicated in women of child-bearing potential.[5,6]

Angiotensin II Receptor Blockers

ARBs are first-line agents for patients with uncomplicated hypertension and for patients with diabetes. They are good alternatives to ACE inhibitors when the latter are specifically indicated but not tolerated. ARBs are contraindicated in women of child-bearing potential.[7]

Long-acting Calcium Channel Blockers

Long-acting dihydropyridine CCBs can be used as first-line agents but are generally used in combination therapy. *Short-acting formulations may produce harm and should not be used.* Elderly patients with isolated systolic hypertension and black patients are particularly responsive to CCBs.

Other Antihypertensive Drugs

In general, other classes of antihypertensive drugs should not be prescribed unless there are specific indications (Table 5), contraindications or intolerance to first-line therapy, or a requirement for additional blood pressure lowering in combination with first-line antihypertensive drugs.

Combination Therapy

About 50% of patients will require more than one antihypertensive agent to achieve goal blood pressure. If goal blood pressure is not achieved with moderate doses of a suitable first-line drug, add, rather than substitute, a second drug. Any combination of a beta-blocker, ACE inhibitor and/or an ARB has less than additive antihypertensive effects in a two drug regimen. These combinations should be avoided unless there is a specific indication, for example, use of an ACE inhibitor and a beta-blocker post-myocardial infarction (Table 5). All possible combinations of first-line agents are rational choices to lower blood pressure when three or four drugs are required, with the possible exception of the simultaneous prescription of ACE inhibitors and ARBs. (However, there is some evidence that this combination may be beneficial in patients with renal dysfunction.)[8,9] Use of a diuretic is desirable in combination with all other drug classes.

Adherence

Adherence should be assessed at each visit. Lack of adherence to therapy is a major cause of poor blood pressure control and is indicated by:

- Admitting nonadherence when questioned in a nonthreatening manner
- Failure to keep scheduled appointments
- Poor blood pressure control
- Lack of secondary physiologic effects, e.g., decreased heart rate on beta-blocker
- Failure to renew prescriptions on time
- Lack of awareness of usual pill-taking routine and prescriptions

Nonadherence can be prevented. Routine care should include the following:

- Ensure patients are well informed about hypertension and its treatment, preferably verbally and with patient information pamphlets (available at www.hypertension.ca in the public education section)
- Include family or social support in lifestyle modification
- Use a simplified regimen of long-acting, once-daily drugs, and use tablets that contain two drugs in combination when appropriate
- Ensure the patient can afford the prescribed drugs
- Advise the patient to establish a daily routine for pill-taking, e.g., putting their pills by their toothbrush and taking them every morning prior to brushing

Treat nonadherence:

- Determine the reason for nonadherence and tailor advice or interventions to the cause
- Increase the frequency of office visits
- Advise use of adherence-enhancing medication dispensers, i.e., dosettes
- Advise self-measurement of blood pressure
- Consider assessing adherence with an electronic pill dispenser
- Advise self-monitoring of adherence with pill counts and marking on a calendar when the prescription needs renewing
- Consider regular telephone contact with the patient if feasible

Resistant Hypertension

Many patients with hypertension require multiple drugs for blood pressure control. In those with resistant hypertension, investigate for a white coat effect, secondary hypertension, renal dysfunction, nonadherence, and in those with a poor response to an adequate combination of medications, consider the possibility of an "interfering lifestyle." Refer those who do not achieve blood pressure targets with medication regimens you feel comfortable prescribing.

Hypertensive Emergencies

It is uncommon for elevated blood pressure alone, without new or progressive target organ damage, to require emergency therapy. Refer true hypertensive emergencies to experienced centres with facilities to continuously monitor blood pressure. In stabilizing patients for transfer, the use of intermediate-acting drugs with close blood pressure monitoring is generally safer than using short-acting drugs that can rapidly produce hypotension with complications.

Therapeutic Tips

- Prescribe a lower starting dose of antihypertensive drugs in elderly patients.

- Recent onset of hypertension or change in blood pressure control suggests an identifiable or secondary cause, such as drugs known to exacerbate hypertension or new onset of significant renal artery stenosis.
- Many drugs ineffective as monotherapy for hypertension are effective components in a rational combination regimen.
- Consider concurrent risk factors and disease states when prescribing therapy (Table 5)
- Cardiovascular risk can vary 10-fold in persons with the same blood pressure. Assess global cardiovascular risk in all hypertensive patients using a risk form, chart or computer program (see back cover).

Table 5: **Individualization of Antihypertensive Therapy**[1]

Risk Factor/Disease	Initial Therapy	Second-line Therapy	Notes/Cautions
Hypertension Without Other Compelling Indications			
Diastolic +/- systolic hypertension	Thiazide diuretic, beta-blocker, ACE inhibitor, ARB or long-acting CCB. Consider ASA and statins in select patients.	Combinations of first-line drugs	Beta-blockers are not recommended as initial therapy in patients over 60 years of age. Avoid hypokalemia in those who are prescribed diuretics by using K^+-sparing agents. ACE inhibitors are not recommended as initial therapy in black patients. ACE inhibitors and ARBs are teratogenic. Marked caution is required if prescribing to women of child-bearing potential.
Isolated systolic hypertension without other compelling indications	Thiazide diuretic, ARB or long-acting dihydropyridine CCB.	Combinations of first-line drugs	See diastolic +/- systolic hypertension above.
Diabetes Mellitus			
Diabetes mellitus with nephropathy	ACE inhibitor or ARB	Add a thiazide diuretic, cardioselective beta-blocker, long-acting CCB or use an ARB/ACE inhibitor combination	If the SCr is >150 µmol/L, use a loop diuretic rather than a low-dose thiazide if volume control is required.
Diabetes mellitus without nephropathy	ACE inhibitor, ARB, long-acting dihydropyridine CCB or thiazide diuretic	Combine first-line drugs. If first line agents are not tolerated add a cardioselective beta-blocker and/or a long-acting nondihydropyridine CCB	Nephropathy is defined as an albumin to creatinine ratio (ACR) < 2.0 mg/mmol in men and < 2.8 mg/mmol in women.

(cont'd)

Table 5: **Individualization of Antihypertensive Therapy[1]** *(cont'd)*

Risk Factor/Disease	Initial Therapy	Second-line Therapy	Notes/Cautions
Cardiovascular and Cerebrovascular Disease			
Angina	Beta-blocker and ACE inhibitor except in low risk revascularized patients	Long-acting CCB	Avoid short-acting nifedipine
Heart failure	ACE inhibitor, ARB or hydralazine/isosorbide dinitrate (ARBs if ACEI-intolerant), beta-blockers and spironolactone	Thiazide or loop diuretic as additive therapy Long-acting dihydropyridine CCB	Avoid nondihydropyridine CCB (diltiazem, verapamil). Monitor serum K^+ and SCr if combining an ACE inhibitor and ARB.
Left ventricular hypertrophy	ACE inhibitor, ARB, long acting dihydropyridine CCB, diuretic Beta-blocker for patients < 55 years	Combinations of first-line drugs	Avoid hydralazine and minoxidil.
Past cerebrovascular accident or TIA	ACE inhibitor/diuretic combination		Does not apply to patients with acute stroke. Blood pressure reduction reduces recurrent cerebrovascular events in patients with stable past cerebrovascular disease.
Nondiabetic Chronic Kidney Disease			
Nondiabetic chronic kidney disease with proteinuria	ACE inhibitor (ARB if not tolerated) diuretics as additive therapy	Combinations of additional agents	Avoid ACE inhibitors or ARBs in patients with bilateral renal artery stenosis or unilateral disease with solitary kidney. Carefully monitor serum K^+ and SCr in patients on an ACE inhibitor or an ARB.
Renovascular disease	Treat similar to diastolic +/- systolic hypertension without compelling indications for other medications	Combinations of first-line drugs	Avoid ACE inhibitors or ARBs in patients with bilateral renal artery stenosis or unilateral disease with solitary kidney.

Risk Factor/Disease	Initial Therapy	Second-line Therapy	Notes/Cautions
Other Conditions			
Peripheral arterial disease	Does not affect initial treatment recommendations	Does not affect initial treatment recommendations	Avoid beta-blockers in patients with severe disease
Dyslipidemia	Does not affect initial treatment recommendations	Does not affect initial treatment recommendations	
Global vascular protection	Statin therapy for patients with 3 or more cardiovascular risk factors or with atherosclerotic disease		
	Low-dose ASA in patients with controlled blood pressure		Exercise caution if blood pressure is not controlled.

Adapted with permission from Canadian Hypertension Education Program. 2007 Hypertension Recommendations, available from http://www.hypertension.ca.

Abbreviations: ACE = angiotensin converting enzyme; ARB = angiotensin II receptor blocker; CCB = calcium channel blocker; SCr = serum creatinine; TIA = transient ischemic attack

Table 6: **Drugs for Hypertension**

Class	Drug	Dose	Adverse Effects	Drug Interactions	Comments	Cost[a]
Diuretics[b]	*hydrochlorothiazide (HCTZ)* generics	Initial: 12.5 mg/day Usual: 25 mg/day Once daily	Hypotension, weakness, muscle cramps, impotence. Hypokalemia, hyponatremia, hyperuricemia, hyperglycemia, hyperlipidemia. Rare: azotemia, blood dyscrasias, allergic reactions (potential cross sensitivity with other sulfonamide derivatives), photosensitivity, fatigue.	↓ Li^+ excretion (monitor Li^+ levels, adjust dose). NSAIDs ↓ hypotensive efficacy. Diuretic-induced hypokalemia ↑ the risk of digoxin toxicity. ↓ efficacy of antihyperglycemic agents.	Particularly effective in ISH, the elderly and black patients. Monitor SCr and K^+. Consider alternatives in patients with or predisposed to arrhythmias. Can exacerbate gout and diabetes (biochemical abnormalities are less frequent at 12.5–25 mg/day). Ineffective in patients with ClCr < 30 to 40 mL/min.	$
	indapamide Lozide, generics	Initial: 1.25 mg/day Usual: 2.5 mg/day Once daily	See HCTZ.	See HCTZ.	See HCTZ.	$
	metolazone Zaroxolyn	Initial: 2.5 mg/day Usual: 5 mg/day Max: 10 mg/day Once daily	See HCTZ.	See HCTZ.	See HCTZ. Metolazone is effective in patients with moderate to severe renal dysfunction.	$
Diuretic Combinations	*HCTZ/amiloride (50/5)* Moduret, generics	½ tab/day Once daily	See HCTZ.	See HCTZ. May exacerbate ACE inhibitor–induced hyperkalemia.	See HCTZ. Lower incidence of hypokalemia than with HCTZ alone.	$

Class	Drug	Dose	Adverse Effects	Drug Interactions	Comments	Cost[a]
	HCTZ/triamterene (25/50) generics	Initial: ½ tab/day Usual: 1 tab/day Once daily	See HCTZ.	See HCTZ/amiloride.	See HCTZ/amiloride.	$
	HCTZ/spironolactone (25/25) Aldactazide, generics	Initial: ½ tab/day Usual: 1 tab/day Once daily	See HCTZ. Gynecomastia in men and breast tenderness in women.	See HCTZ/amiloride.	See HCTZ/amiloride.	$
Beta$_1$-adrenergic Antagonists, nonselective	*nadolol* generics	Initial: 20 mg/day Usual: 160 mg/day Max: 320 mg/day Once daily	Fatigue, bradycardia, decreased exercise capacity, headache, impotence, vivid dreams. Less common: hyperglycemia, depression, heart failure, heart block.	Bradycardia with digoxin or nondihydropyridine CCBs. Cardiodepressant effects with nondihydropyridine CCBs and amiodarone.	Beta-blockers should not be used as initial therapy in patients aged > 60 y. Avoid in patients with asthma.[10] Avoid abrupt withdrawal (may precipitate ischemia). Taper the dose before discontinuation. Avoid in patients with severe peripheral arterial disease (PAD). Contraindicated in patients with 2nd or 3rd degree heart block in the absence of a pacemaker.	$
	propranolol, controlled release Inderal-LA, generics	Initial: 80 mg/day Usual: 320 mg/day Max: 480 mg/day SR (once-daily) formulations are recommended	See nadolol.	See nadolol. CYP2D6 inhibitors ↑ levels of propranolol and metoprolol. Propranolol ↑ serum levels of rizatriptan.	See nadolol. Propranolol is more likely to cause CNS side effects (insomnia, depression, vivid dreams) than other agents because of greater lipid solubility.	$$$

(cont'd)

Table 6: **Drugs for Hypertension** *(cont'd)*

Class	Drug	Dose	Adverse Effects	Drug Interactions	Comments	Cost[a]
	timolol generics	Initial: 5 mg BID Usual: 20 mg BID Max: 30 mg BID	See nadolol.	See nadolol.	See nadolol.	$$
Beta$_1$-adrenergic Antagonists, β_1-selective	*atenolol* Tenormin, generics	Initial: 25 mg/day Usual: 50 mg/day Max: 100 mg/day Once daily or BID	See nadolol.	See nadolol.	See nadolol.	$
	bisoprolol Monocor , generics	Initial: 2.5 mg/day Max: 20 mg/day Once daily	See nadolol.	See nadolol.	See nadolol. See atenolol.	$
	metoprolol Betaloc, Lopresor, generics	Initial: 50 mg/day Usual: 100–200 mg/day Max: 400 mg/day Give regular formulations BID; SR formulations once daily	See nadolol.	See nadolol. CYP2D6 inhibitors increase levels of propranolol and metoprolol.	See nadolol. See atenolol.	$
Beta$_1$-adrenergic Antagonists, nonselective with ISA	*oxprenolol* Trasicor	Initial: 60–80 mg/day Usual: 120–320 mg/day Max: 480 mg/day Give regular formulation BID or TID; SR formulations once daily	See nadolol.	See nadolol.	See nadolol. Agents with ISA have less effect on resting heart rate than those without ISA.	$$$

Class	Drug	Dose	Adverse Effects	Drug Interactions	Comments	Cost[a]
	pindolol Visken, generics	Initial: 5 mg BID Usual: 15 mg BID Max: 60 mg/day	See nadolol.	See nadolol.	See nadolol. See oxprenolol.	$$
$Beta_1$-adrenergic Antagonists, β_1-selective with ISA	*acebutolol* Rhotral, Sectral, generics	Initial: 100 mg/day Usual: 400 mg/day Max: 800 mg/day Once daily or BID	See nadolol.	See nadolol.	See nadolol. Agents with ISA have less effect on resting heart rate than those without ISA.	$
$Beta_1$-adrenergic Antagonists with $alpha_1$-blocking activity	*labetalol* Trandate, generics	Initial: 100 mg/day BID Usual: 200 mg BID Max: 1200 mg/day	See nadolol. Edema, dizziness, and nasal congestion and postural hypotension due to $alpha_1$ antagonism.	See nadolol.	See nadolol.	$
ACE Inhibitors	*benazepril* Lotensin	Initial: 10 mg/day Usual: 20 mg/day Max: 40 mg/day Once daily or BID	Dry cough, hyperkalemia. Unusual: angioedema. Can precipitate renal failure in renovascular disease, volume depletion or those receiving NSAIDs.	Marked ↑ in serum K^+ in patients receiving K^+ supplements and/or K^+-sparing diuretics. ↓ hypotensive effect with NSAIDs and ↑ risk of renal dysfunction. Elevated Li^+ levels (potential toxicity).	**Contraindicated in pregnancy—caution when prescribing to women of child-bearing potential.**[5,6] Use lower (50%) initial doses if on diuretics (↑ risk of hypotension with hypovolemia). Hyperkalemia usually occurs only in those on K^+ supplements or drugs that cause K^+ retention, those with renal impairment or diabetics with high serum K^+ levels. Assess	$$

(cont'd)

Table 6: **Drugs for Hypertension** *(cont'd)*

Class	Drug	Dose	Adverse Effects	Drug Interactions	Comments	Cost[a]
					SCr and K^+ after a few days, then regularly.	
	captopril Capoten, generics	Initial: 25 mg/day Usual: 75 mg/day Max: 150 mg/day Divide BID or TID	See benazepril.	See benazepril.	See benazepril.	$$
	cilazapril Inhibace, generics	Initial: 2.5 mg/day Usual: 2.5–5 mg/day Max: 10 mg/day Once daily or BID	See benazepril.	See benazepril.	See benazepril.	$$
	enalapril Vasotec	Initial: 5 mg/day Usual: 10–40 mg/day Max: 40 mg/day Once daily or BID	See benazepril.	See benazepril.	See benazepril.	$$
	fosinopril Monopril, generics	Initial: 10 mg/day Usual: 20 mg/day Max: 40 mg/day Once daily or BID	See benazepril.	See benazepril.	See benazepril.	$$
	lisinopril Prinivil, Zestril, generics	Initial: 10 mg/day Usual: 20 mg/day Max: 40 mg/day Once daily	See benazepril.	See benazepril.	See benazepril.	$$

Class	Drug	Dose	Adverse Effects	Drug Interactions	Comments	Cost[a]
	perindopril Coversyl	Initial: 4 mg/day Max: 8 mg/day Once daily or BID	See benazepril.	See benazepril.	See benazepril.	$$
	quinapril Accupril	Initial: 10 mg/day Max: 40 mg/day Once daily or BID	See benazepril.	See benazepril.	See benazepril.	$$
	ramipril Altace	Initial: 2.5 mg/day Usual: 10 mg/day Max: 20 mg/day Once daily or BID	See benazepril.	See benazepril.	See benazepril.	$$
	trandolapril Mavik	Initial: 1 mg/day Max: 4 mg/day Once daily	See benazepril.	See benazepril.	See benazepril.	$$
Angiotensin Receptor Blockers (ARB)	*candesartan* Atacand	Initial: 8 mg/day Usual: 8–16 mg/day Once daily	Hyperkalemia. Can precipitate renal failure in susceptible patients (bilateral renovascular disease, those with volume depletion or with concurrent NSAID use). Angioedema has been reported, but a causal association has not been established.	Marked ↑ in serum K^+ in patients receiving K^+ supplements and/or K^+-sparing diuretics. May elevate Li^+ levels (monitor Li^+ levels, adjust dose).	**Contraindicated in pregnancy—caution when prescribing to women of child-bearing potential.**[7] Use lower initial doses in patients who are volume depleted or on diuretics (↑ risk of hypotension in hypovolemia). Hyperkalemia usually occurs only in those on K^+ supplements or drugs that cause K^+ retention, those with renal impairment or diabetics with high serum K^+ levels. Assess	$$

(cont'd)

Table 6: **Drugs for Hypertension** *(cont'd)*

Class	Drug	Dose	Adverse Effects	Drug Interactions	Comments	Cost[a]
					SCr and K^+ after a few days, then regularly.	
	eprosartan Teveten	Initial: 600 mg/day Max: 800 mg/day Once daily or BID	See candesartan.	See candesartan.	See candesartan.	$$
	irbesartan Avapro	Initial: 150 mg/day Usual: 150–300 mg/day Once daily	See candesartan.	See candesartan.	See candesartan.	$$
	losartan Cozaar	Initial: 50 mg/day Usual: 25–100 mg/day Max: 100 mg/day Once daily or BID	See candesartan.	See candesartan.	See candesartan.	$$
	telmisartan Micardis	Initial: 80 mg/day Usual: 80 mg/day Once daily	See candesartan.	See candesartan.	See candesartan.	$$
	valsartan Diovan	Initial: 80 mg/day Usual: 80–320 mg/day Once daily	See candesartan.	See candesartan.	See candesartan.	$$

Class	Drug	Dose	Adverse Effects	Drug Interactions	Comments	Cost[a]
Calcium Channel Blockers, dihydropyridine	*amlodipine* Norvasc	Initial: 2.5 mg/day Max: 10 mg/day Once daily	Ankle edema, flushing, headache and palpitations.	CYP3A4 substrate (many potential interactions). Strong inhibitors include azole antifungals, protease inhibitors, macrolides and quinidine. Grapefruit juice may ↑ serum concentrations.		$$$
	felodipine Plendil, Renedil	Initial: 2.5 mg/day Usual: 10 mg/day Max: 20 mg/day Once daily	See amlodipine.	See amlodipine.	Grapefruit juice causes marked elevations in felodipine serum levels and adverse events.	$$
	nifedipine XL Adalat XL, generics	Initial: 30 mg/day Usual: 60 mg/day Max: 120 mg/day Once daily	See amlodipine.	See amlodipine.	Do not use short-acting nifedipine formulations for treatment of essential hypertension.	$$$
Calcium Channel Blockers, nondihydropyridine	*diltiazem* Cardizem, Cardizem CD, Cardizem SR, Tiazac, generics	Initial: 120 mg/day Usual: 240–360 mg/day Max: 360 mg/day Give CD formulation once daily, SR formulation BID	Headache, dizziness, bradycardia, heart block, new onset or worsening of heart failure.	See amlodipine. Nondihydropyridines inhibit the metabolism of carbamazepine, cyclosporine, lovastatin, simvastatin. Rifampin induces metabolism of nondihydropyridines. Additive negative inotropic effects with amiodarone,	Caution in patients with heart failure, or 2nd or 3rd degree heart block without a functioning pacemaker.	$$$

(cont'd)

Table 6: **Drugs for Hypertension** *(cont'd)*

Class	Drug	Dose	Adverse Effects	Drug Interactions	Comments	Cost[a]
				beta-blockers and digoxin.		
	verapamil Covera HS, Isoptin SR, generics	Initial: 80 mg; maximum 160 mg TID Covera HS (QHS): Initial: 180 mg/day; Usual: 180–360 mg/day; Max: 480 mg/day SR (once daily or BID): Initial: 180 mg/day; Usual: 180–480 mg/day; Max: 480 mg/day	See diltiazem. Constipation.	See amlodipine. See diltiazem. Verapamil ↑ digoxin levels by 50–75% within 1 wk (monitor levels).	See diltiazem.	$$-$$$
Centrally Acting Antihypertensive Agents	*methyldopa* generics	Initial: 500 mg/day Usual: 2000 mg/day Max: 3000 mg/day Divide BID or TID	Drowsiness, dry mouth, nasal congestion, depression, orthostatic hypotension, palpitations, sexual dysfunction, sodium and water retention.	Iron salts ↓ absorption (separate administration). Additive hypotension with levodopa. May exacerbate Li^+ adverse events without increasing Li^+ levels.	Positive Coombs' test is common, but usually unimportant; hemolytic anemia is rare. Drug fever with or without an influenza-like illness; hepatic disorders have occurred.	$
Alpha$_1$-adrenergic Antagonists	*doxazosin* Cardura, generics	Initial: 1 mg/day Usual: 1–8 mg/day Max: 16 mg/day Once daily	Orthostatic hypotension, headache, drowsiness, palpitations, nasal congestion. Syncope usually occurs at the start of therapy, with rapid dose titration or on addition of other	Caution when adding other hypotensive drugs, may cause syncope.	Not for initial therapy.	$

Class	Drug	Dose	Adverse Effects	Drug Interactions	Comments	Cost[a]
			agents. Titrate slowly. If interrupted for several days restart at initial dose.			
	prazosin Minipress, generics	Initial: 0.5 mg with p.m. meal (day 1), then 0.5 mg BID-TID x 3 days Max: 20 mg/day	See doxazosin.	See doxazosin.	Not for initial therapy.	\$-\$\$
	terazosin Hytrin, generics	Initial: 1 mg QHS Usual: 1–5 mg/day Max: 20 mg/day Once daily or BID	See doxazosin.	See doxazosin. Verapamil ↑ serum concentrations of terazosin.	Not for initial therapy.	\$
Beta$_1$-adrenergic Antagonist/ Diuretic Combinations	*atenolol/ chlorthalidone* Tenoretic, generics	50/25 mg, or 100/25 mg once daily[c]	See nadolol. See HCTZ.	See nadolol. See HCTZ.	See nadolol. See HCTZ.	\$-\$\$
	pindolol/HCTZ Viskazide	10/25 mg or 10/50 mg once daily[c]	See nadolol. See HCTZ.	See nadolol. See HCTZ.	See nadolol. See HCTZ.	\$\$

(cont'd)

Table 6: **Drugs for Hypertension** *(cont'd)*

Class	Drug	Dose	Adverse Effects	Drug Interactions	Comments	Cost[a]
ACE Inhibitor/ Calcium Channel Blocker Combinations	*trandolapril/ verapamil* Tarka	Trandolapril 1–4 mg/day plus verapamil 180–480 mg/day. Once daily or BID[c]	See benazepril. See diltiazem. Constipation.	See benazepril. See amlodipine. Inhibits metabolism of carbamazepine, cyclosporine, lovastatin, simvastatin. Rifampin ↑ metabolism of verapamil. Additive inotropic effects with amiodarone, beta-blockers, digoxin. Verapamil ↑ digoxin levels by 50–75% within 1 wk (monitor levels).	See benazepril. See diltiazem.	\$\$\$-\$\$\$\$
ACE Inhibitor/ Diuretic Combinations	*cilazapril/HCTZ* Inhibace Plus	5/12.5 mg once daily[c]	See benazepril. See HCTZ.	See benazepril. See HCTZ.	See benazepril. See HCTZ.	\$\$
	enalapril/HCTZ Vaseretic	5/12.5 mg or 10/25 mg once daily[c]	See benazepril. See HCTZ.	See benazepril. See HCTZ.	See benazepril. See HCTZ.	\$\$
	lisinopril/HCTZ Prinzide, Zestoretic, generics	10/12.5 mg, 20/12.5 mg or 20/25 once daily[c]	See benazepril. See HCTZ.	See benazepril. See HCTZ.	See benazepril. See HCTZ.	\$-\$\$

Class	Drug	Dose	Adverse Effects	Drug Interactions	Comments	Cost[a]
	perindopril/ indapamide Coversyl Plus, Preterax	4/1.25 mg once daily[c]	See benazepril. See HCTZ.	See benazepril. See HCTZ.	See benazepril. See HCTZ.	$$
	quinapril/HCTZ Accuretic	10/12.5 mg, 20/12.5 mg or 20/25 mg once daily[c]	See benazepril. See HCTZ.	See benazepril. See HCTZ.	See benazepril. See HCTZ.	$$
	ramipril/HCTZ Altace HCT	2.5/12.5 mg, 5/12.5 mg, 10/12.5 mg, 5/25, mg or 10/25 mg once daily[c]	See benazepril. See HCTZ.	See benazepril. See HCTZ.	See benazepril. See HCTZ.	$$
ARB/ Diuretic Combina-tions	*candesartan/HCTZ* Atacand Plus	16/12.5 mg once daily[c]	See candesartan. See HCTZ.	See candesartan. See HCTZ.	See candesartan. See HCTZ.	$$
	eprosartan/HCTZ Teveten Plus	600/12.5 mg once daily[c]	See candesartan. See HCTZ.	See candesartan. See HCTZ.	See candesartan. See HCTZ.	$$
	irbesartan/HCTZ Avalide	150/12.5, 300/12.5 or 300/25 mg once daily[c]	See candesartan. See HCTZ.	See candesartan. See HCTZ.	See candesartan. See HCTZ.	$$
	losartan/HCTZ Hyzaar, Hyzaar DS	50/12.5 mg or 100/25 mg once daily[c]	See candesartan. See HCTZ.	See candesartan. See HCTZ.	See candesartan. See HCTZ.	$$
	telmisartan/HCTZ Micardis Plus	80/12.5 mg once daily[c]	See candesartan. See HCTZ.	See candesartan. See HCTZ.	See candesartan. See HCTZ.	$$
	valsartan/HCTZ Diovan-HCT	80/12.5 mg, 160/12.5 mg or 160/25 mg once daily[c]	See candesartan. See HCTZ.	See candesartan. See HCTZ.	See candesartan. See HCTZ.	$$

(cont'd)

Table 6: **Drugs for Hypertension** *(cont'd)*

Class	Drug	Dose	Adverse Effects	Drug Interactions	Comments	Cost[a]
Centrally Acting Antihypertensive/ Diuretic Combinations	*methyldopa/HCTZ* ◗ generics	250/15 mg or 250/25 mg once daily[c]	See methyldopa. See HCTZ.	See methyldopa. See HCTZ.	See methyldopa. See HCTZ.	$
Calcium Channel Blocker/ HMG CoA Reductase Inhibitor Combinations	*amlodipine/atorvastatin* Caduet	Amlodipine 5 or 10 mg plus atorvastatin 10, 20, 40 or 80 mg[c]	See amlodipine. Adverse effects of atorvastatin include constipation, flatulence, dyspepsia, abdominal pain and myalgia.	See amlodipine. Amlodipine and atorvastatin are both substrates of CYP3A4.	For patients with hypertension and an indication for an HMG-Co inhibitor.	$$$$

[a] Cost of 30-day supply of usual dose of drug; includes drug cost only.
[b] Chlorthalidone is also available in Canada. However, the tablet strengths available do not permit use of the preferred low doses.
[c] It is generally recommended that the dose of the each component is titrated before starting a combination product.
◗ Dosage adjustment may be required in renal impairment; see Appendix I.
Abbreviations: CV = cardiovascular; HCTZ = hydrochlorothiazide; IR = immediate release; ISA = intrinsic sympathomimetic activity; ISH = isolated systolic hypertension; PAD = peripheral arterial disease; SR = slow release; TCA = tricyclic antidepressant
Legend: $ < $20 $-$$ < $20–40 $$ $20–40 $$-$$$ $20–60 $$$ $40–60 $$$-$$$$ $40– > 60 $$$$ > $60

Suggested Readings

Adrogue HJ, Madias NE. Sodium and potassium in the pathogenesis of hypertension. *N Engl J Med* 2007;356(19):1966-78.

Canadian Hypertension Society. Canadian recommendations on the management of hypertension are updated annually. A summary of the important and new recommendations can be found at http://www.hypertension.ca/ in the *Public Recommendations* section and is also broadly published in multidisciplinary journals annually.

Khan NA, Hemmelgarn B, Padwal R et al. The 2007 Canadian Hypertension Education Program recommendations for the management of hypertension: Part 2–therapy. *Can J Cardiol* 2007;23(7):539-50.

Padwal RS, Hemmelgarn BR, McAlister FA et al. The 2007 Canadian Hypertension Education Program recommendations for the management of hypertension: Part 1–blood pressure measurement, diagnosis and assessment of risk. *Can J Cardiol* 2007;23(7):529-38.

References

1. Canadian Hypertension Society. *Canadian Hypertension Education Program Recommendations, 2007.* Available from http://www.hypertension.ca/chep/docs/2007RecommendationsSummary.pdf. Accessed May 30, 2007.
2. Khan N, Chockalingam A, Campbell NR. Lack of control of high blood pressure and treatment recommendations in Canada. *Can J Cardiol* 2002;18(6):657-61.
3. ALLHAT Officers and Coordinators for the ALLHAT Collaborative Research Group. The Antihypertensive and Lipid-Lowering Treatment to Prevent Heart Attack Trial. Major outcomes in high-risk hypertensive patients randomized to angiotensin-converting enzyme inhibitor or calcium channel blocker vs diuretic: The Antihypertensive and Lipid-Lowering Treatment to Prevent Heart Attack Trial (ALLHAT). *JAMA* 2002;288(23):2981-97.
4. [No authors listed]. MRC trial of treatment of mild hypertension: principal results. Medical Research Council Working Party. *Br Med J (Clin Res Ed)* 1985;291(6488):97-104.
5. Cooper WO, Hernandez-Diaz S, Arbogast PG et al. Major congenital malformations after first-trimester exposure to ACE inhibitors. *N Engl J Med* 2006;354(23):2443-51.
6. Friedman JM. ACE inhibitors and congenital anomalies. *N Engl J Med* 2006;354(23):2498-500.
7. Alwan S, Polifka JE, Friedman JM. Angiotensin II receptor antagonist treatment during pregnancy. *Birth Defects Res A Clin Mol Teratol* 2005;73(2):123-30.
8. Nakao N, Yoshimura A, Morita H et al. Combination treatment of angiotensin-II receptor blocker and angiotensin-converting-enzyme inhibitor in non-diabetic renal disease (COOPERATE): a randomised controlled trial. *Lancet* 2003;361(9352):117-24.
9. Doulton TW, He FJ, MacGregor GA. Systematic review of combined angiotensin-converting enzyme inhibition and angiotensin receptor blockade in hypertension. *Hypertension* 2005;45(5):880-6.
10. Salpeter SS, Ormiston T, Salpeter E et al. Cardioselective beta-blockers for chronic obstructive pulmonary disease. *Cochrane Database Syst Rev* 2002;(2):CD003566.

Pharmacoeconomic Considerations: Hypertension

Blair Jarvis, MSc, BSP

Epidemiology	
Country (Year)	**Prevalence (%)**
Canada (1992)	27.4% among adults aged 35–64[1]

(cont'd)

Cost of Illness Data		
Country and Year of Estimate	**Direct Costs[a]**	**Indirect Costs[b]**
United States (2000)[2]	US $3072 per person	US $854 per person

Commentary

Hypertension is one of the most common chronic conditions encountered in primary care. Effective treatment prevents morbidity and mortality related to heart failure, myocardial infarction, stroke and end-stage renal disease. Hypertension is generally asymptomatic and does not adversely affect health-related quality of life. Antihypertensive drugs are safe and well tolerated, many inexpensive generic products are available in Canada and comprehensive recommendations are updated annually, yet there is concern that control of blood pressure in hypertensive patients is often suboptimal. The question one must ask is not whether treatment of hypertension is cost-effective, but rather what is the cost of "clinical inertia," which refers to the failure to initiate or intensify therapy when it is indicated.[3,4]

Nonpharmacologic therapy for hypertension is effective and cost-effective. It is estimated that reducing dietary sodium intake by 1840 mg/day would decrease systolic blood pressure by 5 mm Hg, reduce the number of Canadians requiring antihypertensive drugs by 23% and reduce direct medical expenditures on hypertension by $430 million.[5]

As the target blood pressure is lowered, the average medical costs associated with drugs and office visits increase, but these costs are offset, at least partially, by decreased costs associated with hospitalization for cardiovascular causes.[6] Intensive treatment for hypertension is particularly cost-effective in patients with diabetes, where the risk of negative outcomes with poorer control is greater.[7,8]

Most patients with hypertension will require two or more drugs to achieve the recommended target blood pressure.[9] In patients without comorbid conditions, it is the extent of blood pressure lowering, rather than the specific drug, that is correlated with reductions in morbidity and mortality. For this reason, isolated economic comparisons of individual agents are not particularly helpful to the primary care physician.

Many Canadians do not have prescription drug coverage and must pay for chronic medications themselves. The use of older agents (when appropriate), less expensive generic products and combination products may reduce prescription costs for these individuals.

(cont'd)

Commentary

A presumed disadvantage of thiazide diuretics relative to "newer" antihypertensive agents is the need for more frequent laboratory testing to detect and prevent adverse events. A population-based cohort study involving elderly Ontario patients showed that, although laboratory testing was done more frequently in those initially treated with a diuretic, the additional cost of such testing was only $0.63 per patient over six months.[10] Thus, testing for biochemical abnormalities should not be considered an economic barrier to the use of diuretics as first-line agents for hypertension.

[a] Direct costs include those associated with physician services, nursing care, diagnostic procedures, drugs and hospitalization.

[b] Indirect costs include those associated with lost productivity and days off work due to morbidity or premature mortality.

References

1. Wolf-Maier K, Cooper RS, Banegas JR et al. Hypertension prevalence and blood pressure levels in 6 European countries, Canada, and the United States. *JAMA* 2003;289(18):2363-9.
2. Maetzel A, Li LC, Pencharz J et al. The economic burden associated with osteoarthritis, rheumatoid arthritis, and hypertension: a comparative study. *Ann Rheum Dis* 2004;63(4):395-401.
3. Degli EL, Valpiani G. Pharmacoeconomic burden of undertreating hypertension. *Pharmacoeconomics* 2004;22(14):907-28.
4. Phillips LS, Branch WT, Cook CB et al. Clinical inertia. *Ann Intern Med* 2001;135(9):825-34.
5. Joffres MR, Campbell NR, Manns B et al. Estimate of the benefits of a population-based reduction in dietary sodium additives on hypertension and its related health care costs in Canada. *Can J Cardiol* 2007;23(6):437-43.
6. Jonsson B, Hansson L,.Stalhammar NO. Health economics in the Hypertension Optimal Treatment (HOT) study: costs and cost-effectiveness of intensive blood pressure lowering and low-dose aspirin in patients with hypertension. *J Intern Med* 2003;253(4):472-80.
7. CDC Diabetes Cost-effectiveness Group. Cost-effectiveness of intensive glycemic control, intensified hypertension control, and serum cholesterol level reduction for type 2 diabetes. *JAMA* 2002;287(19):2542-51.
8. Clarke PM, Gray AM, Briggs A et al. Cost-utility analyses of intensive blood glucose and tight blood pressure control in type 2 diabetes (UKPDS 72). *Diabetologia* 2005;48(5):868-77.
9. Chobanian AV, Bakris GL, Black HR et al. The Seventh Report of the Joint National Committee on Prevention, Detection, Evaluation, and Treatment of High Blood Pressure: the JNC 7 report. *JAMA* 2003;289(19):2560-72.
10. McAlister FA, Tu K, Majumdar SR et al. Laboratory testing in newly treated elderly hypertensive patients without co-morbidities: a population-based cohort study. *Open Medicine* 2007;1(2):E60–7

CHAPTER 33
Stable Angina

P.J. Devereaux, MD

Angina pectoris is a discomfort in the chest and/or an adjacent area resulting from myocardial ischemia (i.e., inadequate blood supply to the myocardium). Coronary artery disease (CAD) is the most common cause of myocardial ischemia; the therapeutic discussions in this chapter assume CAD is the underlying etiology, unless indicated otherwise. Other conditions that can cause myocardial ischemia should be considered when evaluating a patient with angina pectoris (e.g., critical aortic stenosis, hypertrophic cardiomyopathy, arrhythmia, coronary arterial spasm, anemia). Identifying these less common causes of angina pectoris is important not only to ensure that appropriate treatments are given, but also to ensure that inappropriate treatments are not (e.g., to ensure a patient with angina due to hypertrophic cardiomyopathy is not treated with long-acting nitrate therapy).

Goals of Therapy

- Minimize the risk of cardiovascular death and nonfatal myocardial infarction
- Improve quality of life by decreasing or preventing angina and improving exercise tolerance
- Minimize modifiable risk factors

Investigations

- History
  - a thorough history focusing on the patient's age, sex and discomfort characteristics (i.e., location, precipitating factors and alleviating factors) is the most important tool for estimating the likelihood that significant CAD is the cause of a patient's discomfort (Table 1)
  - modifiable risk factors for CAD (i.e., diabetes mellitus, smoking, hyperlipidemia and hypertension)
- Physical examination to assess for:
  - hypertension
  - evidence of atherosclerotic disease, e.g., arterial bruits
  - evidence of critical aortic stenosis, hypertrophic cardiomyopathy or arrhythmia
- Noninvasive cardiovascular testing:
  - resting ECG
  - exercise stress test, radionuclide myocardial perfusion imaging or stress echocardiography is helpful in revising the probability

of CAD in patients who have a > 10% or < 90% probability of coronary artery disease based on Table 1[1]
- echocardiography if critical aortic stenosis or hypertrophic cardiomyopathy is suspected

- Laboratory tests:
  - nonfasting total cholesterol and fasting cholesterol panel
  - fasting blood glucose
  - serum creatinine and electrolytes
  - hemoglobin if anemia is suspected

Table 1: **Likelihood of Significant Coronary Artery Disease According to Age, Sex and Character of Symptoms**

Age (y)	Nonanginal[a] (%)		Atypical Angina[a] (%)		Typical Angina[a] (%)	
	Men	Women	Men	Women	Men	Women
30–39	5	1	22	4	70	26
40–49	14	3	46	13	87	55
50–59	22	8	59	32	92	79
60–69	28	19	67	54	94	91

[a] The following three questions establish if the discomfort is considered nonanginal chest pain, atypical angina or typical angina.

1. Is the discomfort substernal?
2. Are the symptoms precipitated by exertion?
3. Are the symptoms relieved within ten minutes of rest?

If the patient responds "yes" to all three questions, they have typical angina. If the patient responds "yes" to two of the above, they have atypical angina. If the patient responds "yes" to one or none of these questions, they have nonanginal chest pain.

Adapted with permission from Diamond GA, Forrester JS. Analysis of probability as an aid in the clinical diagnosis of coronary-artery disease. *N Engl J Med* 1979;300(24):1350-8. Copyright © 1979 Massachusetts Medical Society. All rights reserved.

Therapeutic Choices

Nonpharmacologic Choices

- Educate patients about their disease state and treatment options.
- Encourage patients to exercise regularly. Ideally, patients should attend a rehabilitation exercise program with trained personnel. If not available, instruct patients to undertake dynamic exercise (e.g., walking, jogging, cycling, swimming) and not isometric exercise (e.g., weight lifting). The frequency and intensity of exercise should increase gradually over a six- to eight-week period, ultimately targeting 20 to 45 minutes of exercise three to six times a week.
- Encourage patients who are overweight to lose weight and see a dietitian.

Pharmacologic Choices (Figure 1)

Drugs that Decrease the Risk of Cardiovascular Death, Nonfatal Myocardial Infarction or Stroke

There is clear evidence from large randomized controlled trials that patients with angina pectoris benefit from an angiotensin-converting enzyme (ACE) inhibitor, an antiplatelet agent, and an HMG CoA reductase inhibitor (statin therapy).[2,3,4] Therefore, unless there is a significant risk or financial restriction, all patients with angina pectoris due to CAD should be treated with an ACE inhibitor and an antiplatelet agent, and all patients with a nonfasting total cholesterol level ≥ 3.5 mmol/L should receive statin therapy. Current recommendations are to treat all high-risk patients to a target low-density lipoprotein cholesterol (LDL-C) level < 2 mmol/L.[5]

Antiplatelet Agents (Figure 1)

A systematic review of randomized controlled trials demonstrated that antiplatelet agents decrease the relative risk of cardiovascular death, nonfatal myocardial infarction (MI) or nonfatal stroke by 30% compared with placebo. It also showed that **ASA** 80 to 160 mg daily is as effective as higher doses.[2] Randomized controlled trials comparing ASA with **clopidogrel** or **ticlopidine** have not been conducted exclusively in patients with stable angina. Clopidogrel is at least as effective as ASA in patients with a history of MI.[2] The combination of ASA plus clopidogrel offers no advantage over ASA alone in reducing cardiovascular event rates in patients with atherosclerosis.[7] In patients with vascular disease (i.e., patients with a prior stroke/transient ischemic attack, post-angioplasty or with peripheral vascular disease), ticlopidine is at least as effective as ASA therapy.[6] Clopidogrel is appropriate for those who cannot take ASA. Ticlopidine is associated with neutropenia, thrombocytopenia and thrombotic thrombocytic purpura, which is rare but potentially fatal. Thus, the use of ticlopidine should be considered only when a patient cannot take ASA and cannot afford clopidogrel.

ACE Inhibitors

ACE inhibitors have a number of potential anti-ischemic mechanisms including decreasing sympathetic adrenergic transmission, reducing afterload and blood pressure and improving coronary flow reserve. ACE inhibitors prevent major cardiovascular events in patients with stable angina who do not have heart failure or left ventricular systolic dysfunction.[8]

In the HOPE trial, which enrolled patients at high risk of cardiovascular events, **ramipril** 10 mg/day decreased the relative risk of cardiovascular death, nonfatal MI or nonfatal stroke by 20% as compared with placebo in the subgroup of patients with angina.[4]

HMG CoA Reductase Inhibitors (Statins)

The mechanism of action of statins is not limited to reducing cholesterol levels but includes improving endothelial function.

The Heart Protection Study (HPS) trial randomized patients with a nonfasting total cholesterol ≥ 3.5 mmol/L and demonstrated that **simvastatin** 40 mg daily decreased the relative risk of death by 13%, nonfatal MI by 37% and nonfatal stroke by 26% compared with placebo.[3] For more information on statins, see Chapter 31.

Drugs that Decrease or Prevent Angina

There is a paucity of randomized controlled trials comparing anti-ischemic drugs (nitrates, beta-blockers and calcium channel blockers) in patients with angina.[9,10] As such, it is reasonable to use any of these drugs, and the choice of which drug to start with should include consideration of patient–specific factors. For example, a patient with a history of MI should be treated with a beta-blocker as a first choice.

Nitrates (Table 2)

Nitrates are effective for acute and chronic angina. Sublingual nitroglycerin tablets or spray alleviate anginal pain and, if taken in advance, can prevent symptoms that occur with activity. Advise patients to sit when taking sublingual nitrates to reduce the risk of syncope. Long-acting nitrate preparations prevent angina but frequently cause headaches. Tolerance to the anti-anginal effects of nitrates develops unless a nitrate-free period of 10 to 12 hours is prescribed each day.

Beta-blockers (Table 2)

Beta-blockers lower heart rate, blood pressure and free fatty acid levels, and prevent angina by decreasing myocardial oxygen demand. Both selective and nonselective beta-blockers are effective. Beta-blockers reduce the risk of MI and mortality in patients with a prior MI. Avoid beta-blocker therapy in patients with coronary arterial spasm (Prinzmetal's angina).

Calcium Channel Blockers (Table 2)

Verapamil and **diltiazem** lower heart rate and reduce blood pressure, whereas the dihydropyridines (**nifedipine, felodipine, amlodipine**) exert their effects primarily by arteriolar dilatation. Calcium channel blockers are the treatment of choice in patients with coronary arterial spasm.

Short-acting nifedipine has been associated with higher mortality rates when used in the treatment of acute ischemic syndromes and hypertension and should be avoided.[11,12]

Minimize Modifiable Risk Factors

Observational studies demonstrate smoking cessation decreases mortality and morbid cardiac events. Patients who smoke must be made aware of the risk and encouraged to stop smoking (see Chapter 10).

Based on the results of the Heart and Estrogen/progestin Replacement Study (HERS trial) and the Women's Health Initiative trial, avoid hormone therapy (HT) in postmenopausal women when possible.[13,14] If HT is required to prevent symptoms, keep the duration of therapy to a minimum and consider alternative interventions (see Chapter 64).

Although observational studies have suggested lower homocysteine levels and vitamin E therapy are beneficial for patients with angina, large randomized controlled trials have not shown any benefit to folic acid, B vitamins and vitamin E in patients with angina.

Treat hypertension and diabetes according to the current Canadian guidelines (see Chapter 32 and Chapter 27).

Coronary Artery Revascularization

Coronary artery revascularization is indicated for medically refractory angina pectoris to improve patients' quality of life by decreasing frequency of angina. It is also indicated to prolong life in any patient with > 50% stenosis of the left main descending artery, > 70% stenosis of the proximal left anterior descending coronary artery or > 70% stenosis in three coronary arteries.

Therapeutic Tips

- When an ACE inhibitor is prescribed to a patient with renal dysfunction, monitor the serum potassium and creatinine. If a patient with renal dysfunction can tolerate an ACE inhibitor, the drug will preserve renal function.
- Start nitrate therapy at low doses and titrate according to symptoms, ensuring a 10- to 12-hour nitrate-free period each day to avoid tolerance. Schedule the nitrate-free period for a time when minimal symptoms are expected, usually at night.
- If the use of a beta-blocker is desired in a patient with resting bradycardia, try one with intrinsic sympathomimetic activity (e.g., acebutolol).
- Titrate the dose of beta-blockers, diltiazem and verapamil to achieve a resting heart rate between 50 and 60 beats per minute (BPM) and an exercise heart rate that does not exceed 100 to 110 BPM. The dose of dihydropyridines (e.g. amlodipine, nifedipine) should be titrated to achieve maximum symptom relief with minimal adverse effects.
- In patients with left ventricular systolic dysfunction (ejection fraction < 40%), start beta-blocker therapy at very low doses and titrate slowly (e.g., no more frequently than every two weeks).

- Do not withdraw beta-blocker therapy abruptly in patients who have been on chronic high dose beta-blocker therapy, as this may precipitate an acute coronary syndrome. Taper the dose over a 10- to 14-day period.
- Avoid verapamil and diltiazem in patients with left ventricular systolic dysfunction and use with caution in patients with AV nodal disease.
- As a general rule, when adding a calcium channel blocker to the regimen of a patient with persistent angina who is already on a beta-blocker, use a long-acting dihydropyridine.
- Close monitoring of heart rate and AV nodal function is required if verapamil or diltiazem is combined with beta-blocker therapy.
- Cyclooxygenase-2 (COX-2) inhibitors and all traditional nonsteroidal anti-inflammatory drugs (NSAIDs) increase the risk of vascular events and thus physicians should minimize their use in patients with angina.[15]

Figure 1: **Medical Management of Stable Angina Pectoris**

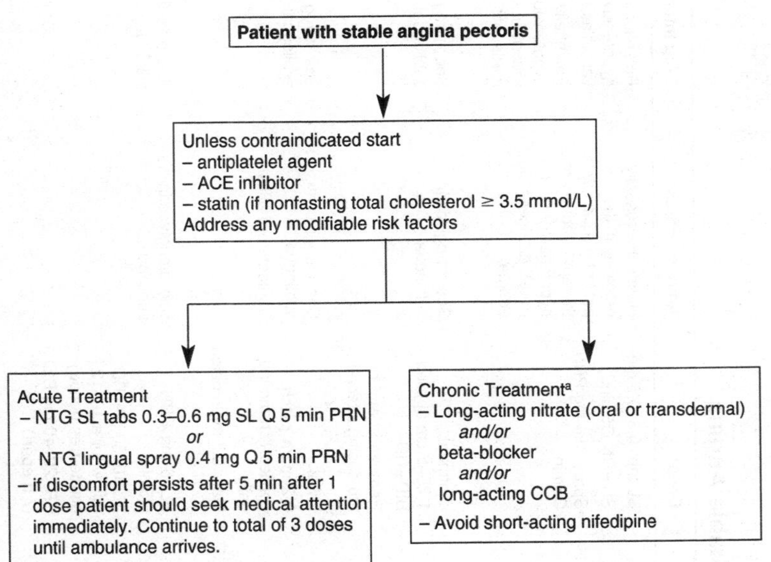

[a] Agents are not listed in order of preference.
Abbreviations: ACE = angiotensin-converting enzyme; CCB = calcium channel blocker; NTG = nitroglycerin

Table 2: **Drugs for Stable Angina**

Class	Drug	Dose	Adverse Effects	Drug Interactions	Comments	Cost[a]
Nitrates	*nitroglycerin, sublingual* Nitrolingual Pumpspray, Nitrostat, Rho-Nitro Pumpspray, generics	SL tab: 0.3–0.6 mg SL PRN Q5min Spray: 0.4 mg PRN Q5min	Headache (usually resolves if the patient persists with therapy), tachycardia, hypotension, syncope (rare), dizziness, flushing edema.	Potentiates the hypotensive effects of vasodilators. Potentially fatal hypotension with sildenafil, tadalafil and vardenafil.	If discomfort persists after 5 min after 1 dose, patient should seek medical attention immediately. Continue to total of 3 doses until ambulance arrives.	$
	nitroglycerin, topical Nitrol	Ointment: 1.25–5 cm applied BID–TID Remove at end of the dosing interval	See nitroglycerin, sublingual.	See nitroglycerin, sublingual.	Ensure a 10–12 h nitrate-free period daily to prevent tolerance.	$
	nitroglycerin, transdermal Minitran, Nitro-Dur, Transderm-Nitro, Trinipatch	Initial: 0.2 mg/h patch applied & removed daily Max: 0.8 mg/h patch	See nitroglycerin, sublingual. Contact dermatitis.	See nitroglycerin, sublingual.	See nitroglycerin, topical.	$$
	isosorbide dinitrate Cedocard CR, generics	SL: 5 mg PRN Q5min IR: 10–30 mg TID (allow for a 10–12 h nitrate-free period) CR: 20–40 mg BID (7 h apart)	See nitroglycerin, sublingual.	See nitroglycerin, sublingual.	See nitroglycerin, topical.	SL: $ IR: $ CR: $$-$$$

Class	Drug	Dose	Adverse Effects	Drug Interactions	Comments	Cost[a]
	isosorbide-5-mononitrate Imdur, generics	Initial: 30 or 60 mg/day Max: 240 mg/day Once daily	See nitroglycerin, sublingual.	See nitroglycerin, sublingual.	To minimize headache, start with 30 mg once daily.	$$
Antiplatelet Agents	*ASA* Aspirin, Bufferin, Coated Aspirin, generics	80–325 mg once daily	Nausea, vomiting, gastritis, bleeding (epistaxis to major GI bleeds), rash.	Increased risk of bleeding when combined with other antiplatelets or anticoagulants.	Serious GI bleeding is less common with lower doses (80–160 mg/day).	$
	clopidogrel Plavix	75 mg once daily	Bleeding, diarrhea, rash.	See ASA.		$$$$
	ticlopidine Ticlid, generics	250 mg BID	Bleeding, diarrhea, rash, purpura, neutropenia.	See ASA.	Monitor neutrophils every 2 wk for the first 3 mo of therapy.	$$
Beta$_1$-adrenergic Antagonists, nonselective	*nadolol* generics	Initial: 20 mg/day Max: 320 mg/day Once daily	Fatigue, hypotension, bradycardia, impotence, sleep disorders. Less common: hyperglycemia, depression, heart failure, heart block.	Bradycardia with digoxin or nondihydropyridine CCBs. Cardiodepressant effects with nondihydropyridine CCBs and amiodarone.	Avoid abrupt withdrawal (may precipitate ischemia). Taper the dose before discontinuation. Avoid in severe peripheral arterial disease. Contraindicated in asthma and in 2nd or 3rd degree heart block in the absence of a pacemaker.	$

(cont'd)

Table 2: **Drugs for Stable Angina** *(cont'd)*

Class	Drug	Dose	Adverse Effects	Drug Interactions	Comments	Cost[a]
	propranolol, immediate release generics	Initial: 40–60 mg QID Usual: 80–320 mg/day (divided BID-QID)	See nadolol.	See nadolol. CYP2D6 inhibitors ↑ levels of propranolol and metoprolol. Propranolol ↑ serum levels of rizatriptan.	See nadolol. More likely to cause CNS side effects (insomnia, depression, vivid dreams) than other agents because of greater lipid solubility.	$
	propranolol, controlled release Inderal-LA	60–320 mg/day	See nadolol.	See propranolol	Initiate therapy with immediate release preparation.	$$$
	timolol generics	Initial: 10 mg BID Max: 30 mg BID	See nadolol.	See nadolol.	See nadolol.	$$
Beta$_1$-adrenergic Antagonists, selective	*atenolol* Tenormin, generics	Initial: 25 mg/day Max: 200 mg/day Once daily or BID	See nadolol.	See nadolol.	See nadolol.	$
	bisoprolol Monocor, generics	Initial: 2.5 mg/day Max: 20 mg/day Once daily	See nadolol.	See nadolol.	See nadolol.	$
	metoprolol Betaloc, Lopresor, generics	Initial: 50 mg/day Max: 400 mg/day Give regular formulations BID; SR once daily	See nadolol.	See nadolol. CYP2D6 inhibitors increase levels of propranolol and metoprolol.	See nadolol.	$

Class	Drug	Dose	Adverse Effects	Drug Interactions	Comments	Cost[a]
$Beta_1$-adrenergic Antagonists, nonselective with ISA	*pindolol* Visken, generics	Initial: 5 mg TID Max: 15 mg TID or QID	See nadolol.	See nadolol.	See nadolol. Agents with ISA have less effect on resting heart rate than those without ISA.	$$
$Beta_1$-adrenergic Antagonists, selective with ISA	*acebutolol* Rhotral, Sectral, generics	Initial: 200 mg BID Max: 400 mg BID	See nadolol.	See nadolol.	See nadolol. Agents with ISA have less effect on resting heart rate than those without ISA.	$
$Beta_1$-adrenergic Antagonists with $alpha_1$-blocking activity	*labetalol* Trandate, generics	Initial: 100 mg BID Max: 1200 mg BID	See nadolol. Edema, dizziness, nasal congestion and postural hypotension due to $alpha_1$ antagonism.	See nadolol.	See nadolol.	$
Calcium Channel Blockers, dihydropyridine	*amlodipine* Norvasc	Initial: 2.5 mg/day Max: 10 mg/day Once daily	Ankle edema, flushing, headache, hypotension and tachycardia.	CYP3A4 substrate (many potential interactions). Strong inhibitors include azole antifungals, protease inhibitors, macrolides and quinidine. Grapefruit juice may ↑ serum concentrations.		$$$
	nifedipine XL Adalat XL, generics	Initial: 30 mg/day Max: 120 mg/day Once daily	See amlodipine.	See amlodipine.		$$$

(cont'd)

Table 2: **Drugs for Stable Angina** *(cont'd)*

Class	Drug	Dose	Adverse Effects	Drug Interactions	Comments	Cost[a]
Calcium Channel Blockers, nondihydropyridine	*diltiazem* Cardizem, Cardizem CD, Tiazac, Tiazac XC, generics	Initial: 120 mg/day Max: 360 mg/day Give CD formulation once daily; XC formulation BID	Headache, dizziness, bradycardia, heart block, new onset or worsening of heart failure.	See amlodipine. Nondihydropyridines inhibit the metabolism of carbamazepine, cyclosporine, lovastatin, simvastatin. Rifampin induces metabolism of nondihydropyridines. Additive negative inotropic effects with amiodarone, beta-blockers and digoxin.	Caution in patients with heart failure or 2nd or 3rd degree heart block without a functioning pacemaker.	$$$
	verapamil Covera HS, Isoptin SR, generics	Initial: 80 mg; Max: 160 mg TID Covera HS (QHS): Initial: 180 mg/day; Max: 480 mg/day SR (once daily or BID): Initial: 180 mg/day; Max: 480 mg/day	See diltiazem. Constipation.	See amlodipine. See diltiazem. Verapamil ↑ digoxin levels by 50–75% within 1 wk (monitor levels).	See diltiazem.	$$–$$$

[a] Cost of a 30-day supply of usual dose of drug; includes drug cost only.

Dosage adjustment may be required in renal impairment; see Appendix I.

Abbreviations: CCBs = calcium channel blockers; IR = immediate release; ISA = intrinsic sympathomimetic activity

Legend: $ < $20 $$ $20–40 $$-$$$ $20–60 $$$ $40–60 $$$$ $ > 60

Suggested Readings

Bennett NM, Paris MC. Coronary artery disease. In: Black ER, Bordley DR, Tape TG et al, editors. *Diagnostic strategies for common medical problems*. 2nd ed. Philadelphia (PA): American College of Physicians; 1999. p.47-60.

Sudlow C, Lonn E, Pignone M, Ness A, Rihal C. Secondary prevention of ischaemic cardiac events. *Clin Evid* 2002;(7):124-60.

References

1. Bennett NM, Paris MC. Coronary artery disease. In: Black ER, Bordley DR, Tape TG et al, editors. *Diagnostic strategies for common medical problems*. 2nd ed. Philadelphia (PA): American College of Physicians; 1999. p.47-60.
2. Antithrombotic Trialists' Collaboration. Collaborative meta-analysis of randomised trials of antiplatelet therapy for prevention of death, myocardial infarction, and stroke in high risk patients. *BMJ* 2002;324(7329):71-86.
3. Heart Protection Study Collaborative Group. MRC/BHF Heart Protection Study of cholesterol lowering with simvastatin in 20,536 high-risk individuals: a randomised placebo-controlled trial. *Lancet* 2002;360(9326):7-22.
4. Yusuf S, Sleight P, Pogue J et al. Effects of an angiotensin-converting-enzyme inhibitor, ramipril, on cardiovascular events in high-risk patients. The Heart Outcomes Prevention Evaluation Study Investigators. *N Engl J Med* 2000;342(3):145-53.
5. McPherson R, Frohlich J, Fodor G et al. Canadian Cardiovascular Society position statement--recommendations for the diagnosis and treatment of dyslipidemia and prevention of cardiovascular disease. *Can J Cardiol* 2006;22(11):913-27.
6. Cairns JA, Theroux P, Lewis HD et al. Antithrombotic agents in coronary artery disease. *Chest* 2001;119(1 Suppl):228S-252S.
7. Bhatt DL, Fox KA, Hacke W et al. Clopidogrel and aspirin versus aspirin alone for the prevention of atherothrombotic events. *N Engl J Med* 2006;354(16):1706-17.
8. Danchin N, Cucherat M, Thuillez C et al. Angiotensin-converting enzyme inhibitors in patients with coronary artery disease and absence of heart failure or left ventricular systolic dysfunction: an overview of long-term randomized controlled trials. *Arch Intern Med* 2006;166(7):787-96.
9. Dargie HJ, Ford I, Fox KM. Total Ischaemic Burden European Trial (TIBET). Effects of ischaemia and treatment with atenolol, nifedipine SR and their combination on outcome in patients with chronic stable angina. The TIBET Study Group. *Eur Heart J* 1996;17(1):104-12.
10. Rehnqvist N, Hjemdahl P, Billing E et al. Effects of metoprolol vs verapamil in patients with stable angina pectoris. The Angina Prognosis Study in Stockholm (APSIS). *Eur Heart J* 1996;17(1):76-81.
11. Alderman MH, Cohen H, Roque R et al. Effect of long-acting and short-acting calcium antagonists on cardiovascular outcomes in hypertensive patients. *Lancet* 1997;349(9052):594-8.
12. Opie LH, Yusuf S, Kubler W. Current status of safety and efficacy of calcium channel blockers in cardiovascular diseases: a critical analysis based on 100 studies. *Prog Cardiovasc Dis* 2000;43(2):171-96.
13. Hulley S, Grady D, Bush T et al. Randomized trial of estrogen plus progestin for secondary prevention of coronary heart disease in postmenopausal women. Heart and Estrogen/progestin Replacement Study (HERS) Research Group. *JAMA* 1998;280(7):605-13.
14. Rossouw JE, Anderson GL, Prentice RL et al. Risks and benefits of estrogen plus progestin in healthy postmenopausal women: principal results from the Women's Health Initiative randomized controlled trial. *JAMA* 2002;288(3):321-33.
15. Kearney PM, Baigent C, Godwin J et al. Do selective cyclo-oxygenase-2 inhibitors and traditional non-steroidal anti-inflammatory drugs increase the risk of atherothrombosis? Meta-analysis of randomised trials. *BMJ* 2006;332(7553):1302-8.

CHAPTER 34

Acute Coronary Syndromes

Michelle Graham, MD, FRCPC

The term "acute coronary syndrome" (ACS) refers to any clinical symptoms compatible with acute myocardial ischemia, from ST segment elevation myocardial infarction (STEMI) to non-ST segment elevation myocardial infarction (which implies nontransmural ischemia and was formerly known as non-Q wave myocardial infarction) and unstable angina.

UNSTABLE ANGINA AND NON-ST SEGMENT ELEVATION MYOCARDIAL INFARCTION (NSTEMI)

Goals of Therapy

- Reduce morbidity and mortality
- Reduce the severity of or eliminate episodes of ischemia
- Prevent further myocardial injury

Investigations

- Careful history with special attention to pain (quality, severity, location, radiation, precipitating and relieving factors), duration of symptoms, previous cardiac history, cardiac risk factors (smoking status, diabetes mellitus, hyperlipidemia, hypertension, family history of premature coronary disease) and effect of nitroglycerin
- Physical examination, with attention to the presence of hypertension, congestive heart failure or valvular heart disease
- Laboratory tests, including ECG, CBC, electrolytes, glucose, creatinine, creatine kinase (CK), troponin and cholesterol profile
- A careful search for secondary causes of ischemia, e.g., anemia, fever, infection, arrhythmia, thyroid disease
- Echocardiography can be used early when clinical history and ECG are nondiagnostic—the presence of regional wall motion abnormalities with chest pain is suggestive of underlying ischemia

The TIMI (Thrombolysis in Myocardial Infarction) Risk Score is a comprehensive risk stratification tool for patients with NSTEMI or unstable angina, using clinical features present at the time of initial assessment in the emergency department (Table 1). It predicts the risk of both death and recurrent ischemic events and is used to target different evidence-based therapies to appropriate patients. As the risk score increases, so too do adverse outcomes; for example there is a 5% risk of major adverse cardiac events in patients with a risk score of 0 or 1, and a 41% risk in those with a risk score of 6 or 7.[1]

Table 1: Clinical Features Used to Calculate TIMI Risk Score[1]

One point is assigned for each of the following clinical features:

- age > 65 y
- ≥ 3 cardiac risk factors
- known coronary disease
- any ASA use within 7 d
- ≥ 2 episodes of angina within the last 24 h
- elevation in cardiac markers (troponin or CK-MB)
- ST segment deviation ≥ 0.5 mm on ECG

Therapeutic Choices (Figure 1)

The management of patients with NSTEMI or unstable angina has evolved significantly. Evidence from randomized clinical trials now strongly supports the use of the "invasive strategy"—coronary angiography followed if possible by revascularization with percutaneous coronary intervention (PCI, angioplasty) or bypass surgery in all high-risk patients. Patients are at high risk if they have one or more of the following: positive cardiac enzymes, ST segment changes, TIMI Risk Score ≥ 3, recurrent ischemic symptoms, heart failure, hemodynamic instability, sustained ventricular tachycardia or a prior revascularization procedure—coronary artery bypass graft (CABG) or PCI.[2]

Nonpharmacologic Choices

All patients admitted with NSTEMI or unstable angina should be placed on bedrest while ischemia is ongoing, then gradually mobilized when symptoms have stabilized. Use supplemental oxygen in patients with inadequate arterial oxygen saturation to keep the SaO_2 above 90%. Continuous ECG monitoring for potentially lethal arrhythmias and ST segment shifts (if available) is indicated in all high-risk patients.

Pharmacologic Choices (Table 2)

Nitrates

Initial attempts at symptom relief should involve the use of **nitroglycerin**, first with sublingual tablets or spray. Intravenous nitroglycerin is indicated in patients whose symptoms are not relieved promptly (i.e., within 15 to 20 minutes). Longer acting oral or topical nitrates can be used when patients are symptom-free, to help prevent recurrent episodes of ischemia. The use of sildenafil, tadalafil or vardenafil in the previous 24 hours or the presence of significant hypotension is a contraindication to the use of nitrates.

Beta-blockers and Calcium Channel Blockers

Start beta-blockers as soon as possible in all patients without contraindications (reactive airways disease, bradycardia, second- or third-degree heart block without a functioning pacemaker, hypotension). The dose should be titrated to a resting heart rate of 50 to 60 beats per minute (BPM). If anginal pain is ongoing at presentation, beta-blockers are initially administered intravenously followed by oral dosing.

Calcium channel blockers can be used to control ongoing symptoms of ischemia in patients who are receiving maximum tolerated doses of beta-blockers and adequate doses of nitrates. In addition, these agents are used in patients who cannot tolerate beta-blockers, and in those with variant angina (coronary spasm). Avoid immediate-release nifedipine because controlled trials suggest increased adverse outcomes.

Angiotensin Converting Enzyme (ACE) Inhibitors

ACE inhibitors reduce mortality in patients with recent myocardial infarction, left ventricular systolic dysfunction or clinical heart failure, diabetes and a broad spectrum of patients with high-risk chronic coronary artery disease.[3,4] Therefore, use these agents in all of these patient groups and in patients with hypertension not controlled with beta-blockers and nitrates.

Antiplatelet and Anticoagulation Therapy

ASA

ASA provides a striking benefit in patients with acute coronary syndromes. If patients with suspected UA/NSTEMI are not already receiving ASA, it should be initiated promptly and continued long term.

Thienopyridines

Clopidogrel is the preferred agent in this class due to its more rapid onset of action and better safety profile compared to ticlopidine. In the CURE (Clopidogrel in Unstable angina to prevent Recurrent ischemic Events) trial, clopidogrel (plus ASA) significantly reduced the incidence of major adverse cardiac events in ACS patients compared with ASA alone, and reduced the incidence of recurrent ischemia, an effect which was evident within a few hours.[5] The benefit of clopidogrel was consistent among patients regardless of TIMI Risk Score.[6] The major benefits were noted at 30 days, with small additional benefits observed over the subsequent treatment period (average eight months). In the CURE trial, there was an excess of both major and minor bleeding in the clopidogrel group, with an insignificant trend towards an increase in life-threatening bleeding. Bleeding risks increase with increasing aspirin dose.[7] Because of this risk, many hospitals with cardiac catheterization facilities do not initiate clopidogrel until it is clear that bypass surgery is not needed for appropriate revascularization. Clopidogrel should be held for a minimum of five days in patients scheduled for bypass surgery.[5,6]

Unfractionated Heparin (UFH) or Low Molecular Weight Heparins (LMWH)

Heparin is a key component in the successful management of patients with ACS. Studies of ASA with either UFH or LMWH have shown 50 to 60% relative reductions (absolute 3–3.5%) in the rate of death or MI in the first week.[8,9] UFH has important limitations due to poor bioavailability and significant variability in anticoagulant response. LMWH have the advantage of ease of administration, predictable anticoagulant response and lack of need for monitoring. Clinical trials have demonstrated the superiority of **enoxaparin** over UFH, but have shown neutral or unfavourable trends with other LMWH (**dalteparin** and **nadroparin**).[10,11,12,13] A direct comparison favoured enoxaparin over **tinzaparin**.[14] Enoxaparin is therefore the preferred agent in patients with UA/NSTEMI who do not have significant renal dysfunction (estimated creatinine clearance > 30 mL/min). In those with an estimated creatinine clearance ≤ 30 mL/min, UFH is appropriate.

Fondaparinux, a direct inhibitor of factor Xa, is as effective as enoxaparin in patients with non-ST segment elevation ACS, but is associated with a lower incidence of major bleeding according to the results of a large randomized trial.[15]

Glycoprotein IIb/IIIa Inhibitors

Numerous trials have demonstrated the efficacy of these agents in the treatment of high-risk patients with UA/NSTEMI undergoing coronary angiography and subsequent PCI. Clinical trials support the use of **eptifibatide** and **tirofiban** at the time of admission or immediately before PCI.[16,17,18,19,20] **Abciximab** is also effective, but its expense limits its use to the cardiac catheterization laboratory. The benefit of these agents is less clear for patients for whom an initial conservative management approach is planned. Patients receiving any of these agents must be carefully monitored for bleeding. However, the combined use of glycoprotein IIb/IIIa inhibitors and heparin does appear to be safe.[21] Thrombocytopenia is an unusual complication of treatment with these agents.

Therapeutic Tips

- The standard dose of **ASA** is 325 mg daily. This dose can be decreased to 80 mg in those patients receiving long-term clopidogrel.
- Discontinue **clopidogrel** five days prior to bypass surgery to decrease the risk of bleeding.

ST SEGMENT ELEVATION MYOCARDIAL INFARCTION (STEMI)

Patients with STEMI represent the extreme of the acute coronary syndrome spectrum, are considered to be a medical emergency and, therefore, require urgent assessment and treatment.

Goals of Therapy

- Decrease mortality and complications
- Reduce or contain infarct size
- Salvage functioning myocardium and prevent remodelling
- Re-establish patency of the infarct-related artery

Investigations

- Rapid, targeted history and physical examination, with particular attention to onset of symptoms, contraindications to use of thrombolytic agents and evidence of high-risk features (tachycardia, hypotension, congestive heart failure)
- ECG STAT, then every eight hours for the first 24 hours, then daily for 3 days. In addition, repeat the ECG with each recurrence of chest pain
- Baseline CK, CK-MB and troponin (Tn) STAT, then every eight hours for the first 24 hours. CK-MB and Tn do not need to be measured after enzymatic confirmation of the diagnosis.
- CBC to rule out the presence of anemia, baseline electrolytes, creatinine, fasting lipid profile and liver function tests
- Portable chest x-ray (CXR) STAT
- Echocardiography to assess LV function after stabilization and treatment. Echocardiography is also used emergently when there is suspicion of acute mechanical complications post-MI

Therapeutic Choices (Figure 2)

Nonpharmacologic Choices

Place all patients on bedrest with supplemental oxygen and continuous ECG monitoring. Begin gradual mobilization after stabilization provided there is no evidence of complications.

Primary Percutaneous Coronary Intervention (PCI)

Urgent coronary angiography with PCI is an excellent alternative to thrombolytics if appropriate high-volume cardiac catheterization facilities exist. Primary PCI is indicated in patients with contraindications to thrombolytic therapy and those with cardiogenic shock. In addition, it is preferred in patients over the age of 75 because of a higher risk of intracranial hemorrhage and higher overall early mortality seen with thrombolytic agents in this age group.[22,23,24]

Pharmacologic Choices (Table 2)

Thrombolytic Therapy

Thrombolytic therapy administered early in the course of STEMI substantially reduces mortality and morbidity, particularly if the patient presents within 6 hours of symptom onset. The benefit is present but less substantial if symptom onset is 6 to 12 hours prior to presentation, and the evidence is much less clear for presentation beyond 12 hours. The greatest absolute benefit is seen where the risk of mortality is highest (i.e., anterior MI, previous MI). **Streptokinase** is preferred in those over 75 years old. In other patients **alteplase (rt-PA), reteplase** or **tenecteplase** are generally preferred.

Heparin

Give intravenous unfractionated heparin to all STEMI patients receiving alteplase, tenecteplase or reteplase. **Enoxaparin** is an alternative, and has been shown to be superior to heparin in patients treated with tenecteplase, but must be used with caution in elderly patients or those with renal insufficiency (estimated ClCr < 30 mL/min) because of increased bleeding risks.[25] The indications for heparin after streptokinase are unclear, but its use can be considered in patients with an anterior MI, atrial fibrillation, heart failure or a history of embolism.

Beta-blockers

These agents are recommended in all STEMI patients without contraindications, and are particularly useful when sinus tachycardia and hypertension are present. They should be initiated once hemodynamic stability is achieved. Titrate doses to a resting heart rate of 50 to 60 BPM.

Calcium Channel Blockers

Calcium channel blockers are not recommended in patients with STEMI as they have been shown to increase morbidity and mortality.[26] They may be used *cautiously* for ischemia or for rate control in patients with atrial fibrillation if beta-blockers are contraindicated.

Nitroglycerin

Unlike NSTEMI or unstable angina, iv, oral or topical nitrates should be used only in the presence of persistent/recurrent ischemia, a large anterior MI, hypertension or heart failure.[27]

ACE Inhibitors

These are recommended for routine use in all patients post-STEMI without contraindications and should ideally be started within 24 hours of the event unless the patient is hypotensive (SBP < 100 mm Hg). Doses should be increased every 24 hours as blood pressure tolerates while in hospital and at one- to two-week intervals as outpatients. Based on the results of the HOPE trial, it is reasonable to continue an ACE inhibitor indefinitely even in those patients with preserved LV function.[4] An angiotensin receptor blocker should be used in STEMI patients who are intolerant of ACE inhibitors and have either clinical or radiological signs of heart failure or documented LV dysfunction.

Aldosterone Antagonists

Long-term use of an aldosterone antagonist (e.g., **spironolactone**, **eplerenone**), reduces morbidity and mortality in STEMI patients with clinical evidence of heart failure, LV ejection fraction < 40%, or both based on the results of two randomized trials.[28,29] Caution must be used in patients with renal insufficiency or pre-existing hyperkalemia, and in those receiving ACE inhibitors concomitantly.[28,29]

Clopidogrel

In patients with STEMI treated with fibrinolysis, clopidogrel increases patency of the affected vessel and decreases ischemic complications according to the results of two randomized trials, and should therefore be considered for routine use in these patients.[30,31]

Complications of STEMI

Recurrent or Ongoing Ischemia

Optimize anti-anginal therapy, and consider all patients with this problem for urgent coronary angiography and possible revascularization.

Heart Failure

Treat heart failure aggressively. In addition, consider angiography and possible revascularization in patients with depressed LV function after MI.

Arrhythmias

Asymptomatic premature ventricular contractions (PVCs) do not require therapy. Symptomatic ectopy may require therapy, usually with a beta-blocker. Class IC agents are contraindicated. Patients with sustained ventricular arrhythmias require investigation to rule out recurrent ischemia, and may require subsequent electrophysiologic assessment.[32] Consider urgent electrical or pharmacologic cardioversion in patients with atrial fibrillation causing ischemia or heart failure. Treat all patients with atrial fibrillation to control ventricular rate (usually with a beta-blocker or digoxin if there is concomitant heart failure), and consider oral anticoagulant therapy with warfarin.

Patients with an ejection fraction of < 30% one month post-MI or three months post-revascularization should be referred for automatic implantable cardioverter-defibrillator therapy (AICD).[33]

Pericarditis

Pericarditis, although uncommon, usually presents within 72 hours post-MI, and symptoms usually resolve within three or four days. Symptomatic pericarditis can be treated by increasing the dose of **ASA** to 650 mg QID for one to two weeks. If ASA is ineffective, a nonsteroidal anti-inflammatory drug (NSAID) or corticosteroid can be added. Discontinuation of anticoagulants is unnecessary if pericarditis occurs early post-infarction, but caution is urged if pericarditis presents weeks or months following MI (Dressler's syndrome) due to the risk of pericardial bleeding and tamponade.[34]

Mechanical Complications

These are devastating problems infrequently encountered post-MI. Ruptured papillary muscle (and severe mitral regurgitation), ventricular septal defects, or ventricular free wall rupture can present with acute cardiac arrest or cardiogenic shock. Patients should be considered for emergency angiography and surgical intervention, but even with urgent treatment the mortality rate associated with these conditions is very high.

Special Consideration: Clopidogrel in PCI

Pretreatment with clopidogrel prior to PCI reduced the risk of death, MI and repeat revascularization in the PCI-CURE substudy.[35] Therapy must be continued for at least one month post-procedure, particularly if a coronary stent is used. However, if drug-eluting stents are used, the duration of thienopyridine therapy must be extended due to delayed endothelialization and an increased risk of late stent thrombosis. For sirolimus-eluting (Cypher) stents, it is recommended that clopidogrel be continued for at least three months, whereas for paclitaxel-eluting (Taxus) stents, clopidogrel therapy is recommended for a minimum of six months.[36] For patients treated with PCI who receive a stent, any elective surgery should be postponed until after the course of clopidogrel is completed. If surgery cannot be postponed, continue clopidogrel throughout the perioperative period. Early discontinuation of clopidogrel results in a high risk of acute stent thrombosis with high morbidity and mortality.

Therapeutic Tips

- The goal for thrombolytic treatment is a door-to-needle time of 30 minutes or less.
- The goal for primary PCI is a door-to-dilatation time of 90 minutes or less.
- Careful attention to maximum pain relief is important.
- In patients with right ventricular infarcts:
  - avoid nitrates and diuretics
  - use fluids and inotropes to treat hypotension
- Administer beta-blockers early to all patients without contraindications, beginning with iv administration. Oral administration can follow soon thereafter. If blood pressure and heart rate allow, doses can be increased every 12 hours (every 24 hours for once-daily beta-blockers) until the patient has reached adequate beta-blockade.
- Start ACE inhibitors early. The choice of agent can depend on practitioner preference, hospital formulary or financial constraints for the individual patient.

- In smokers, the need to quit smoking should be reinforced early (i.e., within 24 hours) and frequently.
- Stool softeners are often used in the immediate post-MI period to prevent straining with bowel movements.
- Anxiolytics are often used on an as-needed basis in the immediate post-MI period.

Figure 1: **Early Management of UA/NSTEMI**

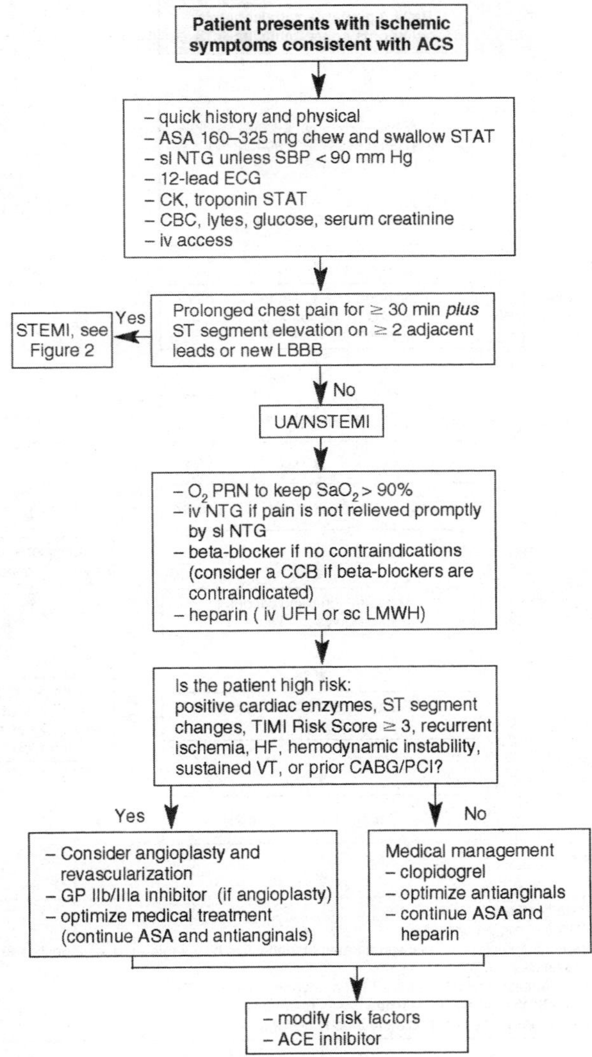

Abbreviations: ACS = acute coronary syndrome; CBC = complete blood count; CK = creatine kinase; CCB = calcium channel blocker; NTG = nitroglycerin; UA = unstable angina; STEMI = ST segment elevation myocardial infarction; UFH = unfractionated heparin; LMWH = low molecular weight heparins; TIMI = Thrombolysis in Myocardial Infarction; HF = heart failure; VT = ventricular tachycardia; PCI = percutaneous coronary intervention; CABG = coronary artery bypass graft; DVT = deep vein thrombosis; LBBB = left bundle branch block.

Figure 2: **Early Management of STEMI**

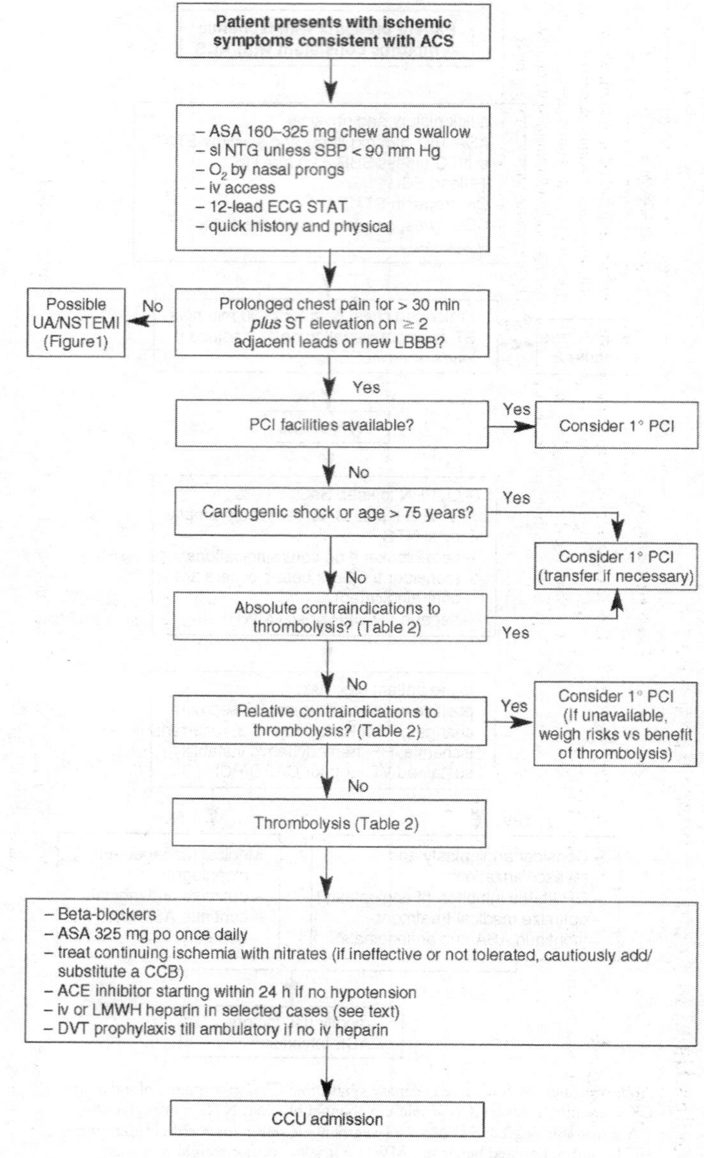

Table 2: **Drugs Used in Acute Coronary Syndromes**

Class	Drug	Dose	Adverse Effects	Drug Interactions	Cost[a]
$Beta_1$-adrenergic Antagonists, selective with ISA	*acebutolol* Rhotral, Sectral, generics	Initial: 100–200 mg BID Usual: 400 mg BID	Bronchospasm, HF, sleep disturbances, dizziness, fatigue, anorexia, nausea, AV block, bradycardia, claudication, Raynaud's, lethargy, drowsiness.	Enhanced cardiodepressant effect with calcium channel blockers, antiarrhythmics, anesthetics. Increased bradycardia with digoxin. Hypertension with alpha-agonists.	$$
$Beta_1$-adrenergic Antagonists, selective without ISA	*atenolol* Tenormin, generics	Initial: 50 mg/day Usual: 100 mg/day	See acebutolol.	See acebutolol.	$
	metoprolol Betaloc, Lopresor, generics	Initial: 50 mg po BID iv: 5 mg over 1–2 min repeat Q5 min (max 15 mg) Usual: 100 mg po BID po can be started 15 min after iv	See acebutolol.	See acebutolol.	$
$Beta_1$-adrenergic Antagonists, nonselective without ISA	*nadolol* generics	Initial: 40–80 mg/day Usual: 120 mg/day	See acebutolol.	See acebutolol.	$
	propranolol generics	Initial: 40 mg BID/TID Usual: 40 mg QID	See acebutolol.	See acebutolol.	$

(cont'd)

Table 2: **Drugs Used in Acute Coronary Syndromes** *(cont'd)*

Class	Drug	Dose	Adverse Effects	Drug Interactions	Cost[a]
	timolol generics	Initial: 5–10 mg BID Usual: 10 mg BID	See acebutolol.	See acebutolol.	$
Calcium Channel Blockers	*amlodipine* Norvasc	5–10 mg/day	Hypotension, flushing, marked peripheral edema.		$$–$$$
	diltiazem Cardizem CD & SR, Tiazac, Tiazac XC, generics	120–360 mg/day Give SR BID; CD and XC once daily	Bradycardia, heart block, edema, hypotension.	Additive effect with β-blockers, digoxin, amiodarone. Monitor for excessive bradycardia.	$–$$$
	verapamil Covera HS, Isoptin SR, generics	180–480 mg/day Give IR formulations TID; SR BID; Covera-HS once daily	Bradycardia, heart block, hypotension, constipation, flushing, edema.	See diltiazem.	$-$$$
Nitrates	*isosorbide dinitrate, IR* generics	Initial: 30–90 mg/day IR: give TID (allow a 12 h nitrate-free period)	Headache (up to 50%; tolerance may develop), tachycardia, palpitation, hypotension, syncope (rare), dizziness, nausea, flushing, weakness.	Potential hypotensive effect with vasodilators. Contraindicated with recent (< 24 h) use of sildenafil, tadalafil or vardenafil; use with caution when hypotension present.	$
	isosorbide dinitrate, SR Cedocard SR	SR: Give two daily doses 6 h apart	See isosorbide dinitrate, IR.	See isosorbide dinitrate, IR.	$
	isosorbide-5-mononitrate Imdur	30–60 mg once daily	See isosorbide dinitrate, IR.	See isosorbide dinitrate, IR.	$

Class	Drug	Dose	Adverse Effects	Drug Interactions	Cost[a]
	nitroglycerin, intravenous generics	Initial: 10–150 µg/min iv (titrate to symptoms and blood pressure)	Hemodynamic monitoring is required for iv nitroglycerin. See isosorbide dinitrate, IR.	See isosorbide dinitrate, IR.	$ [b]
	nitroglycerin transdermal Minitran, Nitro-Dur, Transderm-Nitro, Trinipatch	0.2–0.8 mg/h patch applied daily for 10–12 h	See isosorbide dinitrate, IR.. Contact dermatitis.	See isosorbide dinitrate, IR.	$-$$
ACE Inhibitors	*captopril* Capoten, generics	Initial: 6.25 mg Q8H Target: 37.5 mg Q8H	Proteinuria (1%), neutropenia (rare), rash, angioedema, hypotension, alterations in taste, nausea, anorexia, dizziness, dry cough (common). Caution in patients with renovascular hypertension, renal insufficiency, hyperkalemia, angioedema.	↑ risk of neutropenia with antiarrhythmics, allopurinol, corticosteroids. Hyperkalemia with spironolactone, triamterene, amiloride. Hypotension with diuretics. Avoid concurrent therapy with lithium.	$$
	cilazapril Inhibace, generics	Initial: 0.5 mg once daily Target: 2.5 mg once daily	See captopril.	See captopril.	$
	enalapril Vasotec, generics	Initial: 2.5 mg BID Target: 10 mg BID	See captopril.	See captopril.	$$$
	fosinopril Monopril, generics	Initial: 5 mg once daily Target: 10 mg once daily	See captopril.	See captopril.	$
	lisinopril Zestril, Prinivil, generics	Initial: 2.5 mg once daily Target: 20 mg once daily	See captopril.	See captopril.	$
	quinapril Accupril	Initial: 5 mg once daily Target: 15 mg once daily	See captopril.	See captopril.	$

(cont'd)

Table 2: **Drugs Used in Acute Coronary Syndromes** *(cont'd)*

Class	Drug	Dose	Adverse Effects	Drug Interactions	Cost[a]
	ramipril Altace	Initial: 2.5 mg once daily Target: 5 mg BID or 10 mg once daily	See captopril.	See captopril.	$$
Aldosterone Antagonists	*spironolactone* Aldactone, generics	Initial: 12.5 mg daily Target 25–50 mg daily	Rash, urticaria, gynecomastia, nausea, vomiting, diarrhea, confusion, hyperkalemia, agranulocytosis, SLE.	Hyperkalemia with ACE inhibitors, digoxin, NSAIDs.	$
Antiplatelet Agents	*ASA* Aspirin,Bufferin, Coated Aspirin, Entrophen, generics	80–325 mg/day	Gastritis, gastric/duodenal ulceration (rarely bronchospasm). Nausea, vomiting, GI hemorrhage, tinnitus, vertigo, hypersensitivity.	Heparin, warfarin (bleeding risk with heparin is low); other NSAIDs.	$
	clopidogrel Plavix	Loading dose pre-PCI or STEMI: 300–600 mg, then 75 mg once daily	Bleeding, rash, purpura. Similar tolerability to ASA.	Caution with NSAIDs.	$$$$
	ticlopidine Ticlid, generics	250 mg BID	Diarrhea, rash, neutropenia, purpura. Measure neutrophils Q2 wk × 3 mo initially.	Caution with NSAIDs. May ↑ theophylline levels.	$$
Heparin, Unfractionated	*heparin sodium* Hepalean, Heparin Leo, Heparin Sodium Injection	75 U/kg, then 1250 U/h. Adjust to maintain aPTT at 1.5–2 × control. First aPTT 4 h after bolus Post-lytic: bolus 60 U/kg then 1200 U/hr. Adjust to maintain aPTT at 1.5–2 × control. First aPTT 6 h after bolus	Bleeding, thrombocytopenia.	ASA, warfarin (bleeding risk with ASA is low); aPTT response may be blunted with concurrent iv nitroglycerin (controversial).	$[b]

Class	Drug	Dose	Adverse Effects	Drug Interactions	Cost[a]
Heparins, Low Molecular Weight	*dalteparin* Fragmin	20 IU/kg sc BID Max: 10 000 IU/dose	Hematoma at injection site, bleeding, thrombocytopenia; caution if ClCr < 30 mL/min).	ASA, warfarin (bleeding risk with ASA is low).	\$\$[b]
	enoxaparin Lovenox	1 mg/kg sc BID Max:10 000 IU/dose	See dalteparin. Caution in elderly patients and those with renal insufficiency. Preferred LMWH in ACS.	See dalteparin.	\$\$[b]
Thrombolytics	*alteplase* Activase rt-PA	Bolus: 15 mg iv, then 0.75 mg/kg × 30 min (max 50 mg), then 0.50 mg/kg × 60 min (max 35 mg) Max dose 100 mg Start heparin with infusion	Bleeding (can be fatal). Absolute contraindications: previous intracranial hemorrhage; known malignant intracranial neoplasm, ischemic stroke within 3 mo EXCEPT acute stroke within 3 h; suspected aortic dissection; active bleeding or bleeding diathesis (excluding menses); significant closed head or facial trauma within 3 mo. Relative contraindications: history of chronic severe, poorly controlled HTN, severe uncontrolled HTN(BP > 180/110 mm Hg)[c]; prior CVA greater than 3 mo or known intracerebral pathology not covered above; traumatic or prolonged (> 10 min) CPR or major surgery (< 3 wk); noncompressible venous punctures; recent (2–4 wk) internal bleeding;		\$2746 (100 mg vial) [b]

(cont'd)

Table 2: **Drugs Used in Acute Coronary Syndromes** *(cont'd)*

Class	Drug	Dose	Adverse Effects	Drug Interactions	Cost[a]
			pregnancy; active peptic ulcer; current use of anticoagulants.		
	reteplase Retavase	Bolus: 10 U iv, then 10 U iv 30 min later. Give each bolus over ≤ 2 min. Start heparin.	See alteplase.		\$1900 (2 × 10 unit vials)[b]
	streptokinase Streptase	1.5 million units iv over 1 h	See alteplase.		\$630 (1.5 MU vial)[b]
	tenecteplase TNKase	< 60 kg: 30 mg iv × 1 60–69 kg: 35 mg iv × 1 70–79 kg: 40 mg iv × 1 80–89 kg: 45 mg iv × 1 ≥ 90 kg: 50 mg iv × 1 Given as iv bolus over 5 s	See alteplase.		\$2897 (50 mg vial)[b]
Glycoprotein IIb/IIIa Inhibitors	*eptifibatide* Integrilin	Bolus: 180 μg/kg over 1–2 min, then 2 μg/kg/min Max: 15 mg/h ClCr < 50 mL/min: infuse at 1 μg/kg/min	Bleeding (risk of serious bleeding appears to be low), primarily at puncture sites. Thrombocytopenia. Allergic reactions.	Use caution with other drugs that affect hemostasis.	\$\$\$\$[b]

Class	Drug	Dose	Adverse Effects	Drug Interactions	Cost[a]
	tirofiban Aggrastat	Bolus: 0.4 μg/kg/min then 0.1 μg/kg/min × 48–72 h ClCr < 30 mL/min: Bolus 0.2 μg/kg/min, then 0.05 μg/kg/min × 72 h	See eptifibatide.	See eptifibatide.	$$$$[b]

[a] Cost of 30-day supply, includes drug cost only except where noted.
[b] Cost of average 1-day supply.
[c] Could be an absolute contraindication in low-risk patients with STEMI.
Dosage adjustment may be required in renal impairment; see Appendix I.
Abbreviations: aPTT = activated partial thromboplastin time; HF = heart failure; CVA = cerebrovascular accident; DBP = diastolic blood pressure; GI = gastrointestinal; GU = genitourinary; HTN = hypertension; IR = immediate-release; ISA = intrinsic sympathomimetic activity; NSAIDs = nonsteroidal anti-inflammatory drugs; NTG = nitroglycerin; SBP = systolic blood pressure; SCr = serum creatinine; SR = slow-release; TTP = thrombotic thrombocytopenic purpura; U = units
Legend: $ < $25 $-$$ < $25–50 $$ $25–50 $-$$$ < $25–75 $$-$$$ $25–75 $$$ $50–75 $$$$ $75–100

Suggested Readings

Boersma E, Harrington RA, Moliterno DJ et al. Platelet glycoprotein IIb/IIIa inhibitors in acute coronary syndromes: a meta-analysis of all major randomised clinical trials. *Lancet* 2002;359(9302):189-98.

Braunwald E, Antman EM, Beasley JW et al. ACC/AHA guideline update for the management of patients with unstable angina and non-ST-segment elevation myocardial infarction—2002: summary article: a report of the American College of Cardiology/American Heart Association Task Force on Practice Guidelines (Committee on the Management of Patients With Unstable Angina). *Circulation* 2002;106(14):1893-900.

Ryan TJ, Antman EM, Brooks NH et al. 1999 update: ACC/AHA guidelines for the management of patients with acute myocardial infarction. A report of the American College of Cardiology/American Heart Association Task Force on Practice Guidelines (Committee on Management of Acute Myocardial Infarction). *J Am Coll Cardiol* 1999;34(3):890-911.

References

1. Antman EM, Cohen M, Bernink PJ et al. The TIMI risk score for unstable angina/non-ST elevation MI: a method for prognostication and therapeutic decision making. *JAMA* 2000;284(7):835-42.
2. Cannon CP, Weintraub WS, Demopoulos LA et al. Comparison of early invasive and conservative strategies in patients with unstable coronary syndromes treated with the glycoprotein IIb/IIIa inhibitor tirofiban. *N Engl J Med* 2001;344(25):1879-87.
3. [No authors listed]. Indications for ACE inhibitors in the early treatment of acute myocardial infarction: systematic overview of individual data from 100,000 patients in randomized trials. ACE Inhibitor Myocardial Infarction Collaborative Group. *Circulation* 1998;97(22):2202-12.
4. Yusuf S, Sleight P, Pogue J et al. Effects of an angiotensin-converting-enzyme inhibitor, ramipril, on cardiovascular events in high-risk patients. The Heart Outcomes Prevention Evaluation Study Investigators. *N Engl J Med* 2000;342(3):145-53.
5. Yusuf S, Zhao F, Mehta SR et al. Effects of clopidogrel in addition to aspirin in patients with acute coronary syndromes without ST-segment elevation. *N Engl J Med* 2001;345(7):494-502.
6. Budaj A, Yusuf S, Mehta SR et al. Benefit of clopidogrel in patients with acute coronary syndromes without ST-segment elevation in various risk groups. *Circulation* 2002;106(13):1622-6.
7. Mehta SR, Yusuf S, Peters RJ et al. Effects of pretreatment with clopidogrel and aspirin followed by long-term therapy in patients undergoing percutaneous coronary intervention: the PCI-CURE study. *Lancet* 2001;358(9281):527-33.
8. Holdright D, Patel D, Cunningham D et al. Comparison of the effect of heparin and aspirin versus aspirin alone on transient myocardial ischemia and in-hospital prognosis in patients with unstable angina. *J Am Coll Cardiol* 1994;24(1):39-45.
9. Theroux P, Ouimet H, McCans J et al. Aspirin, heparin, or both to treat acute unstable angina. *N Engl J Med* 1988;319(17):1105-11.
10. [No authors listed]. Comparison of two treatment durations (6 days and 14 days) of a low molecular weight heparin with a 6-day treatment of unfractionated heparin in the initial management of unstable angina or non-Q wave myocardial infarction: FRAX.I.S. (FRAxiparine in Ischaemic Syndrome). *Eur Heart J* 1999;20(21):1553-62.
11. Antman EM, McCabe CH, Gurfinkel EP et al. Enoxaparin prevents death and cardiac ischemic events in unstable angina/non-Q-wave myocardial infarction. Results of the thrombolysis in myocardial infarction (TIMI) 11B trial. *Circulation* 1999;100(15):1593-601.
12. Cohen M, Demers C, Gurfinkel EP et al. A comparison of low-molecular-weight heparin with unfractionated heparin for unstable coronary artery disease. Efficacy and Safety of Subcutaneous Enoxaparin in Non-Q-Wave Coronary Events Study Group. *N Engl J Med* 1997;337(7):447-52.
13. Klein W, Buchwald A, Hillis SE et al. Comparison of low-molecular-weight heparin with unfractionated heparin acutely and with placebo for 6 weeks in the management of unstable coronary artery disease. Fragmin in unstable coronary artery disease study (FRIC). *Circulation* 1997;96(1):61-8.
14. Michalis LK, Katsouras CS, Papamichael N et al. Enoxaparin versus tinzaparin in non-ST-segment elevation acute coronary syndromes: the EVET trial. *Am Heart J* 2003;146(2):304-10.

15. Yusuf S, Mehta SR, Chrolavicius S et al. Comparison of fondaparinux and enoxaparin in acute coronary syndromes. *N Engl J Med* 2006;354(14):1464-76.
16. [No authors listed]. A comparison of aspirin plus tirofiban with aspirin plus heparin for unstable angina. Platelet Receptor Inhibition in Ischemic Syndrome Management (PRISM) Study Investigators. *N Engl J Med* 1998;338(21):1498-505.
17. [No authors listed]. Inhibition of the platelet glycoprotein IIb/IIIa receptor with tirofiban in unstable angina and non-Q-wave myocardial infarction. Platelet Receptor Inhibition in Ischemic Syndrome Management in Patients Limited by Unstable Signs and Symptoms (PRISM-PLUS) Study Investigators. *N Engl J Med* 1998;338(21):1488-97.
18. Labinaz M, Kilaru R, Pieper K et al. Outcomes of patients with acute coronary syndromes and prior coronary artery bypass grafting: results from the platelet glycoprotein IIb/IIIa in unstable angina: receptor suppression using integrilin therapy (PURSUIT) trial. *Circulation* 2002;105(3):322-7.
19. Moliterno DJ, Yakubov SJ, DiBattiste PM et al. Outcomes at 6 months for the direct comparison of tirofiban and abciximab during percutaneous coronary revascularisation with stent placement: the TARGET follow-up study. *Lancet* 2002;360(9330):355-60.
20. O'Shea JC, Hafley GE, Greenberg S et al. Platelet glycoprotein IIb/IIIa integrin blockade with eptifibatide in coronary stent intervention: the ESPRIT trial: a randomized controlled trial. *JAMA* 2001;285(19):2468-73.
21. Braunwald E, Antman EM, Beasley JW et al. ACC/AHA guidelines for the management of patients with unstable angina and non-ST-segment elevation myocardial infarction. A report of the American College of Cardiology/American Heart Association Task Force on Practice Guidelines (Committee on the Management of Patients With Unstable Angina). *J Am Coll Cardiol* 2000;36(3):970-1062.
22. Grines CL, Browne KF, Marco J et al. A comparison of immediate angioplasty with thrombolytic therapy for acute myocardial infarction. The Primary Angioplasty in Myocardial Infarction Study Group. *N Engl J Med* 1993;328(10):673-9.
23. Hochman JS, Sleeper LA, White HD et al. One-year survival following early revascularization for cardiogenic shock. *JAMA* 2001;285(2):190-2.
24. Thiemann DR, Coresh J, Schulman SP et al. Lack of benefit for intravenous thrombolysis in patients with myocardial infarction who are older than 75 years. *Circulation* 2000;101(19):2239-46.
25. Antman EM, Morrow DA, McCabe CH et al. Enoxaparin versus unfractionated heparin with fibrinolysis for ST-elevation myocardial infarction. *N Engl J Med* 2006;354(14):1477-88.
26. Yusuf S, Held P, Furberg C. Update of effects of calcium antagonists in myocardial infarction or angina in light of the second Danish Verapamil Infarction Trial (DAVIT-II) and other recent studies. *Am J Cardiol* 1991;67(15):1295-7.
27. Yusuf S, Collins R, MacMahon S et al. Effect of intravenous nitrates on mortality in acute myocardial infarction: an overview of the randomised trials. *Lancet* 1988;1(8594):1088-92.
28. Pitt B, Zannad F, Remme WJ et al. The effect of spironolactone on morbidity and mortality in patients with severe heart failure. Randomized Aldactone Evaluation Study Investigators. *N Engl J Med* 1999;341(10):709-17.
29. Pitt B, Remme W, Zannad F et al. Eplerenone, a selective aldosterone blocker, in patients with left ventricular dysfunction after myocardial infarction. *N Engl J Med* 2003;348(14):1309-21.
30. Chen ZM, Jiang LX, Chen YP et al. Addition of clopidogrel to aspirin in 45,852 patients with acute myocardial infarction: randomised placebo-controlled trial. *Lancet* 2005;366(9497):1607-21.
31. Sabatine MS, Cannon CP, Gibson CM et al. Addition of clopidogrel to aspirin and fibrinolytic therapy for myocardial infarction with ST-segment elevation. *N Engl J Med* 2005;352(12):1179-89.
32. Moss AJ, Zareba W, Hall WJ et al. Prophylactic implantation of a defibrillator in patients with myocardial infarction and reduced ejection fraction. *N Engl J Med* 2002;346(12):877-83.
33. Gregoratos G, Abrams J, Epstein AE et al. ACC/AHA/NASPE 2002 guideline update for implantation of cardiac pacemakers and antiarrhythmia devices: summary article: a report of the American College of Cardiology/American Heart Association Task Force on Practice Guidelines (ACC/AHA/NASPE Committee to Update the 1998 Pacemaker Guidelines). *Circulation* 2002;106(16):2145-61.
34. Berman J, Haffajee CI, Alpert JS. Therapy of symptomatic pericarditis after myocardial infarction: retrospective and prospective studies of aspirin, indomethacin, prednisone, and spontaneous resolution. *Am Heart J* 1981;101(6):750-3.
35. Mehta SR, Yusuf S, Peters RJ et al. Effects of pretreatment with clopidogrel and aspirin followed by long-term therapy in patients undergoing percutaneous coronary intervention: the PCI-CURE study. *Lancet* 2001;358(9281):527-33.
36. Popma JJ, Berger P, Ohman EM et al. Antithrombotic therapy during percutaneous coronary intervention: the Seventh ACCP Conference on Antithrombotic and Thrombolytic Therapy. *Chest* 2004;126(3 Suppl):576S-599S.

CHAPTER 35
Post-myocardial Infarction

William L. Williams, MDCM, FRCPC

About 70% of patients presenting with myocardial infarction (MI) qualify for acute reperfusion by thrombolysis or primary coronary angioplasty.[1] The reperfused patient with an aborted MI presents a particular challenge with respect to recurrent ischemic complications. Reperfusion therapy has reduced 30-day mortality from 10% to between 3 and 4% and improved overall prognosis.[2] The prognosis of the post-MI patient depends on the interaction between residual left ventricular dysfunction, the potential for recurrent ischemia and the risk of arrhythmia (Table 1).[3] Older patients with comorbid conditions such as diabetes mellitus or renal failure have worse outcomes. Patients who receive timely reperfusion therapy with thrombolysis or primary angioplasty enjoy a much better prognosis than those treated conservatively.[1]

Table 1: Investigation and Therapy of the Post-Infarction Patient to Improve Prognosis

Factor Affecting Prognosis	Investigation	Therapy
Left Ventricular Dysfunction	Ejection fraction: echocardiogram, gated nuclear or contrast ventriculogram	Beta-blockers, ACE inhibitors, ARBs, warfarin for LV thrombus or atrial fibrillation
Ischemia	Low-risk outpatients post-thrombolysis: physiologic stress test using exercise, dipyridamole or dobutamine with ECG; nuclear scintigraphy or echocardiographic wall motion assessment. Perform coronary angiography if the result is abnormal High-risk patients: coronary angiography	Beta-blockers, statins, ACE inhibitors, ARBs, antiplatelet agents
Arrhythmia	Holter monitor, event recorder, implantable arrhythmia detector	Beta-blockers, possibly amiodarone or ICD

Abbreviations: ACE inhibitor = angiotensin converting enzyme inhibitor; ARB = angiotensin receptor blocker; ICD = implantable cardioverter/defibrillator; LV = left ventricle.

Cardiovascular disease in women remains the leading cause of death and accounts for more than half of all deaths among women over the age of 50 years. Sex differences are apparent with respect to prevalence, presentation, treatment and outcome. Some risk factors, for example diabetes mellitus, appear to be more malignant in women than in men. Mortality rates in men have been declining, while those in women have remained stable.[4]

Historically, women have been under-represented in clinical trials, perhaps due to exclusion with advanced age and comorbidities. This has led to a knowledge gap whereby little is known about why cardiovascular disease affects women differently from men.

Investigation and treatment of patients after myocardial infarction should be gender neutral as the vast majority of post-MI interventions benefit patients of both sexes.[4]

Goals of Therapy

- Establish a risk profile
- Prevent death and prevent or delay recurrent events (MI, heart failure and angina)
- Retard progression of coronary disease
- Return patient to a meaningful quality of life
- Target modifiable risk factors that are responsible for 90% of risk

Investigations

A simple algorithm for evaluating post-infarction patients who have been treated with or without fibrinolysis is presented in Figure 1. The higher the risk, the more likely the patient will benefit from an invasive strategy.[5] Identifying patients at high risk begins with an assessment of readily accessible clinical predictors.

- Predictors of early recurrent events (i.e, one to six months post-MI) include:[6]
  - recurrent ischemia or angina with an ST-segment shift
  - bigger infarction as evidenced by: pulmonary congestion, hypotension, tachycardia, higher Killip class (Table 2), azotemia

Table 2: **The Killip Classification**

Killip Class	Patient Characteristics
I	No clinical signs of heart failure
II	Mild heart failure, rales, elevated jugular venous pulse (SBP ≥ 90 mm Hg)
III	Frank pulmonary edema (SBP ≥ 90 mm Hg)
IV	Cardiogenic shock (SBP < 90 mm Hg)

- Predictors of late recurrent events (i.e., one to two years post-MI):[6]
  - residual left ventricular ejection fraction < 30%
  - older age and comorbidity (diabetes, renal failure, other vascular disease)
  - ventricular irritability, as evidenced by resuscitated VF or sustained or nonsustained VT, especially in patients with low ejection fraction

An important determinant of prognosis after MI is left ventricular dysfunction, which is reflected by the left ventricular ejection fraction (LVEF). LVEF can be measured by echocardiography or inferred from clinical signs present at the time of infarction such as pulmonary congestion, resting tachycardia, hypotension, new bundle branch block or recurrent arrhythmia. The extent of the current of injury pattern on ECG and the degree of enzyme release also reflect infarct size. If a low LVEF is suspected (< 40%), refer the patient to a tertiary care centre for further investigation. Otherwise, smaller centres without access to echocardiography can perform a modified treadmill test prior to discharge.

Indications for post-infarction coronary arteriography sanctioned by current guidelines are listed in Table 3. However, in many centres most patients treated with thrombolytics also visit the angiography suite before hospital discharge,[7] as the prognosis is improved among those with demonstrable ischemia.[8]

A decision algorithm for the unique situation presented by post-MI patients following primary angioplasty is illustrated in Figure 2.

Table 3: **Evidence-based Indications for Post-infarction Coronary Angiography[4]**

Spontaneous or provocable ischemia, especially when present after fibrinolysis
LV dysfunction/LVEF ≤ 40%
Hemodynamic instability
Prior repair of a mechanical complication
Malignant ventricular arrhythmia
Patients with non-ST-segment elevation MI

Abbreviations: LV = left ventricle; LVEF = LV ejection fraction.

Select patients may be investigated for arrhythmia (Holter monitor, event recorder, implantable arrhythmia detector); however, this is not routinely recommended.[4]

Therapeutic Choices

Vascular inflammation contributes to the pathogenesis of plaque rupture. Thus agents with anti-inflammatory and antithrombotic properties now have a well-established role in the management of the post-MI patient.

Comprehensive management of the post-MI patient should include treatment of hypertension, dyslipidemia and diabetes mellitus. Smoking cessation decreases the relative risk of death and re-infarction by 50% in patients with MI.[9] The rate of re-infarction and death decreased from 16 to 6% during two years of observation among men who succeeded in stopping smoking.[10] Weight loss and physical activity are also important components of secondary prevention of MI.

Nonpharmacologic Choices

- Essential elements of cardiac rehabilitation are provided in Figure 3.
- Weight loss is indicated if the patient's BMI is > 25 or the waist circumference is > 100 cm in men or > 90 cm in women. The goal is a sustained 5 to 10% decrease in body weight.[9] Nutritional counselling is beneficial for patients attempting to lose weight.[9]
- Regular exercise with an individual prescription that accounts for age, obesity, level of fitness and biomechanical capability. Generally, the goal of burning off 1000 kcal/week can be attained by engaging in 30–45 minutes of moderate aerobic activity three or four times per week.[9]
- Revascularization is indicated in select patients (Figure 1 and Figure 2).
- An implantable cardioverter/defibrillator may be indicated in select patients.

Pharmacologic Choices

Among high-risk patients, antiplatelet agents, beta-blockers, ACE inhibitors and lipid-lowering therapies independently reduce the incidence of vascular events by approximately 25% (Table 4).[11] An overview of individual agents is provided in Table 6.

Table 4: Potential Cumulative Impact of Four Treatments for Secondary Prevention of Cardiovascular Events

	Relative Risk Reduction	2-year Event Rate (death, MI or stroke)
None	—	8%
ASA	25%	6%
Beta-blocker	25%	4.5%
Lipid lowering (↓ LDL-C by 1.5 mmol/L)	30%	3%
ACE inhibitor	25%	2.3%
Cumulative relative risk reduction if all four drugs are used is about 75%		
To calculate the cumulative risk reduction a multiplicative scale was used. For example, two interventions each reducing the risk of an event by 30% would be expected to have about a 50% relative risk reduction (1–[0.7 × 0.7]). No interactions in treatment effects are observed in trials, suggesting that the proportionate risk reduction of a specific drug in the presence or absence of other effective interventions would be expected to be similar. Smoking cessation lowers the risk of recurrent MI by about half after two years. In a smoker with vascular disease, quitting smoking and the use of the four preventive strategies could theoretically have a large potential benefit (approximately 80% relative risk reduction)		

Reprinted from The Lancet. Volume 360(9326). Yusuf S. Two decades of progress in preventing vascular disease. *Lancet* pages 2-3. Copyright 2002. With permission from Elsevier.

Antiplatelet Agents[12,13,14,15]

Antiplatelet agents are effective in preventing vascular events, including nonfatal MI and death, in post-MI patients.[5,16] **ASA** is the antiplatelet agent of choice due to its effectiveness and low cost, and is recommended as chronic therapy in all CAD patients without contraindications, including those who are post-MI. Low doses (80 to 325 mg daily) are usually well tolerated.

Clopidogrel is recommended in patients who have contraindications to or cannot tolerate ASA. Acute and long-term outcomes in patients treated conservatively or with thrombolysis are improved by clopidogrel.[17] Clopidogrel is essential therapy for those undergoing stent deployment. When used with ASA, clopidogrel has been effective in improving coronary patency and reducing the risk of infarction or death among those with unstable angina, ST-segment elevation MI treated with thrombolytics[18] and after stent deployment. When drug-eluting stents are used according to the approved indications, it is recommended that clopidogrel be continued for at least one year after deployment; when these devices are used in more complex, off-label settings, it is recommended that clopidogrel be continued indefinitely.[19]

Beta-Blockers[20,21,22]

Beta-blockers reduce cardiovascular mortality and re-infarction rates, and increase the probability of long-term survival by up to 40%.[5] In the absence of contraindications, these drugs are recommended in all patients post-MI including those with non-ST-segment elevation MI (NSTEMI) and those receiving thrombolytic therapy or primary angioplasty (Figure 2). They should be started within a few days of MI, if not earlier, and therapy should be continued indefinitely.[5] Beta-blockers should be avoided among patients with hypotension, bradycardia and active heart failure.

Higher-risk patients with reduced LV function, especially when associated with heart failure, receive the greatest benefit from beta-blockers provided they can be closely monitored. As a class, all beta-blockers that lower resting heart rate improve outcome. Moreover, this benefit extends to those already on ACE inhibitors.

Beta-blockers are underused in the post-MI population,[5] with less than half of patients receiving long-term therapy. However, the benefit of therapy with these drugs outweighs the risk in patients with type 1 diabetes mellitus, chronic obstructive pulmonary disease (COPD), severe peripheral vascular disease, a PR interval > 0.24 sec and moderate or severe heart failure (Figure 2).[5] Low-dose beta-blockers may be safely administered in some patients with a history of asthma. The appropriate use of beta-blockers after MI is illustrated in Figure 4.

ACE Inhibitors[23,24,25]

ACE inhibitors improve heart failure, reduce mortality and may reduce the likelihood of a recurrent MI.[5] These agents have greater relative and absolute benefits among high-risk patients with LV dysfunction or pulmonary congestion. Start ACE inhibitors early in all patients without contraindications post-STEMI. Long term treatment with ACE inhibitors is recommended for patients with STEMI, with the greatest benefit conferred among the higher-risk subgroup with previous myocardial infarction, heart failure, depressed LVEF and tachycardia.[5] Among patients with evidence of atherosclerosis or multiple risk factors, chronic use of an ACE inhibitor reduces the risk of MI.[25]

Angiotensin Receptor Blockers

Angiotensin receptor blockers (ARBs) have similar benefits to ACE inhibitors. A large randomized trial demonstrated equivalence between the ACE inhibitor captopril and the ARB valsartan in MI patients with heart failure and LV dysfunction.[26] There was no advantage of combined therapy with captopril and valsartan. ARBs may be used instead of ACE inhibitors in patients who do not tolerate the latter due to cough or angioedema. Data are accumulating to suggest that ARBs may be used in lieu of ACE inhibitors as primary therapy, especially among patients with heart failure or an LVEF < 40%.[5]

HMG CoA Reductase Inhibitors (Statins)

There is a linear relationship between LDL-C levels and cardiovascular risk. Lipid-lowering therapy to achieve a 1 mmol/L decrease in LDL-C reduces the absolute risk by 1% and relative risk by 20% over five years.[27] The pleiotropic benefits of statin therapy may extend beyond mere lipid lowering.[28] Aggressive lipid lowering not only decreases the atherosclerotic burden, but may reduce coronary events by stabilizing fragile coronary plaques.[29,30]

Recommended targets for LDL-C have become progressively lower as the safety and efficacy of cholesterol-lowering treatment have become established. Among high-risk patients, attainment of an LDL-C < 2 mmol/L provides optimal benefits.[31] Lipid-lowering therapy should be considered for most individuals with an LDL-C of 5 mmol/L or a total cholesterol to high-density lipoprotein cholesterol ratio (TC:HDL-C) of 6.0.[31] Attainment of more aggressive targets may require more intensive treatment with, for example, atorvastatin 80 mg/day[32] or rosuvastatin 40 mg/day.

Only 1% of patients discontinue therapy due to muscle discomfort, and there is no increase in myopathy with more aggressive therapy.[31]

A small minority of patients may require additional therapy with an agent that inhibits cholesterol absorption (i.e., ezetimibe or a bile acid sequestrant such as cholestyramine).

Recommendations from the Canadian Cardiovascular Society Guidelines are categorized by cardiovascular risk (Table 5).[31] Starting a statin prior to discharge after an acute MI improves both early and late outcomes. The benefit is independent of the lipid level at the start of treatment.[29,33]

Table 5: Canadian Cardiovascular Society 2006 Guidelines for Lipid-lowering Treatment

Risk Level	10-year CAD Risk	Recommendations
High	≥ 20%	Primary treatment target: LDL-C < 2.0 mmol/L Secondary treatment target: TC:HDL-C < 4.0
Moderate	10–19%	Initiate treatment when: LDL-C ≥ 3.5 mmol/L TC:HDL-C ≥ 5.0
Low	< 10%	Initiate treatment when: LDL-C ≥ 5.0 mmol/L TC:HDL-C ≥ 6.0

Adapted from McPherson R et al. *Can J Cardiol* 2006;22(11):913-27.[31]
Abbreviations: HDL-C = high-density lipoprotein cholesterol; LDL-C = low-density lipoprotein cholesterol; TC = total cholesterol

Oral Anticoagulants

Oral anticoagulants are recommended for post-MI patients with persistent or paroxysmal atrial fibrillation, demonstrable LV thrombus, or large infarcts with extensive dyskinetic segments or aneurysm.[34,35]

All post-MI patients seem to benefit modestly from warfarin therapy with a 20% risk reduction relative to ASA in the combined end-point of death, re-infarction or embolic stroke (ARR 3%). Moderate to high intensity anticoagulation with warfarin, administered alone or in combination with ASA, is superior to ASA alone in reducing composite events but is associated with a higher risk of bleeding.[36] The increased risk of bleeding and the demands of adjusting the dose to maintain the INR prevent routine use of warfarin for the secondary prevention of cardiovascular events post-MI. Consequently, warfarin tends to be reserved for select patients at identifiable risk for a thrombotic accident.

Therapeutic Tips

- It is anticipated that a larger proportion of patients receiving timely reperfusion therapy will qualify as low-risk survivors of MI.
- Patients receiving therapy that closely adheres to published guidelines do significantly better than those whose therapy does not.
- Refer motivated patients to cardiac rehabilitation programs, where available, especially those who are older, deconditioned, overweight or have modifiable risk factors.

- Depression is associated with increased mortality post-MI. Maintain a high level of awareness and treat the condition appropriately. Avoid the use of tricyclic antidepressants.
- The return to usual activity can be guided by a baseline exercise stress test undertaken in the fully ambulated patient using a modified rehabilitation protocol. Poor exercise endurance, provocation of angina or ischemic ECG abnormalities may prompt further evaluation and more caution on the path to increased activity. Patients deemed to be at low risk with good exercise characteristics can often progress to full activity and return to work in two or three weeks.
- Give all patients sl **nitroglycerin** with instructions on how to respond to recurrent chest pain.
- Provide an unequivocal recommendation to quit smoking. Encourage the use of nicotine replacement or bupropion as aids to smoking cessation.
- **Hormone therapy** is not indicated for primary or secondary prevention of cardiovascular events in postmenopausal women.
- Routine use of **antioxidant vitamins** (vitamin E, vitamin C, beta carotene) for prevention of cardiovascular events is not recommended
- Selective **Cox-2 inhibitors** and some nonselective **NSAIDs** such as ibuprofen may reduce the protective effects of ASA, resulting in atherothrombotic complications.[37]

Figure 1: Stratifying Post-MI Patients to Conservative or Invasive Therapy

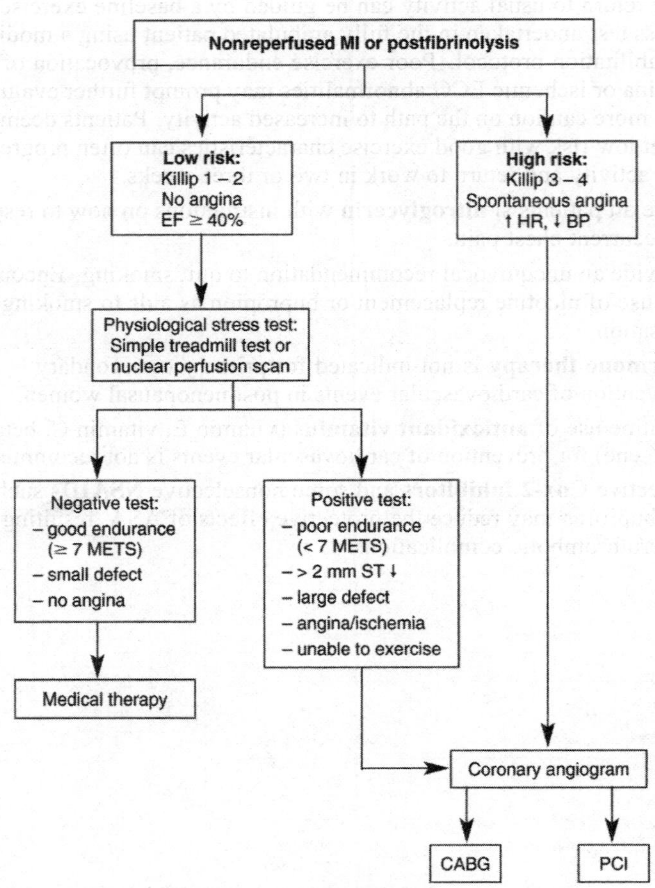

Abbreviations: EF = ejection fraction; HR = heart rate; METS = metabolic equivalents; CABG = coronary artery bypass graft surgery; PCI = percutaneous coronary intervention

Figure 2: **Management of MI Patients After Primary PCI**

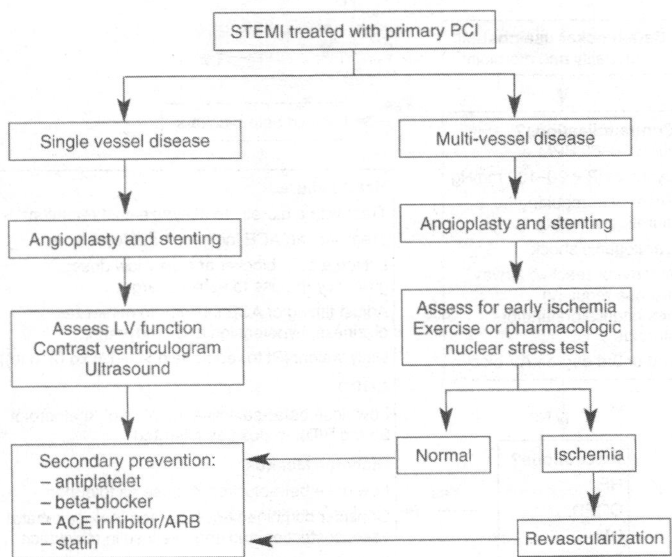

Figure 3: **Elements of Cardiac Rehabilitation**

Inpatient	**Outpatient**			
Identification of Patient	**Evaluation**	**Prescribed Exercise**	**Modification of Risk Factors**	**Specification of Long-Term Goals**
Smoking cessation and prevention of relapse Initial assessment of physical activity Outpatient referral	Medical history Assessment of risk factors Exercise stress test Vocational counselling	Aerobic training (high caloric or interval) Resistance training On-site or at-home exercise program	Education Nutritional counselling Exercise Medication	Physical Vocational Psychological Clinical

Reproduced from Ades PA. Cardiac rehabilitation and secondary prevention of coronary heart disease. *N Engl J Med* 2001;345(12):892-902. With permission. Copyright© 2001 Massachusetts Medical Society.

Figure 4: **Beta-Blockers in the Chronic Post-MI Period**

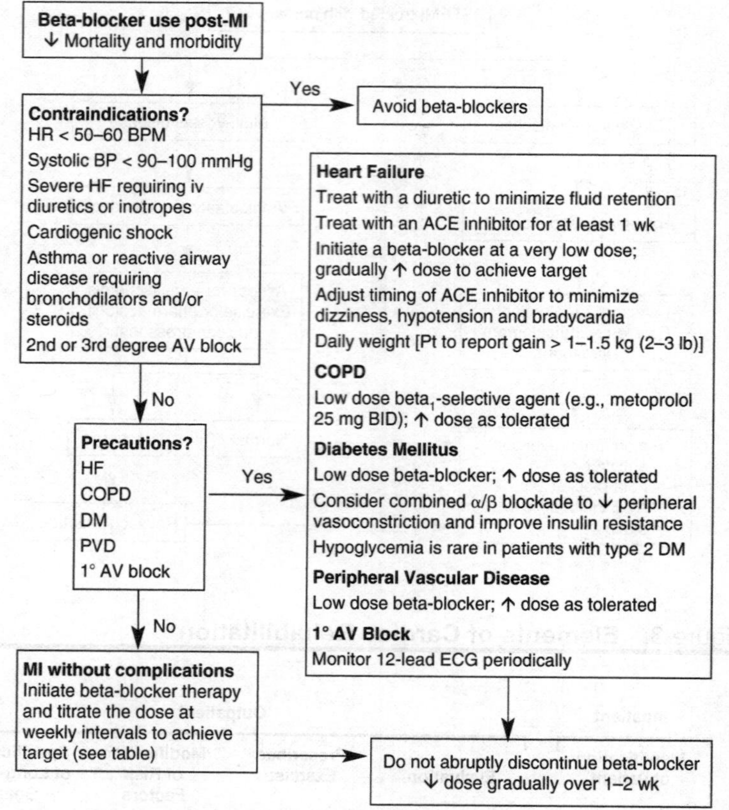

Abbreviations: AV = atrioventricular; BP = blood pressure; DM = diabetes mellitus; HR = heart rate; LV = left ventricular

Adapted with permission from Fig. 2. Gheorghiade M, Goldstein S. Beta blockers in the post-myocardial infarction patient. Circulation 2002;106:394–8.

Table 6: **Drugs Used in the Post-MI Patient**

Drug Class	Drug	Dose	Adverse Effects	Drug Interactions	Comments	Cost[a]
Antiplatelet Agents	*ASA* Aspirin, Bufferin, Coated Aspirin, generics	80–325 mg/day	Nausea, vomiting, GI hemorrhage, tinnitus, vertigo, hypersensitivity.	Increased risk of bleeding when antiplatelets are given with anticoagulants (e.g., warfarin). Caution with NSAIDs.		$
	clopidogrel Plavix	75 mg/day	Rash, purpura, diarrhea, bleeding.	Caution with NSAIDs.		$$$$
	ticlopidine Ticlid, generics	250 mg BID	Diarrhea, rash, bleeding, neutropenia (usually reversible), purpura.	Caution with NSAIDs.	Rarely used. Must monitor neutrophil counts Q 2 wk for the first 3 mo.	$$
Beta$_1$-adrenergic Antagonists, nonselective	*nadolol* generics	Initial: 40–80 mg/day Usual: 120 mg/day	Fatigue, bradycardia, decreased exercise capacity, headache, impotence, vivid dreams. Less common: hyperglycemia, depression, heart failure, heart block.	Bradycardia with digoxin or nondihydropyridine CCBs. Cardiodepressant effects with nondihydropyridine CCBs antiarrhythmics, anesthetics.	See Figure 3.	$

(cont'd)

Table 6: **Drugs Used in the Post-MI Patient** *(cont'd)*

Drug Class	Drug	Dose	Adverse Effects	Drug Interactions	Comments	Cost[a]
	propranolol generics	Initial: 40 mg BID–TID Usual: 40 mg QID	See nadolol.	See nadolol. CYP2D6 inhibitors ↑ levels of propranolol and metoprolol.	See nadolol. Propranolol is more likely to cause CNS side effects (insomnia, depression, vivid dreams) because of greater lipid solubility.	$
	timolol generics	Initial: 5–10 mg BID Usual: 10 mg BID	See nadolol.	See nadolol.	See nadolol.	$
Beta$_1$-adrenergic Antagonists, selective	*atenolol* Tenormin, generics	Initial: 50 mg/day Usual: 100 mg/day	See nadolol.	See nadolol.	See nadolol.	$
	bisoprolol Monocor, generics	Initial: 2.5 mg/day Usual: 10 mg/day	See nadolol.	See nadolol.	See nadolol.	$
	metoprolol Betaloc, Lopresor, generics	Initial: 100 mg/day Usual: 200 mg/day IR: give in 2 divided doses SR: give once daily	See nadolol.	See nadolol. CYP2D6 inhibitors ↑ levels of propranolol and metoprolol.	See nadolol.	$
Beta$_1$-adrenergic Antagonists, selective with ISA	*acebutolol* Rhotral, Sectral, generics	Initial: 100–200 mg BID Usual: 400 mg BID	See nadolol.	See nadolol.	See nadolol. Agents with ISA have less effect on resting heart rate than those without ISA.	$$

Drug Class	Drug	Dose	Adverse Effects	Drug Interactions	Comments	Cost[a]
Beta$_1$-adrenergic Antagonists with alpha$_1$-blocking activity	*carvedilol* Coreg, generics	Initial: 3.125 mg BID Usual: 25 mg BID	See nadolol. Edema, dizziness, nasal congestion and postural hypotension due to alpha$_1$ antagonism.	See nadolol.	See nadolol.	$$
ACE Inhibitors	*captopril* Capoten, generics	Initial: 6.25 mg TID Target dose post-MI: 50 mg TID	Dry cough, hyperkalemia, angioedema (unusual). Can precipitate renal failure in patients with renovascular disease, volume depletion or in those receiving NSAIDs.	Marked ↑ in serum K^+ in patients receiving K^+ supplements and/or K^+-sparing diuretics. ↓ hypotensive effect with NSAIDs ↑ risk of renal dysfunction. Elevated Li^+ levels (potential toxicity).	Use lower (i.e., 50%) initial doses in patients on diuretics (↑ risk of hypotension with hypovolemia). Hyperkalemia usually occurs only in those on K^+ supplements or drugs that cause K^+ retention, those with renal impairment or diabetics with high serum K^+ levels. Assess SCr and K^+ after a few days, then regularly.	$$
	enalapril Vasotec	Initial: 2.5 mg BID Target dose in HF: 10 mg BID	See captopril.	See captopril.	See captopril.	$$$
	lisinopril Zestril, Prinivil, generics	Initial: 2.5 mg/day Target dose: 20–35 mg once daily	See captopril.	See captopril.	See captopril.	$-$$
	perindopril Coversyl	Initial: 2 mg/day Target dose for CAD: 8 mg/day	See captopril.	See captopril.	See captopril.	$$

(cont'd)

Table 6: **Drugs Used in the Post-MI Patient** *(cont'd)*

Drug Class	Drug	Dose	Adverse Effects	Drug Interactions	Comments	Cost[a]
	ramipril Altace	Initial: 2.5 mg/day Target dose post-MI: 5 mg BID or 10 mg daily	See captopril.	See captopril.	See captopril.	$$
	trandolapril Mavik	Initial: 1 mg/day Target dose post-MI: 4 mg daily	See captopril.	See captopril.	See captopril.	$$
Angiotensin Receptor Blockers	*candesartan* Atacand	Initial: 4 or 8 mg/day Target dose in HF: 32 mg/day once daily	Hyperkalemia. Can precipitate renal failure in susceptible patients (bilateral renovascular disease, those with volume depletion or with concurrent NSAID use). Angioedema has been reported, but a causal association has not been established.	Marked ↑ in serum K^+ in patients receiving K^+ supplements and/or K^+-sparing diuretics. May elevate Li^+ levels (potential toxicity).	Use lower (i.e., 50%) initial doses in patients on diuretics (↑ risk of hypotension with hypovolemia). Hyperkalemia usually occurs only in those on K^+ supplements or drugs that cause K^+ retention, those with renal impairment or diabetics with high serum K^+ levels. Assess SCr and K^+ after a few days, then regularly.	$$$
	valsartan Diovan	Initial dose post-MI: 20 mg BID Target dose post-MI:[21] 160 mg BID	See candesartan.	See candesartan.	See candesartan.	$$$$$

Drug Class	Drug	Dose	Adverse Effects	Drug Interactions	Comments	Cost[a]
HMG CoA Reductase Inhibitors	*atorvastatin* Lipitor	Initial: 10 or 20 mg/day Maximum: 80 mg/day Once daily with or without meals	GI disturbances, sleep disturbances, headache, rash, myalgia (with and without ↑ CPK levels), ↑ CPK and transaminase levels (reversible). Rare: myopathy, rhabdomyolysis.	CYP3A4 inhibitors (e.g., amiodarone, cyclosporine, macrolides, protease inhibitors, gemfibrozil, grapefruit juice, azole antifungals, verapamil) increase serum levels of atorvastatin, lovastatin and simvastatin.	Start with 40 mg/day if the desired ↓ in LDL-C is > 45%. Maximum response is usually evident within 4 wk.	$$$$$
	fluvastatin Lescol	Initial: 20 or 40 mg/day Maximum: 80 mg/day Once daily with or without meals	See atorvastatin.	Fluconazole inhibits the metabolism and increases serum levels of fluvastatin.	Start with 40 mg/day if the desired ↓ in LDL-C is > 25%.	$$$$$
	lovastatin Mevacor, generics	Initial: 20 mg/day Maximum: 80 mg/day Take with the evening meal	See atorvastatin.	See atorvastatin.		$$$$$
	pravastatin Pravachol, generics	Initial: 20 mg/day Maximum: 80 mg/day Take at bedtime	See atorvastatin.	Low potential for drug interactions (not metabolized by CYP450 isozymes).		$$

(cont'd)

Table 6: **Drugs Used in the Post-MI Patient** *(cont'd)*

Drug Class	Drug	Dose	Adverse Effects	Drug Interactions	Comments	Cost[a]
	rosuvastatin Crestor	10–40 mg/day	See atorvastatin.	May increase the INR in patients taking warfarin.		$$$
	simvastatin Zocor, generics	10–80 mg/day with the evening meal	See atorvastatin.	See atorvastatin.		$$

[a] Cost of 30-day supply of usual or target doses; includes drug cost only.

Dosage adjustment may be required in renal impairment; see Appendix I.

Abbreviations: IR = immediate release; SR = sustained release; HF = heart failure

Legend: $ < $25 $-$$ < $25–50 $$ $25–50 $$$ $50–75 $$$$ $75–100 $$$$$ > $100

Suggested Readings

Antman EM, Anbe DT, Armstrong PW et al. ACC/AHA guidelines for the management of patients with ST-elevation myocardial infarction. *Circulation* 2004;110(9):e82-292.

Braunwald,E, Antman EM, Beasley JW et al. ACC/AHA guideline update for the management of patients with unstable angina and non-ST-segment elevation myocardial infarction--2002. *Circulation* 2002;106(14):1893-900.

Califf RM, Pieper KS, Lee KL et al. Prediction of 1-year survival after thrombolysis for acute myocardial infarction in the global utilization of streptokinase and TPA for occluded coronary arteries trial. *Circulation* 2000;101(19):2231-8.

Libby P. Current concepts of the pathogenesis of the acute coronary syndromes. *Circulation* 2001;104(3):365-72.

Libby P, Ridker PM. Inflammation and atherothrombosis from population biology and bench research to clinical practice. *J Am Coll Cardiol* 2006;48(9 Suppl):A33-46.

Singh M, Reeder GS, Jacobsen SJ et al. Scores for post-myocardial infarction risk stratification in the community. *Circulation* 2002;106(18):2309-14.

References

1. Barron HV, Bowlby LJ, Breen T et al. Use of reperfusion therapy for acute myocardial infarction in the United States: data from the National Registry of Myocardial Infarction. *Circulation* 1998;97(12):1150-6.
2. Weaver WD, Simes RJ, Betriu A et al. Comparison of primary coronary angioplasty and intravenous thrombolytic therapy for acute myocardial infarction: a quantitative review. *JAMA* 1997;278(23):2093-98.
3. Pitt B. Evaluation of the postinfarct patient. *Circulation* 1995;91(6):1855-60.
4. Pilote L, Dasgupta K, Guru V et al. A comprehensive view of sex-specific issues related to cardiovascular disease. *CMAJ* 2007;176(6):S1-44.
5. Antman EM, Anbe DT, Armstrong PW et al. ACC/AHA guidelines for the management of patients with ST-elevation myocardial infarction--executive summary.*J Am Coll Cardiol* 2004;44(3):671-719.
6. Califf RM, Pieper KS, Lee KL et al. Prediction of 1-year survival after thrombolysis for acute myocardial infarction in the global utilization of streptokinase and TPA for occluded coronary arteries trial. *Circulation* 2000;101(19):2231-8.
7. Forrester JS, Liebson PR, Parrillo JE et al. Risk stratification post-myocardial infarction: is early coronary angiography the more effective strategy? *Prog Cardiovasc Dis* 2002;45(1):49-66.
8. Madsen JK, Bech J, Jorgensen E et al. Yield of 5,536 diagnostic coronary arteriographies: results from a data registry. *Cardiology* 2002;98(4):191-4.
9. Ades PA. Cardiac rehabilitation and secondary prevention of coronary heart disease. *N Engl J Med* 2001;345(12):892-902.
10. Wilhelmsson C, Vedin JA, Elmfeldt D et al. Smoking and myocardial infarction. *Lancet* 1975;1(7904):415-20.
11. Yusuf S. Two decades of progress in preventing vascular disease. *Lancet* 2002;360(9326):2-3.
12. Antithrombotic Trialists' Collaboration. Collaborative meta-analysis of randomised trials of antiplatelet therapy for prevention of death, myocardial infarction, and stroke in high risk patients. *BMJ* 2002;324(7329):71-86.
13. Lauer MS. Clinical practice. Aspirin for primary prevention of coronary events. *N Engl J Med* 2002;346(19):1468-74.
14. Patrono C. Aspirin as an antiplatelet drug. *N Engl J Med* 1994;330(18):1287-94.
15. Yusuf S, Zhao F, Mehta SR et al. Effects of clopidogrel in addition to aspirin in patients with acute coronary syndromes without ST-segment elevation. *N Engl J Med* 2001;345(7):494-502.
16. Harrington RA, Becker RC, Ezekowitz M et al. Antithrombotic therapy for coronary artery disease: the Seventh ACCP Conference on Antithrombotic and Thrombolytic Therapy. *Chest* 2004;126(3 Suppl):513S-548S.
17. Cannon CP. Evolving management of ST-segment elevation myocardial infarction: update on recent data. *Am J Cardiol* 2006;98(12A):10Q-21Q.

18. Sabatine MS, Cannon CP, Gibson CM et al. Addition of clopidogrel to aspirin and fibrinolytic therapy for myocardial infarction with ST-segment elevation. *N Engl J Med* 2005;352(12):1179-89.
19. Grines CL, Bonow RO, Casey DE, et al. Prevention of premature discontinuation of dual antiplatelet therapy in patients with coronary artery stents: a science advisory from the American Heart Association, American College of Cardiology, Society for Cardiovascular Angiography and Interventions, American College of Surgeons, and American Dental Association, with representation from the American College of Physicians. *Circulation* 2007;115(6):813-8.
20. Gottlieb SS, McCarter RJ,.Vogel RA. Effect of beta-blockade on mortality among high-risk and low-risk patients after myocardial infarction. *N Engl J Med* 1998;339(8):489-97.
21. Packer M, Bristow MR, Cohn JN et al. The effect of carvedilol on morbidity and mortality in patients with chronic heart failure. U.S. Carvedilol Heart Failure Study Group. *N Engl J Med* 1996;334(21):1349-55.
22. Yusuf S, Wittes J,.Friedman L. Overview of results of randomized clinical trials in heart disease. I. Treatments following myocardial infarction. *JAMA* 1988;260(14):2088-93.
23. Al-Mallah MH, Tleyjeh IM, Abdel-Latif AA et al. Angiotensin-converting enzyme inhibitors in coronary artery disease and preserved left ventricular systolic function: a systematic review and meta-analysis of randomized controlled trials. *J Am Coll Cardiol* 2006;47(8):1576-83.
24. Pfeffer MA, Braunwald E, Moye LA et al. Effect of captopril on mortality and morbidity in patients with left ventricular dysfunction after myocardial infarction. Results of the survival and ventricular enlargement trial. The SAVE Investigators. *N Engl J Med* 1992;327(10):669-77.
25. Yusuf S, Sleight P, Pogue J et al. Effects of an angiotensin-converting-enzyme inhibitor, ramipril, on cardiovascular events in high-risk patients. The Heart Outcomes Prevention Evaluation Study Investigators. *N Engl J Med* 2000;342(3):145-53.
26. Pfeffer MA, McMurray JJ, Velazquez EJ et al. Valsartan, captopril, or both in myocardial infarction complicated by heart failure, left ventricular dysfunction, or both. *N Engl J Med* 2003;349(20):1893-906.
27. Baigent C, Keech A, Kearney PM et al. Efficacy and safety of cholesterol-lowering treatment: prospective meta-analysis of data from 90,056 participants in 14 randomised trials of statins. *Lancet* 2005;366(9493):1267-78.
28. Libby P. Current concepts of the pathogenesis of the acute coronary syndromes. *Circulation* 2001;104(3):365-72.
29. Cannon CP, Braunwald E, McCabe CH et al. Intensive versus moderate lipid lowering with statins after acute coronary syndromes. *N Engl J Med* 2004;350(15):1495-504.
30. Grundy SM. Statin trials and goals of cholesterol-lowering therapy. *Circulation* 1998;97(15):1436-9.
31. McPherson R, Frohlich J, Fodor G et al. Canadian Cardiovascular Society position statement--recommendations for the diagnosis and treatment of dyslipidemia and prevention of cardiovascular disease. *Can J Cardiol* 2006;22(11):913-7.
32. LaRosa JC, Grundy SM, Waters DD et al. Intensive lipid lowering with atorvastatin in patients with stable coronary disease. *N Engl J Med* 2005;352(14):1425-35.
33. Schwartz GG, Olsson AG, Ezekowitz MD et al. Effects of atorvastatin on early recurrent ischemic events in acute coronary syndromes: the MIRACL study: a randomized controlled trial. *JAMA* 2001;285(13):1711-8.
34. van Es RF, Jonker JJ, Verheugt FW et al. Aspirin and coumadin after acute coronary syndromes (the ASPECT-2 study): a randomised controlled trial. *Lancet* 2002;360(9327):109-13.
35. Hurlen M, Abdelnoor M, Smith P et al. Warfarin, aspirin, or both after myocardial infarction. *N Engl J Med* 2002;347(13):969-74.
36. Hirsh J, Fuster V, Ansell J et al. American Heart Association/American College of Cardiology Foundation guide to warfarin therapy. *Circulation* 2003;107(12):1692-711.
37. Antman EM, Bennett JS, Daugherty A et al. Use of nonsteroidal antiinflammatory drugs: an update for clinicians: a scientific statement from the American Heart Association. *Circulation* 2007;115(12):1634-42.

CHAPTER 36
Heart Failure

Simon de Denus, B. Pharm, MSc and
Michel White, MD, FRCPC, FACC

Heart failure (HF) is associated with a five-year mortality rate of 5–50% depending on the severity of symptoms.[1] HF may require frequent hospitalizations and significantly reduces quality of life and exercise tolerance.[1] Typical symptoms of HF include dyspnea, fatigue and fluid retention.[1]

HF is characterized by impaired left ventricular (LV) function and reduced LV reserve. HF is generally categorized as systolic HF or HF with preserved systolic function (PSF).[2] Less common types of HF will not be discussed. Systolic HF is characterized by decreased pump function, dilatation of the left ventricle and decreased LV ejection fraction (LVEF $\leq$ 40%). Most clinical trials have been conducted in patients with systolic HF. There is no strong consensus on the definition of HF with PSF or its treatment.[1,2,3,4,5] It is variably defined as the presence of signs and symptoms of HF with LVEF > 40 or 50%. HF with PSF can be associated with many conditions (hypertension, arterial stiffness, diabetes mellitus), although abnormal myocardial relaxation, hypertrophy and/or fibrosis are generally present.[1,2,3,4,5]

Goals of Therapy[1,2,3,4,5]

- Treat risk factors
- Prevent disease progression
- Improve symptoms, exercise tolerance and quality of life
- Reduce morbidity and mortality

Table 1: **Laboratory Investigations for Evaluation of Patients with Heart Failure**

All patients	
	Complete blood count
	Serum creatinine, electrolytes, blood urea nitrogen and transaminase levels
	Fasting plasma glucose and serum lipids
	Thyroid function tests
	Urinalysis
Select patients	
	Brain natriuretic peptide (BNP) or N-terminal proBNP (NT-proBNP)[a]
	Iron studies, ferritin and transferrin
	HIV test

[a] BNP or NT-proBNP is potentially useful in the emergency care setting. Value in primary care is not definitive.

Investigations[1] (Figure 1)

- A history, physical examination and select laboratory tests should be performed to establish the diagnosis (Table 1)
- Identify and correct modifiable risk factors and exacerbating factors (Table 2)
- Determine ventricular size and function with transthoracic echocardiography or isotopic ventriculography in all patients with suspected HF. Echocardiography allows for identification of valvular abnormalities and other myocardial problems
- Additional tests should be performed in select individuals to identify the etiology of HF and to guide specific treatment when appropriate
- The New York Heart Association functional classification is commonly used to describe patients with HF (Table 3)

Table 2: **Factors That Can Exacerbate Heart Failure**

Patient-specific factors

- Noncompliance with drug therapy or dietary restrictions
- Anemia
- Arrhythmias
- Infections
- Myocardial ischemia
- Pulmonary embolism
- Renal dysfunction
- Thyroid dysfunction
- Uncontrolled hypertension
- Valvular heart disease

Drugs

Drugs that cause sodium and fluid retention:
- NSAIDs including selective COX-2 inhibitors and high-dose salicylates
- Corticosteroids
- Minoxidil
- Androgens
- Thiazolidinediones (pioglitazone, rosiglitazone)
- Drugs with high sodium content
- Licorice-containing products

Negative inotropes:
- Antiarrhythmic agents except amiodarone and dofetilide
- Beta-blockers at maintenance doses
- Calcium channel blockers: diltiazem, nifedipine, verapamil, but not amlodipine or felodipine
- Itraconazole

Cardiotoxic drugs
- Alcohol
- Anthracyclines (doxorubicin)
- Cocaine
- Cyclophosphamide
- Imatinib
- Trastuzumab

Table 3: **New York Heart Association (NYHA) Functional Classification**

Class	Characteristics
I	No symptoms
II	Symptoms occur with ordinary activity
III	Symptoms occur with less than ordinary activity
IV	Symptoms occur at rest or with minimal activity

Therapeutic Choices

Nonpharmacologic Choices[1,3,4,5]

- Control HF risk factors (hypertension, obesity, diabetes mellitus, supraventricular arrhythmia, dyslipidemia, coronary artery disease and other vascular diseases).
- Recommend moderate regular physical activity in stable patients.
- Recommend no more than moderate alcohol consumption in all patients.
  - avoid completely in alcoholic cardiomyopathy.
- Restrict sodium intake in all patients (< 2–3 g/day; 1–2 g/day in those with severe HF).
- Restrict fluid intake (< 1.5–2 L/day) in patients with fluid retention that is not easily controlled with diuretics, or in patients with hyponatremia.
- Annual influenza vaccination in all patients.
- Pneumococcal vaccination in all patients.
- Daily weight.
  - patients who gain 0.5 kg/day on several consecutive days or 2 kg in 3 days should alert their team or physician.

Device Therapy

Given their high cost, the following devices should generally be reserved for patients who do not have significant comorbidities that are expected to significantly limit survival.

- *Implantable cardioverter defibrillators* (ICD) are recommended for stable patients with a history of sudden cardiac arrest, ventricular fibrillation (VF) or hemodynamically unstable sustained ventricular tachycardia (VT) in the absence of reversible factors; or coronary artery disease with or without mild to moderate symptoms and an LVEF ≤ 30%.[1] An ICD may also be considered for stable patients with nonischemic NYHA class II–III HF and an LVEF ≤ 30%; or ischemic HF and a history of myocardial infarction, NYHA class II–III HF and an LVEF of 31–35% and inducible VT/VF during an electrophysiology study.

- *Cardiac resynchronization therapy* (CRT) should be considered in patients with NYHA class III–IV HF despite optimal medical therapy who are in sinus rhythm and have an LVEF ≤ 35% and a QRS interval ≥ 120 msec.[1]
- *Left ventricular assist devices* (LVAD)[6] should be used as a bridge to transplantation. Use of LVADs as a bridge to recovery is controversial.
- *Continuous positive airway pressure* (CPAP)[4] should be considered in patients with obstructive sleep apnea.

Reperfusion and Surgery

- *Revascularization*, either by percutaneous coronary intervention or coronary artery bypass surgery, should be performed in select patients with symptomatic ischemia.[1]
- *Cardiac transplantation* should be considered in patients with severe refractory HF, despite optimal therapy, who would otherwise have a good life expectancy.[1]

Pharmacologic Choices

Systolic Heart Failure

In the absence of contraindications, the cornerstone of therapy for systolic HF in all patients with an LVEF ≤ 40% (NYHA class I–IV) is long-term treatment with the combination of an angiotensin converting enzyme (ACE) inhibitor and a beta-blocker (Figure 2). Diuretics are used to control signs and symptoms of hypervolemia. Digoxin, angiotensin II receptor blockers (ARBs), aldosterone antagonists or the combination of isosorbide dinitrate/hydralazine are used in select individuals.[5]

Consideration should be given to the use of agents for which mortality and morbidity benefits have been established in large randomized clinical trials (Table 4). Drugs used in the treatment of HF are presented in Table 5. Target doses are those used in such trials.

Consider a patient's comorbid conditions when contemplating the use of a particular class of medication, a specific agent and the target dosage.

ACE Inhibitors

ACE inhibitors are recommended in all patients because they improve symptoms and reduce the risk of hospitalization, myocardial infarction and death in patients with systolic HF.[7,8,9] Start with a low dose and titrate the dose at 7- to 14-day intervals to the target dose, or maximum tolerated dose if the target dose cannot be reached. Treatment with target doses is more effective than low doses.[10] Measure serum creatinine, potassium and blood pressure before initiating an ACE inhibitor or increasing the dose and 7–14 days after any increase in dosage.[5] An increase in serum creatinine of up to 30% is expected and acceptable after initiation of an ACE inhibitor.[1] Patients at greatest risk of hyperkalemia are those with moderate to severe renal dysfunction, high baseline potassium, diabetes mellitus and those receiving potassium-sparing diuretics.[11]

Beta-blockers

Beta-blockers improve symptoms and reduce the risk of hospitalization and death in patients with systolic HF.[12,13,14,15] They are recommended in all patients with an LVEF ≤ 40%.[5] Only beta-blockers that have been shown to reduce mortality should be used: **carvedilol, bisoprolol** and **metoprolol succinate** (not available in Canada).[5] **Metoprolol tartrate** is available in Canada, but has not been shown to reduce mortality in patients with HF. Dose titration should be performed at 2- to 4-week intervals.[5] Monitor blood pressure and heart rate before initiating a beta-blocker and before any increase in dose. Watch for the signs and symptoms of HF decompensation when initiating or increasing the dose of a beta-blocker. Pay particular attention to the daily morning weight.[5] Beta-blockers should not be stopped abruptly.[1] Refer patients with severe HF (NYHA class III–IV) to an HF specialist for initiation of a beta-blocker.[1]

Diuretics

Diuretics are recommended to control signs and symptoms of congestion. **Thiazide diuretics** can be used in patients with minimal fluid retention, but **loop diuretics**, usually **furosemide**, are required in most patients.[1,3,4,5] Use of ethacrynic acid is limited to patients with an allergy to furosemide. Thiazides have poor efficacy as monotherapy in patients with creatinine clearance < 50 mL/min.[16] Higher doses of furosemide are required in patients with renal dysfunction.[16] The lowest effective dose should be used.[5] Serum creatinine and electrolytes should be measured before and 3 to 7 days after initiation of a diuretic and then as indicated (i.e., until serum potassium and renal function are stable) after increasing the dose.

Thiazide and loop diuretics deplete potassium and magnesium. Serum potassium should be maintained at ≥ 4 mmol/L because hypokalemia increases the risk of fatal ventricular arrhythmias and digoxin toxicity.[1] In patients with refractory volume overload, consider the addition of a low-dose thiazide intermittently (e.g., a few times/week) to a loop diuretic.[1,3,4,5] This strategy should be used only by experienced clinicians with close monitoring of weight, renal function and serum potassium because of the risk of severe and potentially fatal dehydration and electrolyte imbalances.[1,3,4,5] When prescribed once a day, diuretics should generally be taken in the morning. When prescribed twice daily or more, the last dose should be taken before 4:00 p.m. to avoid diuresis during the night.

With the exception of spironolactone (see below), the role of **potassium-sparing diuretics** is limited to prevention of hypokalemia and hypomagnesemia in patients treated with thiazides or loop diuretics.[3]

Angiotensin II Receptor Blockers

Angiotensin II receptor blockers (ARBs) are an alternative to ACE inhibitors in patients with ACE inhibitor–induced cough or angioedema. Patient education and follow-up are essential because ARB-induced angioedema has been reported.[4,17] Similar to ACE inhibitors, ARBs are associated with renal dysfunction and hyperkalemia; thus, ARBs should not be substituted for ACE inhibitors specifically for these adverse events.[18] Considerations for initiation, dosage titration and monitoring for ARBs are the same as for ACE inhibitors.

Addition of an ARB may be considered in patients with persistent symptoms despite optimal therapy with an ACE inhibitor and a beta-blocker.[1,19] In this setting, **candesartan** reduced cardiovascular mortality and hospitalizations for HF.[19] Reductions in morbidity but not mortality were obtained with **valsartan** in another trial.[20] Limited data suggest that an ARB may be a valuable addition to an ACE inhibitor in patients not receiving a beta-blocker.[1] Close monitoring of vital signs, serum creatinine and potassium is essential when combining an ACE inhibitor and an ARB. The combination of an ACE inhibitor, an ARB and an aldosterone antagonist is not recommended because of the uncertainty regarding the benefit and safety of this combination.[1]

Aldosterone Antagonists

Aldosterone antagonists reduce the risk of mortality and morbidity in patients with severe HF (NYHA class III–IV and LVEF < 35%) and in post-MI patients with an LVEF ≤ 40% and either HF symptoms or diabetes mellitus.[4,21,22] The benefit of these agents in patients with stable mild to moderate symptoms is unknown.[4] Aldosterone antagonists should not be used in patients with a baseline potassium > 5.0 mmol/L, a serum creatinine > 221 µmol/L or a creatinine clearance < 30 mL/min.[4] In patients with a creatinine clearance of 30–50 mL/min, start **spironolactone** at a dose of 12.5 mg daily or every other day. Monitor vital signs, serum creatinine and potassium 3 days and 1 week after initiating or titrating the dose of spironolactone and repeated as necessary until the potassium level and renal function are stable.[5] Monitoring should then be performed monthly for 3 months and then every 3 months.[5]

Eplerenone is a selective aldosterone antagonist that does not produce gynecomastia (not available in Canada).[5]

Digoxin

Digoxin improves symptoms and reduces the risk of hospitalization for HF, but does not reduce mortality in patients with moderate to severe persistent symptoms (NYHA class II–IV) despite optimal medical therapy.[4,23] It may also be considered for control of the ventricular rate in patients with atrial fibrillation that cannot be controlled by beta-blockers, or in patients who cannot tolerate beta-blockers.[5] The dosage is individualized based on the patient's age, weight, renal function and concomitant drugs, but usually ranges from 0.0625 to 0.25 mg daily. Lower doses may be appropriate in select patients. Given the narrow therapeutic index of digoxin, particular attention should be devoted to identifying and preventing potential drug interactions. Digoxin serum concentrations should be monitored when renal function changes significantly, an interacting drug is added or discontinued, or when digoxin toxicity is suspected. Serum concentrations may also be monitored once steady state is achieved after initiating digoxin, particularly in elderly patients and those with renal dysfunction.[4,24] Measure trough serum concentrations at least 8 hours after administration and adjust the dose to maintain the serum concentration between 0.6 and 1.0 nmol/L, which is associated with greater reductions in hospitalization and, possibly, a reduction in all cause and HF mortality.[25,26]

Nitrates/hydralazine

The combination of isosorbide dinitrate plus hydralazine reduces mortality and morbidity in Black patients with NYHA class III–IV HF and is recommended in addition to standard therapy in this setting.[27] Use of this combination may also be considered in Black patients with NYHA class II HF[1,4,27] and in other HF patients who do not tolerate ACE inhibitors and ARBs.[1]

Nitrate monotherapy is valuable to treat symptoms of exercise-induced dyspnea or angina, paroxysmal nocturnal dyspnea and orthopnea. Nitrates have not been shown to reduce mortality in the absence of hydralazine.[1]

Calcium Channel Blockers

Felodipine and **amlodipine** are safe, but do not reduce mortality or morbidity in patients with systolic HF.[28,29] They may be useful in select patients with persistent angina despite the use of beta-blockers (and nitrates) or in patients with uncontrolled hypertension despite the use of an ACEI, ARB, beta-blocker and a diuretic.[3]

Avoid use of diltiazem and verapamil in patients with systolic HF because of their negative inotropic effects.[1,3,4,5] Avoid nifedipine because of the lack of data and availability of safe alternatives.

Antiarrhythmics[4]

Consider **amiodarone** to maintain sinus rhythm in patients with atrial fibrillation. Amiodarone also reduces the frequency of repetitive ICD discharges. Avoid other antiarrhythmic drugs. Antiarrhythmics are not recommended to prevent sudden cardiac death because they do not reduce mortality.

Heart Failure with Preserved Systolic Function

Treatment of HF with PSF has been studied to a limited extent. Control risk factors (hypertension, diabetes mellitus, ventricular rate in patients with supraventricular arrhythmias), volume status and decrease heart rate to optimize filling time.[1,4] Use of **ACE inhibitors** or **ARBs** should be considered in most patients.[1,4] **Beta-blockers** are recommended in most patients,[1] particularly those with CAD, prior MI, hypertension or atrial fibrillation (Figure 3).[4] **Diuretics** should be used to optimize volume status.[1] Use of **verapamil** or **diltiazem** may be considered to control the ventricular rate in patients with supraventricular arrhythmias[1,4] or angina, in those who cannot tolerate a beta-blocker,[4] and may be particularly useful in patients with hypertrophic cardiomyopathy. CCBs may also be considered in patients with hypertension.[4]

Decompensated Heart Failure

Few large, randomized trials have been performed in patients with decompensated or acute HF. Intravenous **loop diuretics** are recommended in patients with signs and symptoms of fluid retention (e.g., **furosemide** 40–200 mg twice or three times daily based on renal function or the patient's usual dose of furosemide).[1,4,16]

Combinations of diuretics, or the addition of a vasodilator such as **nitroglycerin**, **nesiritide** (not available in Canada) or **nitroprusside** should be given to patients who do not respond to intravenous furosemide.[1,4] Intravenous vasodilators with a loop diuretic can be used initially in patients with moderate to severe symptoms of pulmonary congestion or those with severe hypertension.[1,4] Sublingual nitroglycerin can be given before intravenous nitroglycerin. Invasive monitoring is recommended when administering nitroprusside.[4] Great care should be taken to prevent cyanide and thiocyanide toxicity with nitroprusside; avoid in patients with hepatic or renal failure.[3]

In patients with low cardiac output, **milrinone** or **dobutamine** should be given if the systolic blood pressure is > 90 mm Hg,[1] and dobutamine if the systolic blood pressure is < 90 mm Hg.[1] The use of vasopressors (**dopamine** or **norepinephrine**) should be limited to patients with significant hypotension.[1] Dosages of these agents are based on vital signs, clinical status, comorbidities and the treatment regimen of the patient. In select patients, invasive monitoring of hemodynamic parameters may be used to adjust the dose.

Therapeutic Tips

- The choice of whether to start an ACE inhibitor or a beta-blocker first in a given patient is based on the vital signs, blood pressure and comorbidities. Most clinicians will start both agents simultaneously at low doses.
- If introduced sequentially, it is not necessary to reach the target doses of one agent before starting the other.
- The doses of ACE inhibitors and beta-blockers should generally not be increased simultaneously.
- Hypotension or worsening renal function when initiating or increasing the dose of an ACE inhibitor usually indicates the need to reduce the dose of a diuretic.
- The formulation of metoprolol available in Canada (metoprolol tartrate) has not been shown to reduce mortality in patients with HF, is not available in a commercial dosage form that is suitable for initial treatment of HF and is not included in Canadian guidelines. Mortality and hospital admissions were significantly more frequent in patients treated with metoprolol tartrate (target dose 50 mg BID) than with

carvedilol (25 mg BID) in a large randomized trial.[30] The target dose of metoprolol tartrate used in this trial was lower than the target dose of controlled-release metoprolol succinate that has been shown to significantly decrease mortality in a large placebo-controlled trial.[12]

- In patients with hypotension, consider administering the blood pressure–lowering drugs at different times during the day.
- Cough is a symptom of HF decompensation. Careful evaluation is necessary when evaluating a cough in a patient receiving an ACE inhibitor.
- Electrolyte abnormalities are common in patients with HF. Patients need to be closely monitored, especially when taking combinations that have additive effects, for example, increased serum potassium due to the combination of an ACE inhibitor or ARB plus spironolactone.

Figure 1: **Evaluation of Patients with Heart Failure**

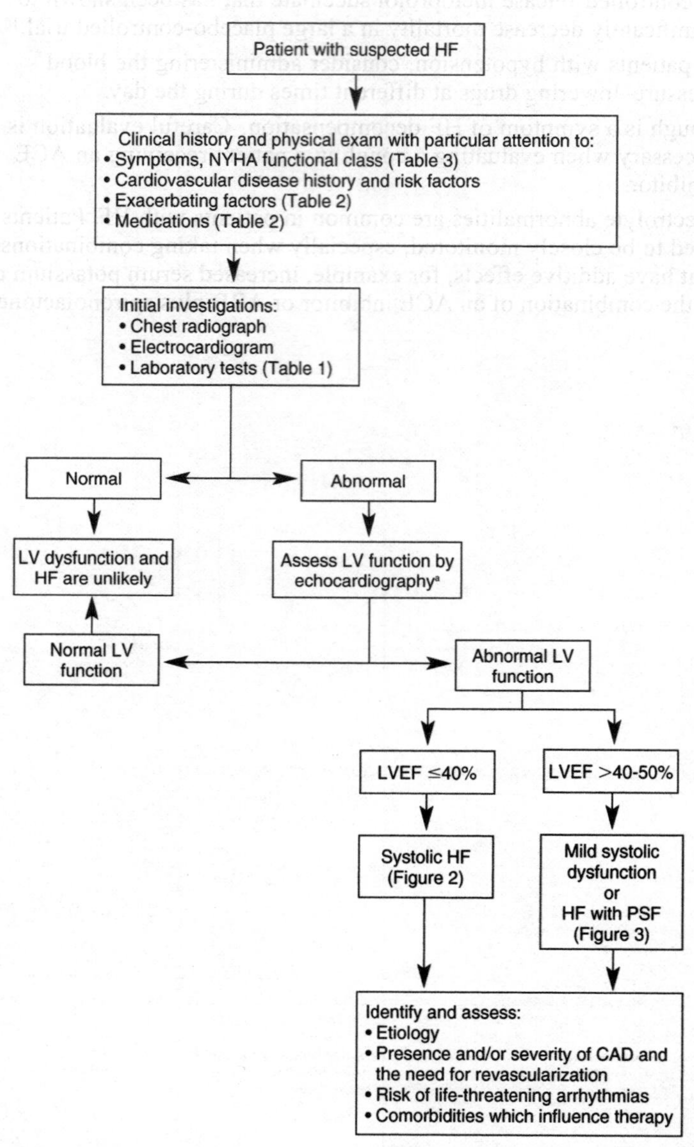

[a] Echocardiography (two dimensional or transthoracic) is used to determine LVEF, chamber size, wall thickness, valve function and presence of pericardial disease. Consider other diagnostic investigations if inconclusive (e.g., magnetic resonance imaging or cardiac catheterization).

Abbreviations: HF = heart failure; LV = left ventricular; LVEF = LV ejection fraction

Figure 2: **Management of Systolic Heart Failure**

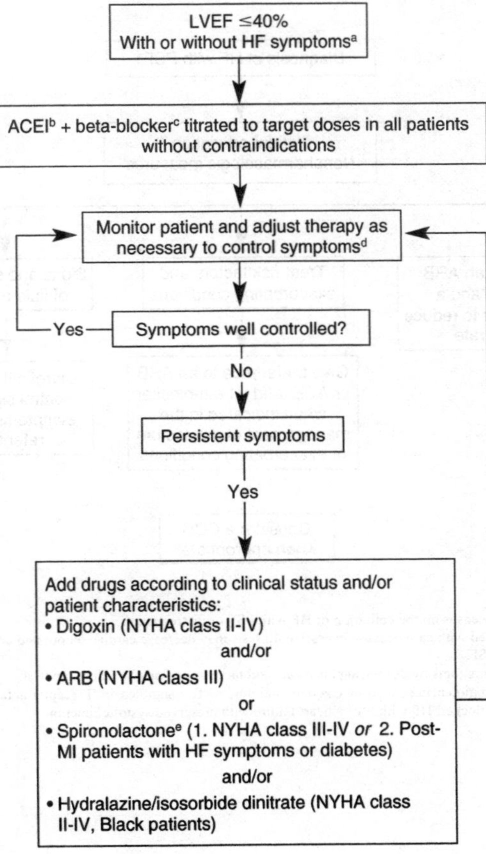

[a] Identify and manage risk factors, educate all patients about their disease and implement nonpharmacologic treatment. Consider ICD and resynchronization therapy in select patients.

[b] Use an ARB in patients with ACEI-induced cough that is intolerable or angioedema (although there is a low risk of angioedema with ARBs). Alternatively, substitute hydralazine/isosorbide dinitrate combination therapy for ACEI and or ARB-induced hyperkalemia, renal dysfunction or angioedema.

[c] Consider using ACEI/ARB combination therapy to prevent disease progression in patients with minimal to moderate symptoms (i.e., NYHA II) who cannot tolerate a beta-blocker.

[d] Use diuretics to minimize fluid retention. Consider combination diuretic therapy in patients with severe symptoms.

[e] Avoid the combination of an ACEI plus an ARB and spironolactone because of the risk of hyperkalemia.

Abbreviations: ACEI = angiotensin converting enzyme inhibitor; ARB = angiotensin II receptor blocker; LVEF = left ventricular ejection fraction; NYHA = New York Heart Association

Figure 3: **Management of Heart Failure with Preserved Systolic Function**

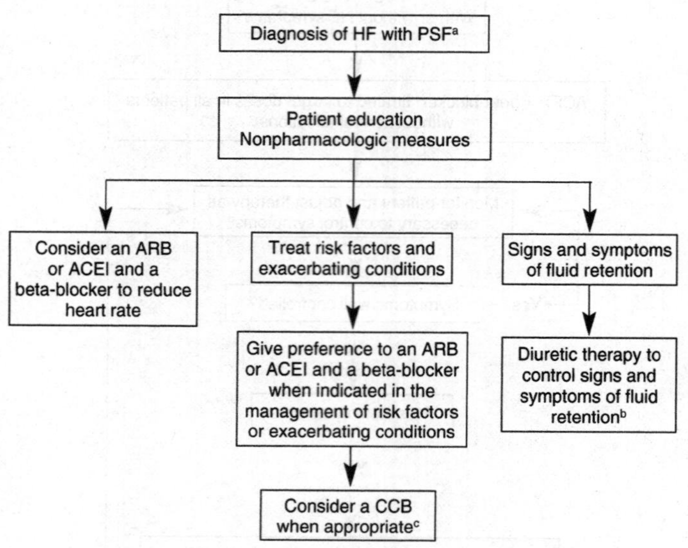

[a] There is no strong consensus on the definition of HF with PSF or its treatment.
[b] Diuretics should be used with care because excessive diuresis may decrease cardiac output and compromise renal function in HF with PSF.
[c] CCBs may improve symptoms by decreasing heart rate and increasing diastolic filling time.
Abbreviations: ACEI = angiotensin converting enzyme inhibitor; ARB = angiotensin II receptor antagonist; CCB = calcium channel blocker; HF with PSF = heart failure with preserved systolic function

Table 4: Outcomes Associated with Drugs Used for Systolic Heart Failure

Outcome	Intervention	Comparator	Relative risk reduction (%)	Absolute risk reduction (%)	Number needed to treat to prevent one outcome
Death prevented	ACE inhibitor[8]	Placebo	16	4.5	23
	Beta-blocker[13]	Placebo	32	5.5	29
	Aldosterone antagonist[22]	Placebo	30	11	10
	Hydralazine/isosorbide dinitrate[27]	Placebo	39	4	25
Hospitalizations avoided	ACE inhibitor[8]	Placebo	30	10.8	9
	Beta-blocker[13]	Placebo	33	6	17
	Digoxin[23]	Placebo	28	7.9	13

Table 5: Drugs Used for Heart Failure

Class	Drug	Dose	Adverse Effects	Drug Interactions	Comments	Cost[a]
ACE Inhibitors[b]	*captopril* Capoten, generics	Initial: 6.25–12.5 mg TID Target: 25–50 mg TID	Hypotension, hyperkalemia, dry cough, renal insufficiency, angioedema (rare), skin rashes, taste disturbance, proteinuria, neutropenia (rare), headache, dizziness.	Diuretics: hypotension (monitor BP). Potassium-sparing diuretics, potassium supplements, ARBs: hyperkalemia (monitor K^+). NSAIDs: decreased hypotensive effect (monitor BP), fluid retention, renal failure. Lithium: lithium toxicity (monitor lithium levels).	Monitor serum creatinine and potassium after initiation of therapy. Some experienced clinicians use doses higher than usual target doses.	$$
	enalapril Vasotec, generics	Initial: 1.25–2.5 mg BID Target: 10 mg BID	See captopril.	See captopril.	See captopril.	$$$
	lisinopril Prinivil, Zestril, generics	Initial: 2.5–5 mg once daily Target: 20–35 mg once daily	See captopril.	See captopril.	See captopril.	$$
	ramipril Altace, generics	Initial: 1.25–2.5 mg BID Target: 5 mg BID	See captopril.	See captopril.	See captopril.	$$
	trandolapril Mavik	Initial: 1 mg once daily Target: 4 mg once daily	See captopril.	See captopril.	See captopril.	$$

Class	Drug	Dose	Adverse Effects	Drug Interactions	Comments	Cost[a]
Angiotensin Receptor Blocker	*candesartan* Atacand	Initial: 4 mg once daily Target: 32 mg once daily	Hypotension, hyperkalemia, renal insufficiency, angioedema (rare, less frequent than with ACE inhibitors), headache, dizziness.	Diuretics: hypotension (monitor BP). Potassium-sparing diuretics and ACE inhibitors: hyperkalemia (monitor K^+). Potassium: hyperkalemia (monitor K^+). NSAIDs: decreased hypotensive effect (monitor BP), fluid retention, renal failure. Lithium: lithium toxicity (monitor lithium levels).		$$$
	valsartan Diovan	Initial: 40 mg BID Target: 160 mg BID	See candesartan.	See candesartan.		$$$$$
Thiazides and Related Diuretics	*chlorthalidone* ❥ generics	50–100 mg once daily Max: 200 mg/day (use lower doses when used in combination with a loop diuretic)	Dehydration, hypokalemia, nausea, hypotension, azotemia, hypomagnesemia, hypercalcemia, hyponatremia, hyperglycemia (more with thiazides), hyperuricemia, rash, increased total cholesterol.	Lithium: lithium toxicity (monitor lithium levels). Digoxin: digoxin toxicity if K^+ depleted (monitor K^+). Corticosteroids: hypokalemia (monitor K^+). NSAIDs: decreased diuretic effect; increased renal toxicity (monitor).	Use in patients with mild HF or with a loop diuretic.	$

(cont'd)

Table 5: **Drugs Used for Heart Failure** *(cont'd)*

Class	Drug	Dose	Adverse Effects	Drug Interactions	Comments	Cost[a]
	hydrochlorothiazide generics	25–100 mg/day given in 1 or 2 divided doses Max: 200 mg/day (use lower doses when used in combination with a loop diuretic)	See chlorthalidone.	See chlorthalidone.	See chlorthalidone.	$
	metolazone Zaroxolyn	2.5–10 mg once daily (use lower doses in combination with a loop diuretic)	See chlorthalidone.	See chlorthalidone.	Use in patients with mild HF or with a loop diuretic in those with refractory HF.	$
Loop Diuretics	*bumetanide* Burinex	1–4 mg/day	Dehydration, hypokalemia, hypocalcemia, nausea, hypotension, azotemia, hypomagnesemia, anorexia, hyperglycemia (less than with thiazides), hyperuricemia, weakness, fatigue, rash, increased total cholesterol, ototoxicity with high doses.	See chlorthalidone.	1 mg = 40 mg furosemide.	$–$$$$
	furosemide Lasix, generics	20–500 mg/day given daily to BID For decompensated HF: may be given BID or TID	See bumetanide.	See chlorthalidone.		$

Class	Drug	Dose	Adverse Effects	Drug Interactions	Comments	Cost[a]
	ethacrynic acid Edecrin	50–200 mg daily or divided BID	See bumetanide.	See chlorthalidone.	An alternative diuretic in patients with allergies to loop diuretics. Higher risk of ototoxicity than furosemide.	$$
Aldosterone Antagonists	*spironolactone* Aldactone, generics	Initial: 12.5 mg daily Target (for mortality benefit): 25–50 mg/day Higher doses can be used for stronger diuretic effects, but rarely used/appropriate, unless patient has severe right HF	Hyperkalemia; dehydration; gynecomastia (usually reversible upon discontinuation).	ACE inhibitors, ARBs, potassium supplements: hyperkalemia. NSAIDs: decreased diuretic effect, worsening renal function, hyperkalemia.		$
Beta$_1$-adrenergic Antagonists	*bisoprolol* Monocor, generics	Initial: 1.25 mg po daily Target: 10 mg daily	Orthostatic hypotension, fluid retention, bronchospasm (less with beta$_1$-selective), dyspnea, bradycardia, malaise, fatigue, asthenia, erectile dysfunction, may mask hypoglycemia.	Digoxin, amiodarone, diltiazem, verapamil: ↑ bradycardia. Nondihydropyridine calcium channel blockers: additive cardiodepressant effect.	Selective beta-blocker.	$

(cont'd)

Table 5: **Drugs Used for Heart Failure** *(cont'd)*

Class	Drug	Dose	Adverse Effects	Drug Interactions	Comments	Cost[a]
	carvedilol Coreg, generics	Initial: 3.125 mg po BID Target: 25 mg BID	See bisoprolol. More likely to cause orthostatic hypotension than bisoprolol.	See bisoprolol. CYP 2D6 inhibitors.	Nonselective beta-blocker with alpha-blocking activity. Has some vasodilating effects.	$$
Vasodilators	*hydralazine*	Initial: 37.5 mg po TID Target: 75 mg TID	Hypotension, gastrointestinal complaints, lupus-like syndrome.		Used in combination with isosorbide dinitrate in Black patients with HF.	$$
	isosorbide dinitrate generics	Initial: 20 mg po TID Target: 40 mg TID	Headache, hypotension.	Sildenafil, vardenafil and tadalafil: severe hypotension.	Use in combination with hydralazine in Black patients with HF.	$
	nitroglycerin generics	5–200 µg/min iv	Hypotension, headache, tachycardia, bradycardia.	See isosorbide dinitrate.		$$$$$
	nitroprusside generics	0.1–5 µg/kg/min iv	Hypotension, cyanide toxicity, thiocyanate toxicity, methemoglobinemia, coronary artery steal, tachycardia, increased intracranial pressure.			$$$$$
Calcium Channel Blockers	*amlodipine* Norvasc	2.5–10 mg daily	Hypotension, constipation, peripheral edema, gingival hyperplasia, headache, dizziness.			$$-$$$

Class	Drug	Dose	Adverse Effects	Drug Interactions	Comments	Cost[a]
	felodipine Plendil, Renedil, generics	2.5–10 mg daily	See amlodipine.			$
Inotropic Agents	*digoxin* [renal] Lanoxin	0.0625–0.25 mg daily (lower doses may be appropriate in select patients)	Anorexia, nausea, vomiting, visual disturbances, fatigue, dizziness, confusion, delirium. Cardiac arrhythmia. Noncardiovascular adverse effects do not always precede potentially fatal arrhythmias.	Amiodarone, quinidine, verapamil, propafenone, erythromycin, clarithromycin, tetracycline, itraconazole, cyclosporine and ritonavir ↑ digoxin levels. Antacids, cholestyramine, colestipol, sulfasalazine, neomycin, rifampin, St. John's wort ↓ digoxin levels. Beta-blockers, amiodarone, verapamil, diltiazem ↑ risk of bradycardia.	Adjust dose based on patient's age, weight, renal function and concomitant drugs.	$
	milrinone generics	0.1 to 0.75 µg/kg/min	Tachyarrhythmias, hypotension, myocardial ischemia, thrombocytopenia.			$$$$$
	dobutamine generics	2 to 20 µg/kg/min	Tachyarrhythmias, hypokalemia, myocardial ischemia.	Beta-blockers: reduce positive inotropic effects of dobutamine.		$$$$$

[a] Cost of 30-day supply for target doses; includes drug cost only. For ACE inhibitors, cost was calculated for the targeted dose.
[b] Only captopril, enalapril, ramipril and trandolapril have been shown to reduce morbidity and prolong survival in heart failure or in patients with LV dysfunction post-MI.
[renal] Dosage adjustment may be required in renal impairment; see Appendix I
Legend: $ < $25 $$ $25–50 $$–$$$ $25–75 $$$ $50–75 $$$$ $75–100 $–$$$$ < $25–100 $$$$$ > $100

Suggested Readings

Arnold JM, Liu P, Demers C et al. Canadian Cardiovascular Society consensus conference recommendations on heart failure 2006: diagnosis and management. *Can J Cardiol* 2006;22(1):23-45.

Heart Failure Society Of America. HFSA 2006 comprehensive heart failure practice guideline. *J Card Fail* 2006;12(1):e1-122.

Hunt SA. ACC/AHA 2005 guideline update for the diagnosis and management of chronic heart failure in the adult: a report of the American College of Cardiology/American Heart Association Task Force on Practice Guidelines (Writing Committee to Update the 2001 Guidelines for the Evaluation and Management of Heart Failure). *J Am Coll Cardiol* 2005;46(6):e1-82.

Jessup M, Brozena S. Heart failure. *N Engl J Med* 2003;348(20):2007-18.

Swedberg K, Cleland J, Dargie H et al. Guidelines for the diagnosis and treatment of chronic heart failure: executive summary (update 2005): The Task Force for the Diagnosis and Treatment of Chronic Heart Failure of the European Society of Cardiology. *Eur Heart J* 2005;26(11):1115-40.

References

1. Arnold JM, Liu P, Demers C et al. Canadian Cardiovascular Society consensus conference recommendations on heart failure 2006: diagnosis and management. *Can J Cardiol* 2006;22(1):23-45.
2. Jessup M, Brozena S. Heart failure. *N Engl J Med* 2003;348(20):2007-18.
3. Swedberg K, Cleland J, Dargie H et al. Guidelines for the diagnosis and treatment of chronic heart failure: executive summary (update 2005): The Task Force for the Diagnosis and Treatment of Chronic Heart Failure of the European Society of Cardiology. *Eur Heart J* 2005;26(11):1115-40.
4. Heart Failure Society Of America. HFSA 2006 comprehensive heart failure practice guideline. *J Card Fail* 2006;12(1):e1-122.
5. Hunt SA. ACC/AHA 2005 guideline update for the diagnosis and management of chronic heart failure in the adult: a report of the American College of Cardiology/American Heart Association Task Force on Practice Guidelines (Writing Committee to Update the 2001 Guidelines for the Evaluation and Management of Heart Failure). *J Am Coll Cardiol* 2005;46(6):e1-82.
6. Ross H, Hendry P, Dipchand A et al. 2001 Canadian Cardiovascular Society Consensus Conference on cardiac transplantation. *Can J Cardiol* 2003;19(6):620-54.
7. [No authors listed]. Effects of enalapril on mortality in severe congestive heart failure. Results of the Cooperative North Scandinavian Enalapril Survival Study (CONSENSUS). The CONSENSUS Trial Study Group. *N Engl J Med* 1987;316(23):1429-35.
8. [No authors listed]. Effect of enalapril on survival in patients with reduced left ventricular ejection fractions and congestive heart failure. The SOLVD Investigators. *N Engl J Med* 1991;325(5):293-302.
9. [No authors listed]. Effect of enalapril on mortality and the development of heart failure in asymptomatic patients with reduced left ventricular ejection fractions. The SOLVD Investigators. *N Engl J Med* 1992;327(10):685-91.
10. Packer M, Poole-Wilson PA, Armstrong PW et al. Comparative effects of low and high doses of the angiotensin-converting enzyme inhibitor, lisinopril, on morbidity and mortality in chronic heart failure. ATLAS Study Group. *Circulation* 1999;100(23):2312-8.
11. de Denus S, Tardif JC, White M et al. Quantification of the risk and predictors of hyperkalemia in patients with left ventricular dysfunction: a retrospective analysis of the Studies of Left Ventricular Dysfunction (SOLVD) trials. *Am Heart J* 2006;152(4):705-12.
12. [No authors listed]. Effect of metoprolol CR/XL in chronic heart failure: Metoprolol CR/XL Randomised Intervention Trial in Congestive Heart Failure (MERIT-HF). *Lancet* 1999;353(9169):2001-7.
13. [No authors listed]. The Cardiac Insufficiency Bisoprolol Study II (CIBIS-II): a randomised trial. *Lancet* 1999;353(9146):9-13.
14. Packer M, Bristow MR, Cohn JN et al. The effect of carvedilol on morbidity and mortality in patients with chronic heart failure. U.S. Carvedilol Heart Failure Study Group. *N Engl J Med* 1996;334(21):1349-55.
15. Packer M, Coats AJ, Fowler MB et al. Effect of carvedilol on survival in severe chronic heart failure. *N Engl J Med* 2001;344(22):1651-8.

16. Brater DC. Diuretic therapy. *N Engl J Med* 1998;339(6):387-95.
17. Granger CB, McMurray JJ, Yusuf S et al. Effects of candesartan in patients with chronic heart failure and reduced left-ventricular systolic function intolerant to angiotensin-converting-enzyme inhibitors: the CHARM-Alternative trial. *Lancet* 2003;362(9386):772-6.
18. Pfeffer MA, McMurray JJ, Velazquez EJ et al. Valsartan, captopril, or both in myocardial infarction complicated by heart failure, left ventricular dysfunction, or both. *N Engl J Med* 2003;349(20):1893-906.
19. McMurray JJ, Ostergren J, Swedberg K et al. Effects of candesartan in patients with chronic heart failure and reduced left-ventricular systolic function taking angiotensin-converting-enzyme inhibitors: the CHARM-Added trial. *Lancet* 2003;362(9386):767-71.
20. Cohn JN, Tognoni G. A randomized trial of the angiotensin-receptor blocker valsartan in chronic heart failure. *N Engl J Med* 2001;345(23):1667-75.
21. Pitt B, Remme W, Zannad F et al. Eplerenone, a selective aldosterone blocker, in patients with left ventricular dysfunction after myocardial infarction. *N Engl J Med* 2003;348(14):1309-21.
22. Pitt B, Zannad F, Remme WJ et al. The effect of spironolactone on morbidity and mortality in patients with severe heart failure. Randomized Aldactone Evaluation Study Investigators. *N Engl J Med* 1999;341(10):709-17.
23. [No authors listed]. The effect of digoxin on mortality and morbidity in patients with heart failure. The Digitalis Investigation Group. *N Engl J Med* 1997;336(8):525-33.
24. Gheorghiade M, van Veldhuisen DJ, Colucci WS. Contemporary use of digoxin in the management of cardiovascular disorders. *Circulation* 2006;113(21):2556-64.
25. Rathore SS, Curtis JP, Wang Y et al. Association of serum digoxin concentration and outcomes in patients with heart failure. *JAMA* 2003;289(7):871-8.
26. Adams KF, Gheorghiade M, Uretsky BF et al. Clinical benefits of low serum digoxin concentrations in heart failure. *J Am Coll Cardiol* 2002;39(6):946-53.
27. Taylor AL, Ziesche S, Yancy C et al. Combination of isosorbide dinitrate and hydralazine in blacks with heart failure. *N Engl J Med* 2004;351(20):2049-57.
28. Cohn JN, Ziesche S, Smith R et al. Effect of the calcium antagonist felodipine as supplementary vasodilator therapy in patients with chronic heart failure treated with enalapril: V-HeFT III. Vasodilator-Heart Failure Trial (V-HeFT) Study Group. *Circulation* 1997;96(3):856-63.
29. Packer M, O'Connor CM, Ghali JK et al. Effect of amlodipine on morbidity and mortality in severe chronic heart failure. Prospective Randomized Amlodipine Survival Evaluation Study Group. *N Engl J Med* 1996;335(15):1107-14.
30. Poole-Wilson PA, Swedberg K, Cleland JG, et al. Comparison of carvedilol and metoprolol on clinical outcomes in patients with chronic heart failure in the Carvedilol Or Metoprolol European Trial (COMET): randomised controlled trial. *Lancet* 2003;362(9377):7–13.

Pharmacoeconomic Considerations: Heart Failure

Blair Jarvis, MSc, BSP

Epidemiology	
Country (Year)	**Prevalence**
Canada (2000-2001)[1]	85 679 people spent a total of 1.4 million days in hospital for heart failure Median length of stay: 7 days
Cost of Illness Data	

(cont'd)

Country and Year of Estimate	Direct Costs[a]
United States (2000)[2]	Direct costs over a 5-year period for: • patients with left ventricular ejection fraction < 50%: US $33 023 • patients with preserved left ventricular ejection fraction: US $32 580

Commentary

Heart failure is the most common cause of hospitalization in the elderly, and 80% of hospitalizations for heart failure and 90% of deaths due to heart failure occur in those older than 65 years.[3] In Canada, the mean age of a person hospitalized for heart failure in 2000–2001 was 76 years and the in-hospital mortality rate was 15.5%.[1] There were more than 100 000 hospital discharges for heart failure in that year, approximately one-third of which were after re-admissions. The burden of heart failure in Canada is projected to increase as the population ages.[4] Measures that stabilize the disease and reduce the rate of hospitalization are likely to be highly cost-effective.

Drug therapy for heart failure reduces symptoms, improves health-related quality of life, retards disease progression, prevents hospitalizations and prolongs life. The most extensive evidence of benefit pertains to the use of ACE inhibitors and beta blockers.

There is evidence of substantial care gaps where the benefits of heart failure therapies are not being realized in routine clinical practice.[5] The difference in impact of interventions in clinical trials and clinical practice has been likened to a "diffusion gradient." Removing this diffusion gradient and increasing adherence with treatment guidelines is likely to be cost-effective. For example, increasing use of ACE inhibitors, beta-blockers, digoxin and spironolactone by 10% would be expected to reduce the rate of hospitalization for heart failure and save as much as $6.6 million in one year based on Alberta data.[6] This would result in a net savings of $2.3 million.[6] Canadian treatment guidelines provide target doses for each medication, so clinicians should be sure not only to prescribe appropriate drugs, but to titrate the dose to a level shown to produce benefits in clinical trials. Programs of follow-up by nurses or pharmacists with patients released from hospital have been shown to reduce re-admissions and hospital costs within six months.[7]

Most pharmacoeconomic studies are conducted from the societal rather than an individual perspective. The relative cost of individual medications for heart failure is inexpensive because of the availability of generic products; however, because patients must take a number of drugs to achieve optimal outcomes, the total cost for an individual may

(cont'd)

Commentary

be substantial. Patients who perceive the medical costs of heart failure to be a burden have worse health status than those without a perceived economic burden.[8] Thus, inquiring about financial constraints and involving other members of the health care team (e.g., nurses, social workers, pharmacists) may be helpful in addressing the needs of patients with diminished health status.

[a] Direct costs include those associated with physician services, nursing care, diagnostic procedures, drugs and hospitalization.

References

1. Tsuyuki RT, Shibata MC, Nilsson C et al. Contemporary burden of illness of congestive heart failure in Canada. *Can J Cardiol* 2003;19(4):436-8.
2. Liao L, Jollis JG, Anstrom KJ et al. Costs for heart failure with normal vs reduced ejection fraction. *Arch Intern Med* 2006;166(1):112-8.
3. Haldeman GA, Croft JB, Giles WH et al. Hospitalization of patients with heart failure: National Hospital Discharge Survey, 1985 to 1995. *Am Heart J* 1999;137(2):352-60.
4. Johansen H, Strauss B, Arnold JM et al. On the rise: The current and projected future burden of congestive heart failure hospitalization in Canada. *Can J Cardiol* 2003;19(4):430-5.
5. Kosiborod M, Lichtman JH, Heidenreich PA et al. National trends in outcomes among elderly patients with heart failure. *Am J Med* 2006;119(7):616-7.
6. Shibata MC, Nilsson C, Hervas-Malo M et al. Economic implications of treatment guidelines for congestive heart failure. *Can J Cardiol* 2005;21(14):1301-6.
7. Tsuyuki RT, Fradette M, Johnson JA et al. A multicentre disease management program for hospitalized patients with heart failure. *J Card Fail* 2004;10(6):473-80.
8. Conard MW, Heidenreich P, Rumsfeld JS et al. Patient-reported economic burden and the health status of heart failure patients. *J Card Fail* 2006;12(5):369-74.

CHAPTER 37
Prevention of Ischemic Stroke

Robert Côté, MD, FRCPC

Identification of high risk individuals based on their vascular risk profile is the most efficient strategy for preventing stroke. Risk factors for a first stroke are classified either as nonmodifiable (e.g., age, sex, family history) or modifiable (hypertension, dyslipidemia, smoking, diabetes mellitus, carotid disease). Primary prevention of stroke is covered in detail elsewhere (see Chapter 30). Secondary prevention of ischemic stroke is the main subject of this chapter.

The occurrence of a first transient ischemic attack (TIA) or ischemic stroke increases the risk of experiencing a second ischemic event. The short-term prognosis after a first TIA may be worse for patients with certain characteristics and a particular constellation of symptoms, of whom 10% will present with a stroke within three months.[1] Adverse prognostic indicators include age > 60 years, diabetes mellitus, speech and/or motor symptoms and duration of the symptoms for > 10 minutes. Accordingly, these higher risk patients should be promptly investigated and treated, optimally within two weeks of the initial ischemic event.

Goals of Therapy

- Prevent disabling neurologic deficits (stroke) and recurrent TIA
- Prevent cerebrovascular and cardiovascular-related mortality

Investigations

- Complete history with attention to:
  - nature, frequency, duration and distribution of symptoms (cerebral localization)
  - identification of vascular risk factors
- Physical examination:
  - complete neurologic assessment
  - visual assessment including eye movements, visual fields, acuity and funduscopy
  - complete vascular examination including auscultation (cranium, cervical, cardiac), palpation (temporal artery, peripheral pulses) and blood pressure in both arms
- Laboratory tests—indicated in most patients with TIAs or mild strokes (without disabling deficits):
  - CT brain scan (to exclude a hemorrhagic process and/or TIA mimics), cervical and transcranial ultrasonography
  - CBC, coagulation parameters, blood glucose, renal, lipid and hepatic enzyme profile

- in select patients (i.e., young patients or older patients with possible arteritis), more specialized blood tests (e.g., ESR, immunologic work-up, testing for hypercoagulable states, antiphospholipid antibodies, homocysteine) should be performed
- baseline ECG (exclude atrial fibrillation)
- other cardiac tests (e.g., transthoracic or transesophageal echocardiography, Holter monitoring) may be indicated (usually have a higher yield in patients with established cardiac disease or in young stroke patients)
- cerebral angiography in select patients to confirm occlusive cerebrovascular disease and to establish appropriateness of endarterectomy. MRI, MR angiography (MRA) or CT angiography may be required to confirm the diagnosis and/or exclude other neurologic conditions mimicking cerebral ischemia.

Therapeutic Choices (Figure 1)

Nonpharmacologic Choices

- Stop smoking (see Chapter 10).
- Control vascular risk factors through weight reduction and diet modification (reducing alcohol, fat and salt consumption).
- Start rehabilitative therapy (physiotherapy, occupational and speech therapy) if indicated.

Carotid Endarterectomy

- The prevalence of asymptomatic carotid disease in patients aged > 65 years can be as high as 10% for the presence of a stenosis (≥ 50%). The risk of ischemic stroke increases with the degree of stenosis and evidence of progression of the stenosis, and with the presence of coronary disease, hypertension and/or peripheral vascular disease.[2] The annual rate of unheralded stroke ipsilateral to a substantial (≥ 50%) stenosis is about 1.5%. In addition, the presence of carotid disease is a marker of concomitant coronary disease which accounts for about half of all ischemic events in these individuals. Presently, no evidence supports the use of ASA for ischemic stroke prevention in this clinical context although it may be required for its cardioprotective effects in patients with evidence of coronary disease.[6] The role of prophylactic carotid endarterectomy for asymptomatic carotid disease may be considered in select individuals with a high degree (i.e., ≥ 60%) of stenosis and when performed by surgeons with low complication rates (≤ 3%).[3] In many cases, however, close follow-up with patient education about potential neurologic symptoms and elimination or control of vascular risk factors is acceptable.
- Consider carotid endarterectomy in addition to long-term antithrombotic therapy for patients with carotid symptoms, ipsilateral to a significant (≥ 70%) carotid stenosis documented by angiography, cervical duplex, MRA or CT angiography.

Pharmacologic Choices (Table 1)

Antiplatelet agents are the drugs of choice for long-term prevention of atherothrombotic events (intra-arterial disease with secondary embolic phenomena).[4,5]

Oral anticoagulants are used to prevent cerebral ischemic events from emboli presumed to be of cardiac origin (see Chapter 39); however, ASA or other antiplatelet medications are preferred for the prevention of noncardioembolic ischemic strokes.[5]

Antihypertensive and lipid-lowering treatments have recently been shown to be effective for patients who have previously experienced a TIA or a stroke, especially those who are hypertensive (BP > 140/90) or have elevated cholesterol (LDL-C > 2.6 mmol/L).[6,7]

Antiplatelet Agents

Acetylsalicylic Acid (ASA)

Often given as initial therapy for stroke prevention, **ASA** reduces vascular events (cardiac and cerebral) by about 25% in high-risk individuals. Its protective effect is more modest in patients with TIA or ischemic stroke with a relative risk reduction of approximately 15% for the prevention of major vascular events.[4] It is well tolerated with few (dose-dependent) side effects. Patient acceptability and low cost are advantages. The recommended dosage for stroke prevention is 50 to 325 mg/day, depending on the patient's tolerance and the clinical situation. For example, in patients with concomitant coronary disease the recommended minimum dosage is 75 mg/day.

When combined with an oral anticoagulant, ASA 100 mg/day provides better protection against cardioembolic events than an anticoagulant alone in patients with prosthetic heart valves.[8,9]

Thienopyridines

Clopidogrel 75 mg daily is somewhat more effective than ASA for the prevention of ischemic events, including stroke, in patients at high risk of ischemic events. The absolute difference in annual rate of ischemic stroke, MI or vascular death between clopidogrel and ASA was 0.5%, corresponding to an 8.7% relative risk reduction in favour of clopidogrel. Thus clopidogrel is an alternative antiplatelet agent, albeit an expensive one, in patients who are allergic to or cannot tolerate ASA.[10] It is as effective as ticlopidine but does not increase the risk of neutropenia, and is administered once daily.

The combination of low-dose ASA and clopidogrel did not significantly reduce the rate of ischemic events, including stroke, in patients with recent stroke or TIA when compared with clopidogrel alone,[11] or in patients with multiple risk factors, when compared with low-dose ASA alone.[12] However, combination therapy significantly increased the risk of bleeding in both trials,[11,12] and the risk of intracranial hemorrhage in the study that enrolled patients with a history of stroke or TIA.[11] Thus, although ASA plus clopidogrel is more effective than ASA alone in patients with acute coronary syndromes,[13] the combination should not be used for long-term secondary prevention of ischemic events in patients with a history of stroke.

Ticlopidine 250 mg twice daily is comparable to ASA for prevention of all vascular events in patients at risk and may be slightly superior for stroke prevention.[14] Diarrhea and skin rash are common adverse events of ticlopidine. Neutropenia occurs infrequently but is potentially serious and requires frequent monitoring (every two weeks for the first three months). For these reasons, ticlopidine is not recommended for routine use in stroke prevention.

Dipyridamole/ASA

The combination of **dipyridamole SR plus low-dose ASA** (200/25 mg) given twice daily reduces the relative risk of stroke by 23% (mostly for ischemic strokes) when compared with ASA in patients with cerebral ischemic symptoms.[15] This finding was confirmed in a recent randomized controlled trial in which the incidence of death, stroke, MI or major bleeding complications occurred significantly less often in patients with cerebral ischemia treated with dipyridamole/ASA than ASA alone (13% vs. 16% over a mean of 3.5 years).[16] No increased risk of cardiac events was reported in the dipyridamole/ASA groups in either study; however, a higher dose of ASA may be desirable in patients with concomitant coronary artery disease. The addition of 81 mg of ASA to the dipyridamole/ASA combination appears to be reasonable in these patients.

Anticoagulants

Warfarin or Nicoumalone

Oral anticoagulants prevent cerebral and systemic emboli in patients with acute MI, valvular and nonvalvular atrial fibrillation and prosthetic cardiac valves. The risk of bleeding is influenced by many factors (e.g., the intensity of anticoagulation, concomitant use of high doses of ASA or other drugs with antiplatelet effects, and the presence of cerebral white matter changes in the elderly).[17] Patients with nonvalvular atrial fibrillation and prior TIA/stroke may require a higher target International Normalized Ratio (INR) of 3.0 instead of 2.5.[18]

Therapeutic Tips

- In most cases antithrombotic treatment should be continued long term, especially in older individuals with atherosclerosis and vascular risk factors.
- The combination of low-dose ASA and slow-release dipyridamole appears to be more protective than ASA alone in patients with a recent cerebral ischemic event.
- It is common practice to switch treatment to dipyridamole/ASA or clopidogrel in patients who experience recurrent attacks of cerebral

ischemia while on low-dose ASA (i.e., 325 mg/day or less), although this has not been validated in clinical trials.

- It is common practice to prescribe the combination of low-dose ASA (81 mg/day) plus an oral anticoagulant in patients who have not responded to an anticoagulant alone and who are at risk for a cardioembolic stroke, although this has not been validated in clinical trials. Such patients should be followed very closely, as the risk for hemorrhagic complications is increased.
- Combination therapy (oral anticoagulant plus low-dose ASA) is superior to anticoagulant alone in patients with prosthetic heart valves but has an increased risk of minor bleeding episodes. For patients intolerant of ASA, dipyridamole (400 mg/day) plus an oral anticoagulant may be used. This approach has not been validated in clinical trials.
- In healthy postmenopausal women, the risks associated with combination **estrogen/progestin** therapy (i.e., increased risk of coronary heart disease, breast cancer and a 40% increase in stroke risk) exceed the beneficial effects on colorectal cancer and hip fracture.[19]
- In postmenopausal women who have suffered a recent stroke or TIA, hormonal therapy with estrogen does not have a protective effect.[20]
- The risk of ischemic stroke is increased in users of **low-dose oral contraceptives** compared with non-users. This translates into a relatively small increase in the absolute risk of stroke,[21] except possibly in the presence of other risk factors such as hypertension, smoking and prior thromboembolic events. In these settings, oral contraceptives should probably be avoided.

Figure 1: **Secondary Prevention of Cerebral Ischemia**

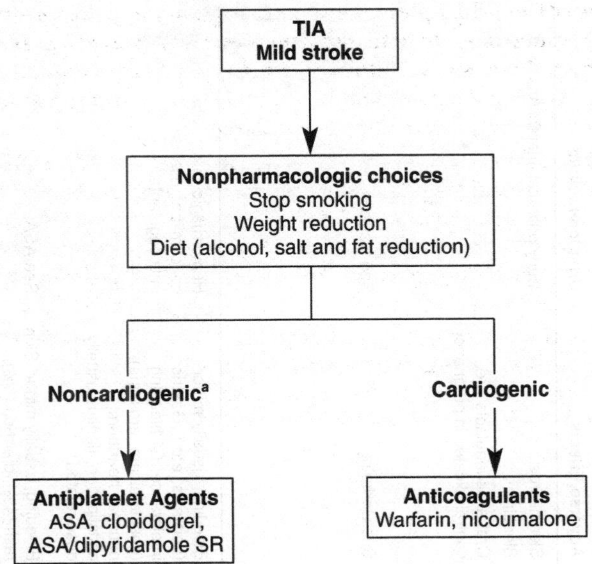

[a] If symptomatic carotid stenosis, consider surgery.
Mild or minor stroke = No substantial impact on activities of daily living.

Table 1: **Drugs Used in Secondary Prevention of Stroke**

Class	Drug	Dose	Adverse Effects	Drug Interactions	Cost[a]
Anticoagulants	*warfarin* Coumadin, generics	Oral: Dose to maintain INR between 2.0 and 3.0 for most cerebrovascular indications; for stroke prevention in patients with **mechanical heart valves**, maintain INR between 2.5 and 3.5	Skin necrosis. Bleeding. Oral anticoagulants are contraindicated in pregnancy.	Many potential interactions.	$
	nicoumalone Sintrom	Oral: Dose to maintain INR between 2.0 and 3.0 for most cerebrovascular indications; for stroke prevention in patients with mechanical heart valves, maintain INR between 2.5 and 3.5	See warfarin.	See warfarin.	$$-$$$
Antiplatelet Agents	*ASA* Aspirin, Bufferin, Coated Aspirin, generics	50–325 mg/day	Bleeding, usually minor (epistaxis, etc.) Gastric intolerance, GI bleeding (gastric ulcers, erosions), nausea, heartburn, constipation, tinnitus usually dose-related.	Hemorrhagic risk ↑ with concomitant use of anticoagulants.	$
	clopidogrel Plavix	75 mg daily	Bleeding, usually minor. Skin rash (4%); diarrhea (5%).	See ASA.	$$$$

Class	Drug	Dose	Adverse Effects	Drug Interactions	Cost[a]
	ticlopidine Ticlid, generics	250 mg BID	Bleeding, usually minor. Diarrhea (up to 20%), skin rash, neutropenia; contraindicated in severe hepatic impairment.	See ASA. ↓ digoxin levels. Absorption ↓ by antacids.	$$$
	dipyridamole/ASA 200/25 mg Aggrenox	1 capsule BID	Bleeding, usually minor. Headache, diarrhea.	See ASA.	$$$

[a] Cost of 30-day supply; includes drug cost only.
Legend: $ < $20 $$ $20–40 $$-$$$ $20–60 $$$ $40–60 $$$$ $60–80

Suggested Readings

Albers GW, Amarenco P, Easton JD et al. Antithrombotic and thrombolytic therapy for ischemic stroke: the Seventh ACCP Conference on Antithrombotic and Thrombolytic Therapy. *Chest* 2004;126(3 Suppl):483S-512S.

Antithrombotic Trialists' Collaboration. Collaborative meta-analysis of randomised trials of antiplatelet therapy for prevention of death, myocardial infarction, and stroke in high risk patients. *BMJ* 2002;324(7329):71-86.

Goldstein LB, Adams R, Alberts MJ et al. Primary prevention of ischemic stroke.*Circulation* 2006;113(24):e873-923.

Sacco RL, Adams R, Albers G et al. Guidelines for prevention of stroke in patients with ischemic stroke or transient ischemic attack. *Stroke* 2006;37(2):577-617.

References

1. Johnston SC, Gress DR, Browner WS et al. Short-term prognosis after emergency department diagnosis of TIA. *JAMA* 2000;284(22):2901-6.
2. Mackey AE, Abrahamowicz M, Langlois Y et al. Outcome of asymptomatic patients with carotid disease. Asymptomatic Cervical Bruit Study Group. *Neurology* 1997;48(4):896-903.
3. Goldstein LB, Adams R, Alberts MJ et al. Primary prevention of ischemic stroke: a guideline from the American Heart Association/American Stroke Association Stroke Council: cosponsored by the Atherosclerotic Peripheral Vascular Disease Interdisciplinary Working Group; Cardiovascular Nursing Council; Clinical Cardiology Council; Nutrition, Physical Activity, and Metabolism Council; and the Quality of Care and Outcomes Research Interdisciplinary Working Group. *Circulation* 2006;113(24):e873-923.
4. Antithrombotic Trialists' Collaboration. Collaborative meta-analysis of randomised trials of antiplatelet therapy for prevention of death, myocardial infarction, and stroke in high risk patients. *BMJ* 2002;324(7329):71-86.
5. Albers GW, Amarenco P, Easton JD et al. Antithrombotic and thrombolytic therapy for ischemic stroke: the Seventh ACCP Conference on Antithrombotic and Thrombolytic Therapy. *Chest* 2004;126(3 Suppl):483S-512S.
6. Amarenco P, Bogousslavsky J, Callahan A et al. High-dose atorvastatin after stroke or transient ischemic attack. *N Engl J Med* 2006;355(6):549-59.
7. Chapman N, Huxley R, Anderson C et al. Effects of a perindopril-based blood pressure-lowering regimen on the risk of recurrent stroke according to stroke subtype and medical history: the PROGRESS Trial. *Stroke* 2004;35(1):116-21.
8. Dentali F, Douketis JD, Lim W et al. Combined aspirin-oral anticoagulant therapy compared with oral anticoagulant therapy alone among patients at risk for cardiovascular disease: a meta-analysis of randomized trials. *Arch Intern Med* 2007;167(2):117-24.
9. Salem DN, Stein PD, Al-Ahmad A et al. Antithrombotic therapy in valvular heart disease--native and prosthetic: the Seventh ACCP Conference on Antithrombotic and Thrombolytic Therapy. *Chest* 2004;126(3 Suppl):457S-482S.
10. CAPRIE Steering Committee. A randomised, blinded, trial of clopidogrel versus aspirin in patients at risk of ischaemic events (CAPRIE). *Lancet* 1996;348(9038):1329-39.
11. Diener HC, Bogousslavsky J, Brass LM et al. Aspirin and clopidogrel compared with clopidogrel alone after recent ischaemic stroke or transient ischaemic attack in high-risk patients (MATCH): randomised, double-blind, placebo-controlled trial. *Lancet* 2004;364(9431):331-7.
12. Bhatt DL, Fox KA, Hacke W et al. Clopidogrel and aspirin versus aspirin alone for the prevention of atherothrombotic events. *N Engl J Med* 2006;354(16):1706-17.
13. Yusuf S, Zhao F, Mehta SR et al. Effects of clopidogrel in addition to aspirin in patients with acute coronary syndromes without ST-segment elevation. *N Engl J Med* 2001;345(7):494-502.
14. Hass WK, Easton JD, Adams HP et al. A randomized trial comparing ticlopidine hydrochloride with aspirin for the prevention of stroke in high-risk patients. Ticlopidine Aspirin Stroke Study Group. *N Engl J Med* 1989;321(8):501-7.
15. Diener HC, Cunha L, Forbes C et al. European Stroke Prevention Study. 2. Dipyridamole and acetylsalicylic acid in the secondary prevention of stroke. *J Neurol Sci* 1996;143(1-2):1-13.
16. ESPRIT Study Group; Halkes PH, van Gijn J et al. Aspirin plus dipyridamole versus aspirin alone after cerebral ischaemia of arterial origin (ESPRIT): randomised controlled trial. *Lancet* 2006;367(9523):1665-73.

17. Singer DE, Albers GW, Dalen JE et al. Antithrombotic therapy in atrial fibrillation: the Seventh ACCP Conference on Antithrombotic and Thrombolytic Therapy. *Chest* 2004;126(3 Suppl):429S-456S.
18. The European Atrial Fibrillation Trial Study Group. Optimal oral anticoagulant therapy in patients with nonrheumatic atrial fibrillation and recent cerebral ischemia. *N Engl J Med* 1995;333(1):5-10.
19. Rossouw JE, Anderson GL, Prentice RL et al. Risks and benefits of estrogen plus progestin in healthy postmenopausal women: principal results From the Women's Health Initiative randomized controlled trial. *JAMA* 2002;288(3):321-33.
20. Viscoli CM, Brass LM, Kernan WN et al. A clinical trial of estrogen-replacement therapy after ischemic stroke. *N Engl J Med* 2001;345(17):1243-9.
21. Gillum LA, Mamidipudi SK,.Johnston SC. Ischemic stroke risk with oral contraceptives: A meta-analysis. *JAMA* 2000;284(1):72-78.

Pharmacoeconomic Considerations: Prevention of Ischemic Stroke

Blair Jarvis, MSc, BSP

Epidemiology

Country (Year)	Incidence
Canada (Quebec 1988-2002)[1]	101 831 persons with ischemic stroke; 11 215 with hemorrhagic stroke

Cost of Illness Data

Region and Year of Estimate	Direct Costs[a]
Europe (1997)[2]	Cost of recurrent cerebral infarction: €18 560 over 18 months

Commentary

The epidemiology of stroke is changing in Canada. Over a 15-year period in Quebec, the rate of ischemic stroke dropped by 32.5% in men and 25.5% in women, and the case fatality rate decreased.[1] The authors of this study speculate that improved preventive measures may be responsible for the change in the incidence of ischemic stroke, but that more aggressive management of risk factors may be responsible for the increase in the incidence of hemorrhagic stroke.[1] Although the overall incidence of stroke is decreasing, the age and extent of comorbid disease in stroke survivors is increasing. This suggests that the burden borne by those caring for stroke survivors in the community may be growing.

The mean lifetime cost resulting from an ischemic stroke is estimated to be US $140 000.[3] A European study concluded that the costs of a first and a recurrent cerebral infarction were similar (approximately €20 000 over 18 months).[2] Therefore, interventions that prevent stroke and recurrence of stroke have the potential to produce significant cost savings for both the health care system and patients.

(cont'd)

Commentary

Antiplatelet agents are highly effective at preventing ischemic stroke. ASA is inexpensive and is recommended as first-line therapy. For patients without contraindications and without a drug plan, ASA is highly affordable and cost-effective.[4] Approximately one-third of patients experience gastrointestinal symptoms when taking ASA, which may limit the clinical effectiveness of the drug, particularly in an aging population with comorbid conditions.[5]

Alternatives to ASA (clopidogrel, dipyridamole/ASA) are more expensive but may offer modest improvements in efficacy. For patients aged > 65 years and older, dipyridamole/ASA is considered to be more effective and cost saving (dominant) when compared with ASA for secondary prevention of stroke or transient ischemic attack.[6,7] In contrast, clopidogrel is more effective than ASA, but the cost per quality-adjusted life-year is considerable (recently estimated to be US $57 714).[7]

Given the expense of these newer medications relative to ASA, the patient's ability to pay is pivotal. Regardless of the agent selected, tolerability and adherence must be closely monitored to ensure that patients receive maximum benefit from antiplatelet drugs.[5]

Other strategies for secondary prevention of stroke that are considered to be cost-effective include smoking cessation and blood pressure and cholesterol reduction.[4]

[a] Direct costs include those associated with physician services, nursing care, diagnostic procedures, drugs and hospitalization.

References

1. Mayo NE, Nadeau L, Daskalopoulou SS et al. The evolution of stroke in Quebec: a 15-year perspective. *Neurology* 2007;68(14):1122-7.
2. Spieler JF, De Pouvourville G, Amarenco P. Cost of a recurrent vs. cost of first-ever stroke over an 18-month period. *Eur J Neurol* 2003;10(6):621-4.
3. Centers for Disease Control and Prevention (CDC). Prevalence of stroke--United States, 2005. *MMWR Morb Mortal Wkly Rep* 2007;56(19):469-74.
4. Hankey GJ, Warlow CP. Treatment and secondary prevention of stroke: evidence, costs, and effects on individuals and populations. *Lancet* 1999;354(9188):1457-63.
5. Morton JA, Newton J, Gray CS. Counting the true cost of antiplatelet therapy for stroke prevention. *Age Ageing* 2005;34(3):212-4.
6. Sarasin FP, Gaspoz JM, Bounameaux H. Cost-effectiveness of new antiplatelet regimens used as secondary prevention of stroke or transient ischemic attack. *Arch Intern Med* 2000;160(18):2773-8.
7. Matchar DB, Samsa GP, Liu S. Cost-effectiveness of antiplatelet agents in secondary stroke prevention: the limits of certainty. *Value Health* 2005;8(5):572-80.

CHAPTER 38

Acute Ischemic Stroke

Stephen J. Phillips, BSc, MBBS, FRCPC and
Gord Gubitz, BSc, MD, FRCPC

Stroke, recognized clinically as the sudden onset of a focal disturbance of central nervous system function, may be caused by cerebral infarction (ischemic stroke, responsible for about 85% of all strokes), intracerebral hemorrhage or subarachnoid hemorrhage.[1]

There is no acute-phase intervention of proven value for intracerebral hemorrhage.[2] Intravenous recombinant activated factor VII has shown promise.[3]

Post-acute treatment of primary intracerebral hemorrhage is similar to that of ischemic stroke except that antithrombotic drugs are avoided. Treatment of subarachnoid hemorrhage is primarily nonpharmacologic (i.e., endovascular and/or surgical ablation of the bleeding source).[4] Refer patients with suspected subarachnoid hemorrhage to a neurosurgical centre.

Goals of Therapy

- Minimize brain damage
- Prevent complications
- Reduce risk of recurrence
- Restore function of the individual

Canadian Stroke Care Recommendations developed by the Best Practices and Standards Working Group of the Canadian Stroke Strategy are now available at http://www.canadianstrokestrategy.ca/technical_docs/StrokeStrategyManual.pdf.

Investigations

- History
  - time of onset, symptoms at onset, course of symptoms since onset
  - antecedent trauma or illness, previous neurovascular events
  - vascular comorbidity (angina, MI, heart failure, atrial fibrillation, peripheral and renal vascular disease)
  - vascular disease risk factors (hypertension, smoking, diabetes mellitus, cholesterol, excessive alcohol intake, body mass index, exercise, family history of vascular disease or hemostatic disorders)
  - other health problems (particularly peptic ulcer disease or other disorders that predispose to bleeding)
  - pre-stroke cognitive and functional status
  - place of residence and social supports

  - medications (particularly warfarin, ASA and other antiplatelet drugs)
- Physical examination to localize the lesion by brain region and vascular territory; determine the syndromic diagnosis, severity and cause; and assess comorbid conditions
- Laboratory tests:
  - CBC, INR, PTT, glucose (to rule out hypoglycemia as a stroke mimic), electrolytes, urea, creatinine, liver function tests, albumin
  - fasting glucose, hemoglobin A_{1c}, cholesterol panel (for risk factor modification)[5]
  - ECG (to look for atrial fibrillation, MI and left ventricular hypertrophy)
  - chest x-ray
  - CT (or MR) brain scan is required for all patients to rule out intracerebral hemorrhage and stroke mimics such as tumor. The urgency depends on the clinical situation (Table 1)
  - urgent (same or next day) vascular imaging (duplex carotid ultrasonography, CT angiography or MR angiography) is required for patients with nondisabling carotid territory strokes who are fit for carotid endarterectomy to determine the degree of carotid stenosis. Urgent referral to a stroke centre is required for patients with carotid stenosis > 50%[6,7]
  - echocardiography (transthoracic +/− transesophageal) is used to search for a cardiac source of emboli in patients with a recent history of MI or cardiac surgery, those aged < 50 years, and any patient with a large-vessel territory (nonlacunar) stroke and neurovascular imaging studies showing no large-vessel disease, provided anticoagulation is not contraindicated[8]
  - other investigations should be undertaken if indicated to rule out endocarditis, vasculitis or thromboembolic disorders

Table 1: **Indications for Immediate Brain Imaging**

Suspected subarachnoid hemorrhage
Potential candidates for thrombolysis within 3 h of stroke onset (Table 2)
Suspected cerebellar stroke (possible need for neurosurgical intervention)
No history available (possible subdural hematoma and need for neurosurgical intervention)
Patients on warfarin or heparin (possible need for reversal of anticoagulation)

Therapeutic Choices (Figure 1, Figure 2)

I. Minimize Brain Damage

Restore Perfusion

- **Alteplase** should be administered (iv) within three hours of stroke onset for patients who meet strict eligibility criteria[9,10] (Table 2, Table 3, Table 4)

Intra-arterial administration of thrombolytic agents is of limited usefulness.[11,12] Eligibility criteria and the time window for thrombolysis may be redefined as more data from randomized trials become available.[13,14]

Nonpharmacologic methods of achieving recanalization are under investigation.[15]

Table 2: **Alteplase in Acute Ischemic Stroke: Eligibility Criteria[10,12]**

Inclusion criteria
< 3 h from onset of symptoms
Disabling neurologic deficit
Symptoms present for ≥ 60 min with no sign of resolution
Consent of patient or legal next-of-kin (if unavailable, document the circumstances in the patient's hospital chart)

Exclusion criteria[a]
Intracranial hemorrhage on CT
Suspected subarachnoid hemorrhage
Previous intracranial hemorrhage
Cerebral infarct or severe head injury within the past 3 mo
Recent pericarditis
Major surgery within the past 14 days
GI or urinary hemorrhage within the past 21 days
Recent lumbar puncture or arterial puncture at a noncompressible site
Pregnancy
BP ≥ 185 mm Hg systolic or ≥ 110 mm Hg diastolic
Bleeding diathesis
Prolonged PTT or INR > 1.7
Platelet count ≤ 100 × 10^9/L
Blood glucose < 2.8 or > 22 mmol/L

If a patient fulfills all inclusion criteria and has no exclusion criteria, alteplase may be given (Table 4)

[a] A score > 22 on the NIH Stroke Scale[9] and CT signs of early ischemia are associated with an increased risk of intracerebral hemorrhage[14] but are not absolute contraindications to alteplase.

Salvage Ischemic Brain

- Provide supplemental oxygen if pulse oximetry shows desaturation.[16,17]
- Elevated body temperature is associated with poor outcome after stroke.[18,19,20] Hypothermia is strikingly beneficial in animal models of stroke. Symptomatic treatment of pyrexia (and investigation of its cause) is recommended.[16]
- Hyperglycemia is associated with poor outcome after stroke, suggesting that strict blood glucose control may be beneficial, but no definitive clinical trial data are available to guide treatment.[21]
- There are no good data to guide blood pressure treatment in the setting of acute stroke.[22,23,24] Transdermal nitroglycerin lowers blood pressure without altering cerebral blood flow in patients with recent stroke.[25]

The impact of blood pressure lowering with nitroglycerin on outcomes is the subject of a large ongoing trial (ENOS).[26]

Neurosurgical Intervention

- *Craniectomy* or *ventricular shunting* is sometimes performed on patients with massive hemispheric or cerebellar infarcts whose level of consciousness is declining. There is no evidence from randomized controlled trials to support this practice, but consensus opinion is that patients with cerebellar strokes, in particular, benefit from surgical intervention in this situation.
- According to an analysis of pooled data from randomized trials, the benefits of *endarterectomy* for symptomatic carotid stenosis are greatest in men, those aged 75 years or older with hemispheric rather than retinal events, and patients operated on soonest after the onset of symptoms.[27] Ideally, the procedure should be done within two weeks of the patient's last symptoms. The benefit of surgery is lost after four weeks for patients with 50–69% stenosis, and after 12 weeks for patients with stenosis >70%.[28]

Table 3: **Alteplase in Acute Ischemic Stroke: Monitoring**[9]

Vital Signs
- Baseline, then Q15min × 2 h after starting alteplase
- Then Q30min × 6 h
- Then Q1h × 4 h
- Then Q2h × 12 h
- Call MD if the systolic BP is > 180 mm Hg or if the diastolic BP is > 110 mm Hg on two or more occasions taken 5–10 min apart

Neurologic Signs
- Q1h × 12 h
- Then Q2h × 12 h
- Stop the infusion and notify MD if there is neurologic deterioration, severe headache, or new onset of nausea or vomiting

Blood Glucose
- Call MD if glucose > 12 mmol/L

Medications
- No ASA, ticlopidine, clopidogrel, heparin or warfarin for 24 h
- Acetaminophen 650 mg po or pr Q4h if body temperature is ≥ 38°C or for analgesia
- O_2 via nasal prongs or face mask to keep O_2 saturation > 90%
- After the alteplase infusion is completed, continue iv normal saline with KCl

Investigations
- CT brain scan after 24 h

II. Prevent Complications

Expert nursing care and early mobilization are the mainstays of treatment.

Aspiration Pneumonia and Malnutrition[29]

- Review the nutritional status (pre-albumin, weight) on admission to identify patients who were malnourished before their stroke.
- Give *nothing by mouth* if any of the following are present: reduced level of consciousness, severe dysarthria, wet voice, weak cough, impaired palatal sensation, inability to sit, or if aspiration is suspected.
- Monitor recovery of dysphagia using serial bedside swallowing assessments. These are best performed by a dietitian and a speech-language pathologist.
- A videofluoroscopic examination (modified barium swallow) may be required to exclude significant aspiration when the results of the bedside examination are ambiguous.
- Tube feeding may be required if significant aspiration is demonstrated or suspected. Initially, this is usually done via a nasogastric tube. If swallowing does not recover, tube feeding via percutaneous endoscopic gastrostomy (PEG) may be necessary. The results of the FOOD trial did not support a policy of early initiation of PEG feeding in dysphagic stroke patients.[30]
- Parenteral nutrition is required only in exceptional circumstances.
- Give a texture-modified diet for dysphagic patients at lower risk of aspiration. Additional iv fluids are often necessary for these patients.

Venous Thromboembolism[31]

- Early mobilization (even if only up in a chair) is recommended (i.e., within the first day of admission to hospital).
- Maintain adequate hydration.
- Graduated *compression stockings* are recommended if mobility is limited by leg weakness.
- **ASA** (75 to 325 mg daily) reduces the risk of thromboembolism.[32]
- Subcutaneous unfractionated **heparin**, **low molecular weight heparins** or **heparinoids** reduce the risk of deep vein thrombosis and pulmonary embolism after acute stroke but increase the risk of intra- and extracranial bleeding. Heparins do not decrease long-term death or disability and are not definitely superior to early mobilization, hydration, support stockings and ASA.[33,34]

III. Reduce the Risk of Stroke Recurrence

Antithrombotic Drug Treatment

Antiplatelet therapy

- Avoid antiplatelet agents for 24 hours in patients who have received thrombolytics.[9,16]
- Give **ASA** 325 mg as soon as intracranial hemorrhage is excluded by CT scan followed by ASA 75–325 mg daily (Table 4).[35] Administer as a suppository or via nasogastric tube to dysphagic patients. Use enteric-coated formulation for patients who can swallow. No evidence

supports the use of ASA doses greater than 325 mg/day for secondary stroke prevention;[32] the GI side effects of ASA are dose related.

- For patients who were taking ASA prior to their stroke, consider other antiplatelet agents, such as **clopidogrel** 75 mg daily[32,36] or a **combination of ASA and sustained-release dipyridamole** 25/200 mg twice daily,[32,37,38] although these regimens have not been tested in acute stroke.
- The combination of **ASA and clopidogrel** is not recommended for long-term secondary stroke prevention.[39,40]

Anticoagulant therapy

- Immediate systemic anticoagulation with unfractionated heparin, low molecular weight heparin, heparinoids or specific thrombin inhibitors is not recommended in the setting of acute ischemic stroke—not even for patients in atrial fibrillation (AF)—because there is no evidence of short- or long-term benefit. Specifically, reduction in early recurrent ischemic stroke is completely offset by an increase in major intracranial and extracranial bleeding.[34]
- ASA is as effective as warfarin for secondary stroke prevention in patients in normal sinus rhythm, and does not require laboratory monitoring.[41]
- For patients in AF, use **warfarin** at a dose to maintain the INR in the range 2.0 to 3.0, provided there are no contraindications to anticoagulation. For patients who cannot take warfarin, use enteric-coated **ASA** 80 to 325 mg daily.[42]
- The best time to initiate anticoagulant therapy is unclear. For patients with minor strokes, start warfarin as soon as intracranial hemorrhage has been excluded by CT scan. For patients with major strokes, delay warfarin until a CT scan done about a week or two after the stroke has excluded hemorrhagic transformation of the infarct.

For post-acute antithrombotic treatment, carotid endarterectomy and risk-factor modification, see Chapter 37.

IV. Restore Function of the Individual

- Outcomes are optimized by care on a stroke unit provided by a coordinated interdisciplinary team.[43,44]
- Start rehabilitation as soon as the patient is medically stable.
- Family and community supports are important for social reintegration.

Therapeutic Tips

- The effectiveness of thrombolytic therapy with alteplase is exquisitely time dependent; delays of any sort *cannot be tolerated.* A minority of patients present to hospital within the first 90 minutes of stroke onset, leaving limited time to act. Immediate contact with the patient, rapid triage, and (most importantly) *staying with the patient* continuously during the clinical assessment, CT scan, blood tests and consent procedures are vital in ensuring that the appropriate steps are being taken as rapidly as possible prior to alteplase administration. For example, it is not necessary to wait for hospital porters to take the patient to the CT scanner.

- Determining the time of stroke onset is critical in deciding to use alteplase, but checking the clock is not a natural reaction in the setting of an acute stroke. Encourage patients and families to think of "time anchors" (e.g., what was on the radio or TV at the time, or at what point in the patient's daily routine did the symptoms first occur).
- Patients with acute stroke are often unable to communicate. When possible, the next-of-kin should travel with the patient to hospital (or between hospitals if the patient is transferred) to provide collateral history and consent for treatment before the time window for intervention closes.
- If the patient is referred to a tertiary care hospital, have the stat blood work (CBC, INR) drawn at the community hospital and the results faxed to the referral centre as soon as possible.
- Signs of infarction on a CT scan done within three hours of stroke onset are usually subtle. If the CT scan of a patient being considered for treatment with alteplase shows a very definite infarct in a location that explains the presenting clinical symptoms and signs, recheck the time of onset.

Figure 1: **Diagnosis and Initial Management of Suspected Acute Stroke**

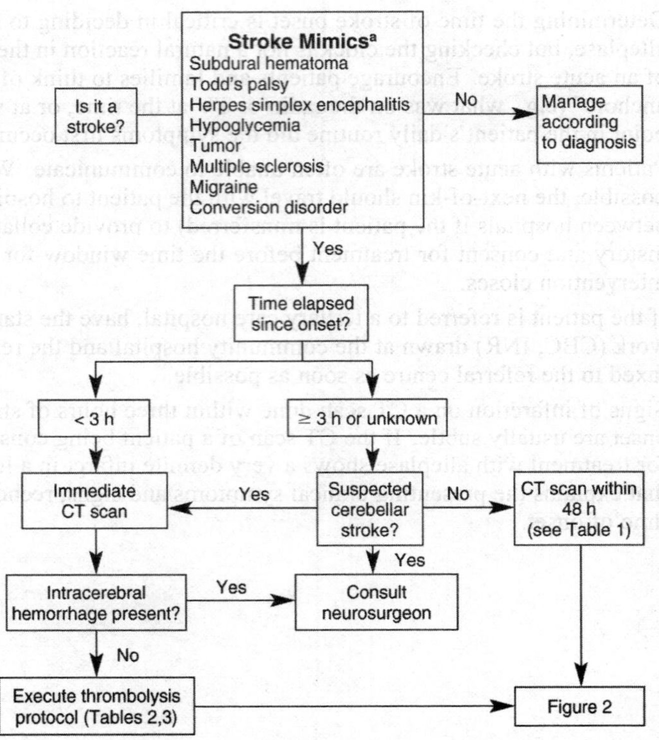

[a] List not exhaustive. Disorders listed are common or require specific treatment or both.

Figure 2: **General Management of the Stroke Patient**

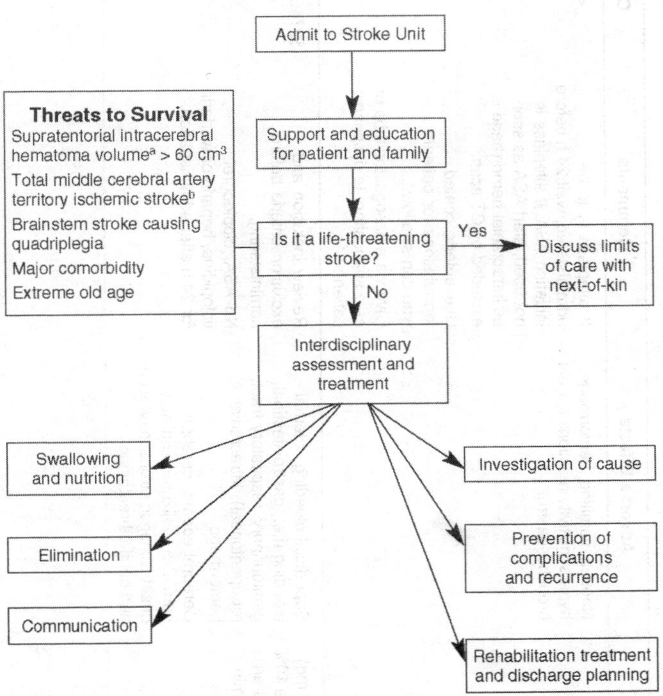

[a] Hematoma volume (cm^3) = A+B+C/2 where A = largest diameter (cm) on CT scan, B = diameter (cm) perpendicular to A, C = number of scan slides (cm) showing hematoma.[5,6]

[b] Hemiparesis and hemianopia with either aphasia or visuospatial deficit.[10]

Table 4: **Drugs Used for Acute Ischemic Stroke**

Class	Drug	Dose	Adverse Effects	Comments	Cost[a]
Antiplatelet Agents	*ASA* Aspirin, Bufferin, Coated Aspirin, generics	Initial: 160 mg Maintenance: 75–325 mg daily	Nausea, vomiting, hemorrhage, hypersensitivity reactions (rarely bronchospasm).	If alteplase is to be administered, wait 24 h before initiating ASA. If alteplase is not used, start ASA as soon as intracranial hemorrhage is excluded by CT scan. Use enteric coated formulations for patients who can swallow. Give via a nasogastric tube or as a suppository to dysphagic patients.	< $1
Fibrinolytic Agents	*alteplase* Activase rt-PA	0.9 mg/kg (max 90 mg) iv over 60 min. Give 10% of the total dose as an initial bolus over 1 min	Superficial bleeding, internal bleeding (i.e., gastrointestinal, genitourinary, respiratory tract, retroperitoneal), intracranial hemorrhage. Cerebral edema, cerebral herniation, seizures and new onset ischemic stroke may occur and be life threatening.	Review inclusion and exclusion criteria before administering. No ASA, clopidogrel, ticlopidine, heparin or warfarin for 24 h after administration.	$2746/100 mg vial

[a] Cost of a 1-day supply; includes drug cost only.

Suggested Readings

Antithrombotic Trialists' Collaboration. Collaborative meta-analysis of randomised trials of antiplatelet therapy for prevention of death, myocardial infarction, and stroke in high risk patients. *BMJ* 2002;324(7329):71-86.

Internet Stroke Center at Washington University School of Medicine. *Stroke Trials Registry*. Available from: http://www.strokecenter.org/trials/ Accessed November 15, 2006.

Stroke Unit Trialists' Collaboration. Organised inpatient (stroke unit) care for stroke. *Cochrane Database Syst Rev* 2002;(1):CD000197.

Wardlaw JM, Zoppo G, Yamaguchi T et al. Thrombolysis for acute ischaemic stroke. *Cochrane Database Syst Rev* 2003;(3):CD000213.

Warlow C, Sudlow S, Dennis M et al. Stroke. *Lancet* 2003;362(9391):1211-24.

References

1. Warlow C, Sudlow S, Dennis M et al. Stroke. *Lancet* 2003;362(9391):1211-24.
2. Broderick JP, Adams HP, Barsan W et al. Guidelines for the management of spontaneous intracerebral hemorrhage: A statement for healthcare professionals from a special writing group of the Stroke Council, American Heart Association. *Stroke* 1999;30(4):905-15.
3. Mayer SA, Brun NC, Begtrup K et al. Recombinant activated factor VII for acute intracerebral hemorrhage. *N Engl J Med* 2005;352(8):777-85.
4. Mayberg MR, Batjer HH, Dacey R et al. Guidelines for the management of aneurysmal subarachnoid hemorrhage. A statement for healthcare professionals from a special writing group of the Stroke Council, American Heart Association. *Stroke* 1994;25(11):2315-28.
5. Phillips S. Risk factors for stroke. *Can J Cardiol* 1999(Suppl G):102G-5G.
6. Barnett HJ, Meldrum HE, Eliasziw M et al. The appropriate use of carotid endarterectomy. *CMAJ* 2002;166(9):1169-79.
7. Rothwell PM, Eliasziw M, Gutnikov SA et al. Analysis of pooled data from the randomised controlled trials of endarterectomy for symptomatic carotid stenosis. *Lancet* 2003;361(9352):107-16.
8. Kapral MK, Silver FL. Preventive health care, 1999 update: 2. Echocardiography for the detection of a cardiac source of embolus in patients with stroke. Canadian Task Force on Preventive Health Care. *CMAJ* 1999;161(8):989-96.
9. [No authors listed]. Tissue plasminogen activator for acute ischemic stroke. The National Institute of Neurological Disorders and Stroke rt-PA Stroke Study Group. *N Engl J Med* 1995;333(24):1581-7.
10. Canadian Stroke Strategy; Canadian Stroke Network; Heart and Stroke Foundation. *Canadian best practice recommendations for stroke care: 2006*. Available from: http://www.strokeconsortium.ca/000b.docs/2007/Canadian_Stroke_Stragegy_Manual.pdf Accessed June 13, 2007.
11. Furlan A, Higashida R, Wechsler L et al. Intra-arterial prourokinase for acute ischemic stroke. The PROACT II study: a randomized controlled trial. Prolyse in Acute Cerebral Thromboembolism. *JAMA* 1999;282(21):2003-11.
12. Adams H, Adams R, Del Zoppo G et al. Guidelines for the early management of patients with ischemic stroke: 2005 guidelines update. A scientific statement from the Stroke Council of the American Heart Association/American Stroke Association. *Stroke* 2005;36(4):916-23.
13. Wardlaw JM, Warlow CP, Counsell C. Systematic review of evidence on thrombolytic therapy for acute ischaemic stroke. *Lancet* 1997;350(9078):607-14.
14. Wardlaw JM, Zoppo G, Yamaguchi T et al. Thrombolysis for acute ischaemic stroke. *Cochrane Database Syst Rev* 2003;(3):CD000213.
15. Gobin YP, Starkman S, Duckwiler GR et al. MERCI 1: a phase 1 study of Mechanical Embolus Removal in Cerebral Ischemia. *Stroke* 2004;35(12):2848-54.
16. Adams HP, Adams RJ, Brott T et al. Guidelines for the early management of patients with ischemic stroke: a scientific statement from the Stroke Council of the American Stroke Association. *Stroke* 2003;34(4):1056-83.
17. Ronning OM, Guldvog B. Should stroke victims routinely receive supplemental oxygen? A quasi-randomized controlled trial. *Stroke* 1999;30(10):2033-7.
18. Jorgensen HS, Reith J, Pedersen PM et al. Body temperature and outcome in stroke patients. *Lancet* 1996;348(9021):193.
19. Jorgensen HS, Reith J, Nakayama H et al. What determines good recovery in patients with the most severe strokes? The Copenhagen Stroke Study. *Stroke* 1999;30(10):2008-12.

20. Reith J, Jorgensen HS, Pedersen PM et al. Body temperature in acute stroke: relation to stroke severity, infarct size, mortality and outcome. *Lancet* 1996;347(8999):422-5.
21. Scott JF, Robinson GM, French JM et al. Glucose potassium insulin infusions in the treatment of acute stroke patients with mild to moderate hyperglycemia: the Glucose Insulin in Stroke Trial (GIST). *Stroke* 1999;30(4):793-9.
22. Bath P, Chalmers J, Powers W, et al. International Society of Hypertension (ISH): statement on the management of blood pressure in acute stroke. *J Hypertens* 2003;21(4):665-72
23. Blood pressure in Acute Stroke Collaboration (BASC). Vasoactive drugs for acute stroke. *Cochrane Database Syst Rev* 2000;(4):CD002839.
24. Blood pressure in Acute Stroke Collaboration (BASC). Interventions for deliberately altering blood pressure in acute stroke. *Cochrane Database Syst Rev* 2001;(3):CD000039.
25. Willmot M, Ghadami A, Whysall B et al. Transdermal glyceryl trinitrate lowers blood pressure and maintains cerebral blood flow in recent stroke. *Hypertension* 2006;47(6):1209-15.
26. The ENOS Trial Investigators. Glyceryl trinitrate vs. control, and continuing vs. stopping temporarily prior antihypertensive therapy, in acute stroke: rationale and design of the Efficacy of Nitric Oxide in Stroke (ENOS) trial (ISRCTN99414122). *Int J Stroke* 2006;1(4):245-9.
27. Rothwell PM, Eliasziw M, Gutnikov SA et al. Endarterectomy for symptomatic carotid stenosis in relation to clinical subgroups and timing of surgery. *Lancet* 2004;363(9413):915-24.
28. Gasecki AP, Ferguson GG, Eliasziw M et al. Early endarterectomy for severe carotid artery stenosis after a nondisabling stroke: results from the North American Symptomatic Carotid Endarterectomy Trial. *J Vasc Surg* 1994;20(2):288-95.
29. Bath PM, Bath FJ, Smithard DG. Interventions for dysphagia in acute stroke. *Cochrane Database Syst Rev* 2000;(2):CD000323.
30. Dennis MS, Lewis SC, Warlow C et al. Effect of timing and method of enteral tube feeding for dysphagic stroke patients (FOOD): a multicentre randomised controlled trial. *Lancet* 2005;365(9461):764-72.
31. Geerts WH, Pineo GF, Heit JA et al. Prevention of venous thromboembolism: the Seventh ACCP Conference on Antithrombotic and Thrombolytic Therapy. *Chest* 2004;126(3 Suppl):338S-400S.
32. Antithrombotic Trialists' Collaboration. Collaborative meta-analysis of randomised trials of antiplatelet therapy for prevention of death, myocardial infarction, and stroke in high risk patients. *BMJ* 2002;324(7329):71-86.
33. Sandercock P, Counsell C, Stobbs SL. Low-molecular-weight heparins or heparinoids versus standard unfractionated heparin for acute ischaemic stroke. *Cochrane Database Syst Rev* 2005;(2):CD000119.
34. Gubitz G, Sandercock P, Counsell C. Anticoagulants for acute ischaemic stroke. *Cochrane Database Syst Rev* 2004;(3):CD000024.
35. Sandercock P, Gubitz G, Foley P et al. Antiplatelet therapy for acute ischaemic stroke. *Cochrane Database Syst Rev* 2003;(2):CD000029.
36. [No authors listed]. A randomised, blinded, trial of clopidogrel versus aspirin in patients at risk of ischaemic events (CAPRIE). CAPRIE Steering Committee. *Lancet* 1996;348(9038):1329-39.
37. ESPRIT Study Group; Halkes PH, van Gijn J et al. Aspirin plus dipyridamole versus aspirin alone after cerebral ischaemia of arterial origin (ESPRIT): randomised controlled trial. *Lancet* 2006;367(9523):1665-73.
38. Leonardi-Bee J, Bath PM, Bousser MG et al. Dipyridamole for preventing recurrent ischemic stroke and other vascular events: a meta-analysis of individual patient data from randomized controlled trials. *Stroke* 2005;36(1):162-8.
39. Bhatt DL, Fox KA, Hacke W et al. Clopidogrel and aspirin versus aspirin alone for the prevention of atherothrombotic events. *N Engl J Med* 2006;354(16):1706-17.
40. Diener HC, Bogousslavsky J, Brass LM et al. Aspirin and clopidogrel compared with clopidogrel alone after recent ischaemic stroke or transient ischaemic attack in high-risk patients (MATCH): randomised, double-blind, placebo-controlled trial. *Lancet* 2004;364(9431):331-7.
41. Mohr JP, Thompson JL, Lazar RM et al. A comparison of warfarin and aspirin for the prevention of recurrent ischemic stroke. *N Engl J Med* 2001;345(20):1444-51.
42. Singer DE, Albers GW, Dalen JE et al. Antithrombotic therapy in atrial fibrillation: the Seventh ACCP Conference on Antithrombotic and Thrombolytic Therapy. *Chest* 2004;126(3 Suppl):429S-456S.
43. Stroke Unit Trialists' Collaboration. Organised inpatient (stroke unit) care for stroke. *Cochrane Database Syst Rev* 2002;(1):CD000197.
44. Hankey GJ, Warlow CP. Treatment and secondary prevention of stroke: evidence, costs, and effects on individuals and populations. *Lancet* 1999;354(9188):1457-63.

Pharmacoeconomic Considerations: Acute Ischemic Stroke

Nicole Mittmann, MSc, PhD

Epidemiology

Country (Year)	Incidence and Prevalence (%)
Canada (2002)[1]	40 000–50 000 strokes per year 300 000 individuals live with the effects of stroke

Cost of Illness Data

Country and Year of Estimate	Direct Costs[a]	Indirect Costs[b]
Canada (Ontario 1994-95)[2]	$529 million	$328 million
Canada (Ontario 1991-92)[3]	$27 500 for acute stroke admission	Not reported
Canada (Ontario 1996)[4]	$9763 for acute stroke admission	Not reported

Commentary

Ischemic stroke is a significant disease in the aging population. From an economic perspective, the impact of stroke on society will increase significantly as the population ages. Of every 100 people hospitalized for stroke, 50 will be discharged home, 20 will die before leaving the hospital, 15 will require long-term care and 10 will enter an inpatient rehabilitation program. Stroke incidence is related to increased age and has an economic impact on the patient, health care system and society.

Direct medical and nonmedical costs associated with stroke are significant. In acute stroke, hospitalization, length of stay and rehabilitation are the cost drivers.[5] Direct nonmedical costs including informal care, out-of-pocket expenses and caregiver time are not well documented but have been estimated to be significant for informal care.[5] Indirect costs have not been well documented. Depending on the severity of the stroke, work productivity and regular daily activities may be severely restricted. Long-term costs are significant.

Quality of life is significantly impaired by stroke.[6] Predictors of poor quality of life included physical impairment, disability and anxiety/depression.

Alteplase, which is used in patients with acute stroke, is expensive and must be administered expeditiously.

(cont'd)

Commentary
Researchers in Australia assessed the relative benefits of various interventions for acute stroke from a community perspective.[7] For every 1000 patients with stroke, death or dependency could be prevented in 46 individuals by management in a stroke unit, in 6 individuals through use of ASA and in 11 individuals through use of alteplase within 3 hours. The authors concluded that the greatest benefit to the community could be provided through the establishment of dedicated stroke units.

[a] Direct costs include those associated with physician services, nursing care, diagnostic procedures, drugs and hospitalization.

[b] Indirect costs include those associated with lost productivity and days off work due to morbidity or premature mortality.

References

1. Heart and Stroke Foundation. 2/4/2002 Stroke Statistics. Available at: http://ww2.heartandstroke.ca/Page.asp?PageID=33=1078=news=SubCategory. Accessed July 4, 2007
2. Chan B, Hayes B. Cost of stroke in Ontario, 1994/95. *CMAJ* 1998;159(6 Suppl):S2-S8.
3. Smurawska LT, Alexandrov AV, Bladin CF et al. Cost of acute stroke care in Toronto, Canada. *Stroke* 1994;25(8):1628-31.
4. Tran C, Nadareishvili Z, Smurawska L et al. Decreasing costs of stroke hospitalization in Toronto. *Stroke* 1999;30(1):185-6.
5. Dewey HM, Thrift AG, Mihalopoulos C et al. Informal care for stoke survivors: results from the north east Melbourne stroke incidence study (NEMESIS). *Stroke* 2002;33(4):1028-33.
6. Sturm JW, Donnan GA, Dewey HM et al. Quality of life after stroke: the North East Melbourne Stroke Incidence Study (NEMESIS). *Stroke* 2004;35(10):2340-5.
7. Gilligan AK, Thrift AG, Sturm JW et al. Stroke units, tissue plasminogen activator, aspirin and neuroprotection: which stroke intervention could provide the greatest community benefit? *Cerebrovasc Dis* 2005;20(4):239-44.

CHAPTER 39

Supraventricular Tachycardia

David Birnie, MD

Supraventricular tachycardia (SVT) includes all tachyarrhythmias arising from above the ventricles. SVT usually has a narrow QRS response. Occasionally the QRS complex during tachycardia is broad because there is co-existent bundle branch block. In this situation the initial step in the differential diagnosis is to exclude ventricular tachycardia (see Figure 1).

The classification of common forms of SVT is shown in Table 1.

Table 1: **Classification of Supraventricular Tachycardia**

Arrhythmia	Clinical Significance of Arrhythmia
Atrial Fibrillation	Significant because of thromboembolic risk
Atrial Flutter	Probably similar thromboembolic risk to atrial fibrillation
Atrioventricular Nodal Re-entry Tachycardia (AVNRT)	Usually benign
Atrioventricular Re-entry Tachycardia (AVRT)	Usually benign. There is a risk of sudden death if AVRT degenerates into pre-excited SVT (rare)
Atrial Tachycardia	Usually benign unless it persists for prolonged period (rare)

The terms "permanent," "persistent" and "paroxysmal" are now used to classify atrial fibrillation and flutter; the older term "chronic atrial fibrillation" is obsolete (Table 2).

Table 2: **Classification of Atrial Fibrillation or Flutter[1]**

Paroxysmal	Recurrent self-limiting episodes (lasting less than 7 days)
Persistent	Episodes lasting more than 7 days and sinus rhythm achievable (spontaneously or by cardioversion)
Permanent	Cardioversion failed or not attempted/planned

Management of atrial fibrillation and atrial flutter is similar. The risk of thromboembolic complications should be assessed in both situations. Many patients will have a combination of both arrhythmias. However, there are some important differences in the management of the two arrhythmias. Firstly, it is often more difficult to achieve heart rate control in patients with atrial flutter than atrial fibrillation. Secondly, the threshold for catheter ablation for atrial flutter is lower than the threshold for considering ablation for atrial fibrillation.

An algorithm for the management of newly discovered atrial fibrillation is provided in Figure 2.

The heart is usually structurally normal in patients with atrioventricular re-entry tachycardia (AVRT), atrioventricular nodal re-entry tachycardia (AVNRT) and focal atrial tachycardia (AT). AVRT is due to a congenital accessory bypass track between the atria and ventricles. The circuit usually follows an antegrade limb through the AV node and a retrograde limb through the accessory pathway, although the opposite occasionally occurs. If the accessory pathway is capable of antegrade conduction during sinus rhythm it usually manifests on the resting ECG as a delta wave and is known as Wolff-Parkinson-White (WPW) syndrome. AVNRT involves a localized short circuit within the AV node. Focal atrial tachycardia (AT) arises from a localized area of atrial myocardium that is capable of accelerated automatic firing.

Goals of Therapy

- In the acute stage the goal is to restore sinus rhythm. Rhythm control should always be possible in re-entrant arrhythmias (AVRT or AVNRT)
- Rhythm control may not be possible or desirable in some patients with atrial fibrillation or atrial flutter or atrial tachycardia. In these situations the goal is to control the rate of the SVT
- In the longer term the goal is to prevent arrhythmia recurrence, or substantially reduce the overall arrhythmia burden
- Reduce the risk of thromboembolic events (stroke) in patients with atrial fibrillation/atrial flutter

Investigations

- Detailed history including a description of the onset, frequency and duration of episodes and identification of possible triggers
- Document the arrhythmia, ideally on 12-lead ECG, but a Holter or loop monitor is also acceptable
- Echocardiography to assess left ventricular function, left atrial size and valvular status

Therapeutic Choices

Nonpharmacologic Choices

Cardioversion

In general, any tachycardia that produces hemodynamic compromise, heart failure or angina, and is resistant to prompt medical management should be terminated electrically. Most supraventricular arrhythmias, with the exception of atrial flutter and fibrillation, are usually responsive to medical therapy and hence cardioversion is seldom necessary. Furthermore, cardioversion can be a useful adjunctive therapy in patients with persistent atrial fibrillation or flutter. A synchronized shock on the R wave is used and there is no evidence that any paddle position is more effective than another. It is normal to start with the anterior-apex position, and if this is unsuccessful, then another position, usually antero-posterior, is tried. The initial success rate of cardioversion for atrial fibrillation is 70–90% but only about 20% of patients will remain in sinus rhythm at 12-months' follow-up. Using additional antiarrhythmic therapy can improve maintenance of sinus rhythm. For example, 50–70% of patients treated with amiodarone are still in sinus rhythm at 12 months. Direct current cardioversion has a low incidence of side effects. Arrhythmias induced by the cardioversion generally are caused by inadequate synchronization.

Catheter Ablation

The success rate for ablation of atrial flutter is usually about 90% with a low rate of complications; hence, catheter ablation should be considered as the first-line treatment for patients with troublesome atrial flutter.

Catheter ablation for atrial fibrillation is an option for patients who have failed at least one antiarrhythmic drug. Ablation is often not a complete cure for atrial fibrillation but can significantly reduce the arrhythmia burden. Success rates vary from 30% to 90% depending on technique, atrial fibrillation subtype and the extent of structural heart disease. The technique involves extensive ablation of the left atrium, primarily focusing on the areas around the pulmonary veins. The success of ablation seems to relate to disconnection of atrial fibrillation triggers arising from the pulmonary veins and/or modification of the arrhythmogenic left atrial substrate. Procedural complications are rare but include about a 1% risk of stroke and a low risk of death, usually due to atrial esophageal fistula.

In patients with re-entrant tachycardias or focal atrial tachycardia, the reported cure rates after catheter ablation range from 90% to 98% and complication rates range from 1% to 3%. Hence the threshold for nonpharmacologic management of these arrhythmias is low. Catheter ablation is strongly recommended for patients with WPW and rapidly conducted pre-excited SVT. Catheter ablation should be considered as a first line treatment option in patients with recurrent symptomatic re-entry tachycardia or focal atrial tachycardia. Catheter ablation is also an option for patients with occasional episodes of AVNRT who desire complete rhythm control and for patients with asymptomatic pre-excitation.

Pharmacologic Choices

Long-term Management of Atrial Fibrillation or Flutter

This first decision is whether to choose rate control (leaving atrial arrhythmia as the permanent rhythm) or to actively pursue sinus rhythm (rhythm control). The AFFIRM Study compared these two treatment strategies in 4060 patients and found no difference in stroke or death rates between the two groups.[2] However, patients in the AFFIRM study were relatively old (mean age 69.7) and were either asymptomatic or had minimal symptoms. Therefore, rhythm control should be actively pursued in patients with more than minimal symptoms, in asymptomatic young patients and in patients with possible tachycardia-related cardiomyopathy. Recent data suggest that this latter diagnosis is a more frequent problem than previously thought.

Heart Rate Control in Patients with Persistent or Permanent Atrial Fibrillation or Flutter

Most patients will need drugs to achieve rate control. Some patients with intrinsic AV nodal disease (usually elderly individuals) will not need drugs for rate control. Pharmacologic control of heart rate should initially be attempted with a **beta-blocker** or a **calcium channel blocker** (**diltiazem** or **verapamil**). The dose should be titrated to achieve a resting heart rate of < 80 bpm and a mean heart rate of < 100 bpm on 24-hour Holter monitoring. **Digoxin** is usually inadequate alone for rate control.

Because of its potential toxicity, **amiodarone** should only be used as a last resort for rate control. Nonpharmacologic rate control with AV nodal ablation and permanent pacemaker implantation should be pursued before considering chronic oral administration of amiodarone for rate control.

Anticoagulation for Paroxysmal and Persistent and Permanent Atrial Fibrillation or Flutter

Antithrombotic agents are indicated for the prevention of thromboembolic stroke in patients with atrial flutter or fibrillation. The choice of agent is based on the presence of risk factors (Table 3). The estimated annual risk of stroke in a patient with a $CHADS_2$ score of 0 not receiving warfarin is 1.9%.[3] In the absence of antithrombotic therapy, the risk of stroke increases by a factor of about 1.5 for each 1 unit increase in $CHADS_2$ score in patients with atrial fibrillation. Most experts recommend **warfarin** (aiming for an INR range of 2–3) for patients with a $CHADS_2$ score of > 1 (Table 3). **ASA** 81 to 325 mg daily is recommended for patients with atrial fibrillation/flutter and a $CHADS_2$ score of 0. Management of patients with a score of 1 is controversial. Recent guidelines[4] suggest that either ASA in the above dosage or warfarin are reasonable choices.

Table 3: **Stroke Risk in Patients with Nonvalvular Atrial Fibrillation or Flutter[3]**

	$CHADS_2$ Risk Criteria	Assigned Score
C	Congestive heart failure	1
H	Hypertension	1
A	Age > 75 years	1
D	Diabetes mellitus	1
S	Prior stroke or transient ischemic attack	2

Management of Re-entrant Tachycardias and Focal Atrial Tachycardia

There have been no large randomized controlled trials in patients with re-entry tachycardias or focal atrial tachycardia. An overview of the acute management of a patient with AVRT, AVNRT and AT is illustrated in Figure 4. Indications for chronic pharmacologic therapy are presented in Table 4.

Table 4: **Medical Therapy of Re-entrant Tachycardias and Focal Atrial Tachycardia**

Arrhythmia	Details	Recommendation
Atrioventricular Re-entry Tachycardia (AVRT)	Asymptomatic WPW	No therapy
	Single or infrequent episode(s)	No therapy Vagal manoeuvres [a]Pill-in-the-pocket verapamil, diltiazem or beta-blocker
	Frequent symptomatic	Any of the following: Flecainide, propafenone Sotalol, beta-blocker Verapamil, diltiazem
Atrioventricular Nodal Re-entry Tachycardia (AVNRT)	Single or infrequent episode(s)	No therapy Vagal manoeuvres [a]Pill-in-the-pocket verapamil, diltiazem or beta-blocker
	Frequent symptomatic	Verapamil, diltiazem, beta-blockers
	Recurrent AVNRT unresponsive to a beta blocker or calcium channel blocker in a patient not desiring radiofrequency ablation	Flecainide, propafenone, or sotalol
Focal Atrial Tachycardia (AT)	Single or infrequent episode(s)	No therapy Pill-in-the-pocket verapamil, diltiazem or beta-blocker
	Recurrent symptomatic	Any of the following: Beta-blocker, verapamil, diltiazem Flecainide/propafenone[b] Sotalol, amiodarone[c]

[a] Single dose oral pill-in-the-pocket approach is an option in carefully selected patients. Suitable candidates should not have significant LV dysfunction or sinus bradycardia. Intermittent single-dose therapy minimizes exposure to unnecessary therapy between events.

[b] Flecainide and propafenone should not be used unless they are combined with an AV-nodal blocking agent such as a beta-blocker, verapamil or diltiazem. Also these drugs should not be used in patients with coronary artery disease or structural heart disease.

[c] Ablation should be considered before amiodarone.

Abbreviations: WPW = Wolff-Parkinson-White

Modified from Circulation 2003;108(15):1871-909 with permission of the American Heart Association.

Therapeutic Tips

- Either rate or rhythm control is reasonable for elderly asymptomatic or mildly symptomatic patients with atrial fibrillation or atrial flutter.
- Rhythm control should be pursued in younger patients or symptomatic elderly patients with atrial fibrillation or atrial flutter.
- Rhythm control for atrial fibrillation should initially be with antiarrhythmic drugs.
- Rhythm control with catheter ablation should be considered second-or third-line in atrial fibrillation and first-line in atrial flutter.
- Rhythm control should *always* be the objective in patients with re-entry tachycardia (AVRT or AVNRT). Rhythm control should be attempted with either antiarrhythmic drugs or catheter ablation.
- Rhythm control should usually be the objective in patients with AT. Rate control is acceptable if rhythm control cannot be achieved.
- Avoid use of flecainide and propafenone in patients with structural heart disease.
- Use only immediate-release dosage forms when prescribing single-dose “pill-in-the-pocket” oral therapy.
- All patients with a possible indication for ablation should be referred to an electrophysiologist.
- All patients with possible tachycardia–mediated cardiomyopathy should be referred to an electrophysiologist.
- Patients in whom it is difficult to achieve rate or rhythm control should be referred to a cardiologist.

Figure 1: **Differential Diagnosis of Supraventricular Tachycardia**

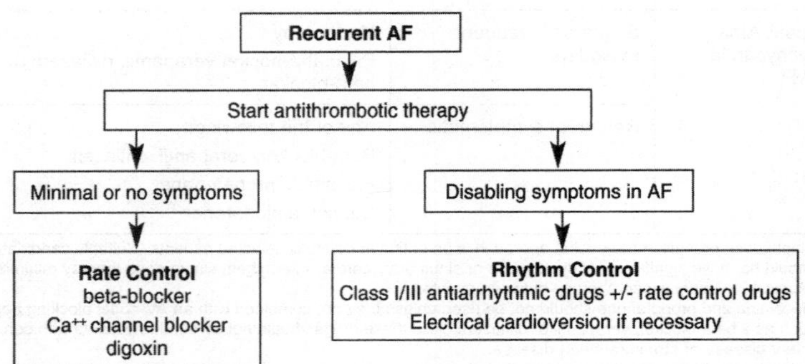

Abbreviations: AV = atrioventricular; AVNRT = atrioventricular nodal re-entry tachycardia; AVRT = atrioventricular re-entry tachy
Modified from Circulation 2003;108(15):1871-909 with permission of the American Heart Association.

Figure 2: Therapy of Newly Discovered Atrial Fibrillation or Flutter

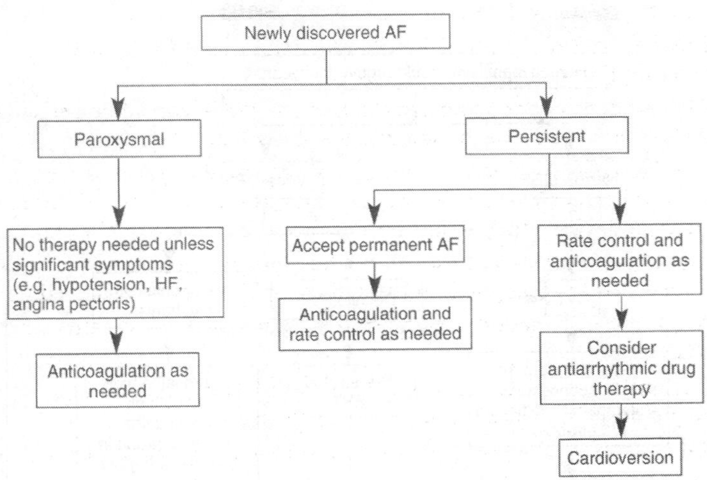

Abbreviations: AF = atrial fibrillation or flutter; HF = heart failure
Modified from Circulation 2006;114:e257-354 with permission of the American Heart Association.

Figure 3: Methods to Maintain Sinus Rhythm in Patients with Atrial Fibrillation

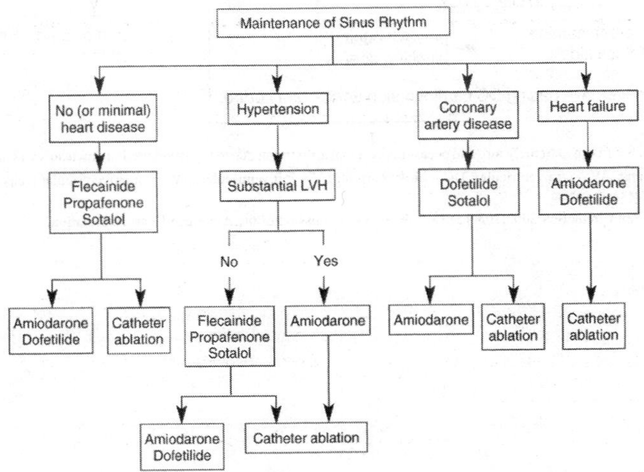

A similar algorithm can be followed for atrial flutter. However, catheter ablation for atrial flutter should be considered first-line. An AV nodal blocking agent should always be co-prescribed with propafenone or flecainide.

Abbreviations: LVH = left ventricular hypertrophy
Modified from Circulation 2006;114:e257-354 with permission of the American Heart Association.

Figure 4: **Acute Management of Atrioventricular Re-entry Tachycardia, Atrioventricular Nodal Re-entry Tachycardia and Atrial Tachycardia**

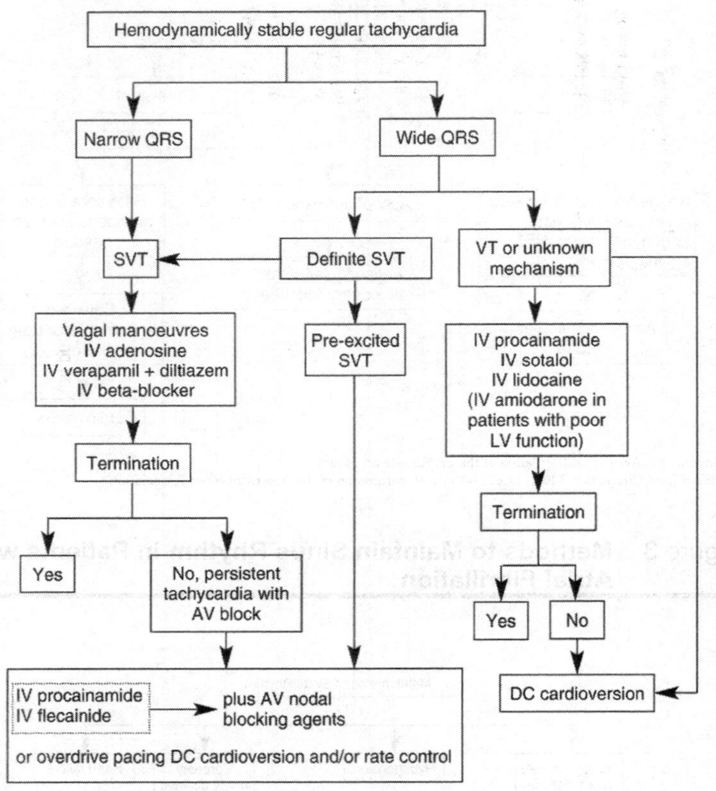

Pre-excited SVT is an extremely rare and occasionally lethal arrhythmia due to rapid conduction down an accessory pathway.

Abbreviations: AV = atrioventricular; DC = direct current; LV = left ventricular; SVT = supraventricular tachycardia; VT = ventricular tachycardia

Modified from Circulation 2003;108(15):1871-909 with permission of the American Heart Association.

Table 5: **Drug Therapy for Control of Heart Rate in Patients with Supraventricular Tachycardia**

Class	Drug	Dose	Adverse Effects	Drug Interactions	Comments	Cost[a]
Cardiac Glycosides	*digoxin* Lanoxin	Loading: 1–1.5 mg po/iv in divided doses Maintenance: 0.125–0.375 mg/day po/iv If patient hypokalemic ↓ dose by 25–50%	Bradycardia, nausea, vomiting, visual disturbances, proarrhythmia.	With beta-blockers, Ca^{++} channel blockers, amiodarone, propafenone, quinidine: ↓ digoxin dose by 25–50%.	Rarely indicated.	$
$Beta_1$-adrenergic Antagonists[b]	*propranolol* Inderal-LA, generics	iv: 4–8 mg po: 80–240 mg/day	Bradycardia, hypotension, dyspnea, fatigue, depression.	With digoxin, Ca^{++} channel blockers, amiodarone: ↓ dose 25–50%. Hypoglycemic agents.	Monitor carefully in diabetic patients; caution in patients with CHF or bronchospastic lung disease.	\$-\$\$
	atenolol Tenormin, generics	po: 50–150 mg/day	See propranolol. Less likely to cause CNS effects, e.g., depression.	See propranolol.	See propranolol. $Beta_1$ selective.	$
	metoprolol Betaloc, Lopresor, generics	iv: 5–15 mg po: 100–400 mg/day	See propranolol.	See propranolol.	See propranolol. $Beta_1$ selective.	$
	nadolol generics	po: 20–160 mg/day	See propranolol. Less likely to cause CNS effects, e.g., depression.	See propranolol.	See propranolol.	$

(cont'd)

Table 5: **Drug Therapy for Control of Heart Rate in Patients with Supraventricular Tachycardia** *(cont'd)*

Class	Drug	Dose	Adverse Effects	Drug Interactions	Comments	Cost[a]
Calcium Channel Blockers, Nondihydropyridine	*verapamil* Isoptin, Isoptin SR, Covera-HS, generics	iv: 5–15 mg po: usual starting dose 120 mg/day; max 480 mg/day IR given TID-QID; SR given daily or BID; Chronovera given QHS	Bradycardia, hypotension, constipation, flushing.	Beta-blockers, digoxin, amiodarone.	Caution in patients with CHF.	$–$$
	diltiazem Cardizem, Cardizem CD, Tiazac, Tiazac XC, generics	iv: 0.25 mg/kg iv. May give another 0.35 mg/kg after 15 min if necessary po: 180–540 mg/day. IR given TID-QID; SR given BID; CD and Tiazac given daily	Bradycardia, hypotension.	See verapamil.	See verapamil.	$$–$$$

[a] Cost of 30-day supply of oral doses; includes drug cost only.
[b] The beta-blockers suggested are examples only. Acebutolol, labetalol and timolol would also be effective. Some agents are available as sustained-release preparations.
Dosage adjustment may be required in renal impairment; see Appendix I.
Abbreviations: IR = immediate release; SR = sustained release
Legend: $ < $30 $–$$ < $30–60 $$ $30–60 $$–$$$ $30–90 $$$ $60–90

Table 6: Drug Therapy for Control of Heart Rhythm in Patients with Supraventricular Tachycardia

Class	Drug	Dose	Adverse Effects	Drug Interactions	Comments	Cost[a]
Antiarrhythmics, Class IC	*flecainide* Tambocor, generics	50 mg Q12H Titration: ↑ by 50 mg increments based on QRS intervals. ↓ dose if QRS increases > 20% from baseline Max: 200 mg po Q12H Renal dysfunction: ↓ initial dose 50%	VT proarrhythmia, tremor, blurred vision, CHF.		In patients with atrial fibrillation and/or atrial flutter, a beta-blocker or nondihydropyridine calcium antagonist *should always be* co-prescribed with a Class IC agent. Not to be used in patients with coronary artery disease or structural heart disease.	$
	propafenone Rythmol, generics	150 mg Q8H ↓ dose if QRS prolonged > 20% from baseline Max: 300 mg po Q8H Renal/hepatic dysfunction: ↓ initial dose 50% and ↑ dosing interval to Q12H	Constipation, headache, metallic taste, VT proarrhythmia.	↓ digoxin dose by 25–50%.	Active metabolites accumulate in rapid metabolizers. Monitor QRS duration carefully. See flecainide.	$$

(cont'd)

Table 6: **Drug Therapy for Control of Heart Rhythm in Patients with Supraventricular Tachycardia** *(cont'd)*

Class	Drug	Dose	Adverse Effects	Drug Interactions	Comments	Cost[a]
Antiarrhythmics, Class III	*sotalol* (renal symbol) generics	80 mg Q12H Titration: ↑ by 80 mg increments if QT_c < 460 msec. ↓ dose if QT_c ≥ 500 msec Max: 240 mg Q12H Elderly: ↓ initial dose to 40 mg Q12H Renal dysfunction: ↓ initial dose in renal failure	Hypotension, bradycardia, wheezing, VT proarrhythmia. Torsades de pointes, especially at higher doses or with renal dysfunction.	Digoxin, diltiazem, verapamil, other beta-blockers: may cause AV block, bradycardia.	Sotalol is a beta blocker. Use with great caution in view of the risk of QT prolongation and torsades de pointes.	$$
	amiodarone Cordarone, generics	200 mg po TID × 2 wk then 200 mg daily Accelerated loading doses may be used by some cardiologists	Various gastrointestinal, dermatologic, neurologic, ophthalmologic and thyroid abnormalities. Pulmonary fibrosis, hepatic dysfunction and aggravation of arrhythmias are rare but potentially life-threatening.	↓ doses of quinidine, procainamide, digoxin, beta-blockers and warfarin by 50%.	Monitor transaminases and thyroid function Q6 months, CXR annually.	$$$
	dofetilide Tikosyn	125–500 μg po BID ↓ dose if QT interval prolonged by 15% after first dose	Headache, nausea, torsades de pointes.	↑ levels with cimetidine, verapamil, ketaconazole, trimethoprim (alone or combined with sulfamethoxazole).	Requires prescription by an electrophysiologist: must be initiated in hospital.	[b]

[a] Cost of 30-day supply; includes drug cost only.
[b] Available through Special Access Programme, Health Canada.
(renal symbol) Dosage modification may be required in renal dysfunction; see Appendix I.
Abbreviations: BPM = beats per minute; CHF = congestive heart failure; HR = heart rate; IR = immediate release; SLE = systemic lupus erythematosus
Legend: $ < $30 $$ $30–60 $$$ $60–90

Suggested Readings

Calkins H. Radiofrequency catheter ablation of supraventricular arrhythmias. *Heart* 2001;85(5):594-600.

Ferguson JD, Dimarco JP. Contemporary management of paroxysmal supraventricular tachycardia. *Circulation* 2003;107(8):1096-9.

Schilling RJ. Which patient should be referred to an electrophysiologist: supraventricular tachycardia. *Heart* 2002;87(3):299-304.

Wellens HJ. Contemporary management of atrial flutter. *Circulation* 2002 6;106(6):649-52.

References

1. Blomstrom-Lundqvist C, Scheinman MM, Aliot EM et al. ACC/AHA/ESC guidelines for the management of patients with supraventricular arrhythmias. *Circulation* 2003;108(15):1871-909.
2. Wyse DG, Waldo AL, DiMarco JP et al. A comparison of rate control and rhythm control in patients with atrial fibrillation. *N Engl J Med* 2002;347(23):1825-1833.
3. Gage BF, Waterman AD, Shannon W et al. Validation of clinical classification schemes for predicting stroke: results from the National Registry of Atrial Fibrillation. *JAMA* 2001;285(22):2864-70.
4. Fuster V, Ryden LE, Cannom DS et al. ACC/AHA/ESC 2006 guidelines for the management of patients with atrial fibrillation. *Europace* 2006;8(9):651-745.

CHAPTER 40
Ventricular Tachyarrhythmias

Paul Dorian, MD, MSc, FRCPC

Ventricular tachycardia (VT) is defined as ≥ 3 consecutive ventricular complexes at a rate > 100 BPM on an ECG recording.

Ventricular fibrillation (VF) is defined as a rapid, disorganized rhythm without recognizable QRS complexes on the ECG. It is invariably associated with cardiovascular collapse and is almost invariably fatal unless the patient is electrically defibrillated.

Goals of Therapy[1,2]

- Relieve symptoms, including restoring a perfusing rhythm as quickly as possible in sustained VT, VF or cardiac arrest
- Prevent the potentially fatal occurrence or recurrence of sustained VT or VF

Investigations[3,4]

- Careful history with special reference to:
  - syncope or severe presyncope
  - angina, heart failure symptoms
  - history suggesting structural heart disease, especially prior MI, or heart failure
  - symptom correlation with exercise or stress
  - recent ingestion of medications that might cause or contribute to arrhythmias
- Physical examination for signs of structural heart disease
- 12-lead ECG:
  - signs of prior MI
  - repolarization abnormalities (prolonged QT interval)
  - *Note:* A 12-lead ECG documenting ventricular tachycardia is very helpful. If available, ECG at tachycardia onset (or offset) is very useful
- Echocardiogram with special reference to:
  - left ventricular size and function
  - right ventricular size
- Consider Holter or loop event recorder monitoring with special reference to:
  - presence and morphology of ventricular ectopy and symptom–rhythm correlation
- Treadmill exercise test with special reference to:

- exercise-induced VT
- ECG signs and symptoms of myocardial ischemia (or scintigraphic evidence of ischemia if necessary)

All wide-complex tachycardias (QRS duration ≥ 0.12 seconds) in patients over the age of 50 years should be considered to be VT until proven otherwise. Wide-complex tachycardia in an older patient with a history of heart disease is *almost always* VT, regardless of the morphology of ECG complexes. Most wide-complex tachycardias in any patient of any age group are due to VT.

Significance of VT/VF

The clinical and prognostic importance and management of VT depend on whether it is sustained or nonsustained and whether there is associated structural heart disease, particularly left ventricular systolic dysfunction.

Asymptomatic: Asymptomatic VT is usually discovered during routine screening ECG or other electrocardiographic monitoring. In the presence of structural heart disease, especially left ventricular dysfunction, asymptomatic VT (usually nonsustained) may indicate a risk of future serious, symptomatic, sustained VT or VF.[3]

Symptomatic: Symptoms may include palpitations, dyspnea, chest discomfort, presyncope, loss of consciousness or cardiac arrest. The severity of symptoms does not determine the prognostic importance of VT and its management (e.g., even severe symptoms in a patient with nonsustained VT and no structural heart disease are prognostically benign; such patients require reassurance, but not necessarily specific antiarrhythmic therapy).[5]

Cardiac arrest: Most episodes of out-of-hospital cardiac arrest are likely the result of VF, although the initial cardiac rhythm documented by first responders is often asystole. VF almost always leads to cardiac arrest, whereas sustained VT may lead to cardiac arrest after a variable duration, usually one to several minutes.

Sustained VT: Lasts ≥ 30 seconds or requires immediate medical intervention. For management decisions, > 15 beats is a reasonable working definition. It is most often associated with structural heart disease, typically coronary disease with previous MI. Sustained VT requires investigation and therapy with antiarrhythmic drugs, an implanted cardioverter defibrillator or antitachycardia surgery.

Nonsustained VT: Lasts < 30 seconds but usually only a few seconds. Most commonly there are < 10 consecutive ventricular complexes. Unless symptomatic, it requires treatment only if the likelihood of subsequent sustained VT or cardiac arrest is high.

VT associated with structural heart disease (e.g., coronary, valvular or hypertensive heart disease): Is usually symptomatic and associated with a high risk of sudden death or recurrence (if sustained), or is asymptomatic and associated with at least a moderate risk of sudden death (if nonsustained). The magnitude of left ventricular dysfunction is the most important prognostic factor.

VT associated with a structurally normal heart: May be symptomatic but rarely is life-threatening even if sustained; it requires no therapy if asymptomatic and nonsustained.[5]

Monomorphic VT: Usually implies an abnormal automatic focus in the ventricle or a fixed reentrant pathway associated with a scar. It does not by itself suggest prognosis or therapy.

Polymorphic VT: Usually presents as long runs of nonsustained VT. Consider myocardial ischemia and abnormalities of repolarization (torsades de pointes VT with QT prolongation).[4]

VF may complicate acute MI. However, the prognosis for resuscitated patients with VF occurring during the first 48 hours post-MI is similar to that in patients with an infarction of equivalent severity uncomplicated by VF. The most common underlying cause is coronary artery disease (CAD), often with prior MI, with or without acute ischemia or infarction.

Most patients with VF are at high risk of recurrence. These individuals should be investigated in a similar fashion to patients with sustained VT and should be treated to prevent recurrences.[1,2,3]

Therapeutic Choices

Immediate Therapy for Sustained VT or VF

For sustained monomorphic VT, if the patient is unstable (e.g., has hypotension, angina, heart failure or marked symptoms), cardioversion is effective and safe.[1,6] A synchronized biphasic shock of 120 J or more is usually effective for VT. If immediate conversion to sinus rhythm is not considered necessary, antiarrhythmic drug therapy can be given.[6]

For polymorphic VT or VF, an immediate nonsynchronized shock of 120 to 200 J (biphasic) is required, repeated as necessary (with minimum interruptions in CPR) until defibrillation is achieved.

Amiodarone: iv amiodarone is effective in terminating VT and is especially effective in preventing early recurrence. It is likely the most effective therapy for electrical storm (characterized by frequent recurrences of VT/VF) and is probably useful in shock-resistant VF.[6,7,8,9] The usual dose is 3 to 5 mg/kg iv over 5 to 10 minutes followed by a 0.5 to 1 mg/min infusion. In most patients this is equivalent to about 300 mg iv over 5 to 10 minutes and 1 to 1.5 g iv over the first 24 hours. There are few randomized studies to guide dosing, but most experts follow the above dosing guideline. Hypotension may occur, especially if the drug is administered very rapidly.

Procainamide: 10 to 15 mg/kg iv over 30 to 45 minutes will often slow VT and terminate tachycardia. Hypotension may occur, especially at more rapid infusion rates, and blood pressure should be carefully monitored.[6,9]

Magnesium: 2 to 5 g iv over 3 to 5 minutes is the treatment of choice for torsades de pointes VT associated with QT prolongation and a characteristic long-short initiating sequence, and may be useful in the presence of myocardial ischemia. It is probably of no benefit in monoform VT.[4,10] Magnesium is generally safe, but may rarely cause hypotension.

Beta-blockers (e.g., **metoprolol, propranolol, esmolol):** iv beta-blockers can prevent VT or VF in the setting of acute myocardial ischemia, recent MI or electrical storm.[1,4,9] Bradycardia or hypotension may occur.

Lidocaine: 1 to 1.5 mg/kg iv followed by a 1 to 3 mg/minute infusion is occasionally effective (i.e. in < 20% of cases of sustained monomorphic VT).[2] If conversion does not occur within 10 to 15 minutes, lidocaine will probably not be effective. There is no good evidence that lidocaine is useful in shock-resistant VF.[2,6,9] Lidocaine rarely causes hypotension and at high doses can cause CNS adverse events.

Chronic Therapy—Prevention of VT/VF Recurrence (Figure 1, Figure 2)

Therapeutic choices for long-term management of sustained VT/VF include both drug therapy (Table 1)[1,2,4,9] and nondrug therapy (implanted cardioverter defibrillator, ICD, map-guided endocardial resection, catheter ablation).[5,11,12,13,14,15]

Sustained monomorphic VT/VF is likely to recur in the absence of treatment. Objective documentation of efficacy (e.g., electrophysiologic testing or reduction of VT episodes on Holter monitoring) can be considered. In patients with LV dysfunction, drug therapy should rarely be used as the only therapy for the prevention of recurrent sustained VT or prevention of first occurrence of VT in at-risk patients (primary prophylaxis).

Indicators of efficacy of drugs in individual patients include: the ability of a drug to prevent induction of VT during an electrophysiologic study or with exercise; and the marked reduction of the frequency or elimination of nonsustained VT episodes or premature ventricular contractions (PVCs). The latter indicator is unproven and not recommended.

Patients with a history of VF or cardiac arrest are at risk of recurrence of VF or VT, since their original arrhythmia may have been VT degenerating to VF. Their treatment is similar to that of patients with sustained VT, although markers to judge drug efficacy (inducible VT or VF; PVCs or nonsustained VT on Holter monitoring) are less often present.[17]

Beta-blockers, if tolerated, should be administered to all patients in whom drug therapy is used (and will be indicated in any event in almost all patients with CAD or severe LV dysfunction). They are particularly useful in patients with exercise-, stress- or ischemia-induced VT.

Amiodarone and **sotalol** are effective in preventing VT or VF but almost all studies show they are less effective than implanted defibrillators in preventing sudden death and decreasing all-cause mortality in patients at high risk for sustained VT or VF.[2,5,11,12,13,14,15,16,17] No randomized study has shown that antiarrhythmic drugs reduce mortality. However, amiodarone or sotalol can be used as an adjunct to ICD implantation to prevent ICD shocks, which are painful.[18]

In patients with multiple, frequent recurrences of VT or VF (electrical storm) resistant to the combination of a beta-blocker and amiodarone, or if amiodarone is ineffective or not tolerated, Class I agents such as **mexiletine**, **quinidine** or **procainamide** can be cautiously added. Such combinations are entirely empiric and should be used only as a last resort.[4] In highly selected cases, empiric combinations of sotalol and quinidine or procainamide,[19] or quinidine and mexiletine,[20] or other combinations of drugs with class Ia, Ib, and III activity can be considered.

Nonpharmacologic Choices for VT

- *An implanted cardioverter defibrillator* (ICD) is very effective in treating VT or VF but requires complex evaluation and follow-up.[11,12,13,14,15,16] The AVID trial reported a 39% reduction in total mortality after one year in ICD-treated patients relative to antiarrhythmic therapy (primarily amiodarone).[14]
- *Map-guided endocardial ablation or surgery* requires careful patient selection, specialized facilities and complex open mapping equipment. It may be very effective in certain patient subsets but is rarely performed as a stand-alone procedure.
- *Catheter ablation* using radiofrequency energy may be especially effective for VT arising from the right or left ventricles in patients with apparently normal hearts. In patients with LV dysfunction, it is usually reserved for patients with an ICD who have frequent VT recurrences despite antiarrhythmic drug therapy.

Figure 1: **Management of Nonsustained Ventricular Tachycardia (< 15 beats)**

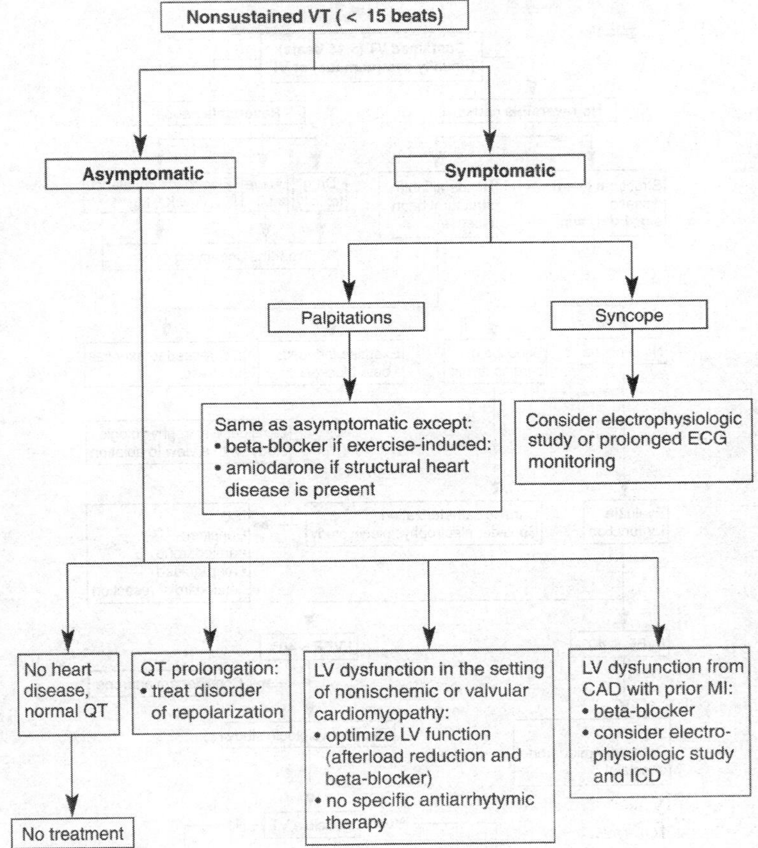

Abbreviations: CAD = coronary artery disease; LV = left ventricular; ICD = implanted cardioverter defibrillator

Figure 2: **Long-term Management of Sustained Ventricular Tachycardia (VT) (> 15 beats), Ventricular Fibrillation (VF), or Resuscitated Cardiac Arrest[a]**

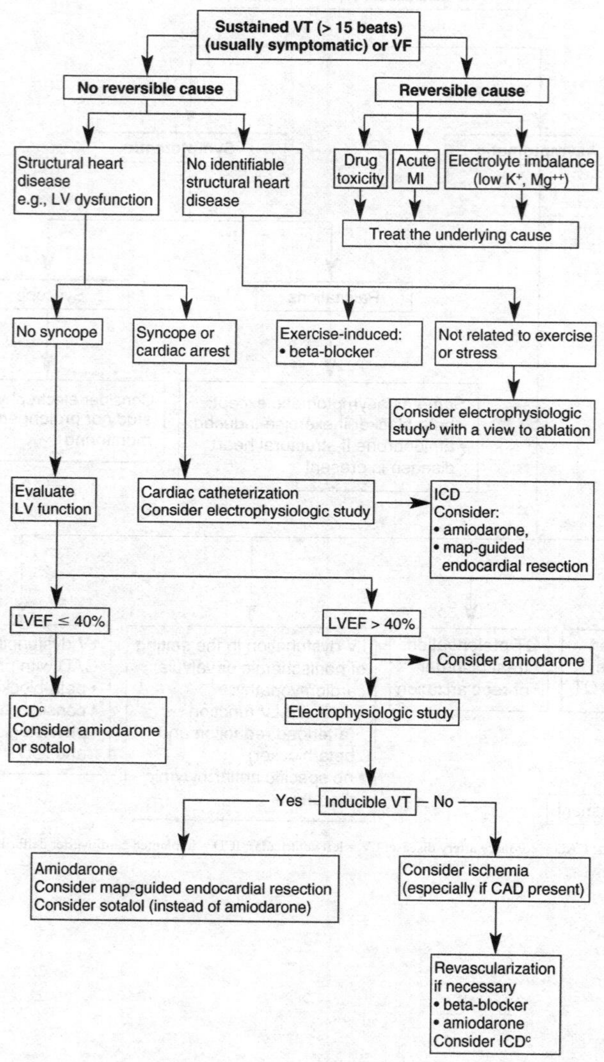

[a] Current guidelines[21] indicate that in most cases an ICD is the preferred therapy for any patient with sustained VT and symptoms in the presence of structural heart disease (with no reversible cause). Electrophysiologic studies are not necessarily indicated in such patients. Cardiac catheterization may be reasonable but is also not necessarily indicated in such patients.

[b] Patients with monomorphic VT.

[c] An ICD may be considered for any patient with sustained VT, and most patients with VF or cardiac arrest. In addition to the therapies listed, all patients should receive beta-blockers unless contraindicated.

Abbreviations: CAD = coronary artery disease; LV = left ventricular; LVEF = LV ejection fraction; ICD = implanted cardioverter defibrillator

Table 1: **Drug Therapy for Ventricular Tachycardia and Ventricular Fibrillation**

Class	Drug	Dose	Drug Interactions	Adverse Effects	Comments	Cost[a]
Class IA Antiarrhythmics[b]	*quinidine* Biquin Durules, generics	Usual: 800–1600 mg/day (sulfate equivalent) Renal dysfunction: ↓ initial dose by 50% and ↑ dosing interval to Q12H	↓ digoxin dose by 50%. Inhibits CYP2D6 (many potential interactions).	Frequent GI intolerance. Rare fever, thrombocytopenia. Torsades de pointes; (proarrhythmic) VT.	Active metabolites accumulate in renal failure, but therapeutic blood monitoring is not readily available. Monitor ECG intervals to guide dosing decisions.	$
	procainamide Procan SR, generics	Usual: 2–4 g/day administer Q6H if using an SR preparation		Frequent arthralgias after long-term use. May cause SLE syndrome. Rare granulocytopenia. Occasional torsades de pointes.	Metabolism depends on rate of acetylation. The active metabolite NAPA accumulates in fast acetylators and in renal failure. Monitor procainamide and NAPA levels; monitor ECG intervals.	$$$–$$$$
Class IB Antiarrhythmics[b]	*mexiletine* generics	Usual: 600–900 mg/day Renal dysfunction: ↓ dose by 50% and ↑ dosing interval to Q12H	Phenytoin and rifampin may ↓ effect (may need to ↑ mexiletine dose).	Frequent CNS side effects.	Rarely used as monotherapy.	$$$$$
Class 1C Antiarrhythmics[b]	*flecainide* Tambocor	Usual: 100–200 mg/day Renal dysfunction: ↓ initial dose by 50% in renal failure		Moderately frequent proarrhythmia.	Titrate dose based on QRS intervals. Do not use in patients with LV dysfunction, especially prior MI (increases mortality in patients who have frequent PVCs after MI).	$$–$$$

(cont'd)

Table 1: **Drug Therapy for Ventricular Tachycardia and Ventricular Fibrillation** *(cont'd)*

Class	Drug	Dose	Drug Interactions	Adverse Effects	Comments	Cost[a]
	propafenone Rythmol, generics	Usual: 600–900 mg/day Renal dysfunction or hepatic failure: ↓ initial dose by 50% and ↑ dosing interval to Q12H	↓ digoxin dose by 25–50%.	Depresses LV function.	Weak beta-blocking effect. Use with great reservation, if at all, in patients with LV dysfunction, especially prior MI. Active metabolites accumulate in rapid metabolizers. Monitor QRS duration.	$$$$$
Class III Antiarrhythmics	*sotalol* generics	Usual: 160–480 mg/day Elderly: ↓ initial dose to 40 mg po Q12H	Digoxin, verapamil, other beta-blockers may cause AV block, bradycardia. See metoprolol.	Torsades de pointes, especially at higher doses or with renal dysfunction. See metoprolol.	Sotalol is a beta blocker. May be especially effective in exercise-related arrhythmias. Likely more effective than other drugs in suppressing inducibility of VT. Contraindicated in asthma.	$$–$$$
	amiodarone Cordarone, generics	Loading dose: 800–1600 mg/day for 7–10 days po Maintenance dose: 200–400 mg/day po Avoid high loading dose in setting of sinus bradycardia (HR < 50 BPM).	↓ digoxin dose by 50%. ↓ beta-blocker dose by 50%. ↓ quinidine or procainamide dose by 50%. ↓ warfarin dose by 50%.	Various gastrointestinal, dermatologic, neurologic, ophthalmologic and thyroid abnormalities. Pulmonary fibrosis, hepatic dysfunction and aggravation of arrhythmias are rare but potentially life-threatening.	Slows conduction, blocks adrenergic activity, blocks Ca^{++} channels. Very long half-life. Likely the most effective antiarrhythmic drug. Usually used empirically.	$$$

Class	Drug	Dose	Drug Interactions	Adverse Effects	Comments	Cost[a]
Beta$_1$-adrenergic Antagonists[c]	*metoprolol* Betaloc, Lopresor, generics	100–400 mg/day	With digoxin, Ca^{++} channel blockers, amiodarone, ↓ dose 25–50%. ↓ dose of hypoglycemic agents by 25–50%.	Fatigue, bradycardia, AV block, decreased exercise capacity, headache, impotence, vivid dreams. Less common: hyperglycemia, depression, heart failure.	Monitor carefully in diabetic patients. Caution in patients with HF. Especially useful in exercise-induced VT, with ischemia, or VT in the absence of structural heart disease. Of probable but unclear benefit in patients with sustained VT and prior MI. May enhance efficacy of other antiarrhythmic drugs in this setting. Very low proarrhythmic risk. Contraindicated in asthma.	$–$$

[a] Cost of 30-day supply; includes drug cost only.

[b] There is no evidence that any drug with primarily class I activity is of long-term benefit in reducing mortality from VT or VF; in particular, Class I drugs are not recommended in patients with VT or VF and structural heart disease (in the absence of an ICD).

[c] The beta$_1$-adrenergic antagonist suggested is an example only. Other beta$_1$-adrenergic antagonists may be used.

Dosage adjustment may be required in renal impairment; see Appendix I.

Abbreviations: HF = heart failure; LV = left ventricular; NAPA = n-acetylprocainamide; PVC = premature ventricular contraction; SLE = systemic lupus erythematosus; VT = ventricular tachycardia

Legend: $ < $15 $-$$ < $15–30 $$ $15–30 $$-$$$ $15–60 $$$ $30–60 $$$-$$$$ $30–90 $$$$ $60–90 $$$$$ > $90

Suggested Readings

2005 American Heart Association guidelines for cardiopulmonary resuscitation and emergency cardiovascular care. Part 5: Electrical therapies: automated external defibrillators, defibrillation, cardioversion, and pacing. *Circulation* 2005;112(24 Suppl):IV35-46. Available from: http://circ.ahajournals.org/cgi/content/full/112/24_suppl/IV-35 Accessed May 8, 2007.

Atkins DL, Dorian P, Gonzalez ER et al. Treatment of tachyarrhythmias. *Ann Emerg Med* 2001;37(4 Suppl):S91-109.

Connolly SJ, Hallstrom AP, Cappato R et al. Meta-analysis of the implantable cardioverter defibrillator secondary prevention trials. AVID, CASH and CIDS studies. *Eur Heart J* 2000;21(24):2071-8.

European Heart Rhythm Association; Heart Rhythm Society; Zipes DP et al. ACC/AHA/ESC 2006 guidelines for management of patients with ventricular arrhythmias and the prevention of sudden cardiac death. *J Am Coll Cardiol* 2006;48(5):e247-346.

Kudenchuk PJ. Advanced cardiac life support antiarrhythmic drugs. *Cardiol Clin* 2002;20(1):79-87.

References

1. Atkins DL, Dorian P, Gonzalez ER et al. Treatment of tachyarrhythmias. *Ann Emerg Med* 2001;37(4 Suppl):S91-109.
2. Dorian P, Philippon F. The management of acute ventricular tachycardia or fibrillation. *Can J Cardiol* 2000;16(Suppl C):16C-9C.
3. Green MS, Ricci J, Wolfe K. The appropriate evaluation of the patient at risk for sudden death from ventricular arrhythmias. *Can J Cardiol* 2000;16(Suppl C):13C-5C.
4. Gillis AM. Intractable ventricular tachyarrhythmias: immediate evaluation and management, role of pharmacological therapy. *Card Electrophysiol Rev* 2001;5:354-8.
5. Gillis AM, Hamilton RM, LeFeuvre CA. Unusual causes of sudden cardiac death due to ventricular tachyarrhythmias. *Can J Cardiol* 2000;16(Suppl C):34C-40C.
6. [No authors listed]. Guidelines 2000 for Cardiopulmonary Resuscitation and Emergency Cardiovascular Care. Part 6: advanced cardiovascular life support: section 1: Introduction to ACLS 2000: overview of recommended changes in ACLS from the guidelines 2000 conference. The American Heart Association in collaboration with the International Liaison Committee on Resuscitation. *Circulation* 2000;102(8 Suppl):I86-9.
7. Dorian P, Cass D, Schwartz B et al. Amiodarone as compared with lidocaine for shock-resistant ventricular fibrillation. *N Engl J Med* 2002;346(12):884-90.
8. Kowey PR, Levine JH, Herre JM et al. Randomized, double-blind comparison of intravenous amiodarone and bretylium in the treatment of patients with recurrent, hemodynamically destabilizing ventricular tachycardia or fibrillation. The Intravenous Amiodarone Multicenter Investigators Group. *Circulation* 1995;92(11):3255-63.
9. Kudenchuk PJ. Advanced cardiac life support antiarrhythmic drugs. *Cardiol Clin* 2002;20(1):79-87.
10. Tzivoni D, Banai S, Schuger C et al. Treatment of torsade de pointes with magnesium sulfate. *Circulation* 1988;77(2):392-7.
11. Buxton AE, Lee KL, Fisher JD et al. A randomized study of the prevention of sudden death in patients with coronary artery disease. Multicenter Unsustained Tachycardia Trial Investigators. *N Engl J Med* 1999;341(25):1882-90.
12. Moss AJ, Zareba W, Hall WJ et al. Prophylactic implantation of a defibrillator in patients with myocardial infarction and reduced ejection fraction. *N Engl J Med* 2002;346(12):877-83.
13. Connolly SJ, Gent M, Roberts RS et al. Canadian implantable defibrillator study (CIDS): a randomized trial of the implantable cardioverter defibrillator against amiodarone. *Circulation* 2000;101(11):1297-302.
14. [No authors listed]. A comparison of antiarrhythmic-drug therapy with implantable defibrillators in patients resuscitated from near-fatal ventricular arrhythmias. The Antiarrhythmics versus Implantable Defibrillators (AVID) Investigators. *N Engl J Med* 1997;337(22):1576-83.
15. Moss AJ, Hall WJ, Cannom DS et al. Improved survival with an implanted defibrillator in patients with coronary disease at high risk for ventricular arrhythmia. Multicenter Automatic Defibrillator Implantation Trial Investigators. *N Engl J Med* 1996;335(26):1933-40.

16. Connolly SJ, Krahn A, Klein G. Long term management of the survivor of ventricular fibrillation or sustained ventricular tachycardia. *Can J Cardiol* 2000;16(Suppl C):20C-2C.
17. Connolly SJ, Hallstrom AP, Cappato R et al. Meta-analysis of the implantable cardioverter defibrillator secondary prevention trials. AVID, CASH and CIDS studies. Antiarrhythmics vs Implantable Defibrillator study. Cardiac Arrest Study Hamburg. Canadian Implantable Defibrillator Study. *Eur Heart J* 2000;21(24):2071-8.
18. Connolly SJ, Dorian P, Roberts RS et al. Comparison of beta-blockers, amiodarone plus beta-blockers, or sotalol for prevention of shocks from implantable cardioverter defibrillators: the OPTIC Study: a randomized trial. *JAMA* 2006;295(2):165-71.
19. Lee SD, Newman D, Ham M et al. Electrophysiologic mechanisms of antiarrhythmic efficacy of a sotalol and class Ia drug combination: elimination of reverse use dependence. *J Am Coll Cardiol* 1997;29(1):100-5.
20. Duff HJ, Mitchell LB, Wyse DG et al. Mexiletine/quinidine combination therapy: electrophysiologic correlates of anti-arrhythmic efficacy. *Clin Invest Med* 1991;14(5):476-83.
21. European Heart Rhythm Association; Heart Rhythm Society; Zipes DP et al. ACC/AHA/ESC 2006 guidelines for management of patients with ventricular arrhythmias and the prevention of sudden cardiac death: a report of the American College of Cardiology/American Heart Association Task Force and the European Society of Cardiology Committee for Practice Guidelines (Writing Committee to Develop Guidelines for Management of Patients With Ventricular Arrhythmias and the Prevention of Sudden Cardiac Death). *J Am Coll Cardiol* 2006;48(5):e247-346.

CHAPTER 41

Syncope

Robert Sheldon, MD, PhD

Syncope is defined as a reversible loss of consciousness not requiring specific resuscitative measures, and not associated with generalized seizures. Probably 40% of people faint at least once in their life, and many faint recurrently.[1] Most people who faint have a benign cause but a few are at risk of death. Common causes of syncope are listed in Table 1.

Table 1: **Common Causes of Syncope**

Volume depletion and drugs

- Volume depletion
  - Diarrhea
  - Diminished oral intake
  - Polyuria
- Drugs
  - ACE inhibitors
  - Alcohol
  - Antiparkinsonian drugs
  - Diuretics
  - Alpha- and beta-adrenergic blockers
  - Vasodilators
  - Nitrates
  - Phosphodiesterase type 5 inhibitors (sildenafil, tadalafil, vardenafil)

Orthostatic intolerance disorders

- Reflex syncope syndromes
  - Carotid sinus hypersensitivity
  - Vasovagal syncope syndromes
- Postural orthostatic tachycardia syndrome (POTS)
- Autonomic neuropathies
  - Pure autonomic failure syndromes
  - Multiple system atrophy syndromes

Arrhythmias

- Bradycardias
  - Sinus node disease
  - Complete (third degree) heart block
- Tachycardias
  - Supraventricular arrhythmias (uncommon)
  - Ventricular tachycardia
  - Torsades de pointes polymorphic ventricular tachycardia

Obstruction

- Aortic stenosis
- Pulmonary emboli
- Many other rare causes

Goals of Therapy

- Identify potentially fatal causes of syncope
- Aggressively investigate and treat high-risk patients
- Remove reversible causes of syncope
- Treat patients with therapies appropriate to the degree of their symptoms

Investigations

- Complete cardiovascular and neurologic history and physical examination.[2,3] Rule out seizures, then screen for life-threatening causes such as obstruction, ventricular tachycardia and asystole or heart block (Figure 1)
- Tailor laboratory investigations to the individual patient:[3]
  - ECG (most patients)[4]
  - older patients (> 55 years) should have ambulatory ECG monitoring unless the history is strongly persuasive for vasovagal syncope
  - ambulatory ECGs and stress tests are of limited use in younger patients
  - echocardiogram or other noninvasive measure of left ventricular function if structural heart disease is suspected
  - coronary angiography as indicated
  - refer patients with structural heart disease for electrophysiologic assessment
  - unless contraindicated, carotid sinus massage should be performed in patients > 50 years old to screen for carotid sinus hypersensitivity
  - implanted patient-activated loop recorders may be useful in patients with infrequent syncope that eludes conventional attempts at diagnosis[5]
  - tilt table testing might be useful in diagnosing vasovagal syncope in patients with atypical symptoms[6,7]
- After potentially fatal causes are eliminated and reversible causes are removed, most patients will have one of several syndromes of orthostatic intolerance:[6]
  - reflex syncope syndromes
    - vasovagal syncope
    - carotid sinus hypersensitivity in the elderly
  - postural orthostatic tachycardia syndrome (POTS)
  - pure autonomic failure syndromes
  - multiple system atrophy syndromes
- The orthostatic intolerance syndromes can be distinguished based on history and a simple *stand test* in the office. To perform the stand test, first measure blood pressure and heart rate after the patient has been

supine for five minutes, then after two and four minutes of standing. These responses are seen:

Normal and vasovagal syncope: modest rises in heart rate (about 10 BPM) and blood pressure (about 10 mm Hg).

Postural orthostatic tachycardia syndrome: > 30 BPM rise or heart rate > 120 BPM with normal blood pressure or mild orthostatic hypotension.

Autonomic failure: progressive fall in blood pressure of ≥ 20 mm Hg systolic or ≥ 10 mm Hg diastolic with development of presyncope; often no increase in heart rate.

Therapeutic Choices

Treatment is directed at the cause of syncope. Treat any reversible causes. Refer patients with syncope secondary to bradycardia (asystole or complete heart block) for a permanent pacemaker. Refer patients with suspected or diagnosed ventricular tachycardia, and all patients with structural heart disease to a cardiologist, preferably an electrophysiologist. The following addresses treatment of syndromes of orthostatic intolerance.

Vasovagal Syncope

Nonpharmacologic Choices

- Reassure the patient that this syndrome is not life threatening and that it is a physical problem, not a psychiatric disorder. Encourage *increased dietary salt* intake of about 3 to 5 g daily, in the absence of contraindications such as hypertension or heart failure.[6,8]
- Teach the patient to use physical counterpressure manoeuvres at the onset of presyncope.[9,10] These include squatting, crossing the legs with isometric contraction if standing, and vigorous hand clenching with upper girdle isometric contraction. All should be tried. The evidence is based on good physiologic studies, but no randomized clinical trials have been published.
- Pacemaker therapy is no longer indicated, based on the results of an adequately powered randomized placebo-controlled trial.[11] The occasional patient with asystole documented during vasovagal syncope might benefit, and these uncommon patients should be assessed at a tertiary referral clinic.

Pharmacologic Choices (Table 2)

Drug therapy may be effective in some, although the evidence is mixed. Few drugs have been evaluated in large randomized trials. Therapy may be unnecessary in patients with infrequent vasovagal syncope who have recognizable premonitory symptoms.

Fludrocortisone can be tried if simple salt supplements are ineffective. The goal is fluid retention, which may precipitate heart failure. A single randomized trial in children was negative.[12] Fludrocortisone has not been evaluated in adults in randomized trials.

Alpha-agonists increase venous return, thereby preventing the onset of vasovagal syncope. **Midodrine** improved symptoms in patients enrolled in small randomized trials,[13,14] including one that showed midodrine to be more effective after six months than salt and fluid supplementation.[13] Supine hypertension may complicate treatment.

Beta-blockers are no longer indicated for vasovagal syncope, and there is little evidence that specific patients who might respond can be identified. This is based on one adequately powered, randomized placebo-controlled trial[15] and two smaller studies.[16,17]

Serotonin reuptake inhibitors may prevent syncope in some patients in whom other therapies are ineffective or poorly tolerated. **Paroxetine** significantly reduced the frequency of spontaneous syncope over two years compared with placebo in a randomized clinical trial.[18] Agents in this class have also been reported to increase the frequency of fainting.[19]

Orthostatic Hypotension

The goal of therapy is to relieve symptoms of cerebral hypoperfusion while avoiding treatment side effects. Orthostatic hypotension is often associated with supine hypertension, which complicates its therapy.

Nonpharmacologic Choices

Remove as many hypotensive and volume-depleting drugs as possible. *Increase dietary salt* intake if not contraindicated. Elevate the head of the bed on blocks or bricks by 15 to 30 cm (this is often not well tolerated). Instruct patients to avoid hemodynamic stress such as getting up quickly, eating large meals, warm environments or hot baths and heavy exertion.

Pharmacologic Choices (Table 2)

Sodium and water retention may be beneficial in patients with orthostatic hypotension. **Fludrocortisone** increases blood volume and sensitizes peripheral alpha receptors. **NSAIDs** promote fluid retention and also indirectly cause vasoconstriction. Try **indomethacin** 25 to 50 mg three times daily or equivalent doses of related drugs.

Midodrine is a pressor amine that causes both venoconstriction (thereby increasing venous return) and arteriolar constriction (which directly increases blood pressure). Midodrine significantly increased standing blood pressure and decreased the severity of symptoms in placebo-controlled trials.[20,21] As noted above, supine hypertension may complicate treatment.

The acetylcholinesterase inhibitor **pyridostigmine**, given alone or in combination with midodrine, significantly improved standing blood pressure without increasing supine blood pressure in a short-term randomized placebo-controlled trial.[22] Further study is needed before this agent can be recommended.

Octreotide, a somatostatin analogue that blocks production of gut vasodilator hormones and reduces splanchnic blood flow,[23] may be useful in postprandial hypotension. The combination of octreotide plus midodrine significantly increased postprandial blood pressure and standing time before onset of symptoms, to a greater extent than either drug alone, in a small randomized crossover study.[24] Octreotide is given by SC injection.

Yohimbine is an $alpha_2$-antagonist that stimulates sympathetic outflow.[25] Adverse effects may limit its use.

Nonselective beta-blockers (e.g., **propranolol**, **timolol**, **nadolol**) block vasodilatory $beta_2$-receptors and reduce or abolish the fall in blood pressure upon standing in patients with orthostatic hypotension.[26]

Postural Orthostatic Tachycardia Syndrome

POTS manifests as a dramatic increase in heart rate and light-headedness upon assuming an upright posture from the supine position. Few rigorous clinical trials have been reported. Salt, fludrocortisone, midodrine and beta-blockers are all reasonable empiric treatments.

Therapeutic Tips

- All physicians treating syncope patients should be familiar with provincial regulations for the ability of syncope patients to drive. The regulations vary with the cause of syncope and with the therapy. The Canadian Cardiovascular Society recently updated its guidelines on the fitness of syncope patients to drive.[27]

Figure 1: **Diagnostic Approach to the Patient with Syncope**

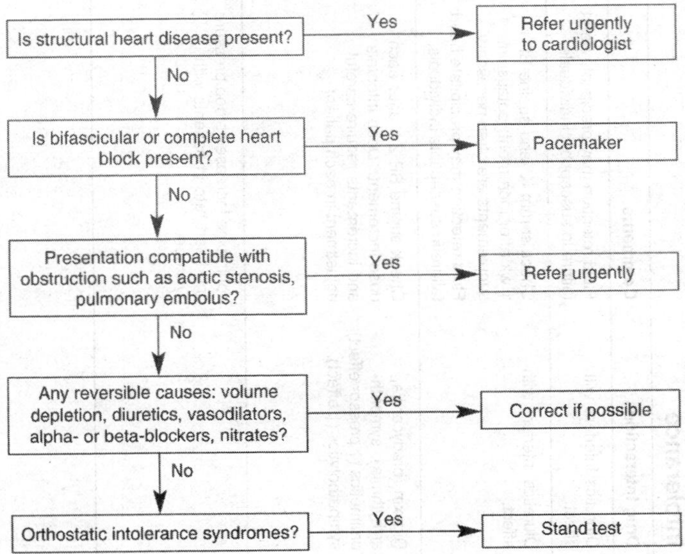

Table 2: **Drugs for Treatment of Syndromes of Orthostatic Intolerance**

Class	Drug	Dose	Adverse Effects	Drug Interactions	Comments	Cost[a]
Electrolytes	*sodium chloride*	3–5 g Na^+ daily	Gastric upset, fluid retention.	Diuretics interfere with effect.	Fluid retention may precipitate heart failure in susceptible individuals.	$
Mineralocorticoids	*fludrocortisone* Florinef	Initial: 0.1 mg daily Increase by 0.1 mg Q1–2 wk to 0.4 mg	Mild edema, supine hypertension, hypokalemia, eczema, thin skin.	Diuretics interfere with effect.	Check serum K^+ and supine BP 1 wk after increment; potassium supplements are often necessary. Fluid retention may precipitate heart failure in susceptible individuals.	$–$$
Alpha$_1$-adrenergic Agonists	*midodrine* Amatine	Initial: 2.5–5 mg TID ac; none after 5 pm Increase by 2.5 mg TID Q1–2 wk to tolerance, effectiveness, or 15 mg TID	Supine hypertension, headache, shivering, paresthesias, piloerection.	Digoxin (bradycardia, arrhythmia); sympathomimetics (↑ pressor effect); sympatholytics (↓ effect).	Check supine BP 2 h after each dose increment. Dose intervals and increments require careful adjustment in each patient.	$$–$$$
Alpha$_2$-adrenergic Antagonists	*yohimbine* Yocon, generics	Initial: 4 mg BID Increase by 2 mg BID Q1–2 wk to tolerance, effectiveness, or 8–14 mg BID	Anxiety, tremor, headache, diarrhea.		Yohimbine increases blood pressure and heart rate in patients with syncope.	$$–$$$

Class	Drug	Dose	Adverse Effects	Drug Interactions	Comments	Cost[a]
Beta$_1$-adrenergic Antagonists	*metoprolol* Betaloc, Lopresor, generics	Initial: 50 mg BID Max: 100 mg BID	Fatigue, bradycardia, hypotension, depression, bronchospasm.	Digoxin (↑ bradycardia); diltiazem, verapamil (↑ cardiodepressant effect).	Other nonselective beta-blockers may be used (e.g. nadolol, timolol). Check heart rate, BP after each dose ↑. Caution in patients with bronchospastic lung disease, diabetes or bradyarrhythmias. Not indicated for vasovagal syncope.	\$–\$\$

[a] Cost of 30-day supply; includes drug cost only.

Dosage adjustment may be required in renal impairment; see Appendix I.

Legend: \$ < \$10 \$-\$\$ < \$10–50 \$\$ \$10–50 \$\$-\$\$\$ \$10–100

Suggested Readings

Benditt DG, Fahy GJ, Lurie KG et al. Pharmacotherapy of neurally mediated syncope. *Circulation* 1999;100(11):1242-8.

Brignole M, Alboni P, Benditt DG et al. Guidelines on management (diagnosis and treatment) of syncope-update 2004. Executive summary. *Eur Heart J* 2004;25(22):2054-72.

Grubb BP, Karas B. Clinical disorders of the autonomic nervous system associated with orthostatic intolerance: an overview of classification, clinical evaluation, and management. *Pacing Clin Electrophysiol* 1999;22(5):798-810.

Sheldon R, Morillo CA, Krahn A. Management of vasovagal syncope: 2004. *Expert Rev Cardiovasc Ther* 2004;2(6):915-23.

References

1. Ganzeboom KS, Colman N, Reitsma JB et al. Prevalence and triggers of syncope in medical students. *Am J Cardiol* 2003;91(8):1006-8, A8.
2. Brignole M, Alboni P, Benditt DG et al. Guidelines on management (diagnosis and treatment) of syncope--update 2004. *Europace* 2004;6(6):467-537.
3. Sheldon R, Rose S, Connolly S et al. Diagnostic criteria for vasovagal syncope based on a quantitative history. *Eur Heart J* 2006;27(3):344-50.
4. Kapoor WN, Karpf M, Wieand S et al. A prospective evaluation and follow-up of patients with syncope. *N Engl J Med* 1983;309(4):197-204.
5. Moya A, Brignole M, Menozzi C et al. Mechanism of syncope in patients with isolated syncope and in patients with tilt-positive syncope. *Circulation* 2001;104(11):1261-7.
6. Bloomfield DM, Sheldon R, Grubb BP et al. Putting it together: a new treatment algorithm for vasovagal syncope and related disorders. *Am J Cardiol* 1999;84(8A):33Q-39Q.
7. Sheldon R. Tilt testing for syncope: a reappraisal. *Curr Opin Cardiol* 2005;20(1):38-41.
8. Benditt DG, Fahy GJ, Lurie KG et al. Pharmacotherapy of neurally mediated syncope. *Circulation* 1999;100(11):1242-8.
9. Brignole M, Croci F, Menozzi C et al. Isometric arm counter-pressure maneuvers to abort impending vasovagal syncope. *J Am Coll Cardiol* 2002;40(11):2053-9.
10. Krediet CT, van Dijk N, Linzer M et al. Management of vasovagal syncope: controlling or aborting faints by leg crossing and muscle tensing. *Circulation* 2002;106(13):1684-9.
11. Connolly SJ, Sheldon R, Thorpe KE et al. Pacemaker therapy for prevention of syncope in patients with recurrent severe vasovagal syncope: Second Vasovagal Pacemaker Study (VPS II): a randomized trial. *JAMA* 2003;289(17):2224-9.
12. Salim MA, Di Sessa TG. Effectiveness of fludrocortisone and salt in preventing syncope recurrence in children: a double-blind, placebo-controlled, randomized trial. *J Am Coll Cardiol* 2005;45(4):484-8.
13. Perez-Lugones A, Schweikert R, Pavia S et al. Usefulness of midodrine in patients with severely symptomatic neurocardiogenic syncope: a randomized control study. *J Cardiovasc Electrophysiol* 2001;12(8):935-8.
14. Ward CR, Gray JC, Gilroy JJ et al. Midodrine: a role in the management of neurocardiogenic syncope. *Heart* 1998;79(1):45-9.
15. Sheldon R, Connolly S, Rose S et al. Prevention of Syncope Trial (POST): a randomized, placebo-controlled study of metoprolol in the prevention of vasovagal syncope. *Circulation* 2006;113(9):1164-70.
16. Sheldon R, Rose S, Flanagan P et al. Effect of beta blockers on the time to first syncope recurrence in patients after a positive isoproterenol tilt table test. *Am J Cardiol* 1996;78(5):536-9.
17. Madrid AH, Ortega J, Rebollo JG et al. Lack of efficacy of atenolol for the prevention of neurally mediated syncope in a highly symptomatic population: a prospective, double-blind, randomized and placebo-controlled study. *J Am Coll Cardiol* 2001;37(2):554-9.
18. Di Girolamo E, Di Iorio C, Sabatini P et al. Effects of paroxetine hydrochloride, a selective serotonin reuptake inhibitor, on refractory vasovagal syncope: a randomized, double-blind, placebo-controlled study. *J Am Coll Cardiol* 1999;33(5):1227-30.
19. Tandan T, Giuffre M, Sheldon R. Exacerbations of neurally mediated syncope associated with sertraline. *Lancet* 1997;349(9059):1145-6.
20. Low PA, Gilden JL, Freeman R et al. Efficacy of midodrine vs placebo in neurogenic orthostatic hypotension. A randomized, double-blind multicenter study. Midodrine Study Group. *JAMA* 1997;277(13):1046-51.
21. Wright RA, Kaufmann HC, Perera R et al. A double-blind, dose-response study of midodrine in neurogenic orthostatic hypotension. *Neurology* 1998;51(1):120-4.

22. Singer W, Sandroni P, Opfer-Gehrking TL et al. Pyridostigmine treatment trial in neurogenic orthostatic hypotension. *Arch Neurol* 2006;63(4):513-8.
23. Hoeldtke RD, Davis KM, Joseph J et al. Hemodynamic effects of octreotide in patients with autonomic neuropathy. *Circulation* 1991;84(1):168-76.
24. Hoeldtke RD, Horvath GG, Bryner KD et al. Treatment of orthostatic hypotension with midodrine and octreotide. *J Clin Endocrinol Metab* 1998;83(2):339-43.
25. Mosqueda-Garcia R, Fernandez-Violante R, Tank J et al. Yohimbine in neurally mediated syncope. Pathophysiological implications. *J Clin Invest* 1998;102(10):1824-30.
26. Cleophas TJ, Kauw FH, Bijl C et al. Effects of beta adrenergic receptor agonists and antagonists in diabetics with symptoms of postural hypotension: a double-blind, placebo-controlled study. *Angiology* 1986;37(11):855-62.
27. Simpson C, Dorian P, Gupta A et al. Assessment of the cardiac patient for fitness to drive: drive subgroup executive summary. *Can J Cardiol* 2004;20(13):1314-20.

CHAPTER 42
Venous Thromboembolism

Alexander G.G. Turpie, MD, FRCP(Lond), FRCP(Glas), FACP, FACC, FRCPC

Treatment of Venous Thromboembolism

Goals of Therapy

Deep Vein Thrombosis (DVT)

- Prevent major pulmonary embolism
- Prevent thrombus extension
- Prevent postphlebitic syndrome
- Reduce morbidity of the acute event

Pulmonary Embolism (PE)

- Prevent death
- Prevent recurrent thromboembolism
- Prevent chronic thromboembolic pulmonary hypertension

Investigations

Because the clinical diagnosis of DVT and PE is insensitive and nonspecific, objective diagnosis using specific procedures is important for optimal management.

- DVT: B-mode compression ultrasound (most practical and useful clinically), ascending venography, impedance plethysmography
- PE: Pulmonary angiography, perfusion lung scan, ventilation lung scan, spiral CT, MRI, tests for DVT as described immediately above
- Patients under the age of 40 with recurrent VTE or a family history should be screened for thrombophilia (see Clinical Risk Categories below)
- D-dimer

Therapeutic Choices

General Measures

The majority of patients with DVT can be treated as outpatients. Likewise, many patients with PE who do not have compromised cardiopulmonary function may be treated as outpatients.

Deep Vein Thrombosis

- Rest if symptoms warrant (reduces pain and swelling).
- Elevate limb (reduces edema and pain).

- Avoid pressure on the swollen leg.
- **Analgesics** for pain (NSAIDs are effective but may increase the risk of bleeding, especially when used with anticoagulants). Acetaminophen is commonly used. Narcotics are not usually required for analgesia.

Pulmonary Embolism

- Oxygen
- Intravenous fluids
- Vasopressor agents
- Other resuscitory measures (depending on the patient's clinical status)

Pharmacologic Choices

Subcutaneous **low molecular weight heparin (LMWH)** or **fondaparinux**, or iv **unfractionated heparin (UFH)** are recommended for the initial treatment of established DVT and/or PE. Oral **warfarin** can be started at the same time and administered concurrently for several days. LMWH, fondaparinux or UFH is continued for a minimum of five days or until the International Normalized Ratio (INR, an indicator of the intensity of anticoagulation induced by warfarin) is therapeutic for at least two days. The duration of oral anticoagulation is dependent on the risk of recurrence of VTE (Table 1). Treatment of a first episode in a patient with a transient risk factor should continue for three months. In those with idiopathic VTE or irreversible risk factors, treatment should continue for a longer period. In these patients, treatment with oral anticoagulants for an indefinite period may be considered because it further reduces the risk of recurrence.[1] LMWH may be used as an alternative to warfarin in some circumstances[2,3] and is particularly useful in cancer-associated thrombosis.

Table 1: **Duration of Secondary Prophylaxis for Venous Thromboembolism**

3 months
First event with reversible or time-limited risk factor such as surgery
6-12 months (consider indefinite treatment)
First idiopathic event[a]
First event with heterozygous activated protein C resistance (APCR)
Protein C or S deficiency
12 months (consider indefinite treatment)
Recurrent disease
Cancer until resolved
Antiphospholipid antibody, two or more thrombophilic conditions

[a] Antithrombotic therapy for venous thromboembolic disease: the Seventh ACCP Conference on Antithrombotic and Thrombolytic Therapy. *Chest* 2004;126(3 Suppl):401S-428S.

Prophylaxis of Venous Thromboembolism

Goals of Therapy

- Prevent deep vein thrombosis (DVT) and pulmonary embolism (PE)
- Reduce mortality
- Prevent the postphlebitic syndrome
- Prevent chronic thromboembolic pulmonary hypertension

Clinical Risk Categories

Venous thromboembolism (VTE) is a common cause of morbidity and mortality in hospitalized patients; the frequency varies according to patients' risk. The risk of VTE is increased in the presence of factors related to venous stasis and coagulopathy (Table 2). Consensus conferences have defined risk categories based on clinical criteria and made specific recommendations for thrombosis prophylaxis according to risk group (Table 5).[4,5]

Table 2: **Risk Factors for Venous Thromboembolism**

Surgery	Myeloproliferative disorders
Trauma (major or lower extremity)	Paroxysmal nocturnal hemoglobinuria
Immobility, paresis	Obesity
Malignancy	Smoking
Cancer therapy (hormonal, chemotherapy or radiotherapy)	Varicose veins
Previous VTE episode	Central venous catheterization
Increasing age	Inherited or acquired thrombophilia:
Pregnancy and the postpartum period	Protein C, protein S or antithrombin deficiency
Estrogen-containing contraceptives or hormone therapy	Prothrombin 20210 gene mutation
Selective estrogen receptor modulators (raloxifene)	Factor V Leiden
Acute medical illness	Antiphospholipid antibody or lupus anticoagulant
Heart or respiratory failure	Hyperhomocysteinemia
Inflammatory bowel disease	Elevated factor VIII
Nephrotic syndrome	

Adapted with permission from Geerts WH et al. Prevention of venous thromboembolism: the Seventh ACCP Conference on Antithrombotic and Thrombolytic Therapy. *Chest* 2004:126(3 Suppl):338S-400S.

Nonpharmacologic Choices

Graduated compression stockings and *intermittent pneumatic compression devices* reduce the risk of VTE and are particularly useful in clinical settings where the risk of bleeding is high (e.g., after neurosurgery).

Caval interruption by filter is rarely indicated for primary prophylaxis but should be considered in patients in whom anticoagulants have failed or are absolutely contraindicated.[5] A variety of removable filters are now available and are preferred over the permanent ones.

Pharmacologic Choices[4,5,6] (Table 6, Table 7)

Low Molecular Weight Heparins

Enoxaparin, dalteparin, tinzaparin and **nadroparin** are approved for both prophylaxis in conjunction with surgery and treatment of VTE (Table 6, Table 7).[8]

The kinetics of LMWHs are more predictable than those of UFH, and their elimination half-life is longer. These properties make weight-adjusted fixed-dose sc dosing of LMWHs an excellent alternative to adjusted-dose iv UFH in the initial treatment of VTE. LMWHs have become the management of choice for initial treatment of DVT for many outpatients. They are also effective in the treatment of PE.

Unfractionated Heparin (UFH)

For treatment of VTE, UFH is most commonly given by iv infusion in a dose adjusted to prolong the activated partial thromboplastin time (aPTT) to 1.5 to 2.5 times control (the target therapeutic range should be determined by an institution's coagulation laboratory). It is also effective by sc injection if a sufficiently high dose is given (generally 15 000 to 25 000 units Q12H). An iv bolus (5000 to 10 000 units) should be given with the sc injection in the initial treatment. Monitoring four to six hours after the sc dose should aim for an aPTT of 2 to 2.5 times control. A practical weight-based nomogram has been developed for adjusting iv heparin (Table 3).[9]

Table 3: **Body Weight–based Dosing of Intravenous Heparin in Adults**[a]

aPTT (seconds)	Dose Change (units/kg/h)	Additional Action	Next aPTT (h)
< 35 (< 1.2 × mean normal)	+4	Rebolus with 80 units/kg	6
35–45 (1.2–1.5 × mean normal)	+2	Rebolus with 40 units/kg	6

(cont'd)

Table 3: **Body Weight–based Dosing of Intravenous Heparin in Adults[a]** *(cont'd)*

aPTT (seconds)	Dose Change (units/kg/h)	Additional Action	Next aPTT (h)
46–70[b] (1.5–2.3 × mean normal)	0	0	6[c]
71–90 (2.3–3 × mean normal)	-2	0	6
> 90 (> 3 × mean normal)	-3	Stop infusion for 1 h	6

[a] Initial dosing: 80 units/kg iv bolus; maintenance infusion of heparin, at a rate dictated by body weight through an infusion apparatus calibrated for low flow rates: 18 units/kg/h (aPTT in 6 hours).
[b] The therapeutic range in seconds should correspond to a plasma heparin level of 0.2 to 0.4 units/mL by protamine sulfate titration. When aPTT is checked at 6 hours or longer, steady-state kinetics can be assumed.
[c] During the first 24 hours, repeat aPTT every 6 hours. Thereafter, monitor aPTT once every morning unless it is outside the therapeutic range.
Adapted with permission from Hyers TM et al. Antithrombotic therapy for venous thromboembolic disease. *Chest* 1998;114(5 Suppl):561S-578S.

Specific Factor Xa Inhibitors

Fondaparinux is the first of a new class of antithrombotic agents, the specific factor Xa inhibitors. It is approved for the prophylaxis of VTE in high-risk orthopedic patients[6] and for the treatment of DVT and PE. Fondaparinux also prevents VTE with minimal risk of bleeding in older acute medical patients,[7] although this is not an approved indication in Canada.

Warfarin

Warfarin therapy is monitored using the INR. It is given in a dose to maintain the INR at 2 to 3.[10] When therapy is initiated the INR is measured frequently, then less often as it stabilizes. It is generally measured daily or every other day for the first three to four days, then every three days for a week, then one or two times weekly, then every two to four weeks when stable. While a less intense level of anticoagulation (INR 1.5–2) has been shown to be effective, it is less so than the standard treatment (INR 2–3).

A common cause of poor anticoagulant control is drug interactions (Table 4). ASA and NSAIDs contribute to bleeding by inhibiting platelet function. Several herbal or alternative products interact with warfarin, for example gingko, ginseng and St. John's wort. Patients should be discouraged from using such products.

Table 4: **Clinically Significant Warfarin Drug Interactions[a]**

Class	Drug
Drugs that increase INR and potentiate the effects of warfarin	
Anti-inflammatory analgesics and immunologics	Acetaminophen,[b] ASA, celecoxib, dextropopoxyphene, interferon, phenylbutazone, piroxicam, sulfinpyrazone, tramadol

(cont'd)

Table 4: **Clinically Significant Warfarin Drug Interactions**[a] *(cont'd)*

Class	Drug
Antimicrobials	
Azole antifungals	Fluconazole, itraconazole, miconazole (including vaginal preparations), voriconazole
Fluoroquinolones	Ciprofloxacin, levofloxacin
Macrolides	Azithromycin, clarithromycin, erythromycin
Other	Amoxicillin/clavulanate, sulfamethoxazole/trimethoprim, isoniazid, metronidazole, ritonavir, tetracycline
Cardiovascular Drugs	
Fibrates	Clofibrate, fenofibrate
Statins	Fluvastatin, simvastatin
Other	Amiodarone, diltiazem, propafenone, propranolol, quinidine
CNS Drugs	
Antiparkinsonian Drugs	Entacapone, ropinirole
SSRI	Citalopram, fluvoxamine, sertraline
Other	Alcohol (large amounts; patients with liver disease), chloral hydrate, disulfiram, phenytoin
Gastrointestinal Drugs	Cimetidine, omeprazole
Foods, Chinese medicines, herbs	Boldo-fenugreek,[c] Danshen,[d] Dong quai,[e] fish oil, grapefruit juice, *Lycium barbarum*, mango fruit, PC-SPES, Quilinggao[f]
Other	Anabolic steroids, fluorouracil, gemcitabine, levamisole/fluorouracil, paclitaxel, tamoxifen, tolterodine, zileuton
Drugs that decrease INR and diminish the effects of warfarin	
Antimicrobials	Griseofulvin, dicloxacillin, nafcillin, ribavirin, rifampin, ritonavir
Cardiovascular Drugs	Bosentan, cholestyramine
CNS Drugs	Barbiturates, carbamazepine, chlordiazepoxide
Gastrointestinal Drugs	Azathioprine, mesalamine, sucralfate
Foods and Herbs	Avocado (large amounts), ginseng, foods, enteral feeds or multivitamins that contain large amounts of vitamin K
Other	Chelation therapy, influenza vaccine, mercaptopurine, raloxifene

a Rated as "highly-probably" or "probably" clinically significant according to a systematic review.[11]
b Doses >2 g/day.[12]
c A herbal combination of boldo (*Peumus boldus*) and fenugreek (*Trigonella foenum-graecum*).
d A Chinese medicine derived from *Salvia miltiorrhiza*.
e A Chinese medicine derived from Chinese Angelica (*Angelica sinensis*).
f A Chinese medicine that contains several herbs. The composition varies between manufacturers.

Parenteral warfarin is now available for iv use. It is used to replace oral warfarin in patients who temporarily cannot take medications by mouth.

Thrombolytic Agents[13]

The use of thrombolytic therapy for the treatment of acute DVT or PE is uncommon as clinical trials have not demonstrated reductions in acute morbidity or improved long-term outcomes. There is also a significant risk of intracranial hemorrhage.

Less than 20% of VTE patients are eligible for thrombolytic therapy (i.e., young patients with massive ileofemoral vein thrombosis or patients with hemodynamically unstable PE). **Streptokinase** (SK) and **alteplase** are approved for treatment of VTE. The best results are obtained with recent thrombi, but substantial lysis may be obtained in patients with symptoms of up to 14 days' duration. Consider use on a case-by-case basis for patients with life- or limb-threatening VTE and no bleeding contraindications.

SK is the least-expensive thrombolytic. However, given the prolonged infusions of SK used in VTE, alteplase, with its short infusion, may be more cost effective.

Anticoagulation in Pregnancy[14]

- UFH or LMWH is the anticoagulant of choice during pregnancy. UFH and LMWHs do not cross the placental barrier.
- SC injections of UFH twice daily achieve therapeutic levels.
- UFH or LMWH should be stopped at the first sign of labour.
- Warfarin or sc UFH may be used for about six weeks after delivery for secondary prevention.
- Women can breastfeed while being treated with warfarin.
- The management of pregnant women with a previous DVT or PE is controversial; UFH 5000 units sc Q12H or LMWH throughout pregnancy is recommended in some women.

Therapeutic Tips

- **Danaparoid, lepirudin** and **argatroban** are approved for treatment of heparin-induced thrombocytopenia (HIT) in Canada. Limited data indicate that **bivalirudin** may also be effective.[15]

Table 5: Risk Categories and Thrombosis Prophylaxis[1,2]

Risk Group	Clinical Criteria	Frequency of VTE: Surgical Patients (without prophylaxis)			Prophylactic Measures
		DVT	Proximal vein thrombosis	Fatal PE	(continue for a minimum of 5–7 days until the patient is fully ambulant)
Low	Minor surgery (< 30 min); no risk factors other than age Major surgery (> 30 min); age < 40 y, no other risk factors Minor trauma or medical illness	10%	1%	0.01%	Mobilize Graduated compression stockings
Moderate	Major general, urologic, gynecologic, cardiothoracic, vascular or neurologic surgery; age ≥ 40 y or other risk factor Major medical illness: heart or lung disease, cancer, inflammatory bowel disease Major trauma or burns Minor surgery, trauma or illness in patients with previous deep vein thrombosis, pulmonary embolism or thrombophilia	10–40%	1–10%	0.1%–1%	Low molecular weight heparin (Table 7) Low-dose heparin (5000 units sc Q12H or Q8H) Graduated compression stockings External pneumatic compression
High	Fracture or major orthopedic surgery of pelvis, hip or lower limb Major pelvic or abdominal surgery for cancer Major surgery, trauma or illness in patients with previous deep vein thrombosis, pulmonary embolism or thrombophilia Lower limb paralysis (e.g., hemiplegic stroke, paraplegia) Major lower limb amputation	40–80%	10–30%	1–10%	Fondaparinux (orthopedic surgery only) Low molecular weight heparin (Table 7) External pneumatic compression Combinations

Abbreviations: DVT = deep vein thrombosis; PE = pulmonary embolism
Adapted with permission from Hyers TM et al. Antithrombotic therapy for venous thromboembolic disease. *Chest* 1998;114(5 Suppl):561S-578S.

Table 6: **Drugs for Treatment of Venous Thromboembolism**

Drug Class	Drug	Dose	Adverse Effects	Comments	Cost[a]
Low Molecular Weight Heparins	*dalteparin* Fragmin	200 IU/kg sc Q24H Max: 18 000 IU/day	Bleeding; HIT and osteoporosis are both less common than with UFH.	Contraindicated in those with a history of HIT; caution in those with renal dysfunction.	$$
	enoxaparin Lovenox	100 IU/kg sc BID or 150 IU sc Q24H Max: 18 000 IU/day	See dalteparin.	See dalteparin. 100 IU = 1 mg.	$$-$$$
	nadroparin Fraxiparine, Fraxiparine Forte	171 IU/kg sc Q24H or 86 IU/kg sc BID Max: 17 100 IU/day	See dalteparin.	See dalteparin.	$$
	tinzaparin Innohep	175 IU/kg sc Q24H Max: 18 000 IU/day	See dalteparin.	See dalteparin.	$$
Specific Factor Xa Inhibitors	*fondaparinux* Arixtra	< 50 kg: 5 mg sc daily 50–100 kg: 7.5 mg daily > 100 kg: 10 mg daily	Bleeding; thrombocytopenia; allergic reactions (rare).	Use caution in patients with renal dysfunction. Use with caution in patients with a history of HIT.	$$$$
Unfractionated Heparin (UFH)	*heparin, unfractionated* Hepalean, Heparin Leo	Treatment: iv infusion most common (see Table 3 for dosing nomogram). Also can use sc 5000–10 000 units iv followed by 15 000–20 000 sc Q12H adjusted to maintain therapeutic aPTT	Bleeding, HIT, osteoporosis.	Monitor platelets closely during first week. Contraindicated in pts with a history of HIT.	$

Drug Class	Drug	Dose	Adverse Effects	Comments	Cost[a]
Oral Anticoagulants	*warfarin* Coumadin, generics	Usual dose: 0.5–5 mg po daily. Adjust dose to maintain INR 2.0–3.0; higher doses may be necessary in some patients IV dose: same as po administered as a slow bolus over 1 to 2 min. Do not give im	Bleeding; hair loss, blue fingers and toes (uncommon); skin necrosis (rare).	See Table 4 for drug interactions. The IV formulation is suitable for patients who cannot take oral drugs.	$

[a] Costs provided are for the first week of therapy, based on 50 kg; includes drug cost only.

Dosage adjustment may be required in renal dysfunction; see Appendix I.

Abbreviations: HIT = heparin-induced thrombocytopenia

Legend: $ < $50 $$ $50-150 $$-$$$ $50–250 $$$ $150-250 $$$$ $250–350 $$$$$ $350–450

Table 7: **Drugs for Prophylaxis of Venous Thromboembolism**

Drug Class	Drug	Dose	Adverse Effects	Comments	Cost[a]
Low Molecular Weight Heparins	*dalteparin* Fragmin	General surgery: 2500 IU sc daily Orthopedics: 5000 IU sc daily	Bleeding, HIT and osteoporosis (less common than UFH).	Contraindicated in those with a history of HIT.	$
	enoxaparin Lovenox	General surgery: 4000 IU sc Q24H Orthopedics: 3000 IU sc Q12H	See dalteparin.	See dalteparin. 100 IU = 1 mg.	$
	nadroparin Fraxiparine, Fraxiparine Forte,	General surgery: 2850 IU sc daily Orthopedics: 38 IU/kg sc Q12H × 2; then 38 IU/kg sc Q24H through postoperative day 3, then 57 IU/kg sc Q24H	See dalteparin.	See dalteparin.	$
	tinzaparin Innohep	General surgery: 3500 IU sc Q24H Orthopedics: 50–75 IU/kg sc Q24H	See dalteparin.	See dalteparin.	$
Specific Factor Xa Inhibitors	*fondaparinux* Arixtra	Patients ≥ 50 kg: 2.5 mg sc daily after high-risk orthopedic surgery Patients < 50 kg: not recommended	Bleeding, allergic reactions (rare).	Not recommended in patients with renal dysfunction.	$$
Unfractionated Heparin (UFH)	*heparin, unfractionated* Hepalean, Heparin Leo	General surgery: 5000 units sc Q12H or Q8H	Bleeding, HIT, osteoporosis.	Monitor platelets closely during first week of therapy. Contraindicated in those with a history of HIT.	$

[a] Costs provided are for 1 day of therapy, based on 50 kg; includes drug cost only.

Dosage adjustment may be required in renal dysfunction; see Appendix I.

Abbreviations: HIT = heparin-induced thrombocytopenia

Legend: $ < $10 $$ $10–20

Suggested Readings

Goldhaber SZ, Turpie AG. Prevention of venous thromboembolism among hospitalized medical patients. *Circulation* 2005;111(1):e1-3.

Kyrle PA, Eichinger S. Deep vein thrombosis. *Lancet* 2005;365(9465):1163-74.

Qaseem A, Snow V, Barry P et al. Current diagnosis of venous thromboembolism in primary care: a clinical practice guideline from the American Academy of Family Physicians and the American College of Physicians. *Ann Fam Med* 2007;5(1):57-62.

Scarvelis D, Wells PS. Diagnosis and treatment of deep-vein thrombosis. *CMAJ* 2006;175(9):1087-92.

Snow V, Qaseem A, Barry P et al. Management of venous thromboembolism: a clinical practice guideline from the American College of Physicians and the American Academy of Family Physicians. *Ann Intern Med* 2007;146(3):204-10.

Wells PS, Owen C, Doucette S et al. Does this patient have deep vein thrombosis? *JAMA* 2006;295(2):199-207.

References

1. Buller HR, Agnelli G, Hull RD et al. Antithrombotic therapy for venous thromboembolic disease: the Seventh ACCP Conference on Antithrombotic and Thrombolytic Therapy. *Chest* 2004;126(3 Suppl):401S-28S.
2. Hyers TM, Agnelli G, Hull RD et al. Antithrombotic therapy for venous thromboembolic disease. *Chest* 2001;119(1 Suppl):176S-93S.
3. Turpie AG. Looking forward in the treatment of deep-vein thrombosis. *Semin Hematol* 2001;38(2 Suppl 5):49-57.
4. [No authors listed]. Risk of and prophylaxis for venous thromboembolism in hospital patients. Thromboembolic Risk Factors (THRIFT) Consensus Group. *BMJ* 1992;305(6853):567-74.
5. Geerts WH, Pineo GF, Heit JA et al. Prevention of venous thromboembolism: the Seventh ACCP Conference on Antithrombotic and Thrombolytic Therapy. *Chest* 2004;126(3 Suppl):338S-400S.
6. Turpie AG, Bauer KA, Eriksson BI et al. Fondaparinux vs enoxaparin for the prevention of venous thromboembolism in major orthopedic surgery: a meta-analysis of 4 randomized double-blind studies. *Arch Intern Med* 2002;162(16):1833-40.
7. Cohen AT, Davidson BL, Gallus AS et al. Efficacy and safety of fondaparinux for the prevention of venous thromboembolism in older acute medical patients: randomised placebo controlled trial. *BMJ* 2006;332(7537):325-9.
8. Weitz JI. Low-molecular-weight heparins. *N Engl J Med* 1997;337(10):688-98.
9. Hirsh J, Fuster V. Guide to anticoagulant therapy. Part 1: Heparin. American Heart Association. *Circulation* 1994;89(3):1449-68.
10. Hirsh J, Fuster V. Guide to anticoagulant therapy. Part 2: Oral anticoagulants. American Heart Association. *Circulation* 1994;89(3):1469-80.
11. Holbrook AM, Pereira JA, Labiris R et al. Systematic overview of warfarin and its drug and food interactions. *Arch Intern Med* 2005;165:1095-106.
12. Gebauer MG, Nyfort-Hansen K, Henschke PJ et al. Warfarin and acetaminophen interaction. *Pharmacother* 2003;23(1):109-12.
13. Dalen JE, Alpert JS, Hirsh J. Thrombolytic therapy for pulmonary embolism: is it effective? Is it safe? When is it indicated? *Arch Intern Med* 1997;157(22):2550-2556.
14. Bates SM, Greer IA, Hirsh J et al. Use of antithrombotic agents during pregnancy: the Seventh ACCP Conference on Antithrombotic and Thrombolytic Therapy. *Chest* 2004;126(3 Suppl):627S-44S.
15. Campbell KR, Mahaffey KW, Lewis BE et al. Bivalirudin in patients with heparin-induced thrombocytopenia undergoing percutaneous coronary intervention. *J Invasive Cardiol* 2000;12(Suppl F):14F-9.

CHAPTER 43
Intermittent Claudication

Richard I. Ogilvie, MD, FRCPC, FACP

Goals of Therapy

- Improve mobility and quality of life
- Increase walking distance and time to claudication
- Increase capacity for regular dynamic leg exercise
- Prevent associated cardiovascular events

Investigations

- History with special attention to cardiovascular disease risk factors and associated conditions:
  - hypertension
  - diabetes mellitus
  - smoking
  - dyslipidemia
  - angina pectoris/MI
  - TIA/stroke
- Define walking time to claudication (*severe* < 1/2 city block; *moderate* 1/2 to 1 block; *mild* > 1 block)
- Define duration of symptoms (6 to 12 months are required to develop collateral circulation)
- Physical examination:
  - signs of hypertension, dyslipidemia, diabetes mellitus, atherosclerosis (aortic aneurysm, bruits), heart failure
  - signs of peripheral artery obstruction (diminished pulses in the femoral, popliteal, posterior tibeal and/or dorsalis pedis arteries)
  - evidence of acute peripheral artery occlusion (acute onset of continuous pain, pale and cool limb or mottled discolouration, thickened, swollen, stiff muscles plus pain over the muscle)
  - resting pain, dependent rubor, cyanosis, muscle atrophy and/or trophic ulcers suggest severe obstruction
- Laboratory tests:
  - fasting blood glucose, serum creatinine and lipid profile
  - hemoglobin (anemia may exacerbate symptoms), hematocrit, platelet count
  - resting Doppler-derived or sphygmomanometric ankle/arm systolic pressure index (ankle-brachial index) (Figure 1)[1]
  - consider invasive angiography for patients with signs of severe limb ischemia (resting pain, muscle atrophy, cyanosis, nonhealing

ischemic ulcers or gangrene) in preparation for possible angioplastic or surgical revascularization

Therapeutic Choices (Figure 1)

Nonpharmacologic Choices

- Discontinuation of smoking (active and passive) (see Chapter 10)
- Time (collateral flow develops over 6 to 12 months)
- Nondrug treatment of obesity (see Chapter 28), lipid disorders (see Chapter 31), hypertension (see Chapter 32) and associated conditions
- Regular dynamic leg exercise (5 times per week for 8 weeks initially).[2] Dynamic leg exercise for 6 to 12 months after the onset of claudication allows collateral circulation to develop; continued exercise 3 or more times a week over 24 to 36 months slows functional decline[3]
- For patients with chronic intermittent claudication, and without signs of severe arterial obstruction, the role of angioplasty remains to be defined
- For patients with severe ischemia, bypass surgery or angioplasty have similar effects on amputation-free survival and all-cause mortality over a 6-month period, although morbidity and costs are higher for patients receiving surgery first rather than angioplasty.[4] Amputation-free survival is higher and all-cause mortality is lower between two and three years after surgery compared with angioplasty according to a post-hoc analysis of a large randomized trial[4]
- Paresthesia and paralysis require immediate surgical revascularization (fibrinolysis may be considered)

Pharmacologic Choices (Table 1)

Pharmacologic options for improving mobility, walking distance and time to claudication are limited. Drug therapy is most effective in reducing the risk of cardiovascular events.

Cardiovascular Risk Reduction

Patients with intermittent claudication are at increased risk of cardiovascular events. For this reason it is essential to optimize treatment of hypertension (see Chapter 32), dyslipidemia (see Chapter 31) and diabetes mellitus (see Chapter 27).[5]

Antiplatelet agents reduce the risk of vascular death in high-risk patients by about 25% and are equally effective in those with coronary artery disease (CAD) and peripheral arterial disease (PAD).[6] **Clopidogrel** may be more effective than **ASA** in patients with peripheral vascular disease (PVD)[7] but is usually reserved for those who cannot tolerate ASA or continue to have events while on ASA. Clopidogrel plus ASA is not significantly better than aspirin alone in patients with atherothrombosis, but combination therapy increases the risk of bleeding,[8] and is therefore not recommended.

ACE inhibitors reduce the risk of ischemic events beyond that expected from lowering blood pressure in patients with PAD.[9] Ramipril demonstrated similar effects in patients with or without PAD in the HOPE study. Ramipril also increases walking time and distance over a 6-month period in patients with PAD, according to the results of a small randomized study.[10]

Beta-blockers reduce the risk of MI and death in patients with atherosclerosis, but use of these agents in patients with PVD was previously discouraged because they were thought to worsen symptoms. Beta-blockers do not affect walking capacity in patients with PVD;[11] thus, it is reasonable to use them to treat hypertension in this population,[12] although they should be used cautiously in those with severe PVD.[12] Beta-blockers are not recommended for the treatment of hypertension in patients over 60 years of age unless there are other compelling indications such as angina or a recent MI.

Lipid-lowering drugs reduce the risk of cardiovascular events in patients with atherosclerosis and may improve symptoms and increase walking distance in patients with intermittent claudication.[13,14]

Specific Therapy for Intermittent Claudication

Pentoxifylline, a methylxanthine derivative, alters erythrocyte deformability and reduces blood viscosity, platelet reactivity and plasma hypercoagulability.[15] Pentoxifylline produces marginal but statistically significant improvement in pain-free and maximal walking distance and thus is not indicated for *mild* claudication. Smoking cessation and regular dynamic leg exercise are probably more beneficial than pentoxifylline for *moderate* claudication. If pentoxifylline is used, a total of 24 weeks of therapy followed by an eight-week drug-free period (as exercise tolerance increases) can decrease or eliminate the need for pentoxifylline.

Pentoxifylline may be beneficial adjunctive therapy for *trophic ulcers* in diabetic and nondiabetic patients.[16] Assess therapy at four-week intervals with a usual maximum duration of 24 weeks due to cost.

Cilostazol inhibits platelet aggregation by selectively inhibiting phosphodiesterase III and is a vasodilator that improves maximal treadmill walking distance.[17,18] It is not available in Canada.

Other Therapies

The role of vasoactive agents, buflomedil,[19] prostaglandin analogues,[20] L-carnitine, or arterial gene therapy[21] has not been defined by adequate clinical trials. Low molecular weight heparin, oral anticoagulants, vitamin E and chelation therapy are not effective for PAD.

Figure 1: **Treatment of Intermittent Claudication**

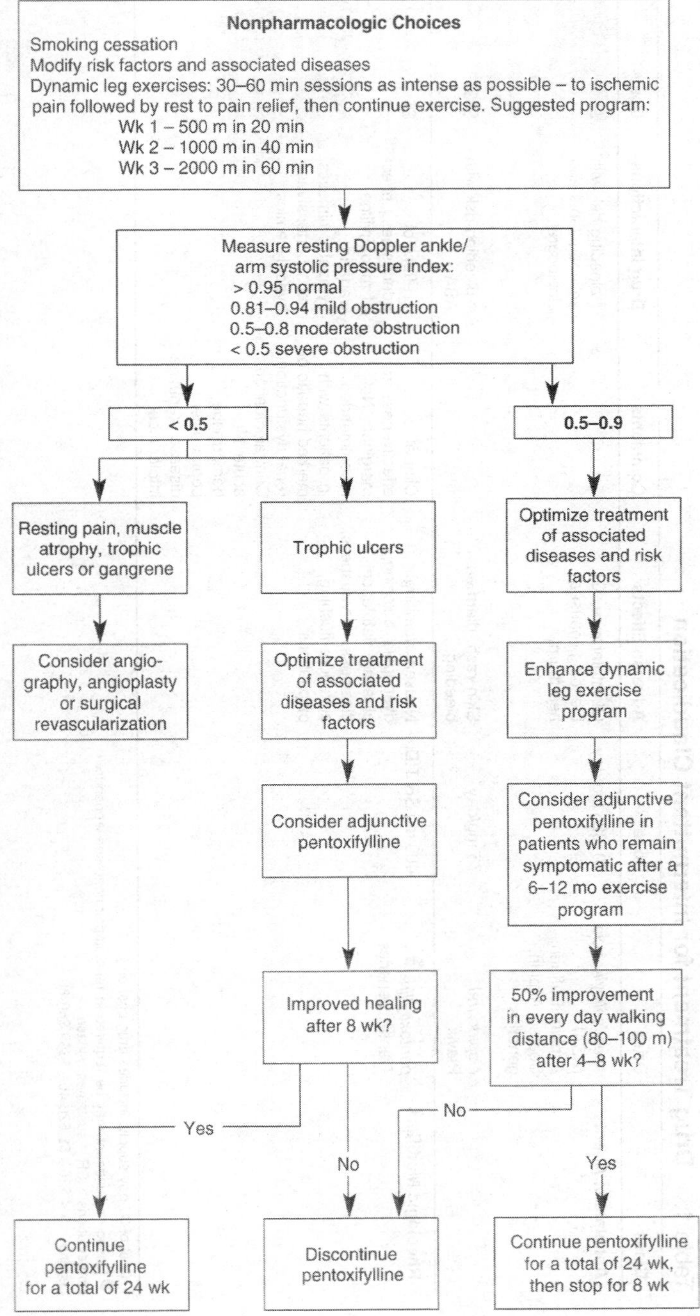

Table 1: **Drug Treatment for Intermittent Claudication**

Class	Drug	Dose	Adverse Effects	Comments	Drug Interactions	Cost[a]
Antiplatelet Agents	*acetylsalicylic acid (ASA)* Aspirin, Bufferin, Coated Aspirin, generics	80–325 mg/day	GI intolerance, GI bleeding, nausea, heartburn.		↑ bleeding risk with anticoagulants and clopidogrel.	$
	clopidogrel Plavix	75 mg/day	Skin rash, diarrhea, bleeding.		↑ bleeding risk with ASA.	$$$$
Rheologic Modifiers	*pentoxifylline* [renal] Trental, generics	400 mg SR TID	Nausea, vomiting, dyspepsia, belching, bloating, flatulence, dizziness, nervousness, agitation, flushing, palpitations.	Clinical effectiveness is marginal. Not recommended in patients with marked hepatic or renal dysfunction. Contraindications: acute MI, hemorrhage, peptic ulcer disease, xanthine intolerance.	↓ effect of adenosine; ↑ effect of theophylline, warfarin, sympathomimetics, antihypertensives, hypoglycemics.	$$

[a] Cost of 30-day supply; includes drug cost only.

[renal] Dosage adjustment may be required in renal impairment; see Appendix I

Abbreviations: SR = sustained release

Legend: $ < $20 $$ $20-40 $$$$ $60-80

Suggested Readings

Abramson BL, Huckell V, Anand S et al. Canadian Cardiovascular Society Consensus Conference: peripheral arterial disease—executive summary. *Can J Cardiol* 2005;21(12):997-1006.

Gardner AW, Poehlman ET. Exercise rehabilitation programs for the treatment of claudication pain. A meta-analysis. *JAMA* 1995;274(12):975-80.

Goy JJ, Urban P. Life and limb: bypass versus angioplasty in the ischaemic limb. *Lancet* 2005;366(9501):1905-6.

Hankey GJ, Norman PE, Eikelboom JW. Medical treatment of peripheral artery disease. *JAMA* 2006;295(5):547-53.

Hirsch AT, Haskal ZJ, Hertzer NR et al. ACC/AHA 2005 Practice Guidelines for the management of patients with peripheral arterial disease (lower extremity, renal, mesenteric, and abdominal aortic). *Circulation* 2006;113(11):e463-654.

References

1. McDermott MM, Greenland P, Liu K et al. The ankle brachial index is associated with leg function and physical activity: the Walking and Leg Circulation Study. *Ann Intern Med* 2002;136(12):873-83.
2. Gardner AW, Poehlman ET. Exercise rehabilitation programs for the treatment of claudication pain. A meta-analysis. *JAMA* 1995;274(12):975-80.
3. McDermott MM, Liu K, Ferrucci L et al. Physical performance in peripheral arterial disease: a slower rate of decline in patients who walk more. *Ann Intern Med* 2006;144(1):10-20.
4. Adam DJ, Beard JD, Cleveland T et al. Bypass versus angioplasty in severe ischaemia of the leg (BASIL): multicentre, randomised controlled trial. *Lancet* 2005;366(9501):1925-34.
5. Hirsch AT, Haskal ZJ, Hertzer NR et al. ACC/AHA 2005 Practice Guidelines for the management of patients with peripheral arterial disease (lower extremity, renal, mesenteric, and abdominal aortic). *Circulation* 2006;113(11):e463-654.
6. Antiplatelet Trialists' Collaboration. Collaborative overview of randomised trials of antiplatelet therapy--I: Prevention of death, myocardial infarction, and stroke by prolonged antiplatelet therapy in various categories of patients. *BMJ* 1994;308(6921):81-106.
7. CAPRIE Steering Committee. A randomised, blinded, trial of clopidogrel versus aspirin in patients at risk of ischaemic events (CAPRIE). *Lancet* 1996;348(9038):1329-39.
8. Bhatt DL, Fox KA, Hacke W et al. Clopidogrel and aspirin versus aspirin alone for the prevention of atherothrombotic events. *N Engl J Med* 2006;354(16):1706-17.
9. Yusuf S, Sleight P, Pogue J et al. Effects of an angiotensin-converting-enzyme inhibitor, ramipril, on cardiovascular events in high-risk patients. *N Engl J Med* 2000;342(3):145-53.
10. Ahimastos AA, Lawler A, Reid CM et al. Brief communication: ramipril markedly improves walking ability in patients with peripheral arterial disease: a randomized trial. *Ann Intern Med* 2006;144(9):660-4.
11. Radack K, Deck C. Beta-adrenergic blocker therapy does not worsen intermittent claudication in subjects with peripheral arterial disease. A meta-analysis of randomized controlled trials. *Arch Intern Med* 1991;151(9):1769-76.
12. Heintzen MP, Strauer BE. Peripheral vascular effects of beta-blockers. *Eur Heart J* 1994;15(Suppl C):2-7.
13. Mohler ER, Hiatt WR,.Creager MA. Cholesterol reduction with atorvastatin improves walking distance in patients with peripheral arterial disease. *Circulation* 2003;108(12):1481-6.
14. Mondillo S, Ballo P, Barbati R et al. Effects of simvastatin on walking performance and symptoms of intermittent claudication in hypercholesterolemic patients with peripheral vascular disease. *Am J Med*2003;114(5):359-64.
15. Hood SC, Moher D,.Barber GG. Management of intermittent claudication with pentoxifylline: meta-analysis of randomized controlled trials. *CMAJ* 1996;155(8):1053-9.
16. Jull A, Waters J,.Arroll B. Pentoxifylline for treatment of venous leg ulcers: a systematic review. *Lancet* 2002;359(9317):1550-4.
17. Dawson DL, Cutler BS, Hiatt WR et al. A comparison of cilostazol and pentoxifylline for treating intermittent claudication. *Am J Med* 2000;109(7):523-30.
18. Money SR , Herd JA, Isaacsohn JL et al. Effect of cilostazol on walking distances in patients with intermittent claudication caused by peripheral vascular disease. *J Vasc Surg* 1998;27(2):267-74.
19. De Backer TL, Vander Stichele RH,.Bogaert MG. Buflomedil for intermittent claudication. *Cochrane Database Syst Rev* 2001;(1):CD000988.

20. Milio G, Mina C, Cospite V et al. Efficacy of the treatment with prostaglandin E-1 in venous ulcers of the lower limbs. *J Vasc Surg* 2005;42(2):304-8.
21. Lederman RJ, Mendelsohn FO, Anderson RD et al. Therapeutic angiogenesis with recombinant fibroblast growth factor-2 for intermittent claudication (the TRAFFIC study): a randomised trial. *Lancet* 2002;359(9323):2053-8.

CHAPTER 44
Raynaud's Phenomenon

André Roussin, MD, FRCPC

Goals of Therapy

- Reduce the frequency and severity of attacks
- Decrease symptoms (cold-induced blanching of the fingers) in patients with primary or secondary Raynaud's phenomenon
- Prevent local and systemic deterioration in secondary Raynaud's phenomenon
- Heal lesions in patients with secondary Raynaud's phenomenon

Investigations (Figure 1)

- Thorough history to differentiate between:
  - *primary* Raynaud's phenomenon (no associated illness or trauma)
  - *secondary* Raynaud's phenomenon (secondary to occupational hazards, vascular diseases, connective tissue diseases [CTD], carpal tunnel syndrome, hypothyroidism or other disorders)
  - possible *drug-induced* Raynaud's phenomenon (see Table 1)

Table 1: **Drugs Implicated in Secondary Raynaud's Phenomenon**

Drug	Comment
Antineoplastic agents	Bleomycin-, vinblastine- and cisplatin-containing regimens have been associated with Raynaud's phenomenon
Cyclosporine	Not dose related
Beta-blockers	Unlikely but controversial. Evidence implicating beta-blockers in Raynaud's phenomenon is equivocal[1]
Ergot derivatives	Bromocriptine, ergonovine maleate, methysergide
Interferon alfa, beta	When used for treatment of cancer, viral hepatitis and multiple sclerosis. May persist for several months after withdrawal

- Physical examination for:
  - altered pulsations
  - abnormal Allen's test, which is done by compressing both the radial and ulnar arteries while clenching the hand, then releasing compression alternately to demonstrate the patency of the arteries
  - local signs of CTD (e.g., sclerodactyly) and carpal tunnel syndrome
  - systemic signs of CTD (e.g., telangiectasis, pulmonary fibrosis), vascular diseases and hypothyroidism
- Laboratory tests:

- nailfold capillary microscopy to detect megacapillaries and other abnormalities suggestive of scleroderma and other CTD. Where available, capillaroscopy will help to diagnose early scleroderma in patients with recent onset of Raynaud's phenomenon, especially when the presentation is atypical or if symptoms suggestive of collagen vascular disease are suspected
- ANA (antinuclear antibodies), ENA (extractable nuclear antibodies), ACA (anticentromere antibodies) and rheumatoid factor to detect CTD
- other tests (ESR, serum electrophoresis, cryoglobulins and all other immunologic tests) are less useful as early markers of secondary Raynaud's phenomenon
- normal test results suggest primary Raynaud's phenomenon

Therapeutic Choices (Figure 1)

Nonpharmacologic Choices

- Minimize cold exposure.
- Avoid prescribing medications with vasoconstrictive potential (e.g., ergot derivatives, beta-blockers) unless there is a compelling reason, e.g., beta-blocker in a patient with coronary artery disease.
- Reassure patients that no complications arise from primary Raynaud's phenomenon.
- Teach warming exercises such as swinging the arms vigorously (windmill effect).
- Instruct patients to dress warmly (including the head and neck) to avoid a sympathetically mediated vasoconstrictive reflex and use warming devices in mittens or boots if appropriate and affordable.
- Encourage patients to stop smoking and to avoid using vibrating tools (grinders, pneumatic hammers, drills, chain saws).
- Acupuncture was ineffective in patients with secondary Raynaud's phenomenon enrolled in a randomized, double-blind, placebo-controlled trial.[2]

Pharmacologic Choices (Table 2)

Dihydropyridine *calcium channel blockers* (CCB) reduce the frequency and severity of attacks and are first-line agents in patients with primary and secondary Raynaud's phenomenon.[3] Nifedipine is the best studied among this class.[4]

Patients with primary or secondary Raynaud's phenomenon may be advised to use a calcium channel blocker (e.g., **nifedipine XL** 30 mg or **felodipine** 5 to 10 mg) 60 minutes before cold exposure, or regularly during the winter months. If nifedipine is not well tolerated, other calcium channel blockers may be considered, although they are less effective for Raynaud's phenomenon. Higher doses may be used in patients with severe primary or secondary Raynaud's phenomenon, or if ulcers are present, e.g., scleroderma.

Peripheral alpha-blockers (e.g., **prazosin**) are less effective than calcium channel blockers, although there are no head-to-head data to substantiate this opinion. Prazosin was more effective than placebo in patients with scleroderma secondary to Raynaud's phenomenon in two randomized trials.[5] However, the dosage is limited by side effects in nonhypertensive patients.[5]

Angiotensin converting enzyme inhibitors, angiotensin II receptor blockers, topical nitrates and pentoxifylline are generally not effective for Raynaud's phenomenon.

Intravenous **iloprost** (PGI_2 analogue) may be useful for short-term treatment of severe secondary Raynaud's phenomenon to reduce the frequency and severity of attacks and, in some cases, increase the rate of digital ulcer healing; oral iloprost is less effective.[6,7] Oral **ketanserin** (a serotonin receptor antagonist) reduces the duration of symptoms somewhat.[8] Neither drug is commercially available in Canada.

Bosentan, an endothelin-1 inhibitor approved for pulmonary hypertension, heals digital ulcers and reduces the Raynaud's phenomenon in select patients with scleroderma.[9]

Phosphodiesterase type 5 inhibitors, which are not approved for Raynaud's phenomenon, reduce the severity of Raynaud's phenomenon according to the results of several small studies.[10] **Sildenafil** 50 mg twice daily reduced the frequency and duration of Raynaud attacks and had acceptable tolerability in patients with severe secondary Raynaud's phenomenon resistant to vasodilator therapy in a randomized, double-blind, placebo-controlled crossover study.[11] **Vardenafil** has also been shown to be effective at a dose of 10 mg twice daily.[12] Several case reports suggest phosphodiesterase inhibitors may be effective in healing digital ulcers.[10]

Surgical Choices

- Extremity sympathectomy, particularly by thoracoscopy, in patients with difficult secondary Raynaud's phenomenon with digital ulcers is not effective in the long term.
- Digital sympathectomy may be more effective, although the evidence is very limited.

Therapeutic Tips

- Many negative studies of pharmacologic therapy for Raynaud's phenomenon have never been published. This complicates the interpretation of the numerous small studies and case reports that report positive outcomes for a variety of drugs.

- There are no evidence-based or consensus-based guidelines for the pharmacologic treatment of Raynaud's phenomenon. Figure 1 is based on the clinical experience of the author.
- Since pharmacologic prophylaxis of Raynaud's phenomenon is effective in only 60% of patients at most (usually 40%), it is important to stress nonpharmacologic approaches and reassure patients. Only about 5% of patients with primary Raynaud's phenomenon will go on to develop secondary Raynaud's phenomenon. It is the underlying disease itself rather than the phenomenon that causes complications.
- Taking medication daily rather than as needed during the winter will increase tolerance to side effects, e.g., headaches.
- If dihydropyridines are ineffective (irrespective of side effects), other vasodilators are not likely to be effective.
- Laboratory cold-induced tests, such as hand immersion with Doppler measurement of the drop in digital blood pressure or blood flow, do not reliably predict a patient's response to any given drug, despite the accentuated response in patients with Raynaud's phenomenon.
- Patients with primary and secondary Raynaud's phenomenon generally respond equally well to medications; it is the frequency of attacks, rather than intensity and duration, that is most likely to be reduced with effective drug therapy.
- Newer, unproven and off-label therapies, such as **bosentan** and **phosphodiesterase type 5 inhibitors**, should be considered only for patients with severe secondary Raynaud's phenomenon, mainly to improve healing of digital ulcers.[9,10] These drugs are not currently approved for this indication, are costly and have a number of contraindications and significant side effects. Specialist consultation is recommended before prescribing such therapies.

Figure 1: **Investigation and Management of Raynaud's Phenomenon**

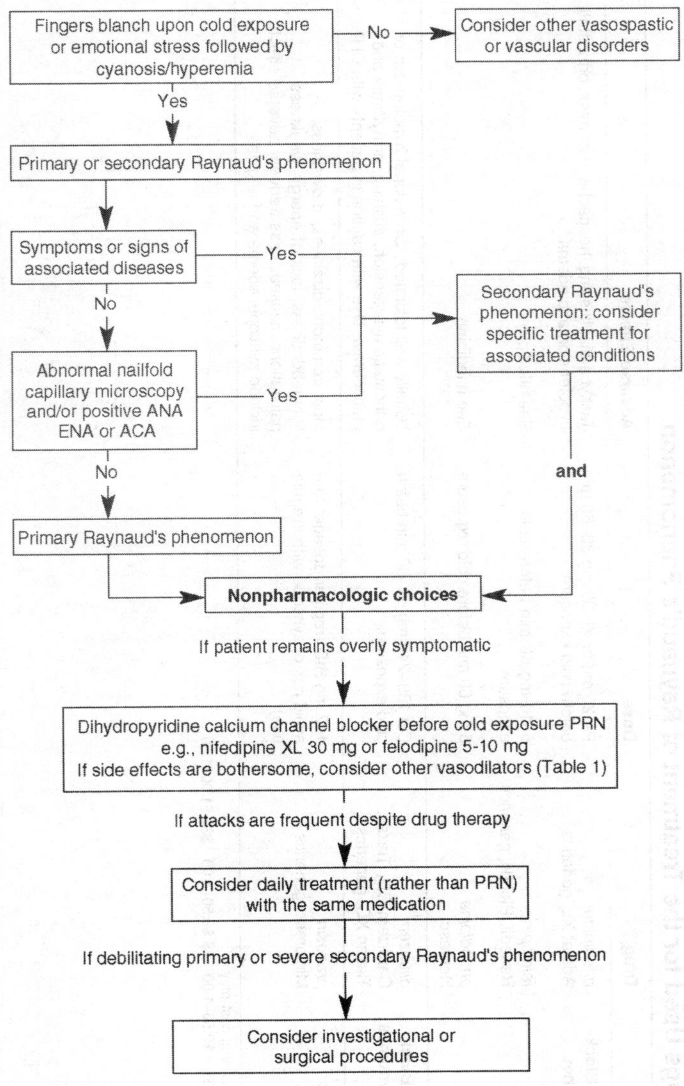

Table 2: Drugs Used for the Treatment of Raynaud's Phenomenon

Class	Drug	Dose	Adverse Effects	Cost[a]
Calcium Channel Blockers, dihydropyridines	*nifedipine* Adalat XL, generics	PA 20 mg or XL 30 mg 30–60 min before cold exposure	Tachycardia, flushing, headache, dizziness, orthostatic hypotension and edema.	$-$$
	felodipine Renedil, Plendil, generics	5–10 mg 60 min before cold exposure	See nifedipine.	$$
	amlodipine Norvasc	5 mg 60 min before cold exposure	See nifedipine.	$$$
Calcium Channel Blockers, nondihydropyridines	*diltiazem* Cardizem CD, Tiazac, Tiazac XC, generics	CD 180–240 mg 60–90 min before cold exposure	Usually well tolerated. Occasional hypotension or orthostatic hypotension, flushing, arrhythmia and bradycardia. Use with caution in patients with CHF.	$$$
Alpha$_1$-Adrenergic Antagonists	*prazosin* Minipress, generics	1–2 mg BID (regular dosage, to avoid risk of syncope with irregular use)	Most common: dizziness, drowsiness, lightheadedness, lack of energy, weakness, palpitations, nausea. Less frequent adverse effects include syncope, edema and angina.	$

[a] Cost per dose; includes drug cost only.
Legend: $ < $0.50 $-$$ < $0.50–1.00 $$ $0.50–1.00 $$$ $1.00–1.50

Suggested Readings

Block JA, Sequeira W. Raynaud's phenomenon. *Lancet* 2001;357(9273):2042-8.

Coffman JD. Vasospastic diseases. In: Young JR, editor. *Peripheral vascular diseases*. St. Louis (MO): Mosby;1996. p.823-9.

Fries R, Shariat K, von-Wilmowsky H et al. Sildenafil in the treatment of Raynaud's phenomenon resistant to vasodilatory therapy. *Circulation* 2005;112(19): 2980-5.

Wigley FM. Clinical practice. Raynaud's phenomenon. *N Engl J Med* 2002;347(13):1001-8.

References

1. Franssen C, Wollersheim H, de Haan A et al. The influence of different beta-blocking drugs on the peripheral circulation in Raynaud's phenomenon and in hypertension. *J Clin Pharmacol* 1992;32(7):652-9.
2. Hahn M, Steins A, Mohrle M et al. Is there a vasospasmolytic effect of acupuncture in patients with secondary Raynaud phenomenon? *J Dtsch Dermatol Ges* 2004;2(9):758-62.
3. Thompson AE, Pope JE. Calcium channel blockers for primary Raynaud's phenomenon: a meta-analysis. *Rheumatology (Oxford)* 2005;44(2):145-50.
4. Thompson AE, Shea B, Welch V et al. Calcium-channel blockers for Raynaud's phenomenon in systemic sclerosis. *Arthritis Rheum* 2001;44(8):1841-7.
5. Pope J, Fenlon D, Thompson A et al. Prazosin for Raynaud's phenomenon in progressive systemic sclerosis. *Cochrane Database Syst Rev* 2000;(2):CD000956.
6. Pope J, Fenlon D, Thompson A et al. Iloprost and cisaprost for Raynaud's phenomenon in progressive systemic sclerosis. *Cochrane Database Syst Rev* 2000;(2):CD000953
7. Wigley FM, Wise RA, Seibold JR et al. Intravenous iloprost infusion in patients with Raynaud phenomenon secondary to systemic sclerosis. A multicenter, placebo-controlled, double-blind study. *Ann Intern Med* 1994;120(3):199-206.
8. Pope J, Fenlon D, Thompson A et al. Ketanserin for Raynaud's phenomenon in progressive systemic sclerosis. *Cochrane Database Syst Rev* 2000;(2):CD000954.
9. Launay D, Diot E, Pasquier E et al. [Bosentan for treatment of active digital ulcers in patients with systemic sclerosis]. *Presse Med* 2006;35(4 Pt 1):587-92. French.
10. Levien TL. Phosphodiesterase inhibitors in Raynaud's phenomenon. *Ann Pharmacother* 2006;40(7-8):1388-93.
11. Fries R, Shariat K, von Wilmowsky H et al. Sildenafil in the treatment of Raynaud's phenomenon resistant to vasodilatory therapy. *Circulation* 2005;112(19):2980-5.
12. Caglayan E, Huntgeburth M, Karasch T et al. Phosphodiesterase type 5 inhibition is a novel therapeutic option in Raynaud disease. *Arch Intern Med* 2006;166(2):231-3.

CHAPTER 45
Allergic Rhinitis

D. William Moote, MD, FRCPC

Goals of Therapy

- Prevent allergic reaction from occurring by avoiding exposure to allergens
- Suppress and control symptoms produced by the allergic response
- Avoid/minimize medication side effects including negative impact on activities of daily living, e.g., minimal interference with school or work performance or attendance, leisure activities, sleep

Investigations

- Clinical history (Table 1) with particular attention to:
  - symptoms, frequency and severity
  - duration and pattern of symptoms (intermittent, persistent)
  - precipitating factors, e.g., environmental allergens such as animal and pollen triggers
  - personal or family history of allergy
- Physical examination (Table 1):
  - View nasal mucosa (e.g., colour, anatomy) using ordinary otoscope
- Objective measurements:
  - Skin testing confirms allergic sensitivity, if present. There is little benefit in measuring serum IgE or eosinophils, which do not correlate well with presence of allergic disease. In vitro measurements of specific allergen sensitivity such as radio-allergosorbent testing (RAST) are acceptable, but more expensive. Skin testing is generally preferred unless conditions exist that make it unsatisfactory, e.g., widespread skin disease. Discontinue antihistamines temporarily three days prior to skin testing

Table 1: **Differential Diagnosis of Rhinitis**

Type	Characteristics
Seasonal or perennial allergic rhinitis	Nasal obstruction and rhinorrhea are common. Often conjunctival symptoms, paroxysmal sneezing, itching of the nasal mucosa and the oropharynx. Seasonal patterns may be recognized, or perennial symptoms may flare up after exposure to allergens like dust mites or animal danders. Nasal mucosa is swollen, often pale or bluish, and moist.

(cont'd)

Table 1: **Differential Diagnosis of Rhinitis** *(cont'd)*

Type	Characteristics
Upper respiratory infections	More episodic, often associated with sore throat or fever and not associated with itch. Nasal mucosa is often red.
Vasomotor rhinitis	Obstruction and rhinorrhea are prominent and other symptoms infrequent. May be triggered by irritant exposures such as smoke, temperature changes, strong odours, cold air and other factors such as exercise, eating hot or spicy foods.
Nasal polyps	Obstruction is the main complaint. Anosmia and reduced taste perception are almost always present. Nasal exam will usually detect a polyp.

Therapeutic Choices (Figure 1)

Nonpharmacologic Choices

- Avoid exposure to allergens to which a patient is sensitized. This allows for reduced medication use.[1,2]
  - Air conditioning reduces pollen exposure.
  - Removing pets from the home will reduce perennial symptoms caused by animal dander.
  - Dust avoidance measures can reduce exposure as much as 60%.

Pharmacologic Choices (Table 2)

Saline nose sprays, available over-the-counter, can help relieve symptoms by washing out mucus and the inhaled allergen. Similarly, **lubricant eyedrops** or cold compresses can reduce *conjunctival symptoms*.

Antihistamines

Antihistamines help relieve all symptoms of acute allergic rhinitis, such as sneezing, rhinorrhea, nasal itch and conjunctivitis, except nasal congestion. **Desloratadine** is an exception to this in that it modestly improved nasal congestion in clinical trials.[3] Antihistamines are most effective if used prophylactically; however, onset of action is fast enough that they are also effective when used on an as-needed basis. Once-daily dosing of the newer antihistamines is usually sufficient.

Although sedation and anticholinergic side effects are common with the older antihistamines, these side effects are usually not seen with newer, more costly agents. Patients who are unaware of sedation may be impaired with respect to attention, memory, vigilance and speed. These effects persist into the next day. Patients whose occupations require vigilance or concentration should receive only second-generation, nonsedating antihistamines, as they do not affect performance and have no anticholinergic effects.[2,4,5,6,7] Patients with hepatic impairment may be at increased risk of adverse effects, and dosage modification may be required. The currently available second- and third-generation, nonsedating antihistamines have not caused QT interval prolongation.[2]

If an antihistamine taken at a recommended dose is not effective, little is gained from changing it to a different chemical class. Although older studies of long-term dosing with first generation antihistamines have demonstrated loss of effectiveness, they are flawed by lack of evidence of compliance. No loss of effectiveness has been shown up to one year.[8] Of the newer antihistamines, cetirizine is more likely to cause some sedation, especially at higher doses.

Decongestants (Alpha-adrenergic Agonists)

Oral decongestants (pseudoephedrine, phenylephrine) relieve nasal obstruction. Some individuals are intolerant of the stimulant side effects of decongestants. Avoid oral decongestants in those receiving monamine oxidase inhibitors. Use them with caution in patients with hypertension, hyperthyroidism or ischemic heart disease, although evidence is weak and circumstantial that use at recommended doses is a problem in these groups when the disease is controlled.[9] Use of **topical nasal decongestants** for more than three to seven days may result in *rhinitis medicamentosa*; thus, they should be avoided in allergic rhinitis because long-term therapy is often required.

Antihistamine–Decongestant Combinations

Antihistamines and decongestants have complementary effects. Patients taking both drugs may find combination tablets convenient, although many combinations include first-generation antihistamines, which may be sedating. Some combinations, e.g., cold preparations, may also contain analgesics and expectorants, which are not helpful in allergic rhinitis.

Intranasal Therapy

Intranasal corticosteroids are the mainstay of therapy for moderate to severe rhinitis symptoms. Aqueous preparations generally have better intranasal deposition than dry powder inhalers, especially when chronic symptoms have caused significant obstruction or there is ciliary dysfunction, as in smokers. Newer preparations have a lower volume spray, which may be preferred by some. Budesonide is available as a dry powder nasal inhaler and offers an alternative for those who dislike aqueous sprays. A 2- to 4-week trial may be needed to determine whether treatment is working.

Topical corticosteroids act locally and are quickly metabolized once absorbed. Adrenal suppression has not been seen at therapeutic dosages.[7,10,11] Data on inhaled corticosteroids in asthma suggest that systemic effects occur at doses in the range of 1000 to 2000 μg of beclomethasone or equivalent — much higher than those recommended for allergic rhinitis. Nasal septal perforation[12] has not been confirmed in controlled studies; however, instruct patients to aim the spray at the turbinates, i.e., inside the nose, pointing upwards and angled laterally towards the tip of the ear, not at the septum.

Sodium cromoglycate (cromolyn sodium) nasal sprays have an excellent safety profile but are less effective than corticosteroids and usually need QID dosing, at least initially.

Levocabastine, an antihistamine nasal spray, has a rapid onset and is effective PRN and for daily use. Systemic effects are minimized compared to oral antihistamines but it is less potent than topical corticosteroids and is not effective for treatment of congestion.

Intranasal **ipratropium**, 0.03% solution, reduces the volume of watery nasal discharge.[15] It may be used when rhinorrhea is the only symptom or when rhinorrhea is refractory to topical intranasal corticosteroids and/or antihistamines. This may be especially helpful in some types of vasomotor rhinitis, e.g. "skier's nose."

Leukotriene Receptor Antagonists

Montelukast has a modest effect in the treatment of allergic rhinitis,[16,17,18] but its role in routine treatment needs to be further defined. It may be especially helpful in patients with concomitant asthma or nasal polyps. Montelukast is approved for the treatment of allergic rhinitis when other medications are ineffective or poorly tolerated.

Ophthalmic Preparations

Oral antihistamines are also useful for conjunctival symptoms. Topical ophthalmic antihistamines such as **levocabastine, olopatadine, emedastine** or **ketotifen,** provide relief in minutes with duration of effect of about 12 hours. Topical mast cell stabilizers such as **cromoglycate, nedocromil** or **lodoxamide,** require several days for onset and are administered QID initially. Regular use of topical vasoconstrictors is discouraged because of development of rebound vasodilation. Once opened, levocabastine and cromoglycate should be discarded within a month. Olopatadine, ketotifen or emedastine eyedrops are more stable once opened.

Immunotherapy

Desensitization or allergy shots are useful, especially for symptoms caused by pollen or dust mites.[19,20] Immunotherapy is indicated only when there is evidence of IgE-mediated sensitivity to a specific antigen the patient cannot effectively avoid and when frequency and severity of symptoms are difficult to control with conventional drug therapy and allergy avoidance.[20,21]

Management of Allergic Rhinitis in Special Populations

Allergic Rhinitis During Pregnancy and Lactation

Rhinitis is common in pregnancy. Pregnant women are also more likely to complain of congestion, even in the absence of allergic rhinitis, i.e., rhinitis of pregnancy.[22,23,24] As with all medications in pregnancy, it is ideal to discuss the relative risks and benefits with the patient. All antihistamines cross the placenta. Unfortunately, there are very few clinical trials in pregnant patients with rhinitis. From historical data and extrapolation from asthma studies, there is satisfactory evidence for use of **beclomethasone,**[25] **budesonide**,[26] **cromoglycate**[27] and **chlorpheniramine.**[28] There are increasing safety data with respect to second-generation antihistamines including cetirizine and loratadine.[28]

The safety of pseudoephedrine during pregnancy has not been established. It concentrates in breast milk although there are no reports of adverse effects on the breastfed infant.

Allergic Rhinitis in Children

Poorly controlled rhinitis impacts significantly on learning performance in children.[29] Treatment of rhinitis symptoms in children is hampered by the difficulty of administering nose sprays of any kind; most children simply don't like the idea of spraying something in their nose. If antihistamines are sufficient, they may be the ideal choice. Second-generation antihistamines are preferred, as first-generation antihistamines are associated with sedation and learning impairment.[2] If sprays are necessary, comparison is difficult. Cromoglycate is almost certainly safe and may be tried. Intranasal corticosteroids are more effective.[2] **Mometasone** or **fluticasone** are usually recommended because of bioavailability and absence of growth suppression with long-term use. However, both are scented and many children prefer unscented preparations. If liquid sprays are not tolerated, dry powder formulations of **budesonide** may be tried (turbuhaler). Once-daily dosing of intranasal corticosteroids in the morning seems to reduce risk of growth suppression.[7] Any risk is increased when total corticosteroid use is increased, e.g., intranasal use plus inhaled corticosteroids for asthma, therefore care must be taken to reduce medication use to the lowest effective dose.

Therapeutic Tips

- Intranasal corticosteroids are the therapy of choice based on cost and effectiveness. Antihistamines are cost effective only for the mildest symptoms. Optimal control of allergic rhinitis may require a combination of intranasal corticosteroids and antihistamines.[30]
- Intranasal corticosteroids will shrink nasal polyps, but long-term treatment is required. Anosmia is not usually improved. If surgery is considered, the use of topical corticosteroids after surgery may decrease the recurrence rate.
- Most antihistamine preparations are available as syrups for children but are not convenient for portable PRN dosing. Loratadine tablets are tasteless and can be chewed.
- Start medications at the maximum dose and then taper to the minimum required for maintenance.

- Patients with predictable seasonal allergic rhinitis can start medications such as intranasal corticosteroids before the allergen exposure period and take them regularly until the end of the season for maximum effectiveness.
- If desired results are not achieved with once-daily dosing of newer topical corticosteroids, a twice-daily regimen may be more effective, even at the same total daily dose.
- Antihistamines are not contraindicated in asthmatic patients; many have a slightly beneficial effect on asthma symptoms.

Figure 1: **Management of Allergic Rhinitis**

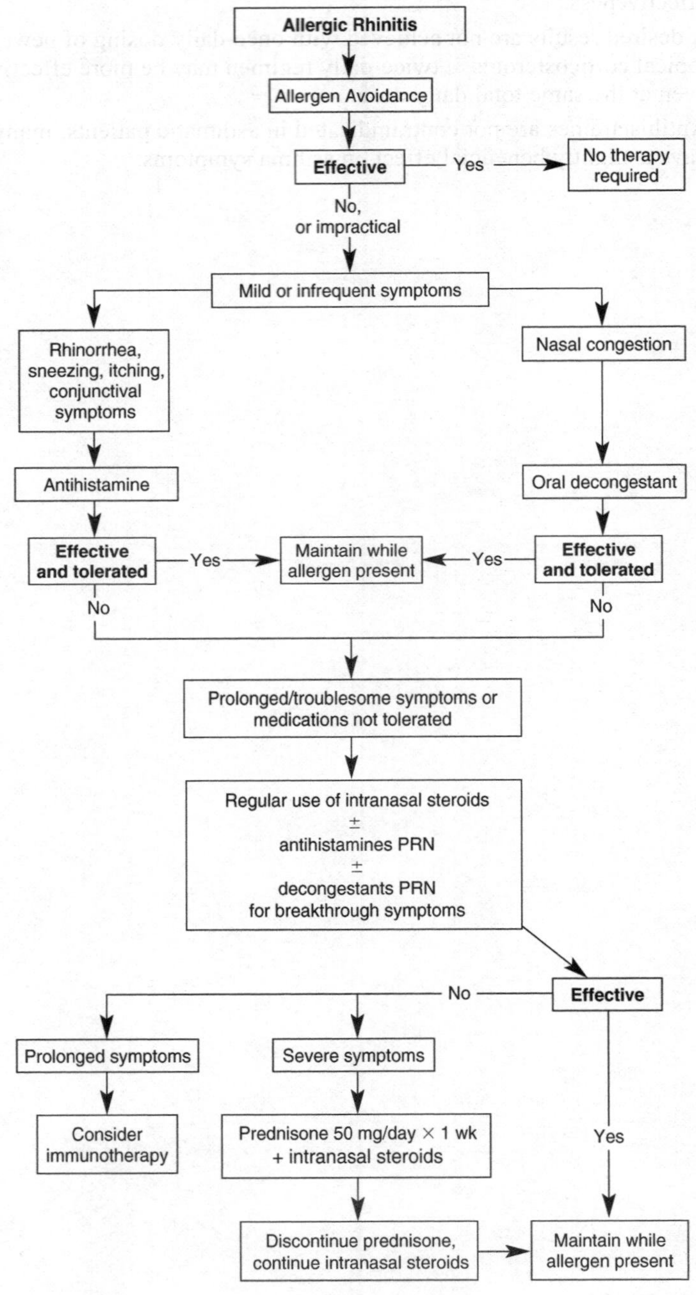

Table 2: **Oral Drugs Used in Allergic Rhinitis**

Class	Drug	Dose	Adverse Effects	Drug Interactions	Comments	Cost[a]
Antihistamines, Alkylamines, first generation	*chlorpheniramine* Novo-Pheniram[b]	Adults and children ≥ 12 y: 4 mg Q4-6H; max dose 24 mg/24 h Children 6–11 y: 2 mg Q4-6H; max dose 12 mg/24 h	CNS: sedation, fatigue, dizziness, impairment of cognition and performance (the patient may be aware of impairment).[2] Anticholinergic: dryness of the mouth and eyes, constipation, inhibition of micturition, potential precipitation of narrow-angle glaucoma.	↑ CNS depression: alcohol, sedatives, tranquilizers, barbiturates. ↑ anticholinergic side effects: TCAs, scopolamine. Phenothiazines: monitor for evidence of ventricular arrhythmias. Moderate CYP3A4 inhibitors, e.g., erythromycin, grapefruit juice: may ↑ chlorpheniramine levels. Strong CYP3A4 inhibitors, e.g., clarithromycin, ketoconazole: avoid combination.	Use with caution in the elderly as they may be more susceptible to side effects such as sedation and syncope. Avoid in patients with narrow-angle glaucoma (↑ IOP), urinary obstruction (prostatic hypertrophy), bladder neck obstruction (can cause urinary retention), GI obstruction. Observe infants and young children for paradoxical excitation. Administer with food to decrease GI distress. Discontinue 2 days before skin testing procedure for allergy.	$
Antihistamines, Ethanolamines, first generation	*diphenhydramine* Benadryl Preparations[b]	Adults and children ≥ 12 y: 25–50 mg TID-QID; max 4 doses/day or 300 mg/24 h	See chlorpheniramine.	See chlorpheniramine. May increase venlafaxine and metoprolol concentrations —	Use with caution in the elderly as they may be more susceptible to side effects such as sedation and syncope.	$

(cont'd)

Table 2: **Oral Drugs Used in Allergic Rhinitis** *(cont'd)*

Class	Drug	Dose	Adverse Effects	Drug Interactions	Comments	Cost[a]
		6–< 12 y: 12.5–25 mg Q4–6H; max 150 mg/day 2–< 6 y: 12.5–25 mg Q12H		clinical significance not established.	Avoid in patients with narrow-angle glaucoma (↑ IOP), urinary obstruction (prostatic hypertrophy), bladder neck obstruction (can cause urinary retention), GI obstruction. Observe infants and young children for paradoxical excitation. Thickening of bronchial secretions. Available in chewable tablets, elixir and liquid.	
Antihistamines, Piperidines, first generation	*azatadine* Optimine	Adults: 1 mg in a.m. and p.m.; can ↑ to 2 mg BID in refractory or more severe cases	See chlorpheniramine.	Monoamine oxidase inhibitors may prolong effects of antihistamines resulting in severe hypotension. ↑ CNS depression: alcohol, sedatives, tranquilizers, barbiturates.	Avoid in narrow-angle glaucoma (↑ IOP), urinary obstruction (prostatic hypertrophy), bladder neck obstruction (can cause urinary retention), GI obstruction. Avoid in patients who pilot planes, drive extensively or operate heavy or dangerous machinery. Observe infants and young children for paradoxical excitation. Discontinue 4 days before skin testing procedure for allergy. Use with caution in the elderly (≥ 60 y) as they are more	$$

Class	Drug	Dose	Adverse Effects	Drug Interactions	Comments	Cost[a]
					susceptible to dizziness, sedation, ↓ bp.	
Antihistamines, Piperidines, second generation	*cetirizine* Reactine[b], generics	> 12 y: 5–10 mg/day dependent on symptom severity; max dose is 20 mg/day 6–12 y: 10 mg/day in single or divided doses Children 2–6 y: 2.5 mg/day, can ↑ to 5 mg/day in single or divided doses 6 mo–< 2 y: 2.5 mg once daily 12–23 mo: max 2.5 mg BID Infants 6–11 mo: 0.25 mg/kg Q12H[31]	Somnolence (with ↑ dose), fatigue, dry mouth, dizziness, headache, diarrhea, nausea, vomiting, pharyngitis.		Metabolite of hydroxyzine. Avoid in patients with a hypersensitivity to hydroxyzine.	$-$$
	fexofenadine Allegra[b]	Adults and children ≥ 12 y: 60 mg Q12H; max 180 mg daily 6–11 y: 30 mg BID Renal impairment: ≥ 12 y: initial dose 60 mg once daily 6–11 y: initial dose 30 mg once daily	Headache, nausea.	↓ fexofenadine level: aluminum- and magnesium-containing antacids; ingestion of fruit juices such as apple, grapefruit, orange or pineapple may ↓ bioavailability.		$$-$$$

(cont'd)

Table 2: **Oral Drugs Used in Allergic Rhinitis** *(cont'd)*

Class	Drug	Dose	Adverse Effects	Drug Interactions	Comments	Cost[a]
	loratadine Claritin[b], generics	Adults and children > 10 y (> 30 kg): 10 mg once daily Children 2–9 y (≤ 30 kg): 5 mg once daily ClCr < 30 mL/min in ≥ 6 y: initial dose 10 mg every other day	≥ 12 y: headache, fatigue, xerostomia. 6–12 y: nervousness, wheezing, fatigue.	↑ loratadine levels: cimetidine, protease inhibitors such as amprenavir, ritonavir. Cimetidine, erythromycin and ketoconazole may ↑ loratadine levels; clinical effect probably minimal. Loratadine–CYP2C19 inhibitor: may ↑ levels or effects of medications such as citalopram, diazepam, propranolol, phenytoin.	Clearance ↓ in patients with severe liver impairment — use lower initial doses. Patients with renal impairment — drug accumulation and increased risk of CNS side effects. May take on an empty stomach. Food delays absorption.	$
Antihistamines, Piperidines, third generation	*desloratadine* Aerius[b]	Adults and children ≥ 12 y: 5 mg daily 6–11 y: 2.5 mg daily 12 mo–5 y: 1.25 mg daily 6–11 mo: 1 mg daily Renal or hepatic impairment: initial dose 5 mg Q2d	Headache, pharyngitis, dyspepsia.	Cimetidine may ↑ desloratidine levels.	Avoid in patients with hypersensitivity to loratadine.	$$

Class	Drug	Dose	Adverse Effects	Drug Interactions	Comments	Cost[a]
Decongestants	*pseudoephedrine* Contac Cold 12 Hour Relief, Eltor 120, Sudafed[b]	Adults and children ≥ 12 y: 60 mg Q4–6H or 120 mg SR Q12H or 240 mg CR Q24H; max 240 mg/24h. Children 6–11 y: 30 mg Q4–6H PRN; max 120 mg/24h Children 2–5 y: 15 mg Q4-6H PRN; max 60 mg/24h Slow-release formulations are not recommended in children < 12 y	Insomnia, tremor, irritability, headache, palpitations, tachycardia, urinary retention.	Beta-blockers: antihypertensive effects may be reduced. MAOIs: concurrent use and use within 14 days of discontinuation of MAOIs is contraindicated.	There is no published evidence to support use of antihistamines, decongestants or combinations in children < 5 y. In addition, accidental ingestion and dosing errors of these products can do much harm. Contraindicated in patients with severe hypertension and coronary artery disease. Use with caution in cardiovascular disease, diabetes, hyperthyroidism, prostatic hypertrophy and angle-closure glaucoma.	$$
	phenylephrine Sudafed PE Extra Strength[b] also available in combination products: Dimetane, Dimetapp Cold Liquids, Dimetapp-C Syrup, Dimetapp Daytime/Nighttime Cold Extra Strength, Novahistex DH, Novahistine DH[b]	Adults and children ≥ 12 y: 10–20 mg Q4H; max 120 mg/24 h Children 6–11 y: 10 mg Q4H; max 60 mg/24 h	See pseudoephedrine.	See pseudoephedrine.	See pseudoephedrine.	$$

(cont'd)

Table 2: **Oral Drugs Used in Allergic Rhinitis** *(cont'd)*

Class	Drug	Dose	Adverse Effects	Drug Interactions	Comments	Cost[a]
Antihistamine/ Decongestant Combinations (first generation)	*azatadine/ pseudoephedrine* Trinalin	Adults and children ≥ 12 y: 1 tab (1 mg/60 mg) BID	Azatadine: common: headache and somnolence. Decongestant: insomnia, tremor, irritability, headache, palpitations, tachycardia, urinary retention.	Antihistamine: additive CNS depressive effects with alcohol and other CNS depressants. Decongestant: antihypertensive effect of beta-blockers may be ↓. MAOIs: concurrent use and use within 14 days of discontinuation of MAOIs is contraindicated.	Azatadine is a first-generation antihistamine and is much more sedating than all of the second- or third-generation antihistamines. See pseudoephedrine.	$$
	triprolidine/ pseudoephedrine Actifed[b]	Adults and children ≥ 12 y: 1 tab (2.5 mg/60 mg) Q4–6H; max 4 doses/24h Children 6–11 y: ½ tab Q4–6H; max 4 doses/24 h	Antihistamine: drowsiness, fatigue, anticholinergic effects such as dry eyes, dry mouth and urinary retention. Paradoxical stimulatory effects may occur in children and the elderly. Decongestant: insomnia, tremor, irritability, headache, palpitations, tachycardia, urinary retention.	See azatadine/ pseudoephedrine.	Triprolidine is a first-generation antihistamine and is much more sedating than all the second- or third-generation antihistamines. See pseudoephedrine.	$$-$$$

Class	Drug	Dose	Adverse Effects	Drug Interactions	Comments	Cost[a]
Antihistamine/ Decongestant Combinations (second generation)	*cetirizine/ pseudoephedrine* Reactine Allergy & Sinus[b]	Adults and children ≥ 12 y: 1 tab (5 mg/120 mg) Q12H	Cetirizine: common: headache and somnolence (with ↑ dose). Decongestant: insomnia, tremor, irritability, headache, palpitations, tachycardia, urinary retention.	See azatadine/ pseudoephedrine.	See pseudoephedrine.	$$
	fexofenadine/ pseudoephedrine Allegra-D[b]	Adults and children ≥ 12 y: 1 tab (60 mg/120 mg) BID	Fexofenadine: common: headache. Decongestant: insomnia, tremor, irritability, headache, palpitations, tachycardia, urinary retention.	↓ fexofenadine level: concurrent aluminum- and magnesium-containing antacids; concurrent ingestion of fruit juices such as apple, grapefruit, orange or pineapple may ↓ bioavailability. See azatadine/ pseudoephedrine.	To be taken on an empty stomach. See pseudoephedrine.	$$

(cont'd)

Table 2: **Oral Drugs Used in Allergic Rhinitis** *(cont'd)*

Class	Drug	Dose	Adverse Effects	Drug Interactions	Comments	Cost[a]
	loratadine/ pseudoephedrine Claritin Allergy & Sinus, Claritin Allergy & Sinus Extra Strength[b]	Adults and children ≥ 12 y: 5 mg/120 mg: 1 tab BID 10 mg/240 mg: 1 tab daily, preferably upon waking	Loratadine: common: headache, fatigue, xerostomia. Decongestant: insomnia, tremor, irritability, headache, palpitations, tachycardia, urinary retention.	↑ loratadine levels: protease inhibitors such as amprenavir, ritonavir, nelfinavir. Loratadine–CYP2C19 inhibitor: may ↑ levels or effects of medications metabolized by CYP2C19 such as citalopram, diazepam, propranolol, phenytoin. See azatadine/ pseudoephedrine	See pseudoephedrine.	$$$
Leukotriene Receptor Antagonists	*montelukast* Singulair	≥ 15 y: 10 mg QHS	Headache, abdominal pain, flu-like symptoms.	↓ montelukast levels: carbamazepine, rifampin, phenobarbital, phenytoin.		$$$

[a] Cost of 10-day supply; includes drug cost only.
[b] Available without a prescription.

Abbreviations: bp = blood pressure; CNS = central nervous system; IOP = intraocular pressure; GI = gastrointestinal; MAOIs = monoamine oxidase inhibitors; TCAs = tricyclic antidepressants

Legend: $ < $10 $-$$ < $10–20 $$ $10–20 $$-$$$ $10–30 $$$ $20–30

Table 3: **Intranasal Drugs Used in Allergic Rhinitis**

Class	Drug	Dose	Adverse Effects	Comments	Cost[a]
Antihistamines	*levocabastine* Livostin Nasal Spray	12–65 y: 2 sprays (50 μg/spray) per nostril BID, may ↑ to 2 sprays TID-QID	Nasal irritation.	Shake well before use. Priming necessary for first time. Discontinue if improvement not seen for 3 days.	$$
Anticholinergics	*ipratropium* Atrovent Nasal Spray	0.03%: 2 sprays per nostril BID-TID	Nosebleeds, nasal dryness, dry mouth or throat, headache.	Avoid accidental release of nasal spray into eyes. Optimal dose based on specific patient's symptoms and response.	$$$
Mast Cell Stabilizers	*sodium cromoglycate* Cromolyn[b], generics	Adults and children ≥ 2 y: 1 spray in each nostril QID, may ↑ to 6 times daily Use lowest effective dose for maintenance therapy	Nasal stinging, burning, irritation, sneezing.	Must cover entire nasal lining. Instruct patient to clear nasal passages before administration. Dosing must be repeated at 6 h intervals to maintain the effect.	$$
Corticosteroids	*beclomethasone* Gen-Beclo AQ., generics	Adults and children ≥ 6 y: (50 μg/spray): use 2 sprays in each nostril BID Adults: max 12 sprays/day Children: max 8 sprays/day Use lowest effective dose for maintenance therapy	Burning or stinging, nosebleeds.	Use at regular intervals. Slow onset (7-14 days for maximal effect). Drug may fail to reach the site of action if excessive nasal mucus secretion or edema of the nasal mucosa is present. May use a vasoconstrictor 2–3 days prior to the suspension. Aim spray up towards turbinates and away from septum. Liquid forms may be more effective than metered-dose inhalers.	$$

(cont'd)

Table 3: **Intranasal Drugs Used in Allergic Rhinitis** *(cont'd)*

Class	Drug	Dose	Adverse Effects	Comments	Cost[a]
	budesonide Rhinocort Aqua, Rhinocort Turbuhaler	Nasal suspension: adults and children ≥ 6 y (64 μg/metered dose): initial dose 2 sprays in each nostril daily or 1 spray in each nostril BID; may ↓ maintenance dose to 1 spray in each nostril daily	See beclomethasone.	See beclomethasone.	\$\$-\$\$\$
	flunisolide Rhinalar, generics	Adults (25 μg/metered spray): 2 sprays in each nostril BID, may ↑ to TID if needed; max 300 μg/day Children 6–14 y: 1 spray in each nostril TID; max 150 μg/day	See beclomethasone.	See beclomethasone.	\$\$
	fluticasone Flonase	Adults and children ≥ 12 y (50 μg/spray): 2 sprays in each nostril daily, may ↑ to BID in severe situations; max 400 μg/day Children 4–11 y: 1–2 sprays in each nostril daily; max 200 μg/day	See beclomethasone.	See beclomethasone.	\$\$\$

Class	Drug	Dose	Adverse Effects	Comments	Cost[a]
	mometasone Nasonex	Adults and children ≥ 12 y (50 µg/spray): 2 sprays in each nostril daily, may ↓ to 1 spray in each nostril daily for maintenance, may ↑ to BID in severe situations 3–11 y: 1 spray in each nostril daily	See beclomethasone.	See beclomethasone. Initial priming needed. Reprime if not used ≥ 14 days.	$$$
	triamcinolone Nasacort AQ	Adults and children ≥ 12 y (55 µg/spray): 2 sprays in each nostril once daily, may ↓ to 1 spray in each nostril once daily	See beclomethasone.	See beclomethasone.	$$$

[a] Cost of 1 unit (spray pump); includes drug cost only.
[b] Available without a prescription.
Legend: $ < $10 $$ $10–20 $$-$$$ $10–30 $$$ $20–30

Table 4: **Ophthalmic Preparations Used in Allergic Conjunctivitis**

Class	Drug	Dose	Adverse Effects	Comments	Cost[a]
Antihistamines	*levocabastine* Livostin[b]	≥ 12 y: 1 drop into affected eye BID, may ↑ to 1 drop TID–QID	Transient ocular effects, eye irritation, stinging or burning, headache.	Quick onset of relief. Shake well prior to use. Discontinue if no improvement seen within 3 days of use. Discard after 1 month of opening bottle. Instruct patients on techniques used to avoid contamination.	$$$
	emedastine Emadine	≥ 3 y: 1 drop into affected eye BID, may ↑ to 1 drop TID–QID	Mild transient ocular discomfort – burning and stinging, pruritus, headache.		$$
Antihistamines & Mast Cell Stabilizers	*ketotifen* Zaditor[b]	1 drop into affected eye Q8–12H	Conjunctival injection, headache.		$$$
	olopatadine Patanol[b]	≥ 3 y: 1–2 drops into affected eye BID	Mild transient burning or stinging, pruritus, hyperemia, photophobia, headache.		$$$
Mast Cell Stabilizers	*lodoxamide* Alomide[b]	> 4 y: 1–2 drops into affected eye QID at regular intervals	Mild and transient discomfort upon instillation — burning, stinging, itching, tearing.	Improvement in signs and symptoms in response to therapy evident in a few days; longer treatment for up to 4 weeks may be required.	$$

Class	Drug	Dose	Adverse Effects	Comments	Cost[a]
	nedocromil Alocril	≥ 3 y: 1 drop into each eye BID	Headache, eye burning, eye stinging, taste perversion.	Use regularly to ensure optimal control of symptoms. Initiate treatment at the start of the symptoms. Contains benzalkonium chloride. Do not use soft contact lenses during the treatment period. Remove hard or gas permeable contact lenses prior to instillation of drops and wait at least 5 minutes after instilling the solution before inserting the contact lenses.	$$$
	sodium cromoglycate Opticrom[b,c]	≥ 5 y: 2 drops in each eye QID at regular intervals	Transient ocular stinging, eye burning.	Use regularly to ensure optimal control of symptoms. Initiate treatment at the start of the symptoms. Onset of symptomatic improvement occurs in 2–3 days.	$

[a] Cost of smallest available pack size; includes drug cost only.
[b] Contains benzalkonium chloride. Remove soft contact lenses prior to instillation of drops and wait at least 10 minutes after instilling the solution before inserting the contact lenses.
[c] Available without a prescription.
Legend: $ < $10 $$ $10–20 $$$ $20–30

Suggested Readings

Bousquet J, Van Cauwenberge P, Khaltaev N et al. Allergic rhinitis and its impact on asthma. *J Allergy Clin Immunol* 2001;108(5 Suppl):S147-334.

Dykewicz MS, Fineman S, Skoner DP et al. Diagnosis and management of rhinitis: complete guidelines of the Joint Task Force on Practice Parameters in Allergy, Asthma and Immunology. American Academy of Allergy, Asthma, and Immunology. *Ann Allergy Asthma Immunol* 1998;81(5 Pt 2):478-518.

Juniper EF, Stahl E, Doty RL et al. Clinical outcomes and adverse effect monitoring in allergic rhinitis. *J Allergy Clin Immunol* 2005;115(3 Pt 2):S390-413.

Milgrom H, Bender B. Adverse effects of medications for rhinitis. *Ann Allergy Asthma Immunol* 1997;78(5):439-44.

Plaut M, Valentine MD. Clinical practice. Allergic rhinitis. *N Engl J Med* 2005;353(18):1934-44.

References

1. Asher I, Baena-Cagnani C, Boner A et al. World Allergy Organization guidelines for prevention of allergy and allergic asthma. *Int Arch Allergy Immunol* 2004;135(1):83-92.
2. Bousquet J, Van Cauwenberge P, Khaltaev N et al. Allergic rhinitis and its impact on asthma. *J Allergy Clin Immunol* 2001;108(5 Suppl):S147-334.
3. Horak F, Stubner UP, Zieglmayer R et al. Effect of desloratadine versus placebo on nasal airflow and subjective measures of nasal obstruction in subjects with grass pollen-induced allergic rhinitis in an allergen-exposure unit. *J Allergy Clin Immunol* 2002 Jun;109(6):956-61
4. Kay GG. The effects of antihistamines on cognition and performance. *J Allergy Clin Immunol* 2000;105(6 Pt 2):S622-7.
5. O'Hanlon JF, Ramaekers JG. Antihistamine effects on actual driving performance in a standard test: a summary of Dutch experience, 1989-94. *Allergy* 1995;50(3):234-42.
6. Howarth PH. Assessment of antihistamine efficacy and potency. *Clin Exp Allergy* 1999;29(Suppl 3):87-97.
7. Juniper EF, Stahl E, Doty RL et al. Clinical outcomes and adverse effect monitoring in allergic rhinitis. *J Allergy Clin Immunol* 2005;115(3 Pt 2):S390-413.
8. Simons KJ, Simons FE. The effect of chronic administration of hydroxyzine on hydroxyzine pharmacokinetics in dogs. *J Allergy Clin Immunol* 1987;79(6):928-32.
9. Radack K, Deck CC. Are oral decongestants safe in hypertension? An evaluation of the evidence and a framework for assessing clinical trials. *Ann Allergy* 1986;56(5):396-401.
10. Boner AL. Effects of intranasal corticosteroids on the hypothalamic-pituitary-adrenal axis in children. *J Allergy Clin Immunol* 2001;108(1 Suppl):S32-9.
11. Wilson AM, Sims EJ, McFarlane LC et al. Effects of intranasal corticosteroids on adrenal, bone, and blood markers of systemic activity in allergic rhinitis. *J Allergy Clin Immunol* 1998;102(4 Pt 1):598-604.
12. Soderberg-Warner ML. Nasal septal perforation associated with topical corticosteroid therapy. *J Pediatr* 1984;105(5):840-1.
13. LaForce C. Use of nasal steroids in managing allergic rhinitis. *J Allergy Clin Immunol* 1999;103(3 Pt 2):S388-94.
14. Edwards TB. Effectiveness and safety of beclomethasone dipropionate, an intranasal corticosteroid, in the treatment of patients with allergic rhinitis. *Clin Ther* 1995;17(6):1032-41.
15. Grossman J, Banov C, Boggs P et al. Use of ipratropium bromide nasal spray in chronic treatment of nonallergic perennial rhinitis, alone and in combination with other perennial rhinitis medications. *J Allergy Clin Immunol* 1995;95(5 Pt 2):1123-7.
16. Rodrigo GJ, Yanez A. The role of antileukotriene therapy in seasonal allergic rhinitis: a systematic review of randomized trials. *Ann Allergy Asthma Immunol* 2006;96(6):779-86.
17. Wilson AM, O'Byrne PM, Parameswaran K. Leukotriene receptor antagonists for allergic rhinitis: a systematic review and meta-analysis. *Am J Med* 2004 Mar 1;116(5):338-44.
18. Saengpanich S, deTineo M, Naclerio RM et al. Fluticasone nasal spray and the combination of loratadine and montelukast in seasonal allergic rhinitis. *Arch Otolaryngol Head Neck Surg* 2003;129:557–562.
19. Durham SR, Walker SM, Varga EM et al. Long-term clinical efficacy of grass-pollen immunotherapy. *N Engl J Med* 1999;341(7):468-75.

20. Joint Task Force on Practice Parameters. Allergen immunotherapy: a practice parameter. American Academy of Allergy, Asthma and Immunology. American College of Allergy, Asthma and Immunology. *Ann Allergy Asthma Immunol* 2003;90(1 Suppl 1):1-40.
21. [No authors listed]. Guidelines for the use of allergen immunotherapy. Canadian Society of Allergy and Clinical Immunology. *CMAJ* 1995;152(9):1413-9.
22. Incaudo GA, Takach P. The diagnosis and treatment of allergic rhinitis during pregnancy and lactation. *Immunol Allergy Clin North Am* 2006;26(1):137-54.
23. Ellegard EK. Pregnancy rhinitis. *Immunol Allergy Clin North Am* 2006;26(1):119-35, vii.
24. Ellegard EK. Clinical and pathogenetic characteristics of pregnancy rhinitis. *Clin Rev Allergy Immunol* 2004;26(3):149-59.
25. Piette V, Daures JP, Demoly P. Treating allergic rhinitis in pregnancy. *Curr Allergy Asthma Rep* 2006;6(3):232-8.
26. Norjavaara E, de Verdier MG. Normal pregnancy outcomes in a population-based study including 2,968 pregnant women exposed to budesonide. *J Allergy Clin Immunol* 2003;111(4):736-42.
27. Schatz M, Zeiger RS, Harden K et al. The safety of asthma and allergy medications during pregnancy. *J Allergy Clin Immunol* 1997;100(3):301-6.
28. Diav-Citrin O, Shechtman S, Aharonovich A et al. Pregnancy outcome after gestational exposure to loratadine or antihistamines: a prospective controlled cohort study. *J Allergy Clin Immunol* 2003;111(6):1239-43.
29. Meltzer EO. Quality of life in adults and children with allergic rhinitis. *J Allergy Clin Immunol* 2001;108(1 Suppl):S45-53.
30. Di Lorenzo G, Pacor ML, Pellitteri ME et al. Randomized placebo-controlled trial comparing fluticasone aqueous nasal spray in mono-therapy, fluticasone plus cetirizine, fluticasone plus montelukast and cetirizine plus montelukast for seasonal allergic rhinitis. *Clin Exp Allergy* 2004;34(2):259-67.
31. Simons FE, Silas P, Portnoy JM et al. Safety of cetirizine in infants 6 to 11 months of age: a randomized, double-blind, placebo-controlled study. *J Allergy Clin Immunol* 2003;111(6):1244-8.

CHAPTER 46
Viral Rhinitis

Timothy P. Lynch, MD, FRCPC

Goals of Therapy

- Lessen interference with activities of daily living
- Improve the discomfort and emotional distress of rhinorrhea
- Improve the discomfort of nasal congestion
- Minimize the potential adverse effects of pharmacologic agents

Investigations

- Diagnosis of the common cold, which is most commonly due to a rhinovirus infection, requires no specific laboratory investigation.
- History with particular attention to intensity, frequency and severity of symptoms.
  - Early symptoms of a cold include headache, chills, sneezing and sore throat. Later symptoms include nasal discharge, nasal obstruction, cough and malaise. Symptoms may last from a few days to a couple of weeks.[1]
  - Symptoms of the flu are more severe than those of colds and typically include abrupt onset of fever, severe myalgias, anorexia, sore throat, headache and cough.[2]
  - Symptoms of sinus headache, difficulty breathing, chest pain or productive cough with yellow-green sputum suggest bacterial infection.

Therapeutic Choices (Figure 1)

Viral rhinitis is usually a benign, self-limited condition. Typical symptoms of rhinorrhea and nasal congestion resolve untreated in 7 to 10 days. There is no evidence that treatment of the rhinitis lessens the risk of developing a complication[3], such as middle ear effusion, otitis media, sinusitis, a febrile seizure or an asthma exacerbation. To improve these symptoms and the patient's quality of life, nonpharmacologic and pharmacologic approaches are available. Each pharmacologic agent employed should be directed against a specific symptom.

Nonpharmacologic Choices

- Avoiding close contact with someone with a cold is key to prevention.[3]
- Strict hand-washing techniques[4], abstaining from touching eyes or nose, and sneezing or coughing into a facial tissue, which is then discarded immediately, may limit risk of inoculation and transmission.
- Normal healthy fluid intake should be encouraged.[5]

Pharmacologic Choices (Figure 1, Table 1, Table 2)

Decongestants (Alpha-adrenergic Agents)

Decongestants are used specifically to relieve nasal congestion and improve rhinorrhea. They help most adults by improving nasal air flow.[6] Both short- and long-acting topical agents are available. A single dose is effective for the short-term (3–10 h) relief of congestion in adults. There is insufficient evidence to support their longer use in children under 12.[7] **Pseudoephedrine** is an effective treatment for nasal congestion.[8,9] Multiple doses of pseudoephedrine over a three-day period are safe.[9]

Anticholinergic Agents

Intranasal **ipratropium** blocks cholinergic-mediated vasodilatation. It is effective in treating rhinorrhea and providing relief of sneezing but does not improve nasal congestion.[10]

Antihistamines

The anticholinergic effects of some first-generation antihistamines may reduce nasal secretions, but there is no evidence in children or adults that they improve recovery time from colds when used as monotherapy. In addition, the incidence of sedation is higher than placebo with these medications.[11] **Antihistamine–decongestant** combinations have been shown to improve short-term nasal symptoms in adolescents and adults.[12]

Second-generation or nonsedating antihistamines have no anticholinergic activity.[3] There is no evidence to support their use alone in controlling rhinorrhea or nasal congestion.[13]

Vitamin C

Daily vitamin C (ascorbic acid) supplementation is not effective in the prevention of colds. However, daily supplementation (1 g) is associated with a reduction in duration and possibly the severity of symptoms.[14] The ingestion of high doses (4 to 8 g) at the onset of cold symptoms has not been shown to reduce either the duration of cold symptoms or their severity.[14]

Zinc Lozenges

Zinc gluconate lozenges may reduce the symptoms and duration of the common cold; however, current evidence remains inconclusive.[15,16,17] Improved benefit has been noted when they are started with the onset of symptoms. No significant adverse effects related to the use of zinc have been described, although it may have an unpleasant taste and may cause nausea.

Antibiotics

Routine antibiotic use is not effective in the treatment of the common cold in children or adults. Gastrointestinal adverse effects are significantly increased in adults who take antibiotics for their colds.[18]

Natural Health Products

Echinacea

A Cochrane review of 16 studies concluded that *Echinacea purpurea* probably can be effective in the prevention and treatment of the common cold in adults.[19] However, no specific product or preparation could be recommended.[19] A recent, well-designed study, which tested extracts of *E. angustifolia* roots, demonstrated that these preparations did not have clinically significant effects on rhinovirus infection or illness.[20] A double-blind, randomized, controlled trial testing *E. purpurea* 100 mg versus placebo, given three times daily until cold symptoms were relieved or until the end of 14 days, demonstrated lack of efficacy in reducing symptoms and duration of the common cold.[21] Echinacea may reduce the severity of symptoms among healthy children if given early.[22]

North American Ginseng Extract (Table 2)

A recent study of a standardized North American ginseng extract, given daily starting in November for four months, showed a significant reduction, compared to placebo, in the number, severity and duration of colds in test subjects.[23] The benefit was demonstrated in individuals who got two or more colds per season.[23]

Appropriate Treatment for Specific Age Groups

Acetaminophen or **ibuprofen** may be helpful for fever or headache in *preschool children*. ASA should not be used in children due to the increased incidence of Reye's syndrome associated with its use during influenza virus infections. Breast- or bottle-fed infants who are obligate nose breathers may benefit from regular administration of **normal saline drops,** which aid in cleaning the nose and which may improve mucociliary clearance in young infants.[24] There is no published evidence to support the use of antihistamines, decongestants or antihistamine–decongestant combinations in children less than 5 years of age.[12,25] In addition, accidental ingestion and dosing errors of these products can do much harm.

There have been few trials in *school-aged children*. It has been shown that an antihistamine–decongestant–antitussive combination was superior to an antihistamine–expectorant combination in reducing nasal symptoms.[12] There are no published trials that evaluate topical nasal decongestants in children.

Antihistamine-decongestant combinations may be of benefit but risks of treatment should be carefully considered.[11]

In *adolescents and adults*, decongestants (topical or oral) and antihistamine–decongestant combinations have been shown to improve short-term nasal symptoms.[12] Oral decongestants are associated with an increased number of adverse effects.[12] Prolonged use (usually over five days) of topical nasal decongestants is associated with rebound congestion (*rhinitis medicamentosa*).[26] Anticholinergic agents have also been shown to improve rhinorrhea.[13] A short course of topical decongestants or topical anticholinergic agents should be considered first-line therapy.

Therapeutic Tips

- There is insufficient evidence to support the use of inhaling steam.[27]
- Single-dose oral or topical decongestants demonstrate evidence for the relief of congestion in adults.

Figure 1: **Management of Viral Rhinitis**

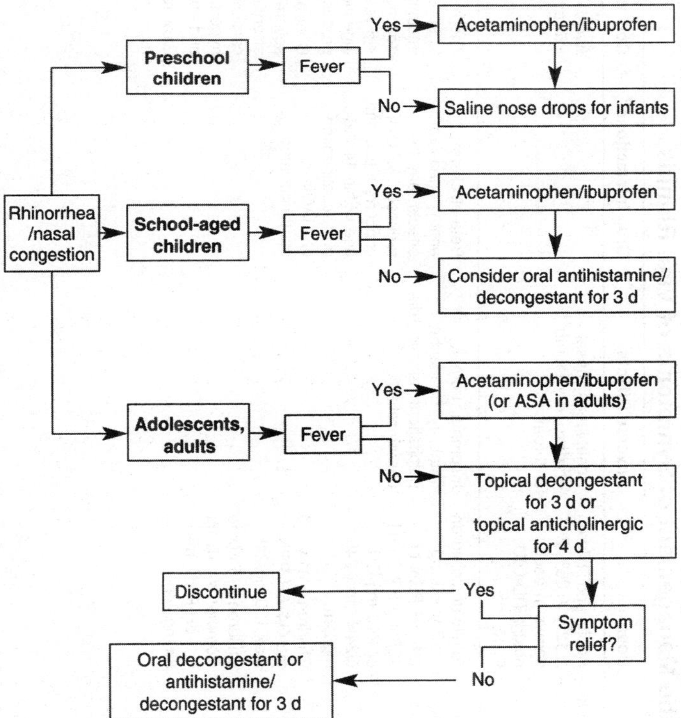

Table 1: Drugs Used in the Management of Symptoms of Viral Rhinitis

Class	Drug	Dose	Adverse Effects	Drug Interactions	Comments	Cost[a]
Anticholinergic Agents	*ipratropium bromide* Atrovent Nasal Spray	Adults and children ≥ 12 y: 0.06% 2 sprays in each nostril TID-QID PRN.	Nosebleeds, nasal dryness, dry mouth or throat.		Avoid accidental release of nasal spray into eyes.	$$
Decongestants, systemic	*pseudoephedrine* Drixoral, Eltor 120, Sudafed, Triaminic Oral Pediatric Drops, generics	Adults and children ≥ 12 y: 60 mg Q4–6H PRN or 120 mg SR Q12H or 240 mg CR Q24H, max 240 mg/24h. Children 6–11 y: 30 mg Q4–6H PRN, max 120 mg/24h. Children 2–5 y (*see Comments*): 15 mg Q4–6H PRN, max 60 mg/24h.	Insomnia, tremor, irritability, headache, palpitations, tachycardia, urinary retention.	Beta-blockers: antihypertensive effects may be reduced. MAOIs: concurrent use and use within 14 days of discontinuation of MAOIs is contraindicated.	There is no published evidence to support use of antihistamines, decongestants or antihistamine-decongestant combinations in children < 5 years of age. In addition, accidental ingestion and dosing errors of these products can do much harm. Contraindicated in patients with severe hypertension and coronary artery disease. Use with caution in cardiovascular disease, diabetes, hyperthyroidism, prostatic hypertrophy and angle-closure glaucoma. Slow-release formulations are not recommended in children < 12 y.	$

Class	Drug	Dose	Adverse Effects	Drug Interactions	Comments	Cost[a]
	phenylephrine, oral – ingredient in combination products Dimetane, Dimetapp Cold Liquids, Dimetapp-C Syrup, Dimetapp Daytime/Nightime Cold Extra Strength, Novahistex DH, Novahistine DH	Adults: 10–20 mg Q4H, max 120 mg/24h. Children 6–11 y: 10 mg Q4H, max 60 mg/24h.	See pseudoephedrine.	See pseudoephedrine.	See pseudoephedrine.	\$-\$\$
Decongestants, topical	*oxymetazoline* Afrin, Claritin Allergic Congestion Relief, Dristan Long Lasting Nasal Spray, generics	Adults and children ≥ 6 y: 0.05% 2 or 3 sprays in each nostril Q10–12H PRN, max 2 doses/24h.	Transient burning, stinging and dryness of nasal mucosa. Rebound congestion may occur with > 3–5 days of continuous use. Topical products are associated with fewer systemic adverse effects than oral decongestants.		Use with caution in patients with hypertension, diabetes, cardiovascular disease or hyperthyroidism.	\$
	xylometazoline Balminil Nasal Decongestant, Otrivin, generics	Adults: 0.1% 1–2 sprays or 2–3 drops each nostril Q8–10H PRN, max 3 doses/24h. Children > 2 y: 0.05% 1 spray or 2–3 drops each	See oxymetazoline.		See oxymetazoline.	\$

(cont'd)

Table 1: **Drugs Used in the Management of Symptoms of Viral Rhinitis** *(cont'd)*

Class	Drug	Dose	Adverse Effects	Drug Interactions	Comments	Cost[a]
		nostril Q8–10H PRN, max 3 doses/24h.				
	phenylephrine, nasal – ingredient in combination products Dristan Decongestant Nasal Spray, Soframycin Nasal Spray	Adults and children ≥ 12 y: 0.25%, 0.5%, 1% 2–3 sprays in each nostril no more than Q4H, max 6 doses/24h. Children 6–11 y: 0.25% 2–3 sprays in each nostril no more than Q4H, max 6 doses/24h. Children 2–5 y: 0.125% 2–3 drops in each nostril no more than Q4H, max 6 doses/24h.	See oxymetazoline.		See oxymetazoline.	$$
Antihistamine/ Decongestant Combinations, first generation	*azatadine/ pseudoephedrine* Trinalin	Adults and children ≥ 12 y: 1 tab (1 mg/60 mg) BID.	Azatadine: common: headache and somnolence. Decongestant: See pseudoephedrine.	Antihistamine: additive CNS depressive effects with alcohol and other CNS depressants. Decongestant: See pseudoephedrine.	Azatadine is more sedating than the second- or third-generation antihistamines. See pseudoephedrine.	$

Class	Drug	Dose	Adverse Effects	Drug Interactions	Comments	Cost[a]
	triprolidine / pseudoephedrine Actifed	Adults and children ≥ 12 y: 1 tab (2.5 mg/60 mg) Q4–6H, max 4 doses/24h. Children 6–11 y: ½ tab Q4–6H, max 4 doses/24h.	Antihistamine: drowsiness, fatigue, anticholinergic effects such as dry eyes, dry mouth and urinary retention. Paradoxical stimulatory effects may occur in children and the elderly. Decongestant: See pseudoephedrine.	Antihistamine: additive CNS depressive effects with alcohol and other CNS depressants. Decongestant: See pseudoephedrine.	See pseudoephedrine.	$
Antihistamine/ Decongestant Combinations, second generation	*cetirizine/ pseudoephedrine* Reactine Allergy & Sinus	Adults and children ≥ 12 y: 1 tab (5 mg/120 mg) Q12H.	Cetirizine: common: headache and somnolence (with ↑ dose). Decongestant: See pseudoephedrine.	Antihistamine: additive CNS depressive effects with alcohol and other CNS depressants. Decongestant: See pseudoephedrine.	See pseudoephedrine.	$
	fexofenadine/ pseudoephedrine Allegra-D	Adults and children ≥ 12 y: 1 tab (60 mg/120 mg) BID.	Fexofenadine: common: headache. Decongestant: See pseudoephedrine.	↓ fexofenadine level: concurrent aluminum- and magnesium-containing antacids or ingestion of fruit juices such as apple, grapefruit, orange or pineapple. Antihistamine: additive CNS depressive effects with alcohol and other CNS depressants.	To be taken on an empty stomach. See pseudoephedrine	$

(cont'd)

Table 1: **Drugs Used in the Management of Symptoms of Viral Rhinitis** *(cont'd)*

Class	Drug	Dose	Adverse Effects	Drug Interactions	Comments	Cost[a]
				Decongestant: See pseudoephedrine.		
	loratadine/ pseudoephedrine Claritin Allergy & Sinus, Claritin Allergy + Sinus Extra Strength	Adults and children ≥ 12 y: 5 mg/120 mg: 1 tab BID. 10 mg/240 mg: 1 tab daily, preferably upon waking.	Loratadine: common: headache, somnolence, fatigue, xerostomia. Decongestant: See pseudoephedrine.	↑ loratadine levels: protease inhibitors such as amprenavir, ritonavir, nelfinavir. Loratadine may ↑ levels of medications metabolized by CYP2C19 such as citalopram, diazepam, propranolol, phenytoin. Antihistamine: additive CNS depressive effects with alcohol and other CNS depressants. Decongestant: See pseudoephedrine.	See pseudoephedrine.	$$

[a] Cost of one unit (spray pump, drops) or 12 tablets; includes drug cost only.
Legend: $ < $10 $-$$ < $10–20 $$ $10–20

Table 2: Natural Health Products Used in the Prevention of Viral Rhinitis

Class	Drug	Dose	Drug Interactions	Comments	Cost[a]
Natural Health Products	*North American ginseng — panax quinquefolium* Cold-fX	Prevention: 2 caps daily for 4 months on an empty stomach at the onset of cold season.[23]	↓ INR with concomitant warfarin use.	May cause hypoglycemia; use with caution in diabetics. Benefit seen in individuals who get ≥ 2 colds/y.	$

[a] Cost of one unit (spray pump, drops) or 12 tablets; includes drug cost only.
Legend: $ < $10

Suggested Readings

Arroll B. Non-antibiotic treatments for upper-respiratory tract infections (common cold). *Respir Med* 2005;99(12):1477-84.

Clemens CJ, Taylor JA, Almquist JR et al. Is an antihistamine-decongestant combination effective in temporarily relieving symptoms of the common cold in preschool children? *J Pediatr* 1997;130(3):463-6.

Gentile DA, Skoner DP. Viral rhinitis. *Curr Allergy Asthma Rep* 2001;1(3):227-34.

Hayden FG, Diamond L, Wood PB, Korts DC, Wecker MT. Effectiveness and safety of intranasal ipratropium bromide in common colds. A randomized, double-blind, placebo-controlled trial. *Ann Intern Med* 1996;125(2):89-97.

Luks D, Anderson MR. Antihistamines and the common cold. A review and critique of the literature. *J Gen Intern Med* 1996;11(4):240-4.

Smith MB, Feldman W. Over-the-counter cold medications. A critical review of clinical trials between 1950 and 1991. *JAMA* 1993;269(17):2258-63.

References

1. Eccles, R. Understanding the symptoms of the common cold and influenza. *Lancet Infect Dis* 2005;5:718–725.
2. Monto AS, Gravenstein S, Elliott M et al. Clinical signs and symptoms predicting influenza infection. *Arch Intern Med* 2000;160:3243–3247.
3. Fireman P. Pathophysiology and pharmacotherapy of common upper respiratory diseases. *Pharmacotherapy* 1993;13(6 Pt 2):101S-9S.
4. Ryan MA, Christian RS, Wohlrabe J. Handwashing and respiratory illness among young adults in military training. *Am J Prev Med* 2001;21(2):79-83.
5. Guppy MP, Mickan SM, Del Mar CB. Advising patients to increase fluid intake for treating acute respiratory infections. *Cochrane Database Syst Rev* 2005;(4):CD004419.
6. Akerlund A, Klint T, Olen L, Rundcrantz H. Nasal decongestant effect of oxymetazoline in the common cold: an objective dose-response study in 106 patients. *J Laryngol Otol* 1989;103(8):743-6.
7. Taverner D, Latte J, Draper M. Nasal decongestants for the common cold. *Cochrane Database Syst Rev* 2004;(3):CD001953.
8. Latte J, Taverner D, Slobodian P, Shakib S. A randomized, double-blind, placebo-controlled trial of pseudoephedrine in coryza. *Clin Exp Pharmacol Physiol* 2004;31(7):429-32.
9. Eccles R, Jawad MS, Jawad SS et al. Efficacy and safety of single and multiple doses of pseudoephedrine in the treatment of nasal congestion associated with common cold. *Am J Rhinol* 2005;19(1):25-31.
10. Hayden FG, Diamond L, Wood PB, Korts DC, Wecker MT. Effectiveness and safety of intranasal ipratropium bromide in common colds. A randomized, double-blind, placebo-controlled trial. *Ann Intern Med* 1996;125(2):89-97.
11. Sutter AI, Lemiengre M, Campbell H, Mackinnon HF. Antihistamines for the common cold. *Cochrane Database Syst Rev* 2003;(3):CD001267.
12. Smith MB, Feldman W. Over-the-counter cold medications. A critical review of clinical trials between 1950 and 1991. *JAMA* 1993;269(17):2258-63.
13. Luks D, Anderson MR. Antihistamines and the common cold. A review and critique of the literature. *J Gen Intern Med* 1996;11(4):240-4.
14. Douglas RM, Hemila H, D'Souza R, Chalker EB, Treacy B. Vitamin C for preventing and treating the common cold. *Cochrane Database Syst Rev* 2000;(2):CD000980.
15. Garland ML, Hagmeyer KO. The role of zinc lozenges in treatment of the common cold. *Ann Pharmacother* 1998;32(1):63-9.
16. Jackson JL, Lesho E, Peterson C. Zinc and the common cold: a meta-analysis revisited. *J Nutr* 2000;130(5S Suppl):1512S-5S.
17. Turner RB, Cetnarowski WE. Effect of treatment with zinc gluconate or zinc acetate on experimental and natural colds. *Clin Infect Dis* 2000;31(5):1202-8.
18. Arroll B, Kenealy T. Antibiotics for the common cold and acute purulent rhinitis. *Cochrane Database Syst Rev* 2005;(3):CD000247.

19. Melchart D, Linde K, Fischer P, Kaesmayr J. Echinacea for preventing and treating the common cold. *Cochrane Database Syst Rev* 2000;(2):CD000530.
20. Turner RB, Bauer R, Woelkart K, Hulsey TC, Gangemi JD. An evaluation of Echinacea angustifolia in experimental rhinovirus infections. *N Engl J Med* 2005;353(4):341-8.
21. Yale SH, Liu K. Echinacea purpurea therapy for the treatment of the common cold: a randomized, double-blind, placebo-controlled clinical trial. *Arch Intern Med* 2004;164(11):1237-41.
22. Vohra S, Rieder M. Efficacy of echinacea for upper respiratory tract infections in children. *Paediatrics & Child Health* 2005;10(4):224. Available from: http//www.pulsus.com/Paeds/10 04/vohr ed.htm Accessed March 1, 2006.
23. Predy GN, Goel V, Lovlin R et al. Efficacy of an extract of North American ginseng containing poly-furanosyl-pyranosyl-saccharides for preventing upper respiratory tract infections: a randomized controlled trial. *CMAJ* 2005;173(9):1043-8.
24. Jones NS. Current concepts in the management of paediatric rhinosinusitis. *J Laryngol Otol* 1999;113(1):1-9.
25. Clemens CJ, Taylor JA, Almquist JR et al. Is an antihistamine-decongestant combination effective in temporarily relieving symptoms of the common cold in preschool children? *J Pediatr* 1997;130(3):463-6.
26. Graf P. Rhinitis medicamentosa: aspects of pathophysiology and treatment. *Allergy* 1997;52(40 Suppl):28-34.
27. Singh M. Heated, humidified air for the common cold. *Cochrane Database Syst Rev* 2004;(2):CD001728.

CHAPTER 47
Adult Asthma

David G. McCormack, MD, FRCPC

Asthma is a respiratory disorder characterized by:

- Paroxysmal or persistent symptoms (dyspnea, chest tightness, wheezing, sputum production and cough)
- Variable airflow limitation
- Airway inflammation
- Airway hyper-responsiveness

Goals of Therapy

- Maintain normal activity levels e.g., avoiding absenteeism from work or school
- Prevent daytime and nocturnal symptoms (cough, wheezing, dyspnea)
- Maintain normal (or near normal) spirometry
- Prevent exacerbations
- Provide optimal pharmacotherapy and avoid side effects

Investigations

- Thorough history with particular attention to:
  - symptoms, frequency and severity
  - pattern of symptoms (seasonal, perennial, diurnal variation, etc.)
  - precipitating factors (environmental allergens, occupational exposures, irritants such as smoke, exercise, drugs such as ASA or beta-blockers, preservatives such as sulfites, viral respiratory infections, rhinitis, sinusitis, gastroesophageal reflux)
  - previous hospitalizations, emergency room visits and intensive care admissions
- Physical examination: wheezing, nasal polyps
- Objective measurements needed to confirm diagnosis and assess severity include:
  - spirometry (preferred method of diagnosis): reduced expiratory flow rates
  - home peak flow monitoring can be used to diagnose asthma or to monitor patients with severe asthma or poor perception of airway obstruction
  - bronchoprovocation challenge test, using methacholine or histamine, if diagnosis in doubt

Therapeutic Choices

Nonpharmacologic Choices

- Identify and avoid precipitating factors such as environmental allergens and occupational irritants.
- Smoking cessation is essential[1] (see Chapter 10).
- Hyposensitization therapy to allergens generally is not useful in the management of asthma.[2]
- An annual flu shot is recommended unless contraindicated.
- Use of home air cleaners/purifiers is not supported by evidence.[3]

Pharmacologic Choices

Choose the initial level of treatment with medication after an assessment of asthma severity and previous treatment (Figure 1).[4] Review treatment every three to six months and if control is achieved, try a stepwise reduction in treatment.

Inhaled therapy that maximizes delivery of drugs to the respiratory tract and minimizes systemic side effects is the cornerstone of asthma management. Metered dose inhalers (pMDI) with spacers or dry powder inhalers (DPI) deliver drugs as effectively as nebulized therapy. Medications include bronchodilators and anti-inflammatory agents (Table 2).

Bronchodilators

Short-acting Inhaled Beta$_2$-agonists (SABA)

Salbutamol, terbutaline and **fenoterol** are selective beta$_2$-agonists that are agents of first choice for treatment of acute exacerbations and for prevention of exercise-induced asthma. They are used as required rather than on a fixed schedule. Although potent bronchodilators, they have little effect on the late (inflammatory) phase of an exacerbation. If patients use a short-acting beta$_2$-agonist more than three times per week (excluding one dose per day before exercise), initiate therapy with an anti-inflammatory agent. Isoproterenol and epinephrine are not recommended for the treatment of asthma because of lack of beta$_2$-selectivity and potential of excessive cardiac stimulation especially at high doses.

Long-acting Inhaled Beta$_2$-agonists (LABA)

Salmeterol and **formoterol** are long-acting beta$_2$-agonists intended for regular twice daily treatment of asthma. Salmeterol has a slow onset of action and should not be used for immediate symptomatic relief of bronchospasm. Formoterol is rapid acting and can be utilized for rescue therapy. They should be used only in patients already taking inhaled corticosteroids and may be particularly useful for the prevention of nocturnal symptoms. These drugs also aid in the prevention of *exercise-induced bronchospasm*. Adding long acting beta$_2$-agonists to inhaled corticosteroids can aid in decreasing the latter's dose.

Oral Beta$_2$-agonists

Oral orciprenaline, salbutamol and terbutaline offer less bronchodilation, more systemic side effects and a slower onset of action than the inhaled preparations and are therefore not recommended.

Anticholinergic Agents

Ipratropium is a useful alternative for patients who are unusually susceptible to tremor or tachycardia from beta$_2$-agonists. Although the onset of action is delayed compared to beta$_2$-agonists, the bronchodilator effect lasts longer. It may also be useful in beta-blocker-induced bronchospasm.[5]

Tiotropium is an attractive alternative to ipratropium bromide although it has identical indications. The advantage over ipratropium bromide is that tiotropium is administered once a day instead of three or four times a day. Unlike ipratropium bromide, tiotropium should not be used for relief of acute bronchospasm but more as maintenance therapy.

Theophylline Products

Oral **theophylline, oxtriphylline** and **aminophylline** are uncommonly used due to systemic toxicity and only mild bronchodilator activity. Administer carefully according to standard regimens and monitor blood levels. In naïve patients, titrate the dose slowly to minimize side effects.

Anti-inflammatory Agents

Inhaled Corticosteroids

Inhaled **budesonide, beclomethasone, ciclesonide** and **fluticasone** are safe, effective, and cost-effective drugs that treat the inflammatory component of asthma.[6] They should be used regularly at the lowest effective dose rather than "as needed" to maintain good asthma control. They have a higher ratio of topical to systemic activity than do oral corticosteroids. The incidence of pharyngeal candidiasis from deposition of the inhaled corticosteroid in the pharynx can be reduced by rinsing the mouth after use and/or using a spacer device. Dose equivalencies for inhaled corticosteroids are listed in Table 1.

Table 1: **Comparative Dose Equivalencies for Inhaled Corticosteroids**[7]

Class	Drug	Dose
Inhaled Corticosteroids	*beclomethasone pMDI (HFA)* Qvar, generics	Low: ≤ 250 μg/day Moderate: 251–500 μg/day High: > 500 μg/day
	budesonide DPI Pulmicort Turbuhaler	Low: ≤ 400 μg/day Moderate: 401–800 μg/day High: > 800 μg/day

(cont'd)

Table 1: **Comparative Dose Equivalencies for Inhaled Corticosteroids[7]** *(cont'd)*

Class	Drug	Dose
	budesonide nebulizer Pulmicort Nebuamp	Low: ≤ 1000 μg/day Moderate: 1001–2000 μg/day High: > 2000 μg/day
	ciclesonide pMDI Alvesco	Low: ≤ 200 μg/day Moderate: 201–400 μg/day High: > 400 μg/day
	fluticasone DPI or pMDI plus spacer Flovent Diskus, Flovent HFA	Low: ≤ 250 μg/day Moderate: 251–500 μg/day High: > 500 μg/day

Abbreviations: pMDI = pressurized metered dose inhaler; DPI = dry powder inhaler; HFA = hydrofluoroalkane

Systemic Corticosteroids

These are useful in both preventing and treating acute exacerbations. Optimal dosage has not been established. Side effects are significant: glucose intolerance, increased appetite, weight gain, mood alterations, fluid retention and hypertension in the short term and adrenal axis suppression, dermal thinning, glaucoma, diabetes, osteoporosis, hypertension, cataracts and myopathy in the long term. Reduce side effects by limiting treatment to short periods (one to two weeks) following an acute exacerbation. Side effects with long-term use may be minimized by using alternate-day dosing regimens.

Leukotriene Receptor Antagonists (LTRAs)

Zafirlukast and **montelukast** have anti-inflammatory properties; however, current evidence suggests that LTRAs are not as effective as beclomethasone dipropionate 400 μg/day or equivalent in improving symptoms or preventing exacerbations. In general, LTRAs may be considered as alternatives to increasing doses of inhaled steroids in patients not controlled on low-moderate doses or may be used in conjunction with higher doses of inhaled steroids to achieve control of persistent symptoms.[6] Mild asthmatics who cannot take or refuse to take an inhaled corticosteroid may be tried on an LTRA.

IgE-Neutralizing Antibody

Omalizumab, a new monoclonal antibody, is indicated for patients with moderate to severe persistent asthma in those who have had a positive skin test or in vitro reactivity to a perennial aeroallergen and whose symptoms are inadequately controlled with inhaled corticosteroids. In these patients, it has been shown to significantly decrease the incidence of asthma exacerbations and improve overall asthma control.

Other Therapies

Antihistamines are not useful. The place of ketotifen in the treatment of adults has not been established. Methotrexate and gold have been used in some chronic steroid-dependent asthmatics but should be limited to centres experienced with this therapy.

Asthma in Pregnancy

The best outcome for pregnancy complicated by asthma occurs with optimal management of asthma. Short-acting inhaled $beta_2$-agonists, theophylline, cromolyn and inhaled corticosteroids (particularly budesonide) have been used extensively and are considered safe for use in pregnancy. However, theophylline may worsen gastroesophageal reflux and can cause nausea, so avoid if possible. There is limited experience with the use of LTRAs and long-acting $beta_2$-agonists during pregnancy. The risk of using medications to control asthma during pregnancy appears to be much less than the risk of adverse outcomes related to severe uncontrolled asthma.[8]

Emergency Treatment (Figure 2)

- Priorities include oxygenation, rehydration, bronchodilation and use of anti-inflammatory medications.
- Bronchodilation with a metered dose inhaler and a spacer is equivalent to nebulized therapy.[9,10]
- Additional bronchodilator effect of ipratropium bromide and the $beta_2$-agonists supports administering these two medications concomitantly.[11]
- Use oral or parenteral steroids early in most patients.[12]
- Avoid aminophylline in acute asthma.[13,14]

Therapeutic Tips

- Avoid ASA, NSAIDs and COX-2 inhibitors in ASA-induced asthmatics and in high-risk patients (i.e., severe asthma symptoms, nasal polyps, urticaria or chronic rhinitis).[15] Exercise caution in all patients.
- Exercise caution with beta-blockers.
- Treat conditions that may affect asthma control such as rhinitis, sinusitis and GERD.
- Patient education about asthma symptoms and therapy is essential for optimal management.
  - Develop a written action plan for self-management based on peak expiratory flow rates and/or signs and symptoms for each patient.
  - Review inhaler technique regularly.

Figure 1: Continuum of Asthma Management

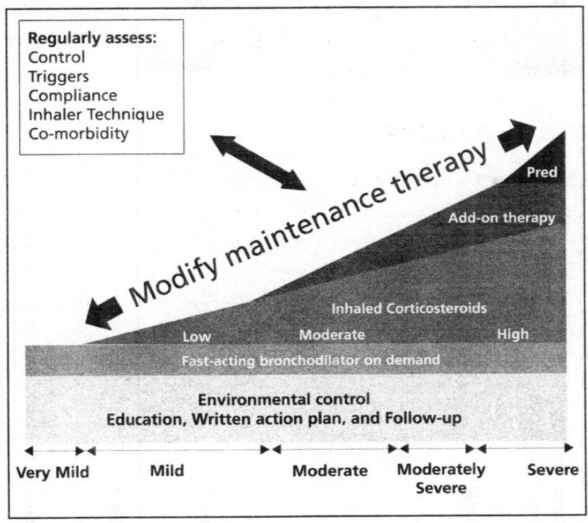

Continuum of asthma management. Very mild asthma is treated with short-acting beta$_2$-agonists, taken as needed. Inhaled corticosteroids (ICSs) may be introduced as the initial maintenance treatment for asthma, even in subjects who report asthma symptoms less than three times per week. For patients who cannot or will not use ICSs, leukotriene receptor antagonists are an alternative, although they are less effective than low doses of ICSs. If asthma is not adequately controlled by low doses of ICSs, additional therapy should be considered. Addition of long-acting beta$_2$-agonists should be considered as the first option. As an alternative, addition of leukotriene receptor antagonists or increasing ICSs to a moderate dose of may be considered. Theophylline may be considered as a third therapeutic option. Severe asthma may require additional treatment with prednisone (Pred). Asthma control should be assessed at each visit, and maintenance therapy should be altered if necessary. Any alteration in medication therapy should be considered a trial, and effectiveness should be re-evaluated after a reasonable period of time. After achieving full control, the medication should be reduced to the minimum necessary to maintain control

Reproduced with permission of Canadian Respiratory Journal 2004;11(Suppl A):9A-18A.

Figure 2: Emergency Treatment of Asthma

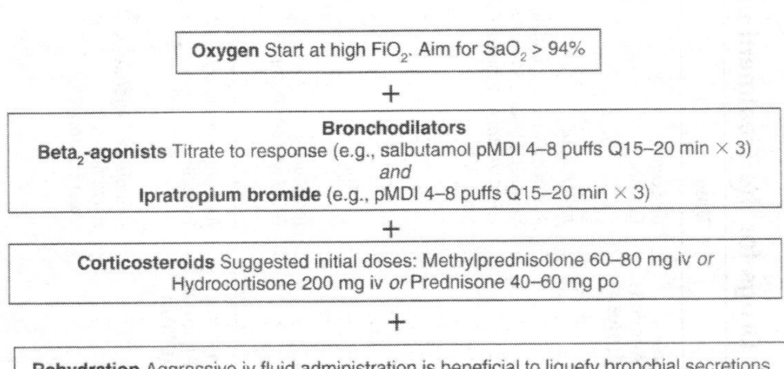

Abbreviations: FiO_2 = fraction of inspired oxygen; SaO_2 = arterial oxygen percent saturation; pMDI = pressurized metered dose inhaler

Table 2: **Drugs for the Treatment of Chronic Asthma in Adults**

Class	Drug	Dose	Adverse Effects	Comments	Cost[a]
Inhaled Beta$_2$-adrenergic Agonists, short-acting (SABA)	*fenoterol* Berotec	pMDI 100 μg/puff: 1 puff TID-QID PRN; max 8 puffs/day	Nervousness, tremor, tachycardia, palpitations.		$
	salbutamol Airomir pMDI, Ventodisk, Ventolin Diskus, Ventolin HFA, Ventolin Nebules P.F., generics	Blisters: 200–400 μg TID-QID PRN; max 1600 μg/day pMDI 100 μg/puff: 1–2 puffs TID-QID PRN; max 8 puffs/day Diskus: 200 μg TID-QID PRN; max 800 μg/day Nebules: 2.5–5 mg QID PRN	See fenoterol.		pMDI$ DPI$$
	terbutaline Bricanyl Turbuhaler	DPI 0.5 mg/puff: 1 puff Q4–6H PRN; max 6 puffs/day	See fenoterol.		$
Inhaled Beta$_2$-adrenergic Agonists, long-acting (LABA)	*formoterol fumarate* Foradil	DPI 12 μg/capsule: 1 capsule BID; max 48 μg/day	See fenoterol.		$$$
	formoterol fumarate dihydrate Oxeze Turbuhaler	DPI: 6–12 μg Q12H; max 48 μg/day	See fenoterol.		$$$

Class	Drug	Dose	Adverse Effects	Comments	Cost[a]
	salmeterol Serevent	Diskhaler 50 µg/blister: 1 blister BID Diskus 50 µg/puff: 1 puff BID	See fenoterol.		$$$$
Anticholinergic Agents, short acting	*ipratropium* Atrovent HFA	pMDI 20 µg/puff: 2 puffs Q6–8H PRN; max 240 µg/day	Dry mouth, metallic taste; mydriasis and glaucoma if released into eye.		$
Anticholinergic Agents, long acting	*tiotropium* Spiriva	DPI 18 µg/puff: 1 puff QD	See ipratropium.		$$$$
Anticholinergic/SABA Combinations	*ipratropium/ salbutamol* Combivent	Nebules: 2.5 mL (0.5 mg/2.5 mg) Q6H PRN	See ipratropium. See fenoterol.		$$
	ipratropium/ fenoterol Duovent UDV	Nebules: 4 mL (0.5/1.25 mg)Q6H PRN	See ipratropium See fenoterol.		$
Corticosteroids, inhaled	*beclomethasone* Qvar, generics	pMDI: 100–800 µg/day divided BID	Sore mouth, sore throat, dysphonia, oral thrush (can be reduced by rinsing mouth or using spacer).	Bone densitometry is suggested in patients who require high doses or have risk factors for osteoporosis. Patients with personal or family history of glaucoma (and need high-dose inhaled corticosteroids) should have IOP checked soon after starting therapy and periodically thereafter.	$$$$

(cont'd)

Table 2: **Drugs for the Treatment of Chronic Asthma in Adults** *(cont'd)*

Class	Drug	Dose	Adverse Effects	Comments	Cost[a]
	budesonide Pulmicort	DPI: 400–2400 µg/day divided BID Nebules: 0.125–2 mg/dose; dose is individualized	See beclomethasone.	See beclomethasone.	$$$$
	ciclesonide Alvesco	pMDI: 100–800 µg daily Individualize dose; max 800 µg daily divided BID	See beclomethasone.	See beclomethasone.	$$$-$$$$
	fluticasone Flovent HFA, Flovent Diskus	pMDI/DPI: 200–1000 µg/day divided BID; may ↑ to 1000 µg BID if very severe	See beclomethasone.	See beclomethasone.	$$$-$$$$
Corticosteroid/LABA Combinations	*budesonide/ formoterol fumarate dihydrate* Symbicort	DPI 100/6 µg or 200/6 µg: 1–2 puffs daily-BID; max 4 puffs/day	See budesonide See fenoterol.	Fixed dose combination inhalers are more convenient, enhance compliance, ensure the patient receives their inhaled corticosteroid with their LABA, and are less expensive than the individual agents combined. A disadvantage is a loss in dosing flexibility.	$$$$

Class	Drug	Dose	Adverse Effects	Comments	Cost[a]
	fluticasone/ salmeterol Advair pMDI, Advair Diskus	pMDI 125/25 µg or 250/25 µg: 2 puffs BID Diskus 100/50 µg or 250/50 µg or 500/50 µg: 1 puff BID	See fluticasone See fenoterol.	See budesonide.	$$$$
Leukotriene Receptor Antagonists	*montelukast* Singulair	10 mg po QHS	Headache (common), abdominal pain, flu-like symptoms.	↓ montelukast levels: carbamazepine, rifampin, phenobarbital, phenytoin.	$$$$
	zafirlukast Accolate	20 mg po BID, at least 1 h before or 2 h after meals	Headache (common), nausea, diarrhea.	↑ zafirlukast levels by ASA; may potentiate effect of warfarin; may ↑ theophylline levels; ↓ zafirlukast levels: erythromycin, theophylline, carbamazepine, rifampin, phenobarbital, phenytoin.	$$$
Theophylline Preparations	*aminophylline* Phyllocontin, generics	225–350 mg po Q12H.	Nausea, vomiting, abdominal cramps, headache, palpitations CNS stimulation.	Monitor serum levels Multiple drug interactions: phenytoin, carbamazepine, rifampin, oral contraceptives, quinolones and macrolides.	$
	oxtriphylline Choledyl elixir, generics	Initial: 200 mg QID. Maintenance dose: 800–1200 mg/day po given in 2 to 4 divided doses depending on preparation used.	See aminophylline.	Available as elixir and tablets. See aminophylline.	$

(cont'd)

Table 2: **Drugs for the Treatment of Chronic Asthma in Adults** *(cont'd)*

Class	Drug	Dose	Adverse Effects	Comments	Cost[a]
	theophylline Uniphyl, generics	Initial: 400–600 mg/day, given in 1 to 3 divided doses depending on preparation used.	See aminophylline.	See aminophylline	$
IgE-Neutralizing Antibody	*omalizumab* Xolair	150–375 mg sc every 2–4 weeks (based on patient's weight and pretreatment serum IgE level)	Injection site reactions (45%), viral infections (24%), upper respiratory tract infections (19%), headache (15%), sinusitis (16%), pharyngitis (10%). Rare: urticaria.	Store at 2–8°C. Reconstituted product may be stored for up to 8 hours at 2–8°C. Do not inject more than 150 mg at one site. After start of treatment, do not use serum IgE for dose adjustment. Omalizumab raises IgE levels which may persist for up to a year after ending the treatment.	$600/vial

[a] Includes drug cost only. Cost of inhaled agents is per unit; cost of oral medications is per 30-day supply.
Legend: $ < $15 $$ $15–30 $$-$$$ $15–45 $$$ $30–45 $$$-$$$$ $30– >45 $$$$ > $45
Abbreviations: DPI = dry powder inhaler; pMDI = pressurized metered dose inhaler; IOP = intraocular pressure; SABA = short-acting inhaled $beta_2$-agonists; LABA = long-acting inhaled $beta_2$-agonists

Suggested Readings

Boulet LP, Becker A, Berube D et al. Summary of recommendations from the Canadian Asthma Consensus Report, 1999. Canadian Asthma Consensus Group. *CMAJ* 1999;161:1-12. Available from: http://www.cmaj.ca/cgi/content/full/161/11_suppl_2/S1. Accessed June 7, 2005.

Global Initiative for Asthma. *Global strategy for asthma management and strategy*. 2002. Available from: http://www.ginasthma.com. Accessed June 7, 2005.

Lemiere C, Bai T, Balter M et al. Adult Asthma Consensus Guidelines Update 2003. *Can Respir J* 2004;11(Suppl A):9A-18A.

References

1. Chaudhuri R, Livingston E, McMahon AD et al. Effects of smoking cessation on lung function and airway inflammation in smokers with asthma. *Am J Respir Crit Care Med* 2006;174(2):127-33.
2. Adkinson NF, Eggleston PA, Eney D et al. A controlled trial of immunotherapy for asthma in allergic children. *N Engl J Med* 1997;336(5):324-31.
3. Boulet LP, Becker A, Berube D et al. Summary of recommendations from the Canadian Asthma Consensus Report, 1999. Canadian Asthma Consensus Group. *CMAJ* 1999;161:1-12.
4. Lemiere C, Bai T, Balter M et al. Adult Asthma Consensus Guidelines Update 2003. *Can Respir J* 2004;11(Suppl A):9A-18A.
5. Ind PW, Dixon CMS, Fuller RW et al. Anticholinergic blockade of beta-blocker induced bronchoconstriction. *Am Rev Respir Dis* 1989;139:1390-1394.
6. Boulet LP, Becker A, Berube D et al. Canadian Asthma Consensus Report, 1999. Canadian Asthma Consensus Group. *CMAJ* 1999;161(11 Suppl):S1-61.
7. Respiratory Review Panel. Respiratory (Asthma and COPD) Guidelines for Family Practice. Toronto: MUMS Guidelines Clearinghouse; 2007.
8. Schatz M. Interrelationships between asthma and pregnancy: a literature review. *J Allergy Clin Immunol* 1999;103(2 Pt 2):S330-6.
9. Turner MO, Patel A, Ginsburg S et al. Bronchodilator delivery in acute airflow obstruction. A meta-analysis. *Arch Intern Med* 1997;157(15):1736-44.
10. Cates CJ, Bara A, Crilly JA et al. Holding chambers (spacers) versus nebulizers for beta-agonist treatment of acute asthma. *Cochrane Database System Rev* 2006;(3):CD000052.
11. Rodrigo GJ, Castro-Rodriguez JA. Anticholinergics in the treatment of children and adults with acute asthma: a systematic review with meta-analysis. *Thorax* 2005;60:740-746.
12. Rowe BH, Spooner CH, Ducharme FM et al. Early emergency department treatment of acute asthma with systemic corticosteroids. *Cochrane Database System Rev* 2001;(1):CD002178.
13. Littenberg B. Aminophylline treatment in severe, acute asthma. A meta-analysis. *JAMA* 1988;259(11):1678-84.
14. Parameswaran K, Belda J, Rowe BH. Addition of intravenous aminophylline to beta-agonists in adults with acute asthma. *Cochrane Database System Rev* 2000;(4):CD002742.
15. Jenkins C, Costello J, Hodge L. Systematic review of prevalence of aspirin induced asthma and its implications for clinical practice. *BMJ* 2004;328(7437):434-41.

Pharmacoeconomic Considerations: Adult Asthma

Nicole Mittmann, MSc, PhD

Epidemiology	
Country	**Prevalence (%)**
Canada (2005)[1]	8.3% (2 249 703) of those aged ≥ 12 years were diagnosed with asthma

(cont'd)

Cost of Illness Data		
Country and Year of Estimate	**Direct Costs[a]**	**Indirect Costs[b]**
Canada (2004)[2]	$162 million annually for exacerbations	Not reported
Canada (1990)[3]	$306 million	$200 million

Commentary

There is a significant societal burden associated with the management of asthma. The largest component of direct costs is drugs ($124 million) and the largest component of indirect costs is illness-related disability ($76 million). Poorly controlled asthma leads to exacerbations, which are associated with large costs due to hospitalization (63%) and physician visits (20%).[2,3]

The 1996/97 National Population Health Survey (NPHS) Asthma Supplement Survey found that 43% of individuals with asthma visited their doctor one to three times and 17% visited their doctor four or more times in the previous year because of asthma. The same survey found that 18% of individuals with active asthma had visited the emergency department at least once in the previous year.[4]

A number of asthma treatments are considered to be cost-effective. Long-acting beta agonists/corticosteroids and leukotriene receptor antagonists (LTRA) reduce the frequency of exacerbations in patients who are not controlled with short-acting beta-agonists. These agents are also cost-effective in terms of their effects on lung function (FEV_1) and in reducing exacerbations.[5,6,7,8] LTRAs by themselves have not uniformly shown benefit in terms of corticosteroid-sparing effects or cost savings.[9]

Outpatient and community pharmacy interventions in patients with asthma have been shown to reduce costs associated with physician visits, emergency room visits and hospitalizations.[10,11,12]

[a] Direct costs include those associated with physician services, nursing care, diagnostic procedures, drugs and hospitalization.

[b] Indirect costs include those associated with lost productivity and days off work due to morbidity or premature mortality.

References

1. Statistics Canada. Canadian Community Health Survey. *Table 105-0401: Asthma, by age group and sex, household population aged 12 and over, Canada, provinces, territories, health regions (June 2005 boundaries) and peer groups, every 2 years*; and *Catalogue no. 82-221-X*. Ottawa (ON): Statistics Canada; 2007.
2. Seung SJ, Mittmann N. Urgent care costs of uncontrolled asthma in Canada, 2004. *Can Respir J* 2005;12(8):435-6.
3. Krahn MD, Berka C, Langlois P et al. Direct and indirect costs of asthma in Canada, 1990. *CMAJ* 1996;154(6):821-31.
4. Health Canada. *National Population Health Survey (NPHS) Asthma Supplement 1996/97 (Health Canada)*. Ottawa (ON): Health Canada.
5. Sheth K, Borker R, Emmett A et al. Cost-effectiveness comparison of salmeterol/fluticasone propionate versus montelukast in the treatment of adults with persistent asthma. *Pharmacoeconomics* 2002;20(13):909-18.

6. O'Connor RD, Nelson H, Borker R et al. Cost effectiveness of fluticasone propionate plus salmeterol versus fluticasone propionate plus montelukast in the treatment of persistent asthma. *Pharmacoeconomics* 2004;22(12):815-25.
7. Rutten-van Molken MP, Van Doorslaer EK, Jansen MC et al. Costs and effects of inhaled corticosteroid in asthma and chronic obstructive pulmonary disease. *Am J Respir Crit Care Med* 1995;151(4):975-82.
8. Johansson G, Andreasson EB, Larsson PE et al. Cost effectiveness of budesonide/formoterol for maintenance and reliever therapy versus salmeterol/fluticasone plus salbutamol in the treatment of asthma. *Pharmacoeconomics* 2006;24(7):695-708.
9. Scow DT, Luttermoser GK, Dickerson KS. Leukotriene inhibitors in the treatment of allergy and asthma. *Am Fam Physician* 2007;75(1):65-70.
10. Statistics Canada; Health Canada; Canadian Lung Association et al. *Respiratory disease in Canada.* Ottawa (ON): Statistics Canada; 2001. Available from: http://www.phac-aspc.gc.ca/publicat/rdc-mrc01/pdf/rdc0901e.pdf Accessed June 28, 2007.
11. Rupp MT, McCallian DJ, Sheth KK. Developing and marketing a community-based asthma management program. *J Am Pharm Assoc (Wash)* 1997;NS37:694-9.
12. McLean W, Gillis J, Waller R. The BC Community Pharmacy Asthma Project: a study of clinical, economic and holistic outcomes influenced by asthma care protocol provided by specially trained community pharmacists in British Columbia. *Can Respir J* 2003;10(4):195-202.

CHAPTER 48
Asthma in Infants and Children

Mark Montgomery, MD, FRCPC

Goals of Therapy

- Prevent cough, wheeze or shortness of breath which interferes with daytime activities, exercise, school attendance or sleep
- Reduce use of $beta_2$-agonists for symptom relief to < 4 doses/week
- Avoid emergency room visits or hospitalizations
- Achieve normal measures of expiratory airflow, such as peak flows or pulmonary function studies, e.g., forced expiratory volume in one second (FEV_1)
- Avoid/minimize medication side effects, especially on growth and development

Investigations

- Diagnosis of asthma in children under the age of 6 years depends on history and physical examination since pulmonary function tests are not easily obtained[1]
- History:
  - evidence suggesting airway hyperreactivity, e.g., wheeze or chest tightness that limits activities, cough that is worse at night, cough with duration longer than usual for an upper respiratory tract infection (URTI)
  - evidence of inherited hyperreactivity, e.g., eczema, multiple food or inhalant allergies, positive family history of asthma, atopy
  - consider features that suggest the cough or respiratory concern is related to conditions other than asthma:
    - associated evidence of malabsorption or failure to thrive, e.g., cystic fibrosis
    - associated swallowing difficulties or choking, e.g., vascular compression of the airway
    - shortness of breath associated with weak voice and/or absent at night or with sleep, e.g., vocal cord dysfunction[2]
    - recurrent otitis media and sinusitis, e.g., primary ciliary dyskinesia
- Physical examination:
  - presence of eczema and allergic rhinitis suggest that the child has inherited the atopic tendency and that the cause of cough or wheeze is related to asthma

- nasal polyps in a prepubertal child or finger clubbing in an individual of any age suggest that the primary cause of the cough is more likely related to cystic fibrosis, not asthma
- localized findings on exam, particularly if the wheeze or cough had a sudden onset, suggest aspiration of a foreign body
- other physical findings: hyperexpansion of thorax, sounds of wheezing during normal breathing or a forced exhalation, increased nasal secretion, pale mucosal swelling

- Objective measurements needed to confirm diagnosis and assess severity include:
  - perform spirometry at least annually on all children over 6 years of age who are using asthma medication regularly to maintain asthma control. Peak flow rates in children are an insensitive indicator of airflow limitation. There may be significant airflow limitation in the presence of normal peak flows
  - explore specific allergies to inhalants by history and/or skin testing[3]

Therapeutic Choices

Nonpharmacologic Choices

- Avoid exposure to cigarette smoke.[4,5,6,7,8]
- Avoid known allergens.[4,5,9] Evaluate and individualize environmental control measures.
- Recommend annual influenza vaccine for children with asthma.[10]
- Educate patients and children regarding chronicity of asthma.

Pharmacologic Choices (Figure 1, Table 2)

Principles of Management

Asthma symptoms are due to narrowing and hyperreactivity of airways. Airway obstruction is due to bronchospasm and airway inflammation. **Beta-agonists** provide short-term relief from bronchospasm and have no effect on airway inflammation. If wheeze and shortness of breath are not relieved by a beta-agonist, consider the contribution of airway inflammation. Regular use of an **inhaled corticosteroid** to treat airway inflammation is required if there is inadequate relief of wheeze or shortness of breath following use of a beta-agonist. Inhaled corticosteroids control airway obstruction within weeks of initiation of therapy. Regular use for months or years is required to control airway inflammation.[11,12] The episodic use of inhaled corticosteroids for a few weeks at a time may reduce airway obstruction, but is unlikely to have a lasting impact on airway hyperreactivity. Symptom control generally occurs with low doses (e.g., budesonide 200 µg/day).[13,14,15,16] The vast majority of children with asthma experience good asthma control with doses of fluticasone 500 µg/day or equivalent. Reconsider diagnosis in children whose asthma is poorly controlled at these doses.

Drug Delivery Devices

Inhalation is the preferred route of administration because therapeutic effect is maximized and systemic side effects minimized. The hydrofluoroalkane propellants (HFA) used in *pressurized metered dose inhalers (pMDIs)* demonstrate excellent lung deposition.[17]

Review *inhalation technique* regularly. For infants and young children (< 5 years), a pMDI and spacer device with mask attachment is useful. Assess very young infants for their ability to produce sufficient respiratory effort to open and close the valves of a spacer device. Consider a switch to wet nebulization if there is evidence that they cannot effectively use the spacer device. Drug deposition with a pMDI and spacer in infants and young children is generally 10 to 20% of the deposition in adults.[18] Therefore, adult doses may be required in children.[19] In older children (≥ 5 years), either a dry powder system (e.g., Diskus, Turbuhaler) or a pMDI with spacer device may be used. Compliance may be enhanced if the child selects the device that works best for them.

Wet nebulization is a less attractive alternative due to difficulties with portability and time required for therapy.[20] Furthermore, lung deposition of drug is compromised if technique is not meticulous, for example when the mask is not on the child's face, if tubing is used rather than the mask or if a soother is in the infant's mouth.

Incentive spirometers provide visual feedback to children about their inspiratory flows and can be invaluable teaching devices.

Bronchodilator Agents

Short-acting Inhaled Beta$_2$-agonists (SABA)

Short-acting beta$_2$-agonists (**salbutamol**, **terbutaline**) effectively relieve smooth muscle spasm, but do not reduce airway reactivity or inflammation. Use on an as-needed basis provides both rapid relief and valuable information on underlying asthma control. Regular use of beta$_2$-agonists, four or more times per week, indicates suboptimal long-term control.[21] Assess children who derive inadequate relief from beta$_2$-agonists or relief for less than two hours; a course of systemic corticosteroids may be required. Beta$_2$-agonists are very effective at providing relief from wheeze or shortness of breath. Consider alternate diagnoses in all children who do not benefit from beta$_2$-agonist use.

Administration of a SABA 5 to 10 minutes before exercise prevents exercise-induced bronchospasm for up to 2 to 4 hours.[22]

Long-acting Inhaled Beta$_2$-agonists (LABA)

Long-acting beta$_2$-agonists (**salmeterol**, **formoterol**) provide up to 12 hours of symptom control and protection from exercise-induced bronchospasm.[23] Do not use these agents as maintenance monotherapy in asthma. Formoterol has a rapid onset of action similar to that of salbutamol. In adults, regular use of a long-acting beta$_2$-agonist combined with an inhaled corticosteroid enhances asthma control more than the use of the inhaled corticosteroid alone.[24,25,26] The safety and efficacy of this combination in children is still undetermined.[27,28] At present it should be reserved as add-on therapy if asthma is uncontrolled by moderate to high doses of inhaled corticosteroids.[5]

Oral Beta$_2$-agonists

Oral beta-agonists for asthma management in children have largely been supplanted by the inhalation form due to vastly improved efficacy and reduction in systemic side effects.

Anticholinergic Agents

Restrict use of **ipratropium** to adjunctive therapy in acute severe asthma in children.

Methylxanthines

Theophylline preparations, used as add-on therapy, may have an additional anti-inflammatory role in patients already using inhaled corticosteroid therapy.[29,30] The anti-inflammatory effect of theophylline occurs at serum levels lower than those employed in an attempt to relieve bronchospasm.[31] Theophylline is rarely used for routine maintenance of asthma because of the potential for toxicity, numerous drug interactions and the need for monitoring serum levels.

Anti-inflammatory Agents

Inhaled Corticosteroids

Inhaled corticosteroids (ICS) (**beclomethasone**, **budesonide**, **fluticasone**) are the cornerstone of asthma management in infants and children, both to reduce and control symptoms and to prevent airway remodeling.[3] Regular use of ICS reduces mortality and asthma exacerbations, improves pulmonary function and controls symptoms, reduces the need for rescue bronchodilator treatment, reduces the need for oral steroids to treat exacerbations and may decrease airway remodeling. ICS do not prevent development of asthma in preschool children at high risk.[32] ICS do not cure asthma. Cessation following months of regular use may result in return of airway hyperreactivity to the previous status.

Symptom control generally occurs within days with low doses (e.g., budesonide 200 µg/day);[33] however, reduction in airway hyperreactivity may require months of regular use.[11,12] The vast majority of children with asthma experience good asthma control with doses of fluticasone 500 µg/day or equivalent.[13,14,15,16] Reconsider the diagnosis in children whose asthma is poorly controlled at these doses.

The practice of doubling the dose of an ICS in response to a viral respiratory tract infection or to control an exacerbation of asthma is controversial.[34,35,36,37] Review the effectiveness of this strategy for each patient.

Doses of budesonide < 400 μg/day or equivalent have minimal systemic side effects. Studies indicate that there is an initial decrease in growth rate during the first year of ICS use, but it is not sustained with long-term therapy. ICS use does not affect final adult height.[38,39,40,41]

Table 1: **Comparative Dose Equivalencies for Inhaled Corticosteroids[4] in Children < 12 y**

Drug	Low Dose	Moderate Dose	High Dose
Beclomethasone dipropionate pMDI	100–200 μg	201–400 μg	> 400 μg
Budesonide DPI	100–200 μg	201–400 μg	> 400 μg
Budesonide nebulizer	250–500 μg	501–1000 μg	> 1000 μg
Fluticasone propionate DPI or pMDI plus spacer	100–200 μg	201–400 μg	> 400 μg

Abbreviations: pMDI = pressurized metered dose inhaler; DPI = dry powder inhaler

Leukotriene Receptor Antagonists (LTRAs)

LTRAs (**zafirlukast, montelukast**) may provide bronchoprotection in ASA-sensitive asthmatics and with exercise.[3,11] However, ASA-sensitive asthmatics should still avoid the use of NSAIDs when on LTRAs. These agents may have steroid-sparing properties, allowing improved control of asthma at a reduced dose of inhaled corticosteroid.[42,43,44] As monotherapy, they exert the equivalent control on airway inflammation of about fluticasone 100 μg/day.[45] Monotherapy with montelukast has resulted in improved asthma control and reduced asthma exacerbations in preschool children.[46,47] Due to insufficient evidence, LTRAs are not recommended as first choice for monotherapy in children.[5]

LTRAs can be used as adjunct therapy with moderate to high doses of inhaled corticosteroids to achieve control of persistent asthma or in patients who cannot or will not use inhaled corticosteroids.

There are reports of development of Churg-Strauss syndrome, an eosinophilic vasculitis, with use of LTRAs but these most likely represent an unmasking of the vasculitis as doses of systemic corticosteroids are reduced.[48,49,50]

Anti-IgE Therapy

Omalizumab, a recombinant humanized monoclonal antibody that binds IgE receptors impeding the IgE-mediated allergic response, is indicated for allergic asthma. The agent has demonstrated reduced asthma exacerbations and allowed reduction in the dose of inhaled corticosteroid with improved asthma symptom control. The dose is titrated based on body weight and serum IgE level. Administer by subcutaneous injection every 2 to 4 weeks.[51,52]

Adjunctive Anti-inflammatory Therapy

Ketotifen has largely been supplanted by the regular use of low-dose inhaled corticosteroids and/or LTRAs. This agent is safe and primarily used for the management of mild asthma. Antihistamines will assist in control of allergic rhinoconjunctivitis and/or eczema but have minimal impact on asthma control or symptoms.

Acute Asthma Management (Figure 2)

An exacerbation of asthma requiring an emergency room visit, unscheduled doctor visit or hospitalization is a failure of long-term management. Immediate care for respiratory distress, evaluation of the cause of the exacerbation and intensification of long-term management are indicated.

Manage acute severe asthma as a pediatric emergency. Initial therapy should be aggressive and then reduced as the exacerbation settles. Ideally, a child with asthma should not deteriorate once in hospital.

Perform pulse oximetry or an arterial blood gas and initiate supplemental oxygen in all asthmatic children with respiratory distress.

The cornerstones of therapy are supplemental oxygen, frequent high-dose inhaled beta$_2$-agonist and systemic corticosteroids (e.g, prednisolone). Ipratropium bromide may provide additional bronchodilation.[53,54] Intravenous magnesium or salbutamol are adjunctive therapies.[55,56,57] There is no evidence that aminophylline provides additional bronchodilation beyond that produced by frequent high-dose beta$_2$-agonists and systemic corticosteroids.[58,59] Avoid sedation. Correct mild to moderate dehydration if present.

Close observation and reassessment of all children with acute severe asthma is mandatory. Closely follow up all children discharged home from the emergency department.

Therapeutic Tips

- Use agents for long-term control (i.e., inhaled corticosteroids) for a minimum of several months after symptoms have resolved to ensure that airway hyperreactivity is controlled.
- pMDIs and DPIs are as effective as nebulizers in acute severe asthma. Choice of delivery device depends on familiarity with use and availability of health care providers.
- Review inhaler technique regularly to ensure optimal use of devices.
- Provide written instructions that describe signs of worsening asthma: cough, wheeze or shortness of breath that interferes with sleep; cough, wheeze or shortness of breath that interferes with activities; regular use of beta$_2$-agonist for relief; drop in peak flow rates.
- Provide written instructions for the family regarding actions to take when signs of worsening asthma are detected.

- If there is little improvement with $beta_2$-agonists or systemic steroids, the diagnosis of asthma is in doubt. Inadequate response to appropriate therapy mandates reassessment of the patient to establish the appropriate diagnosis or identify concomitant conditions, e.g., gastroesophageal reflux, postnasal drip/sinusitis, vocal cord dysfunction.

Figure 1: **Maintenance Therapy of Asthma in Children**

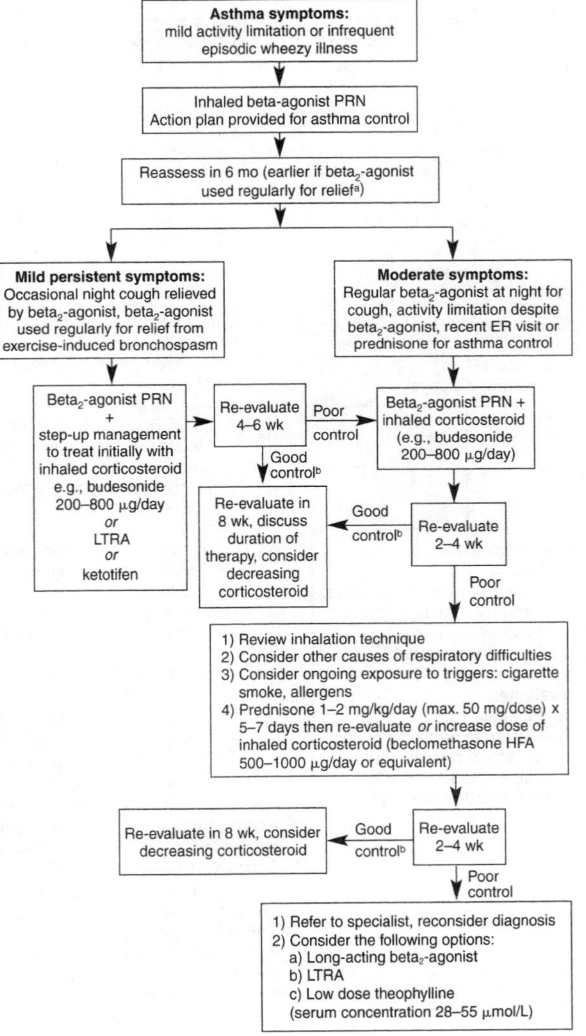

[a] Regular use of beta$_2$-agonist: use > 4 times/week for relief
[b] Good asthma control: see Goals of Therapy
Abbreviations: LTRA = leukotriene receptor antagonist

Figure 2: **Treatment of Acute Asthma in Children**

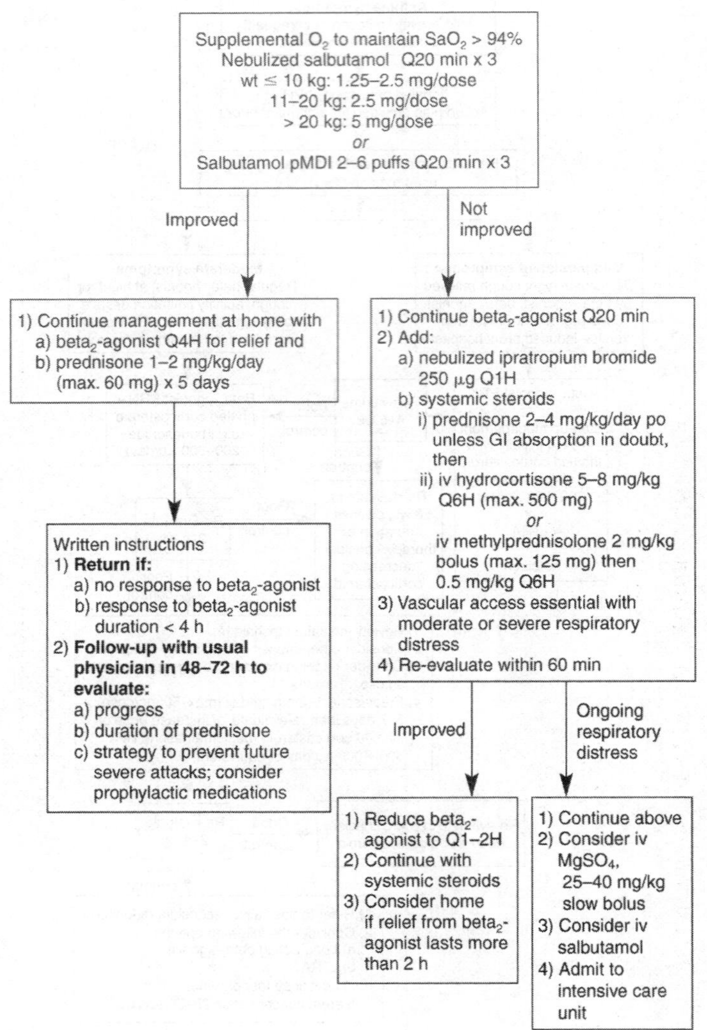

Abbreviations: SaO_2 = arterial oxygen percent saturation; pMDI = pressurized metered dose inhaler

Table 2: **Drugs Used for Maintenance Therapy for Asthma in Children**

Class	Drug	Dose	Adverse Effects	Comments	Cost[a]
Inhaled Beta$_2$-agonists, short-acting (SABA)	*salbutamol* Airomir MDI, Ventodisk, Ventolin Diskus, Ventolin HFA MDI, Ventolin Nebules P.F., generics	Blisters/Diskhaler: ≥ 6 y: 200 µg TID–QID; max 800 µg/day pMDI 100 µg/puff: adult doses may be required due to poor deposition[19,20,21] 4–11 y: 1 inhalation TID–QID; max 400 µg/day ≥ 12 y: 1–2 inhalations TID–QID; max 800 µg/day Diskus 200 µg/blister: ≥ 4 y: 1 inhalation TID–QID; max 800 µg/day Nebules: 5–12 y: 1.25–2.5 mg as a single dose; max 5 mg. May repeat QID	Tachycardia, palpitations, nervousness, tremor, hypokalemia.	Prevents exercise-induced bronchospasm for up to 2–4 h. Provides relief and information on asthma control in that regular use indicates poor control, use of ≥ 1 canister per month associated with increased risk of asthma mortality.	\$–\$\$
	terbutaline Bricanyl Turbuhaler	DPI 0.5 mg/puff: ≥ 6 y: 1 inhalation PRN. Max 6 puffs/24 h	See salbutamol.	See salbutamol.	\$\$

(cont'd)

Table 2: **Drugs Used for Maintenance Therapy for Asthma in Children** *(cont'd)*

Class	Drug	Dose	Adverse Effects	Comments	Cost[a]
Inhaled Beta$_2$-agonists, long-acting (LABA)	*formoterol fumarate* Foradil Aerolizer	DPI 12 µg/capsule: 6–16 y: 1 capsule inhaled Q12H in the morning and evening; max 48 µg/day	See salbutamol. Possibility of tolerance with regular use.	Not to be used as monotherapy. Provides protection from exercise-induced bronchospasm for 10 h.	$$$
	formoterol fumarate dihydrate Oxeze Turbuhaler	DPI: 6–16 y: 6–12 µg Q12H; max 24 µg/daily	See salbutamol. Possibility of tolerance with regular use.	Not to be used as monotherapy. Provides protection from exercise-induced bronchospasm for 10 h.	$$$
	salmeterol Serevent	Diskhaler 50 µg/blister: ≥ 4 y: 1 blister Q12H Diskus 50 µg/puff: ≥ 4 y: 1 inhalation Q12H	See salbutamol. Possibility of tolerance with regular use.	Not for immediate relief. Not to be used as monotherapy. Provides protection from exercise-induced bronchospasm for 10 h.	$$$$
Corticosteroids, inhaled	*beclomethasone* Qvar, generics	Individualize dose. Adult doses may be required due to poor deposition.[19,20,21] pMDI: 100–800 µg/day divided BID 5–11 y: 50 µg BID; max 100 µg BID	Oral thrush, dysphonia.	Follow linear growth every 3–6 mo with regular asthma reassessments. Short-term growth rate may be slowed during first y of inhaled corticosteroid use but is not shown to be sustained. No evidence to date that inhaled corticosteroids impact final adult height. Dysphonia and candidiasis can be decreased by use of spacer with pMDI and rinsing after use. Dose response studies show majority of corticosteroid effect on asthma control is achieved with doses under 800 µg/day of beclomethasone dipropionate or equivalent;[15] children requiring more than this on a regular basis should be assessed by a specialist.	$–$$$$

Class	Drug	Dose	Adverse Effects	Comments	Cost[a]
				Regular re-evaluation required to ensure that lowest effective dose of inhaled corticosteroid being used to maintain control.	
	budesonide Pulmicort Turbuhaler	Individualize dose. DPI: 6–12 y: 200–400 µg/day divided BID Nebules: Individualize dose. 3 mo–12 y: 0.25–0.5 mg BID; may ↑ to 1 mg BID	See beclomethasone.	See beclomethasone.	$$$–$$$$
	fluticasone Flovent HFA, Flovent Diskus	Individualize dose. Adult doses may be required due to poor deposition.[19,20,21] pMDI, DPI: > 16 y: 100–500 µg BID; max 1000 µg BID 4–16 y: 50–100 µg BID; may ↑ to 200 µg BID pMDI: 12 mo–4 y: 50–100 µg BID	See beclomethasone.	See beclomethasone.	$$–$$$$

(cont'd)

Table 2: **Drugs Used for Maintenance Therapy for Asthma in Children** *(cont'd)*

Class	Drug	Dose	Adverse Effects	Comments	Cost[a]
Corticosteroid/ LABA Combinations	*budesonide/ formoterol fumarate dihydrate* Symbicort	DPI 100/6 μg or 200/6 μg: ≥ 12 y: 1–2 inhalations once or BID; max 4 inhalations daily for maintenance therapy, may ↑ temporarily to 4 inhalations BID for worsening asthma	See formoterol fumarate dihydrate. See budesonide.	Fixed-dose combination inhalers are more convenient, enhance compliance, ensure the patient receives their inhaled corticosteroid with their LABA and are less expensive than the individual agents combined. A disadvantage is a loss in dosing flexibility.	$$$$
	fluticasone/ salmeterol Advair MDI, Advair Diskus	pMDI 125/25 μg or 250/25 μg: ≥ 12 y: 2 inhalations BID Diskus 100/50 μg: 4–11 y: 1 inhalation BID	See salmeterol. See fluticasone.	See budesonide/formoterol fumarate dihydrate.	$$$$
Leukotriene Receptor Antagonists	*montelukast* Singulair	≥ 15 y: 10 mg at HS 6–14 y: 5 mg, chewable at HS 2–5 y: 4 mg, chewable or granules at HS	Headache, abdominal pain, flu-like symptoms.	Levels may ↑ by carbamazepine, rifampin, phenytoin.	$$$–$$$$
	zafirlukast Accolate	≥ 12 y: 20 mg BID 1 h before or 2 h after meals	Headache, nausea, diarrhea.	May ↑ levels by ASA; may potentiate effect of warfarin, monitor INR and adjust dose as necessary; may ↑ theophylline levels; levels may ↓ by erythromycin, carbamazepine, rifampin, phenobarbital, phenytoin.	$$$

Class	Drug	Dose	Adverse Effects	Comments	Cost[a]
Anti-inflammatories, miscellaneous	*ketotifen* [renal icon] Zaditen, generics	< 3 y: 0.5 mg po BID ≥ 3 y: 1 mg po BID	Sedation, weight gain.	May require 8–12 wk for effect. Clinical effectiveness, i.e., reduction in use of rescue bronchodilator, rescue oral steroids and in exacerbations, most noted in children aged 4 mo to 18 y with mild asthma.	$$–$$$$
IgE-Neutralizing Antibody	*omalizumab* Xolair	≥12 y: Variable dosing depending on serum IgE and body weight	Common: injection site reactions, viral infections, upper respiratory tract infections, headache, sinusitis, pharyngitis. Rare: urticaria.	Store at 2–8°C. Reconstituted product may be stored for up to 8 h at 2–8°C. Not to inject more than 150 mg at one site. After start of treatment, do not use serum IgE for dose adjustment. Omalizumab raises IgE levels which may persist for up to a year after end of treatment.	$635/ 150 mg vial

[a] Includes drug cost only. Cost of inhaled agents is per unit; cost of inhalation capsules or oral medications is per 30-day supply.

[renal icon] Dosage adjustment may be required in renal dysfunction; see Appendix I.

Legend: $ < $15 $-$$ < $15–30 $$ $15–30 $$$ $30–45 $-$$$$ < $15– > 45 $$-$$$$ $15– > 45 $$$-$$$$ $30– > 45 $$$$ > $45

Abbreviations: DPI = dry powder inhaler; pMDI = pressurized metered dose inhaler

Suggested Readings

Donnell AT, Kumar R. Pediatric asthma: principles and treatment. *Allergy Asthma Proc* 2004;25(4 Suppl 1):S23-5.

FitzGerald JM, editor. *Evidence-based asthma management.* Hamilton (ON): B.C. Decker; 2001.

Global Initiative for Asthma. *Pocket guide for asthma management and prevention in children: a pocket guide for physicians and nurses* (updated 2006). Available from: http://www.ginasthma.com/Guidelineitem.asp?l1=2&l2=1&intID=49 Accessed January 24, 2007.

References

1. Respiratory Review Panel. Respiratory (Asthma and COPD) Guidelines for Family Practice. Toronto: MUMS Guidelines Clearinghouse; 2007.
2. Tilles SA. Vocal cord dysfunction in children and adolescents. *Curr Allergy Asthma Rep* 2003;3(6):467-72.
3. Djukanovic R. Airway inflammation in asthma and its consequences: implications for treatment in children and adults. *J Allergy Clin Immunol* 2002;109(6 Suppl):S539-48.
4. Global Initiative for Asthma. *Pocket guide for asthma management and prevention in children: a pocket guide for physicians and nurses* (updated 2006). Available from: http://www.ginasthma.com/Guidelineitem.asp?l1=2&l2=1&intID=49 Accessed January 24, 2007.
5. Becker A, Berube D, Chad Z et al. Canadian Pediatric Asthma Consensus guidelines, 2003 (updated to December 2004): introduction. *CMAJ* 2005;173(6 Suppl):S12-4.
6. Strachan DP, Cook DG. Health effects of passive smoking. 5. Parental smoking and allergic sensitisation in children. *Thorax* 1998;53(2):117-23.
7. Cook DG, Strachan DP. Health effects of passive smoking. 3. Parental smoking and prevalence of respiratory symptoms and asthma in school age children. *Thorax* 1997;52(12):1081-94.
8. Strachan DP, Cook DG. Health effects of passive smoking. 1. Parental smoking and lower respiratory illness in infancy and early childhood. *Thorax* 1997;52(10):905-14.
9. Morgan WJ, Crain EF, Gruchalla RS et al. Results of a home-based environmental intervention among urban children with asthma. *N Engl J Med* 2004;351(11):1068-80.
10. National Advisory Committee on Immunization (NACI). Statement on influenza vaccination for the 2006-2007 season. An Advisory Committee Statement (ACS). *Can Commun Dis Rep* 2006;32(ACS-7):1-27.
11. Haahtela T, Jarvinen M, Kava T et al. Comparison of a beta 2-agonist, terbutaline, with an inhaled corticosteroid, budesonide, in newly detected asthma. *N Engl J Med* 1991;325(6):388-92.
12. Nielsen KG, Bisgaard H. The effect of inhaled budesonide on symptoms, lung function, and cold air and methacholine responsiveness in 2- to 5-year-old asthmatic children. *Am J Respir Crit Care Med* 2000;162(4 Pt 1):1500-6.
13. Bisgaard H. Delivery of inhaled medication to children. *J Asthma* 1997;34(6):443-67.
14. Bisgaard H, Gillies J, Groenewald M et al. The effect of inhaled fluticasone propionate in the treatment of young asthmatic children: a dose comparison study. *Am J Respir Crit Care Med* 1999;160(1):126-31.
15. Pedersen S, Hansen OR. Budesonide treatment of moderate and severe asthma in children: a dose-response study. *J Allergy Clin Immunol* 1995;95(1 Pt 1):29-33.
16. Visser MJ, Postma DS, Arends LR et al. One-year treatment with different dosing schedules of fluticasone propionate in childhood asthma. Effects on hyperresponsiveness, lung function, and height. *Am J Respir Crit Care Med* 2001;164(11):2073-7.
17. Pedersen S, Warner J, Wahn U et al. Growth, systemic safety, and efficacy during 1 year of asthma treatment with different beclomethasone dipropionate formulations: an open-label, randomized comparison of extrafine and conventional aerosols in children. *Pediatrics* 2002;109(6):e92.
18. Salmon B, Wilson NM, Silverman M. How much aerosol reaches the lungs of wheezy infants and toddlers? *Arch Dis Child* 1990;65(4):401-3.
19. Tal A, Golan H, Grauer N et al. Deposition pattern of radiolabeled salbutamol inhaled from a metered-dose inhaler by means of a spacer with mask in young children with airway obstruction. *J Pediatr* 1996;128(4):479-84.
20. Castro-Rodriguez JA, Rodrigo GJ. beta-agonists through metered-dose inhaler with valved holding chamber versus nebulizer for acute exacerbation of wheezing or asthma in children under 5 years of age: a systematic review with meta-analysis. *J Pediatr* 2004;145(2):172-7.
21. Boulet LP, Becker A, Berube D et al. Canadian Asthma Consensus Report, 1999. Canadian Asthma Consensus Group. *CMAJ* 1999;161(11 Suppl):S1-61.

22. Anderson SD, Seale JP, Rozea P et al. Inhaled and oral salbutamol in exercise-induced asthma. *Am Rev Respir Dis* 1976;114(3):493-500.
23. Green CP, Price JF. Prevention of exercise induced asthma by inhaled salmeterol xinafoate. *Arch Dis Child* 1992;67(8):1014-7.
24. Greening AP, Ind PW, Northfield M et al. Added salmeterol versus higher-dose corticosteroid in asthma patients with symptoms on existing inhaled corticosteroid. Allen & Hanburys Limited UK Study Group. *Lancet* 1994;344(8917):219-24.
25. Pauwels RA, Lofdahl CG, Postma DS et al. Effect of inhaled formoterol and budesonide on exacerbations of asthma. Formoterol and Corticosteroids Establishing Therapy (FACET) International Study Group. *N Engl J Med* 1997;337(20):1405-11.
26. Shrewsbury S, Pyke S, Britton M. Meta-analysis of increased dose of inhaled steroid or addition of salmeterol in symptomatic asthma (MIASMA). *BMJ* 2000;320(7246):1368-73.
27. Simons FE. A comparison of beclomethasone, salmeterol, and placebo in children with asthma. Canadian Beclomethasone Dipropionate-Salmeterol Xinafoate Study Group. *N Engl J Med* 1997;337(23):1659-65.
28. Verberne AA, Frost C, Roorda RJ et al. One year treatment with salmeterol compared with beclomethasone in children with asthma. The Dutch Paediatric Asthma Study Group. *Am J Respir Crit Care Med* 1997;156(3 Pt 1):688-95.
29. Evans DJ, Taylor DA, Zetterstrom O et al. A comparison of low-dose inhaled budesonide plus theophylline and high-dose inhaled budesonide for moderate asthma. *N Engl J Med* 1997;337(20):1412-8.
30. Ukena D, Harnest U, Sakalauskas R et al. Comparison of addition of theophylline to inhaled steroid with doubling of the dose of inhaled steroid in asthma. *Eur Respir J* 1997;10(12):2754-60.
31. Weinberger M, Hendeles L. Theophylline in asthma. *N Engl J Med* 1996;334(21):1380-8.
32. Guilbert TW, Morgan WJ, Zeiger RS et al. Long-term inhaled corticosteroids in preschool children at high risk for asthma. *N Engl J Med* 2006;354(19):1985-97.
33. Shapiro G, Bronsky EA, LaForce CF et al. Dose-related efficacy of budesonide administered via a dry powder inhaler in the treatment of children with moderate to severe persistent asthma. *J Pediatr* 1998;132(6):976-82.
34. Doull IJ, Lampe FC, Smith S et al. Effect of inhaled corticosteroids on episodes of wheezing associated with viral infection in school age children: randomised double blind placebo controlled trial. *BMJ* 1997;315(7112):858-62.
35. Garrett J, Williams S, Wong C et al. Treatment of acute asthmatic exacerbations with an increased dose of inhaled steroid. *Arch Dis Child* 1998;79(1):12-7.
36. Hendeles L, Sherman J. Are inhaled corticosteroids effective for acute exacerbations of asthma in children? *J Pediatr* 2003;142(2 Suppl):S26-32.
37. Wilson N, Sloper K, Silverman M. Effect of continuous treatment with topical corticosteroid on episodic viral wheeze in preschool children. *Arch Dis Child* 1995;72(4):317-20.
38. Agertoft L, Pedersen S. Effect of long-term treatment with inhaled budesonide on adult height in children with asthma. *N Engl J Med* 2000;343(15):1064-9.
39. Pedersen S. Do inhaled corticosteroids inhibit growth in children? *Am J Respir Crit Care Med* 2001;164(4):521-35.
40. Silverstein MD, Yunginger JW, Reed CE et al. Attained adult height after childhood asthma: effect of glucocorticoid therapy. *J Allergy Clin Immunol* 1997;99(4):466-74.
41. Leone FT, Fish JE, Szefler SJ et al. Systematic review of the evidence regarding potential complications of inhaled corticosteroid use in asthma: collaboration of American College of Chest Physicians, American Academy of Allergy, Asthma, and Immunology, and American College of Allergy, Asthma, and Immunology. *Chest* 2003;124(6):2329-40.
42. Ducharme FM. Anti-leukotrienes as add-on therapy to inhaled glucocorticoids in patients with asthma: systematic review of current evidence. *BMJ* 2002;324(7353):1545.
43. Lofdahl CG, Reiss TF, Leff JA et al. Randomised, placebo controlled trial of effect of a leukotriene receptor antagonist, montelukast, on tapering inhaled corticosteroids in asthmatic patients. *BMJ* 1999;319(7202):87-90.
44. Tamaoki J, Kondo M, Sakai N et al. Leukotriene antagonist prevents exacerbation of asthma during reduction of high-dose inhaled corticosteroid. The Tokyo Joshi-Idai Asthma Research Group. *Am J Respir Crit Care Med* 1997;155(4):1235-40.
45. Busse W, Raphael GD, Galant S et al. Low-dose fluticasone propionate compared with montelukast for first-line treatment of persistent asthma: a randomized clinical trial. *J Allergy Clin Immunol* 2001;107(3):461-8.
46. Bisgaard H, Zielen S, Garcia-Garcia ML et al. Montelukast reduces asthma exacerbations in 2- to 5-year-old children with intermittent asthma. *Am J Respir Crit Care Med* 2005;171(4):315-22.
47. Straub DA, Moeller A, Minocchieri S et al. The effect of montelukast on lung function and exhaled nitric oxide in infants with early childhood asthma. *Eur Respir J* 2005;25(2):289-94.
48. Boccagni C, Tesser F, Mittino D et al. Churg-Strauss syndrome associated with the leukotriene antagonist montelukast. *Neurol Sci* 2004;25(1):21-2.
49. Tang MB, Yosipovitch G. Acute Churg-Strauss syndrome in an asthmatic patient receiving montelukast therapy. *Arch Dermatol* 2003;139(6):715-8.

50. Turvey SE, Vargas SO, Phipatanakul W. Churg-Strauss syndrome in a 7-year-old receiving montelukast and inhaled corticosteroids. *Ann Allergy Asthma Immunol* 2003;90(2):274.
51. Milgrom H. Is there a role for treatment of asthma with omalizumab? *Arch Dis Child* 2003;88(1):71-4.
52. Ruffin CG, Busch BE. Omalizumab: a recombinant humanized anti-IgE antibody for allergic asthma. *Am J Health Syst Pharm* 2004;61(14):1449-59.
53. Rodrigo GJ, Castro-Rodriguez JA. Anticholinergics in the treatment of children and adults with acute asthma: a systematic review with meta-analysis. *Thorax* 2005;60(9):740-6.
54. Plotnick LH, Ducharme FM. Should inhaled anticholinergics be added to beta2 agonists for treating acute childhood and adolescent asthma? A systematic review. *BMJ* 1998;317(7164):971-7.
55. Browne GJ, Penna AS, Phung X et al. Randomised trial of intravenous salbutamol in early management of acute severe asthma in children. *Lancet* 1997;349(9048):301-5.
56. Ciarallo L, Brousseau D, Reinert S. Higher-dose intravenous magnesium therapy for children with moderate to severe acute asthma. *Arch Pediatr Adolesc Med* 2000;154(10):979-83.
57. Markovitz B. Does magnesium sulphate have a role in the management of paediatric status asthmaticus? *Arch Dis Child* 2002;86(5):381-2.
58. DiGiulio GA, Kercsmar CM, Krug SE et al. Hospital treatment of asthma: lack of benefit from theophylline given in addition to nebulized albuterol and intravenously administered corticosteroid. *J Pediatr* 1993;122(3):464-9.
59. Strauss RE, Wertheim DL, Bonagura VR et al. Aminophylline therapy does not improve outcome and increases adverse effects in children hospitalized with acute asthmatic exacerbations. *Pediatrics* 1994;93(2):205-10.

CHAPTER 49

Chronic Obstructive Pulmonary Disease

R. Andrew McIvor, MD, FRCPC

Chronic obstructive pulmonary disease is a chronic, systemic disease largely caused by smoking and characterized by progressive, partially reversible airway limitation, systemic manifestations, e.g., altered nutrition, and increasing frequency and severity of exacerbations. The cardinal symptoms are shortness of breath and activity limitation.[1,2]

Goals of Therapy[3]

- Prevent disease progression
- Decrease or abolish breathlessness and other respiratory symptoms
- Improve exercise tolerance
- Reduce the frequency and severity of exacerbations
- Improve health-related quality of life
- Reduce impairment, disability, handicap and mortality

Investigations

- History with particular attention to:
  - symptoms and their pattern: dyspnea (insidious at onset and progressive), cough (seldom entirely nocturnal), sputum production, limitations to physical activity
  - assess degree of shortness of breath and disability: use the Medical Research Council's Dyspnea Scale (Table 1)[2,4]
  - precipitating factors and triggers: cigarette smoking, heavy exposure to occupational dusts and chemicals, air pollution
  - signs/symptoms that suggest other comorbidities or systemic manifestations, e.g., skeletal muscle dysfunction, right heart failure, secondary polycythemia, depression, altered nutrition
  - previous history of acute exacerbations of COPD: hospitalizations, emergency room visits, oral corticosteroids ± antibiotic prescriptions
- Physical examination is relatively insensitive for diagnosis
  - late clinical findings: signs of hyperinflation, hypoxemia and pulmonary hypertension
- Objective measurements needed to confirm diagnosis and assess severity include:
  - spirometry, the gold standard for the diagnosis and risk stratification[1] of COPD. Baseline post-bronchodilator $FEV_1 < 80\%$ of the predicted value and an $FEV_1/FVC < 0.70$ are both necessary to establish the diagnosis.[1,2,5,6] Approximately 30% of patients

thought to have COPD will have an increase of 12% and > 200 mL in FEV_1 after salbutamol
- CBC to assess for anemia that can worsen dyspnea
- chest x-ray to rule out lung cancer, bronchiectasis, tuberculosis
- pulse oximetry ± arterial blood gases if FEV_1 < 50% predicted or clinical signs of respiratory failure or right heart failure[1]
- $alpha_1$-antitrypsin level if patient < 45 years old presents with COPD or has a strong family history of COPD[1]

Table 1: **Modified Medical Research Council Questionnaire for Assessing the Severity of Breathlessness[a,b]**

Statement	
I only get breathless with strenuous exercise.	□
I get short of breath when hurrying on the level or walking up a slight hill.	□
I walk slower than people of the same age on the level because of breathlessness, or I have to stop for breath when walking on my own pace on the level.	□
I stop for breath after walking about 100 meters or after a few minutes on the level.	□
I am too breathless to leave the house or I am breathless when dressing or undressing.	□

[a] Patient can only tick one response at one time.
[b] The MRC scale can be used on follow-up visits to monitor progress or response to therapy. Spirometry is the gold standard for diagnosis of COPD.

Reproduced with permission from Global Initiative for Chronic Obstructive Lung Disease (GOLD). *Global strategy for the diagnosis, management, and prevention of chronic obstructive pulmonary disease, 2006.* Available from: http://goldcopd.com Accessed December 15, 2006. All rights reserved

Therapeutic Choices

Nonpharmacologic Choices

- Recommend smoking cessation to stop COPD progression, reduce the risk of developing COPD[1,2,7,8,9,10,11] and decrease mortality[12] (see Chapter 10).
- Minimize/eliminate exposure to air pollution and occupational dusts and chemicals.[13,14]
- Educate patients and their families to enhance patient outcomes and reduce costs by improving skills, ability to cope with the illness and health status.[1,15]
- Encourage physical activity to prevent decrease in mobility and increase in dyspnea. Patients with a lower activity level at one month after hospital discharge were more likely to be readmitted in the following year.[16]
- Consider early referral of symptomatic patients to pulmonary rehabilitation programs providing respiratory, physical and occupational therapy, exercise conditioning, nutritional assistance and psychosocial and vocational rehabilitation. Although a limited resource, patients benefit from pulmonary rehabilitation in all stages of COPD.[17,18,19,20]

Pharmacologic Choices (Figure 1, Table 3, Table 4, Table 5)

A small improvement in airflow in COPD patients with severe obstruction may be of significant clinical benefit. Initial therapy commences with a short-acting beta$_2$-agonist as needed and may be supplemented by regular long-acting bronchodilators.[1,2,21] Maximum bronchodilation may be obtained with a combination of long-acting beta$_2$-agonists and anticholinergics.[1,2]

Delivery Systems

Inhaled bronchodilators are delivered via *pressurized metered-dose inhaler* (pMDI) (with or without a *spacer device*), *dry powder inhaler* (DPI) or *nebulizer*.[22] If pMDI technique is inadequate or ineffective, consider a spacer device to improve deposition of the medication to the lower respiratory tract and to avoid problems in coordinating the time of inhaler actuation and inhalation. Dry powder devices overcome problems with hand–breath coordination seen with pMDIs. Appropriate use of pMDIs with or without spacer devices or dry powder devices provides optimal drug delivery and should be encouraged over nebulizers. Nebulizers may be used in patients who remain symptomatic despite maximal treatment with handheld inhalers.

The choice of delivery device (pMDI or DPI) for patients with COPD depends on the patient's age and preference, the patient's ability to correctly use the device, convenience, ease of use and affordability.[22,23]

The proper use of inhalers is not intuitive. Careful instruction and demonstration of correct inhaler technique is essential before therapy is initiated and should be reinforced at each visit.

Stable COPD

Bronchodilators, the mainstay of pharmacotherapy, decrease air trapping, improve FEV$_1$, reduce symptoms (e.g., dyspnea), improve exercise capacity and quality of life in stable COPD and in acute exacerbations of COPD. Inhaled bronchodilators can be used as needed for occasional symptoms or regularly for symptom prevention and/or reduction. Canadian guidelines[2] favour the regular use of anticholinergic agents as the foundation of COPD bronchodilator management.

Anticholinergic Agents

The short-acting anticholinergic **ipratropium bromide** has a slower onset of action than inhaled beta$_2$-agonists but a longer duration of action (up to 8 h).[1] The recommended dose of 40 µg, three to four times per day, produces less than maximal bronchodilation and may be doubled or tripled without notable side effects.

Tiotropium bromide is a long-acting anticholinergic available as a breath activated, dry powder inhaler. Compared with ipratropium, it deposits more successfully in the airways of patients with very low inspiratory flow rates. A single daily 18 µg dose gives maximal anticholinergic activity for a full 24 hours.[24] More sustained effects on pulmonary function, activity-related dyspnea and quality of life are noted when compared to ipratropium. In addition, tiotropium decreases rate of exacerbations and hospitalization.[2,25] When given in combination with pulmonary rehabilitation, tiotropium improved treadmill walking endurance time.[26]

Beta$_2$-adrenergic Agonists

The inhaled short-acting beta$_2$-agonists (SABA) **salbutamol**, **terbutaline** and **fenoterol** have approximately equal efficacy, side effects and onset and duration (4–6 h)[1] of bronchodilator effect. Recommended doses of beta$_2$-agonists result in less than maximal bronchodilation; the dose may be doubled or tripled, although tremor and potential hypokalemia must be recognized and monitored in patients at risk.

The inhaled long-acting beta$_2$-agonists (LABA) **salmeterol** and **formoterol** offer sustained improvements in pulmonary function, dyspnea and quality of life compared with SABA.[2,27,28] Unlike salmeterol, formoterol has the added advantage of rapid onset of bronchodilation in addition to the 12 h duration of action.[27,29]

Oral beta$_2$-agonists offer few advantages and are associated with increased side effects. They have no role in the routine management of COPD.

Salbutamol and ipratropium combination produces greater and more sustained improvements in FEV_1 and increased degree of bronchodilation for less or similar side effect profile compared to either drug alone.[1] It confers greater improvement in lung function than either drug given alone or doubling the dose of a single bronchodilator.[30,31]

Theophylline

The use of oral theophylline for treatment of COPD is controversial. Clinically, little bronchodilator effect is observed beyond that of optimal dosing of inhaled bronchodilators. Theophylline may be used as an adjunct to other bronchodilators. Because of its narrow therapeutic index and complex pharmacokinetics, serum levels should be measured and adjusted to the low therapeutic range (55 to 85 µmol/L) to minimize adverse effects. Theophylline has significant drug interactions, e.g., levels may be doubled if the patient stops smoking or by the addition of medications such as antibiotics, e.g., clarithromycin, commonly used during acute exacerbations of COPD.

Inhaled Corticosteroids

The inhaled corticosteroids (ICS) **beclomethasone**, **budesonide** and **fluticasone** effectively reduce the rate and severity of acute exacerbations of COPD in patients with severe airflow obstruction who experience frequent exacerbations.[32] Studies suggest that ICS reduce the frequency of exacerbations in advanced symptomatic disease[33,34] and cardiovascular mortality.[35]

Ensure optimal bronchodilator therapy before considering ICS therapy to prevent exacerbations. ICS may be used in patients presenting for the first time with an exacerbation of COPD. ICS is recommended in those with an $FEV_1 < 50\%$ predicted and repeated exacerbations (three or more per year),[1] especially if these require treatment with oral steroids. ICS may also be considered in patients with severe COPD who remain breathless despite being on optimal bronchodilator therapy.[1,2]

Recently, a three year mortality study in moderate to severe COPD failed to show a mortality benefit for the combination product of fluticasone/salmeterol versus placebo, although it did reduce the rate of exacerbations.[36] A one year Canadian study adding salmeterol/fluticasone combination product to tiotropium in moderate to severe COPD showed no reduction in exacerbation rates; however addition of the combination did improve lung function and decrease hospitalizations.[37]

Oxygen Therapy

Oxygen therapy reduces the risk of death in select patients. In COPD patients with significant hypoxemia ($PaO_2 \leq 55$ mm Hg or $SaO_2 < 88\%$), long-term oxygen therapy may prolong life by six to seven years.[1] Improved survival has been seen only when oxygen is administered for at least 15 hours per day, including nocturnally.[39] The greatest survival benefit is with continuously administered oxygen. A patient whose PaO_2 is between 55 and 59 mm Hg may benefit from oxygen therapy if there is indirect evidence of hypoxemia or organ damage. Oxygen therapy is usually administered via Venturi facemask or nasal prongs at a flow rate sufficient to produce a resting PaO_2 between 65 and 80 mm Hg. Flow rates are often increased by 1 or 2 L/min during exercise and sleep. If hypoventilation ($PaCO_2 > 45$ mm Hg) is present, the titration of oxygen may worsen hypercarbic hypoxia, thus monitoring is advised.

Vaccines

Vaccinate annually against *influenza* early in the fall. Flu vaccine reduces exacerbations and death in patients with COPD.[40,41] Recommend *pneumococcal vaccination* to all patients with COPD without contraindications.[42] Pneumococcal vaccination is effective in patients ≥ 65 years with COPD and those < 65 years with $FEV_1 < 40\%$ predicted, as they are at increased risk of hospitalization and mortality from pneumonia; consider repeating pneumococcal vaccine, in high-risk patients, in 5–10 years.[1,2,43,44]

Acute Exacerbations of COPD

Acute exacerbations are the most frequent cause of medical visits, hospital admissions and death among COPD patients. They contribute to the accelerated rate of decline in lung function. In acute exacerbations of COPD, bronchodilation is optimized by increasing the dose and/or frequency of existing bronchodilator treatment.[1] Treat dyspnea with **combination short-acting beta$_2$-agonist** and **ipratropium**. Apart from optimizing the bronchodilator, patients with purulent acute exacerbations benefit from antibiotics. Severe COPD patients gain additional benefit from a short course of systemic corticosteroids.[1,2]

Systemic Corticosteroids

A two-week course of **oral corticosteroids** is beneficial in improving lung function and shortening length of hospital stay in all patients. There is no advantage to using intravenous steroids. A two-week course of oral **prednisone** 25–50 mg/day or equivalent is sufficient.[2,45,46] Tapering for oral steroid courses that last < 2 weeks is unnecessary. There is no role for oral steroid maintenance therapy for patients with COPD.

Antibiotics (Table 2, Table 5)

The most common infectious agents in exacerbations are viral. Empiric use of antibiotics in acute exacerbations of COPD is based on the prevalence of antimicrobial resistance and the changing patterns of pathogens. Antibiotics are indicated when exacerbations of COPD are accompanied by two to three of the following cardinal signs: increased dyspnea, increased sputum or increased sputum purulence[1,47] and in patients with severe exacerbations of COPD requiring invasive mechanical ventilation.

The common bacterial pathogens causing acute exacerbations of COPD are *Streptococcus pneumoniae, Haemophilus influenzae* and *Moraxella catarrhalis*.[48] In complicated patients, *Klebsiella* species and other gram-negatives including *Pseudomonas aeruginosa* can also appear.[48]

Concerns are constantly raised about whether empiric use of antibiotics in acute exacerbations of COPD is appropriate. These concerns are based on the increasing prevalence of antimicrobial resistance and the changing patterns of pathogens.

Empiric choice of an antibiotic should take into account individual risk stratification and previous use of antibiotics. Consider a change in antibiotic class if the same antibiotic class has been used within the previous three months. Re-evaluate patients who do not respond within 24 to 36 hours.

Oxygen Therapy

Arterial blood gas determination is the gold standard to assess oxygenation and ventilation during an exacerbation.

Table 2: **Empiric Antibiotic Therapy for Acute Exacerbation of COPD[49,50]**

Clinical State	Signs/Risk Factors	Probable Pathogens	Antibiotic of First Choice	Alternatives
Acute tracheobronchitis	↑ dyspnea, ↑ sputum production or ↑ sputum purulence	Virus	Antibiotics not recommended unless symptoms persist for > 10–14 days	Macrolide or tetracycline
Chronic bronchitis without risk factors[a]	≥ 2 of ↑ dyspnea, ↑ sputum production, ↑ sputum purulence	*H. influenzae, M. catarrhalis, S. pneumoniae*	Extended spectrum macrolides, 2nd or 3rd generation cephalosporins, amoxicillin, doxycycline or TMP/SMX	Fluoroquinolone, amoxicillin/ clavulanate or telithromycin
Chronic bronchitis with risk factors[a]	As for chronic bronchitis without risk factors + ≥ 1 of FEV_1 < 50% predicted, > 4 exacerbations/year, cardiac disease, use of home O_2, chronic oral corticosteroid use, antibiotic use in the past 3 months	As for chronic bronchitis without risk factors + *Klebsiella* + other gram-negative pathogens Increased probability of β-lactam resistance	Fluoroquinolone or amoxicillin/ clavulanate	Refer to specialist May require iv therapy
Chronic suppurative bronchitis	As for chronic bronchitis with risk factors + constant purulent sputum FEV_1 usually < 35% predicted	As for chronic bronchitis with risk factors + *P. aeruginosa*, multiresistant *Enterobacteriaceae*	Ambulatory: tailor treatment to airway pathogen Hospitalized patients: iv therapy usually required	

[a] Risk factors: comorbidities, severe COPD, frequent exacerbations (> 3/year), antimicrobial use within the last 3 months.

Abbreviations: TMP/SMX = trimethoprim/sulfamethoxazole

Therapeutic Tips

- Promote smoking cessation at each visit.
- Perform spirometry with bronchodilator assessment in patients such as:[5]
  - all smokers ≥ 35 y
  - past smokers with a ≥ 20-pack/year history of smoking whether or not the patient complains of symptoms

- patients with recurrent or chronic respiratory symptoms including cough and breathlessness on exertion
- patients with a family history of COPD
- patients who have significant occupational exposure to respiratory irritants

- Encourage physical activity to prevent a vicious cycle of decreasing mobility and increasing dyspnea.
- Ensure patient and family are aware of warning signs of a COPD exacerbation and have an action plan for initial management.
- Review inhaler technique at each visit.
- Encourage compliance with therapy by using a step-wise approach to treatment with positive reinforcement at all stages.
- Consider combining tiotropium and LABA for maximal bronchodilation in patients with moderate to severe persistent symptoms and exercise intolerance.[3] Add SABA PRN for acute symptom relief and to improve exercise tolerance.[3]
- ICS and LABA combination is more effective than either drug alone in terms of exercise endurance, symptom control and lung function.[51,52]
- Involve helpline groups including the Lung Association (New Patient Information number 1-866-717–COPD [2673]).

Figure 1: **Pharmacologic Management of COPD[3]**

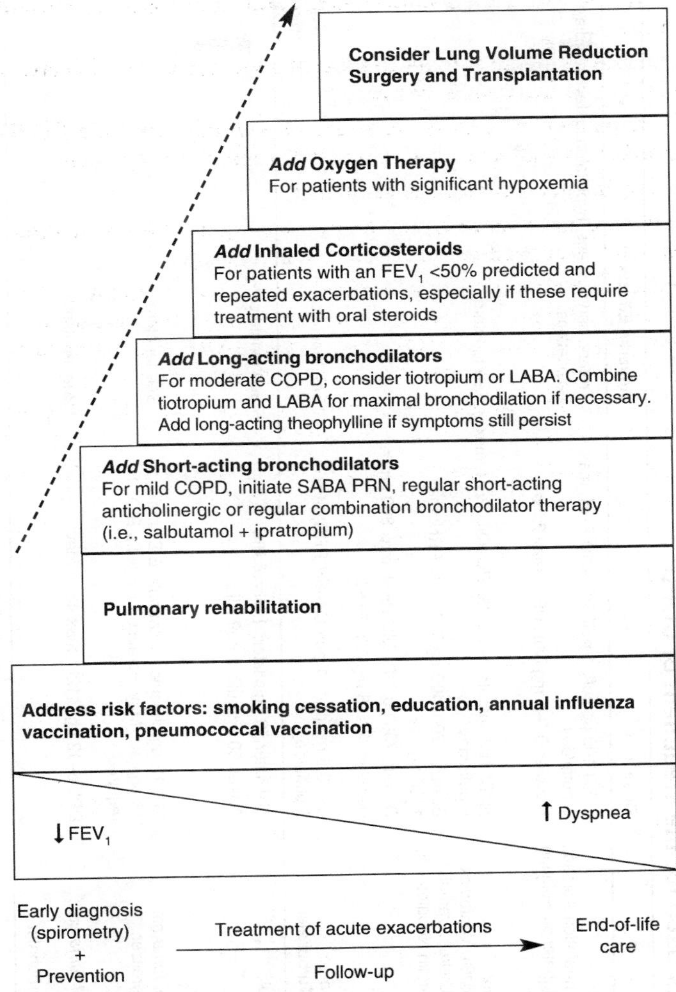

Abbreviations: COPD = chronic obstructive pulmonary disease; FEV_1 = forced expiratory volume in 1 sec; LABA = long-acting $beta_2$-agonist; SABA = short-acting $beta_2$-agonist.
Adapted with permission from O'Donnell DE, Aaron S, Bourbeau J et al. Canadian Thoracic Society recommendations for management of chronic obstructive pulmonary disease-2003. *Can Respir J* 2003;10(Suppl A):11A-65A.

Table 3: **Inhaled Drugs Used for the Treatment of COPD**

Class	Drug	Dose	Adverse Effects	Cost[a]
Inhaled Beta$_2$-adrenergic Agonists, short-acting (SABA)	*fenoterol* Berotec Inhalation Aerosol, Berotec Inhalation Solution	pMDI 100 µg/puff: 1 puff TID–QID PRN; max 8 puffs/day Nebules 0.5–1 mg Q6H PRN; max 2.5 mg	Tremor, nervousness, hypokalemia, tachycardia, palpitations.	$
	salbutamol Airomir pMDI, Ventodisk, Ventolin Diskus, Ventolin HFA, Ventolin Nebules P.F., generics	pMDI 100 µg/puff: 1–2 puffs TID–QID PRN; max 8 puffs/day Blisters: 200–400 µg TID–QID PRN; max 1600 µg/day Diskus: 200 µg TID–QID PRN; max 800 µg/day Nebules: 2.5–5 mg QID PRN	See fenoterol.	$-$$
	terbutaline Bricanyl Turbuhaler	DPI 0.5 mg/puff: 1 puff Q4–6H PRN; max 6 puffs/day	See fenoterol.	$
Inhaled Beta$_2$-adrenergic Agonists, long-acting (LABA)	*salmeterol* Serevent	Diskhaler 50 µg/blister: 1 blister BID Diskus 50 µg/puff: 1 puff BID	See fenoterol.	$$$$
	formoterol fumarate Foradil Aerolizer	DPI 12 µg/capsule: 1 capsule BID; max 48 µg/day. May increase to 2 puffs BID, if required	See fenoterol.	$$$$
	formoterol fumarate dihydrate Oxeze Turbuhaler	DPI: 6–12 µg Q12H; max 48 µg/day	See fenoterol.	$$$-$$$$

Class	Drug	Dose	Adverse Effects	Cost[a]
Anticholinergics, short-acting	*ipratropium bromide* Atrovent HFA, Atrovent Inhalation Solution	pMDI 20 µg/puff: 2–4 puffs Q6–8H up to 6–8 puffs Q6–8H, if tolerated; max 12 puffs/day. May use PRN or regularly scheduled Nebules: 250–500 µg TID-QID	Dry mouth, metallic taste, mydriasis and glaucoma if released into eye, urinary retention.	$$
Anticholinergics, long-acting	*tiotropium* Spiriva	DPI 18 µg (1 capsule) inhaled once daily	See ipratropium.	$$$$
Anticholinergic/ SABA Combinations	*ipratropium bromide/ fenoterol* Duovent UDV	Nebules 0.5 mg /1.25 mg: 4 mL Q6H PRN	See fenoterol. See ipratropium.	$$$$
	ipratropium/salbutamol , Combivent Inhalation Solution	Nebules 0.5 mg/2.5 mg: 2.5 mL Q6H PRN	See fenoterol. See ipratropium.	$$
Corticosteroids, inhaled	*beclomethasone dipropionate* Qvar, generics	pMDI: 100–800 µg divided BID	Oropharyngeal candidiasis and hoarseness can be decreased by using a spacer and rinsing mouth or by using dry powder inhaler. Skin bruising.[53] Accelerated cataracts. Possible worsening of glaucoma. May ↓ bone mineral density and ↑ fractures, consider monitoring bone mineral density in individuals at high risk, e.g., osteoporosis.	$–$$$
	budesonide Pulmicort Turbuhaler	DPI: 400–2400 µg divided BID	See beclomethasone.	$$$-$$$$
	fluticasone Flovent HFA, Flovent Diskus	200–1000 µg divided BID	See beclomethasone.	$$-$$$$

(cont'd)

Table 3: **Inhaled Drugs Used for the Treatment of COPD** *(cont'd)*

Class	Drug	Dose	Adverse Effects	Cost[a]
Corticosteroid/ LABA Combinations	*budesonide/ formoterol fumarate dihydrate* Symbicort Turbuhaler	DPI 100/6 µg or 200/6 µg: 2 puffs BID; max 4 puffs/day	See fenoterol. See beclomethasone.	$$$$
	fluticasone/ salmeterol Advair pMDI, Advair Diskus	pMDI 125/25 or 250/25 µg: 2 puffs BID Diskus 100/50 µg or 250/50 µg or 500/50 µg: 1 puff BID	See fenoterol. See beclomethasone.	$$$$

[a] Cost of inhaled agents is per unit; cost of oral medications is per 30-day supply; cost of inhaled solutions is per 20 vials; includes drug cost only.
Legend: $ < $15 $-$$ < $15–30 $$ $15–30 $-$$$ < $15–45 $$$ $30–45 $$-$$$$ $15–> 45 $$$-$$$$ $30– > 45 $$$$ > $45
Abbreviations: BMD = bone mineral density; pMDI = pressurized metered dose inhaler; DPI = dry powder inhaler

Table 4: **Oral Drugs Used in the Treatment of COPD**

Class	Drug	Dose	Adverse Effects	Drug Interactions	Cost[a]
Corticosteroids, systemic	*prednisone* generics	0.6 mg/kg/day; max 50 mg/day × 10–14 days	Glucose intolerance, ↑ appetite, weight gain, mood alteration, hypertension, osteoporosis, adrenal suppression, cataracts, myopathy, avascular necrosis of the hip (rare).	Oral antihyperglycemic agents: glucocorticoids may ↑ blood glucose concentrations; monitor blood glucose. NSAIDs: may ↑ the risk of GI ulceration with corticosteroids. Potassium-depleting drugs (e.g., thiazides) can deplete potassium as can corticosteroids; monitor serum potassium.	$
Theophylline Preparations	*aminophylline* Phyllocontin, generics	225–350 mg po Q12H. Monitor and adjust based on serum levels	Nausea, vomiting, abdominal cramps, headaches, nervousness, tremor, insomnia, tachycardia.	↑ theophylline serum levels: alcohol, carbamazepine, phenobarbital, phenytoin, rifampin, tobacco smoking. ↓ theophylline serum levels: amiodarone, cimetidine, ciprofloxacin, clarithromycin, erythromycin, fluvoxamine, isoniazid, mexiletine, propranolol, verapamil.	$
	oxtriphylline Choledyl, generics	Initial: 200 mg QID Monitor and adjust based on serum levels Available as elixir and tablets	See aminophylline.	See aminophylline.	$$$

(cont'd)

Table 4: **Oral Drugs Used in the Treatment of COPD** *(cont'd)*

Class	Drug	Dose	Adverse Effects	Drug Interactions	Cost[a]
	theophylline Uniphyl, generics	Initial: 400–600 mg/day with food, given in 1–3 divided doses depending on the preparation used. Monitor and adjust based on serum levels	See aminophylline.	See aminophylline.	$$

[a] Cost of inhaled agents is per unit; cost of oral medications is per 30-day supply; cost of inhaled solutions is per 20 vials; includes drug cost only.
Legend: $ < $15 $$ $15–30 $$$ $30–45
Abbreviations: NSAIDs = non-steroidal anti-inflammatory agents

Table 5: **Antibiotics for Acute Exacerbations of COPD**

Class	Drug	Dose[54]	Adverse Effects	Drug Interactions	Cost[a]
Cephalosporins	*cefprozil* Cefzil, generics	500 mg po Q12H × 7–10 days	Gastrointestinal intolerance, anaphylaxis (rare), rash.		$$$$
	cefuroxime axetil Ceftin, generics	500 mg po Q12H × 7–10 days	See cefprozil.		$$
Macrolides, extended spectrum	*azithromycin* Zithromax, generics	500 mg × 1 day then 250 mg once daily × 4 days 500 mg po Q24H × 3 days	Gastrointestinal intolerance.	Coadministration with pimozide contraindicated. ↑ concentrations of digoxin.	$$
	clarithromycin Biaxin BID, Biaxin XL	Biaxin BID: 500 mg po BID × 7–14 days Biaxin XL: 1000 mg once daily × 7–14 days	Bitter taste, gastrointestinal intolerance.	Coadministration with pimozide contraindicated. Rifampin ↓ macrolide concentrations. May ↑ warfarin effect; ↑ concentrations of some benzodiazepines, buspirone, carbamazepine, cyclosporine, digoxin, disopyramide, ergots, statins, theophylline.	$$$-$$$$
Fluoroquinolones	*ciprofloxacin* Cipro, generics	500–750 mg BID × 7–14 days	Usually well tolerated. Headache, dizziness may occur. Tendon rupture (rare).	Antacids, sucralfate, metal cations ↓ fluoroquinolone absorption. ↑ theophylline and cyclosporine levels; may ↑ warfarin effect.	$$$-$$$$

(cont'd)

Table 5: **Antibiotics for Acute Exacerbations of COPD** *(cont'd)*

Class	Drug	Dose[54]	Adverse Effects	Drug Interactions	Cost[a]
	gemifloxacin Factive	320 mg daily × 5 days	See ciprofloxacin.	Antacids, sucralfate, metal cations ↓ fluoroquinolone absorption. Avoid in patients on Class IA or III antiarrhythmics.	$$$
	levofloxacin Levaquin, generics	500 mg Q24H × 7 days 750 mg Q24H × 5 days	See ciprofloxacin.	Antacids, sucralfate, metal cations ↓ fluoroquinolone absorption. May ↑ warfarin effect. Avoid in patients on Class IA or III antiarrhythmics.	$$-$$$
	moxifloxacin Avelox	400 mg daily × 5 days	See ciprofloxacin.	See gemifloxacin	$$$
Ketolides	*telithromycin* Ketek	400 mg/tablet: 800 mg po Q24H × 5 days	Diarrhea, nausea, vomiting, elevated liver enzymes, hepatotoxicity.[55]	Not considered first line. Contraindicated in myasthenia gravis because of reports of exacerbation.[56] Coadministration with pimozide and cisapride is contraindicated. Coadministration with ergot alkaloids is not recommended. ↑ telithromycin levels: atorvastatin, itraconazole, ketoconazole, lovastatin, simvastatin. ↑ theophylline levels: monitor theophylline levels, may take 1 h apart to decrease GI side effects. ↑ digoxin levels: monitor digoxin levels and side effects.	$$$

Class	Drug	Dose[54]	Adverse Effects	Drug Interactions	Cost[a]
Penicillins	*amoxicillin* (kidney symbol) generics	500 mg TID × 7–10 days	Rash, anaphylaxis (rare).		$
	amoxicillin/clavulanate (kidney symbol) Clavulin, generics	500 mg po TID or 875 mg po BID × 7–10 days	Anaphylaxis, gastrointestinal upset, diarrhea.		$$
Sulfonamide Combinations	*sulfamethoxazole/ trimethoprim* (kidney symbol) generics	1 DS tablet BID or 2 tabs BID × 7–10 days	Nausea, skin rash, Stevens-Johnson syndrome (rare).	↑ warfarin effect, ↑ phenytoin levels.	$
Tetracyclines	*doxycycline* Vibra-Tabs, Vibramycin, generics	100 mg BID × 1 day then 100 mg daily once daily for 7–10 days	Gastrointestinal upset, photosensitivity.	Iron or antacids ↓ doxycycline absorption. Alcohol, barbiturates, phenytoin, rifampin, carbamazepine may ↓ doxycycline levels.	$

[a] Cost is for one course of therapy; includes drug cost only.

(kidney symbol) Dosage adjustment may be required in renal impairment; see Appendix I.

Abbreviations: DS = double strength

Legend: $ < $10 $$ $10–25 $$-$$$ $10–40 $$$ $25–40 $$$-$$$$ $25– >40 $$$$ >$40–50

Suggested Readings

Anzueto A. Clinical course of chronic obstructive pulmonary disease: review of therapeutic interventions. *Am J Med* 2006;119(10 Suppl 1):46-53.

Bourbeau J, Julien M, Maltais F et al. Reduction of hospital utilization in patients with chronic obstructive pulmonary disease: a disease-specific self-management intervention. *Arch Int Med* 2003:163(5):585-91.

Global Initiative for Chronic Obstructive Lung Disease (GOLD). *Global strategy for the diagnosis, management, and prevention of chronic obstructive pulmonary disease, 2006.* Available from: http://goldcopd.com Accessed December 15, 2006.

McIvor A. Chronic obstructive pulmonary disease in the older adult: new approaches to an old disease. *Geriatrics & Aging* 2007;10(4):213-220.

McIvor A, Little P. Chronic obstructive pulmonary disease. *BMJ* 2007;334(7597):798.

O'Donnell DE, Aaron S, Bourbeau J et al. State of the Art Compendium: Canadian Thoracic Society recommendations for the management of chronic obstructive pulmonary disease. *Can Respir J* 2004;11(Suppl B):7B-59B.

References

1. Global Initiative for Chronic Obstructive Lung Disease (GOLD). *Global strategy for the diagnosis, management, and prevention of chronic obstructive pulmonary disease, 2006.* Available from: http://goldcopd.com Accessed December 15, 2006.
2. O'Donnell DE, Aaron S, Bourbeau J et al. State of the Art Compendium: Canadian Thoracic Society recommendations for the management of chronic obstructive pulmonary disease. *Can Respir J* 2004;11(Suppl B):7B-59B.
3. O'Donnell DE, Aaron S, Bourbeau J et al. Canadian Thoracic Society recommendations for management of chronic obstructive pulmonary disease--2003. *Can Respir J* 2003;10(Suppl A):11A-65A.
4. Bestall JC, Paul EA, Garrod R et al. Usefulness of the Medical Research Council (MRC) dyspnoea scale as a measure of disability in patients with chronic obstructive pulmonary disease. *Thorax* 1999;54(7):581-6.
5. McIvor RA, Tashkin DP. Underdiagnosis of chronic obstructive pulmonary disease: a rationale for spirometry as a screening tool. *Can Respir J* 2001;8(3):153-8.
6. Johannessen A, Lehmann S, Omenaas ER et al. Post-bronchodilator spirometry reference values in adults and implications for disease management. *Am J Respir Crit Care Med* 2006;173(12):1316-25.
7. Kanner RE, Connett JE, Williams DE et al. Effects of randomized assignment to a smoking cessation intervention and changes in smoking habits on respiratory symptoms in smokers with early chronic obstructive pulmonary disease: the Lung Health Study. *Am J Med* 1999;106(4):410-6.
8. Stang P, Lydick E, Silberman C et al. The prevalence of COPD: using smoking rates to estimate disease frequency in the general population. *Chest* 2000;117(5 Suppl 2):354S-9S.
9. Wagena EJ, van der Meer RM, Ostelo RJ et al. The efficacy of smoking cessation strategies in people with chronic obstructive pulmonary disease: results from a systematic review. *Respir Med* 2004;98(9):805-15.
10. Scanlon PD, Connett JE, Waller LA et al. Smoking cessation and lung function in mild-to-moderate chronic obstructive pulmonary disease. The Lung Health Study. *Am J Respir Crit Care Med* 2000;161(2 Pt 1):381-90.
11. Anthonisen NR, Connett JE, Kiley JP et al. Effects of smoking intervention and the use of an inhaled anticholinergic bronchodilator on the rate of decline of FEV1. The Lung Health Study. *JAMA* 1994;272(19):1497-505.
12. Anthonisen NR, Skeans MA, Wise RA et al. The effects of a smoking cessation intervention on 14.5-year mortality: a randomized clinical trial. *Ann Intern Med* 2005;142(4):233-9.
13. Becklake MR. Occupational exposures: evidence for a causal association with chronic obstructive pulmonary disease. *Am Rev Respir Dis* 1989;140(3 Pt 2):S85-91.
14. Matheson MC, Benke G, Raven J et al. Biological dust exposure in the workplace is a risk factor for chronic obstructive pulmonary disease. *Thorax* 2005;60(8):645-51.

15. Bourbeau J, Julien M, Maltais F et al. Reduction of hospital utilization in patients with chronic obstructive pulmonary disease: a disease-specific self-management intervention. *Arch Intern Med* 2003;163(5):585-91.
16. Pitta F, Troosters T, Probst VS et al. Physical activity and hospitalization for exacerbation of COPD. *Chest* 2006;129(3):536-44.
17. Lacasse Y, Wong E, Guyatt GH et al. Meta-analysis of respiratory rehabilitation in chronic obstructive pulmonary disease. *Lancet* 1996;348(9035):1115-9.
18. Lacasse Y, Goldstein R, Lasserson TJ et al. Pulmonary rehabilitation for chronic obstructive pulmonary disease. *Cochrane Database Syst Rev* 2006;(4):CD003793.
19. Nici L, Donner C, Wouters E et al. American Thoracic Society/European Respiratory Society statement on pulmonary rehabilitation. *Am J Respir Crit Care Med* 2006;173(12):1390-413.
20. Man WD, Polkey MI, Donaldson N et al. Community pulmonary rehabilitation after hospitalisation for acute exacerbations of chronic obstructive pulmonary disease: randomised controlled study. *BMJ* 2004;329(7476):1209.
21. Tashkin DP, Cooper CB. The role of long-acting bronchodilators in the management of stable COPD. *Chest* 2004;125(1):249-59.
22. Dolovich MB, Ahrens RC, Hess DR et al. Device selection and outcomes of aerosol therapy: evidence-based guidelines: American College of Chest Physicians/American College of Asthma, Allergy, and Immunology. *Chest* 2005;127(1):335-71.
23. Rau JL. Practical problems with aerosol therapy in COPD. *Respir Care* 2006;51(2):158-72.
24. Littner MR, Ilowite JS, Tashkin DP et al. Long-acting bronchodilation with once-daily dosing of tiotropium (Spiriva) in stable chronic obstructive pulmonary disease. *Am J Respir Crit Care Med* 2000;161(4 Pt 1):1136-42.
25. Niewoehner DE, Rice K, Cote C et al. Prevention of exacerbations of chronic obstructive pulmonary disease with tiotropium, a once-daily inhaled anticholinergic bronchodilator: a randomized trial. *Ann Intern Med* 2005;143(5):317-26.
26. Casaburi R, Kukafka D, Cooper CB et al. Improvement in exercise tolerance with the combination of tiotropium and pulmonary rehabilitation in patients with COPD. *Chest* 2005;127(3):809-17.
27. Mahler DA, Donohue JF, Barbee RA et al. Efficacy of salmeterol xinafoate in the treatment of COPD. *Chest* 1999;115(4):957-65.
28. Rennard SI, Anderson W, Zuwallack R et al. Use of a long-acting inhaled beta2-adrenergic agonist, salmeterol xinafoate, in patients with chronic obstructive pulmonary disease. *Am J Respir Crit Care Med* 2001;163(5):1087-92.
29. Maesen BL, Westermann CJ, Duurkens VA et al. Effects of formoterol in apparently poorly reversible chronic obstructive pulmonary disease. *Eur Respir J* 1999;13(5):1103-8.
30. Ikeda A, Nishimura K, Koyama H et al. Bronchodilating effects of combined therapy with clinical dosages of ipratropium bromide and salbutamol for stable COPD: comparison with ipratropium bromide alone. *Chest* 1995;107(2):401-5.
31. Campbell S. For COPD a combination of ipratropium bromide and albuterol sulfate is more effective than albuterol base. *Arch Intern Med* 1999;159(2):156-60.
32. Burge PS, Calverley PM, Jones PW et al. Randomised, double blind, placebo controlled study of fluticasone propionate in patients with moderate to severe chronic obstructive pulmonary disease: the ISOLDE trial. *BMJ* 2000;320(7245):1297-303.
33. Gartlehner G, Hansen RA, Carson SS et al. Efficacy and safety of inhaled corticosteroids in patients with COPD: a systematic review and meta-analysis of health outcomes. *Ann Fam Med* 2006;4(3):253-62.
34. Burge PS, Calverley PM, Jones PW et al. Randomised, double blind, placebo controlled study of fluticasone propionate in patients with moderate to severe chronic obstructive pulmonary disease: the ISOLDE trial. *BMJ* 2000;320(7245):1297-303.
35. Macie C, Wooldrage K, Manfreda J et al. Inhaled corticosteroids and mortality in COPD. *Chest* 2006;130(3):640-6.
36. Calverley PM, Anderson JA, Celli B et al. Salmeterol and fluticasone propionate and survival in chronic obstructive pulmonary disease. *N Engl J Med* 2007 Feb 22;356(8):775-89.
37. Aaron SD, Vandemheen KL, Fergusson D et al. Tiotropium in combination with placebo, salmeterol, or fluticasone-salmeterol for treatment of chronic obstructive pulmonary disease: a randomized trial. *Ann Intern Med.* 2007;146(8):545-55.
38. Hansten PD, Horn JT. *Drug interactions analysis and management: a clinical perspective and analysis of current developments*. St. Louis (MO): Wolter Kluwer; 2007.
39. Ringbaek TJ. Continuous oxygen therapy for hypoxic pulmonary disease: guidelines, compliance and effects. *Treat Respir Med* 2005;4(6):397-408.
40. Poole PJ, Chacko E, Wood-Baker RW et al. Influenza vaccine for patients with chronic obstructive pulmonary disease. *Cochrane Database Syst Rev* 2006;(1):CD002733.
41. Wongsurakiat P, Maranetra KN, Wasi C et al. Acute respiratory illness in patients with COPD and the effectiveness of influenza vaccination: a randomized controlled study. *Chest* 2004;125(6):2011-20.
42. Respiratory Review Panel. *Respiratory (asthma and COPD) guidelines for family practice*. Toronto (ON): MUMS Guidelines Clearinghouse; 2007.

43. Jackson LA, Neuzil KM, Yu O et al. Effectiveness of pneumococcal polysaccharide vaccine in older adults. *N Engl J Med* 2003;348(18):1747-55.
44. Alfageme I, Vazquez R, Reyes N et al. Clinical efficacy of anti-pneumococcal vaccination in patients with COPD. *Thorax* 2006;61(3):189-95.
45. Davies L, Angus RM, Calverley PM. Oral corticosteroids in patients admitted to hospital with exacerbations of chronic obstructive pulmonary disease: a prospective randomised controlled trial. *Lancet* 1999;354(9177):456-60.
46. Niewoehner DE, Erbland ML, Deupree RH et al. Effect of systemic glucocorticoids on exacerbations of chronic obstructive pulmonary disease. Department of Veterans Affairs Cooperative Study Group. *N Engl J Med* 1999;340(25):1941-7.
47. Anthonisen NR, Manfreda J, Warren CP et al. Antibiotic therapy in exacerbations of chronic obstructive pulmonary disease. *Ann Intern Med* 1987;106(2):196-204.
48. Saint S, Bent S, Vittinghoff E et al. Antibiotics in chronic obstructive pulmonary disease exacerbations. A meta-analysis. *JAMA* 1995;273(12):957-60.
49. Martinez FJ, Anzueto A. Appropriate outpatient treatment of acute bacterial exacerbations of chronic bronchitis. *Am J Med* 2005;118(Suppl 7A):39S-44S.
50. Balter MS, La FJ, Low DE et al. Canadian guidelines for the management of acute exacerbations of chronic bronchitis. *Can Respir J* 2003;10(Suppl B):3B-32B.
51. Calverley P, Pauwels R, Vestbo J et al. Combined salmeterol and fluticasone in the treatment of chronic obstructive disease: a randomised controlled trial. *Lancet* 2003;361(9356):449-56.
52. O'Donnell DE, Sciurba F, Celli B et al. Effect of fluticasone propionate/salmeterol on lung hyperinflation and exercise endurance in COPD. *Chest* 2006 Sep;130(3):647-56.
53. Tashkin DP, Murray HE, Skeans M et al. Skin manifestations of inhaled corticosteroids in COPD patients: results from Lung Health Study II. *Chest* 2004;126(4):1123-33.
54. Rosser WW, Pennie RA, Pilla NJ; Anti-infective Review Panel. *Anti-infective guidelines for community-acquired infections*. Toronto (ON): MUMS Guideline Clearinghouse; 2005.
55. Clay KD, Hanson JS, Pope SD et al. Brief communication: severe hepatotoxicity of telithromycin: three case reports and literature review. *Ann Intern Med* 2006;144(6):415-20.
56. Perrot X, Bernard N, Vial C et al. Myasthenia gravis exacerbation or unmasking associated with telithromycin treatment. *Neurology* 2006;67(12):2256-8.

Pharmacoeconomic Considerations: Chronic Obstructive Pulmonary Disease

Nicole Mittmann, MSc, PhD

Epidemiology		
Country (Year)	**Prevalence (%)**	
Canada (1995)[1]	4.6–6.8% of adults aged ≥ 55 years	
Cost of Illness Data		
Country and Year of Estimate	**Direct Costs[a]**	**Indirect Costs[b]**
Canada (2001)[2]	$2000 per patient	$1200 per patient
Commentary		
COPD has a major impact on health care utilization, with hospitalizations due to exacerbations being the primary cost driver in this disease.[3] The annual direct medical cost per patient is higher for COPD than asthma. In Canada, the direct costs of COPD have been estimated to be approximately $2000 per patient annually, with indirect costs accounting for one-third of the total cost of COPD to society.[2]		

(cont'd)

Commentary

The anticholinergic bronchodilators, ipratropium and tiotropium, reduce the overall number of COPD exacerbations per patient per year. Reductions in the frequency of exacerbations and hospitalizations will likely decrease the overall direct medical costs of COPD. The newest agent, tiotropium, is considered to be cost-effective relative to ipratropium by reducing the frequency of exacerbations. This leads to fewer physician visits and hospitalizations.[4]

Quality of life is related to the frequency of COPD exacerbations.[5] Patients reporting a poor quality of life are more likely to be rehospitalized for COPD.[6] Effective pharmacotherapy improves quality of life, although inhaled corticosteroid use has been associated with a decreased quality of life.[7,8]

[a] Direct costs include those associated with physician services, nursing care, diagnostic procedures, drugs and hospitalization.

[b] Indirect costs include those associated with lost productivity and days off work due to morbidity or premature mortality.

References

1. Lacasse Y, Brooks D, Goldstein RS. Trends in the epidemiology of COPD in Canada, 1980 to 1995. COPD and Rehabilitation Committee of the Canadian Thoracic Society. *Chest* 1999;116(2):306-13.
2. Chapman KR, Bourbeau J, Rance L. The burden of COPD in Canada: results from the Confronting COPD survey. *Respir Med* 2003;97(Suppl C):S23-31.
3. Miravitlles M, Murio C, Guerrero T et al. Pharmacoeconomic evaluation of acute exacerbations of chronic bronchitis and COPD. *Chest* 2002;121(5):1449-55.
4. Vincken W, van Noord JA, Greefhorst AP et al. Improved health outcomes in patients with COPD during 1 yr's treatment with tiotropium. *Eur Respir J* 2002;19(2):209-16.
5. Seemungal TA, Donaldson GC, Paul EA et al. Effect of exacerbation on quality of life in patients with chronic obstructive pulmonary disease. *Am J Respir Cri. Care Med* 1998;157(5):1418-22.
6. Osman IM, Godden DJ, Friend JA et al. Quality of life and hospital re-admission in patients with chronic obstructive pulmonary disease. *Thorax* 1997;52(1):67-71.
7. Esteban C, Moraza J, Quintana JM et al. Use of medication and quality of life among patients with COPD. *Respir Med* 2006;100(3):487-95.
8. Aaron SD,Vandemheen KL, Fergusson D et al. Tiotropium in combination with placebo, salmeterol, or fluticasone for treatment of chronic obstructive pulmonary disease: a randomized trial. *Ann Intern Med* 2007;146(8):545-55.

CHAPTER 50

Croup

David W. Johnson, MD

Croup (laryngotracheobronchitis) is a common cause of upper airway obstruction in children. The annual incidence is 1.5–6 per 100 in children < 6 years.[1] Croup is most prevalent in the late fall to early winter months. Though common in children between 6 months and 3 years of age, it can also occur in children as young as 3 months and as old as 15 years.[1] It is rarely reported in adults.[2] Boys are affected more often than girls. Common causes are parainfluenza types 1 and 3. Influenza A and B, adenovirus, respiratory syncytial virus (RSV), metapneumovirus and mycoplasma have also been isolated.[3]

The majority of affected children can be safely managed at home. Very few require artificial support of their airway.[4] More than 60% of children diagnosed with croup have mild symptoms, about 4% are hospitalized and approximately 1 in 5000 children are intubated (approximately 1 in 200 hospitalized children).[4]

Goals of Therapy

- Decrease the duration and severity of symptoms
- Minimize anxiety of the child and parent(s)
- Decrease intubations, hospitalizations and return visits to physicians

Investigations

- Diagnosis of croup, which is most commonly due to a viral infection, requires no specific laboratory or radiologic investigation (see Table 1 for Differential Diagnosis)
- History with particular attention to symptoms:
  - nonspecific cough, rhinorrhea and fever (up to 40°C) may precede characteristic seal-like barky cough
  - substantially worse at night and improves during the day, aggravated by agitation and crying
  - obstructive symptoms generally resolve within 48 hours; a small percentage of children remain asymptomatic for up to 5–6 days[5]
- Physical examination for stridor, chest wall retractions, respiratory distress:
  - stridor: typically occurs during inspiration but may occur during expiration if severe
  - respiratory distress: increased heart rate, initial increase in respiratory rate, then falls

- respiratory failure occurs over several hours. Signs are reduced respiratory effort, lethargy, pallor, cyanosis, dusky appearance, breath sounds
- Objective measurements:
  - lateral and anteroposterior (AP) soft tissue neck films may clarify diagnosis in patients with atypical croup-like disease
  - pulse oximetry is indicated in patients with more severe croup
  - Westley croup score[6] stratifies croup severity into mild (1-2), moderate (3-8) or severe (>8)

Table 1: **Alternative Diagnoses (Other than Croup) for Children Who Present with Acute Onset of Stridor**

Differential Diagnosis	Characteristics
Bacterial tracheitis most common diagnosis after croup	High fever, toxic appearance, poor response to nebulized epinephrine
Epiglottitis relatively rare since introduction of *Haemophilus influenzae* type b vaccine	Absence of barky cough, sudden onset of high fever, dysphagia, drooling, toxic appearance, anxious appearance, and sitting slightly forward in the "sniffing" position
Occult foreign object very rare	Acute onset of stridor, presence of occult foreign body, most commonly lodged in the upper esophagus

Therapeutic Choices (Figure 1)

Patients with mild croup can be managed in the office setting, while those with moderate or severe croup should be referred to an emergency department for treatment and observation.

Nonpharmacologic Choices

- Keep children calm by ensuring a calm and reassuring atmosphere. This will minimize oxygen demand and respiratory muscle fatigue.
- There is insufficient evidence to support the use of mist therapy,[7,8] i.e., mist wanes, bedside humidifiers, mist tents. Placing children in mist tents, a wet, cold, "caged" environment separated from their parents, may provoke anxiety and agitation and should be avoided.[9]
- Oxygen therapy, in conjunction with corticosteroids and epinephrine, is reserved for children with hypoxia and significant respiratory distress. It should never be forced on a child, especially if it results in significant agitation. "Blow-by" administration of oxygen through a plastic hose with the end opening held near the child's nose and mouth, is often the most beneficial way of administering oxygen.
- Helium-oxygen mixtures (heliox) may benefit children with severe respiratory distress.[10,11,12,13] The lower density of a helium oxygen mixture potentially allows laminar flow in narrowed airways, thus improving ventilation and reducing respiratory distress. There

is insufficient evidence to advocate its use outside this setting. Administration of helium to children with croup has been proposed because of the potential of the lower density gas (relative to nitrogen) to decrease turbulent airflow in a narrowed airway.

Pharmacologic Choices (Table 2)

Corticosteroids

Corticosteroids are the mainstay of therapy for croup, regardless of clinical severity.[13] Corticosteroids have been shown to reduce intubations, the duration of intubation, the need for reintubation, the duration of hospitalization, the rate of hospitalization, the need for additional inhaled racemic epinephrine and the rate of return to a health care practitioner for persistent croup symptoms.[14,15,16,17,18,19,20,21,22,23] Dexamethasone and budesonide relieve symptoms of croup as early as 3 hours after treatment.[24]

Dexamethasone, 0.6 mg/kg, is effective when given orally or parenterally.[25,26] While one study suggests lower doses of dexamethasone such as 0.15 mg/kg are effective,[27] a meta-analysis of controlled trials suggests higher doses of corticosteroids yield a clinically important response in a greater proportion of patients.[17] It is not known whether multiple doses of corticosteroids provide greater benefit than a single dose. Given the short duration of croup symptoms in the majority of patients, a single dose of corticosteroid may be sufficient.

Inhaled **budesonide** is effective and equivalent to oral dexamethasone.[18,28,29] Routine use of inhaled budesonide is limited by cost. Patients with severe croup or who are near respiratory failure may benefit from the simultaneous administration of inhaled budesonide and nebulized epinephrine. The combination may be more effective than epinephrine alone.

Corticosteroids should be avoided in children with a known immunodeficiency or recent exposure to varicella.[30,31]

Epinephrine (Adrenergic Agonist)

Based on historical data, the administration of nebulized **epinephrine** in children with severe croup substantially reduces the number requiring an artificial airway.[32] Epinephrine substantially reduces respiratory distress within 10 minutes of administration and lasts for more than an hour.[33,34,35,36,37,38]

Effects of epinephrine administration wear off within two hours of administration.[36] Though patients treated with epinephrine may return to their "baseline" severity, they do not routinely develop worse symptoms (the so-called rebound effect).[36] Both retrospective and prospective studies suggest that patients treated with epinephrine may be safely discharged as long as their symptoms do not recur for at least two to three hours after treatment.[18,39,40,41,42,43]

L-epinephrine 1:1000 is comparably as effective and safe as the racemate form.[44] A single size dose (0.5 mL of 2.25% racemic epinephrine or 5 mL of epinephrine 1:1000) is used in all children regardless of size. Children's relative size of tidal volume is thought to modulate the dose of drug actually delivered to the upper airway.

Back-to-back administration of epinephrine can be used in children with near respiratory failure. There is one report of an otherwise normal child with severe croup treated with three nebulizations of epinephrine within one hour who developed ventricular tachycardia and a myocardial infarction.[45] Repeat doses of epinephrine should never be used unless a child is near respiratory failure. If back-to-back epinephrine is considered necessary, the treating physician should contact a pediatric intensivist as soon as possible regarding further treatment and transport.

Analgesics

Analgesics may provide some degree of increased comfort by reducing fever and pain.

Antitussives and Decongestants

No experimental studies have been published regarding the potential benefit of antitussives or decongestants in children with croup. There is no rational basis for their use.

Antibiotics

Antibiotics are not effective in the treatment of croup but may be used in suspected cases of bacterial superinfection. Intravenous antibiotics are generally recommended because of the potential for rapid deterioration.

Figure 1: **Management of Croup in the Outpatient Setting**

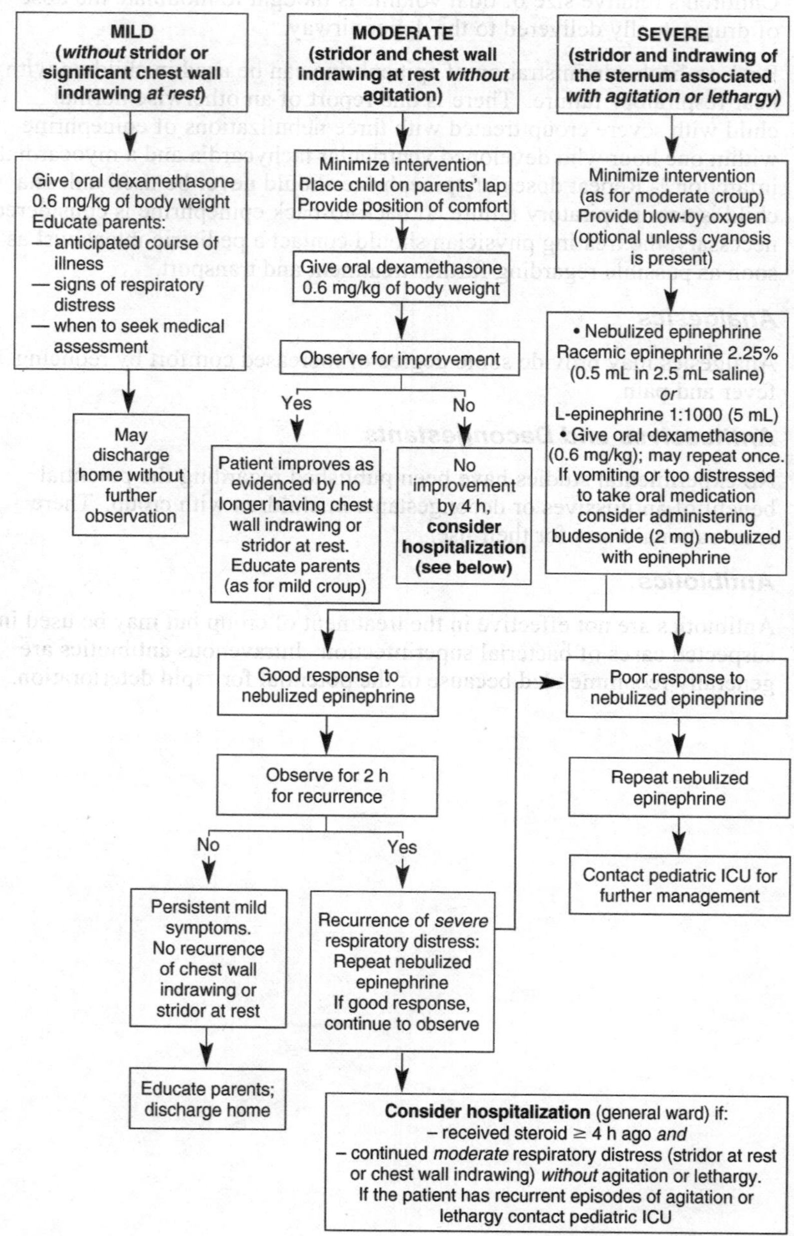

Table 2: Drugs Used for Croup

Drug Class	Drug	Dose and Duration	Comments	Cost[a]
Adrenergic Agonists	*epinephrine, racemic* Vaponefrin	0.5 mL of 2.25% solution diluted in 2.5 mL of NS or sterile water via nebulizer	Racemic epinephrine and L-epinephrine are equivalent in terms of effect and safety. Epinephrine has no effect on clinical symptoms beyond 2 h, consequently patients should not be discharged from medical care before 2 h following treatment.	$
	L-epinephrine Adrenalin	5 mL of 1:1000 (1 mg/mL) solution via nebulizer	See epinephrine, racemic.	$
Corticosteroids	*dexamethasone* generics	0.6 mg/kg po/im/iv once[30,47] May repeat dose in 6 to 24 h	Oral dexamethasone is well absorbed and achieves peak serum concentrations as rapidly as with im administration (without the pain). Several controlled trials suggest oral and im administration yield equivalent results. Experience suggests clinical improvement will begin as early as 2 to 3 h after treatment. No evidence to suggest multiple doses provide additional benefit over a single dose. Reduces rate and duration of intubation, rate and duration of hospitalization and rate of return to medical care.	$
	budesonide Pulmicort Nebuamp	2 mg (2 mL) solution via nebulizer	Inhaled budesonide has been shown in several studies to be equivalent to oral dexamethasone but is substantially more expensive. May be useful in patients with vomiting and severe respiratory distress. Can administer budesonide and epinephrine simultaneously.	$$

[a] Cost of one dose; includes drug cost only.
Abbreviations: NS = normal saline
Legend: $ < $1 $$ $1–5

Suggested Readings

Brown JC. The management of croup. *Br Med Bull* 2002;61:189-202.

Bjornson CL, Johnson DW. Croup-treatment update. *Pediatr Emerg Care* 2005;21(12):863-73.

Johnson D. Croup. *Clin Evid* 2006;15:380-97.

References

1. Denny FW, Murphy TF, Clyde WA et al. Croup: an 11-year study in a pediatric practice. *Pediatrics* 1983;71(6):871-6.
2. Tong MC, Chu MC, Leighton SE et al. Adult croup. *Chest* 1996;109(6):1659-62.
3. Ho HK. Human metapneumovirus and lower respiratory tract disease in children. *N Engl J Med* 2004;350(17):1788-90.
4. Brown JC. The management of croup. *Br Med Bull* 2002;61:189-202.
5. Johnson D, Williamson J. Croup: duration of symptoms and impact on family functioning. *Pediatr Res* 2001;49:83A.
6. Westley CR, Cotton EK, Brooks JG. Nebulized racemic epinephrine by IPPB for the treatment of croup. *Am J Dis Child* 1978;132(5):484-7.
7. Chin R, Browne GJ, Lam LT et al. Effectiveness of a croup clinical pathway in the management of children with croup presenting to an emergency department. *J Paediatr Child Health* 2002;38(4):382-7.
8. Lavine E, Scolnik D. Lack of efficacy of humidification in the treatment of croup: why do physicians persist in using an unproven modality? *Can J Emerg Med* 2001;3(3):209-12.
9. Scolnik D, Coates AL, Stephens D et al. Controlled delivery of high vs low humidity vs mist therapy for croup in emergency departments: a randomized controlled trial. *JAMA* 2006;295(11):1274-80.
10. Henry R. Moist air in the treatment of laryngotracheitis. *Arch Dis Child* 1983;58(8):577.
11. Duncan PG. Efficacy of helium-oxygen mixtures in the management of severe viral and post-intubation croup. *Can Anaesth Soc J* 1979;26(3):206-12.
12. McGee DL, Wald DA, Hinchliffe S. Helium-oxygen therapy in the emergency department. *J Emerg Med* 1997;15(3):291-6.
13. Terregino CA, Nairn SJ, Chansky ME et al. The effect of heliox on croup: a pilot study. *Acad Emerg Med* 1998;5(11):1130-3.
14. Weber JE, Chudnofsky CR, Younger JG et al. A randomized comparison of helium-oxygen mixture (Heliox) and racemic epinephrine for the treatment of moderate to severe croup. *Pediatrics* 2001;107(6):E96.
15. Russel K, Wiebe N, Saenz A et al. Glucocorticoids for croup. *Cochrane Database Syst Rev* 2004;(1): CD001955.
16. Ausejo M, Saenz A, Pham B et al. The effectiveness of glucocorticoids in treating croup: meta-analysis. *BMJ* 1999;319(7210):595-600.
17. Kairys SW, Olmstead EM, O'Connor GT. Steroid treatment of laryngotracheitis: a meta-analysis of the evidence from randomized trials. *Pediatrics* 1989;83(5):683-93.
18. Johnson DW, Jacobson S, Edney PC et al. A comparison of nebulized budesonide, intramuscular dexamethasone, and placebo for moderately severe croup. *N Engl J Med* 1998;339(8):498-503.
19. Bjornson C, Klassen T, Williamson J et al. A randomized trial of a single dose of oral dexamethasone for mild croup. *N Engl J Med* 2004;351(13):1306-13.
20. Tibballs J, Shann FA, Landau LI et al. Placebo-controlled trial of prednisolone in children intubated for croup. *Lancet* 1992;340(8822):745-8.
21. Geelhoed GC. Sixteen years of croup in a Western Australian teaching hospital: effects of routine steroid treatment. *Ann Emerg Med* 1996;28(6):621-6.
22. Geelhoed GC, Turner J, Macdonald WB. Efficacy of a small single dose of oral dexamethasone for outpatient croup: a double blind placebo controlled clinical trial. *BMJ* 1996;313(7050):140-2.
23. Luria JW, Gonzalez-del-Rey JA, DiGiulio GA et al. Effectiveness of oral or nebulized dexamethasone for children with mild croup. *Arch Pediatr Adolesc Med* 2001;155(12):1340-5.
24. Klassen TP, Feldman ME, Watters LK et al. Nebulized budesonide for children with mild-to-moderate croup. *N Engl J Med* 1994;331(5):285-9.
25. Johnson DW, Jacobson S, Edney PC et al. A comparison of nebulized budesonide, intramuscular dexamethasone, and placebo for moderately severe croup. *N Engl J Med* 1998;339(8):498-503.
26. Johnson DW, Schuh S, Koren G et al. Outpatient treatment of croup with nebulized dexamethasone. *Arch Pediatr Adolesc Med* 1996;150(4):349-55.
27. Patel H, Macarthur C, Johnson D et al. Recent corticosteroid use and the risk of complicated varicella in otherwise immunocompetent children. *Arch Pediatr Adolesc Med* 1996;150(4):409-14.
28. Donaldson D, Poleski D, Knipple E et al. Intramuscular versus oral dexamethasone for the treatment of moderate-to-severe croup: a randomized, double-blind trial. *Acad Emerg Med* 2003;10(1):16-21.
29. Rittichier KK, Ledwith CA. Outpatient treatment of moderate croup with dexamethasone: intramuscular versus oral dosing. *Pediatrics* 2000;106(6):1344-8.

30. Geelhoed GC, Macdonald WB. Oral dexamethasone in the treatment of croup: 0.15 mg/kg versus 0.3 mg/kg versus 0.6 mg/kg. *Pediatr Pulmonol* 1995;20(6):362-8.
31. Klassen TP, Craig WR, Moher D et al. Nebulized budesonide and oral dexamethasone for treatment of croup: a randomized controlled trial. *JAMA* 1998;279(20):1629-32.
32. Geelhoed GC, Macdonald WB. Oral and inhaled steroids in croup: a randomized, placebo-controlled trial. *Pediatr Pulmonol* 1995;20(6):355-61.
33. Adair JC, Ring WH, Jordan WS et al. Ten-year experience with IPPB in the treatment of acute laryngotracheobronchitis. *Anesth Analg* 1971;50(4):649-55.
34. Fanconi S, Burger R, Maurer H et al. Transcutaneous carbon dioxide pressure for monitoring patients with severe croup. *J Pediatr* 1990;117(5):701-5.
35. Gardner HG, Powell KR, Roden VJ et al. The evaluation of racemic epinephrine in the treatment of infectious croup. *Pediatrics* 1973;52(1):52-5.
36. Westley CR, Cotton EK, Brooks JG. Nebulized racemic epinephrine by IPPB for the treatment of croup: a double-blind study. *Am J Dis Child* 1978;132(5):484-7.
37. Fogel JM, Berg IJ, Gerber MA et al. Racemic epinephrine in the treatment of croup: nebulization alone versus nebulization with intermittent positive pressure breathing. *J Pediatr* 1982;101(6):1028-31.
38. Corkey CW, Barker GA, Edmonds JF et al. Radiographic tracheal diameter measurements in acute infectious croup: an objective scoring system. *Crit Care Med* 1981;9(8):587-90.
39. Taussig LM, Castro O, Beaudry PH et al. Treatment of laryngotracheobronchitis (croup). Use of intermittent positive-pressure breathing and racemic epinephrine. *Am J Dis Child* 1975;129(7):790-3.
40. Rizos JD, DiGravio BE, Sehl MJ et al. The disposition of children with croup treated with racemic epinephrine and dexamethasone in the emergency department. *J Emerg Med* 1998;16(4):535-9.
41. Corneli HM, Bolte RG. Outpatient use of racemic epinephrine in croup. *Am Fam Physician* 1992;46(3):683-4.
42. Kelley PB, Simon JE et al. Racemic epinephrine use in croup and disposition. *Am J Emerg Med* 1992;10(3):181-3.
43. Ledwith CA, Shea LM, Mauro RD. Safety and efficacy of nebulized racemic epinephrine in conjunction with oral dexamethasone and mist in the outpatient treatment of croup. *Ann Emerg Med* 1995;25(3):331-7.
44. Kunkel NC, Baker MD. Use of racemic epinephrine, dexamethasone, and mist in the outpatient management of croup. *Pediatr Emerg Care* 1996;12(3):156-9.
45. Waisman Y, Klein BL, Boenning DA et al. Prospective randomized double-blind study comparing L-epinephrine and racemic epinephrine aerosols in the treatment of laryngotracheitis (croup). *Pediatrics* 1992;89(2):302-6.
46. Butte MJ, Nguyen BX, Hutchison TJ et al. Pediatric myocardial infarction after racemic epinephrine administration. *Pediatrics* 1999;104(1):e9.
47. Kairys SW, Olmestead EM, O'Connor GT. Steroid treatment of laryngotracheitis: a meta-analysis of the evidence from randomized trials. *Pediatrics* 1989;83(5):683-93.

CHAPTER 51
Chronic Liver Diseases

Mark G. Swain, MD, MSc, FRCPC

This chapter discusses hepatic encephalopathy, ascites, spontaneous bacterial peritonitis, cholestatic disease (including symptom management), autoimmune chronic hepatitis, alcoholic liver disease (including alcoholic hepatitis), hemochromatosis and Wilson's disease. Management of esophageal varices is discussed in Chapter 55. Management of viral hepatitis is discussed in Chapter 52.

Goals of Therapy

- Manage symptoms associated with chronic liver conditions
- Treat complications of chronic disease, e.g., infection
- Prevent recurrence
- Delay or prevent disease progression
- Decrease liver-related mortality

Ascites (Portal Hypertension)

Investigations

- Thorough history with special attention to documented liver disease; rule out other causes of ascites
- Physical examination for features of chronic liver disease (e.g., cutaneous stigmata), hepatosplenomegaly, degree of ascites accumulation (shifting dullness, abdominal protuberance, eversion of umbilicus), signs of portal hypertension (caput medusae, venous hum) or other features of liver failure and related complications (gastrointestinal bleeding, asterixis)
- Laboratory tests:
  - ascitic tap (all patients) for neutrophil count, culture, protein/albumin, amylase, lactate dehydrogenase, glucose
  - calculate serum-ascites albumin gradient (SAAG)[1]

Therapeutic Choices (Figure 1, Table 1)

High plasma aldosterone levels in patients with ascites result in sodium and fluid retention; thus, **spironolactone** (a specific aldosterone antagonist) is the diuretic of choice. **Furosemide** should be added to enhance diuresis and/or control serum potassium levels. **Metolazone** can be added if ascites is refractory to spironolactone and furosemide. The combination of furosemide and metolazone can produce profound diuresis, causing volume depletion and electrolyte abnormalities.

Start with low doses and titrate up. **Amiloride** can be substituted for spironolactone if intolerable side effects develop.

Spontaneous Bacterial Peritonitis (SBP)

Investigations

- History of fever, abdominal pain or clinical deterioration
- Physical examination, other than to confirm the presence of ascites, is often unhelpful
- Laboratory tests: culture and polymorphonuclear (PMN) cell count of ascitic fluid; repeat after treatment to ensure resolution of the infection

Therapeutic Choices (Table 2)

If the ascitic fluid PMN cell count is >0.25 × 10^9/L (250 cells/μL), treat with a third-generation cephalosporin (e.g., **cefotaxime** or **ceftriaxone**) for 5 days and commence intravenous infusion of **albumin** (1.5 g/kg of body weight at the time of diagnosis and 1.0 g/kg on day 3 of treatment).

Use prophylactic antibiotics only after a patient has experienced one episode of SBP. A patient with one episode of SBP has a 69% chance of recurrence within one year. Treatment with **sulfamethoxazole/trimethoprim (cotrimoxazole)**[2] or **norfloxacin**[3] decreases the rate of SBP recurrence, but does not improve survival. Due to overall cost, sulfamethoxazole/trimethoprim is the drug of choice. Prophylactic antibiotics should be started after the completion of intravenous antibiotic therapy for the acute episode and continue until resolution of ascites, transplantation or death.

Hepatic Encephalopathy

See Figure 2 and Table 3.

Cholestatic Disease

Goals of Therapy

- Improve or prevent progression of disease
- Improve symptoms, e.g., fatigue, pruritus
- Improve survival and reduce the need for liver transplantation
- Manage fat-soluble vitamin deficiencies

Investigations

- Clinical/biochemical evidence of cholestasis (↑ alkaline phosphatase and gamma glutamyl transferase [GGT], and later bilirubin) with:
  - for *primary biliary cirrhosis (PBC):* positive antimitochondrial antibody (> 95% of cases); can be confirmed by liver biopsy,

although this is not absolutely required if a patient has a positive antimitochondrial antibody test and a cholestatic biochemical profile
  - for *primary sclerosing cholangitis (PSC):* ductular abnormalities (strictures, beading, etc.) on endoscopic retrograde cholangiopancreatography (ERCP) or magnetic resonance imaging (MRCP).
- Identify vitamin deficiencies by:
  - prothrombin time (↑ if vitamin K deficient)
  - serum calcium and 25(OH)-vitamin D levels
  - serum vitamin A and/or carotene levels

Therapeutic Choices (Figure 3, Table 4)

Primary Biliary Cirrhosis (PBC) and Primary Sclerosing Cholangitis (PSC)

Ursodeoxycholic acid (UDCA) 13 to 15 mg/kg/day improves serum liver biochemical tests in patients with PBC[4,5,6] and PSC. It appears to have limited efficacy in preventing disease progression in PSC although high-dose UDCA (20 to 30 mg/kg/day) may be of benefit.[7,8] In PBC, a combined analysis of three trials suggested that UDCA significantly reduced the probability of transplantation and/or death after a median of nearly four years. It slows disease progression but is not curative.[9] Its effect on symptoms (i.e., fatigue, pruritus) is controversial but likely minimal. Episodes of cholangitis require treatment with appropriate antibiotics (e.g., oral ciprofloxacin in outpatients for early mild episodes; intravenous ampicillin + gentamicin + metronidazole for hospitalized patients).

Vitamin Deficiencies

Vitamin A, D or K supplements may be required to treat deficiencies (usually only in chronic cholestasis). The need for **vitamin E** supplements in adults has not been assessed in well-designed clinical trials.

Management of Pruritus

Rule out local cutaneous causes of pruritus, e.g., eczema. **Cholestyramine** will benefit about 90% of patients; it must be continued as long as pruritus is present. **Antihistamines** (e.g., hydroxyzine) are of no proven benefit, but their sedative properties may help. For patients who do not respond, **naltrexone**[10] or **rifampin**[11] may be tried. Numerous other therapies have been evaluated, but all are investigational.

Autoimmune Chronic Active Hepatitis

Investigations

- Marked ↑ in serum transaminases and hypergammaglobulinemia; antinuclear antibody (ANA) is present in about 70% of patients (Type I autoimmune hepatitis)
- Diagnosis confirmed by liver biopsy

The classic patient is a young woman who presents with either an acute or chronic illness characterized by lethargy, arthralgia, oligomenorrhea, fluctuating jaundice, and who has a cushingoid appearance with striae, hirsutism and acne.

Therapeutic Choices (Table 5)

Immunosuppression with **glucocorticoids**, with or without **azathioprine**, prolongs life, decreases symptoms, improves serum biochemical abnormalities and diminishes hepatic inflammation on liver biopsy. The goal is to induce remission, defined as a decrease in serum aminotransferase levels to within the normal range, but at least to ≤ 2 × the upper limit of normal, and a follow-up liver biopsy that is normal or shows only chronic persistent hepatitis. Most patients will require therapy for up to two years before attempts at discontinuing prednisone should be considered; the majority will require lifelong therapy. If the dose of prednisone cannot be decreased below 10 mg/day, azathioprine may be added to the regimen. The combination of **mycophenolate mofetil** (up to 1 g po BID) and **prednisone** may be used in patients resistant to or intolerant of azathioprine.[12]

Alcoholic Liver Disease

Investigations

- An AST to ALT ratio ≥ 2:1 and GGT ≥ 2 × the upper limit of normal strongly suggests alcohol abuse

Therapeutic Choices (Table 5)

Chronic Alcohol-related Liver Disease

There is no universally accepted medical therapy except *abstention from alcohol*. Long-term treatment with propylthiouracil or colchicine has been studied but results have not been encouraging.[13,14]

Alcoholic Hepatitis

Corticosteroids[15] and **pentoxifylline**[16] improve short-term survival in patients with severe biopsy-proven alcoholic hepatitis. Severe alcoholic hepatitis can be documented by calculating the Maddrey discriminant function: values > 32 denote severe alcoholic hepatitis with a mortality rate approaching 50%.[17] Corticosteroid therapy for severe alcoholic hepatitis has been examined in numerous studies with variable results, whereas the beneficial effects of pentoxifylline have been documented in a single study (reviewed by Haber et al).[17]

Hemochromatosis

Investigations

- Elevated serum ferritin (> 300 μg/L for males; > 200 μg/L for females), fasting percent transferrin saturation index (serum iron level/total iron binding capacity) > 60% for males or > 50% for females
- Confirmed iron overload on liver biopsy or positive C282Y (most commonly) genetic test.

  The classic patient is a middle-aged man who presents with hyperpigmentation, fatigue, abdominal pain, joint pain, diminished libido, loss of body hair and diabetes mellitus

Therapeutic Choices (Table 6)

Reduce dietary iron intake. Phlebotomy (500 mL of whole blood weekly or biweekly as tolerated) will ultimately normalize body iron stores: when repeated weekly, this may take up to two years. If the patient is unable to tolerate phlebotomy due to other causes of iron overload (e.g., transfusions for thalassemia), chelation with **deferoxamine** can be tried.

Wilson's Disease

Investigations

- Hepatic presentations include fulminant hepatitis, chronic active hepatitis and cirrhosis. The diagnosis is confirmed by liver biopsy with hepatic copper concentrations and/or a positive genetic test. Genetic testing is positive in only about 65% of patients
- Laboratory tests: ↑ aminotransferase, ↓ serum ceruloplasmin and total copper, ↑ 24 h urinary copper excretion (> 100 μg/day)
- Family history; most patients are diagnosed before age 30

Therapeutic Choices (Table 7)

Copper chelating agents (**penicillamine** or **trientine**) are the treatment of choice for Wilson's disease, and treatment is lifelong. Trientine may be better tolerated, but is only available through the Special Access Programme; thus, penicillamine is the first–line agent in Canada. **Pyridoxine**, 25 mg daily, should be given with penicillamine to counteract its antipyridoxine effect. Twenty-four hour urinary copper excretion and serum free copper levels can be monitored to ensure adequate removal of copper. Trientine may be used in patients intolerant of penicillamine. Elemental **zinc** is an option in patients intolerant of penicillamine and trientine. Foods high in copper should be avoided (e.g., peanuts, chocolate, liver, shellfish, mushrooms).

Figure 1: **Management of Ascites Secondary to Portal Hypertension**

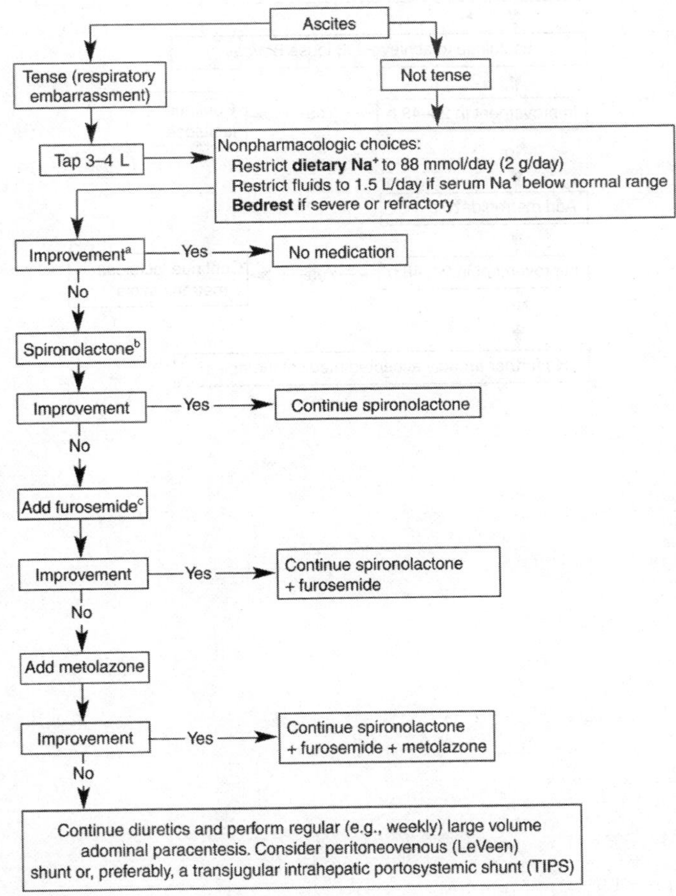

a Aim for weight loss of 1–1.5 kg/day in patients with peripheral edema, and 0.5–1 kg/day in patients without edema.

b If side effects occur (e.g., painful gynecomastia) switch to another potassium-sparing diuretic (e.g., amiloride).

c Spironolactone and furosemide can be started simultaneously, which often provides more predictable diuresis with better electrolyte balance.

Give diuretics as single morning doses. Use the lowest effective dose to achieve adequate diuresis and monitor serum electrolytes, BUN and creatinine before therapy, weekly until stabilized, then monthly. Doses can be reduced after diuresis is initiated.

Abbreviations: TIPS = transjugular intrahepatic portosystemic shunt

Figure 2: **Management of Hepatic Encephalopathy**

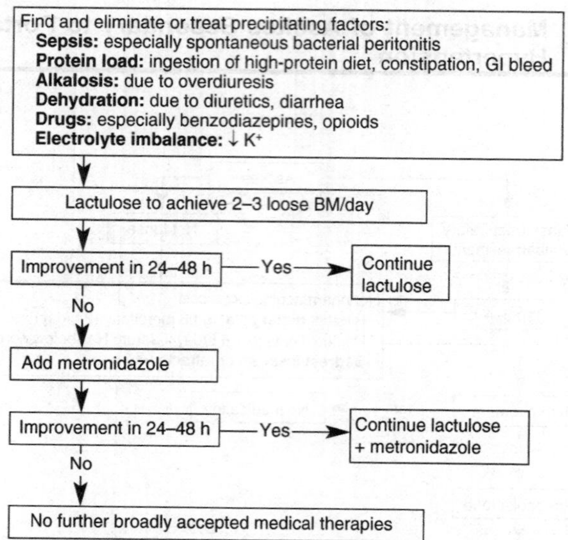

Figure 3: **Management of Cholestatic Symptoms**

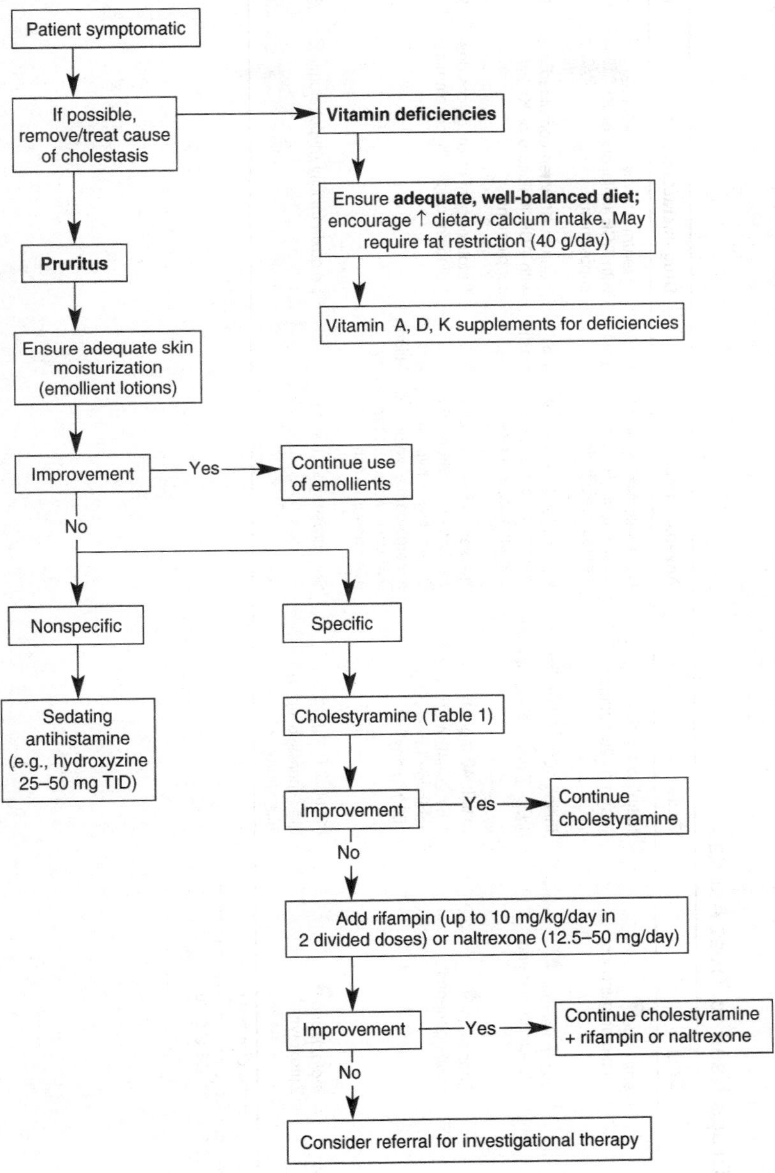

Specific therapies refer to those directed at the possible cause of pruritus, whereas nonspecific therapies cause sedation.

Table 1: Drugs Used to Treat Ascites

Drug Class	Drug	Dose	Adverse Effects	Drug Interactions	Cost[a]
Diuretics	*amiloride*[b] Midamor, generics	Initial: 5 mg/day May ↑ to 20 mg/day	Hyperkalemia, gynecomastia, muscle cramps, hyperchloremic metabolic acidosis.	↑ serum K^+ when combined with ACE inhibitors or K^+ supplements.	$$$
	spironolactone[b] Aldactone, generics	Initial: 100–200 mg/day ↑ Q5–7 days to 400 mg/day	Hyperkalemia, hyperchloremic metabolic acidosis, gynecomastia and mastalgia in men.	↑ serum K^+ when combined with ACE inhibitors or K^+ supplements.	$$$
	furosemide[b] Lasix, generics	Initial: 40 mg/day ↑ by 20–40 mg/day to achieve diuresis (up to 160 mg/day)	Nausea, anorexia, fatigue, weakness, ↓ serum Na^+, Cl^-, K^+, Mg^{++}, hyperuricemia, hyperglycemia, volume depletion, metabolic acidosis, ototoxicity (high doses), rash.	↑ ototoxicity of aminoglycosides; ↑ digoxin toxicity (hypokalemia).	$
	metolazone[b] Zaroxolyn	Initial: 2.5 mg/day May increase up to 10 mg/day	See furosemide.	↑ digoxin toxicity (hypokalemia).	$$

[a] Cost of 30-day supply; includes drug cost only.

[b] Dosage adjustment may be required in renal impairment.

Legend: $ < $10 $$ $10–20 $$$ $20–30

Table 2: Drugs Used for Spontaneous Bacterial Peritonitis

Drug Class	Drug	Dose	Adverse Effects	Drug Interactions	Cost[a]
Cephalosporins, 3rd generation	*cefotaxime* (kidney symbol) Claforan	Treatment: 2 g iv Q8H × 5 days	GI disturbances, hypersensitivity.		$$$$
	ceftriaxone Rocephin	Treatment: 2 g iv Q24H × 5 days	GI disturbances, hypersensitivity, biliary pseudolithiasis (sludging).		$$$$
Sulfonamide Combinations	*sulfamethoxazole/trimethoprim (cotrimoxazole)* (kidney symbol) generics	Prophylaxis: 1 DS tablet 5 × weekly	Nausea, vomiting, fever, hypersensitivity reactions (may be severe), blood dyscrasias.	↑ effect of sulfonylureas and warfarin. ↑ phenytoin levels. ↑ nephrotoxicity of cyclosporine.	$
Fluoroquinolones	*norfloxacin* (kidney symbol) generics	Prophylaxis: 400 mg/day	GI disturbances, CNS effects, skin rash.	Absorption ↓ by antacids, calcium and iron (separate administration). ↑ theophylline levels.	$$

[a] Cost of 30-day supply unless specified otherwise; includes drug cost.

(kidney symbol) Dosage adjustment may be required in renal impairment.

Legend: $ < $10 $$ $10–50 $$$ $50–250 $$$$ $250–350

Table 3: **Drugs Used to Treat Hepatic Encephalopathy**

Drug Class	Drug	Dose	Adverse Effects	Drug Interactions	Cost[a]
Hyperosmotic Agents	*lactulose* generics	30 mL 1–4 × daily; titrate to produce 2–3 loose BM/day	Bloating, flatulence, cramps, diarrhea.		$$
Nitroimidazole Antibiotics	*metronidazole* Flagyl, generics	250–500 mg TID	GI disturbances, headache, metallic taste.	Disulfiram-like reaction with alcohol: ↑ INR with warfarin; barbiturates, phenytoin may ↑ metabolism.	$

[a] Cost of 30-day supply; includes drug cost only.
Legend: $ < $15 $$ $15–50

Table 4: Drugs Used to Treat Cholestatic Liver Disease

Drug Class	Drug	Dose	Adverse Effects	Drug Interactions	Cost[a]
Bile Acid Sequestrants	*cholestyramine* generics	Cholestatic pruritus: Initial: 4 g before breakfast; ↑ in 4 g increments first after breakfast, then at night and then at lunch	Constipation, heartburn, nausea, vomiting.	May bind other drugs given concurrently; separate doses (1 h before or 4–6 h after resin).	$$$$
Opiate Receptor Antagonists	*naltrexone* ReVia	Cholestatic pruritus: 50 mg daily × 4 weeks	Nausea, vomiting, headache, insomnia, dysphoria.	Precipitates opioid withdrawal in dependent patients.	$$$$$
Vitamins, fat-soluble	*vitamin K*	Deficiency in patients with chronic cholestasis: 10 mg im monthly		Antagonizes warfarin (↓ INR); mineral oil ↓ absorption.	$$
	vitamin A	Deficiency in patients with chronic cholestasis: 5000–10 000 IU/day po (aqueous). Use the minimum effective dose.		mineral oil ↓ absorption.	$
	vitamin D	Deficiency in patients with chronic cholestasis: 1000 IU Q2 day po (with 2–3 g elemental calcium/day)			$
Bile Acids	*ursodiol* (ursodeoxy-cholic acid) Urso	Primary biliary cirrhosis: 13–15 mg/kg/day in 2–4 divided doses	Occasional diarrhea, leukopenia, rash.	Do not give with antacids.	$$$$$[b]

[a] Cost of 30-day supply unless specified otherwise; includes drug cost only.
[b] Based on 750 mg/day × 30 days.
Legend: $ < $10 $$ $10–30 $$$ $30–80 $$$$ $80–110 $$$$$ $110–150

Table 5: **Drugs Used in Autoimmune Chronic Active Hepatitis and Alcoholic Hepatitis**

Drug Class	Drug	Dose	Adverse Effects	Drug Interactions	Cost[a]
Corticosteroids	*prednisone* generics	Autoimmune chronic active hepatitis: 60 mg/day × 1 wk, then 40 mg/day × 1 wk, then 30 mg/day × 2 wk, then 20 mg/day. Gradually taper from 20 mg/day over weeks to months using serum aminotransferase levels and clinical status as a guide. Alcoholic hepatitis: 40 mg/day x 28 days. Taper over 2 wk	Fluid/electrolyte imbalance, suppression of pituitary-adrenal function, hyperglycemia, peptic ulcer, behavioural disturbances, ocular cataracts, glaucoma, cushingoid syndrome, aseptic necrosis of hip.	↑ GI ulceration with NSAID; ↓ efficacy with barbiturates, phenytoin, rifampin; ↓ effect of vaccines.	$
Xanthines	*pentoxifylline* ❥ Trental, generics	Alcoholic hepatitis: 400 mg TID × 4 wk	Dizziness, headache, nausea, vomiting, heartburn, chest pain, rash, tremor, flushing.	Cimetidine and quinolones ↑ pentoxifylline levels; ↑ theophylline levels.	$$
Immunosuppressants	*azathioprine* ❥ Imuran, generics	Autoimmune hepatitis: 50–150 mg/day	↓ appetite, leukopenia, thrombocytopenia (monitor CBC monthly), infection, biliary stasis, hypersensitivity reactions, rash, rare veno-occlusive disease, nausea, vomiting.	↑ toxicity with allopurinol.	$$
	mycophenolate mofetil Cellcept	Autoimmune hepatitis: 500–1000 mg BID	Anemia, leucopenia, thrombocytopenia.	Antacids, iron and cholestyramine ↓ absorption.	$$$

[a] Cost of 30-day supply unless specified otherwise; includes drug cost only.

❥ Dosage adjustment may be required in renal impairment.

Legend: $ < $10 $$ $10–50 $$$ $ >200

Table 6: Drugs Used in Iron Overload in Hemochromatosis

Drug Class	Drug	Dose	Adverse Effects	Drug Interactions	Cost[a]
Chelating Agents	*deferoxamine*[b] Desferal, generics	1–4 g sc by minipump over 12 h, adjusted on an individual basis	Allergic reactions, auditory/ocular toxicity, tachycardia, flushing, abdominal discomfort, pain at injection site, hypotension, skin rash, convulsions.	Loss of consciousness with prochlorperazine; cardiac impairment with vitamin C (> 500 mg/day).	$800–3500

[a] Cost of 30-day supply; includes drug cost only.
[b] Phlebotomy is the preferred treatment for iron overload in hemochromatosis. Chelation with deferoxamine can be tried in patients unable to tolerate phlebotomy.

Table 7: Drugs Used in Wilson's Disease

Drug Class	Drug	Dose	Adverse Effects	Drug Interactions	Cost[a]
Chelating Agents	*penicillamine* (renal symbol) Cuprimine	1–2 g/day in 4 divided doses on an empty stomach	Proteinuria, hematologic effects, positive ANA, mouth ulcers, diarrhea, ↓ taste sense, ↓ appetite, nausea, vomiting, hypersensitivity.	↓ effect with antacids, iron, zinc; ↓ levels of digoxin.	$$
	trientine Syprine	1–2 g/day in 4 divided doses	Anemia.	↓ effect with iron.	[b]
	zinc generics	50 mg (elemental zinc) TID between meals	GI disturbances.	↓ levels of quinolones, tetracycline, penicillamine.	$

[a] Cost of 30-day supply; includes drug cost only.
[b] Available through the Special Access Programme, Therapeutic Products Directorate, Health Canada.
(renal symbol) Dosage adjustment may be required in renal impairment.
Abbreviations: ANA = antinuclear antibody
Legend: $ < $15 $$ $100–200

Suggested Readings

Adams PC. Review article: the modern diagnosis and management of haemochromatosis. *Aliment Pharmacol Ther* 2006;23(12):1681-91.

Ala A, Walker AP, Ashkan K et al. Wilson's disease. *Lancet* 2007;369(9559):397-408.

Arroyo V, Colmenero J. Ascites and hepatorenal syndrome in cirrhosis: pathophysiological basis of therapy and current management. *J Hepatol* 2003;38(Suppl 1):S69-89.

Czaja AJ, Freese DK; American Association for the Study of Liver Disease. Diagnosis and treatment of autoimmune hepatitis. *Hepatology* 2002;36(2):479-97.

Das SK, Ray K. Wilson's disease: an update. *Nat Clin Pract Neurol* 2006;2(9):482-93.

Heathcote EJ. Management of primary biliary cirrhosis. The American Association for the Study of Liver Diseases practice guidelines. *Hepatology* 2000;31(4):1005-13.

McCullough AJ, O'Connor JF. Alcoholic liver disease: proposed recommendations for the American College of Gastroenterology. *Am J Gastroenterol* 1998;93(11):2022-36.

References

1. Runyon BA, Montano AA, Akriviadis EA et al. The serum-ascites albumin gradient is superior to the exudate-transudate concept in the differential diagnosis of ascites. *Ann Intern Med* 1992;117(3):215-20.
2. Singh N, Gayowski T, Yu VL et al. Trimethoprim-sulfamethoxazole for the prevention of spontaneous bacterial peritonitis in cirrhosis: a randomized trial. *Ann Intern Med* 1995;122(8):595-8.
3. Gines P, Rimola A, Planas R et al. Norfloxacin prevents spontaneous bacterial peritonitis recurrence in cirrhosis: results of a double-blind, placebo-controlled trial. *Hepatology* 1990;12(4 Pt 1):716-24.
4. Heathcote EJ, Cauch-Dudek K, Walker V et al. The Canadian Multicenter Double-blind Randomized Controlled Trial of ursodeoxycholic acid in primary biliary cirrhosis. *Hepatology* 1994;19(5):1149-56.
5. Lindor KD, Dickson ER, Baldus WP et al. Ursodeoxycholic acid in the treatment of primary biliary cirrhosis. *Gastroenterology* 1994;106(5):1284-90.
6. Poupon RE, Balkau B, Eschwege E et al. A multicenter, controlled trial of ursodiol for the treatment of primary biliary cirrhosis. UDCA-PBC Study Group. *N Engl J Med* 1991;324(22):1548-54.
7. Harnois DM, Angulo P, Jorgensen RA et al. High-dose ursodeoxycholic acid as a therapy for patients with primary sclerosing cholangitis. *Am J Gastroenterol* 2001;96(5):1558-62.
8. Mitchell SA, Bansi DS, Hunt N et al. A preliminary trial of high-dose ursodeoxycholic acid in primary sclerosing cholangitis. *Gastroenterology* 2001;121(4):900-7.
9. Poupon RE, Lindor KD, Pares A et al. Combined analysis of the effect of treatment with ursodeoxycholic acid on histologic progression in primary biliary cirrhosis. *J Hepatol* 2003;39(1):12-6.
10. Wolfhagen FH, Sternieri E, Hop WC et al. Oral naltrexone treatment for cholestatic pruritus: a double-blind, placebo-controlled study. *Gastroenterology* 1997;113(4):1264-9.
11. Bachs L, Pares A, Elena M et al. Effects of long-term rifampicin administration in primary biliary cirrhosis. *Gastroenterology* 1992;102(6):2077-80.
12. Richardson PD, James PD, Ryder SD. Mycophenolate mofetil for maintenance of remission in autoimmune hepatitis in patients resistant to or intolerant of azathioprine. *J Hepatol* 2000;33(3):371-5.
13. Rambaldi A, Gluud C. Colchicine for alcoholic and non-alcoholic liver fibrosis and cirrhosis. *Cochrane Database Syst Rev* 2005;(2):CD002148.
14. Rambaldi A, Gluud C. Propothiouracil for alcoholic liver disease. *Cochrane Database Syst Rev* 2005;(4):CD002800.
15. Ramond MJ, Poynard T, Rueff B et al. A randomized trial of prednisolone in patients with severe alcoholic hepatitis. *N Engl J Med* 1992;326(8):507-12.
16. Akriviadis E, Botla R, Briggs W et al. Pentoxifylline improves short-term survival in severe acute alcoholic hepatitis: a double-blind, placebo-controlled trial. *Gastroenterology* 2000;119(6):1637-48.
17. Haber PS, Warner R, Seth D et al. Pathogenesis and management of alcoholic hepatitis. *J Gastroenterol Hepatol* 2003;18(12):1332-44.

CHAPTER 52

Viral Hepatitis

Kevork M. Peltekian, MD and
Geralynn Hirsch, RN-NP, MSN

Hepatitis A virus (HAV), hepatitis B virus (HBV), hepatitis C virus (HCV), hepatitis D virus (HDV) (which requires coexisting HBV infection) and hepatitis E virus (HEV) cause 95% of acute viral hepatitis cases observed in North America (Table 1).[1] Other causes of viral hepatitis include adenovirus, Coxsackie virus, cytomegalovirus, Epstein-Barr virus and, rarely, herpes simplex virus or parvovirus B19 infection.

This chapter focuses on the prevention of acute viral hepatitis and the management of chronic viral hepatitis, which may lead to the development of liver cirrhosis, hepatocellular carcinoma and liver failure requiring liver transplantation if untreated.

Table 1: **Summary of Viral Hepatitis**

	HAV	HBV	HCV	HDV	HEV
Virus type	RNA	DNA	RNA	RNA	RNA
Incubation (days)	15–45	30–180	15–60	21–140	15–65
Transmission	Fecal-oral	Percutaneous, venereal, perinatal	Percutaneous, perinatal (uncommon)	Percutaneous, venereal, perinatal	Fecal-oral
Acute hepatitis progressing to chronic disease	No	Adults 2–7%, preschoolers 25%, neonates 90%	70–80%	In superinfection; rare in co-infection	No
Prevention	Pre/post-exposure immunization	Pre/post-exposure immunization	Blood donor screening, risk behaviour modification	HBV immunization prevents HDV infection	Ensure safe drinking water

Goals of Therapy

General

- Prevent spread of infection
- Improve quality of life
- Minimize liver damage, prevent cirrhosis, hepatic failure and hepatocellular carcinoma

Specific

- Sustained suppression of viral replication and induction of HBe seroconversion in patients with chronic hepatitis B.[2]
- Eradicate the virus in the case of acute or chronic hepatitis C infection.[3] The desired outcome in chronic hepatitis C is sustained virologic response (SVR), defined as undetectable serum HCV RNA (< 50 IU/mL) 24 weeks after the end of treatment.

Prevention of Viral Hepatitis

Specific vaccines are available for *hepatitis A and B viruses* but not for *hepatitis C, D or E viruses*. HDV is a defective RNA virus that requires HBsAg for entry into and exit from hepatocytes; thus, vaccination against HBV confers immunity against co-infection with HBV and HDV.

Individuals at high risk of contracting hepatitis A or B should be vaccinated (Table 2). Hepatitis A immunoglobulin and hepatitis B immunoglobulin provide immediate short-term passive immunity against HAV and HBV, respectively. Active and passive immunizing agents used for hepatitis A and B are presented in Table 4.

Hepatitis A vaccine (inactivated) is the preferred agent for pre-exposure prophylaxis. It is very effective (up to 10 years) and is recommended for high-risk groups. Detectable antibody is present at one month in 96 to 100% of recipients after the first dose and in 100% after the booster dose, given 6 to 12 months later. Hepatitis A vaccines are well tolerated and safe.

Hepatitis A immune globulin with or without **hepatitis A vaccine** protects against HAV when administered before exposure or during the incubation period. It can be given with the vaccine to persons at risk of contracting HAV before adequate anti-HAV antibody titres are achieved.

Hepatitis B vaccines induce anti-HBs production. Antibody response in general decreases with age. Children between 2 and 19 years of age have the highest response rate (99%). The response rate for those older than 60 years is 70%. In most preparations, the antigen is adsorbed onto aluminum hydroxide with thimerosal as a preservative. A preparation of Recombivax HB without thimerosal is recommended for immunization of infants at birth. Hepatitis B vaccines are well tolerated and safe.

Hepatitis B immune globulin is prepared from pooled human plasma from select donors who have a high level of anti-HBs and are seronegative for bloodborne infections. It provides immediate short-term passive immunity. HBIg administered concurrently with the vaccine, but at a different site, does not interfere with the antibody response to the vaccine.

Table 2: **Recommendations for Hepatitis A and B Vaccinations[4]**

	Hepatitis A Vaccine	Hepatitis B Vaccine
Persons with end-stage renal disease or recipients of hemodialysis		x
Persons with clotting factor disorders	x	x
Persons with HIV infection		x
Persons with chronic liver disease including HCV	x	x
Health care and emergency service workers who have exposure to blood in the workplace		x
Persons handling HAV-infected primates or involved in research on HAV	x	
Persons in training in schools of dentistry, laboratory technology, medicine, nursing and other allied health professions		x
Users of illicit drugs, e.g., snorting cocaine, injection drug use		x
Persons with multiple sex partners and all clients in STI clinics		x
Men who have sex with men	x	x
Household and sexual contacts of persons with chronic HBV		x
Staff and inmates of long-term correctional facilities	?	x
Clients and staff of institutions for the developmentally challenged	?	x
International travellers to HAV- or HBV-endemic areas	x	x

x Highly recommended.
? Recommended when there is evidence for sustained HAV transmission.

Acute Viral Hepatitis

Acute viral hepatitis is a systemic viral infection that, by definition, has been present for less than six months and causes inflammatory necrosis of the liver. Most cases are asymptomatic; however, fulminant hepatitis occurs in 1% of patients (higher in pregnant women).[5] Patients with a prolonged INR, jaundice and encephalopathy should be referred immediately to a liver transplantation centre since massive necrosis may lead to liver failure and death.

Investigations (Figure 1)

- Check for risk factors such as injection drug use, high-risk sexual behaviour, travel history or daycare exposure.
- Rule out drug-induced hepatitis, including that caused by acetaminophen or herbal products, autoimmune hepatitis and Wilson's disease (especially in children and young adults).
- Identify hepatitis viruses by the presence of serologic markers.
- The presence of antibodies to hepatitis B core antibody (IgM) may indicate acute HBV, although it is often impossible to distinguish a flare-up of chronic HBV infection from an acute case. Only time will identify the chronic carriers.
- Acute hepatitis C can be identified by a positive HCV RNA test as early as 2 to 3 weeks after infection. Anti-HCV antibodies may not be detected for up to 20 weeks after exposure to the virus.
- Monitor liver transaminases (ALT, AST) and liver function tests (total bilirubin, serum albumin and INR).

Therapeutic Choices

In most cases specific antiviral therapy is not indicated (Figure 1). Provided with appropriate supportive care, the majority of patients with acute hepatitis A or B recover completely and do not experience chronic complications. Unfortunately, this is not the case with hepatitis C: most patients with acute hepatitis C become chronic carriers.

Nonpharmacologic Choices

- Avoid alcohol for at least three months or until complete normalization of liver enzymes and hepatic function.
- No dietary restrictions are necessary.
- No restraint of physical activities is needed.

Pharmacologic Choices

Stop all hepatotoxic drugs. For patients with a prolonged INR, administer vitamin K 10 mg subcutaneously (avoid frozen plasma unless there is active bleeding). If the patient develops encephalopathy heralding fulminant liver failure, start lactulose to achieve two to three loose bowel movements per day.

Effective and specific antiviral therapy is available only for acute hepatitis C (see the discussion of peginterferon alfa in the section on chronic hepatitis C and in Table 7). Most cases of acute HCV infection are asymptomatic and are usually diagnosed under three circumstances—documented seroconversion, known exposure (e.g., needle-stick exposure) and acute clinical hepatitis with jaundice.

Women, younger patients and icteric patients are more likely to clear the virus than other patients with acute hepatitis C. A single negative HCV

RNA test result is insufficient to confirm viral clearance in a patient with acute hepatitis C, and the test should be repeated at least once. If HCV RNA persists beyond 12 weeks, antiviral treatment should be considered. Treatment is most effective if started by 24 weeks. SVR rates of > 90% have been obtained with peginterferon monotherapy. Patients infected with HCV genotypes 2 or 3 should be treated for 12 weeks; those infected with other genotypes should be treated for 24 weeks.[6]

Chronic Viral Hepatitis

Viral hepatitis is chronic when present for six months or longer. It can progress to cirrhosis, decompensation (liver failure) and hepatoma (primary liver cancer). HBV and HCV are the most common causes.

Chronic Hepatitis B

HBV infection becomes chronic in less than 5% of healthy individuals who are infected as adults (but up to 90% of those infected as children). Among those with chronic hepatitis B, one percent will seroconvert spontaneously each year from an HBsAg–positive to an anti-HBs–positive state (i.e. become immune).

Investigations

- Persistence of detectable levels of HBsAg for more than six months implies chronic hepatitis B infection.
- Since HBV and HIV are acquired by the same transmission routes, patients with HBV should be tested for HIV co-infection, especially when considering nucleos(t)ide analogues for HBV
- Check for HDV co-infection in patients with elevated ALT levels but low serum HBV DNA concentrations especially in those who may have become infected through injection drug use or if they are from endemic areas for HDV, i.e., sub-Saharan Africa, Romania, Central Asia, Eastern Mediterranean and the Amazon.
- Check HBeAg and anti-HBe and serum transaminase (ALT, AST) values to determine the replicative state of HBV. The presence of HBeAg indicates a high rate of viral replication (potentially treatable with antiviral agents).
- Measurement of HBV DNA virus in serum is not routinely available but is helpful when transaminase levels are high in HBeAg-negative and anti-HBe-positive patients. It is recommended that HBV DNA levels be monitored every three to six months.[2]
- Liver biopsy is recommended, especially in those older than 40 years with normal liver enzymes.

Therapeutic Choices (Table 5)

Nonpharmacologic Choices

- Advise against all but modest alcohol consumption (less than four drinks weekly).

Pharmacologic Choices (Table 6)

Peginterferon alfa

Peginterferon alfa is used to treat patients with chronic hepatitis B who are persistently HBeAg-positive and have elevated serum transaminase values. It promotes seroconversion from an HBeAg-positive to anti-HBe-positive state, which is associated with normalization of serum transaminases. Due to the reduced frequency of administration (i.e., once weekly) and documented efficacy, peginterferon alfa is recommended instead of standard interferon alfa, which must be administered at least thrice weekly, for the management of chronic hepatitis B.[7]

Most patients with hepatitis D co-infection relapse after peginterferon alfa therapy. HIV-positive and other immunosuppressed patients with chronic hepatitis B respond poorly to peginterferon alfa.

Nucleos(t)ide Analogues

Nucleoside analogues effectively inhibit replication of HBV in patients who are HBeAg-positive or HBeAg-negative and should be given only to patients who have ongoing hepatitis (persistent ALT and HBV DNA elevations). Inhibition of HBV replication with nucleoside analogues is associated with significant reductions in hepatic necroinflammation and increased rates of HBe seroconversion.

Resistance to nucleos(t)ide analogues is an important issue. Among these agents, lamivudine is associated with the highest rates of resistance and entecavir is associated with the lowest rates of resistance. Lamivudine-resistant HBV is cross-resistant to telbivudine and emtricitabine (an antiretroviral agent with activity against HBV). Mutations that confer resistance to lamivudine do not by themselves confer resistance to entecavir; however, they are a prerequisite for the development of entecavir resistance, and entecavir resistance rates are considerably higher when the drug is initiated in patients with lamivudine-refractory or -resistant strains of HBV. Adefovir has activity against lamivudine-resistant HBV. Conversely, both lamivudine and entecavir have activity against adefovir-resistant HBV.

After three years of treatment with **lamivudine** the HBeAg seroconversion rate is reported to be 40%.[8] Lamivudine-resistant HBV emerges in about 15 to 25% of patients after one-year of treatment and in up to 70% after five-years of therapy.[9] Lamivudine improves outcomes in patients with decompensated cirrhosis and may be used to prevent disease flares in patients on immunosuppressive therapy.

Adefovir dipivoxil has activity against wild-type, precore mutant and lamivudine-resistant HBV. The expected HBeAg seroconversion rate is 12% after one year.[10] Adefovir dipivoxil in high doses is associated with nephrotoxicity. Monitoring of liver function tests may be necessary immediately after discontinuation since severe acute exacerbations of hepatitis have been reported in patients stopping treatment.

Entecavir[11,12] and **telbivudine**[13] produce significantly greater reductions in HBV DNA levels than lamivudine in both HBeAg-positive and HBeAg-negative patients. HBeAg seroconversion was reported in 21% of entecavir-treated patients and 22% of telbivudine-treated patients after one year (similar to lamivudine).[3] The HBeAg seroconversion rate after three years of treatment with entecavir was 39%.[3] Among nucleoside-naïve patients the rate of resistance was < 1% after three years of treatment with entecavir.[14] Limited data are as yet available for telbivudine, but preliminary reports suggest that the rate of resistance may be as high as 20% after two years (vs. 30% with lamivudine).[13]

Tenofovir is a nucleotide analogue that is active against HIV and HBV and is approved only for treatment of HIV. It has activity against lamivudine-resistant HBV, but has only been studied in patients with HIV-HBV co-infection receiving combination antiretroviral regimens.

Chronic Hepatitis C

Over 80% of acute infections with HCV become chronic (the rate is lower in children). HCV is acquired most frequently through illicit drug use (e.g., snorting cocaine, injection drug use), blood transfusion (prior to 1992), tattooing and needle-stick injuries. Risk factors for progressive fibrosis in patients with chronic hepatitis C are male gender, age > 40 years at acquisition, alcohol consumption > 50 g daily and co-infection with HIV or immune suppression.

Investigations

- Anti-HCV is a marker of infection, not immunity; tests are false-positive in less than 4% of patients, but may be false-negative in up to 40% of immunocompromised individuals (in this group the presence of HCV may be detected only by HCV RNA assay).
- HCV RNA by PCR to confirm the diagnosis.
- Liver biopsy to determine inflammatory grade and fibrosis stage is preferred but may not be necessary in all patients prior to initiation of treatment.
- Measure HCV RNA viral load (quantitation) and genotype prior to starting treatment.

Therapeutic Choices

Nonpharmacologic Choices

- Advise against all but modest alcohol consumption (less than four drinks weekly).
- Cannabis may accelerate fibrosis in patients with chronic hepatitis and use should be discouraged.

Pharmacologic Choices

The pharmacologic management of patients with chronic hepatitis C is outlined in Table 6. An overview of the properties of antiviral agents used for chronic hepatitis C is provided in Table 7. SVR is associated with clinically significant outcomes including improvements in liver histology and health-related quality of life, reductions in liver-related morbidity and mortality, and is durable.[16]

Combination Peginterferon plus Ribavirin

The combination of peginterferon alfa plus ribavirin is the recommended treatment for chronic hepatitis C in Canada.[3] Pegylation reduces the clearance of interferon and allows for once-weekly administration. Peginterferon alfa monotherapy is significantly less effective than combination therapy and is appropriate only for patients who have a contraindication to ribavirin and those who cannot tolerate ribavirin. Ribavirin monotherapy is ineffective, thus ribavirin should never be administered alone. The duration of therapy and dose of ribavirin depend on the viral genotype (Table 6, Table 7). Patients most likely to have an SVR are those infected with genotype 2 or 3, individuals with a low baseline HCV RNA level and those without advanced hepatic fibrosis.

For patients infected with HCV genotypes 2 or 3, the standard duration of treatment has traditionally been 24 weeks and the standard dose of ribavirin is 800 mg/day. For patients infected with HCV genotype 1, the standard duration of treatment has traditionally been 48 weeks and the standard dose of ribavirin is 1000 or 1200 mg/day.

Ideally, HCV RNA should be tested at week 4 and week 12 of therapy. Patients with a rapid virologic response (RVR), defined as negative HCV RNA (< 50 IU/mL by qualitative PCR) at week 4, have a very high chance of achieving an SVR, and the duration of therapy may be abbreviated in these select individuals.[3]

Consideration may be given to shortening the duration of treatment from 24 to 16 weeks for genotype 2 or 3 patients who have an RVR. Similarly, the duration of treatment may be shortened from 48 to 24 weeks in genotype 1 patients who have an RVR.[3,17] Abbreviated regimens are most effective in patients with low baseline HCV RNA levels (< 400 000 IU/mL). A 36-week abbreviated regimen is as effective as a 48-week regimen in patients with minimal fibrosis and low baseline HVC RNA levels who are infected with genotype 4.[3]

If HCV RNA is detectable at week 4, treatment should be continued until week 12, at which point serum HCV RNA is reassessed by quantitative assay. Patients without a $\geq$ 2-$\log_{10}$ drop in HCV RNA relative to baseline or undetectable HCV RNA at week 12 are very unlikely to achieve an SVR, thus treatment may be discontinued.

Genotype 1 and 4 patients with undetectable HCV RNA at week 12 should complete 48 weeks of combination therapy. Genotype 1 patients with a $\geq$ 2-$\log_{10}$ drop but detectable HCV RNA at week 12 should continue to week 24, at which time HCV RNA is reassessed by qualitative HCV RNA assay. If HCV RNA is still detectable, treatment should be stopped because of the low probability of SVR. If HCV RNA is undetectable at week 24, continue for 48 weeks and give consideration to prolonging treatment for up to 72 weeks (if funding is available). Preliminary data has shown better outcomes with prolonged treatment in individuals who are "late" responders.[3]

All patients who complete treatment must be advised to return 24 weeks after completion of therapy for a qualitative HCV RNA test to determine SVR status.

Patients who have not responded or who have relapsed after treatment with standard interferon alone or in combination with ribavirin may be retreated successfully with peginterferon plus ribavirin. However, the lack of a virologic response at week 12, as outlined above, indicates a very low likelihood of an SVR, and treatment should be stopped.[3]

Expected SVR rates with the recommended regimens for genotypes 1, 2 and 3 are shown in Table 3. Infection with genotypes other than 1–3 are much less common and outcomes are less well defined. SVR rates in these individuals are more similar to genotype 1 than 2 or 3, thus they should be managed in a manner similar to genotype 1.

Table 3: **Expected SVR Rates in Patients with Chronic Hepatitis C After Treatment with Peginterferon alfa Plus Ribavirin**

Genotype	Patients	Duration of Treatment	SVR Rate
Genotype 1	Unselected	48 weeks	42–52%[17,18,19]
	RVR	24 weeks	88–89%[20,21]
	No RVR	72 weeks	44%[22]
Genotype 2 or 3	Unselected	24 weeks	72–80%[17,18,19]
	RVR	12–16 weeks	82–85%[23,24]

Therapeutic Tips

- Avoid immunosuppressive drugs, including prednisone. Fifty per cent of hepatitis B carriers experience a flare-up upon withdrawal of immunosuppressive drugs with a rise in serum transaminases and conversion from an anti-HBe to HBeAg-positive state. This is especially a problem in those undergoing cancer chemotherapy. Short-term lamivudine use is recommended in this setting.[11]

- Safe sex is recommended for those with multiple sexual partners. The precise sexual transmission rate is unknown, but the prevalence of anti-HCV in partners of HCV-infected patients is only 1.5% (most partners have other risk factors).[25] Presence of HIV co-infection appears to increase the probability of sexual transmission of HCV.[26]
- Nucleoside analogues should not be used as monotherapy for HBV in HIV-positive patients because of the potential for development of resistant HIV strains.
- Treatment of HBV and HCV in patients with decompensated cirrhosis or post–liver transplantation should be handled by transplant hepatologists only.
- In patients with addiction problems, delay treatment of HCV until appropriate interventions have been initiated by addiction medicine specialists.
- Co-infection with HCV and/or HBV in HIV-positive patients should be handled by infectious disease specialists.[27]
- Adherence is very important.
- Depression is a side effect of peginterferon alfa , but antidepressants are effective for peginterferon-induced depression. Monitor patients for depression and treat proactively.
- Hemolytic anemia is a common and dose-limiting side effect of ribavirin that is managed by dose reductions. As dose reductions reduce the likelihood of achieving an SVR, erythropoietin is advocated by some as a means of maintaining the dose of ribavirin (see Chapter 87).[28]

Figure 1: Treatment of Acute Viral Hepatitis

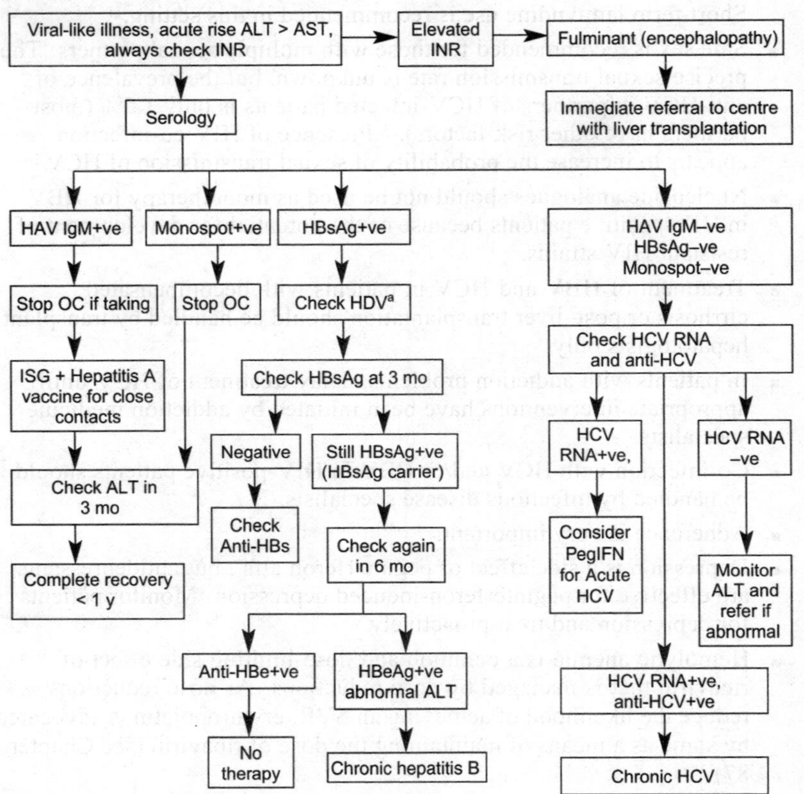

[a] Note: co-infection with HDV does not change treatment course, but is generally more severe.

Abbreviations: HAV IgM = Hepatitis A IgM; HBsAg = Hepatitis B surface antigen; HDV = Hepatitis D (delta) virus; ISG = Immune Serum Globulin; Anti-HCV = Antibody to HCV; OC = Oral contraceptive; PegIFN = peginterferon alfa.

Table 4: **Hepatitis A and Hepatitis B Immunizing Agents**

Class	Vaccine	Dose	Cost[a]
Viral Vaccines, Single Component	*hepatitis A vaccine* Avaxim, Avaxim-Pediatric, Epaxal Berna, Havrix 1440, Havrix 720 Junior, Vaqta, Vaqta pediatric	**Avaxim: Adults and children aged ≥ 12 y:** 0.5 mL (160 AU) im × 2 at 0 and 6–12 months **Avaxim-Pediatric: Children aged 1 to 15 y:** 0.5 mL (80 AU) im × 2 at 0 and 6–12 months **Epaxal: Adults and children aged ≥ 1 y:** 0.5 mL (500 RIA units) im × 2 at 0 and 12 months **Havrix 1440: Adults aged ≥ 19 y:** 1.0 mL (1440 ELISA units) im × 2 at 0 and 6–12 months **Havrix 720 Junior: Children 1 to 18 y:** 0.5 mL (720 ELISA units) im at time 0 and 6–12 mo **Vaqta: Adults aged ≥ 18 y:** 1.0 mL (50 units) im × 2 at 0 and 6 months **Vaqta pediatric: Children aged 1 to 17 y:** 0.5 mL (25 units) im × 2 at 0 and 6–18 months	\$–\$\$
	hepatitis B vaccine Engerix-B, Recombivax HB	**Engerix-B:** **Adults aged ≥ 20 y:** 1.0 mL (20 µg HbsAg) im × 3 at 0, 1 and 6 months *or* × 4 at 0, 1, 2 and 12 months, or 0, 7, 21 and 365 days **Adults (dialysis ≥ 16 y):** 2.0 mL (40 µg HbsAg) im × 4 at 0, 1, 2 and 6 months **Children aged 0 to 19 y:** 0.5 mL (10 µg HbsAg) im × 3 at 0, 1 and 6 months *or* × 4 at 0, 1, 2 and 12 months **Adolescents aged 11 to 15 y (alternative 2 dose schedule):** 1.0 mL (20 µg HbsAg) im × 2 at 0 and 6 months **Immunocompromised patients:** 2.0 mL (40 µg HbsAg) im. Monitor anti-HbsAg titre annually and give boosters as needed **Recombivax HB:** **Adults aged ≥ 20 y:** 1.0 mL (10 µg HbsAg) im × 3 at 0, 1 and ≥ 2 months **Adults (predialysis or dialysis):** 1.0 mL (40 µg HbsAg) im × 3 at 0, 1 and 6 months **Adolescents aged 11 to 19 y:** 0.5 mL (5 µg HbsAg) im × 3 at 0, 1 and ≥ 2 months **Infants and children aged 0 to < 11 y:** 0.25 mL (2.5 µg HbsAg) im × 3 at 0, 1 and ≥ 2 months **Adolescents aged 11 to 15 y (alternative 2 dose schedule):** 1.0 mL (10 µg HbsAg) im × 2 at 0 and 4–6 months	Energix-B: \$ Recombivax HB Adults: \$\$\$ Pediatric: \$

(cont'd)

Table 4: **Hepatitis A and Hepatitis B Immunizing Agents** *(cont'd)*

Class	Vaccine	Dose	Cost[a]
Viral Vaccines, Combinations	*combined hepatitis A and B* Twinrix	**Adults aged ≥ 19 y:** 1.0 mL (720 ELISA units plus 20 μg HbsAg) im × 3 at 0, 1 and 6 months *or* × 4 at 0, 7, 21 and 365 days **Children aged 1 to 18 y:** 0.5 mL (360 ELISA units plus 10 μg HbsAg) im × 3 at 0, 1 and 6 months **Adolescents aged 1 to 15 y (alternative 2 dose schedule):** 1.0 mL (720 ELISA units plus 20 μg HbsAg) im × 2 at 0 and 6–12 months	$$
	combined hepatitis A and Salmonella Typhi Vivaxim	**Adults aged ≥ 16 y:** 1.0 mL (160 AU plus 25 μg *S. typhi* Vi capsular polysaccharide) im × 2 at 0 and 6–12 months	$$$
Passive Immunizing Agents	*hepatitis B immune globulin* Hyperhep B S/D	**Post-exposure prophylaxis for hepatitis B:** 0.06 mL/kg im	$$$$[b]
	hepatitis A immune globulin GamaSTAN S/D	**Post-exposure prophylaxis for hepatitis A within 2 weeks of exposure (If exposure is continuous, repeat in 5 mo):** Adults: 0.08–0.12 mL/kg im Children: 0.02–0.04 mL/kg im	$$[b]

[a] Vaccine cost only.
[b] Available through Canadian Blood Services.
Legend: $ < $25 $$ $25–50 $–$$ < $25–50 $$$ $50–75 $$$$ > $75
Abbreviations: AU = antigen units; ELISA = enzyme-linked immunosorbent assay; RIA = radioimmunoassay

Table 5: **Management of Chronic Hepatitis B[2]**

Patient Characteristics		HBV Serum Markers					Recommended Management[a]
		Anti-HBs	HBsAg	Anti-HBe	ALT Status	HBV DNA, IU/mL	
Immune		+	–	+	↔	–	Antiviral therapy is not indicated
Low-replicating		–	+	+/–	↔	< 1000	No antiviral therapy. Monitor ALT Q6 months
Immune-tolerant	HBeAg(+)	–	+	–	↔	> 10 000	No antiviral therapy. Monitor ALT Q3 months × 1 year, then Q6–12 months thereafter
High-replicating	Wild type	–	+	–	↑	> 10 000	Consider peginterferon or nucleoside analogue therapy (adefovir, entecavir, lamivudine, telbivudine). The goal is to suppress HBV DNA replication below the limit of detection until HBe seroconversion occurs
	Precore mutant	–	+	+	↑	> 1000	Consider long-term nucleoside analogue therapy: adefovir, entecavir or lamivudine
	Lamivudine-resistant[b]	–	+	+/–	↑	> 10 000	Switch to entecavir 1 mg/day; or continue lamivudine and add either adefovir or tenofovir
Decompensated cirrhosis		–	+	+/–	↑	> 100	Lamivudine
Post–liver transplant		–	+	+/–	↔/↑	+	Lamivudine plus HBIg[c]

[a] Where more than one nucleoside analogue is presented, the presentation is alphabetical and does not imply the order of choice. Drug doses are presented in Table 7.

[b] HBV species with mutations in the tyrosine-methionine-aspartate-aspartate (YMDD) locus of the HBV-RNA-dependent DNA polymerase resulting in resistance to lamivudine.

[c] HBIg is generally given during the anhepatic phase (10 000 IU iv bolus), then daily during the first week to ensure an anti-HBs titre > 100 IU/mL, and then either at a dose of 5 mL im monthly or adjusted to maintain an anti HBs titre > 100 IU/mL.

+ = positive (marker is present); – = negative (marker is absent); ↔ = not elevated above the upper limit of normal; ↑ = elevated above the upper limit of normal; HBIg = hepatitis B immune globulin

Table 6: Management of Chronic Hepatitis C[3]

Patient Characteristics	Anti-HCV	HCV RNA	Serum ALT	HCV Genotype	Fibrosis on Liver Biopsy	Recommended Management
Chronic hepatitis C	+	+	↔/↑	1,4,5,6	+	PegIFN + ribavirin × 24 to 72 weeks
	+	+	↔/↑	2,3	+/–	PegIFN + ribavirin × 16 to 24 weeks
Extrahepatic disease[a]	+	+	↔/↑	1-6	+/–	Same as for chronic disease according to HCV genotype
Renal failure[b]	+	+	↔/↑	1-6	+/–	PegIFN monotherapy × at least 48 weeks
No viremia	+	–	↔[c]	1-6	+/–	Antiviral therapy is not indicated

[a] Mixed cryoglobinemia, membranoproliferative glomerulonephritis.
[b] Ribavirin is contraindicated in patients with renal failure.
[c] May be elevated due to other causes.

Table 7: **Drugs Used in Viral Hepatitis**

Class	Drug	Indication and Dose	Adverse Effects	Comments	Cost[a]
Nucleoside Analogues	*adefovir dipivoxil* Hepsera	**Chronic hepatitis B:** 10 mg po daily	Elevated transaminase levels, nephrotoxicity (increased serum creatinine).	Do not use nucleoside analogues as monotherapy for HBV in patients with HIV co-infection: can select resistant HIV variants. Acute exacerbations of HBV disease evidenced by marked ALT elevations have occurred after discontinuing nucleoside analogues.	$$$
	entecavir Baraclude	**Chronic hepatitis B:** Nucleoside–naïve patients: 0.5 mg po daily Lamivudine-experienced patients: 1 mg po daily	Elevated transaminase levels.	See adefovir.	$$$
	lamivudine Heptovir	**Chronic hepatitis B:** 100 mg po daily	Elevated transaminase levels.	See adefovir.	$
	telbivudine Sebivo	**Chronic hepatitis B:** 600 mg po daily	Elevated transaminase levels. Elevated creatine kinase levels.	See adefovir.	$$$
Immuno-modulatory Agents	*peginterferon alfa-2a* Pegasys	**Chronic hepatitis B:** 180 µg sc once/wk for 48 wk	Flu-like syndrome, fatigue, fever, muscle aches, asthenia, weight loss, headaches, irritability, depression, hair loss, soreness and redness at injection site, neutropenia and thrombocytopenia.	Neutropenia ($< 0.75 \times 10^9$/L) and thrombocytopenia ($< 50 \times 10^9$/L) are managed by dose reductions. Neutropenia associated with peginterferon does not appear to increase susceptibility to infection.[29] Contraindications include pregnancy, decompensated liver disease, severe cardiac disease, solid organ transplant (except liver), ongoing/untreated alcohol abuse or injection drug use, severe/untreated major depression or psychosis, renal failure[3]	$$$$

(cont'd)

Table 7: **Drugs Used in Viral Hepatitis** *(cont'd)*

Class	Drug	Indication and Dose	Adverse Effects	Comments	Cost[a]
Combination Nucleoside Analogues/ Immuno-modulatory Agents	*ribavirin/peginterferon alfa-2a* Pegasys RBV	**Chronic hepatitis C** peginterferon alfa-2a 180 μg sc once/wk with ribavirin: (Genotype 1, 4, 5, 6:) • 1000 mg/day if < 75 kg; • 1200 mg/day BID if ≥ 75 kg (Genotype 2 or 3:) • 800 mg/day Give BID with food	Ribavirin: Hemolytic anemia (reduce dose), rash. See peginterferon alfa-2a.	Monotherapy with peginterferon should only be used in patients with contraindications or intolerance to ribavirin. Contraindicated in pregnancy (teratogenic); effective contraception during treatment is mandatory. Anemia (Hgb < 100 g/L) is managed by dose reductions. See peginterferon alfa-2a.	$$$$[b]
	ribavirin/peginterferon alfa-2b Pegetron	**Chronic hepatitis C** peginterferon alfa-2b 1.5 μg/kg sc once/wk with ribavirin 13.5 mg/kg (600–1200 mg/day) Give BID with food.	See ribavirin/peginterferon alfa-2a.	See ribavirin/peginterferon alfa-2a.	$$$$[b]

[a] Cost of 30-day supply; includes drug cost only.
[b] Ribavirin is sold only in combination with peginterferon alfa-2a or peginterferon alfa-2b.
Dosage adjustment may be required in renal impairment; see Appendix I.
Legend: $ < $250 $$ $250–750 $$$ $750–1250 $$$$ $1250–1750

Suggested Readings

Hoofnagle JH, Seeff LB. Peginterferon and ribavirin for chronic hepatitis C. *N Engl J Med* 2006;355(23):2444–2451.

Koziel MJ, Peters MG. Viral hepatitis in HIV infection. *N Engl J Med* 2007;356(14):1445–1454.

Lok AS, McMahon BJ. Chronic hepatitis B. *Hepatology* 2007;45(2):507-39.

National Advisory Committee on Immunization. *Canadian immunization guide*. 7th ed. Ottawa (ON): Public Health Agency of Canada; 2006. Available from: http://www.phac-aspc.gc.ca/publicat/cig-gci/pdf/cig-gci-2006_e.pdf Accessed May 15, 2007.

Scott JD Gretch DR. Molecular diagnostics of hepatitis C virus infection: a systematic review. *JAMA* 2007;297(7):724-32.

References

1. Alter MJ, Mast EE. The epidemiology of viral hepatitis in the United States. *Gastroenterol Clin North Am* 1994;23(3):437-55.
2. Sherman M, Shafran S, Burak K et al. *Management of chronic hepatitis B: consensus guidelines* [in press]. Available from: http://hepatology.ca/cm/ Accessed May 15, 2007.
3. Sherman M, Shafran S, Burak K, et al. *Management of chronic hepatitis C: consensus guidelines* [in press]. Available from: http://hepatology.ca/cm/ Accessed May 15, 2007.
4. National Advisory Committee on Immunization. *Canadian immunization guide*. 7th ed. Ottawa (ON): Public Health Agency of Canada; 2006. Available from: http://www.phac-aspc.gc.ca/publicat/cig-gci/pdf/cig-gci-2006_e.pdf Accessed May 15, 2007.
5. Ryder SD, Beckingham IJ. ABC of diseases of liver, pancreas, and biliary system: acute hepatitis. *BMJ* 2001;322(7279):151-3.
6. Irving WL. Acute hepatitis C virus infection: a neglected disease? *Gut* 2006;55(8):1075-7.
7. Coffin CS, Lee SS. Chronic hepatitis B—who should be treated? *MedGenMed* 2006;8(1):75.
8. Leung NW, Lai CL, Chang TT et al. Extended lamivudine treatment in patients with chronic hepatitis B enhances hepatitis B e antigen seroconversion rates: results after 3 years of therapy. *Hepatology* 2001;33(6):1527-32.
9. Lai CL, Chien RN, Leung NW et al. A one-year trial of lamivudine for chronic hepatitis B. Asia Hepatitis Lamivudine Study Group. *N Engl J Med* 1998;339(2):61-8.
10. Marcellin P, Chang TT, Lim SG et al. Adefovir dipivoxil for the treatment of hepatitis B e antigen-positive chronic hepatitis B. *N Engl J Med* 2003;348(9):808-16.
11. Chang TT, Gish RG, de Man R et al. A comparison of entecavir and lamivudine for HBeAg-positive chronic hepatitis B. *N Engl J Med* 2006;354(10):1001-10.
12. Lai CL, Shouval D, Lok AS et al. Entecavir versus lamivudine for patients with HBeAg-negative chronic hepatitis B. *N Engl J Med* 2006;354(10):1011-20.
13. Dienstag J, Easley C,.Kirkpatrick P. Telbivudine. *Nat Rev Drug Discov* 2007;6(4):267-8.
14. Colonno RJ, Rose R, Baldick CJ et al. Entecavir resistance is rare in nucleoside naive patients with hepatitis B. *Hepatology* 2006;44(6):1656-65.
15. Manns MP, Wedemeyer H,.Cornberg M. Treating viral hepatitis C: efficacy, side effects, and complications. *Gut* 2006;55(9):1350-9.
16. Dienstag JL, McHutchison JG. American Gastroenterological Association technical review on the management of hepatitis C. *Gastroenterology* 2006;130(1):231-64.
17. Manns MP, McHutchison JG, Gordon SC et al. Peginterferon alfa-2b plus ribavirin compared with interferon alfa-2b plus ribavirin for initial treatment of chronic hepatitis C: a randomised trial. *Lancet* 2001;358(9286):958-65.
18. Fried MW, Shiffman ML, Reddy KR et al. Peginterferon alfa-2a plus ribavirin for chronic hepatitis C virus infection. *N Engl J Med* 2002;347(13):975-82.
19. Hadziyannis SJ, Sette H, Morgan TR et al. Peginterferon-alpha2a and ribavirin combination therapy in chronic hepatitis C: a randomized study of treatment duration and ribavirin dose. *Ann Intern Med* 2004;140(5):346-55.
20. Jensen DM, Morgan TR, Marcellin P et al. Early identification of HCV genotype 1 patients responding to 24 weeks peginterferon alpha-2a (40 kd)/ribavirin therapy. *Hepatology* 2006;43(5):954-60.
21. Zeuzem S, Buti M, Ferenci P et al. Efficacy of 24 weeks treatment with peginterferon alfa-2b plus ribavirin in patients with chronic hepatitis C infected with genotype 1 and low pretreatment viremia. *J Hepatol* 2006;44(1):97-103.

22. Sanchez-Tapias JM, Diago M, Escartin P et al. Peginterferon-alfa2a plus ribavirin for 48 versus 72 weeks in patients with detectable hepatitis C virus RNA at week 4 of treatment. *Gastroenterology* 2006;131(2):451-60.
23. Mangia A, Santoro R, Minerva N et al. Peginterferon alfa-2b and ribavirin for 12 vs. 24 weeks in HCV genotype 2 or 3. *N Engl J Med* 2005;352(25):2609-17.
24. von Wagner M, Huber M, Berg T et al. Peginterferon-alpha-2a (40KD) and ribavirin for 16 or 24 weeks in patients with genotype 2 or 3 chronic hepatitis C. *Gastroenterology* 2005;129(2):522-7.
25. Alter MJ. The epidemiology of acute and chronic hepatitis C. *Clin Liver Dis* 1997;1(3):559-68, vi-vii.
26. Filippini P, Coppola N, Scolastico C et al. Does HIV infection favor the sexual transmission of hepatitis C? *Sex Transm Dis* 2001;28(12):725-9.
27. Adeyemi OM. Hepatitis C in HIV-positive patients—treatment and liver disease outcomes. *J Clin Gastroenterol* 2007;41(1):75-87.
28. Sherman M, Cohen L, Cooper MA et al. Clinical recommendations for the use of recombinant human erythropoietin in patients with hepatitis C virus being treated with ribavirin. *Can J Gastroenterol* 2006;20(7):479-85.
29. Cooper CL, Al-Bedwawi S, Lee C et al. Rate of infectious complications during interferon-based therapy for hepatitis C is not related to neutropenia. *Clin Infect Dis* 2006;42(12):1674-8.

CHAPTER 53
Gastroesophageal Reflux Disease

Eldon A. Shaffer, MD, DABIM, FACP, FRCPC

Gastroesophageal reflux disease (GERD) refers to symptoms (commonly heartburn and/or regurgitation) resulting from excessive reflux of caustic, primarily acidic gastric secretions from the stomach into the esophagus. Reflux may lead to inflammation termed reflux or peptic esophagitis. Hence, *reflux esophagitis* is a subset of GERD with endoscopic or histopathologic evidence of esophageal inflammation. GERD with no demonstrable esophageal disease (i.e., a normal esophagus at endoscopy while not on any treatment) is termed *nonerosive reflux disease* (NERD) or *endoscopic-negative reflux disease* (ENRD).

Goals of Therapy

- Relieve symptoms, particularly heartburn, and improve quality of life
- Promote healing of esophagitis
- Prevent complications (stricture formation, bleeding or progression to Barrett's epithelium)
- Prevent recurrences

Table 1: **Classification of Symptom Severity[a]**

Severity of GERD	Criteria
Trivial to mild	Reflux symptoms infrequent (< 3 times/wk) Symptoms of low intensity and short duration • Not nocturnal • Do not interfere with daily activity • Pain (retrosternal heartburn) severity rated as modest (e.g., 1–3 out of 10) No major complications
Severe	Reflux symptoms more frequent and intense; greater impact on quality of life • present for > 6 mo • regularly interfere with daily activity • can awaken patient at night • more severe retrosternal pain (e.g., 7–10 out of 10) • Takes patient to physician Complications arise from the acidic refluxate

[a] Classification does not necessarily correspond to histological severity. Prevalence of esophagitis is low: the majority of patients with GERD (55% to 80%) have no erosive disease on endoscopy. The severity of symptoms and esophageal mucosal injury correlate with the total time the esophageal mucosa is in direct contact with acid (at pH < 4) per 24-hour period.[1]

Investigations

- History — identify:
  - common symptoms of GERD: heartburn, regurgitation of acid or bile, or hypersalivation (water brash). The history is usually sufficient for diagnosis. Heartburn or acid regurgitation has a high specificity (89% and 95%, respectively), but a low sensitivity (38% and 6%) for GERD[2]
  - noncardiac extraesophageal manifestations: chest pain, aspiration (cough, asthma, pneumonia), oropharyngeal symptoms (globus sensation, hoarseness) or ulceration, dental caries, burning mouth syndrome
  - complications: dysphagia from a stricture, or peptic ulceration causing GI bleeding or pain on swallowing (odynophagia)
  - predisposing/associated conditions: pregnancy, obesity, scleroderma
- Endoscopy is indicated in patients with heartburn refractory to optimal therapy with a proton pump inhibitor (Figure 1) or "alarm features" such as:
  - dysphagia, especially for solids
  - vomiting
  - odynophagia
  - atypical noncardiac chest pain
  - GI bleeding, anemia
  - extraesophageal symptoms (respiratory, oropharyngeal)
  - weight loss > 5%
- Ambulatory 24-hour pH monitoring is indicated in patients with atypical reflux symptoms, for those who fail standard medical therapy (but have a normal endoscopy), and as preoperative evaluation (especially with ENRD) before antireflux surgery
- *Helicobacter pylori* infection does not play a causative role in the pathogenesis of GERD. Testing for *H. pylori* is not necessary. *H. pylori* does not alter the effectiveness of PPI therapy nor does it influence reflux symptoms

Therapeutic Choices (Figure 1)

Nonpharmacologic Choices

There is little evidence to support the effectiveness of lifestyle changes, except as initial therapy in mild cases. However, recommending them provides broad health care benefits and carries no risk.

- Dietary modifications (avoid chocolate, caffeine, acidic citrus juices, large fatty meals)
- Weight loss if obese (BMI > 25 to 30 kg/m^2)
- No snacks within three hours before bedtime

- No lying down after meals
- Reduce alcohol intake
- Elevate legs under the head of the bed on 10 to 15 cm blocks
- Stop smoking (see Chapter 10)
- Avoid tight clothing

Pharmacologic Choices (Table 2, Table 3 and Table 4)

When possible, eliminate drugs that impair esophageal motility and lower esophageal sphincter tone (e.g., calcium channel blockers, theophylline, tricyclic antidepressants, beta-blockers, anticholinergic agents).

Trivial-to-Mild GERD

Most people with mild symptoms do not seek medical attention and will obtain symptomatic relief with **antacids**, **alginates** or nonprescription strength **H_2-receptor antagonists** (H_2RAs). The latter are expensive and yield quite modest acid reduction and symptom control. Additional therapy becomes necessary if GERD severity increases.

Moderate-to-Severe GERD

Antacids or nonprescription strength H_2RAs alone are *not* effective. The most effective and common approach in treating either reflux esophagitis or nonerosive reflux disease is to reduce acid secretion with a **proton pump inhibitor** (PPI). The goal is to raise the intragastric pH > 4, the level above which any reflux is unlikely to elicit symptoms or cause esophageal damage.[1]

H_2-receptor Antagonists

Cimetidine, ranitidine, famotidine and **nizatidine** are equally effective. Twice daily doses relieve symptoms in 60% and heal histologically mild esophagitis in over 40% of patients. Their safety profile is excellent. Their efficacy is limited by the rapid development of tachyphylaxis and the inability to properly suppress meal-related acid secretion.

This class of drugs is inefficient for severe esophagitis, being best reserved for GERD when symptoms are mild and infrequent (< 3 times per week). *Step-down therapy*, where H_2RAs are instituted after symptomatic relief has been achieved with PPIs, can be successful without adversely affecting quality of life and reduces costs.[3]

When initial therapy is beneficial, maintenance will be necessary if/when symptoms recur and cannot be controlled by nonpharmacologic means. Use the lowest dose possible to control symptoms and prevent complications. This is usually effective in mild GERD.

Proton Pump Inhibitors (PPIs)

PPIs are superior to H_2RAs for the reduction of heartburn and healing of esophagitis. PPIs heal all grades of esophagitis in most patients (up to 90% by 12 weeks).[1] PPIs provide more rapid relief of symptoms and twice the healing rates compared to H_2RAs,[1,4,5] which makes PPIs more cost effective as initial therapy.[3] Therefore, PPIs are the drug of choice in most GERD patients with or without mucosal injury and for extraesophageal manifestations.

H_2RAs may be instituted after achieving symptomatic relief with PPIs. Such *step-down therapy* begins with potent antisecretory agents (PPIs) to achieve rapid symptom control. The intensity of acid suppressive therapy is then gradually decreased until breakthrough symptoms occur, which indicates the extent of therapy necessary to control ongoing symptoms.

Though PPIs heal ulceration they do not reverse epithelial changes in patients with Barrett's esophagus. Tachyphylaxis is not a problem, but acid rebound occurs with discontinuation.

For ENRD, PPIs are clearly superior to H_2RAs in relieving symptoms.[6] Generally, therapy aims at controlling symptoms.

At equivalent doses, available PPIs offer similar symptom relief, mucosal healing, tolerability and safety.[7,8] Apparent differences in bioavailability and antisecretory potency upon initial dosing have no apparent clinical importance in most settings. However, the results of a meta-analysis suggest that esomeprazole may confer a modest advantage over other agents for severe erosive esophagitis.[9] Consider cost in the initial selection of a PPI.[10] Less clear is the effectiveness of substituting one PPI for another in patients who have been stabilized on therapy. More important is optimal dosing: PPIs should be ingested ½ hour before meals for the most effective acid suppression.

Helicobacter pylori infection does not cause and has little impact on GERD.[11] Testing for *H. pylori* is not necessary. *H. pylori* eradication has only modest effects on GERD symptoms, resulting in a slight worsening in patients with corpus-predominant gastritis and improvement in those with antral-predominant gastritis.

Table 2: **Efficacy of Drugs Used to Treat GERD**

	Acute Treatment		
	Symptoms	**Esophagitis**	**Prevention of Recurrences**
Antacids	+	–	–
Alginates/antacids	+	–	–
H_2-receptor antagonists	++	+	±
Proton pump inhibitors	+++	+++	+++

+ Drug of proven value (controlled trials)
– Not established (negative trial or not tested)

Prokinetic Agents

Although the basis for acid reflux is incompetence of the antireflux barrier, impaired esophageal clearance of acid and delayed gastric emptying, no effective motility agent is available at this time.

Maintenance Therapy for Severe GERD

The recurrence rate following discontinuation of successful therapy is extremely high (75% to 90%), particularly for erosive/severe esophagitis.[12] PPIs maintain remission far more effectively than H_2RAs and are cost-effective.[12,13] Maintenance therapy for such severe disease appears to be long term.

On-demand (intermittent) medical therapy is the daily intake of a drug for a period of time sufficient to achieve resolution of the reflux symptoms at which time the patient discontinues the drug. PPIs frequently can be so discontinued, with a subsequent drug-free remission lasting for months,[14] particularly in patients with ENRD. Conversely, many patients take their medication prophylactically to prevent occurrence of reflux symptoms. Such periodic therapy is less successful in severe erosive esophagitis.

Use of low-dose or half-dose PPIs is less effective than standard doses. Patients should be maintained on the lowest dose that provides symptom relief. The safety record of PPIs is excellent, even with long-term use over many years. Potential concerns relate to the development of nosocomial pneumonia, *C. difficile* diarrhea, hip fractures and malabsorption of vitamin B_{12}.

Management of the Refractory Patient

PPIs, though potent antisecretory agents, may not provide symptomatic relief or heal esophagitis in all patients. PPI failure may relate to:

- incorrect diagnosis, e.g., esophageal hypersensitivity (visceral hyperalgesia), functional dyspepsia, achalasia
- other causes of esophagitis: alkali (bile) reflux, eosinophilic esophagitis, pill esophagitis
- inadequate acid suppression (twice-daily dosing is sometimes necessary)
- improper use
  - nonadherence
  - taking PPI with meals or in combination with H_2RAs (PPI bioavailability is highest with secretion of gastric acid)
  - genetic rapid metabolism via CYP2C19 (less common)
  - gastric acid hypersecretion (less common)

Additional investigations such as endoscopy with biopsies, 24–hour pH monitoring, or esophageal motility studies may be warranted to identify the cause of refractory esophagitis

Nocturnal acid breakthrough with gastric pH < 4, and symptoms can occur in up to 70% of patients on twice daily PPI therapy. Supplementary bedtime H_2RA therapy may temporarily improve symptoms, but tolerance limits its use, making such therapy no better than placebo.[15] Another option for patients refractory to a PPI, though not completely substantiated, is to switch to another PPI as some individuals may be more responsive to one PPI or another.[16]

Antireflux Surgery

Failure of optimal medical therapy suggests intuitively that refractory patients would benefit from surgery to restore the physiological equivalent of the lower esophageal sphincter. In fact, complete response to medical therapy is the best predictor of surgical success. Antireflux surgery is effective for reflux control in well-selected cases. Indications include intractable reflux esophagitis (particularly in a young person) despite medical therapy, or complications such as severe erosive esophagitis, stricture formation or recurrent lung disease (e.g., aspiration pneumonia). Long-term outcome studies show little difference in surgically versus medically treated patients.[17] In fact, drug therapy may be less expensive than surgery.[18,19] Laparoscopic approaches and natural orifice transluminal endoscopic surgery (NOTES) have not been critically assessed.[20]

Therapeutic Tips

- For patients with mild symptomatic GERD, nonprescription H_2RAs are expensive and yield quite modest acid reduction and symptom control.
- PPIs are superior to H_2RAs for reduction of heartburn and healing of esophagitis in patients with moderate to severe GERD. H_2RAs may be instituted after achieving symptomatic relief with PPIs.
- The recurrence rate of GERD is extremely high and long term maintenance therapy is often necessary. PPIs maintain remission far more effectively than H_2RAs. On demand (intermittent) therapy with PPIs may be effective in select patients.

Figure 1: **Management of GERD**

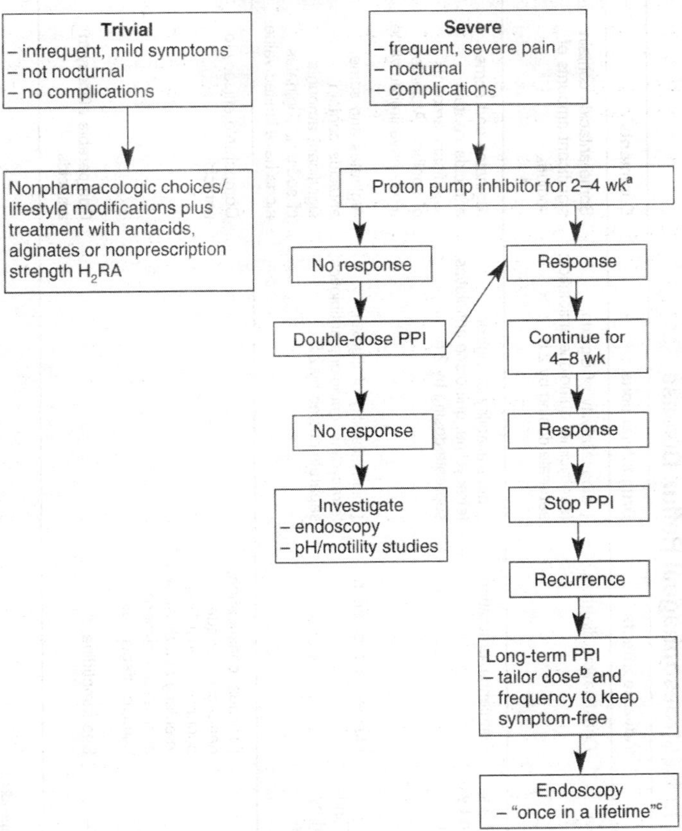

[a] For suspected GERD, an empiric trial of PPI BID for two weeks also can be diagnostic.
[b] May be able to step down to H_2RA in some with nonerosive GERD.
[c] For those on long-term PPI, indicating severe GERD, it is reasonable to evaluate for the presence of Barrett's epithelium (a premalignant lesion) and assess for erosive esophagitis (which requires PPIs) vs a normal esophagus (the "hypersensitive" esophagus, which sometimes can be controlled with H_2RA).
Abbreviations: PPI = proton pump inhibitor

Table 3: **Nonprescription Drugs Used in Gastroesophageal Reflux Disease**

Class	Drug	Dose	Adverse Effects	Drug Interactions	Comments	Cost[a]
Antacids	*aluminum hydroxide/magnesium hydroxide combinations* (renal symbol)	30 mL (regular strength) 1 h PC and QHS	Constipation, diarrhea.	↓ bioavailability of digoxin, tetracycline, quinolone antibiotics; separate dosing by 2 h.	Some antacids contain significant amounts of sodium.	$$
Alginates	*alginate (sodium salt)/aluminum hydroxide* (renal symbol) Gaviscon Liquid	10–20 mL PC and QHS, followed by glass of water	Flatulence, eructation.	↓ bioavailability of digoxin, tetracycline, quinolone antibiotics; separate dosing by 2 h.	Alginates and some antacids contain significant amounts of sodium. Alginates alone have limited value.	$-$$
	alginic acid/magnesium carbonate (renal symbol) Gaviscon Tablets	2–4 tablets (chewed) PC and QHS, followed by glass of water	Flatulence, eructation.	↓ bioavailability of digoxin, tetracycline, quinolone antibiotics; separate dosing by 2 h.	Alginates and some antacids contain significant amounts of sodium. Alginates alone have limited value.	$-$$
H_2-antagonists	*famotidine* (renal symbol) Pepcid AC, generics	10 mg BID	Diarrhea, constipation, headache, fatigue, confusion (most likely in elderly and those with poor renal function), cardiac effects, rash.		Comparable efficacy to antacids.	$
	ranitidine (renal symbol) Zantac-75, generics	75 mg BID	See famotidine.		Comparable efficacy to antacids.	$

[a] Cost of 30-day supply.

(renal symbol) Dosage adjustment may be required in renal impairment; see Appendix I.

Legend: $ < $20 $-$$ < $20–40 $$ $20–40

Table 4: Prescription Drugs Used in Gastroesophageal Reflux Disease

Class	Drug	Dose	Adverse Effects	Drug Interactions	Comments	Cost[a]
H_2-antagonists	*cimetidine* various generics	600 mg BID	Diarrhea, constipation, headache, fatigue, confusion (most likely in elderly and those with poor renal function), cardiac effects, rash. Also gynecomastia, impotence (rare).	Cimetidine ↓ CYP450-mediated metabolism of several agents (e.g., warfarin, phenytoin, theophylline) — use another H_2RA.		$
	ranitidine Zantac, generics	150 mg BID	Diarrhea, constipation, headache, fatigue, confusion (most likely in elderly and those with poor renal function), cardiac effects, rash.	Minor decrease in CYP450-mediated metabolism of several agents (e.g., warfarin, phenytoin, theophylline) — monitor.		$$
	famotidine Pepcid, generics	20 mg BID	See ranitidine.			$$
	nizatidine Axid, generics	150 mg BID	See ranitidine.			$$

(cont'd)

Table 4: **Prescription Drugs Used in Gastroesophageal Reflux Disease** *(cont'd)*

Class	Drug	Dose	Adverse Effects	Drug Interactions	Comments	Cost[a]
Proton Pump Inhibitors	*omeprazole* Losec Capsules, Losec MUPS, Losec Tablets, generics	Usual: 20 mg once daily ½ hour before food[b]	Abdominal pain, nausea, headache.	Monitor for ↓ efficacy of drugs requiring an acid medium for absorption from the stomach (e.g., itraconazole, atazanavir, indinavir). Omeprazole may interfere with cytochrome P450-metabolized agents (e.g., diazepam, warfarin, phenytoin). When omeprazole is added or removed, these drugs may require dosage adjustment.	If partial or no response, give usual dose BID AC so total daily dose is doubled. Giving half the usual dose may be useful for maintenance of some patients with less severe symptoms or who have gone into remission on standard dosages.	$$
	esomeprazole Nexium	20–40 mg once daily ½ hour before food Usual: 40 mg once daily before food	Abdominal pain, diarrhea, headache.	Monitor for ↓ efficacy of drugs requiring an acid medium for absorption from the stomach (e.g., itraconazole, atazanavir, indinavir).	Commonly used at 40 mg daily.	$$$$
	lansoprazole Prevacid	30 mg once daily ½ hour before food	Diarrhea, abdominal pain, headache.	See esomeprazole.	See omeprazole.	$$$
	pantoprazole Pantoloc	40 mg once daily ½ hour before food	Diarrhea, headache, dizziness, pruritus.	See esomeprazole.	See omeprazole.	$$$
	rabeprazole Pariet	20 mg once daily ½ hour before food	Diarrhea, headache.	See esomeprazole Digoxin levels may increase moderately in some patients.	See omeprazole.	$$

[a] Cost of 30-day supply, includes drug cost only.
[b] Not to exceed 20 mg/day in hepatic impairment.
Dosage adjustment may be required in renal impairment; see Appendix I.
Legend: $ < $20 $$ $20–40 $$$ $40–60 $$$$ $60–80

Suggested Readings

Armstrong D, Marshall JK, Chiba N et al. Canadian Consensus Conference on the management of gastroesophageal reflux disease in adults - update 2004. *Can J Gastroenterol* 2005;19(1):15-35.

DeVault KR, Castell DO. Updated guidelines for the diagnosis and treatment of gastroesophageal reflux disease. *Am J Gastroenterol* 2005;100(1):190-200.

Fass R. Towards a consensus in symptomatic gastroesophageal reflux disease. *Am J Gastroenterol* 2003;98(3 Suppl 1):S1-S55.

Moayyedi P, Talley NJ. Gastro-oesophageal reflux disease. *Lancet* 2006;367(9528):2086-100.

Wo JM, Mendez C, Harrell S et al. Clinical impact of upper endoscopy in the management of patients with gastroesophageal reflux disease. *Am J Gastroenterol* 2004;99(12):2311-6.

References

1. Hunt RH. Importance of pH control in the management of GERD. *Arch Intern Med* 1999;159(7):649-57.
2. Klauser AG, Schindlbeck NE, Muller-Lissner SA. Symptoms in gastro-oesophageal reflux disease. *Lancet* 1990;335(8683):205-8.
3. Inadomi JM, Jamal R, Murata GH et al. Step-down management of gastroesophageal reflux disease. *Gastroenterology* 2001;121(5):1095-100.
4. Chiba N, De Gara CJ, Wilkinson JM et al. Speed of healing and symptom relief in grade II to IV gastroesophageal reflux disease: a meta-analysis. *Gastroenterology* 1997;112(6):1798-810.
5. van Pinxteren B, Numans ME, Lau J et al. Short-term treatment of gastroesophageal reflux disease. *J Gen Intern Med* 2003;18(9):755-63.
6. Richter JE, Campbell DR, Kahrilas PJ et al. Lansoprazole compared with ranitidine for the treatment of nonerosive gastroesophageal reflux disease.*Arch Intern Med* 2000;160(12):1803-9.
7. Vakil N, Fennerty MB. Direct comparative trials of the efficacy of proton pump inhibitors in the management of gastro-oesophageal reflux disease and peptic ulcer disease. c0045n00154 2003;18(6):559-68.
8. FDC reports. *Pharmaceutica; approval monthly* 2001;6:34.
9. Gralnek IM, Dulai GS, Fennerty MB et al. Esomeprazole versus other proton pump inhibitors in erosive esophagitis: a meta-analysis of randomized clinical trials. *Clin Gastroenterol Hepatol* 2006;4(12):1452-8.
10. Nelson WW, Vermeulen LC, Geurkink EA et al. Clinical and humanistic outcomes in patients with gastroesophageal reflux disease converted from omeprazole to lansoprazole. *Arch Intern Med* 2000;160(16):2491-6.
11. Raghunath AS, Hungin AP, Wooff D et al. Systematic review: the effect of Helicobacter pylori and its eradication on gastro-oesophageal reflux disease in patients with duodenal ulcers or reflux esophagitis. *Aliment Pharmacol Ther* 2004;20(7):733-44.
12. Harris RA, Kuppermann M, Richter JE. Prevention of recurrences of erosive reflux esophagitis: a cost-effectiveness analysis of maintenance proton pump inhibition. *Am J Med* 1997;102(1):78-88.
13. Vigneri S, Termini R, Leandro G et al. A comparison of five maintenance therapies for reflux esophagitis. *N Engl J Med* 1995;333(17):1106-10.
14. Talley NJ, Lauritsen K, Tunturi-Hihnala H et al. Esomeprazole 20 mg maintains symptom control in endoscopy-negative gastro-oesophageal reflux disease: a controlled trial of 'on-demand' therapy for 6 months. *Aliment Pharmacol Ther* 2001;15(3):347-54.
15. Orr WC, Harnish MJ. The efficacy of omeprazole twice daily with supplemental H2 blockade at bedtime in the suppression of nocturnal oesophageal and gastric acidity.*Aliment Pharmacol Ther* 2003;17(12):1553-8.
16. Hatlebakk JG. *Am J Gastroenterol* 1998;93:1636.
17. Spechler SJ, Lee E, Ahnen D et al. Long-term outcome of medical and surgical therapies for gastroesophageal reflux disease: follow-up of a randomized controlled trial. *JAMA* 2001;285(18):2331-8.
18. Myrvold HE, Lundell L, Miettinen P et al. The cost of long term therapy for gastro-oesophageal reflux disease: a randomised trial comparing omeprazole and open antireflux surgery.*Gut* 2001;49(4):488-94.
19. Romagnuolo J, Meier MA, Sadowski DC. Medical or surgical therapy for erosive reflux esophagitis: cost-utility analysis using a Markov model. *Ann Surg* 2002;236(2):191-202.

20. Wallace MB. Take NOTES (Natural Orifice Transluminal Endoscopic Surgery). *Gastroenterology* 2006;131(1):11-2.

Pharmacoeconomic Considerations: Gastroesophageal Reflux Disease

Nicole Mittmann, MSc, PhD

Epidemiology	
Country	**Prevalence (%)**
Canada[1]	9% of population with GERD symptoms once a week or more
US[2]	20% of population with GERD symptoms once a week or more
Australia[3]	18% of population with GERD symptoms once a week or more

Cost of Illness Data		
Country and Year of Estimate	**Direct Costs[a]**	**Indirect Costs[b]**
US (1998)[4]	US $9.3 billion annually	US $479 million annually

Commentary

The direct and indirect medical costs of gastroesophageal reflux disease (GERD) are significant. Medication costs are the major cost driver in the overall economic burden of GERD and account for more than 50% of direct medical costs.[5] Between 6% and 48% of patients with GERD report lost work productivity, which is severity dependent.[4,5,6]

A number of agents are available for the treatment of GERD. Proton pump inhibitors (PPIs) are more cost-effective than histamine H_2-receptor blockers.[7,8,9] There are relatively few economic evaluations available that directly compare different PPIs.[10] PPIs have relatively similar efficacy and safety profiles and branded products are generally priced similarly. The availability of generic PPIs will have an important impact on direct medical costs.

[a] Direct costs include those associated with physician services, nursing care, diagnostic procedures, drugs and hospitalization.

[b] Indirect costs include those associated with lost productivity and days off work due to morbidity or premature mortality.

References

1. Frank L, Kleinman L, Ganoczy D et al. Upper gastrointestinal symptoms in North America: prevalence and relationship to health care utilization and quality of life. *Dig Dis Sci* 2000;45(4):809-18.
2. Locke GR, Talley NJ, Fett SL et al. Prevalence and clinical spectrum of gastroesophageal reflux: a population-based study in Olmsted County, Minnesota. *Gastroenterology* 1997;112(5):1448-56.

3. Talley NJ, Boyce P, Jones M. Identification of distinct upper and lower gastrointestinal symptom groupings in an urban population. *Gut* 1998;42(5):690-5.
4. Dean BB, Crawley JA, Schmitt CM et al, The burden of illness of gastro-oesophageal reflux disease: impact on work productivity. *Aliment Pharmacol Ther* 2003;17(10):1309-17.
5. Sandler RS, Everhart JE, Donowitz M et al. The burden of selected digestive disease in the United States. *Gastroenterology* 2002;122(5):1500-11.
6. Wahlqvist P, Carlsson J, Stalhammar NO et al. Validity of a Work Productivity and Activity Impairment questionnaire for patients with symptoms of gastro-esophageal reflux disease (WPAI-GERD) — results from a cross-sectional study. *Value Health* 2002;5(2):106-13.
7. Wahlqvist P, Junghard O, Higgins A et al. Cost effectiveness of proton pump inhibitors in gastro-oesophageial reflux disease without oesophagitis: comparison of on-demand esomeprazole with conventional omeprazole strategies. *Pharmacoeconomics* 2002;20(4):267-77.
8. Ofman JJ, Gralnek IM et al. Clinical and economic assessment of the omeprazole test in patients with symptoms suggestive of gastroesophageal reflux disease. *Arch Intern Med.* 1999;159(18):2161-8.
9. Bardhan KD. The role of proton pump inhibitos in the treatment of gastro-oesophageal reflux disease. *Aliment Pharmacol Ther* 1995;9(Suppl 1):15-25.
10. Dean BB, Siddique RM, Yamashita BD et al. Cost-effectiveness of proton-pump inhibitors for maintenance therapy of erosive reflux esophagitis. *Am J Health Syst Pharm* 2001;58(14):1338-46.

CHAPTER 54
Peptic Ulcer Disease

A.B.R. Thomson, MD, PhD, FRCPC, FACG

Dyspepsia, defined as pain or discomfort in the upper abdomen, is one of the most common complaints bringing patients to consult their family physician. The most common causes of dyspepsia include nonulcer dyspepsia (NUD), gastroesophageal reflux disease (GERD) (Chapter 53), duodenal ulcer (DU) and gastric ulcer (GU). DU and GU are considered to be two of the *Helicobacter pylori*-associated diseases, and both are components of the gastroenteropathy associated with nonsteroidal anti-inflammatory drugs (NSAIDs).

Goals of Therapy

- Relieve dyspepsia and heal the ulcer
- Prevent complications, e.g., bleeding, perforation
- Prevent recurrence

Investigations

- History and physical examination
  - exclude nongastrointestinal sources of pain or discomfort in the upper abdomen, e.g., ischemic heart disease
  - inquire into possible alarm symptoms (vomiting, bleeding, dysphagia, anemia or weight loss) and confirm patient age (potential risk factor for cancer)
  - determine the character of the dyspeptic symptoms to establish if heartburn and/or regurgitation are predominant symptoms:
    - — ulcer-like (pain, relief with food)
    - — reflux-like (heartburn, regurgitation) (See Chapter 53 GERD)
    - — dysmotility-like (bloating, fullness)
  - take a drug history for NSAID/ASA use, including low-dose ASA for cardioprotection, as well as other medications that may cause or aggravate dyspepsia, e.g., bisphosphonates, tetracyclines, calcium channel blockers
  - physical examination will usually be normal. Epigastric tenderness is a common but nonspecific finding; an abdominal mass is an alarm sign
- *H. pylori* infection
  - ^{14}C or ^{13}C urea breath test (UBT) in selected individuals (Figure 1). The ^{13}C (nonradioactive) UBT is recommended for use in children and women of child-bearing age.[1]
  - Serology is appropriate if there is no access to UBT or endoscopy. If the serology is negative, the patient is truly *H. pylori* negative,

but if serology is positive, there is about a 20% risk that the test is falsely positive. Serology is not useful for confirming eradication.

- Esophagogastroduodenoscopy (or endoscopy): Investigation of choice in patients with: dyspepsia over the age of 50, alarm symptoms (such as vomiting, bleeding, anemia, weight loss, dysphagia), GU reported on an upper GI series (to obtain biopsies to exclude gastric cancer); also following 8 to 12 weeks' treatment of a GU to confirm healing, or to diagnose an *H. pylori* infection when UBT is not available.
- *Prompt endoscopy*: the most sensitive and specific means to diagnose the cause of dyspepsia is endoscopy. It permits the diagnosis of erosive esophagitis, Barrett's epithelium, GU or DU, gastric or duodenal erosions, *H. pylori* infection and gastric or esophageal cancer. The patient and physician will be reassured as to the cause of dyspepsia, and future use of medications and health care resources may be lessened.

  The disadvantages of prompt endoscopy are self-evident. In many Canadian communities, the average waiting time to consult a gastroenterologist to arrange for an endoscopy is at least eight weeks and may be as long as six months. Time is lost from work, the procedure is expensive to the health care system (total cost approximately $500), and there is a very small but real risk of a complication (about 1 per 5000 procedures) such as aspiration or perforation.
- Upper GI Barium Study: The upper GI series has an approximately 20% false-positive and false-negative rate for ulcer disease and is generally not recommended. However, barium studies are often more available than UBT or endoscopy and are still used to reassure the physician that nothing serious has been missed as a cause of the dyspepsia. Because of the relatively low sensitivity and specificity of the upper GI series, perform endoscopy if the patient is over 50 or has alarm features, rather than performing a barium study.[2] An upper GI series should not be performed in the patient with bleeding from the upper GI tract as this may obscure the diagnosis when endoscopy is performed.

Therapeutic Choices (Figure 1)

Nonpharmacologic Choices

- Bland diets are no longer prescribed. A simple rule of thumb is to use moderation if a food or beverage makes dyspepsia worse. Common offenders are coffee, orange juice, spicy foods, fatty foods, large meals or eating on the run.
- Smoking cessation improves ulcer healing and reduces recurrence of ulcers not related to *H. pylori* infection. See Chapter 10 for more information on smoking cessation.

Pharmacologic Choices (Table 2)

Management of PUD

If the patient has dyspepsia with suspected ulcer (i.e, dyspepsia where heartburn and regurgitation are not the predominant symptoms), the following are commonly used approaches:[3]

- *Empiric therapy* – treat with a proton pump inhibitor (PPI) once a day before breakfast or an H_2-receptor antagonist (H_2RA) twice a day for four to eight weeks. This duration is sufficient to heal the erosive esophagitis present in about 50% of all patients with uninvestigated dyspepsia.[4] However, PPIs are much superior.[5] See the patient in follow-up, and for those who remain symptomatic, consider switching to another PPI or dosing with twice daily PPI. If dyspepsia persists, or if there are frequent recurrences, investigate with a UBT for *H. pylori* infection, or with prompt endoscopy. The patient should not have taken a PPI or H_2RA for at least one week before performing the UBT, since these may suppress the growth of the *H. pylori* sufficiently to render the UBT falsely negative. Noninvasive testing for *H. pylori* is as safe and effective as endoscopy and more comfortable and less distressing for the patient,[6] although fewer patients are satisfied with their treatment.[7] Most patients with dyspepsia and an abnormal endoscopy will have erosive esophagitis (45%), and far fewer (5%) will have DU or GU.

  The advantage of empiric therapy is that it is an office-based approach that does not require initial investigations such as UBT or endoscopy. The disadvantage is that some patients continue with dyspepsia, or the symptoms recur and there is no diagnosis.

- *Test-and-treat* – a diagnostic test is performed for *H. pylori*, and a positive test result is treated with triple therapy (Table 1). This approach assumes that if the patient's dyspepsia is caused by DU/GU, they will be positive for *H. pylori*. About 90% of DU and 70% of GU may be *H. pylori*-positive, although the association may be less striking in community practice, or in patients with a past history of an ulcer complicated by bleeding.

  The advantage of this approach is that the investigations needed to diagnose *H. pylori*, when available in the community, can be readily used by the family physician and the results are rapidly available. The disadvantage is that serology and UBT are not universally available in all communities in Canada, and the cost of these tests is not usually covered by provincial health care plans.

  Note that in dyspeptic nonulcer patients with an *H. pylori* infection, the benefit of eradication is small (7% to 15% symptom resolution).[8,9,10]

Modest Acid Inhibition

Over-the-counter (OTC) therapy with antacids or H_2 RAs are commonly used by patients before seeking medical advice. They provide moderate benefit for mild symptoms of dyspepsia.

Prescription doses of H_2 RAs may be used for symptom relief but are much less effective for pain relief or ulcer healing than PPIs, and must be used twice a day and for longer periods (4 to 8 weeks for duodenal ulcer and 8 to 12 weeks for gastric ulcer). Tachyphylaxis (loss of effectiveness over time) may develop quickly, and the H_2 RAs have no role to play in the approved regimens used to eradicate *H. pylori*.

Extensive Acid Inhibition

The duration of use of PPI needed to heal a DU is shortened to one week when triple therapy is used to eradicate an associated *H. pylori* infection.[11] For those individuals with a DU or GU not associated with either *H. pylori* infection or use of NSAIDs, once in the morning PPI should be used for two to four weeks, and maintenance therapy must be considered on an individualized basis. Patients with a GU must have a follow-up endoscopy to prove ulcer healing in order to avoid the rare initial misdiagnosis of a gastric cancer.

As a class of medications, the five PPIs available in Canada are all very effective. There are minor pharmacokinetic and pharmacodynamic differences, but the variations in healing rates are only about 5% (NNT, 20). A recent Canadian Consensus Conference suggested that there were no clinically significant differences between the PPIs.[12] Note that some PPIs are as much as 40% less costly than others.

Maintenance Therapy

Continuous use of acid inhibition, preferably with a PPI, may be needed in selected patients with DU/GU not associated with *H. pylori* infection, especially when the ulcer is complicated by bleeding or perforation, or when the patient suffers from frequent recurrences of dyspepsia.

It is controversial whether some ulcer patients cured of their *H. pylori* infection may develop *de novo* reflux-like dyspepsia, and require intermittent or continuous PPI. Some high-risk patients requiring continuous use of NSAIDs may need to be maintained on PPIs to reduce the risk of recurrent GU/DU.

Eradication of H. pylori Infection (Table 1)

Eradication of *H. pylori* infection is more cost-effective than maintenance therapy with acid-lowering medications and reduces the risk of developing gastric cancer or mucosa-associated lymphoid tissue (MALT) lymphoma.

Treatment regimens approved by the Canadian Helicobacter Study Group achieve a minimum eradication rate (on an intention-to-treat basis) of at least 80%. First-line therapy includes *triple therapy* PPI plus two antibiotics (**clarithromycin** and either **amoxicillin** or **metronidazole**) twice daily for one week (Table 1). *Quadruple therapy* is also considered first-line treatment.[1] Ranitidine bismuth citrate, which was previously recommended, is no longer available in Canada. Because the prevalence of metronidazole resistance in Canada is about 20% and resistance to amoxicillin is less than 1%,[1] increasing use is made of the amoxicillin-containing regimen. Prepacked combinations of triple therapy are available.

Table 1: ***H. pylori* Eradication Regimens**

Regimen	Dosage	Treatment Period	Cost[a]
Triple Therapy			
PPI *clarithromycin* *amoxicillin* Hp-PACLosec 1-2-3 A	BID 500 mg BID 1 g BID	7 days	$$$
PPI *clarithromycin* *metronidazole* Losec 1-2-3 M	BID 250 mg BID 500 mg BID	7 days	$$$
Quadruple Therapy			
PPI *bismuth subsalicylate* *metronidazole* *tetracycline* ❥	BID 2 tabs QID 250 mg QID 500 mg QID	7 days	$$$

[a] Cost per treatment period; includes drug cost only.
Legend: $ < $20 $$ $20–40 $$$ $40–60
Abbreviations: PPI = proton pump inhibitor
❥ Dosage adjustment may be required in renal impairment; see Appendix I.

If the patient fails one triple-therapy regimen, repeat treatment with a different antibiotic combination, or treat for two weeks rather than one, or use quadruple therapy (PPI, bismuth, metronidazole plus tetracycline). After successful *H. pylori* eradication, the risk of reinfection is only about 1% per year.

Repeated testing by UBT or endoscopic biopsies to prove eradication is necessary in patients with a complicated ulcer (bleeding or perforation) to ensure healing and prevent recurrence. In the occasional patient who experiences recurrent dyspepsia after the use of an approved eradication regimen, it may be necessary to prove successful eradication before looking for new causes of dyspepsia.

NSAID-associated Ulcers

Unlike *H. pylori*-associated ulcers, GU/DU caused by ASA or NSAIDs are more likely to be painless, and patients often present for the first time with a complication such as bleeding or perforation.[13,14] Over a one-year interval, about 3% of NSAID users will develop a GU/DU. Controversy exists regarding the extent to which COXIBs may reduce the risk of serious GI events, but the risk is not eliminated by use of these drugs.[15,16,17] Recent reports of cardiovascular complications with use of COXIBs have limited their use and challenged their safety.

The risk of developing an NSAID ulcer is greater in persons over the age of 65, and with use of more than one NSAID, higher doses of NSAID, concomitant use of steroids or anticoagulants, a past history of ulcer disease and coexisting ischemic heart disease. Patients taking ASA with an NSAID are also at higher risk of ulcer complications. Discuss the risk of NSAID-induced gastric complications with patients, including signs and symptoms associated with GI bleed, e.g., dyspepsia, coffee ground emesis, melena. At-risk patients may be offered gastric protective therapy with standard doses of PPI. Alternatively, misoprostol 200 μg QID may be offered, but use may be limited by GI adverse effects.[18]

An NSAID-induced ulcer should be treated like a non-NSAID-induced ulcer. Whenever possible, the NSAID should be stopped.

There is an additive effect between *H. pylori* infection and NSAID use on the development of peptic ulcer and ulcer bleeding.[19] For this reason, many experts recommend that persons beginning long-term NSAIDs should be screened for *H. pylori* and treated if found to be positive.[1]

Figure 1: **Management of Suspected Peptic Ulcers**[2]

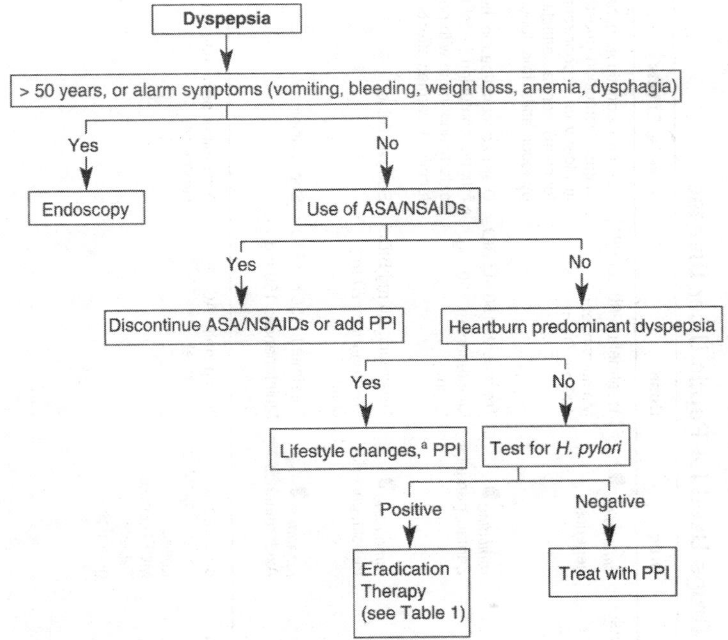

[a] Treat symptoms; lifestyle changes, diet, short courses (no more than 4 wks) of OTC antacids/H_2-receptor antagonist (H_2RA) and therapeutic doses of H_2RA, or preferentially a proton pump inhibitor.

Adapted with permission from Thomson ABR. A suggested approach to patients with dyspepsia. *Can J Gastroenterol* 1997;11:135–140.

Table 2: **Drugs Used for Peptic Ulcer Disease**

Class	Drug	Dose	Adverse Effects	Drug Interactions	Cost[a]
H_2-antagonists[b]	*cimetidine* generics	Treatment: 300 mg BID Maintenance: 400 mg Q pm	Diarrhea, constipation, headache, fatigue, confusion (most likely in elderly or in poor renal function), cardiac effects, rash, gynecomastia, impotence (rare).	Cimetidine ↓ cytochrome P450 metabolism of several agents (e.g., warfarin, phenytoin, theophylline). Use another H_2-antagonist; ranitidine or famotidine have minor effect.	$
	ranitidine Zantac, generics	Treatment: 150 mg BID Maintenance: 150 mg Q pm	Diarrhea, constipation, headache, fatigue, confusion (most likely in elderly and those with poor renal function), cardiac effects, rash.		$$
	famotidine Pepcid, generics	Treatment: 20 mg BID Maintenance: 20 mg Q pm	See ranitidine.		$$
	nizatidine Axid, generics	Treatment: 150 mg BID Maintenance: 150 mg Q pm	See ranitidine.		$$
Proton Pump Inhibitors	*omeprazole* Losec Capsules, Losec MUPS, Losec Tablets, generics	20 mg daily AC breakfast	Abdominal pain, nausea, headache.	Monitor for ↓ efficacy of drugs requiring an acid medium for absorption from the stomach (e.g., itraconazole). Omeprazole may interfere with cytochrome P450-metabolized agents (e.g., diazepam, warfarin, phenytoin). When omeprazole is added or removed, these drugs may require dosage adjustment.	$$

Class	Drug	Dose	Adverse Effects	Drug Interactions	Cost[a]
	esomeprazole Nexium	Treatment: 40 mg daily AC breakfast Maintenance: 20 mg daily AC breakfast	Abdominal pain, diarrhea, headache.	Metabolized via cytochrome P450. No significant drug interactions with warfarin, phenytoin or diazepam.	$$$$
	lansoprazole Prevacid	Treatment: 30 mg daily AC breakfast Maintenance: 15 mg daily AC breakfast	Diarrhea, abdominal pain, headache.	Metabolized via cytochrome P450. No significant interactions with warfarin, ASA, phenytoin, prednisone, antacids, diazepam.	$$$
	pantoprazole Pantoloc	40 mg daily AC breakfast	Diarrhea, headache, dizziness, pruritus.	Metabolized via cytochrome P450. No interactions with diazepam, phenytoin, nifedipine, theophylline, warfarin, digoxin, oral contraceptives or antacids.	$$$
	rabeprazole Pariet	20 mg daily AC breakfast	Diarrhea, headache.	Metabolized via cytochrome P450. No clinically significant drug interactions with drugs metabolized by the CYP450 system.	$$
Mucosal Protective Agents	*misoprostol* generics	Treatment: 200 μg QID	Diarrhea (dose-related), abdominal cramps, flatulence. **Contraindicated in pregnancy** – abortifacient.		$$

[a] Cost of 30-day (treatment dosages) supply; includes drug cost only.
[b] Duration of treatment for DU is 4–8 wk; Duration of treatment for GU is 8–12 wk.
Dosage adjustment may be required in renal impairment; see Appendix I.
Legend: $ < $20 $-$$ < $20–40 $$ $20–40 $$$ $40–60 $$$-$$$$ $40–80 $$$$ $60–80

Suggested Readings

Huang JQ, Sridhar S, Hunt RH. Role of Helicobacter pylori infection and non-steroidal anti-inflammatory drugs in peptic-ulcer disease: a meta-analysis. *Lancet* 2002;359(9300):14-22.

Hunt R, Thomson AB. Canadian Helicobacter pylori consensus conference. Canadian Association of Gastroenterology. *Can J Gastroenterol* 1998;12(1):31-41.

Lassen AT, Pedersen FM, Bytzer P, Schaffalitzky de Muckadell OB. Helicobacter pylori test-and-eradicate versus prompt endoscopy for management of dyspeptic patients: a randomised trial. *Lancet* 2000;356(9228):455-60.

References

1. Hunt R, Fallone C, Veldhuyzan van Zanten S et al. Canadian Helicobacter Study Group Consensus Conference: Update on the management of Helicobacter pylori – an evidence-based evaluation of six topics relevant to clinical outcomes in patients eradicated for H pylori infection. *Can J Gastroenterol* 2004;18(9):547-54.
2. Veldhuyzen van Zanten SJ, Flook N, Chiba N et al. An evidence-based approach to the management of uninvestigated dyspepsia in the era of Helicobacter pylori. *CMAJ* 2000;162(12 Suppl):S3-23.
3. Spiegel BM, Vakil NB, Ofman JJ. Dyspepsia management in primary care: a decision analysis of competing strategies. *Gastroenterology* 2002;122(5):1270-85.
4. Thomson AB, Barkun AN, Armstrong D et al. The prevalence of clinically significant endoscopic findings in primary care patients with uninvestigated dyspepsia: the Canadian Adult Dyspepsia Empiric Treatment - Prompt Endoscopy (CADET-PE) study. *Aliment Pharmacol Ther* 2003;17:1481-91.
5. Edwards SJ, Lind T, Lundell L. Systematic review of proton pump inhibitors for the acute treatment of reflux oesophagitis. *Aliment Pharmacol Ther* 2001;15(11):1729-36.
6. McColl KE, Murray LS, Gillen D et al. Randomised trial of endoscopy with testing for Helicobacter pylori compared with non-invasive H pylori testing alone in the management of dyspepsia. *BMJ* 2002;324(7344):999-1002.
7. Lassen AT, Pedersen FM, Bytzer P, Schaffalitzky de Muckadell OB. Helicobacter pylori test-and-eradicate versus prompt endoscopy for management of dyspeptic patients: a randomised trial. *Lancet* 2000;356(9228):455-60.
8. Chiba N, Van Zanten SJ, Sinclair P et al. Treating Helicobacter pylori infection in primary care patients with uninvestigated dyspepsia: the Canadian adult dyspepsia empiric treatment-Helicobacter pylori positive (CADET-Hp) randomized controlled trial. *BMJ* 2002 324(7344):1012-6.
9. Moayyedi P, Deeks J, Talley NJ et al. An update of the Cochrane systematic review of Helicobacter pylori eradication therapy in nonulcer dyspepsia: resolving the discrepancy between systematic reviews. *Am J Gastroenterol* 2003;98(12):2621-6.
10. Moayyedi P, Soo S, Deeks J et al. Pharmacological interventions for non-ulcer dyspepsia. *Cochrane Database Syst Rev* 2003;(1):CD001960.
11. Hunt R, Thomson AB. Canadian Helicobacter pylori consensus conference. Canadian Association of Gastroenterology. *Can J Gastroenterol* 1998;12(1):31-41.
12. Armstrong D, Marshall JK, Chiba N et al. Canadian Consensus Conference on the management of gastroesophageal reflux disease in adults – update 2004. *Can J Gastroenterol* 2005;19(1):15-35.
13. Laine L. Approaches to nonsteroidal anti-inflammatory drug use in the high-risk patient. *Gastroenterology* 2001;120(3):594-606.
14. Hawkey CJ. Nonsteroidal anti-inflammatory drug gastropathy. *Gastroenterology* 2000;119(2):521-35.
15. Wright JM, Perry TL, Bassett KL et al. Reporting of 6-month vs 12-month data in a clinical trial of celecoxib. *JAMA* 2001;286(19):2398-400.
16. McCormack JP, Rangno R. Digging for data from the COX-2 trials. *CMAJ* 2002;166(13):1649-50.
17. Chan FK, Hung LC, Suen BY et al. Celecoxib versus diclofenac and omeprazole in reducing the risk of recurrent ulcer bleeding in patients with arthritis. *N Engl J Med* 2002;347(26):2104-10.
18. Rostom A, Dubé C, Jolicoeur E, Boucher M, Joyce J. Gastroduodenal ulcers associated with the use of non-steroidal anti-inflammatory drugs: a systematic review of preventative pharmacological interventions. Ottawa (ON): Canadian coordinating Office for Health Technology Assessment; 2004. Technology overview No 12.
19. Huang JQ, Sridhar S, Hunt RH. Role of Helicobacter pylori infection and non-steroidal anti-inflammatory drugs in peptic-ulcer disease: a meta-analysis. *Lancet* 2002;359(9300):14-22.

Pharmacoeconomic Considerations: Peptic Ulcer Disease

Nicole Mittmann, MSc, PhD

Epidemiology		
Country (Year)	**Prevalence**	
United States (1998)[1]	An estimated 6 730 000 Americans have peptic ulcer disease	
Cost of Illness Data		
Country and Year of Estimate	**Direct Costs**[a]	**Indirect Costs**[b]
United States (1998)[1]	US $3.1 million	US $0.2 million
Commentary		
Outpatient physician office visits account for the majority (70%) of direct medical costs associated with peptic ulcer disease (PUD).[2] PUD is associated with significant lost work productivity; 42% of patients miss work because of physician visits and sick days or are less productive because of PUD.[2] Some authors have speculated that economic losses due to indirect costs, namely lost productivity, are almost as large as the direct medical costs of PUD.[2] Screening for *Helicobacter pylori* and eradication with antibiotics is cost-effective.[3,4] In terms of symptomatic treatment for PUD, there are few direct comparative trials for histamine (H_2) receptor antagonists (H_2 RAs) and proton pump inhibitors. A meta-analysis found proton pump inhibitors to be more effective than placebo for dyspeptic symptoms.[5] Because H_2 RAs can be purchased over-the-counter, the cost is borne by the patient. In contrast, proton pump inhibitors are prescription-only medicines and thus the cost may be covered by third-party payers.		

[a] Direct costs include those associated with physician services, nursing care, diagnostic procedures, drugs and hospitalization.

[b] Indirect costs include those associated with lost productivity and days off work due to morbidity or premature mortality.

References

1. Sandler RS, Everhart JE, Donowitz M et al. The burden of selective digestive disease in the United States. *Gastroenterology* 2002;122(5):1500-11.
2. Henke CJ, Levin TR, Henning JM et al. Work loss costs due to peptic ulcer disease and gastroesophageal reflux disease in a health maintenance organization. *Am J Gastroenterol* 2000;95(3):788-92.
3. Mason J, Axon AT, Forman D et al. The cost-effectiveness of population Helicobacter pylori screening and treatment: a Markov model using economic data from a randomized controlled trial. *Aliment Pharmacol Ther* 2002;16(3):559-68.
4. Ford AC, Delaney BC, Forman D et al. Eradication therapy in Helicobacter pylori positive peptic ulcer disease: systematic review and economic analysis. *Am J Gastroenterol* 2004;99(9):1833-55.
5. Shiau JY, Shukla VK, Dube C. *The efficacy of proton pump inhibitors in adults with functional dyspepsia*. Ottawa (ON): Canadian Coordinating Office for Health Technology Assessment (CCOHTA); 2002. Technology report no 22.

CHAPTER 55
Upper Gastrointestinal Bleeding

A.B.R. Thomson, MD, PhD, FRCPC, FACG

Upper gastrointestinal bleeding (UGIB) is a common medical emergency, with a mortality rate of about 7%, especially in older persons with comorbid conditions. Common causes include duodenal ulcer (DU), gastric ulcer (GU), gastric or esophageal erosions and esophageal varices. Rarely, bleeding may result from an eroded gastric blood vessel (Dieulafoy's lesion) or, less commonly, from a tear of the gastroesophageal junction (Mallory-Weiss tear).[1]

Goals of Therapy

- Resuscitate and save the patient's life
- Prevent hypoxia-related damage to other organs
- Heal the underlying lesion
- Prevent recurrences of UGIB

Investigations

- History and physical examination:
  - resuscitate immediately to ensure the patient is breathing and to restore circulating blood volume, while quickly taking a focused history and performing a physical examination
  - cause of bleeding may be suggested by history: *ulcer disease* – present history of pain, past history of ulcer, use of ASA/NSAIDs; *varices* – signs of liver disease (jaundice, ascites, hepatosplenomegaly, coagulopathy, skin changes suggestive of liver disease) in patients at risk (e.g., alcohol abuse, infectious hepatitis B or C); retching or vomiting followed by bleeding is suggestive of a Mallory-Weiss tear
  - prognosis is usually worse if the patient is vomiting fresh red blood or passing red blood per rectum, or has tachycardia or hypotension
  - coffee-ground emesis or melena stools imply slower loss of a smaller volume of blood, but may still be dangerous in the older patient or one with comorbidities such as COPD or coronary artery disease
- Draw venous blood for "stat" type and cross match (usually four units of packed red blood cells or more depending on the severity of bleeding), hemoglobin concentration or hematocrit, electrolytes, renal function (creatinine or BUN) and coagulation studies (platelet count, INR and PTT)

- Rapid estimate of blood loss can be made at the bedside: 50% loss of blood volume is suggested by systolic pressure < 100 mm Hg, pulse rate > 100 BPM and Hgb < 10 g/dl
- Nasogastric lavage:
  - if the patient is observed, or previously witnessed, to vomit blood there is no need to pass a nasogastric (NG) tube
  - in patients with melena or hematochezia, the discovery of fresh, red blood in the NG tube aspirate indicates more severe bleeding and points to the cause being in the upper GI tract
  - absence of fresh blood in the NG tube aspirate may be a false negative finding if the tip of the NG tube has not been placed in the pool of blood in the stomach or duodenum, or if the source of bleeding is beyond a closed pylorus
- An electrocardiogram is useful in older patients with suspected or possible ischemic heart disease
- Barium swallow. An upper GI series must not be performed in the patient with UGIB. The diagnostic accuracy is poor in this setting, it may obscure a clear field for subsequent esophagogastroduodenoscopy (EGD), and endoscopic hemostatic therapy (EHT) cannot be performed if the field of vision is obscured by barium
- Esophagogastroduodenoscopy
  - all patients with UGI bleeding should be referred for EGD after they are stabilized. The timing will depend on the suspected severity of bleeding, the likely cause and the patient's general condition
  - use of a prokinetic (iv **erythromycin** 250 mg) 20 to 90 minutes prior to EGD clears blood from the stomach, which improves the field of vision
  - prompt EGD will identify the lesion in about 90% of patients. Inability to make a diagnosis is usually due to profuse bleeding. Tc-labelled red blood cell scanning, angiography, or repeat EGD after saline lavage of the stomach may be necessary
  - prognosis may be established at the time of EGD. If there is a clean-based ulcer in an otherwise healthy person with reliable and available family support, the stable patient may be discharged home from the emergency room after endoscopy
  - biopsies for *H. pylori*: obtain two biopsies from the gastric antrum, plus two biopsies from the gastric body in the patient who has recently been on acid suppression therapy

Therapeutic Choices (Figure 1, Table 1)

Nonpharmacologic Choices

Protect the airway, provide supplementary nasal oxygen and place at least two large bore (#18 or larger) iv lines. Fluid resuscitation and hemodynamic stability are essential before attempting endoscopy.

Endoscopic Treatment

In the more serious lesions seen in EGD, such as an ulcer with an adherent clot, visible vessel or active bleeding, EHT must be used.[2] EHT involves coaptive thermal coagulation, injection of epinephrine or a sclerosing agent and/or a mechanical technique (banding, clips, staples, sutures).[1]

In *nonvariceal bleeding*, injection therapy, thermal therapy or a combination of the two may be used, although combination therapy is recommended.[1]

Gastric and duodenal ulcers are the most common lesions in Canadian patients with nonvariceal UGIB. After EHT, the rates of rebleeding, surgery and mortality are reported to be 14.1%, 6.5% and 5.4%, respectively.[3]

In *bleeding esophageal varices*, endoscopic variceal band ligation or sclerotherapy are both highly effective in stopping bleeding and preventing rebleeding;[4,5] band ligation is preferred because there are fewer complications. For bleeding gastric varices, the tissue adhesive cyanoacrylate, (e.g., Krazy Glue) may be carefully applied.

Pharmacologic Choices

Nonvariceal UGIB

Optimal therapy for nonvariceal UGIB includes early EGD (within 24 hours of the initial bleeding episode), EHT (depending on the nature of the bleeding site) and acid inhibition with an iv **proton pump inhibitor** (PPI) to stabilize the clot and to reduce ulcer bleeding. Use of oral or iv H_2-receptor antagonists is not recommended.

PPIs significantly reduce rebleeding and the need for surgery in patients with nonvariceal UGIB. PPI use is associated with significant reductions in mortality when used with EHT in patients with high-risk stigmata (active bleeding or a nonbleeding visible vessel).[6,7,8,9] Oral PPIs may be as effective as iv PPIs in nonvariceal UGIB, although this is controversial.[10]

Pantoprazole and **omeprazole** are the most extensively studied parenteral PPIs for UGIB, but iv omeprazole is not approved in Canada. IV pantoprazole is administered by continuous infusion (see Table 1). After two to three days of iv therapy, switch to an oral PPI to heal the associated ulcer or esophagitis. Where EHT or iv PPIs are not available, oral **omeprazole** 40 mg (or the equivalent dose of another oral PPI) may be administered twice daily. Most episodes of recurrent bleeding occur during the first three days.[10]

If the patient is *H. pylori*-negative, treat them with a PPI for four weeks. If the ulcer is associated with *H. pylori* or use of ASA or NSAIDs, continue PPI maintenance therapy for life to reduce the risk of rebleeding.

Bleeding Esophageal Varices

For bleeding esophageal varices, EHT (banding/sclerotherapy) may be supplemented with pharmacologic agents aimed at reducing portal pressure. The long-acting somatostatin analogue, **octreotide**, reduces portal pressure and bleeding, and is given intravenously for up to two days after the bleeding stops.[11] **Vasopressin** reduces splanchnic blood flow and portal pressure, but causes vasoconstriction in other vascular beds. Thus, caution is advised in patients with myocardial ischemia or peripheral vascular disease. Where octreotide or banding/sclerotherapy are not available, vasopressin may be used. IV **nitroglycerin** mitigates the adverse vasoconstrictive effects of vasopressin.

Prevention of Variceal Bleeding

Nonselective beta-blockers (e.g., **propranolol, nadolol**) may be used to prevent an initial bleed or to reduce the risk of recurrent bleeding in patients with *portal hypertension* and *esophageal varices*. However, beta-blockers do not prevent the development of varices in patients with cirrhosis.[12] Prophylaxis must be continued indefinitely as the risk of hemorrhage returns to that of an untreated patient if beta-blocker therapy is stopped.[13] In patients with high-risk (large) esophageal varices, endoscopic ligation of the varices is more effective than propranolol for the primary prevention of variceal bleeding.[14]

Therapeutic Tips

- Rapid diagnosis of UGIB using EGD is important to institute appropriate therapy. Patients with UGIB should be hemodynamically stable prior to EGD.
- Bleeding associated with gastric or duodenal ulcers should be treated empirically with a PPI.
- The patient should be assessed for *H. pylori* and treated with triple therapy for one week if indicated. A follow-up urea breath test (not serology) is essential in this setting to prove successful eradication of *H. pylori* and thereby reduce the risk of ulcer recurrence and recurrent bleeding.

Figure 1: **Management of Acute Upper GI Bleeding**[1]

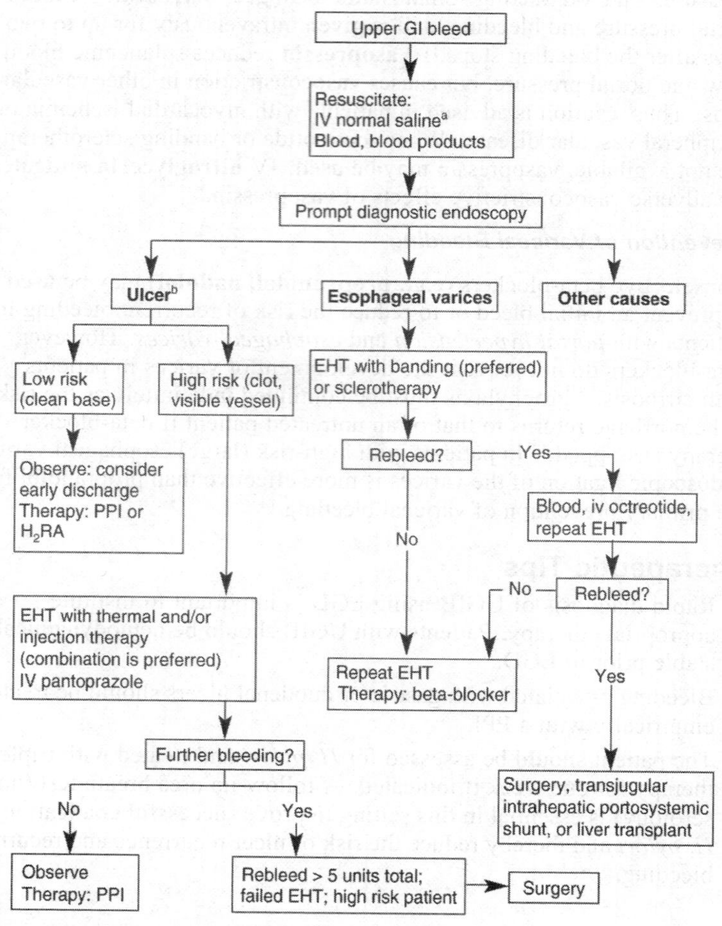

[a] Avoid normal saline in patients with suspected liver disease because of the risk of precipitating ascites.

[b] Antral biopsies may be taken at endoscopy to determine *H. pylori* status.
If not done initially, wait two weeks after stopping PPI before repeating endoscopy for biopsy.
If *H. pylori* positive, treat, repeat *H. pylori* testing and retreat if necessary.
If bleeding DU not associated with *H. pylori* or NSAIDuse, offer PPI maintenance therapy to minimize risk of recurrent DU and bleeding.
Patient with GU, biopsy to rule out gastric cancer.

Abbreviations: EHT=endoscopie hemostatic therapy; PPI=proton pump inhibitor.

Table 1: **Parenteral Drugs Used in the Management of Upper Gastrointestinal Bleeding**

Class	Drug	Indication	Dose	Adverse Effects	Comments	Cost[a]
Proton Pump Inhibitors	*pantoprazole* Panto IV	Nonvariceal bleeding	80 mg bolus over 2 h then 4–8 mg/h continuous infusion x 1–3 days[b]	Abdominal pain, chest pain, rash, pruritus, anaphylaxis.	Metabolized via the cytochrome P-450 system. Switch to oral PPI as soon as possible.	$100
Somatostatin Analogues	*octreotide* Sandostatin	Bleeding esophageal varices	50–100 µg bolus in 0.9% NaCl, then 25–50 µg/h infusion for up to 2 days after bleeding stops (mix 500 µg in 500 mL 0.9% NaCL and infuse at 50 mL/h)	Abdominal pain, nausea, diarrhea, hyperglycemia, headache, flushing.	May inhibit morphine analgesia.	$300
Vasopressin Receptor Agonists	*vasopressin* Pressyn, Pressyn AR, generics	Bleeding esophageal varices	20 units in 20 mL D5W bolus over 20 minutes then 0.2–0.4 units/min infusion for up to 2 days	Tremor, sweating, vertigo, nausea, anaphylaxis, water intoxication (early signs are drowsiness, listlessness, headache). Vascular disease patients may experience angina or even myocardial infarction.	Consider use of iv nitroglycerin to minimize ischemia. Ganglionic blocking agents may increase sensitivity to pressor effects.	$1200

[a] Cost for bolus and 48 h infusion.
[b] May be infused over 15 minutes.

Suggested Readings

Barkun A, Bardou M, Marshall JK et al. Consensus recommendations for managing patients with nonvariceal upper gastrointestinal bleeding. *Ann Intern Med* 2003;139(10):843-57.

Barkun A, Fallone CA, Chiba N et al. A Canadian clinical practice algorithm for the management of patients with nonvariceal upper gastrointestinal bleeding. *Can J Gastroenterol* 2004;18(10):605-9.

Barkun A, Sabbah S, Enns R et al. The Canadian Registry on Nonvariceal Upper Gastrointestinal Bleeding and Endoscopy (RUGBE): Endoscopic hemostasis and proton pump inhibition are associated with improved outcomes in a real-life setting. *Am J Gastroenterol* 2004;99(7):1238-46.

Dallal HJ, Palmer KR. ABC of the upper gastrointestinal tract: Upper gastrointestinal haemorrhage. *BMJ* 2001;323(7321):1115-7.

Sharara AI, Rockey DC. Gastroesophageal variceal hemorrhage. *N Engl J Med* 2001;345(9):669-81.

References

1. Dallal HJ, Palmer KR. ABC of the upper gastrointestinal tract: Upper gastrointestinal haemorrhage. *BMJ* 2001;323(7321):1115-7.
2. Lau JY, Sung JJ, Lam YH et al. Endoscopic retreatment compared with surgery in patients with recurrent bleeding after initial endoscopic control of bleeding ulcers. *N Engl J Med* 1999;340(10):751-6.
3. Barkun AN, Thomson A, Marshall J et al. Response to "Potentially flawed interpretation of data by Andriulli et al." *Am J Gastroenterol* 2005;100(9):2133.
4. Sharara AI, Rockey DC. Gastroesophageal variceal hemorrhage. *N Engl J Med* 2001;345(9):669-81.
5. Ferguson JW, Tripathi D, Hayes PC. Review article: the management of acute variceal bleeding. *Aliment Pharmacol Ther* 2003;18(3):253-62.
6. Andriulli A, Annese V, Caruso N et al. Proton-pump inhibitors and outcome of endoscopic hemostasis in bleeding peptic ulcers: a series of meta-analyses. *Am J Gastroenterol* 2005;100(1):207-19.
7. Bardou M, Toubouti Y, Benhaberou-Brun D et al. Meta-analysis: proton-pump inhibition in high-risk patients with acute peptic ulcer bleeding. *Aliment Pharmacol Ther* 2005;21(6):677-86.
8. Khuroo MS, Yattoo GN, Javid G et al. A comparison of omeprazole and placebo for bleeding peptic ulcer. *N Engl J Med* 1997;336(15):1054-8.
9. Leontiadis GI, Sharma VK, Howden CW. Proton pump inhibitor treatment for acute peptic ulcer bleeding. *Cochrane Database Syst Rev* 2006;(1):CD002094.
10. Lau JY, Sung JJ, Lee KK et al. Effect of intravenous omeprazole on recurrent bleeding after endoscopic treatment of bleeding peptic ulcers. *N Engl J Med* 2000;343(5):310-6.
11. Gotzsche PC, Hrobjartsson A. Somatostatin analogues for acute bleeding oesophageal varices. *Cochrane Database Syst Rev* 2005;(1):CD000193.
12. Groszmann RJ, Garcia-Tsao G, Bosch J et al. Beta-blockers to prevent gastroesophageal varices in patients with cirrhosis. *New Engl J Med* 2005;353(21):2254-61.
13. Abraczinkas DR, Ookubo R, Grace ND et al. Propranolol for the prevention of first esophageal variceal hemorrhage: a lifetime commitment? *Hepatology* 2001;34(6):1096-102.
14. Garcia-Tsao G. Portal hypertension. *Curr Opin Gastroenterol* 2002;18(3):351-9.

CHAPTER 56
Inflammatory Bowel Disease

Brian G. Feagan, MD, FRCPC

The idiopathic inflammatory bowel diseases consist of Crohn's disease, ulcerative colitis and ulcerative proctitis. Crohn's disease may involve any part of the gastrointestinal tract while ulcerative colitis is restricted, with a variable extent of involvement, to the colon. Ulcerative proctitis is a variant of ulcerative colitis, involving less than 30 cm of the distal colon.

Investigations

- History:
  - diarrhea, abdominal pain, rectal bleeding and weight loss are the most important symptoms
  - presence of nocturnal diarrhea usually indicates "organic" pathology in distinction to functional disorders such as irritable bowel syndrome
  - extraintestinal manifestations, e.g., aphthous ulcers, arthritis, erythema nodosum, iritis, perianal disease, fever
  - genetics: increased risk in patients with a family history, Ashkenazi Jews, and those with the NOD-2\CARD 15 gene (patients with Crohn's disease), the first susceptibility gene identified for inflammatory bowel disease
  - previous endoscopic/radiologic test results
  - previous medical (e.g., drugs, dose, duration) or surgical treatment (e.g., type and number of surgeries)
- Physical examination: weight, abdominal tenderness, presence of abdominal mass, malnutrition, perianal disease (fistulae, abscess)
  - growth failure in children (chart height and weight, growth curve Tanner stage)
  - extraintestinal manifestations
- Precise diagnosis and extent of disease:
  - colonoscopy or upper gastrointestinal endoscopy
  - barium radiocontrast studies
  - biopsy/histopathology, small bowel x-rays
  - presence of small bowel involvement; granulomata are pathognomonic for Crohn's disease
- 10% of cases with colonic disease cannot be classified and are termed *indeterminate colitis*
- A definitive diagnosis is important since:
  - colectomy cures ulcerative colitis; Crohn's disease recurs after surgery

  - the conditions respond differently to drug therapy (especially aminosalicylates)
- Precise anatomic localization is necessary for selecting drug therapy and planning surgery
- Laboratory tests:
  - measures of inflammation (WBC, Hgb, ESR, C-reactive protein, albumin)
  - stool cultures, *C. difficile* toxin assay

Goals of Therapy

- Relieve symptoms and improve patients' quality of life
- Improve nutritional status and growth (children/adolescents)
- Prevent disease recurrence
- Prevent development of cancer of the colon, which is associated with ulcerative colitis and colonic Crohn's disease
- Identify and treat extraintestinal manifestations (e.g., arthritis, arthralgia, iritis, uveitis)

Therapeutic Choices

Therapy is determined by the site and extent of disease, and by the severity of symptoms. Patients with mild to moderate disease activity are managed as outpatients, whereas those with severe symptoms may require hospitalization. Therapy is sequential in first inducing and then maintaining remission.

Pharmacologic Choices (Table 1)

Pharmacologic management of inflammatory bowel disease includes the use of aminosalicylates, corticosteroids, immunosuppressives, antidiarrheals, antibiotics and, to a limited degree, opioid analgesics. In selecting therapy consider, in addition to efficacy, the route of administration (oral, iv, rectal) and potential adverse events.

Aminosalicylates

Preparations containing **5-aminosalicylic acid** (5-ASA) are formulated to release the drug at specific sites in the gastrointestinal tract, since efficacy is dependent on luminal concentration. Salofalk, Mesasal and Pentasa release 5-ASA in the small bowel. Sulfasalazine, olsalazine and Asacol release 5-ASA primarily in the colon.

All 5-ASA compounds are highly effective for the treatment of ulcerative colitis. However, sulfasalazine has only modest efficacy in active Crohn's disease (approximately 40% efficacy for induction of remission versus 30% with placebo[1,2]) and is generally used in patients with mild disease. Pentasa and Asacol have been evaluated in active Crohn's disease with equivocal results, and their widespread use for both induction and maintenance of remission is coming under increasing scrutiny. Although these compounds are often used interchangeably in clinical practice, evidence favours use of sulfasalazine for mildly active colonic Crohn's disease.[1,2] Sulfasalazine has the least-favourable adverse effect profile, which includes nausea, headache, rash, hemolytic anemia and hepatotoxicity. However, many of these effects are minor and dose related. The majority of these events (> 90%) are related to the sulfapyridine moiety which is not present in 5-ASA preparations. Reversible oligospermia has been reported with sulfasalazine, but has not been associated with 5-ASA.

Corticosteroids

Patients with a moderately severe exacerbation of Crohn's disease or ulcerative colitis are treated initially with oral **prednisone** 40 to 60 mg/day.[2] In those with severe disease, hospitalization and treatment with iv corticosteroids (e.g., hydrocortisone, methylprednisolone) may be necessary. Patients who respond to iv therapy are switched to prednisone once stabilized. Taper the prednisone dose as improvement occurs (total duration of therapy is 12 to 16 weeks for Crohn's disease; 8 to 12 weeks for ulcerative colitis).[2,3]

Long-term use of glucocorticoids should be avoided and is restricted to patients unresponsive to other drugs. Make patients aware of the possible side effects and obtain informed consent. Osteoporosis is a concern with long-term therapy. Supplemental calcium and vitamin D intake, smoking cessation, exercise and, in select individuals, treatment with bisphosphonates are useful interventions. Use of glucocorticoids is also associated with avascular necrosis of the femoral head.

Budesonide is rapidly inactivated in the liver, resulting in lower systemic bioavailability and a reduced effect on the hypothalamic-pituitary-adrenal axis. It is available as an oral controlled-release capsule for the treatment of terminal ileal/right-sided colonic Crohn's disease[4,5] and as an enema for treatment of ulcerative colitis. In clinical trials, response rates for oral budesonide are marginally lower than those for prednisone in patients with active Crohn's disease (50 to 60% versus 70%). An important advantage of budesonide over prednisone is that the manifestations of Cushing's syndrome occur less frequently.[6] Budesonide enemas are as effective as other steroid enemas and have a lower incidence of side effects, but are more costly.[7]

Immunosuppressive Agents

Azathioprine, **6-mercaptopurine (6-MP)** or **methotrexate** are used in patients with refractory Crohn's disease to control symptoms or to reduce the dose of prednisone.[8,9,10] All immunosuppressive drugs have important side effects (e.g., bone marrow suppression, cytopenias and infections). Hypersensitivity pneumonitis and hepatotoxicity are the most important adverse effects of methotrexate. Coadministration of folic acid is recommended with methotrexate (1 mg daily). Pancreatitis occurs in approximately 3% of patients treated with azathioprine or 6-MP.[11]

Development of lymphoma is an uncommon complication of treatment with purine antimetabolites, whereas no strong evidence exists to support a similar relationship with methotrexate.

Biologic Response Modifiers

Infliximab, a chimeric (murine/human) antibody directed towards tumor necrosis factor-alpha (TNF-α), is effective for induction of remission[12,13] and closure of fistulas[14] in patients with active Crohn's disease refractory to other treatments, and in patients with active ulcerative colitis who do not respond to conventional therapy. Infusion reactions may be minor (headache, flushing, lightheadedness) or major (manifestations of anaphylaxis). Formation of anti-nuclear antibodies, a rare lupus-like syndrome, serum sickness and lymphoma are important concerns. Opportunistic infections such as tuberculosis, histoplasmosis and aspergillosis may occur. Screen for tuberculosis by obtaining a history of exposure, a chest x-ray and tuberculin skin testing prior to treatment. Manage patients who are infected with tuberculosis collaboratively with an infectious disease physician.

Antibiotics

Short courses (two to four weeks) of **metronidazole** and/or **ciprofloxacin** are useful as a treatment for patients with Crohn's disease and perianal fistulae.[15] Metronidazole has a potent disulfiram-like activity if alcohol is ingested and neuropathy may occur with long-term use. Avoid the use of metronidazole in pregnant patients.

Antidiarrheals

Use antidiarrheals with caution and avoid in severe disease because of the risk of toxic megacolon. **Diphenoxylate with atropine** is a combination of an opiate and an anticholinergic drug which can cause CNS side effects. **Loperamide** acts on both cholinergic and opiate receptors, but has a lower incidence of adverse effects than diphenoxylate.

Patients who develop diarrhea after extensive bowel resection often respond well to resins that bind bile salts (e.g., cholestyramine).

Opiate Analgesics

Opiates decrease gastrointestinal motility. Chronic use may lead to narcotic bowel syndrome, the risk for habituation is high and, in some individuals, may worsen symptoms.

Codeine is useful for pain control and decreasing the number of bowel movements (although approximately 10% of patients may not respond to the drug because of a genetic polymorphism, see the section on analgesics in Chapter 72). Avoid use of morphine or meperidine; restrict use to short-term treatment in select patients.

Crohn's Disease

Therapeutic Choices (Figure 1)

Nonpharmacologic Choices

- Encourage the patient to stop smoking (limited evidence suggests smoking worsens Crohn's disease).[16]
- Advise patients not to arbitrarily limit food groups. The goal is to ensure an adequate caloric intake. Nutritional supplements or parenteral nutrition may be necessary in select patients who are malnourished.
- Surgery may be necessary to treat strictures, abscesses, fistulae or for patients refractory to medical management. Recurrence after surgery is almost universal, so conservative surgical management with resection of a minimum amount of bowel is favoured.
- Psychological and social support is important, especially for adolescents.

Pharmacologic Choices (Table 1)

See the previous general discussion of pharmacologic choices in inflammatory bowel diseases.

- **Corticosteroids** are most effective for the *induction of remission* (70% response rate). Prednisone (40 to 60 mg/day for 12 to 16 weeks) is the most commonly used drug.[2]
- Chronic low-dose corticosteroid therapy is ineffective for the *maintenance of remission*.[17] However, some patients with chronically active disease may require continuous low-dose prednisone (10 to 15 mg/day) to suppress their symptoms.
- **Sulfasalazine** (6 to 8 g/day) is only marginally effective for the induction of remission (approximately 40% response rate versus 30% with placebo in patients with mild disease).[2] It is not clear whether 5-ASA is effective for treatment of active disease.[18]
- The value of **5-ASA** as a maintenance therapy for Crohn's disease is controversial (in contrast to its status in ulcerative colitis). A recent synthesis of available data concluded that maintenance therapy provided no benefit.[19]
- Patients who receive purine antimetabolites and methotrexate should use effective contraception as these drugs may be teratogenic.[20]
- In *pregnancy*, methotrexate is absolutely contraindicated and purine antimetabolites are often discontinued (although this is controversial). Despite earlier concerns regarding a potential risk of kernicterus, sulfasalazine has been used in pregnancy with relative safety. Aminosalicylates and corticosteroids are considered to be safe and may be continued in pregnancy if indicated.[20]
- **Infliximab** is effective for patients who are refractory to antimetabolite therapy.[12,22] Infliximab is considered to be a primary therapy for

patients with moderate to severe disease with fistulae.[14,21] Most gastroenterologists coadminister antimetabolites to prevent the development of antibodies to infliximab and potentially to enhance efficacy. Limited experience supports the use of infliximab in pregnancy.[20] Infusions should not be given late in the third trimester since the antibody is actively transported across the placenta, resulting in measurable concentrations of infliximab in the neonate.

Therapeutic Tips

- A rare hypersensitivity reaction to 5-ASA preparations can worsen symptoms.
- 5-ASA does not have a corticosteroid-sparing effect.
- Bile salt–induced diarrhea may occur in patients who have had resection of their terminal ileum. This usually responds to **cholestyramine** or **antidiarrheals**. Vitamin B_{12} deficiency may occur in this setting.
- Infusion reactions from infliximab may require treatment with epinephrine, antihistamines and corticosteroids.
- NSAIDs may exacerbate symptoms and should be avoided.
- Perform colonoscopy to screen for colon cancer according to published guidelines.[23]

Ulcerative Colitis

Therapeutic Choices (Figure 2)

Nonpharmacologic Choices

- Maintain a well-balanced diet with supplements. Total parenteral nutrition may be necessary in a minority of patients with severe disease.
- Surgery (colectomy) may be used to treat patients who are refractory to medical therapy or who have cancerous changes in the colon.
- Colonoscopic surveillance programs in patients at high risk for cancer (early age of onset, extensive disease, long disease duration, concomitant sclerosing cholangitis) is recommended starting seven years from the time of diagnosis.[20]
- Although colectomy "cures" ulcerative colitis, pouchitis, a chronic inflammatory condition which occurs after ileal-anal reservoir construction, can be troublesome.[15] Symptoms of pouchitis include tenesmus, diarrhea and bleeding.

Pharmacologic Choices (Table 1)

See the previous general discussion of pharmacologic choices in inflammatory bowel diseases.

Aminosalicylates are highly effective for inducing and maintaining remission in patients with ulcerative colitis compared with placebo.

Sulfasalazine is the least expensive preparation available and is well tolerated by most patients. Although the newer 5-ASA products are better tolerated than sulfasalazine, they do not possess superior efficacy. Only 20% of patients will be unable to tolerate sulfasalazine. Continuous use of **corticosteroids**, **immunosuppressive agents** or **infliximab** is reserved for patients with refractory disease who decline surgery. Use the lowest possible dose of prednisone to control disease activity.

The efficacy of the **purine antimetabolites** in ulcerative colitis is less well established than in Crohn's disease. **Methotrexate** is not effective for the treatment of ulcerative colitis.[22] High-dose iv **cyclosporine** may be effective in up to 80% of patients with severe ulcerative colitis, but is associated with a 1% one-year mortality rate.[24] It should only be offered to patients who refuse surgery and are informed of the potential for toxicity. Recent studies have confirmed the efficacy of **infliximab** for the treatment of refractory ulcerative colitis.

Therapeutic Tips

- Use extreme caution when prescribing narcotics and anticholinergic drugs for patients with active ulcerative colitis due to the risk of toxic megacolon. Use these drugs only when all other alternatives have failed.
- Weak evidence suggests that folate supplementation and high compliance with aminosalicylate maintenance therapy may reduce the risk of colon cancer.[25,26]
- Patients with severe colitis often will not tolerate tube feeds due to diarrhea.
- NSAIDs may exacerbate symptoms or precipitate relapse and should be avoided.

Ulcerative Proctitis

Therapeutic Choices (Figure 3)

Pharmacologic Choices (Table 1)

Given the limited extent of the inflammation (rectum/sigmoid colon), the focus is on topical therapy. **5-ASA** preparations (suppositories, enemas) administered at bedtime are the initial treatment of choice. Alternatively, **topical corticosteroids** can be used. If a response is not achieved with one of these strategies, switching to the other is advised. Suppositories are effective only for proctosigmoiditis, whereas enemas can be used to treat disease in the descending colon and rectum from the splenic flexure distally.

If a remission is not induced within two to four weeks, oral 5-ASA can be added. Limited data suggest that there is an additive benefit of combined oral and topical 5-ASA induction therapy. Switch patients unresponsive to these measures to prednisone or (rarely) iv corticosteroids. Patients who are brought into remission easily after a first episode (i.e., within four to eight weeks) should have all medications discontinued. Follow-up is essential; patients with a recurrence of symptoms should receive chronic maintenance therapy with 5-ASA. Most patients prefer oral maintenance therapy, although in practice many will require prolonged topical 5-ASA therapy.

Patients brought into remission with difficulty should continue on long-term oral or topical 5-ASA preparations or corticosteroid enemas, without an attempt to discontinue therapy.

Patients rarely require chronic treatment with low-dose prednisone or purine antimetabolites. Colectomy may be necessary in some patients despite the limited extent of the disease. Infliximab has not been specifically evaluated in this group of patients, although it may be considered before surgery is recommended.

Therapeutic Tips

- Topical therapy is preferred.
- In patients who are difficult to manage, perform a repeat sigmoidoscopy to ensure that the inflammation is still confined to the lower bowel and has not developed into more extensive colitis.

Figure 1: **Management of Crohn's Disease**

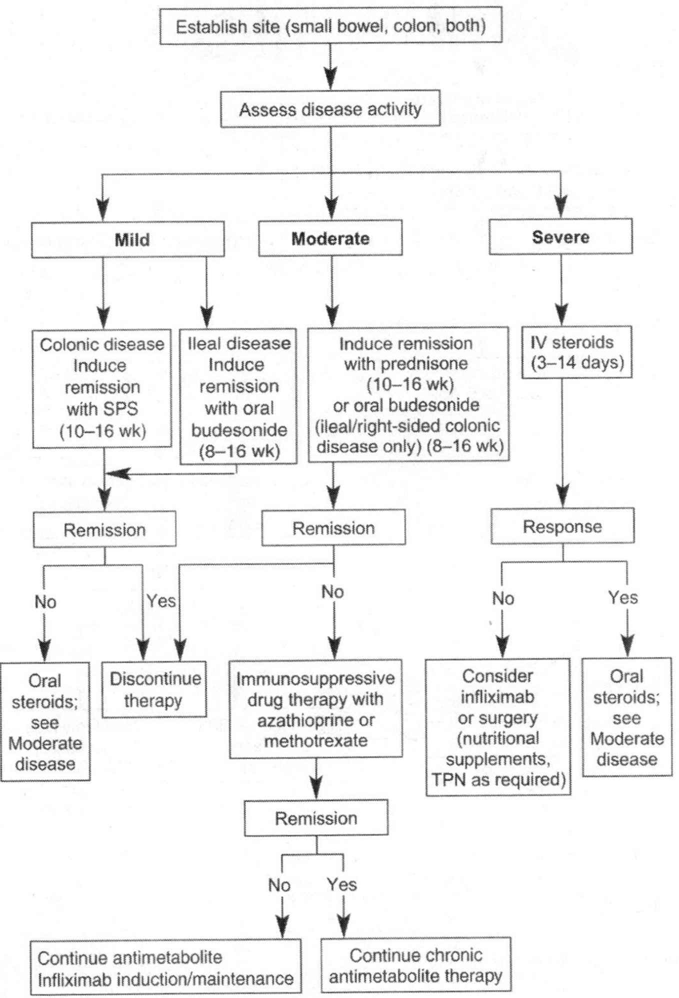

Abbreviations: SPS = sulfasalazine; TPN = total parenteral nutrition

Figure 2: **Management of Ulcerative Colitis**

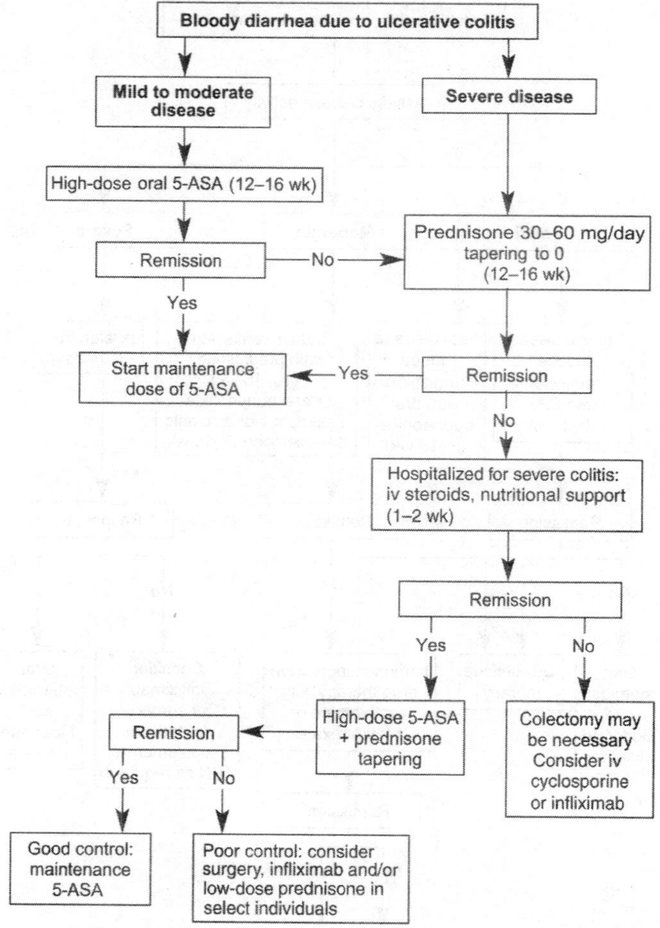

Abbreviation: 5–ASA = 5–aminosalicylic acid

Figure 3: **Management of Ulcerative Proctitis**

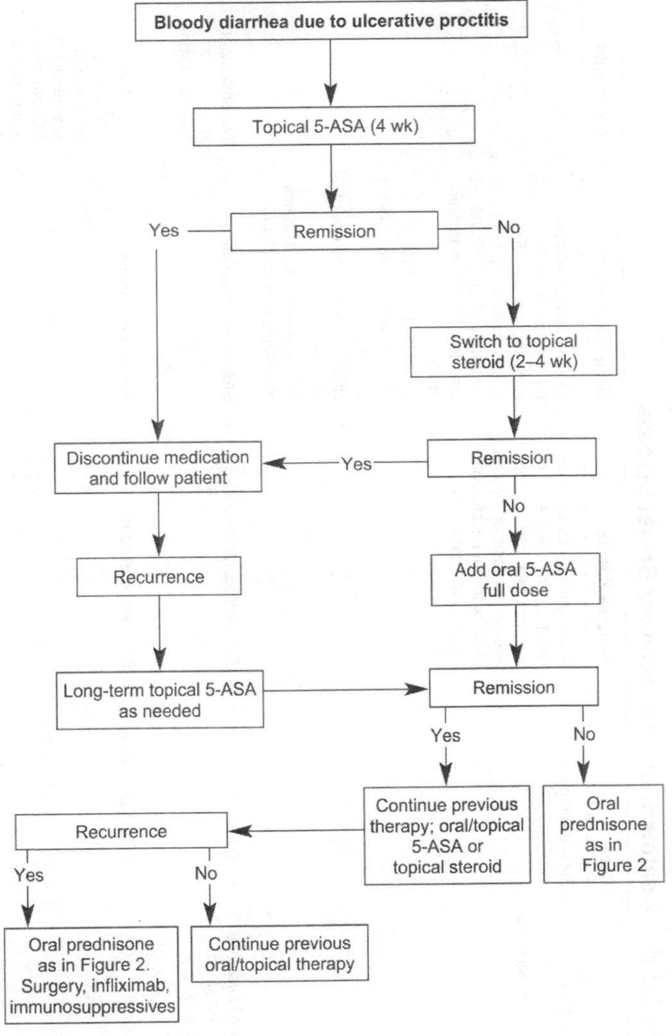

Abbreviation: 5–ASA = 5–aminosalicylic acid

Table 1: **Drugs Used for the Treatment of Inflammatory Bowel Disease**

Class	Drug	Dose	Adverse Effects	Drug Interactions	Comments	Cost[a]
Corticosteroids, systemic	*hydrocortisone sodium succinate* Solu-Cortef, generics	300–400 mg/day iv	Acne, glucose intolerance, weight gain, hypertension, hypokalemia, osteoporosis, aseptic necrosis of femoral head, adrenal insufficiency with sudden cessation.	Cyclosporine: although corticosteroids and cyclosporine are often used concurrently, both are metabolized by CYP3A4; be alert to ↑ response to both drugs. Antidiabetic agents: glucocorticoids may ↑ blood glucose. NSAIDs: may ↑ the risk of GI ulceration. Thiazide and loop diuretics also deplete potassium.		$$$
	methylprednisolone sodium succinate Solu-Medrol, generics	40–60 mg/day iv	See hydrocortisone.	See hydrocortisone.	No advantage over hydrocortisone.	$$
	prednisone generics	30–60 mg po (QAM)	See hydrocortisone.	See hydrocortisone.	Useful in moderately severe and severe UC and CD. No role in maintenance therapy.	$

Class	Drug	Dose	Adverse Effects	Drug Interactions	Comments	Cost[a]
	budesonide, oral Entocort Capsules	Acute exacerbation: 9 mg/day po Maintenance: 3–6 mg/day po	See hydrocortisone.	See hydrocortisone.	Controlled-release capsule for treating CD in the ileum and/or ascending colon. Rapidly metabolized, somewhat fewer adverse effects than conventional corticosteroids.	$
Corticosteroids, topical	*hydrocortisone, enema* Cortenema, Cortifoam, Hycort	80–100 mg QHS as enema	Topical therapy, in general, has less severe adverse effects than systemic therapy.		Enemas effective in UP. Useful in UC; role in CD not well established.	$$
	betamethasone, enema Betnesol	5 mg QHS as enema	See hydrocortisone enema.			$$
	budesonide, enema Entocort Enema	2 mg QHS as enema	See hydrocortisone enema.			$$
Aminosalicylates	*sulfasalazine* Salazopyrin, generics	Active[b]: ≥ 4 g/day divided Maintenance[c]: 2–3 g/day divided	Dose-related adverse effects: nausea, vomiting, diarrhea, anorexia, headache. Hypersensitivity reaction (rash, fever), aplastic anemia, oligospermia (reversible).	Sulfasalazine may ↓ GI absorption of digoxin. It is unknown whether 5-ASA also ↓ digoxin absorption.	All aminosalicylates are equally effective in UC.	$

(cont'd)

Table 1: **Drugs Used for the Treatment of Inflammatory Bowel Disease** *(cont'd)*

Class	Drug	Dose	Adverse Effects	Drug Interactions	Comments	Cost[a]
	olsalazine Dipentum	Active[b]: > 1 g/day divided Maintenance[c]: 1 g/day divided	Diarrhea; may be minimized by increasing dose gradually.			$
	5-aminosalicylic acid (5–ASA) Asacol, Asacol 800, Mesasal, Pentasa, Salofalk, generics	Asacol – Active[b]: > 1.6 g/day divided. Maintenance[c]: 0.8–1.6 g/day divided Mesasal – Active[b]: > 1.5 g/day divided Maintenance[c]: 1–1.5 g/day divided Pentasa – Active[b]: > 2 g/day divided Maintenance[c]: 1.5–2 g/day divided Salofalk – Active[b]: 3–4 g/day divided Maintenance[c]: 1–2 g/day divided	Rare hypersensitivity reactions, including pneumonitis, hepatitis and worsening of colitis. Abdominal pain, cramps or discomfort as well as rash, pruritus and anal irritation can occur with rectal administration.	See sulfasalazine.	All aminosalicylates are equally effective in UC. The value of 5-ASA as maintenance therapy in CD is controversial. Best evidence for Asacol 2.4 g/day and Pentasa 3 g/day.	$
	5-aminosalicylic acid, rectal Salofalk , Pentasa	Enema: 1–4 g/day Suppositories: 0.5–1 g/day	See 5-ASA.		Enemas and suppositories effective in UP.	$

Class	Drug	Dose	Adverse Effects	Drug Interactions	Comments	Cost[a]
Immunosuppressives	*azathioprine* Imuran, generics	2.5 mg/kg/day po	Major adverse effects: cytopenias and rarely, pancreatitis, hepatotoxicity. Common adverse effects: nausea, stomatitis, GI discomfort, arthralgias diarrhea, anorexia, increased risk of opportunistic infection.	Allopurinol may ↑ azathioprine toxicity; dosage adjustment may be necessary (1/4 of regular dose); similar interaction with mercaptopurine. ACE inhibitors may ↑ the likelihood of neutropenia when combined with azathioprine or mercaptopurine.	Not for use in pregnant women. Metabolism of azathioprine and mercaptopurine is influenced by a genetic polymorphism.	$
	6-mercaptopurine Purinethol	100 mg/day po	Major adverse effects: blood dyscrasias, and rarely pancreatitis, hepatotoxicity. See azathioprine.	Oral anticoagulants: mercaptopurine may inhibit hypoprothrombinemic response to warfarin and possibly other anticoagulants. See azathioprine.	See azathioprine.	$$
	methotrexate Methotrexate, generics	25 mg im weekly	Nausea, flu-like aches, headache, oral ulcers, bone marrow and liver toxicity, pneumonitis, immunosuppression, lymphoma.	Alcohol restriction may minimize hepatotoxicity. NSAIDs may ↑ MTX serum concentrations (probably not significant with low once-weekly MTX doses). Some penicillins may ↓ MTX clearance.	Methotrexate is potentially hepatotoxic. Oral methotrexate has not been evaluated in controlled trials. See azathioprine.	$$

(cont'd)

Table 1: **Drugs Used for the Treatment of Inflammatory Bowel Disease** *(cont'd)*

Class	Drug	Dose	Adverse Effects	Drug Interactions	Comments	Cost[a]
	cyclosporine (renal symbol) Sandimmune	4 mg/kg/day iv	Renal toxicity, hypertension, hypertrichosis, cytopenia, gum hyperplasia, electrolyte imbalances, nausea, diarrhea. Seizures. Opportunistic infection.	Metabolized by cytochrome P450: many possible drug interactions (e.g., erythromycin, ketoconazole, rifampin, St. John's wort).	See azathioprine.	$$$$
Biologic Response Modifiers[c]	*infliximab* Remicade	Crohn's Disease: Luminal CD: 5 mg/kg iv × 1–2–3 doses Fistulizing CD: 5 mg/kg iv × 3 at wks 0, 2 and 6 Maintenance therapy every 8 weekly infusions.	Nausea, infusion/hypersensitivity reactions. Development of anti-DNA antibodies and rarely a reversible lupus-like syndrome. Use with antimetabolites may potentiate response and reduce the formation of human antichimeric antibodies. Possible development of lymphoma.	The manufacturer recommends that patients receiving infliximab not receive live vaccines.		$$$$

[a] Cost of 1-day supply for 70 kg person; includes drug cost only.
[b] Active dose is for CD and UC.
[c] Maintenance dose is for UC only.
(renal symbol) Dosage adjustment may be required in renal impairment; see Appendix I.
Abbreviations: UC = ulcerative colitis; CD = Crohn's disease; UP = ulcerative proctitis
Legend: $ < $5 $$ $5–10 $$$ $10–15 $$$$ > $15

Suggested Readings

Bamias G, Nyce MR, De La Rue SA et al. New concepts in the pathophysiology of inflammatory bowel disease. *Ann Intern Med* 2005;143(12):895-904.

Collins P, Rhodes J. Ulcerative colitis: diagnosis and management. *BMJ* 2006;333(7563):340-3.

Hanauer SB. Inflammatory bowel disease: epidemiology, pathogenesis, and therapeutic opportunities. *Inflamm Bowel Dis* 2006:12(Suppl 1):S3-9.

Lichtenstein GR, Abreu MT, Cohen R et al. American Gastroenterological Association Institute medical position statement on corticosteroids, immunomodulators, and infliximab in inflammatory bowel disease. *Gastroenterology* 2006;130(3):935-9.

Mahadevan U, Kane S. American Gastroenterological Association Institute medical position statement on the use of gastrointestinal medications in pregnancy. *Gastroenterology* 2006;131(1):278-82.

Su C, Lewis JD, Goldberg B, Brensinger C et al. A meta-analysis of the placebo rates of remission and response in clinical trials of active ulcerative colitis. *Gastroenterology* 2007;132(2):516-26.

References

1. Malchow H, Ewe K, Brandes J et al. European Cooperative Crohn's Disease Study (ECCDS): results of drug treatment. *Gastroenterology* 1984;86(2):249-66.
2. Summers RW, Switz DM, Sessions JT et al. National Cooperative Crohn's Disease Study: results of drug treatment. *Gastroenterology* 1979;77(4 Pt 2):847-69.
3. Jani N, Regueiro MD. Medical therapy for ulcerative colitis. *Gastroenterol Clin North Am* 2002;31(1):147-66.
4. Greenberg GR, Feagan BG, Martin F et al. Oral budesonide for active Crohn's disease. Canadian Inflammatory Bowel Disease Study Group. *N Engl J Med* 1994;331(13):836-41.
5. Rutgeerts P, Lofberg R, Malchow H et al. A comparison of budesonide with prednisolone for active Crohn's disease. *N Engl J Med* 1994;331(13):842-5.
6. Kane SV, Schoenfeld P, Sandborn WJ et al. The effectiveness of budesonide therapy for Crohn's disease. *Aliment Pharmacol Ther* 2002;16(8):1509-17.
7. Hanauer SB, Robinson M, Pruitt R et al. Budesonide enema for the treatment of active, distal ulcerative colitis and proctitis: a dose-ranging study. U.S. Budesonide enema study group. *Gastroenterology* 1998;115(3):525-32.
8. Candy S, Wright J, Gerber M et al. A controlled double blind study of azathioprine in the management of Crohn's disease. *Gut* 1995;37(5):674-8.
9. Feagan BG, Rochon J, Fedorak RN et al. Methotrexate for the treatment of Crohn's disease. The North American Crohn's Study Group Investigators. *N Engl J Med* 1995;332(5):292-7.
10. Pearson DC, May GR, Fick GH et al. Azathioprine and 6-mercaptopurine in Crohn disease. A meta-analysis. *Ann Intern Med* 1995;123(2):132-42.
11. Present DH, Meltzer SJ, Krumholz MP et al. 6-Mercaptopurine in the management of inflammatory bowel disease: short- and long-term toxicity. *Ann Intern Med* 1989;111(8):641-9.
12. Hanauer SB, Feagan BG, Lichtenstein GR et al. Maintenance infliximab for Crohn's disease: the ACCENT I randomised trial. *Lancet* 2002;359(9317):1541-9.
13. Targan SR, Hanauer SB, van Deventer SJ et al. A short-term study of chimeric monoclonal antibody cA2 to tumor necrosis factor alpha for Crohn's disease. Crohn's Disease cA2 Study Group. *N Engl J Med* 1997;337(15):1029-35.
14. Present DH, Rutgeerts P, Targan S et al. Infliximab for the treatment of fistulas in patients with Crohn's disease. *N Engl J Med* 1999;340(18):1398-405.
15. Shen B, Achkar JP, Lashner BA et al. A randomized clinical trial of ciprofloxacin and metronidazole to treat acute pouchitis. *Inflamm Bowel Dis* 2001;7(4):301-5.
16. Sutherland LR, Ramcharan S, Bryant H et al. Effect of cigarette smoking on recurrence of Crohn's disease. *Gastroenterology* 1990;98(5 Pt 1):1123-8.
17. Steinhart AH, Ewe K, Griffiths AM et al. Corticosteroids for maintenance of remission in Crohn's disease. *Cochrane Database Syst Rev* 2003;(4):CD000301.
18. Hanauer SB, Stromberg U. Oral Pentasa in the treatment of active Crohn's disease: a meta-analysis of double-blind, placebo-controlled trials. *Clin Gastroenterol Hepatol* 2004;2(5):379-88.

19. Akobeng AK, Gardener E. Oral 5-aminosalicylic acid for maintenance of medically-induced remission in Crohn's Disease. *Cochrane Database Syst Rev* 2005;(1):CD003715.
20. Mahadevan U, Kane S. American Gastroenterological Association Institute technical review on the use of gastrointestinal medications in pregnancy. *Gastroenterology* 2006;131(1):283-311.
21. Lichtenstein GR, Abreu MT, Cohen R et al. American Gastroenterological Association Institute technical review on corticosteroids, immunomodulators, and infliximab in inflammatory bowel disease. *Gastroenterology* 2006;130(3):940-87.
22. Oren R, Arber N, Odes S et al. Methotrexate in chronic active ulcerative colitis: a double-blind, randomized, Israeli multicenter trial. *Gastroenterology* 1996;110(5):1416-21.
23. Winawer S, Fletcher R, Rex D et al. Colorectal cancer screening and surveillance: clinical guidelines and rationale. Update based on new evidence. *Gastroenterology* 2003;124(2):544-60.
24. Lichtiger S, Present DH, Kornbluth A et al. Cyclosporine in severe ulcerative colitis refractory to steroid therapy. *N Engl J Med* 1994;330(26):1841-5.
25. Bernstein CN, Eaden J, Steinhart AH et al. Cancer prevention in inflammatory bowel disease and the chemoprophylactic potential of 5-aminosalicylic acid. *Inflamm Bowel Dis* 2002;8(5):356-61.
26. Lashner BA, Heidenreich PA, Su GL et al. Effect of folate supplementation on the incidence of dysplasia and cancer in chronic ulcerative colitis. A case-control study. *Gastroenterology* 1989;97(2):255-9.

Pharmacoeconomic Considerations: Inflammatory Bowel Disease

Nicole Mittmann, MSc, PhD

Epidemiology		
Country	**Incidence and Prevalence (%)**	
Canada (1987-1996)[1]	Ulcerative colitis: 15.6 cases per 100 000 person-years Crohn's disease: 15.6 cases per 100 000 person-years	
Cost of Illness Data		
Country and Year of Estimate	**Direct Costs**[a]	**Indirect Costs**[b]
United States (1990)[2]	US $0.4 to $0.6 billion	US $1.4 to $2.0 billion
Commentary		
Inflammatory bowel disease (IBD) refers collectively to ulcerative colitis (UC) and Crohn's disease (CD). Wages lost from UC and CD are significant, and are more than double the direct costs of treatment.[2] In one study from the United Kingdom, lost wages accounted for £230 to £299 per patient over a six-month period.[3] Although hospitalization for IBD is not common,[4] it accounted for almost 50% of the overall costs associated with IBD over six months in a university hospital setting, while medications accounted for less than 25% of the remainder.[2] Surgery accounts for a significant portion (40% to 60%) of the costs associated with hospitalization.[5,6]		

(cont'd)

Commentary

In terms of therapeutic choices, infliximab is more expensive than methotrexate, but reduces costs associated with hospitalizations.[7] Infliximab is cost-effective when combined with methotrexate for the episodic management of CD, but long-term maintenance therapy exceeds conventional benchmarks for cost-effectiveness.[8,9,10] Economic evaluations of infliximab have generally considered patients refractory to standard therapies with few other treatment options. However, direct head-to-head comparative trials of infliximab with other biological agents are not yet available and would be helpful in determining with greater certainty the place of infliximab in the management of IBD.[8]

[a] Direct costs include those associated with physician services, nursing care, diagnostic procedures, drugs and hospitalization.

[b] Indirect costs include those associated with lost productivity and days off work due to morbidity or premature mortality.

References

1. Blanchard JF, Bernstein CN, Wajda A et al. Small-area variations and sociodemographic correlates for the incidence of Crohn's disease and ulcerative colitis. *Am J Epidemiol* 2001;154(4):328-35.
2. Hay JW, Hay AR. Inflammatory bowel disease: costs of illness. *J Clin Gastroenterol* 1992;14(4):309-17.
3. Bassi A, Dodd S, Williamson P et al. Cost of illness of inflammatory bowel disease in the UK: a single centre retrospective study. *Gut* 2004;53(10):1471-8.
4. Feagan BG, Vreeland MG, Larson LR et al. Annual cost of care for Crohn's disease: a payor perspective. *Am J Gastroenterol* 2000;95(8):1955-60.
5. Bernstein CN, Papineau N, Zajaczkowski J et al. Direct hospital costs for patients with inflammatory bowel disease in a Canadian tertiary care university hospital. *Am J Gastroenterol* 2000;95(3):677-83.
6. Cohen RD, Larson LR, Roth JM et al. The cost of hospitalization in Crohn's disease. *Am J Gastroenterol* 2000;95(2):524-30.
7. Jewell DP, Satsangi J, Lobo A et al. Infliximab use in Crohn's disease: impact on health care resources in the UK. *Eur J Gastroenterol Hepatol* 2005;17(10):1047-52.
8. Jaisson-Hot I, Flourie B, Descos L et al. Management for severe Crohn's disease: a lifetime cost-utility analysis. *Int J Technol Assess Health Care* 2004;20(3):274-9.
9. Bodger K. Economic implications of biological therapies for Crohn's disease: review of infliximab. *Pharmacoeconomics* 2005;23(9):875-88.
10. Marshall JK, Blackhouse G, Goeree R et al. *Clinical and economic assessment: infliximab for the treatment of Crohn's disease.* Ottawa (ON): Canadian Coordinating Office for Health Technology Assessment (CCOHTA); 2002. Technology overview no 8.

CHAPTER 57
Irritable Bowel Syndrome

W. Grant Thompson, MD, FRCPC

The irritable bowel syndrome (IBS) is a collection of symptoms attributed to the intestine, related to defecation and unpredictable bowel habit (Table 1). Since there is no known pathology or pathophysiology, IBS can only be recognized by its characteristic pattern of abdominal pain and discomfort, which is invariably relieved by defecation. In Canadian adults, the one-year prevalence is about 12%,[1] and females with IBS outnumber males 4:1. Because the symptoms come and go, the lifetime prevalence is much higher. Most people who have these symptoms do not consult physicians. Nevertheless, IBS accounts for 30% of gut complaints in primary care (2% of all adult patients), and the few that are referred to specialists are a fifth of a gastroenterologist's practice. While the syndrome occurs at all ages, more young IBS sufferers see physicians. IBS is the ninth most costly gastrointestinal (GI) disorder, and in the year 2000, US direct and indirect expenditure was over $1.5 billion.

Goals of Therapy

- Establish caring doctor–patient relationship
- Conduct a thorough interview and examination to establish the diagnosis and rule out serious pathology
- Reassure the patient through a confident diagnosis. Address fears of serious disease
- Alleviate symptoms while establishing realistic expectations. Patients have greater expectation of benefit from lifestyle modification than drugs[2]
- Promote coping and normal social and occupational functioning
- Treat psychosocial comorbidity if present

Investigations

The history should note the abdominal pain and its relationship with diet, defecation, and altered stool frequency and form (Table 1). Pelvic pain (actually lower abdominal pain) may be due to IBS rather than a gynecologic cause.[3] However, potential gynecologic causes of pain must be ruled out. Physical findings or alarm symptoms such as rectal bleeding, anemia, fever or profound weight loss are not explained by IBS (Table 2). The history should also explore the patient's psychosocial circumstances and the reasons that the patient has chosen to consult a physician.

Tests may be unnecessary in a young person with chronic and typical symptoms (Table 1), no alarm symptoms and no family history of colon cancer, inflammatory bowel disease (IBD) or celiac disease (Table 2).[3,4] If the patient is over the age of 50 years, and/or has risk factors for cancer or recent onset of atypical symptoms, further investigation with a barium enema or colonoscopy is recommended.[5,6] A recent history of bacterial gastroenteritis may explain self-limiting IBS-like symptoms. Difficult, chronic constipation or persistent diarrhea are not likely due to IBS, and raise different diagnostic and treatment issues that are discussed elsewhere (see Chapter 114 and Chapter 115).

Table 1: **Diagnostic Criteria[a,b] (Rome III)[c] for IBS[7]**

Recurrent abdominal pain or discomfort[d] at least 3 days per month in the last 3 months associated with two or more of the following: 1. Improvement with defecation 2. Onset associated with a change in frequency of stool 3. Onset associated with a change in form (appearance) of stool

[a] Criteria fulfilled for the last 3 months with symptom onset at least 6 months prior to diagnosis
[b] Supportive symptoms that are not part of the diagnostic criteria include abnormal stool frequency (a) fewer than three bowel movements per week, or (b) greater than three bowel movements per day; abnormal stool form (c) lumpy/hard stool, or (d) loose/watery stool; (e) defecation straining; (f) urgency, or also feeling of incomplete bowel movement, passing mucus and bloating.
[c] In the absence of structural or metabolic abnormalities to explain the symptoms.
[d] "Discomfort" means an uncomfortable sensation not described as pain.

Table 2: **Alarm Symptoms That Cannot be Explained by IBS**

Fever
Anemia
Bleeding from the gut
Significant weight loss
Family history of cancer, IBD or celiac disease
Recent consistent change in bowel habit
Persistent, daily diarrhea or constipation
Abnormal physical findings, for example, abdominal mass or malnutrition

Abbreviations: IBD = inflammatory bowel disease; IBS = irritable bowel syndrome

Therapeutic Choices (Table 3)

Nonpharmacologic Choices

- Discuss the diagnosis and prognosis with the patient.
- Address the patient's fears and provide reassurance.
- A good doctor–patient relationship maximizes placebo effects[8] and improves long-term outcomes.[9]
- Patients generally derive more benefit from lifestyle modification than drug therapy.
- Encourage consumption of a healthy diet (*Canada's Food Guide to Healthy Eating*)[4] and sufficient fluid intake.
- Avoid food fads, excessive caffeine, alcohol, sorbitol (in gums and candies) and fructose (in preserves).
- Encourage the patient to keep a diary of foods that trigger or relieve symptoms and to note any stressors.

- Many treatments proposed by alternative practitioners or the media have no proven efficacy. Some diets may be nutritionally unsound.
- Be alert to gut symptoms that may be caused by adverse effects of drugs or alternative health products, for example, herbal medicines.
- If constipated, ensure sufficient dietary fibre.
- Lifestyle adjustment: stress management, relaxation advice, quiet time for eating and defecation.
- Treat comorbid conditions: depression,[10] anxiety,[10] panic, life stress.[11,12]
- Psychological treatments may require the involvement of a mental health professional, and the benefits in patients with IBS are difficult to prove.[13] The following may help in refractory cases, or when psychopathology is evident: psychopharmacology,[14] individual or group psychotherapy,[15] cognitive-behavioural therapy,[16] hypnosis[17] (if available) and stress management or relaxation techniques including audio and video tapes.
- Avoid inappropriate referral and unnecessary surgery. IBS symptoms are sometimes mistaken for gynecologic or gallbladder diseases.

Pharmacologic Choices (Table 4)

- For the purposes of treatment, patients are grouped by their predominant bowel habit: constipation-predominant, diarrhea-predominant or alternating between constipation and diarrhea.
- When nonpharmacologic measures fail, target the most troublesome symptom (Table 3).
- The *Bristol Stool Form Scale* (Figure 1)[18] can be used to identify patients who suffer from constipation or diarrhea.[2,19] Selection of pharmacotherapy depends largely upon the predominant symptom.
- For patients with predominant diarrhea (Bristol Stool Form Scale type 6 or 7): **loperamide** PRN[20] may be recommended, especially if the patient is concerned about incontinence.[21]
- For patients with predominant constipation (pellety stools, Bristol Stool Form Scale type 1): recommend two to four tablespoonsful of raw bran or **psyllium** daily with plenty of fluids.
- For patients with chronic abdominal pain that impairs normal functioning: **amitriptyline**[22] or **desipramine**[16,22] may be useful, and may be effective in lower-than-antidepressant doses.[23]
- **Tegaserod** (a 5-HT_4 partial agonist) was approved for women with IBS who have constipation on the basis of eight randomized, controlled trials.[24] With a dosage of 6 mg twice daily, the number of patients that must be treated to provide global relief of GI symptoms in one patient (NNT) is 14 (RR 1.19 vs. placebo). The manufacturer suspended sales of the drug on March 30, 2007 in Canada and the US citing data from all randomized, controlled trials that showed those receiving tegaserod to be statistically significantly more likely to suffer ischemic

cardiovascular events than placebo recipients (0.11% vs. 0.01%, p=0.024).[25] Clinical investigation is continuing, and it is possible that restricted access to the drug may eventually be allowed in Canada.

There is much interest in the use of **probiotics** for IBS, but the quality (bioavailability) of the products and the supporting evidence is meagre. Promising results were demonstrated using *Bifidobacterium infantis* in a small study of IBS patients where symptomatic improvement after eight weeks correlated with normalization of the IL-10/IL-12 ratio. The IL-10/IL-12 ratio is an indicator of a pro-inflammatory state and was elevated at baseline in this study.[26]

Bacterial overgrowth is a supposed cause of IBS, but a recent consensus questions the evidence for this hypothesis and recommends against the use of antibiotics with their attendant potential for harm.[2]

Prognosis[27]

- Usually lifelong and recurrent—no effect upon life expectancy.
- A diagnosis of IBS is associated with a low risk of structural disease when carefully made.
- No predisposition to structural disease such as diverticular disease, cancer or IBD.

The Difficult-to-Treat Patient

Complicated patients that tend to be referred to specialists often have comorbid conditions such as depression, or a history of serious emotional trauma such as sexual abuse. Such patients are best managed with regularly scheduled visits for a sympathetic discussion.[28] If necessary, a gastroenterology consultation may support the primary care physician's diagnosis and management plan, and reduce future IBS-related costs.[29] A mental health professional may assist with a severe comorbid psychological disorder. Long-term cure is unlikely, so the emphasis should be on coping and normal occupational and social functioning.

Therapeutic Tips

- The efficacy of many drugs proposed for IBS is unproven or varies greatly.[30,31,32] "Colonic spasm" does not explain IBS symptoms and therefore drugs that "relieve spasm" are unlikely to be helpful. Antispasmodic drugs approved by Health Canada for IBS before 2002 include dicyclomine, hyoscyamine, trimebutine and pinaverium. If used at all, these drugs should only be taken for a few weeks at a time. This author endorses none of them. These drugs differ from those approved in other countries, reflecting a lack of agreement about efficacy among regulatory authorities.[27]
- No single drug has been shown to be beneficial for the entire IBS symptom complex.
- No medication has proven beneficial for bloating.

Table 3: **Management of Irritable Bowel Syndrome (IBS)**

Diagnosis: It is essential to make a positive diagnosis, rather than a diagnosis of exclusion, and to convincingly convey this to the patient
Education/reassurance: explain the pathophysiology and natural history of IBS
• Physiological abnormalities include altered intestinal motility and visceral hypersensitivity • IBS can be precipitated by a previous enteric infection • Diet has no causal role, but may exacerbate IBS • Emotional stress does not cause IBS, but psychosocial factors may exacerbate IBS and/or contribute to the distress it causes • Validate symptoms. The symptoms are real, not imagined. Gut and brain interact to alter motility (muscle contractions) and/or increase bowel sensation • **IBS is a chronic, relapsing, but benign disorder**
Healthy lifestyle: provide advice regarding the importance of a balanced diet, exercise and time for toilet each morning
Diet
• Follow Canada's Food Guide to Healthy Eating (http://www.hc-sc.gc.ca/fn-an/food-guide-aliment/fg_rainbow-arc_en_ciel_ga_e.html) • Limit intake of alcohol, caffeine, fat and sorbitol. They do not cause IBS, but may exacerbate the symptoms • Restrict lactose consumption only in patients with proven lactase deficiency • Refer problem eaters to a dietitian
Psychosocial issues: explore in select patients
"Indicators" of difficulty coping with IBS: • Poor insight • Inability to express emotions • Comorbid conditions • History of physical or sexual abuse or other major life stresses • Multiple somatic complaints or abnormal illness behaviour • "Catastrophizing" symptoms, e.g., "First sign of pain means my day is ruined" • Poor coping mechanisms • Inadequate social supports A 2-week symptom diary may assist select patients to connect diet and stress with aggravation of symptoms Consider cognitive-behavioural therapy or hypnosis and relaxation therapy for patients with severe IBS
Drug Therapy
• Most patients will not require drug therapy • No single drug has been shown to be beneficial for the IBS symptom complex • *Specific* IBS symptoms may be amenable to drug therapy (Table 4) – first identify the predominant symptom (Figure 1)

Adapted with permission from Paterson WG et al. *CMAJ* 1999;161(2):154-60.

Figure 1: **Bristol Stool Form Scale**

Stool form	Appearance	Type
Separate hard lumps like nuts, (hard to pass). Result of slow transit.	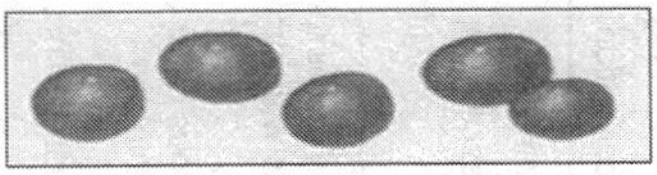	1
Sausage-shaped but lumpy.	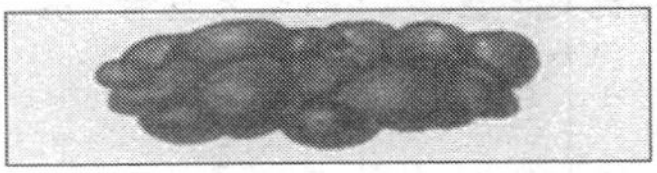	2
Like a sausage but cracks on its surface.	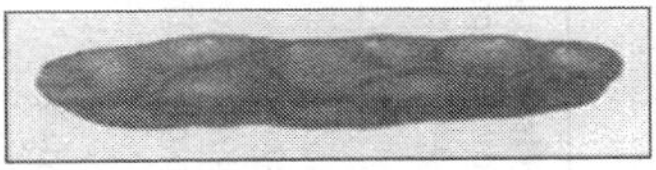	3
Like a sausage or snake — smooth and soft.	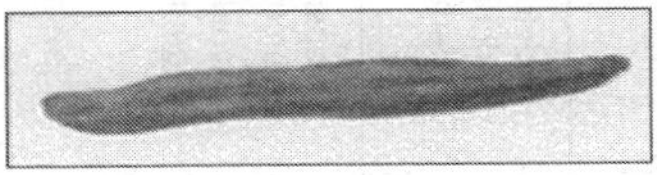	4
Soft blobs with clear cut edges (easy to pass).	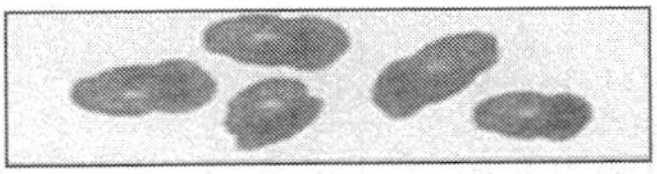	5
Fluffy pieces with ragged edges, a mushy stool.	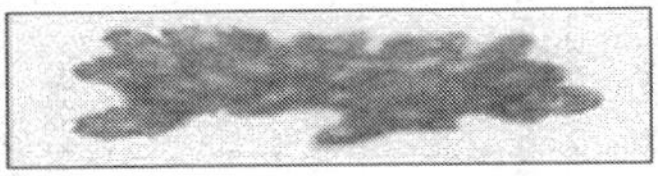	6
Watery, no solid pieces. Result of very fast transit.	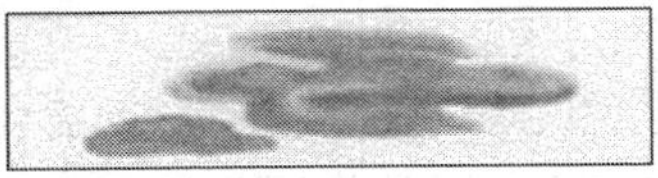	7

Reproduced with permission from Thompson WG, Heaton KW. Fast fact: irritable bowel syndrome. 2nd edition. Oxford: Health Press Limited; 2003.

Table 4: **Drugs Used for the Management of Irritable Bowel Syndrome**

Symptom	Drug	Dose	Adverse Effects	Drug Interactions	Comments	Cost[a]
Antidiar-rheals	*loperamide* Imodium, generics	**For diarrhea:** 2–4 mg as needed (max. 12 mg/day)	Abdominal cramps, dizziness, dry mouth.		For short-term control of diarrhea. Nonprescription.	$-$$
Bulk-forming Agents	*psyllium hydrophilic mucilloid* Metamucil, Prodiem Plain, generics	**For constipation:** 15 mL BID with meals, then adjust (varies with product)	Cramps, bloating, flatulence.	Advise patients not to take psyllium within 3 h of other drugs to minimize interference with absorption.	Take with fluids. Nonprescription.	$
Tricyclic Antidepres-sants	*amitriptyline* Elavil, generics	**For abdominal pain:** 25–100 mg QHS	Drowsiness, dry mouth, headache.	Possible CNS excitation with serotonergic agents. Avoid combined use with other agents that prolong QTc.	Use low doses for select patients with intractable pain. Numerous other agents are available.	$
	desipramine Norpramin, generics	**For abdominal pain:** 25–100 mg QHS	See amitriptyline.	See amitriptyline.	See amitriptyline.	$

[a] Cost per day includes drug cost only.
Legend: $ < $1 $-$$ < $1–2 $$ $1–2

Suggested Readings

Burstall D, Vallis TM, Turnbull GK. *I.B.S. relief: a doctor, a dietitian, and a psychologist provide a team approach to managing irritable bowel syndrome*. Minneapolis (MN): Chronimed;1998.

Longstreth GF, Thompson WG, Chey WD et al. Functional bowel disorders. *Gastroenterology* 2006;130(5):1480-91.

Paterson WG, Thompson WG, Vanner SJ et al. Recommendations for the management of irritable bowel syndrome in family practice. IBS Consensus Conference Participants. *CMAJ* 1999;161(2):154-60.

Thompson WG. *The placebo effect in health: combining science & compassionate care*. Amherst (NY): Prometheus Books; 2005.

Thompson WG. The treatment of irritable bowel syndrome. *Aliment Pharmacol Ther* 2002;16(8):1395-406.

References

1. Thompson WG, Irvine EJ, Pare P et al. Functional gastrointestinal disorders in Canada: first population-based survey using Rome II criteria with suggestions for improving the questionnaire. *Dig Dis Sci* 2002;47(1):225-235.
2. Whitehead WE, Levy RL, Von Korff M et al. The usual medical care for irritable bowel syndrome. *Aliment Pharmacol Ther* 2004;20(11-12):1305-15.
3. Thompson WG, Heaton KW, Smyth GT et al. Irritable bowel syndrome in general practice: prevalence, characteristics, and referral. *Gut* 2000;46(1):78-82.
4. Paterson WG, Thompson WG, Vanner SJ et al. Recommendations for the management of irritable bowel syndrome in family practice. IBS Consensus Conference Participants. *CMAJ* 1999;161(2):154-60.
5. Winawer S, Fletcher R, Rex D et al. Colorectal cancer screening and surveillance: clinical guidelines and rationale-Update based on new evidence. *Gastroenterology* 2003;124(2):544-60.
6. Winawer SJ, Fletcher RH, Miller L et al. Colorectal cancer screening: clinical guidelines and rationale. *Gastroenterology* 1997;112(2):594-642.
7. Longstreth GF, Thompson WG, Chey WD et al. Functional bowel disorders. *Gastroenterology* 2006;130(5):1480-91.
8. Thompson WG. Placebos: a review of the placebo response. *Am J Gastroenterol* 2000;95(7):1637-43.
9. Owens DM, Nelson DK, Talley NJ. The irritable bowel syndrome: long-term prognosis and the physician-patient interaction. *Ann Intern Med* 1995;122(2):107-12.
10. Tollefson GD, Tollefson SL, Pederson M et al. Comorbid irritable bowel syndrome in patients with generalized anxiety and major depression. *Ann Clin Psychiatry* 1991;3215-222.
11. Craig TK, Brown GW. Goal frustration and life events in the aetiology of painful gastrointestinal disorder. *J Psychosom Res* 1984;28(5):411-21.
12. Creed F. Life events and appendicectomy. *Lancet* 1981;1(8235):1381-5.
13. Talley NJ, Owen BK, Boyce P et al. Psychological treatments for irritable bowel syndrome: a critique of controlled treatment trials. *Am J Gastroenterol* 1996;91(2):277-83.
14. Potter WZ, Rudorfer MV, Manji H. The pharmacologic treatment of depression. *N Engl J Med* 1991;325(9):633-42.
15. Guthrie E, Creed F, Dawson D et al. A randomised controlled trial of psychotherapy in patients with refractory irritable bowel syndrome. *Br J Psychiatry* 1993;163:315-21.
16. Drossman DA, Toner BB, Whitehead WE et al. Cognitive-behavioral therapy versus education and desipramine versus placebo for moderate to severe functional bowel disorders. *Gastroenterology* 2003;125(1):19-31.
17. Gonsalkorale WM, Houghton LA, Whorwell PJ. Hypnotherapy in irritable bowel syndrome: a large-scale audit of a clinical service with examination of factors influencing responsiveness. *Am J Gastroenterol* 2002;97(4):954-61.
18. Heaton KW, O'Donnell LJ. An office guide to whole-gut transit time. Patients' recollection of their stool form. *J Clin Gastroenterol* 1994;19(1):28-30.
19. Thompson WG, Heaton KW. *Irritable bowel syndrome*. 2nd ed. Oxford: Health Press; 2003.
20. Thompson WG. Nonulcer dyspepsia. *Can Med Assoc J* 1984;130(5):565-9.
21. Read M, Read NW, Barber DC et al. Effects of loperamide on anal sphincter function in patients complaining of chronic diarrhea with fecal incontinence and urgency. *Dig Dis Sci* 1982;27(9):807-14.
22. Jackson JL, O'Malley PG, Tomkins G et al. Treatment of functional gastrointestinal disorders with antidepressant medications: a meta-analysis. *Am J Med* 2000;108(1):65-72.
23. Halpert A, Dalton CB, Diamant NE et al. Clinical response to tricyclic antidepressants in functional bowel disorders is not related to dosage. *Am J Gastroenterol* 2005;100(3):664-71.

24. Evans BW, Clark WK, Moore DJ et al. Tegaserod for the treatment of irritable bowel syndrome. *Cochrane Database Syst Rev* 2004;(1):CD003960.
25. Health Canada; Novartis Pharmaceuticals Canada Inc. *Marketing and sales suspension notice for Zelnorm tablets, 6 mg*. Available from: http://hc-sc.gc.ca/dhp-mps/alt_formats/hpfb-dgpsa/pdf/medeff/zelnorm_hpc-cps_2_e.pdf Accessed April 4, 2007.
26. O'Mahony L, McCarthy J, Kelly P et al. Lactobacillus and bifidobacterium in irritable bowel syndrome: symptom responses and relationship to cytokine profiles. *Gastroenterology* 2005;128(3):541-51.
27. Thompson WG. The treatment of irritable bowel syndrome. *Aliment Pharmacol Ther* 2002;16(8):1395-406.
28. Drossman DA. Struggling with the "controlling" patient. *Am J Gastroenterol* 1994;89(9):1441-6.
29. Ilnyckyj A, Graff LA, Blanchard JF et al. Therapeutic value of a gastroenterology consultation in irritable bowel syndrome. *Aliment Pharmacol Ther* 2003;17(7):871-80.
30. Akehurst R, Kaltenthaler E. Treatment of irritable bowel syndrome: a review of randomised controlled trials. *Gut* 2001;48(2):272-82.
31. Klein KB. Controlled treatment trials in the irritable bowel syndrome: a critique. *Gastroenterology* 1988;95(1):232-41.
32. Quartero AO, Meineche-Schmidt V, Muris J et al. Bulking agents, antispasmodic and antidepressant medication for the treatment of irritable bowel syndrome. *Cochrane Database Syst Rev* 2005;(2):CD003460.

CHAPTER 58
Lower Urinary Tract Symptoms and Benign Prostatic Hyperplasia

Richard W. Norman, MD, FRCSC

Goals of Therapy

- Improve or abolish lower urinary tract symptoms (LUTS)
- Prevent or delay clinical progression of benign prostatic hyperplasia (BPH)
- Reduce the risk of surgical intervention
- Prevent the sequelae of long-term bladder outlet obstruction (urinary tract infections, bladder stones, hydronephrosis)

Investigations

- Thorough history with attention to:
  - voiding (weak/interrupted stream, dribbling, hesitancy, straining) and storage (nocturia, frequency, urgency) symptoms
  - onset and progression of LUTS and degree of inconvenience or bother to the patient (International Prostate Symptom Score is recommended — available at http://universityurologists.com/ipss1.doc)
  - details of urethral infection, injury or instrumentation
  - episodes of urinary tract infection, hematuria or urinary retention
- Physical examination:
  - abdomen (bladder distention, flank tenderness)
  - external genitalia (phimosis, meatal stenosis, urethral mass/induration)
  - digital rectal examination (DRE) (document prostate size, consistency, symmetry and tenderness)
- Laboratory tests:
  - urinalysis (and urine culture if pyuria)
  - serum creatinine
  - prostate specific antigen (PSA); optional but recommended when a diagnosis of prostate cancer would alter treatment in otherwise healthy men between 50 and 70 years of age with a life expectancy of at least 10 years; start obtaining annual PSA levels at age 45 when there is a positive family history and/or patient is of African descent; PSA can be used as a surrogate marker of prostate size in benign disease[1]

- Other diagnostic tests are occasionally required when the history is not clear, there are abnormalities of the physical examination or laboratory tests or the response to treatment is unsatisfactory:
  - cystoscopy
  - urodynamic studies
  - renal/bladder/transrectal ultrasonography
  - iv pyelography

Therapeutic Choices (Figure 1)

Nonpharmacologic Choices

- Manage minimal symptoms with reassurance and active surveillance (i.e., regular reassessment). Phytotherapeutic agents may provide some benefit in these patients (see Pharmacologic Choices).
- Advise patients with problematic nocturia to avoid caffeine-containing beverages and alcohol in the evening.

Pharmacologic Choices (Table 1)

The alpha$_1$-adrenergic blockers, alfuzosin, doxazosin, tamsulosin and terazosin, and the 5-alpha-reductase inhibitors, dutasteride and finasteride, are all useful in improving symptoms.

Alpha$_1$-adrenergic Blocking Agents

Alfuzosin, **doxazosin**, **tamsulosin** and **terazosin** are the agents most commonly used to block alpha$_1$-adrenergic receptors that mediate muscular activity in the bladder neck, prostate and prostatic capsule, reducing the dynamic component of bladder outlet obstruction. Over a period of days to weeks, this may improve urinary flow rates by 1 to 3 mL/sec and symptom scores by 1 to 3 points. The effectiveness of the alpha$_1$-adrenergic blockers is not influenced by prostate size.

To avoid first-dose syncope, doxazosin and terazosin must be started at a low dosage and gradually increased until symptomatic improvement or intolerance occurs. Dose titration is not necessary with alfuzosin and tamsulosin because of their greater selectivity for the alpha$_{1A}$-receptor subtype which predominates in the prostate, bladder neck and urethra.

Side effects of alpha-blockers include dizziness (10 to 20%), headaches (15%), asthenia (5 to 15%) and nasal congestion (5 to 10%). Retrograde ejaculation develops in 5 to 10% of men taking tamsulosin. These drugs may potentiate other antihypertensive medications, and caution should be used when they are added to an ongoing regimen, particularly in the elderly. Doxazosin and sildenafil, taken within hours of each other, may result in an undesirable hypotensive effect in some patients.[2] Alfuzosin and tamsulosin have fewer systemic side effects because of their greater selectivity for the alpha$_{1A}$-receptor subtype, and because their administration with meals produces more constant serum drug concentrations. Side effects of terazosin and doxazosin may be reduced by taking them at bedtime.

Terazosin and doxazosin may cause a small decrease in total cholesterol and low-density lipoprotein fraction. The clinical importance of this is unknown.

Although there are differences in the adverse event profiles of these agents, all four have equal clinical effectiveness. Choice of agent should depend upon the side effect profile and on the patient's comorbidities and individual tolerance. In patients with no significant cardiovascular or cerebrovascular disease and with the ability to understand and carry out dose titration, terazosin and doxazosin are cost-effective $alpha_1$-blockers.

5-Alpha-reductase Inhibitors

Finasteride inhibits the type II and **dutasteride** the type I and II isoenzymes of 5-alpha-reductase, which blocks the metabolism of testosterone to dihydrotestosterone. The net effect is a decrease in intraprostatic dihydrotestosterone and a progressive reduction in prostatic volume. This reduces the static component of bladder outlet obstruction over a period of several weeks to months and may be accompanied by an improvement in urinary flow rates of 1 to 2 mL/sec and symptom scores of 1 to 2 points.

5-alpha-reductase inhibitors work best in men with a large prostate.[3] Because of their site specificity, there is a low incidence of side effects (e.g., 3 to 4% sexual dysfunction) and little risk of significant drug interactions. Within six months of initiation, these drugs decrease serum PSA levels by approximately 50% in men with BPH and may partially suppress serum PSA in men with prostate cancer.

BPH patients who are concerned about prostate cancer may be counselled on the proven benefits (beyond reducing symptoms and progression of BPH) of using a 5-alpha-reductase inhibitor for reduction of overall prostate cancer risk. As part of the discussion, inform them of the possibility that those who do develop prostate cancer while taking these drugs may be at increased risk of developing a higher grade of the disease.[4]

Combination Alpha-blocker and 5-Alpha-reductase Inhibitor Therapy

The combination of an $alpha_1$-adrenergic receptor blocker and a 5-alpha-reductase inhibitor is an appropriate and effective treatment for patients with LUTS associated with demonstrable prostatic enlargement. Note: In patients without prostate cancer, PSA value may be useful as an estimate of prostate size.[3]

Give patients who are successfully treated with combination therapy the option of discontinuing the alpha-blocker after 6–12 months.[5] If symptoms recur, the alpha-blocker should be restarted.

Phytotherapeutic Agents

Saw palmetto (*Serenoa repens*) and **African plum tree** (*Pygeum africanum*) are examples of plant extracts used by patients to reduce symptoms related to BPH. Some data suggest they may produce a favourable response. Identification and pharmacokinetics of active ingredients are often unclear in these mixtures; until more information regarding their mode of action and long-term efficacy and safety becomes available, their role in management will remain unclear.[6]

Procedures (Table 2)

While transurethral resection of the prostate (TURP) and retropubic prostatectomy are traditional means of dealing with an enlarged and obstructing prostate gland, transurethral incision of the prostate (TUIP) and various forms of laser prostatectomy are useful in some patients. Newer forms of minimally invasive surgical therapies (MIST) are under investigation and may play a larger role as knowledge of these technologies, including their long-term efficacy and side effects, becomes more widespread.[7] Long-term catheter drainage is appropriate for patients who are not candidates for any other intervention.

Therapeutic Tips

- Patients with minimal symptoms that do not interfere with their normal activities should be managed by active surveillance and regular follow-up.
- Patients starting to develop progressive symptoms or who are moderately inconvenienced or bothered by them are candidates for pharmacologic intervention.
- Continue drug therapy indefinitely since symptoms recur when medication is stopped.
- Complicating factors or unexpected (or lack of) response to any intervention are indications for urologic consultation.
- Avoid decongestants and other drugs with alpha-adrenergic activity because they can stimulate smooth muscle in the bladder neck and prostate, and increase obstruction.
- Drugs with anticholinergic activity may reduce detrusor contractility. Use these agents with caution in patients with symptoms of bladder outlet obstruction.

Figure 1: **Management of Benign Prostatic Hyperplasia**

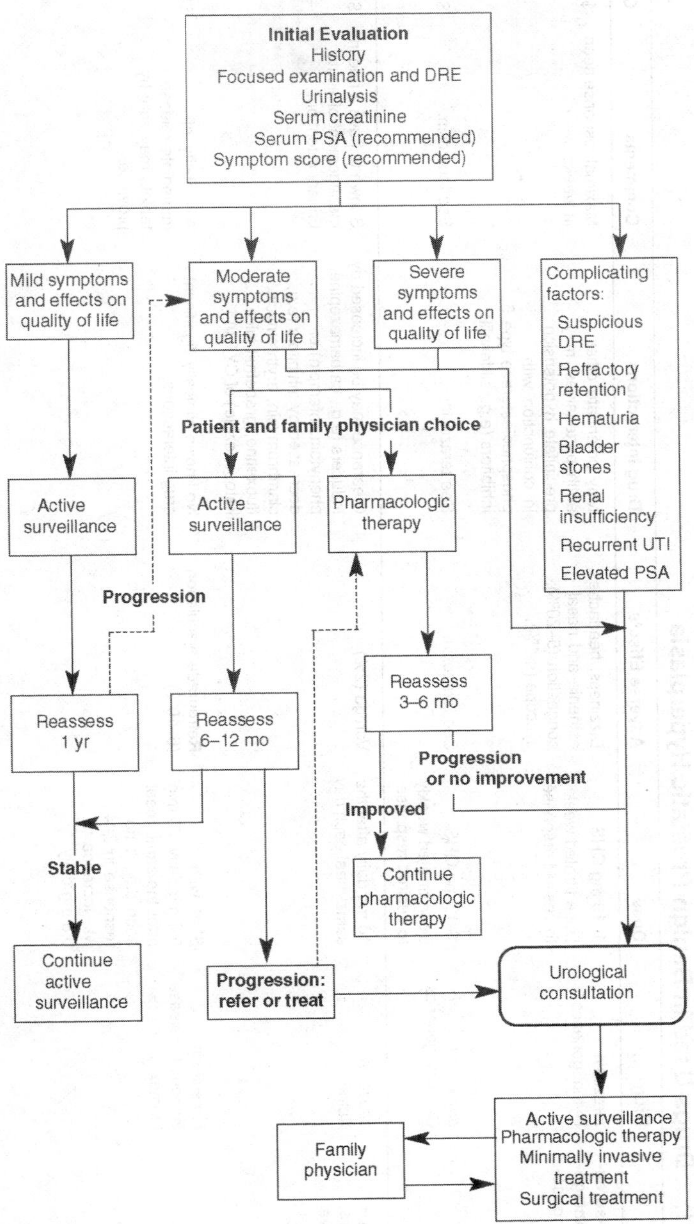

Abbreviations: DRE = digital rectal examination; PSA = prostate specific antigen

Table 1: **Drugs Used in Benign Prostatic Hyperplasia**

Class	Drug	Dose	Adverse Effects	Drug Interactions	Comments	Cost[a]
Alpha$_1$-adrenergic Antagonists, nonselective	*terazosin* Hytrin, generics	1–10 mg QHS Dose titrated weekly to desired response	Dizziness, headaches, asthenia and nasal congestion (5–20%); syncope (< 1%).	May potentiate other antihypertensives; may precipitate hypotension in conjunction with phosphodiesterase type 5 inhibitors (e.g., sildenafil).	Maximal response seen in weeks.	$-$$
	doxazosin Cardura, generics	1–12 mg QHS Dose titrated weekly to desired response	See terazosin.	See terazosin.	See terazosin.	$-$$$
Alpha$_{1A}$–blockers, selective	*alfuzosin* Xatral	10 mg daily after the same meal each day	Vertigo (2%).	Clearance may be increased by inducers (e.g., carbamazepine, phenytoin, rifampin) or decreased by inhibitors (e.g., clarithromycin, erythromycin, fluoxetine, grapefruit juice, ketoconazole) of CYP3A4.	Shown to have a role in management of acute urinary retention.	$$
	tamsulosin immediate-release Flomax	Start with 0.4 mg daily, 30 min after the same meal each day; if no response in 2–4 wk, increase to 0.8 mg daily	Retrograde ejaculation (5–10%).	No known clinically significant drug interactions.	Availability of immediate-release tablets may vary by province.	$$-$$$

Class	Drug	Dose	Adverse Effects	Drug Interactions	Comments	Cost[a]
	tamsulosin controlled-release Flomax CR	0.4 mg once daily at the same time each day, with or without food	Retrograde ejaculation (5–10%).	No known clinically significant drug interactions.	Swallow tablets whole; do not crush or chew.	$$
5-Alpha-reductase Inhibitors	*dutasteride* Avodart	0.5 mg daily	Sexual dysfunction (3–4%).	Clearance may be increased by inducers (e.g., carbamazepine, phenytoin, rifampin) or decreased by inhibitors (e.g., clarithromycin, erythromycin, fluoxetine, grapefruit juice, ketoconazole) of CYP3A4.	Blocks types I and II isoenzymes. Prostate-specific antigen (PSA) decreases in patients taking 5-alpha-reductase inhibitors; maximal response seen in 6 mo.	$$$$
	finasteride Proscar	5 mg daily	See dutasteride.	See dutasteride.	Blocks type I isoenzyme. Prostate-specific antigen (PSA) decreases in patients taking 5-alpha-reductase inhibitors; maximal response seen in 6 mo.	$$$$

[a] Cost of 30-day supply; includes drug cost only.
Legend: $ < $15 $-$$ < $15–30 $$ $15–30 $-$$$ < $15–45 $$-$$$ $15–45 $$$ $30–45 $$$$ > $45

Table 2: **Procedures for BPH**

Procedure	Description/Efficacy	Adverse Effects	Comments
Transurethral resection of prostate (TURP)	1–2 days in hospital; gold standard for efficacy (85–90% reduction in symptoms).	Retrograde ejaculation (50–95%), urethral strictures (3%), bladder neck contracture (3–10%), re-resection (3–8%).	For moderately enlarged prostates.
Retropubic prostatectomy	Open surgery; 3–5 days in hospital; similar efficacy to TURP.	Retrograde ejaculation (80–90%); bladder neck contraction (2–3%).	For very enlarged prostates or when required to correct other bladder pathology.
Transurethral incision of prostate (TUIP)	Outpatient; 80% reduction in symptoms.	Retrograde ejaculation (6–55%).	Useful for smaller prostates.
Laser prostatectomy (various types)	1-day hospital stay; 80% reduction in symptoms.	Little or no bleeding.	Preferred technique for patients requiring anticoagulants or with uncorrected coagulopathies; long-term data awaited.
Transurethral microwave thermotherapy (TUMT)	Outpatient; 30–40% reduction in symptoms.	Prolonged postoperative catheterization and risk of infection.	Variable patient responses; not reimbursed or widely available.
Urethral stents (various types and compositions)	Temporary or permanent procedure for poor surgical candidates.	Encrustation, migration, breakage, stress incontinence.	Biodegradable stents (and indications for stents in general) under investigation.
Transurethral needle ablation of prostate (TUNA)	Outpatient; intraprostatic placement of needle electrodes causes heating and necrosis of tissue; 60% reduction in symptoms.	Temporary postoperative urinary retention (13–42%); irritative voiding symptoms (40%); re-operation (14%).	Long-term data awaited; not reimbursed or widely available.

Suggested Readings

Burnett AL and Wein AJ. Benign prostatic hyperplasia in primary care: what you need to know. *J Urol* 2006;175(3 Pt 2):S19-24.

Carson CC. Combination of phosphodiesterase-5 inhibitors and alpha-blockers in patients with benign prostatic hyperplasia: treatments of lower urinary tract symptoms, erectile dysfunction, or both? *BJU Int* 2006;97(Suppl 2):39-43.

Fitzpatrick JM. The natural history of benign prostatic hyperplasia. *BJU Int* 2006;97(Suppl 2):3-6.

Reich O, Gratzke C, Stief CG. Techniques and long-term results of surgical procedures for BPH. *Eur Urol* 2006;49(6):970-8.

References

1. Nickel JC, Herschorn S, Corcos J et al. Canadian guidelines for the management of benign prostatic hyperplasia. *Can J Urol* 2005;12(3):2677-83.
2. *Viagra (sildenafil citrate) tablets*. Available from: http://pfizer.com/pfizer/download/uspi_viagra.pdf Accessed November 30, 2006.
3. McConnell JD, Roehrborn CG, Bautista OM et al. The long-term effect of doxazosin, finasteride, and combination therapy on the clinical progression of benign prostatic hyperplasia. *N Engl J Med* 2003;349(25):2387-98.
4. Thompson IM, Goodman PJ, Tangen CM et al. The influence of finasteride in the development of prostate cancer. *N Engl J Med* 2003;349(3):215-24.
5. Baldwin KC, Ginsberg PC, Roehrborn CG et al. Discontinuation of alpha-blockade after initial treatment with finasteride and doxazosin in men with lower urinary tract symptoms and clinical evidence of benign prostatic hyperplasia. *Urology* 2001;58(2):203-9.
6. Dreikorn K. The role of phytotherapy in treating lower urinary tract symptoms in benign prostatic hyperplasia. *World J Urol* 2002;19(6):426-35.
7. Tunuguntla HS, Evans CP. Minimally invasive therapies for benign prostatic hyperplasia. *World J Urol* 2002;20(4):197-206.

Pharmacoeconomic Considerations: Benign Prostatic Hyperplasia

Nicole Mittmann, MSc, PhD

Epidemiology	
Country	**Prevalence (%)**
Worldwide[1]	50% of men aged ≥ 50 years in the general population
Cost of Illness Data	
Country and Year of Estimate	**Direct Costs[a]**
United Kingdom (1990)[2]	£62–91 million

(cont'd)

Commentary

The symptoms of benign prostatic hyperplasia (BPH) interfere with activities of daily living.[2,4] Direct costs associated with this condition are dependent on the management choice for BPH, namely surgery or medical. With respect to surgery or transurethral prostatectomy (TURP), length of stay is the major cost driver.[3]

In general, medical management is more cost-effective than surgical management.[3,4] Patient preference is important, with most men preferring medical over surgical management.[4] Surgery is associated with higher indirect costs than medical management.[5]

A number of economic evaluations for the management of BPH have been conducted but the results are inconsistent. Terazosin and finasteride, reported to be equivalent in terms of efficacy, have both been shown to be more cost-effective than TURP (with and without complications).[6] Other studies have indicated that the costs per patient treated were similar for terazosin and placebo (i.e., a strategy of watch and wait), but the lower medication costs in the watch and wait group were offset by higher inpatient costs in the terazosin group.[6] Tamsulosin is reported to be more cost-effective than finasteride, but comparable to surgical management.[7] A simple decision analytic model comparing tamsulosin, doxazosin and terazosin reported that tamsulosin was more cost-effective than the comparators.[8]

A number of non-drug treatments for BPH, including photoselective vaporization and high intensity focused ultrasound, exist for patients who may not be eligible for surgery. The costs of photoselective vaporization are comparable to surgery (TURP)[9] but sustainable and economic benefit have not yet been demonstrated.

[a] Direct costs include those associated with physician services, nursing care, diagnostic procedures, drugs and hospitalization.

References

1. Napalkov P, Maisonneuve P, Boyle P. Worldwide patterns of prevalence and mortality from benign prostatic hyperplasia. *Urology* 1995;46(3 Suppl A):41-6.
2. Drummond MF, McGuire AJ, Black NA et al. Economic burden of treated benign prostatic hyperplasia in the United Kingdom. *Br J Urol* 1993;71(3):290-6.
3. Manyak MJ, Ackerman SJ, Blute ML et al. Cost effectiveness of treatment for benign prostatic hyperplasia: an economic model for comparison of medical, minimally invasive, and surgical therapy. *J Endourol* 2002;16(1):51-6.
4. Cockrum PC, Finder SF, Ries AJ et al. A pharmacoeconomic analysis of patients with symptoms of benign prostatic hyperplasia. *Pharmacoeconomics* 1997;11(6):550-65.
5. Lowe FC, McDaniel RL, Chmiel JJ et al. Economic modeling to assess the costs of treatment with finasteride, terazosin and transurethral resection of the prostate for men with moderate to severe symptoms of benign prostatic hyperplasia. *Urology* 1995;46(4):477-83.
6. Plosker GL, Goa KL. Terazosin. A pharmacoeconomic evaluation of its use in benign prostatic hyperplasia. *Pharmacoeconomics* 1997;11(2):184-97.
7. Nickel JC, Herschorn S, Corcos J et al. Canadian guidelines for the management of benign prostatic hyperplasia. *Can J Urol* 2005;12(3):2677-83.
8. Oshfeldt RL, Kreder KJ, Klein RW et al. Cost-effectiveness of tamsulosin, doxazosin, and terazosin in the treatment of benign prostatic hyperplasia. *J Manag Care Pharm* 2004;10(5):412-22.
9. Ruszat R, Sulser T, Seifert HH et al. Photoselective vaporisation (PVP) vs. transurethral electroresection of the prostate (TURP): a comparing cost analysis. *Eur Urol Suppl* 2006;5(2):271.

CHAPTER 59
Urinary Incontinence in Adults

R. E. Grymonpré, PharmD

Stress incontinence is the loss of urine due to an increase in intra-abdominal pressure (e.g., cough, exercise) and is more common in women. Urethral hypermobility and/or intrinsic sphincter deficiency (ISD) are commonly present and often have been caused by weakness in pelvic musculature (e.g., due to childbirth, abdominal obesity) or postmenopausal urogenital atrophy. *Urge incontinence*, often referred to synonymously as (or as a symptom of) *overactive bladder*, involves leakage of moderate to large amounts of urine due to inability to delay voiding when an urge is perceived. Causes include bladder wall hyperactivity or instability and CNS disorders (e.g., parkinsonism, stroke). *Overflow incontinence* involves leakage of urine due to an overdistended bladder, commonly resulting from outlet obstruction (e.g., prostatic hyperplasia) or neurogenic causes (e.g., diabetic neuropathy, multiple sclerosis). *Functional incontinence* is the loss of urine caused by the inability to get to a toilet. Causes include physical constraints (e.g., restricted mobility, difficulty removing clothing), cognitive factors (e.g., depression, dementia) and environmental barriers (distance to toilet, positioning).

Goals of Therapy

- Relieve urinary symptoms
- Increase functional capacity of the bladder

Investigations[1,2,3]

Screening questions:

- Do you ever lose urine when you don't want to?
- Do you ever leak urine when you cough, laugh or exercise?
- Do you ever leak urine on the way to the bathroom?
- Do you ever use pads, tissue or cloth in your underwear to catch urine?
- Do you ever feel that you are unable to completely empty your bladder?

If positive:

- Thorough history with attention to:
  - possible causes such as diabetes, depression, mobility or cognitive limitations, previous bladder surgeries or neurologic conditions such as multiple sclerosis, stroke or spinal cord injury
  - modifiable risk factors (Table 1)

  - bladder diary to determine frequency, timing and amount of voiding and urine leakage
  - cough test (to detect stress incontinence)
  - urinalysis (to rule out infection, glucosuria, hematuria)
  - pelvic examination (to rule out pelvic masses, organ prolapse, latent stress incontinence)
- Supplemental investigations:
  - renal function tests (BUN, serum creatinine, glucose and calcium) if renal dysfunction suspected or polyuria present
  - urodynamic testing to measure detrusor compliance and contractility, postvoid residual volume and bladder capacity

Table 1: **Modifiable Risk Factors for Urinary Incontinence in Adults**

Caffeine intake
Bowel problems (constipation, fecal impaction)
Fluid intake (1.5–2 L/day is considered appropriate)
Morbid obesity
Smoking
High-impact physical activities
Medications (diuretics, anticholinergics, alpha-agonists, alpha-antagonists, psychotropics, alcohol)
Restricted mobility (includes dexterity in clothing removal, accessibility to toilets)

Stress Incontinence

Therapeutic Choices (Figure 1, Table 3)

Nonpharmacologic Choices

When secondary causes have been ruled out or treated, initiate behavioural therapy:[4]

- *Bladder training (timed voiding)*: maintain a voiding schedule (e.g., one-hour voiding interval) which is gradually (e.g., weekly) increased to a reasonable interval (e.g., voiding every two to three hours) with minimal incontinence episodes
- *Pelvic floor muscle training (*also known as *Kegel exercises)*: a daily minimum of 30 to 45 pelvic floor muscle contractions (goal of 10 seconds for each contraction); done in two or three sets; may take six to eight weeks to see results
- *Biofeedback* and/or *electrical stimulation therapy*: stimulation that teaches the patient to isolate and control pelvic floor muscles

Surgical options depend on the etiology. For urethral hypermobility in females, retropubic suspension is superior to anterior vaginal repair.[5] For ISD in females, sling procedures (including tension-free vaginal tape) or urethral bulking injections can be done. For males postprostatectomy, urethral bulking injections or artificial sphincters are available.

Pharmacologic Choices

Due to limited evidence of pharmacologic efficacy, surgery may be recommended first-line.[2,6] The current literature on estrogen therapy in the treatment of postmenopausal stress incontinence is inconclusive, although long-term oral therapy is not recommended.[7,8,9,10,11] A Cochrane review determined that three to six months of unopposed estrogen therapy resulted in a 43% perceived cure/improvement of stress incontinence symptoms compared to a 27% placebo response, with reduced efficacy when estrogen was opposed with progesterone.[9] In contrast, a secondary analysis of the Women's Health Initiative trial[10] found an increased risk of stress incontinence with opposed and unopposed estrogen. Vaginal estrogen for women with postmenopausal urogenital atrophy may be a viable option as an adjunct to behavioural or pharmacologic treatment in stress incontinence.[11] The decision to use estrogen therapy must be discussed with the patient in the context of her individual health needs and risk factors (e.g., cancer, DVT, MI).

Few well-designed studies have evaluated the efficacy of **imipramine**, and evidence supporting its role in the management of stress incontinence is not strong.[8,12]

The efficacy of **pseudoephedrine** in stress incontinence has been extrapolated from studies involving phenylpropanolamine, an agent that has been withdrawn from the Canadian market due to concerns of cerebral hemorrhage. There is no direct evidence supporting the use of pseudoephedrine in the management of stress incontinence.

Duloxetine, a serotonin-norepinephrine reuptake inhibitor awaiting approval from Health Canada for the treatment of stress incontinence, influences the micturition reflex centrally.[13]

Urge Incontinence

Therapeutic Choices (Figure 1, Table 3)

Nonpharmacologic Choices

When secondary causes have been ruled out or treated, initiate behavioural therapy:[4]

- *Bladder training (timed voiding)*: as described under stress incontinence
- *Pelvic floor muscle training*: as described under stress incontinence.
- *Biofeedback training*: as described under stress incontinence

Maintaining vigilance in the management of urge incontinence is critical to minimizing associated adverse sequelae, especially in older adults. One study found an increased risk of falling and nonvertebral fractures in older women experiencing weekly or more frequent urge incontinence episodes.[14]

Consider surgical options only after failure of noninvasive treatments, including pharmacotherapy.

Pharmacologic Choices

Anticholinergics such as **oxybutynin** and **tolterodine** are recommended as first-line treatment as they have been shown to increase bladder capacity and diminish frequency of uninhibited detrusor contractions.[2,12,15] Both are now available as once-daily, controlled-release tablets, and oxybutynin is available as a transdermal patch; these dosage forms may reduce side effects and improve adherence.[8,12,16,17,18,19] As a nonselective muscarinic antagonist, tolterodine may be a useful alternative in patients experiencing dry mouth or constipation from oxybutynin, which has more M3 receptor selectivity compared to tolterodine, although the newly available dosage forms of oxybutynin minimize this advantage.[2,16,19,20] **Darifenacin**, **solifenacin** and **trospium** are anticholinergics now available in Canada. Darifenacin and solifenacin are both M3 selective agents; trospium is a nonselective quaternary ammonium compound. There is insufficient evidence to substantiate any advantage of these agents over previously available therapies for urge incontinence.[19,21,22,23]

A Cochrane review determined that anticholinergic therapy resulted in a 56% perceived cure/improvement of incontinence symptoms compared to 41% placebo response. The treatment group reported four fewer leakage episodes and five fewer voids per week compared to the placebo group. The clinical significance of these benefits has been questioned.[25]

The current literature on **estrogen** therapy in the treatment of postmenopausal urge incontinence is inconclusive, although long-term oral therapy is not recommended.[8,9,10,11] A Cochrane review determined that three to six months of unopposed estrogen therapy resulted in a 57% perceived cure/improvement of urge incontinence symptoms compared to a 28% placebo response, with reduced efficacy when estrogen was opposed with progesterone.[9] A reduction in leakage/micturition episodes was also reported (two fewer episodes per 24 hours compared to placebo).[9] In contrast, a secondary analysis of the Women's Health Initiative trial[10] found an increased risk of urge incontinence with opposed and unopposed estrogen. Vaginal estrogen for women with postmenopausal urogenital atrophy may be a viable option as an adjunct to behavioural or pharmacologic treatment.[11] The decision to use estrogen therapy must be discussed with the patient in the context of her individual health needs and risk factors (e.g., cancer, DVT, MI).

The direct smooth muscle relaxant **flavoxate** has limited efficacy.[8,12,15] Tricyclic antidepressants (e.g., **imipramine**, **doxepin**, **desipramine**, **nortriptyline**) should be reserved for patients with concurrent depression or those unresponsive to first-line therapies.[2,8,12,15] Doxepin has strong anticholinergic side effects and is not recommended in older adults.[26]

Overflow Incontinence

Therapeutic Choices (Figure 1, Table 3)

Nonpharmacologic Choices

- Overflow incontinence due to acontractile bladder is poorly responsive to behavioural or surgical therapy.[27]
- Surgery is the treatment of choice in many men with moderate to severe overflow incontinence due to benign prostatic hyperplasia (see Chapter 58).[27]

Table 2: **Drugs that May Cause or Aggravate Urinary Retention[28]**

Antiarrhythmics	**Antiparkinsonian Agents**	**Sympathomimetics (alpha-agonists)**
disopyramide	amantadine	ephedrine
procainamide	benztropine	phenylephrine
quinidine	bromocriptine	pseudoephedrine
Anticholinergics	levodopa	**Sympathomimetics (beta-agonists)**
flavoxate	trihexyphenidyl	isoproterenol
oxybutynin	**Antipsychotics**	orciprenaline
scopolamine	chlorpromazine	terbutaline
Antidepressants	prochlorperazine	**Miscellaneous**
amitriptyline	thioridazine	carbamazepine
doxepin	**Muscle Relaxants**	indomethacin
imipramine	baclofen	nifedipine
Antihistamines	cyclobenzaprine	
chlorpheniramine	**Sedative/Hypnotics**	
diphenhydramine	diazepam	
hydroxyzine	flurazepam	

- Catheterization is associated with urinary tract infections (UTIs) and sepsis and should only be used for well-documented indications. For individuals who are either waiting for surgery or are not surgical candidates, catheterization may be a temporary or permanent option:
  - intermittent catheterization (use *clean* technique for all except immunocompromised patients; use *sterile* technique for elderly and immunocompromised patients)
  - indwelling catheter: for terminally ill patients or patients with pressure ulcers requiring short-term treatment
- Discontinue drugs reported to induce or aggravate urinary retention (Table 2) if at all possible.

Pharmacologic Choices

Overflow incontinence due to acontractile bladder is poorly responsive to pharmacologic therapy.[8,27] For management of BPH, see Chapter 58.

Therapeutic Tips

- Treat all secondary causes (e.g., UTI, lifestyle factors, medications or poor mobility) either before or concurrently with other management strategies.
- Several weeks of therapy may be required to achieve maximum effect. If no subjective improvement occurs after four to six weeks, increase the drug dose or switch/discontinue the drug.
- Provide patient education regarding management alternatives (risks, benefits, realistic outcomes), determine patient expectations and involve the patient in the decision-making process.
- As initial therapy, recommend the strategy that is the least invasive, is reversible and has the fewest side effects.
- For various reasons (physical or cognitive impairment, medications), many individuals will never achieve complete bladder control. Scheduled toileting (at fixed times every two to four hours, based on individual toilet habits), habit training (toileting based on individual voiding patterns) and prompted voiding (checking for dryness, regular reminders and praising) are toileting assistance strategies that will help to keep chronically incontinent patients drier.
- Protective products such as pads that absorb and contain leaked urine, or devices such as vaginal pessaries that support the bladder neck and prevent leakage, may be useful at different stages of management. Stress the importance of using absorbent products designed specifically for bladder problems, as they reduce odour and prevent skin breakdown. They should not be considered first-line management but rather as a supportive adjunct to other treatment measures. A thorough assessment is the mainstay of continence care.
- Be attentive to medication nonadherence. The anticholinergic side effect of dry mouth is a common cause of patient-initiated dosage reduction or drug discontinuation.

Figure 1: **Management of Urinary Incontinence in Adults**

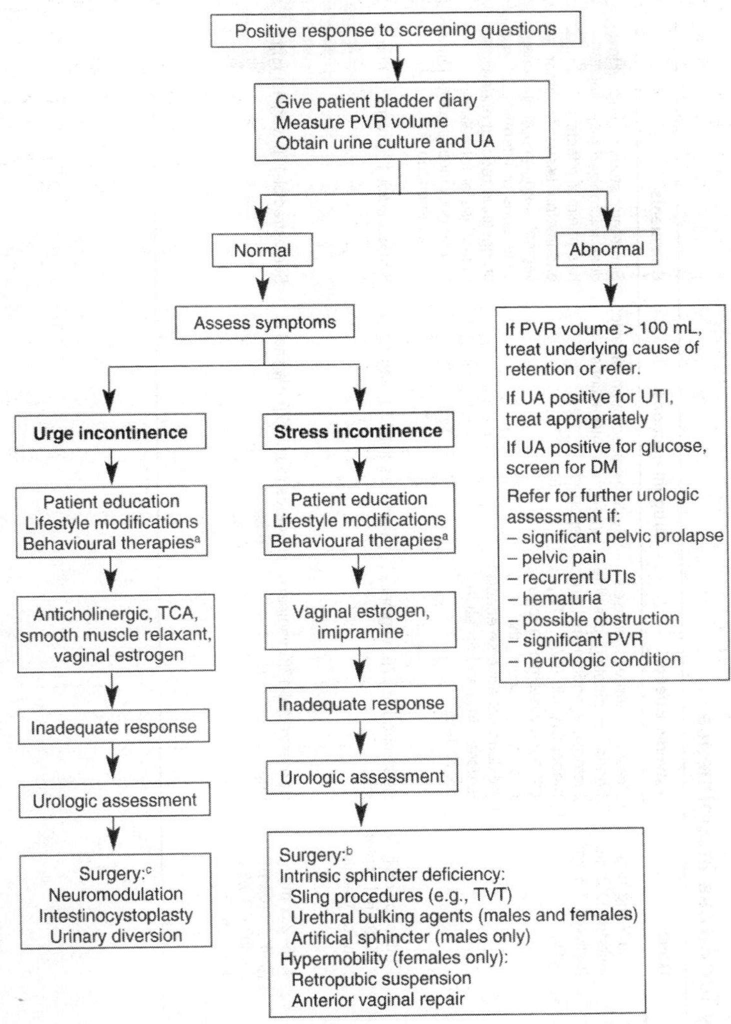

[a] In most circumstances it is appropriate to initiate treatment without referral for urologic testing.

[b] In the management of stress incontinenence, surgery may be recommended first-line due to limited efficacy of pharmacotherapy.[3]

[c] In the management of urge incontinence, surgical options should only be considered after failure with noninvasive treatments, including pharmacotherapy.

Abbreviations: PVR=postvoid residual; UA=urinalysis; DM=diabetes mellitus; TCA=tricyclic antidepressant; TVT=tension-free vaginal tape.

Adapted with permission from Culligan PJ. Urinary incontinence in women: Evaluation and management. *Am Fam Phys* 2000; 62:2433–44,2447,2452.

Table 3: **Drug Therapy for Stress Incontinence**

Class	Drug	Dose	Adverse Effects	Drug Interactions	Comments	Cost[a]
Estrogens, vaginal	*estradiol-17β, vaginal ring* Estring	One 2 mg ring inserted Q 3 mo (delivers 7.5 µg daily)	Breast tenderness, nausea, headache, bloating; possible increase in endometrial and breast CA, MI, CVA, VTE; although systemic estrogen absorption occurs, the incidence of adverse effects is dose, drug and duration dependent.	Systemic absorption variable; no serious interactions reported.	Short-term studies suggest low dose micronized estradiol-17β has minimal effects on endometrial tissue; for other vaginal estrogen preparations, continuous or intermittent progestin is recommended; regardless of formulation, routine endometrial surveillance is recommended.[29]	$$$$
	estradiol-17β, vaginal tablet 25 µg Vagifem	1 tablet pv daily X 2 wk then 1 tablet pv twice weekly	See estradiol-17β, vaginal ring.	See estradiol-17β, vaginal ring.	See estradiol-17β, vaginal ring.	$$$
	conjugated estrogens, vaginal cream 0.625 mg/g Premarin Vaginal Cream	1.25–2.5 mg (2–4 g cream) pv daily, 3 wk on / 1 wk off	See estradiol-17β, vaginal ring.	See estradiol-17β, vaginal ring.	See estradiol-17β, vaginal ring.	$$-$$$

Class	Drug	Dose	Adverse Effects	Drug Interactions	Comments	Cost[a]
Tricyclic Antidepressants	*imipramine* Tofranil, generics	25–100 mg HS	Orthostatic hypotension, dizziness, arrhythmias, cognitive impairment.	Potential additive anticholinergic effects with other drugs; mania, excitation, hyperpyrexia with MAOIs; enzyme inducers (e.g., barbiturates, carbamazepine, dexamethasone, phenytoin, rifampin) may ↓ TCA levels/efficacy; enzyme inhibitors (e.g., amiodarone, cimetidine, erythromycin, fluconazole, itraconazole, ketoconazole, quinidine, ritonavir, SSRIs) may ↑ TCA levels/effects.		$

[a] Cost of 30-day supply; includes drug cost only.
Legend: $ < $5 $$ $5–20 $$-$$$ $5–50 $$$ $20–50 $$$$ $50–75
Abbreviations: CA = carcinoma; MI = myocardial infarction; CVA = cerebrovascular accident; VTE = venous thromboembolism; TCA = tricyclic antidepressant

Table 4: Drug Therapy for Urge Incontinence

Class	Drug	Dose	Adverse Effects	Drug Interactions	Comments	Cost[a]
Anticholinergics	*darifenacin, extended-release* Enablex	7.5 mg daily; after 2 weeks, may increase to 15 mg daily if necessary	Primarily anticholinergic effects (dry mouth, constipation, cognitive dysfunction, tachycardia).	Potential additive anticholinergic effects with other drugs. Do not exceed 7.5 mg daily with potent inhibitors of CYP3A4 such as erythromycin, itraconazole, ketoconazole, nelfinavir, ritonavir. Caution with other substrates of CYP2D6 that have narrow therapeutic indices (e.g., TCAs as their clearance may be ↓.	Avoid in patients with severe hepatic insufficiency.	$$$
	oxybutynin, immediate-release Ditropan, generics	2.5–5 mg BID-QID	See darifenacin, extended-release.	Potential additive anticholinergic effects with other drugs.	In older adults, prescribe the lowest recommended starting dose; when switching from immediate-release to extended-release formulation, use closest equivalent dose.	$$-$$$
	oxybutynin, extended-release Ditropan XL, Uromax	5–30 mg daily	See darifenacin, extended-release.	See oxybutynin, immediate-release.	See oxybutynin, immediate-release. Extended-release formulation must not be divided, chewed or crushed.	$$$$-$$$$$

Class	Drug	Dose	Adverse Effects	Drug Interactions	Comments	Cost[a]
	oxybutynin, transdermal patch Oxytrol	1 patch applied twice weekly (alternating sites); delivers 3.9 mg per day	See darifenacin, extended-release.	See oxybutynin, immediate-release.	In older adults, prescribe the lowest recommended starting dose.	$$$$
	solifenacin VESIcare	5 mg daily; may ↑ to 10 mg daily if tolerated	See darifenacin, extended-release.	See oxybutynin, immediate-release. Do not exceed 5 mg daily with potent CYP3A4 inhibitors, e.g., erythromycin, itraconazole, nelfinavir, ritonavir.	Avoid in patients with severe hepatic insufficiency.	$$$$
	tolterodine, immediate-release Detrol	1–2 mg BID	See darifenacin, extended-release.	Potential additive anticholinergic effects with other drugs. CYP3A4 metabolism becomes significant in CYP2D6 poor metabolizers — maximum dose of 2 mg per day in patients taking potent inhibitors of CYP3A4 (e.g., erythromycin, itraconazole, ketoconazole, nelfinavir, ritonavir).	In older adults, prescribe the lowest recommended starting dose.	$$$$

(cont'd)

Table 4: Drug Therapy for Urge Incontinence *(cont'd)*

Class	Drug	Dose	Adverse Effects	Drug Interactions	Comments	Cost[a]
	tolterodine, extended-release Detrol LA	2–4 mg once daily	See darifenacin, extended-release.	See tolterodine, immediate-release. Coadministration of Detrol LA with antacid results in $\uparrow C_{max}$ of tolterodine and the potential for 'dose-dumping.' It is not known whether a similar interaction exists with concurrent use of acid-suppressing agents.[30]	In older adults, prescribe the lowest recommended starting dose.	$$$$
	trospium Trosec	20 mg BID on an empty stomach or 1 h before meals In older patients an initial dose of 20 mg HS is recommended.	See darifenacin, extended-release.	See oxybutynin, immediate-release.		$$$$
Smooth Muscle Relaxants	*flavoxate* Urispas, generics	200–400 mg TID-QID	GI: nausea, vomiting. CNS: nervousness, vertigo, headache, drowsiness. Ocular: blurred vision, increased ocular tension. Anticholinergic: dry mouth, tachycardia.	Potential additive anticholinergic effects with other drugs.	Limited efficacy.	$$$$-$$$$$

Class	Drug	Dose	Adverse Effects	Drug Interactions	Comments	Cost[a]
TCAs	*imipramine* Tofranil, generics	10–100 mg HS	CV: orthostatic hypotension, tachycardia, quinidine-like cardiotoxicity. CNS: dizziness, cognitive impairment. Anticholinergic: see oxybutynin, immediate-release.	Potential additive anticholinergic effects with other drugs; mania, excitation, hyperpyrexia with MAOIs; enzyme inducers (e.g., barbiturates, carbamazepine, dexamethasone, phenytoin, rifampin) may ↓ TCA levels/efficacy; enzyme inhibitors (e.g., amiodarone, cimetidine, erythromycin, fluconazole, itraconazole, ketoconazole, quinidine, ritonavir, SSRIs) may ↑ TCA levels/effects.	In older adults, desipramine and nortriptyline have a lower incidence of adverse effects than other TCAs and are preferable; however, they may also be less effective than imipramine.	$
	doxepin Sinequan, generics	10–100 mg HS	See imipramine.	See imipramine.	See imipramine.	$-$$
	desipramine Norpramin, generics	10–100 mg HS	See imipramine.	See imipramine.	See imipramine.	$$-$$$
	nortriptyline Aventyl, generics	10–100 mg HS	See imipramine.	See imipramine.	See imipramine.	$$-$$$

[a] Cost of 30-day supply; includes drug cost only.
Legend: $ < $5 $-$$ < $5–20 $$ $5–20 $$-$$$ $5–50 $$$ $20–50 $$$$ $50–75 $$$$-$$$$$ $50– > $75 $$$$$ > $75
Abbreviations: TCA = tricyclic antidepressant

Suggested Readings

Corcos J, Gajewski J, Heritz D et al. Canadian Urological Association guidelines on urinary incontinence. *Can J Urol* 2006;13(3):3127-3138.

Geneva Foundation for Medical Education and Research. For access to up-to-date guidelines and reviews on urinary incontinence: Urogynecology, urinary and fecal incontinence. Available from: http://www.gfmer.ch/Guidelines/Urogynecology_urinary_and_fecal_incontinence/Urogynecology_urinary_and_fecal_incontinence.htm Accessed June 8, 2006

Khan IJ, Tariq SH. Urinary incontinence: behavioral modification therapy in older adult. *Clin Geriatr Med* 2004;20(3):499-509.

Schuessler B, Baessler K. Pharmacologic treatment of stress urinary incontinence: expectations for outcome. *Urology* 2003;62 (4 Suppl 1):31-8.

Scottish Intercollegiate Guidelines Network. *Management of urinary incontinence in primary care: a national clinical guideline.* Edinburgh, Scotland: SIGN; 2004.

References

1. Association of Women's Health, Obstetric and Neonatal Nurses. *Evidence-based clinical practice guideline: continence for women.* Washington (DC): AWHONN; 2000.
2. The Canadian Continence Foundation. *Canadian Consensus Conference on Urinary Incontinence: clinical practice guidelines for adults*; 2001. Available from: http://www.continence-fdn.ca/hp-guidelines.htm Accessed June 8, 2006.
3. Farrell SA, Epp A, Flood C et al. The evaluation of stress incontinence prior to primary surgery. *J Obstet Gynaecol Can* 2003;25(4):313-24.
4. Khan IJ, Tariq SH. Urinary incontinence: behavioral modification therapy in older adult. *Clin Geriatr Med* 2004;20(3):499-509.
5. Hendrix SL. Urinary incontinence and menopause: an evidence-based treatment approach. *Dis Mon* 2002;48(10):622-36.
6. Alhasso A, Glazener CMA, Pickard R, N'Dow J. Adrenergic drugs for urinary incontinence in adults. *Cochrane Database Syst Rev*2005;(3):CD001842.
7. Al-Badr A, Ross S, Soroka D et al. What is the available evidence for hormone replacement therapy in women with stress urinary incontinence? *J Obstet Gynaecol Can* 2003;25(7): 567-74.
8. Andersson K-E. *Pharmacological treatment of urinary incontinence.* Plymouth (UK): Health Publication Ltd; 2002.
9. Moehrer B, Hextall A, Jackson S. Oestrogens for urinary incontinence in women. *Cochrane Database Syst Rev* 2003;(2):CD001405.
10. Hendrix SL, Cochrane BB, Nygaard IE et al. Effects of estrogen with and without progestin on urinary incontinence. *JAMA* 2005;293(8):935-48.
11. DuBeau CE. Estrogen treatment for urinary incontinence: never, now, or in the future? *JAMA* 2005;293(8):998-1001.
12. Scottish Intercollegiate Guidelines Network. *Management of urinary incontinence in primary care: a national clinical guideline.* Edinburgh, Scotland: SIGN; 2004.
13. McCormack PL, Keating GM. Duloxetine: in stress urinary incontinence. *Drugs* 2004;64(22):2567-73.
14. Brown JS, Vittinghoff E, Wyman JF et al. Urinary incontinence: does it increase risk for falls and fractures? Study of Osteoporotic Fractures Research Group. *J Am Geriatr Soc* 2000;48(7):721-5.
15. Haeusler G, Leitich H, van Trotsenburg M et al. Drug therapy of urinary urge incontinence: a systematic review. *Obstet Gynecol* 2002;100(5 Pt 1):1003-16.
16. Weiss BD. Selecting medications for the treatment of urinary incontinence. *Am Fam Physician* 2005;71(2):315-22.
17. Thomas DR. Pharmacologic management of urinary incontinence. *Clin Geriatr Med* 2004;20(3):511-23.
18. Dull P. Transdermal oxybutynin (oxytrol) for urinary incontinence. *Am Fam Physician* 2004;70(12):2351-2.
19. Hay-Smith J, Herbison P, Ellis G et al. Which anticholinergic drug for overactive bladder symptoms in adults. *Cochrane Database Syst Rev* 2005(3):CD005429.

20. Hegde SS. Muscarinic receptors in the bladder: from basic research to therapeutics. *Br J Pharmacol* 2006;147(Suppl 2):S80-7.

21. Guay DR. Darifenacin: another antimuscarinic for overactive bladder. *Consult Pharm* 2005;20(5):424-31.

22. Chapple CR, Abrams P. Comparison of darifenacin and oxybutinin in patients with overactive bladder: assessment of ambulatory urodynamics and impact on salivary flow. *Eur Urol* 2005;48(1):102-9.

23. Erdem N, Chu FM. Management of overactive bladder and urge urinary incontinence in the elderly patient. *Am J Med* 2006;119(3 Suppl 1):29-36.

24. Corcos J, Gajewski J, Heritz D et al. Canadian Urological Association guidelines on urinary incontinence. *Can J Urol.* 2006 Jun;13(3):3127-38.

25. Nabi G, Cody JD, Ellis G et al. Anticholinergic drugs versus placebo for overactive bladder syndrome in adults.*Cochrane Database Syst Rev* 2006;(4):CD003781.

26. Fick DM, Cooper JW, Wade WE et al. Updating the Beers criteria for potentially inappropriate medication use in older adults: results of a US consensus panel of experts. *Arch Intern Med* 2003;163(22):2716-24.

27. Johnson TM, Ouslander JG. Urinary incontinence in the older man. *Med Clin North Am* 1999;83(5):1247-66.

28. Curtis LA, Dolan TS, Cespedes RD. Acute urinary retention and urinary incontinence. *Emerg Med Clin North Am* 2001;19(3):591-619.

29. Willhite LA, Dolan TS, Cespedes RD. Urogenital atrophy: prevention and treatment. *Pharmacotherapy* 2001;21(4):464-80.

30. Sathyan G, Dmochowski RR, Appell RA et al. Effect of antacid on the pharmacokinetics of extended-release formulations of tolterodine and oxybutynin. *Clin Pharmacokinet* 2004;43(14):1059–1068.

CHAPTER 60

Enuresis in Children

Fabian P. Gorodzinsky, MD, AAPd, FRCP

Enuresis is defined as the repeated voiding of urine into the bed or clothes at least twice per week for at least three consecutive months in a child who is at least 5 years of age.[1] Most children are successfully toilet trained by around the age of 3, with a very wide range of 0.75 to 5.25 years. Girls are usually trained earlier than boys.[2]

Nocturnal enuresis is bedwetting, or wetting during sleep (e.g., nap time), more than twice weekly beyond the age of 5 for girls and 6 for boys. In primary nocturnal enuresis, bladder control has never been achieved and in secondary nocturnal enuresis, loss of bladder control occurs after at least six months without bedwetting.[3] Primary nocturnal enuresis, which is more common in boys, occurs in 10 to 15% of 5-year-olds and 6 to 8% of 8-year-olds and declines to < 2% by age 15. Two subtypes of primary nocturnal enuresis are volume-dependent enuresis (associated with nocturnal polyuria; a normal nocturnal rise in antidiuretic hormone secretion may not occur in these children) and detrusor-dependent enuresis (associated with diurnal frequency, urgency or incontinence).[4] Possible causes of nocturnal enuresis include developmental delay (immaturity of CNS control over bladder contractions and/or responsiveness to bladder filling), genetics (molecular linkage to chromosome 8q, 12q, 13q) and obstructive sleep apnea[5,6] (very rare). Lack of sufficient arginine-vasopressin (AVP, antidiuretic hormone) release, bladder overactivity and inability to wake can also cause nocturnal enuresis.[3]

Diurnal enuresis (daytime wetting) occurs in about 10% of children 4 to 6 years old, declining to 4% in adolescents. Girls are affected twice as often as boys. It is considered a problem in a child 4 years or older who wets daily (primary) or who relapses after three consecutive months without daytime wetting (secondary). Possible functional or organic causes of diurnal enuresis are listed in Table 1.

There is no evidence that enuresis is associated with any specific behavioural or psychological problems, yet most affected children are clearly distressed by their condition. The parents' supportive role in treatment is crucial; an intolerant attitude on the part of the parents predicts early drop-out from treatment.[7]

Table 1: **Possible Causes of Diurnal Enuresis**

Functional	Constipation
	Deferral of voiding ("holding it in until the last minute")
	Fusion of labia minora
	Urinary tract infection
	Urge syndrome (unstable bladder; sudden attacks of uncontrollable urge to void; characteristic squatting to avoid detrusor contractions)
	Stress incontinence
	Giggle incontinence
	Emotional stress
	Daytime frequency syndrome
Organic	Neurogenic bladder
	Partial urethral obstruction, e.g., posterior urethral valve, congenital strictures
	Ectopic ureter

Goals of Therapy

- Identify and/or manage serious causes
- Minimize symptoms
- Provide reassurance and guidance

Investigations

- History with attention to:
  - family history (often present for nocturnal enuresis)
  - bowel function; constipation is frequently associated with enuresis that is due to decreased bladder capacity
  - pattern of wetting
  - history of urinary tract infections (UTI) or urologic surgery
  - psychological status of child and family dynamics
- Physical examination with attention to:
  - perineal sensation, perineal reflexes, sphincter tone (to rule out neurogenic bladder)
  - genitalia, particularly the urethral meatus (to rule out anatomical causes such as meatal stenosis in boys or labial fusion in girls)
  - possible occult spinal dysraphism such as tethered cord (congenital spinal cord abnormality that can cause progressive neurologic damage); signs include the presence of a hair tuft, dimple, pigmented lesion or subcutaneous lipoma over the lower spine, or asymmetry of the gluteal cleft (refer to pediatric neurosurgeon)
  - direct observation of voiding, if possible, to rule out abnormalities of urinary stream
- Other investigations as indicated:
  - diary to record voiding pattern and/or bowel movements

- urinalysis and urine culture; no other investigations necessary for primary nocturnal enuresis
- voiding cystourethrogram (to detect vesicoureteral reflux, partial urethral obstruction, or neurogenic bladder) as well as ultrasound of kidneys and bladder are recommended if history of UTI
- if voiding cystourethrogram is abnormal, a referral to a urologist is likely indicated[3]

Therapeutic Choices (Figure 1)

Tailor therapy to the etiologic factors. Combinations of different interventions may be useful.

Nonpharmacologic Choices

- Advise parents to avoid humiliation and punishment, and to support the child's efforts with positive reinforcement, e.g., reassurance, diary of dry days, facilitated access to bathroom at home and school.
- Have the child avoid excessive intake of fluids within two hours of bedtime and empty the bladder before going to bed.
- Encourage the child to avoid deferral of micturition.
- *Enuresis alarms* are effective for nocturnal enuresis when used properly for three to four months.[8] Enuresis alarms, which are highly sensitive to moisture, attach to underpants or an absorbent pad and either vibrate or produce sound at the first sign of voiding. Because children with enuresis are usually very deep sleepers, the parent must often be the one to wake the child when the alarm sounds. The child then completes voiding in the toilet and then returns to sleep after changing the underwear or bedding. Alarm therapy may be effective in children with a normal urine output but with small bladder capacity.[9] Enuresis alarms work best in children 7 years or older, require consistent parental involvement and support, and are available at medical supply stores. Relapse rates were lower when overlearning, dry bed training or reward systems were added to alarm treatment.[8]
- Encourage bladder training exercises for diurnal enuresis, e.g., scheduled voiding routine, abdominal or pelvic floor muscle exercises.

Pharmacologic Choices (Table 2)

Antidiuretic Hormone (ADH) Analogues

Desmopressin (DDAVP), an analogue of human ADH, decreases urine production when given at bedtime and reduces the number of wet nights in 75% of children, with complete cessation in about 50% of those who respond.[10] Desmopressin is used when a rapid response is required. There is limited evidence of long-term success with desmopressin use.[8] If successful, consider a one-week interruption every three months to see if treatment is no longer needed.[11] DDVAP may be most effective in children with a normal bladder capacity but with a large urine output.[11]

Responders to desmopressin produce large amounts of dilute urine and concentrate urine poorly.[12]

Available as a nasal spray, oral tablets and meltaways, desmopressin has a good long-term safety record with up to two years' continuous use.[13] If cost is a concern, reserve DDAVP for special occasions such as overnight visits or camp. The risk of overhydration and hyponatremia associated with desmopressin necessitates limiting excess fluid intake.

Smooth Muscle Relaxants

Oxybutynin, a smooth muscle relaxant, is useful for reducing bladder contractions in children with detrusor overactivity (e.g., urge syndrome or neurogenic bladder); efficacy was 67% in a select group of children with detrusor overactivity.[10] A combination of DDAVP and oxybutynin can be tried in children with both detrusor overactivity and increased urine production.

Reserve **oxybutynin plus desmopressin** for refractory cases.[14] A lower dose of oral DDAVP (200 μg) is required when used in combination.[15]

Other therapies

Imipramine has been used in the past but is not recommended because it is not more effective than DDAVP and has a narrow therapeutic window.

There is no evidence of effectiveness for complementary therapies such as hypnosis, acupuncture, chiropractic, faradization, homeopathy or diet or restricted foods.[16]

Therapeutic Tips

- Predictors of positive treatment outcome include a motivated child, supportive family and age over 10 years.
- Predictors of treatment failure include developmental delay, low self-esteem, a history of behaviour problems or multiple wetting at night, frequent daytime voiding, parental intolerance or annoyance, unstable family dynamics and poor maternal education.[17]
- The cause of most cases of diurnal enuresis is uncovered by noninvasive investigations (history, physical exam, urinalysis, urine culture and ultrasound of kidney and bladder).
- Relative to desmopressin, enuresis alarms are effective in reducing nocturnal enuresis episodes during treatment and after discontinuation of treatment.[8] The effects of desmopressin are immediate whereas enuresis alarms make take longer to reduce bedwetting.

Figure 1: **Management of Enuresis in Children**

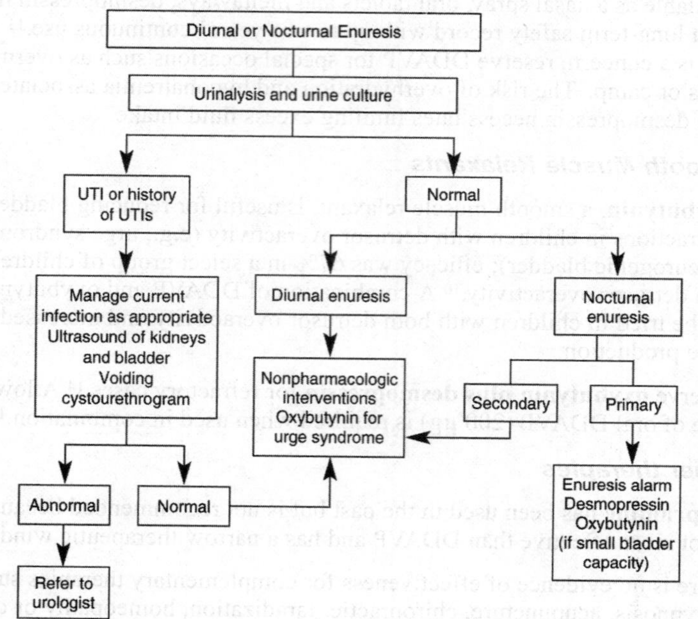

Abbreviation: UTI = urinary tract infection.

Table 2: Drug Therapy for Enuresis in Children ≥ 5 years of age

Class	Drug	Dose	Adverse Effects	Comments	Cost[a]
Antidiuretic Hormone Analogues	*desmopressin* DDAVP Melt, DDAVP Spray, DDAVP Tablets, Minirin, generics	Dose is individualized. Spray: 10–40 µg HS; initial dose: 10 µg one hour before HS, ↑ by 10 µg increments every 3 days if no response. Tablets: 200–600 µg po HS; initial dose: 200 µg one hour before HS; ↑ by 200 µg increments every 3 days if no response. Fast-melting formulation: 120 to 360 µg sl; initial dose: 120 µg sl one hour before HS, ↑ by 120 µg sl increments every 3 days if no response. May continue treatment for up to 3 mo.	Headache (transient), abdominal pain, water intoxication, hyponatremia-related seizures (rare). Nasal spray only: nasal congestion, nasal irritation, epistaxis.	For nocturnal enuresis. Used in conjunction with nonpharmacologic treatment. 20 µg of nasal spray is approximately equivalent to a 200 µg tablet. Nasal formulation may be less effective in children with symptomatic allergic rhinitis or colds. Instruct patients who are using the nasal formulation to close the treated nostril while breathing through the untreated nostril for optimal absorption. Do not shake the bottle. Do not sniff or inhale the contents. Desmopressin should not be used in children with kidney disease, heart failure, diabetes, ileitis or cystic fibrosis. The fast-melting formulation of DDAVP is effective for 7 to 11 h.[18]	$$$–$$$$
Smooth Muscle Relaxants	*oxybutynin* Ditropan, generics	Dose is individualized. 5–12 y: 5 mg daily–TID > 12 y: 5 mg po daily–QID	Dry mouth, constipation, flushing and occasional mood changes.[10]	Available as syrup.	$

[a] Cost of 30-day supply; includes drug cost only.
Legend: $ < $30 $$ $30–60 $$$ $60–90 $$$–$$$$ $60– > 90 $$$$ > $90

Suggested Readings

Bernard-Bonnin AC. Diurnal enuresis in childhood. *Can Fam Physician* 2000;46:1109-15.

Canadian Paediatric Society. Management of primary nocturnal enuresis. *Paediatr Child Health* 2005;10(10):611-4. Available from: http://www.cps.ca/english/statements/CP/cp05-02.pdf Accessed April 2, 2007.

Hjalmas K, Arnold T, Bower W et al. Nocturnal enuresis: an international evidence based management strategy. *J Urol* 2004;171(6 Pt 2):2545-61.

Russell K, Kiddoo D. The Cochrane Library and nocturnal enuresis; an umbrella review. *Evidenced-Based Child Health* 2006;1(1):5-8.

References

1. Fritz G, Rockney R, Bernet W et al. Practice parameter for the assessment and treatment of children and adolescents with enuresis. *J Am Acad Child Adolesc Psychiatry* 2004;43(12):1540-50.
2. Schulpen TW. The burden of nocturnal enuresis. *Acta Paediatr* 1997;86(9):981-4.
3. Bloom DA, Butler RJ, Djurhuus JC et al. *Conservative management in children.* In Incontinence. First International Consultation on Incontinence; 1998 June 28-July 1. Monaco: World Health Organization, International Union Against Cancer (UICC); 1999.
4. Canadian Paediatric Society. Management of primary nocturnal enuresis. *Paediatr Child Health* 2005;10(10):611-4. Available from: http://www.cps.ca/english/statements/CP/cp05-02.pdf Accessed April 2, 2007.
5. Alexopoulos EI, Kaditis AG, Kostadima E, Gourgoulianis K. Resolution of nocturnal enuresis in snoring children after treatment with nasal budesonide. *Urology* 2005;66(1):194.
6. Basha S, Bialowas C, Ende K et al. Effectiveness of adenotonsillectomy in the resolution of nocturnal enuresis secondary to obstructive sleep apnea. *Laryngoscope* 2005;115(6):1101-3.
7. Butler RJ, Redfern EJ, Forsythe I. The Maternal Tolerance Scale and nocturnal enuresis. *Behav Res Ther* 1993;31(4):433-6.
8. Glazener CM, Evans JH, Peto RE. Alarm interventions for nocturnal enuresis in children. *Cochrane Database Syst Rev* 2005;(2):CD002911.
9. Hjalmas K, Arnold T, Bower W et al. Nocturnal enuresis: an international evidence based management strategy. *J Urol* 2004;171(6 Pt 2):2545-61.
10. Butler R, Stenberg A. Treatment of childhood nocturnal enuresis: an examination of clinically relevant principles. *BJU Int* 2001;88(6):563-71.
11. Hjalmas K, Hanson E, Hellstrom AL et al. Long-term treatment with desmopressin in children with primary monosymptomatic nocturnal enuresis: an open multicentre study. Swedish Enuresis Trial (SWEET) Group. *Br J Urol* 1998;82(5):704-9.
12. Neveus T. Osmoregulation and desmopressin pharmacokinetics in enuretic children. *Scand J Urol Nephrol Suppl* 1999;202:52.
13. Zaontz MR, Dean GE, Glazier DB et al. *Long-term experience with desmopressin acetate in children.* Paper presented at: American Academy of Pediatrics 2000 Annual Meeting; October 28, 2000; Chicago. Abstract 51.
14. Vermandel A, de Wachter S, Wyndaele JJ. Refractory monosymptomatic nocturnal enuresis: a combined stepwise approach in childhood and follow-up into adolescence, with attention to the clinical value of normalizing bladder capacity. *BJU Int* 2005;96(4):629-33.
15. Lee T, Suh HJ, Lee HJ et al. Comparison of effects of treatment of primary nocturnal enuresis with oxybutynin plus desmopressin, desmopressin alone or imipramine alone: a randomized controlled clinical trial. *J Urol* 2005;174(3):1084-7.
16. Glazener CM, Evans JH, Cheuk DK. Complementary and miscellaneous interventions for nocturnal enuresis in children. *Cochrane Database Syst Rev* 2005;(2):CD005230.
17. Moffatt ME, Cheang M. Predicting treatment outcome with conditioning alarms. *Scand J Urol Nephrol Suppl* 1995;173:119-22.
18. Vande Walle JG, Bogaert GA, Mattsson S et al. A new fast-melting oral formulation of desmopressin: a pharmacodynamic study in children with primary nocturnal enuresis. *BJU Int* 2006;97(3):603-9.

CHAPTER 61
Contraception

Gillian Graves, MD, FRCSC

Goals of Therapy

- Prevent pregnancy
- Individualize contraceptive method to specific needs, lifestyle, age, parity and desire for future fertility

Therapeutic Choices

Assess the woman's contraceptive needs. Effective contraception and education reduces rates of maternal and child mortality, as well as population growth. Individual contraceptive needs change over time. Preferred contraceptive methods for young women are reversible, affordable and have good safety profiles and low failure rates. The method chosen should not interfere with other physiologic processes, such as vaginal lubrication, spontaneity or pleasure of either partner. Present contraceptive choices along with appropriate counselling to each individual.

Nonpharmacologic Choices

Nonhormonal contraceptive options such as natural timing, barrier methods, spermicides, IUDs and surgical sterilization are included in Table 3.

Pharmacologic Choices (Table 4)

Combined Estrogen- and Progestin-containing Contraceptives

Combined Oral Contraceptives (COCs)

COCs combined with condoms (for STI protection) are the method of choice for most young couples, including teens. COCs containing synthetic estrogen and progestin have been modified as a result of synthesis of more potent steroids. This has led to dose reduction, increased safety and reliability and decreased adverse effects. Absolute contraindications of COCs are listed in Table 1.

Significant differences between monophasic and triphasic COCs in regard to bleeding pattern or efficacy have not been shown.[3] Fixed dose COCs are easier to manipulate than triphasic COCs. Products containing third-generation progestins (e.g., desogestrel) are less androgenic and may be useful in acne. Most oral contraceptives, however, are effective in improving mild to moderate acne (see Chapter 77). **Cyproterone acetate** combined with **ethinyl estradiol** (EE) is very effective for controlling moderate to severe acne.

Table 1: **Absolute Contraindications to Combined Oral Hormonal Contraception**[1,2]

• Breast cancer • Cerebrovascular disease • Complicated valvular heart disease • Current or past history of venous thromboembolism • Diabetes with microvascular complications • History of MI or ischemic heart disease • Known coagulation-factor deficiency • < 6 weeks postpartum if breastfeeding • Liver tumour • Migraines with aura • Hypertension (SBP ≥ 160 mm Hg or DBP ≥ 100 mm Hg) • Severe cirrhosis • Smoker > 35 years of age (≥ 15 cigarettes/day)

Low dose COCs with 20-25 μg EE have been shown to be effective contraceptive agents with pregnancy rates between 0.07 and 2.1 pregnancies per 100 woman-years of treatment.[4] They demonstrate reduced symptoms of bloating and breast tenderness.[5] These COCs may be used in individuals who experience adverse effects with higher EE doses.

Drospirenone, the newest progestin, is related to the aldosterone antagonist spironolactone. It may lead to fewer premenstrual symptoms and less bloating than some other COCs. It has both progestational and antiandrogenic activity.[6]

Progestins can be classified according to their steroid structure and to their first appearance on the market (Table 2).

Transdermal Contraceptives

A transdermal estrogen/progestin patch (Evra) has similar contraceptive efficacy, cycle control and ovulation suppression to COCs.[9,10] Proposed advantages are better compliance (88% vs 78% for COCs)[11] and theoretically less risk of DVT.[12] The pregnancy rate is between 0.70 and 0.88 pregnancies per 100 woman-years of treatment.[4,13]

For women weighing 90 kg or more, this method may not be effective. Obesity may affect metabolism sufficiently to compromise contraceptive efficacy of oral contraceptives as well.[14,15]

Contraceptive Vaginal Ring

An estrogen/progestin-releasing vaginal ring (NuvaRing) provides a more uniform contraceptive hormone concentration throughout the day,[16] thus avoiding daily hormonal fluctuations. Because both hepatic first-pass and gastrointestinal metabolism are avoided, lower doses of hormones can be used. Cycle control is good, with irregular bleeding in 5.5% of cycles and withdrawal bleeding in 98.5% of cycles.[17,18] There has been one case of mesenteric vein thrombosis reported.[19] Failure rate is 0.65 per 100 woman-years.[4]

Table 2: **Progestins: Estrogenic, Progestational and Androgenic Activity[7,8]**

Steroid Structure	Name of Progestin	Activity		
		Estrogenic[a]	Progestational[b]	Androgenic[c]
Estrane	norethindrone acetate	+	+	+
	ethynodiol diacetate	+++	++	+
Gonanes, 2nd generation	dl-norgestrel	-	+++	+++
	levonorgestrel	-	++++	++++
Gonanes, 3rd generation	desogestrel	+/-	++++	++/+
	norgestimate	-	+++	++
Aldosterone antagonist derivative	drospirenone	-	+/-	+

[a] associated adverse effects: nausea, vomiting, bloating, fluid retention, breast fullness, irritability, cyclical weight gain, headache, bleeding irregularities, breakthrough bleeding, chloasma
[b] associated adverse effects: mastalgia, headache
[c] associated adverse effects: acne, oily skin, hirsutism, weight gain, fatigue, mood swings, depression, rash, alterations in lipids, alterations in glucose
Legend:++++ = highest; +++ = high; ++ = intermediate; + = low; +/- = low to none; - = none

Progestin-only Contraceptives

Oral Progestin

Norethindrone (Micronor) inhibits cervical sperm penetration by thickening the cervical mucus. Regular and consistent use is necessary to maintain contraceptive efficacy since effect on cervical mucus decreases rapidly 22 hours after dosing. A backup method for the first month of use is essential. If a dose is missed by more than three hours, a backup method is required. It can be used in women over 35 years of age who smoke, those who cannot tolerate estrogen, have unwanted side effects with COCs, experience migraine headaches with neurologic symptoms and in women who are breastfeeding.

Injectable Medroxyprogesterone Acetate (MPA)

MPA, given by depot injection (Depo-Provera), produces amenorrhea in the majority of women, but some women experience irregular bleeding and side effects such as bloating, weight gain or loss and mood swings. Depot MPA can be used in the postabortal state (five days postpartum) or during lactation (six weeks postpartum). It may be a viable option for women over 35 who smoke and in women who cannot tolerate estrogen. When depot MPA is discontinued, ovulation and regular menstrual periods may not resume for up to a year after the last injection. Failure rate is < 0.3% per year.[13]

A large cross-sectional study of women (18 to 54 years of age) noted a 7.2% lower spinal bone mineral density (BMD) in users of Depo-Provera than in nonusers. The rate of loss was higher for women who started using Depo-Provera before age 21 and in those using it for longer duration (≥ 15 years). Because the loss may not be completely reversible, the clinical significance of low BMD, especially in adolescents who have not yet reached peak bone mass, needs to be elucidated.[20] Continuous losses at both hip and spine were seen in a small study of adolescent women (14 to 18 years of age) over 36 months of MPA use, but significant gains postdiscontinuation indicate this is likely reversible.[21] Small double-blind trials suggest that estrogen supplementation is protective of bone in adolescents who are on depot MPA.[22]

Intrauterine System (IUS)

After insertion of the progestin-releasing intrauterine device (Mirena) into the uterus, a low dose of **levonorgestrel** is released continuously over a period of at least five years. It is associated with low systemic levels of levonorgestrel and is highly efficacious (≤ 0.2 pregnancy rate per year[4]). It can reduce menstrual blood loss, fibroid growth and dysmenorrhea. This method requires a clinician visit for initiation and discontinuation. Normal menstruation restarts within one to three months of IUS removal.

Risks associated with Hormonal Contraception

Cardiovascular Risks

Long-term studies are required to quantify cardiovascular risk for users of third-generation combined oral contraceptives (COCs) compared to COCs containing older progestins. All cardiovascular risks are appreciably higher in pregnancy compared to taking COCs containing < 50 µg ethinyl estradiol (see Table 4).

Smoking and hypertension increase the risk of *ischemic stroke* in COC users.[23,24,25,26,27] Women who have migraine with aura are at a higher risk of ischemic stroke than women who have migraine without aura.[26,28,29,30,31] The risk of stroke does not differ between generations of progestins contained in COCs.[32] Consider alternative contraceptive methods in women who suffer from migraines with focal neurologic signs, smoke cigarettes or are hypertensive.[1,33,34]

The risk of *acute myocardial infarction (AMI)* is compounded in COC users 35 years and older who have other cardiovascular disease risk factors such as smoking, hypertension and diabetes[20,23,35,36] and in those whose blood pressure has not been effectively screened.[20,23,24,29,27] There is an increased risk of MI associated with increasing number of cigarettes smoked per day.[34] No increase in risk of AMI is found in women under 35 years of age who have no additional cardiovascular risk factors.[24] Consider alternative contraceptive methods in women older than 35 years who have additional cardiovascular risk factors.

The risk of *venous thromboembolism (VTE)* increases with age[37,38] and for both short- and long-term COC users, but is less than the 6- to 10-fold increased risk associated with pregnancy.[39] The risk of VTE increases with higher estrogen doses[40,41] but the VTE risk associated with COCs containing 20 µg EE is equivalent to that of COCs containing 30 to 35 µg EE.[30] Inherited hypercoagulable states such as Factor V Leiden mutation, protein C or S deficiency[34] or acquired conditions such as immobility, trauma or surgery are associated with an increased risk of VTE. Obese COC users are at an increased risk of VTE compared to obese nonusers.[42,43] Women with Factor V Leiden who use COCs experience a VTE risk 30 times higher than that of COC users without the mutation.[40,44,45] Broad-based screening for this or other thrombophilias (protein C or S deficiency) is not appropriate because of the rarity of these conditions and the high screening costs. If there is a strong family or personal history of VTE, screening is recommended.[46,47] COCs are contraindicated in women with a history of VTE and hypercoagulable states.

In summary, the risk of cardiovascular disease in nonsmoking normotensive women under the age of 35 is so small that there is no health impact related to the choice of a second- versus third-generation progestin. Individualize COC selection based on history. Control the individual's risk factors for cardiovascular disease such as *obesity*, *smoking* and *hypertension*. Noncontraceptive benefits should also be considered.

Breast Cancer Risk

The risk of breast cancer in COC users is controversial. Most studies of COC use and breast cancer find no overall risk or a slight increase in risk.[1] In women under the age of 35, the risk is 2 in 1000. COC use increases the risk 1.5-fold to 3 in 1000. As women age the risk increases. One of the risk factors for breast cancer is not having a baby by the age of 25. It is uncertain whether the risk is associated with use of an OC or the delay in pregnancy. In women with a positive family history of breast cancer, COC use has been associated with increase in baseline risk;[48] thus early screening is advised.

Emergency Postcoital Contraception (see Table 5)

Levonorgestrel (Plan B: two separate doses of 0.75 mg taken 12 hours apart or a single dose of 1.5 mg[49]) used within 24 hours of unprotected intercourse prevents 95% of expected pregnancies. The Yuzpe method (two separate doses of EE 100 µg with levonorgestrel 0.5 mg taken 12 hours apart) prevents 75% of expected pregnancies.[50] The efficacy of both regimens is highest if treatment is provided within 24 hours. Both regimens can be taken up to five days after unprotected intercourse though the effectiveness declines with increasing delay between unprotected intercourse and treatment initiation.[51] Unprotected intercourse is defined as no contraceptive method used, condom breakage, more than 2 pills of OC missed any time during the cycle, 1 pill missed in the first week, more than 7 day pill-free interval, depot MPA given longer than 13 weeks after previous injection, ejaculation on external genitalia or sexual assault. The incidence of side effects such as nausea, vomiting, dizziness and fatigue is lower with levonorgestrel alone than with the Yuzpe method.[52] Delaying the first dose of either treatment by 12 hours increases the odds of pregnancy by almost 50%.[53]

The progestin-only method (Plan B) has a good safety record. There was no diagnosis of DVT or PE within 45 days of the prescription in a large UK study of emergency contraceptive users.[54] The combined OC (Yuzpe) method is relatively contraindicated in patients with a history of thromboembolism and should not be used in those with a history of migraine with aura.[28] Plan B may be preferred in patients who have contraindications to the estrogens in combined contraceptives. Emergency contraception has no effect on an established postimplantation pregnancy.

Postcoital insertion of a copper IUD can be considered up to seven days after unprotected intercourse. Prior to insertion, it is important to exclude pre-existing pregnancy. A meta-analysis demonstrated a failure rate of 0.1% from more than 8400 insertions of postcoital IUDs.[55] Though the exact mechanism of action is unknown, it is postulated to hamper egg motility and implantation.[56]

Contraception in Special Populations

Breastfeeding and Contraception

There are insufficient data to establish an effect of hormonal contraception, if any, on milk quality or quantity.[57] Avoid use of COCs in lactating women during the first six weeks postpartum and use with caution in the first six months postpartum.[57] Current Canadian Contraception Consensus guidelines recommend progestin-only methods for postpartum women regardless of breastfeeding status. Progestin-only methods can be introduced immediately after delivery.[13] Progestin-only OCs can be used during lactation, without increasing thromboembolic rates in the puerperium. Oral formulations must be taken every day at the same time, without missing a pill, to minimize spotting and maintain contraceptive efficacy.

Low-dose COCs can be used once the milk supply is well established (i.e., six weeks postpartum). There is some decrease in milk quantity noted; however, no negative effect on the infant has been described.

Barrier contraceptives plus spermicide can provide lubrication to the hypoestrogenic vagina but are not as effective for contraception as other methods.

IUDs can be inserted four to six weeks postpartum once involution has occurred and the uterus is firm enough to minimize the risk of insertional perforation. It is important to ensure good fundal placement within a larger uterine cavity, since efficacy of current copper-T devices requires the IUD arms to be near the fundus.

HIV and Contraception

Correct and consistent use of male condoms is the most effective way to reduce risk of acquisition and transmission of HIV. Regardless of formulation or dosage, spermicides containing nonoxynol-9 do not provide any protection against HIV.[58,59]

IUDs do not confer any greater risk of acquiring HIV than if no contraceptive method is used.[58] Although there is concern about the theoretical risk of pelvic infection in women with HIV/AIDS who use IUDs and about transmission to uninfected partners, evidence is lacking. People who engage in sexual intercourse with partners who may be HIV-infected should consistently and correctly use *latex condoms* without nonoxynol-9 regardless of other contraceptive methods used.

No studies of hormone use have directly addressed whether OC use enhances disease progression in women with HIV/AIDS. There is no strong evidence of association between use of OCs or depot MPA and HIV-1 infection.[20]

Therapeutic Tips

- OCs help regulate cycles and decrease menstrual flow. This may help to control anemia in women with heavy or irregular periods.
- Noncontraceptive health benefits attributed to OC use include a decrease in the frequency of endometrial cancer, fibroids, endometriosis pain, benign breast disease, functional ovarian cysts, ectopic pregnancy, dysmenorrhea, pelvic inflammatory disease and perimenopausal symptoms.
- Hormonal contraception does not protect against acquisition of sexually transmitted infections. Educate patients on use of barrier methods.
- Compared to cyclical use, continuous use of monophasic pills results in fewer bleeding days, decreased likelihood of side effects such as pelvic pain, headache, bloating, swelling and tenderness and aids in improving symptoms of endometriosis and polycystic ovary syndrome. With fewer bleeding days, use may benefit women undergoing chemotherapy. Long-term safety data is lacking, however.
- In nonsmoking women with no cardiovascular risk factors, COCs may be considered for contraception or control of dysfunctional uterine bleeding until menopause.
- COC use is associated with a reduced incidence of endometrial and ovarian cancers compared to nonusers.[4]

Table 3: Nonhormonal Contraceptive Methods

Class	Contraceptive Method	Contraindications	Adverse Effects	Comments	Cost[a]
Natural Methods	*Coital Timing*	Relative: irregular cycle.	None.	*Failure rate:* Typical use: 20% Perfect use: 1–9% Requires high motivation; depends on identification of mucus and temperature patterns to identify fertile time; very difficult if there is an irregular cycle or ovulation defects; high pregnancy rates.	N/A
Barrier Methods	*Condoms, Male – latex, polyurethane, lambskin* Trojan, Aventi, various	Relative: hypersensitivity to latex, polyurethane, lanolin (in case of lambskin condoms).	Common: hypersensitivity to latex in either partner.	*Failure rate:* Typical use: 14% in 1st y Perfect use: 3% in 1st y Protect against STIs including HIV (latex only); best suited to infrequent intercourse; may use with a separately provided vaginal spermicide; lambskin condoms do not protect against STI; check expiry date; latex condom integrity degraded by oil-based lubricants—use water-based lubricants.	$0.45–0.70/ male condom
	Condoms, Female Reality	Relative: hypersensitivity to polyurethane, vaginal anatomical abnormalities that make fitting difficult.	Discomfort.	*Failure rate:* Typical use: 20% Perfect use: 5% Not to be used with male condoms, potential for displacement; best suited for women who find spermicide irritating or who dislike messiness of other vaginal barrier methods. Inserted up to 8 h prior to intercourse and removed immediately after; shelf-life of up to 5 y.	$2.60/female condom

Class	Contraceptive Method	Contraindications	Adverse Effects	Comments	Cost[a]
	Diaphragm Ortho Diaphragm Coil, Wide Seal	Relative: hypersensitivity, inability to insert. Absolute: inability to achieve proper fit, marked uterine prolapse, large cystocele/rectocele, vaginal deformity, recurrent UTIs.	Common: hypersensitivity to diaphragm and/or spermicide. Infection if not used/cleaned properly (diaphragm), toxic shock syndrome. Less common: use of spermicide ↑s incidence of *E. coli* UTI due to changes in the vaginal flora.[60] Rare: toxic shock syndrome.	*Failure rate:* Typical use: 20% in 1st y Perfect use: 6% in 1st y Refitting necessary after childbirth, surgery, or if lose/gain 4 kg. Best suited to infrequent intercourse. Use with spermicide. Can be inserted 6 h before intercourse. Can be used in breastfeeding women. For women allergic to latex, silicone diaphragm available.	$40/diaphragm
	Sponge Protectaid Sponge, Today	Relative: hypersensitivity, inability to insert. Absolute: inability to achieve proper fit, recurrent UTIs.	Rare: toxic shock syndrome.	*Failure rate:* Typical use: 9–18% (nulliparous), 20–36% (parous) Perfect use: 10–20% (nulliparous), 20–40% (parous) Spermicide is released in a sustained fashion for up to 12 h. May enhance HIV transmission by damaging vaginal mucosa. Do not use during menstruation.[61]	$6.30/4 sponges

(cont'd)

Table 3: **Nonhormonal Contraceptive Methods** *(cont'd)*

Class	Contraceptive Method	Contraindications	Adverse Effects	Comments	Cost[a]
	Cervical Cap	Relative: abnormal cervical cytology, chronic cervicitis, recurrent salpingitis. Absolute: cervical deformity (i.e., inability to obtain suitable fit), current PID, current vaginal or cervical infection, cervical or uterine cancer, dysplasia, recurrent vaginal, urinary tract or cervical infections.	Common: vaginal discharge, vaginal odour, cervical or fornices ulceration, hypersensitivity (cap or spermicide). Infection if not used/cleaned properly, vaginitis. Rare: toxic shock syndrome.	*Failure rate*: Typical use: 20% (nulliparous), 40% in 1st y (multiparous) Perfect use: 9% (nulliparous), 26% in 1st y (multiparous) Use with spermicide, placed inside the cap prior to insertion. Protects against STI including HIV. Can be left in place for up to 48 h for multiple acts of intercourse. Can be used in breastfeeding women. Not to be used within 6 wk of delivery. Manufacturer recommends refitting after miscarriage, term delivery, abortion, or if lose/gain 3 kg.	$35/cap
Spermicides	*nonoxynol-9* Vaginal Contraceptive Film, others	Relative: hypersensitivity.	Common: hypersensitivity.	*Failure rate:* Typical use: 26% in 1st y Perfect use: 6% in 1 st y May use with condom, diaphragm or cervical cap. Less effective if used alone. Not effective against HIV or STI. ↑ risk of genital lesions resulting in ↑ risk of HIV transmission.[62]	$3/unit

Class	Contraceptive Method	Contraindications	Adverse Effects	Comments	Cost[a]
Intrauterine Devices (IUD)	*Copper-T IUD* Nova-T, Flexi-T	Absolute: pregnancy, undiagnosed vaginal bleeding, stenosed cervix, copper allergy, current PID or STI, cervical or endometrial cancer, copper allergy.	Major: salpingitis, uterine perforation, cervical perforation, endometrial embedding, menorrhagia, pain, infection, ectopic pregnancy.	*Failure rate:* 1–5% in 1st y Excellent for spacing children in a stable relationship; risk of PID and tubal infections is too high for nullipara; immediate risks are insertional infection or perforation; late risks are infection and ectopic pregnancy.	$51 for copper IUD (lasts 3–5 y)
Sterilization, Surgical	*Tubal Ligation*	Pregnancy, systemic conditions (e.g., cardiopulmonary) that can be aggravated by general anesthesia, pelvic infection.	Cumulative 10-year probability of ectopic pregnancy post tubal ligation: 7.3 per 1000.[63]	*Failure rate:* 0.5% Method of choice for couples with completed family. Reversible only if salpingectomy not performed and sufficient length of undamaged tubal remnants remain.	Cost-insured service in Canada. Cost of reversal surgery $3000–$5000
	Vasectomy	Systemic conditions (e.g., acute infectious diseases), local infection, sexual dysfunction, local genital abnormalities (e.g., hernia).	Local pain, scrotal ecchymosis, swelling.	*Failure rate:* < 2.2% Method of choice for couples with completed family; reversible with more surgery if < 10 y since procedure.	Cost-insured service in Canada. Cost of reversal surgery $3000–$5000

[a] Approximate cost per unit (condom, tube, canister, package); includes drug or contraceptive cost only. Mark-up is not included.

Abbreviations: IUD = intrauterine device; IUS = intrauterine system; N/A = not applicable; PID = pelvic inflammatory disease ; STI = sexually transmitted infection

Table 4: **Hormonal Contraceptive Methods**

Class	Drug	Contraindications	Adverse Effects	Drug Interactions	Comments	Cost[a]
Contraceptives, oral – combined estrogen (50 µg EE) and progestin	*EE 50 µg / norgestrel 0.25 mg* Oval	Relative: estrogen hypersensitivity, migraine, gallbladder disease, high BMI/weight. Absolute: history of MI or ischemic heart disease, cerebrovascular disease, complicated valvular heart disease, current or past history VTE, severe cirrhosis, liver tumour, breast cancer, diabetes with microvascular complications, migraines with aura, < 6 wk postpartum if breastfeeding, smoker > 35 y (≥ 15 cigarettes/day), hypertension (SBP ≥ 160 mm Hg or DBP ≥ 100 mm Hg), known coagulation-factor deficiency.	Major: thromboembolism (rare), stroke, retinal artery thrombosis, myocardial infarction, benign liver tumour, cholelithiasis, hypertension. Common: breakthrough bleeding/spotting, amenorrhea, nausea/vomiting, bloating, chloasma, breast tenderness, mood changes such as depression, headaches.	May ↓ lamotrigine levels, may ↑ cyclosporine levels. ↓ EE serum concentrations: carbamazepine, griseofulvin, modafinil, phenobarbital, phenytoin, protease inhibitors, St. John's wort, topiramate. Significant pharmacokinetic interaction with rifampin and griseofulvin; advise backup barrier method during therapy. Reports of failure of COCs with concomitant ampicillin, tetracycline, erythromycin, sulfamethoxazole/trimethoprim or nitrofurantoin. Monitor INR with concurrent oral anticoagulant use.	*Failure rate:* Typical use: 3–8% Perfect use: ≤ 0.1% Method of choice for most young couples, especially for teens, if combined with condoms; lower dose estrogen products have increased safety and decreased side effects; condoms needed for STI protection. Watch for danger signals: ACHES – abdominal pain, chest pain, headaches, eye problems, severe leg pain. Advise physician consult. Patients with diarrhea or breakthrough bleeding may be at higher risk of contraceptive failure.	$$

Class	Drug	Contraindications	Adverse Effects	Drug Interactions	Comments	Cost[a]
Contraceptives, oral – combined estrogen (< 50 µg EE) and progestin, Monophasic	*EE 35 µg / norethindrone 1 mg* Brevicon 1/35, Ortho 1/35, Select 1/35	See EE 50 µg / norgestrel 0.25 mg.	See EE 50 µg / norgestrel 0.25 mg.	See EE 50 µg / norgestrel 0.25 mg.	See EE 50 µg / norgestrel 0.25 mg.	$$
	EE 35 µg / norethindrone 0.5 mg Brevicon 0.5/35, Ortho 0.5/35	See EE 50 µg / norgestrel 0.25 mg.	See EE 50 µg / norgestrel 0.25 mg.	See EE 50 µg / norgestrel 0.25 mg.	See EE 50 µg / norgestrel 0.25 mg.	$$
	EE 35 µg / cyproterone 2 mg Diane-35	See EE 50 µg / norgestrel 0.25 mg.	See EE 50 µg / norgestrel 0.25 mg.	See EE 50 µg / norgestrel 0.25 mg.	See EE 50 µg / norgestrel 0.25 mg. Diane-35 is indicated for severe acne. It should be discontinued 3 to 4 months after signs of acne have completely resolved. Not promoted or prescribed as a method of birth control.	$$$
	EE 35 µg / norgestimate 0.25 mg Cyclen	See EE 50 µg / norgestrel 0.25 mg.	See EE 50 µg / norgestrel 0.25 mg.	See EE 50 µg / norgestrel 0.25 mg.	See EE 50 µg / norgestrel 0.25 mg.	$$

(cont'd)

Table 4: **Hormonal Contraceptive Methods** *(cont'd)*

Class	Drug	Contraindications	Adverse Effects	Drug Interactions	Comments	Cost[a]
	EE 30 μg / desogestrel 0.15 mg Marvelon, Ortho-Cept	See EE 50 μg / norgestrel 0.25 mg.	See EE 50 μg / norgestrel 0.25 mg.	See EE 50 μg / norgestrel 0.25 mg.	See EE 50 μg / norgestrel 0.25 mg.	$$
	EE 30 μg / ethynodiol diacetate 2 mg Demulen 30	See EE 50 μg / norgestrel 0.25 mg.	See EE 50 μg / norgestrel 0.25 mg.	See EE 50 μg / norgestrel 0.25 mg.	See EE 50 μg / norgestrel 0.25 mg.	$$
	EE 30 μg / norethindrone acetate 1.5 mg Loestrin 1.5/30	See EE 50 μg / norgestrel 0.25 mg.	See EE 50 μg / norgestrel 0.25 mg.	See EE 50 μg / norgestrel 0.25 mg.	See EE 50 μg / norgestrel 0.25 mg.	$$
	EE 30 μg / drospirenone 3 mg Yasmin	See EE 50 μg / norgestrel 0.25 mg.	See EE 50 μg / norgestrel 0.25 mg.	See EE 50 μg / norgestrel 0.25 mg.	See EE 50 μg / norgestrel 0.25 mg.	$$
	EE 20 μg / norethindrone acetate 1 mg Minestrin 1/20	See EE 50 μg / norgestrel 0.25 mg.	See EE 50 μg / norgestrel 0.25 mg.	See EE 50 μg / norgestrel 0.25 mg.	See EE 50 μg / norgestrel 0.25 mg.	$$
	EE 20 μg / levonorgestrel 0.1 mg Alesse	See EE 50 μg / norgestrel 0.25 mg.	See EE 50 μg / norgestrel 0.25 mg.	See EE 50 μg / norgestrel 0.25 mg.	See EE 50 μg / norgestrel 0.25 mg.	$$

Class	Drug	Contraindications	Adverse Effects	Drug Interactions	Comments	Cost[a]
Contraceptives, oral – combined estrogen (< 50 μg EE) and progestin, Triphasic	*EE 25 μg × 21 days / desogestrel 0.1 mg × 7 days, 0.125 mg × 7 days, 0.15 mg × 7 days* Linessa	See EE 50 μg / norgestrel 0.25 mg.	See EE 50 μg / norgestrel 0.25 mg.	See EE 50 μg / norgestrel 0.25 mg.	See EE 50 μg / norgestrel 0.25 mg.	$$
	EE 35 μg × 21 days / norethindrone 0.5 mg × 7 days, 0.75 mg × 7 days, 1 mg × 7 days Ortho 7/7/7	See EE 50 μg / norgestrel 0.25 mg.	See EE 50 μg / norgestrel 0.25 mg.	See EE 50 μg / norgestrel 0.25 mg.	See EE 50 μg / norgestrel 0.25 mg.	$$
	EE 35 μg × 21 days / norethindrone 0.5 mg × 7 days, 1 mg × 9 days, 0.5 mg × 5 days Synphasic	See EE 50 μg / norgestrel 0.25 mg.	See EE 50 μg / norgestrel 0.25 mg.	See EE 50 μg / norgestrel 0.25 mg.	See EE 50 μg / norgestrel 0.25 mg.	$$

(cont'd)

Table 4: **Hormonal Contraceptive Methods** *(cont'd)*

Class	Drug	Contraindications	Adverse Effects	Drug Interactions	Comments	Cost[a]
	EE 35 µg × 21 days / norgestimate 0.18 mg × 7 days, 0.215 mg × 7 days, 0.25 mg × 7 days Tri-Cyclen	See EE 50 µg / norgestrel 0.25 mg.	See EE 50 µg / norgestrel 0.25 mg.	See EE 50 µg / norgestrel 0.25 mg.	See EE 50 µg / norgestrel 0.25 mg.	$$
	EE 25 µg × 21 days / norgestimate 0.18 mg × 7 days, 0.215 mg × 7 days, 0.25 mg × 7 days Tri-Cyclen Lo	See EE 50 µg / norgestrel 0.25 mg.	See EE 50 µg / norgestrel 0.25 mg.	See EE 50 µg / norgestrel 0.25 mg.	See EE 50 µg / norgestrel 0.25 mg.	$$
	EE 30 µg × 6 days, 40 µg × 5 days, 30 µg × 10 days / levonorgestrel 0.05 mg × 6 days, 0.075 mg × 5 days, 0.125 mg × 10 days Triphasil, Triquilar	See EE 50 µg / norgestrel 0.25 mg.	See EE 50 µg / norgestrel 0.25 mg.	See EE 50 µg / norgestrel 0.25 mg.	See EE 50 µg / norgestrel 0.25 mg.	$$

Class	Drug	Contraindications	Adverse Effects	Drug Interactions	Comments	Cost[a]
Contra-ceptives, Transder-mal	*EE 20 μg/day / norelgestromin 150 μg/day*[64] Evra	See EE 50 μg / norgestrel 0.25 mg. Relative: body weight ≥ 90 kg.	See EE 50 μg / norgestrel 0.25 mg. Common: breast discomfort (19%) is more common than COC in first 2 mo, headache (22%), skin reaction under patch (20%), nausea (20%), dysmenorrhea.	See EE 50 μg / norgestrel 0.25 mg.	*Failure rate:* Typical use: 0.88 per 100 woman-years Perfect use: 0.7 per 100 woman-years Condoms needed for STI protection. Unknown if the incidence of VTE is similar to OCs. Apply to dry intact skin of buttock, abdomen, upper outer arm, or upper torso. Apply a new patch once a wk on the same day of the wk for 3 wk, followed by a patch-free wk. If off for > 24 h, start new patch and use backup for 7 days. When switching from COCs, apply the first patch on the first day of withdrawal bleeding. If later than the first day of withdrawal bleeding, use a backup method of contraception for 7 days. Similar contraceptive efficacy, cycle control and ovulation suppression as COCs.[9] Evra adheres well to the skin with a 2 to 3% detachment rate. Start on day of scheduled injection when switching from depot MPA to patch.	$$

(cont'd)

Table 4: **Hormonal Contraceptive Methods** *(cont'd)*

Class	Drug	Contraindications	Adverse Effects	Drug Interactions	Comments	Cost[a]
Contraceptives, Vaginal Ring	*EE 15 μg/day /etonorgestrel 120 μg/day* NuvaRing	Relative: uterovaginal prolapse, vaginal stenosis (prevent retention of ring). Absolute: history of MI or ischemic heart disease, cerebrovascular disease, complicated valvular heart disease, current or past history VTE, severe cirrhosis, liver tumour, breast cancer, diabetes with microvascular complications, migraines with aura, < 6 wk postpartum if breastfeeding, smoker > 35 y (≥ 15 cigarettes/day), hypertension (SBP ≥ 160 mm Hg or DBP ≥ 100 mm Hg), known coagulation-factor deficiency.	See EE 50 μg / norgestrel 0.25 mg. Common: vaginal discomfort, vaginitis (5%), headache (6.6%), leukorrhea (5.3%), decreased libido, nausea, breast tenderness.	See EE 50 μg / norgestrel 0.25 mg. May interfere with the correct placement and position of a diaphragm or cervical cap – do not use these methods as backup. Concurrent use of vaginal tampons is not recommended; can use tampons after vaginal ring is removed.	*Failure rate:* Typical use: 0.65–1.18 per 100 woman-years Perfect use: 0.4–0.77 per 100 woman-years Prior to insertion: NuvaRing can be left at room temperature for 4 mo. It is worn vaginally continuously for 3 wk then removed for a 1-wk break. Systemic absorption occurs. NuvaRing can be self-inserted and removed. May not provide protection against pregnancy if left in place for more than 4 wk. Can be expelled from the vagina while removing a tampon, or emptying bladder or bowel, especially during severe straining. If left out for up to 3 h contraceptive efficacy is not reduced. Use a backup method for 7 days if left out longer than 3 h.	$$

Class	Drug	Contraindications	Adverse Effects	Drug Interactions	Comments	Cost[a]
Contraceptives, progestin-only, oral	*norethindrone* Micronor	Relative: active viral hepatitis, liver tumours. Absolute: pregnancy, current breast cancer.	Higher incidence of ectopic pregnancy compared to COCs. Irregular bleeding (~12% of users in the first mo, < 3% in 18 mo).	None.	*Failure rate:* 0.2 per 100 woman-years[65] Perfect use: 0.5%[13] Typical use: 5–10%[13] Preferred in lactating women or if contraindication to estrogen. Contains 28 tablets of active drug.	$$
Contraceptives, progestin-only, injectable	*medroxyprogesterone acetate* Depo-Provera	Relative: severe cirrhosis, active viral hepatitis, benign hepatic adenoma. Absolute: pregnancy, unexplained vaginal or urinary tract bleeding, current diagnosis of breast cancer, known sensitivity to medroxyprogesterone acetate or to the vehicle.	Breast tenderness, insomnia or somnolence, fatigue, mood changes such as depression or irritability, weight gain, menstrual irregularities, ↓ libido, skin sensitivity reactions, hyperpyrexia, acne. Long-term: ↓ in BMD, delayed return of fertility.	None.	*Failure rate:* 0.44 per 100 woman-years (100 mg im Q3MO).[66] Canadian contraception guidelines state: < 0.3%/y[13] Injectable contraceptive that is safe and effective (99.7%); excellent for women who should avoid high estrogen doses, such as migraine sufferers; condoms needed for STI protection. Consider other options in women with risk factors for osteoporosis. Injected within first 5 days of onset of menses to be effective immediately. Interval between injections must not exceed 13 wk.	$25/3 mo

(cont'd)

Table 4: **Hormonal Contraceptive Methods** *(cont'd)*

Class	Drug	Contraindications	Adverse Effects	Drug Interactions	Comments	Cost[a]
Contraceptives, progestin-only, intrauterine system (IUS)	*levonorgestrel 20 μg/day* Mirena	Pregnancy, current or recurrent PID, genital infection, postpartum endometritis, undiagnosed abnormal uterine bleeding, uterine or cervical malignancy, cervicitis, acute liver disease, hypersensitivity to components of system, hematologic malignancies, uterine anomaly.	Spotting for first 3 mo after insertion; menstrual changes such as amenorrhea.	None	*Failure rate:* ≤ 0.2 per 100 woman-years Condoms needed for STI protection. Remains in place for 5 y. Inserted within 7 days of onset of menses to be effective immediately.	$290 (lasts 5 y)

[a] Approximate cost per 1 package for 1 month unless otherwise indicated ; includes drug or contraceptive cost only. Mark-up is not included.
$ < $10 $$ $10–20 $$$ > $20

Abbreviations: BMD = bone mineral density; COC = combined oral contraceptive; MPA = medroxyprogesterone acetate; EE = ethinyl estradiol; IUD = intrauterine device; IUS = intrauterine system; PID = pelvic inflammatory disease; STI = sexually transmitted infection; UTI = urinary tract infection

Table 5: **Emergency Contraceptive Methods**

Class	Drug	Contraindications	Adverse Effects	Drug Interactions	Comments	Cost
Contraceptives, oral – combined estrogen (50 µg EE) and progestin: emergency postcoital	*EE 50 µg plus levonorgestrel 0.25 mg per dose* Ovral	See EE 50 µg / norgestrel 0.25 mg.	See EE 50 µg / norgestrel 0.25 mg. Nausea (50.5%), vomiting (18.8%), dizziness, fatigue.	Efficacy of ECPs unknown when administered concomitantly with rifampin or anticonvulsants.	Dose: 2 doses – 2 tabs Q12H. The 1st dose should be taken as soon as possible after unprotected intercourse (up to 5 days), followed by a 2nd dose 12 h later.	$3.00/4 tablets
Contraceptives, oral progestin: emergency postcoital	*levonorgestrel 0.75 mg per dose* Plan B	Pregnancy.	Nausea (23.1%), vomiting (5.6%), dizziness, fatigue.	See Ovral.	Dose: 2 doses – 1 tab Q12H or 2 tabs taken together. 2nd dose can be taken up to 24 h after the first dose without significant change in pharmacokinetics.[67]	$16
Contraceptives, IUD: emergency postcoital	*Copper-T IUD* Nova-T	See Nova-T.	See Nova-T.		Can be used as ongoing method of contraception. Use within 7 days of unprotected intercourse as an emergency contraceptive. Interferes with implantation after fertilization.	$52

Abbreviations: EE = ethinyl estradiol; IUD = intrauterine device

Suggested Readings

Black A, Francoeur D, Rowe T et al. Canadian contraception consensus. *J Obstet Gynaecol Can* 2004; 26(2):143-56, 158-74.

Black A, Francoeur D, Rowe T et al. Canadian contraception consensus. *J Obstet Gynaecol Can* 2004;26(4):347-87, 389-436.

Black A, Francoeur D, Rowe T et al. SOGC clinical practice guidelines: Canadian contraception consensus. *J Obstet Gynaecol Can* 2004;26(3):219-96.

Faculty of Family Planning & Reproductive Health Care. FFPRHC Guidance (July 2004). Contraceptive choices for breastfeeding women. *J Fam Plann Reprod Health Care* 2004; 30(3):181-9.

Farmer RD, Lawrenson RA, Thompson CR et al. Population-based study of risk of venous thromboembolism associated with various oral contraceptives. *Lancet* 1997;349(9045):83-8.

Peterson HB, Xia Z, Hughes JM et al. The risk of ectopic pregnancy after tubal sterilization. U.S. Collaborative Review of Sterilization Working Group. *N Engl J Med* 1997;336(11):762-7.

References

1. Seibert C, Barbouche E, Fagan J et al. Prescribing oral contraceptives for women older than 35 years of age. *Ann Intern Med* 2003;138(1):54-64.
2. Boukes FS, Beijderwellen L, van der Does FE et al. Summary of the practice guideline "Hormonal contraception" (second revision) from the Dutch College of General Practitioners. *Ned Tijdschr Geneeskd* 2004;148(26):1285-9. Dutch.
3. Van Vliet HA, Grimes DA, Helmerhorst FM et al. Biphasic versus monophasic oral contraceptives for contraception. *Cochrane Database Syst Rev* 2003;(2):CD002032.
4. Practice Committee of the American Society for Reproductive Medicine. Hormonal contraception: recent advances and controversies. *Fert Steril* 2004;82(Suppl 1):S26-32.
5. Rosenberg MJ, Meyers A, Roy V. Efficacy, cycle control and side effects of low- and lower-dose oral contraceptives: a randomized trial of 20 micrograms and 35 micrograms estrogen preparations. *Contraception* 1999;60(6):321-9.
6. Keam SJ, Wagstaff AJ. Ethinylestradiol/drospirenone: a review of its use as an oral contraceptive. *Treat Endocrinol* 2003;2(1):49-70.
7. Kulier R, Helmerhorst FM, Maitra N et al. Effectiveness and acceptability of progestogens in combined oral contraceptives-systematic review. *Reprod Health* 2004;1(1):1.
8. Edwards LA. An update on oral contraceptive options. *Formulary* 2004;39(2):104-21.
9. Sicat BL. Ortho Evra, a new contraceptive patch. *Pharmacotherapy* 2003; 23(4):472-80.
10. Gallo MF, Grimes DA, Schulz KF. Skin patch and vaginal ring versus combined oral contraceptives for contraception. *Cochrane Database Syst Rev* 2003;(1):CD003552.
11. Audet MC, Moreau M, Koltun WD et al. Evaluation of contraceptive efficacy and cycle control of a transdermal contraceptive patch vs an oral contraceptive: a randomized controlled trial. *JAMA* 2001;285(18):2347-54.
12. Gomes MP, Deitcher SR. Risk of venous thromboembolic disease associated with hormonal contraceptives and hormone replacement therapy: a clinical review. *Arch Intern Med* 2004;164(18):1965-76.
13. Black A, Francoeur D, Rowe T et al. SOGC clinical practice guidelines: Canadian contraception consensus. *J Obstet Gynaecol Can* 2004;26(3): 219-96.
14. Holt VL, Cusing-Haugen KL, Daling JR. Body weight and risk of oral contraceptive failure. *Obstet Gynecol* 2002;99(5 Pt 1):820-7.
15. Holt VL, Scholes D, Wicklund KG et al. Body mass index, weight and oral contraceptive failure risk. *Obstet Gynecol* 2005;105(1):46-52.
16. Oddsson K, Leifels-Fischer B, de Melo NR et al. Efficacy and safety of a contraceptive vaginal ring (NuvaRing) compared with a combined oral contraceptive: a 1-year randomized trial. *Contraception* 2005;71(3):176-82.
17. Roumen FJ, Apter D, Mulders TM et al. Efficacy, tolerability and acceptability of a novel contraceptive vaginal ring releasing etonogestrel and ethinyl oestradiol. *Hum Reprod* 2001;16(3):469-75.
18. Dieben TO, Roumen FJ, Apter D. Efficacy, cycle control, and user acceptability of a novel combined contraceptive vaginal ring. *Obstet Gynecol* 2002;100(3):585-93.

19. Voora D, Vijayan A. Mesenteric vein thrombosis associated with intravaginal contraceptives: a case report and review of the literature. *J Thromb Thrombolysis* 2203;15(2):105-8.
20. Curtis KM, Chrisman CE, Peterson HB et al. Contraception for women in selected circumstances. *Obstet Gynecol* 2002;99(6):1100-12.
21. Scholes D, LaCroix AZ, Ichikawa LE et al. Change in bone mineral density among adolescent women using and discontinuing depot medroxyprogesterone acetate contraception. *Arch Pediatr Adolesc Med* 2005;159(2):139-44.
22. Cromer BA, Lazebnik R, Rome E et al. Double-blinded randomized controlled trial of estrogen supplementation in adolescent girls who receive depot medroxyprogesterone acetate for contraception. *Am J Obstet Gynecol* 2005;192(1):42-7.
23. Farley TM, Collins J, Schlesselman JJ. Hormonal contraception and risk of cardiovascular disease. An international perspective. *Contraception* 1998;57(3):211-30.
24. Acute myocardial infarction and combined oral contraceptives: results of an international multicentre case-control study. WHO Collaborative Study of Cardiovascular Disease and Steroid Hormone Contraception. *Lancet* 1997;349(9060):1202-9.
25. Chan WS, Ray J, Wai EK, Ginsburg S et al. Risk of stroke in women exposed to low-dose oral contraceptives: a critical evaluation of the evidence. *Arch Intern Med* 2004;164(7):741-7.
26. Schwartz SM, Petitti DB, Siscovick DS et al. Stroke and use of low-dose oral contraceptives in young women: a pooled analysis of two US studies. *Stroke* 1998;29(11):2277-84.
27. Schwartz SM, Siscovick DS, Longstreth WT et al. Use of low-dose oral contraceptives and stroke in young women. *Ann Intern Med* 1997;127(8 Pt 1):596-603.
28. Chang CL, Donaghy M, Poulter N. Migraine and stroke in young women: case-control study. The World Health Organisation Collaborative Study of Cardiovascular Disease and Steroid Hormone Contraception. *BMJ* 1999;318(7175):13-8.
29. Curtis KM, Mohllajee AP, Peterson HB. Use of combined oral contraceptives among women with migraine and nonmigrainous headaches: a systematic review. *Contraception* 2006;73(2):189-94.
30. Spitzer WO, Faith JM, MacRae KD. Myocardial infarction and third generation oral contraceptives: aggregation of recent studies. *Hum Reprod* 2002;17(9):2307-14.
31. Etminan M, Takkouche B, Isorna FC et al. Risk of ischaemic stroke in people with migraine: systematic review and meta-analysis of observational studies. *BMJ* 2005;330(7482):63.
32. Kemmeren JM, Tanis BC, van den Bosch MA et al. Risk of Arterial Thrombosis in Relation to Oral Contraceptives (RATIO) study: oral contraceptives and the risk of ischemic stroke. *Stroke* 2002;33(5):1202-8.
33. Schiff I, Bell WR, Davis V et al. Oral contraceptives and smoking, current considerations: recommendations of a consensus panel. *Am J Obstet Gynecol* 1999;180(6 Pt 2):S383-4.
34. World Health Organization. *Medical eligibility criteria for contraceptive use*. Geneva (SZ): WHO; 2004. Available from : http://www.who.int/reproductive-health/publications/mec/mec.pdf Accessed September 12, 2006.
35. Petitti DB. Clinical practice. Combination estrogen-progestin oral contraceptives. *N Engl J Med* 2003;349(15):1443-50.
36. Ahmed SB, Hovind P, Parving HH et al. Oral contraceptives, angiotensin-dependent renal vasoconstriction, and risk of diabetic nephropathy. *Diabetes Care* 2005;28(8):1988-94.
37. Farmer RD, Lawrenson RA, Thompson CR et al. Population-based study of risk of venous thromboembolism associated with various oral contraceptives. *Lancet* 1997;349(9045):83-8.
38. Farmer RD, Lawrenson RA, Todd JC et al. A comparison of the risks of venous thromboembolic disease in association with different combined oral contraceptives. *Br J Clin Pharmacol* 2000;49(6):580-90.
39. Kujovich JL. Hormones and pregnancy: thromboembolic risks for women. *Br J Haematol* 2004;126(4):443-54.
40. Bloemenkamp KW, Rosendaal FR, Buller HR et al. Risk of venous thrombosis with use of current low-dose oral contraceptives is not explained by diagnostic suspicion and referral bias. *Arch Intern Med* 1999;159(1):65-70.
41. Lidegaard O, Edstrom B, Kreiner S. Oral contraceptives and venous thromboembolism: a five-year national case-control study. *Contraception* 2002;65(3):187-96.
42. Middeldorp S. Oral contraceptives and the risk of venous thromboembolism. *Gend Med* 2005;2(Suppl A):S3-S9.
43. Nightingale AL, Lawrenson RA, Simpson EL et al. The effects of age, body mass index, smoking and general health on the risk of venous thromboembolism in users of combined oral contraceptives. *Eur J Contracept Reprod Health Care* 2000;5(4):265-74.
44. Vandenbroucke JP, Koster T, Briet E et al. Increased risk of venous thrombosis in oral-contraceptive users who are carriers of factor V Leiden mutation. *Lancet* 1994;344(8935):1453-7.
45. Bloemenkamp KW, Rosendaal FR, Helmerhorst FM et al. Enhancement by factor V Leiden mutation of risk of deep-vein thrombosis associated with oral contraceptives containing a third-generation progestagen. *Lancet* 1995;346(8990):1593-6.
46. Wu O, Robertson L, Twaddle S et al. Screening for thrombophilia in high-risk situations: systematic review and cost-effectiveness analysis. The Thrombosis: Risk and Economic Assessment of Thrombophilia Screening (TREATS) study. *Health Technol Assess* 2006;10(11):1-110.

47. Wu O, Robertson L, Twaddle S et al. Screening for thrombophilia in high-risk situations: a meta-analysis and cost-effectiveness analysis. *Br J Haematol* 2005;131(1):80-90.
48. Borgelt-Hansen L. Oral contraceptives: an update on health benefits and risks. *J Am Pharm Assoc (Wash)* 2001;41(6):875-86.
49. von Hertzen H, Piaggio G, Ding J et al. Low dose mifepristone and two regimens of levonorgestrel for emergency contraception: a WHO multicenter randomised trial. *Lancet* 2002;360(9348):1803-10.
50. Trussell J, Rodriguez G, Ellertson C. Updated estimates of the effectiveness of the Yuzpe regimen of emergency contraception. *Contraception* 1999;59(3):147-51.
51. Rodrigues I, Grou F, Joly J. Effectiveness of emergency contraceptive pills between 72 and 120 hours after unprotected sexual intercourse. *Am J Obstet Gynecol* 2001;184(4):531-7.
52. Randomised controlled trial of levonorgestrel versus the Yuzpe regimen of combined oral contraceptives for emergency contraception. Task Force on Postovulatory Methods of Fertility Regulation. *Lancet* 1998;352(9126):428-33.
53. Piaggio G, von Hertzen H, Grimes DA et al. Timing of emergency contraception with levonorgestrel or the Yuzpe regimen. Task Force on Postovulatory Methods of Fertility Regulation. *Lancet* 1999;353(9154):721.
54. Vasilakis C, Jick SS, Jick H. The risk of venous thromboembolism in users of postcoital contraceptive pills. *Contraception* 1999;59(2):79-83.
55. Trussell J, Ellerston C. Efficacy of emergency contraception. *Fertil Cont Rev* 1995;4:8-11.
56. Thomas MA. Postcoital contraception. *Clin Obstet Gynecol* 2001;44(1):101-5.
57. Truitt ST, Fraser AB, Grimes DA et al. Combined hormonal versus nonhormonal versus progestin-only contraception in lactation. *Cochrane Database Syst Rev* 2003;(2):CD003988.
58. Cates W. Review of non-hormonal contraception (condoms, intrauterine devices, nonoxynol-9 and combos) on HIV acquisition. *J Acquir Immune Defic Syndr* 2005;38(suppl 1):S8-10.
59. Roddy RE, Zekeng L, Ryan RA et al. A controlled trial of nonoxynol-9 film to reduce male-to-femal transmisssion of sexually transmitted diseases. *N Engl J Med* 1998;339(8):504-510.
60. Hooton T, Scholes D, Hughes JP et al. A prospective study of risk factors for symptomatic urinary tract infection in young women. *N Engl J Med* 1996;335(7):468-474.
61. Faich G, Pearson K, Fleming D et al. Toxic shock syndrome and the vaginal contraceptive sponge. *JAMA* 1986;255(2):216-218.
62. Nonoxynol-9 and the risk of HIV transmission. HIV/AIDS Epi Update April 2003. Ottawa, ON: Public Health Agency of Canada; 2003. Available at: http://www.phac-aspc.gc.ca/publicat/epiu-aepi/hiv-vih/nonoxynol_e.html. Accessed September 22, 2006.
63. Peterson HB, Xia Z, Hughes JM et al. The risk of pregnancy after tubal sterilization: findings from the U.S. Collaborative Review of Sterilization. *Am J Obstet Gynecol* 1996;174(4):1161-8.
64. Creasy GW, Abrams LS, Fisher AC. Transdermal contraception. *Semin Reprod Med* 2001;19(4):373-80.
65. Broome M, Fotherby K. Clinical experience with the progestogen-only pill. *Contraception* 1990 ;42(5):489-95.
66. Said S, Omar K, Koetsawang S et al. A multicentered phase III comparative clinical trial of depot-medroxyprogesterone acetate given three-monthly at doses of 100 mg or 150 mg: 1. Contraceptive efficacy and side effects. World Health Organization task force on long-acting systemic agents for fertility regulation. Special programme of research, development and research training in human reproduction. *Contraception* 1986;34(3):223-35.
67. Tremblay D, Gainer E, Ulmann A. The pharmacokinetics of 750 microg levonorgestrel following administration of one single dose or two doses at 12- or 24-h interval. *Contraception* 2001;64(6):327-31.

CHAPTER 62

Dysmenorrhea

Glenn H. Gill, MD, CCFP, FRCSC

Dysmenorrhea is menstrual pain, which affects over 50% of menstruating women to some degree, 15% of whom are incapacitated for one to three days per month.[1,2]

Goals of Therapy

- Decrease or abolish menstrual pain that interferes with everyday activities
- Rule out organic causes of pain that may require alternative therapies

Investigations

- A thorough history to differentiate *primary* from *secondary* dysmenorrhea (Table 1)
- In primary dysmenorrhea:
  - pain starts within several hours before menstruation and up to a few hours after the start of menses[1]
  - pain lasts at most three days
  - pain is described as crampy, located in the lower abdomen and pelvis and is present with each menstrual period
  - other symptoms of prostaglandin excess may be present, e.g., nausea, vomiting, diarrhea, backache, thigh pain, headache, dizziness
- Physical examination for primary dysmenorrhea should reveal:
  - normal abdominal examination, i.e., no evidence of hernia, constipation and other abdominal pathology
  - normal external genitalia
  - no evidence of vaginal anomalies with outflow obstruction
  - normal pelvic examination with no evidence of adnexal tenderness, masses or nodules
- No laboratory tests required unless *secondary* dysmenorrhea suspected; then pelvic ultrasound, laparoscopy, hysteroscopy or hysterosalpingogram (HSG) may be indicated

Table 1: **Characteristics of Dysmenorrhea[1,2,3]**

Primary	Secondary
• Absence of identifiable pelvic pathology • Occurs in ovulatory cycles • Onset within 2 y after menarche and may be accompanied by other symptoms including headache, nausea, dizziness, constipation and diarrhea • Pain due to myometrial contractions induced by prostaglandin production in the secretory endometrium	• Associated with pelvic pathology (e.g., endometriosis, adenomyosis, uterine myomas, endometrial polyps, intrauterine device, pelvic inflammatory disease, obstructed uterine outflow, congenital mullerian malformations, irritable bowel syndrome, simple chronic constipation) • Diagnostic clues include pain onset premenstrually (or lasting throughout the cycle, back pain and pain radiating down the anterior thighs is often found with endometriosis), infertility, dyspareunia, premenstrual or intermenstrual bleeding • Onset immediately at menarche or after age 25 suggests a possible pelvic abnormality • A component of pain may be due to endometrial prostaglandins; therefore partial response to therapy for primary dysmenorrhea may be seen

Therapeutic Choices (Figure 1)

Nonpharmacologic Choices

- Explain that primary dysmenorrhea is a common, natural but exaggerated phenomenon.
- Reassure patient that pain does not indicate an organic process or abnormality in most cases.
- Suggest the use of topical heat therapy.
- Explain that regular exercise may provide some relief by decreasing stress.

Pharmacologic Choices

NSAIDs (Table 2)

Primary dysmenorrhea is caused by abnormal uterine contractions as a result of increased prostaglandin (PG) production by the endometrium in ovulatory cycles. NSAIDs (PG synthetase inhibitors) inhibit endometrial PG production and are the treatment of choice.

All NSAIDs, except ASA which has minimal effect, are effective in about 80% of cases of dysmenorrhea.[4,5] In practice, there appears to be minimal difference among NSAIDs.[4] The choice depends more on tolerance of side effects and cost.

With short-term use, side effects of all NSAIDs are generally minor. NSAIDs should be taken with food, starting immediately at the onset of menses and continued on a regular schedule for 48 to 72 hours. They should not be taken PRN, and are not more effective if started premenstrually.[2]

Combined Oral Contraceptives

Combined oral contraceptives (COCs) inhibit ovulation, which limits endometrial growth and decreases menstrual blood flow, thereby suppressing PG production at menses. COCs have effectively treated dysmenorrhea; however, no large, well-designed studies have been undertaken to prove the effectiveness of low-dose COCs.[6] COCs are the ideal first-line choice for those wishing contraception. Continuous or extended cycle regimens may decrease the frequency of menstrual periods and the incidence of pain. For prescribing information on COCs, see Chapter 61.

Progestin-only Contraceptives

Levonorgestrel intrauterine system (LNG IUS) reduces menstrual bleeding and improves dysmenorrhea.[3,7,8] The release of a low dose of levonorgestrel continuously over a period of at least five years causes the endometrium to become atrophic and inactive[9] (see Chapter 61). Consider LNG IUS as a treatment option in the management of primary dysmenorrhea.[3]

Medroxyprogesterone (MPA), given by a depot injection, suppresses ovulation, induces endometrial atrophy and produces amenorrhea (see Chapter 61). Consider depot MPA as a treatment option in the management of primary dysmenorrhea[3] in women who cannot tolerate estrogen and in women who are over 35 years who smoke. Use with caution in adolescents aged 12 to 18 years due to its effect of reducing bone mineral density.

Therapeutic Tips

- A therapeutic trial of three to six months of either an NSAID or a COC is usually sufficient to demonstrate effectiveness; if either fails, the other may be tried before further investigation.
- Continuous use of COCs is often successful if cyclic use fails.
- Levonorgestrel IUS is highly effective for primary dysmenorrhea and for pain secondary to endometriosis.
- Pharmacotherapy fails in 20% of patients. These patients often have secondary dysmenorrhea and require further investigation. Diagnostic laparoscopy is the most useful to differentiate primary from secondary dysmenorrhea. Therapy can then be directed and may involve surgery, such as laser ablation or electrofulguration of endometriosis.
- In a small percentage of patients in whom pharmacotherapy fails, extensive investigation will not identify a specific cause. Consider other diagnoses (such as a GI or musculoskeletal problem) when pharmacotherapy fails.
- Calcium channel blockers, magnesium, clonidine, transcutaneous electrical nerve stimulation, acupuncture, hypnosis, levonorgestrel-releasing intrauterine system, vitamin B_1, magnesium, omega-3 fatty acids, transdermal nitroglycerin and

chiropractor spinal manipulation have been studied,[10,11,12] but have not been compared to NSAIDs or COCs.

Figure 1: Management of Dysmenorrhea

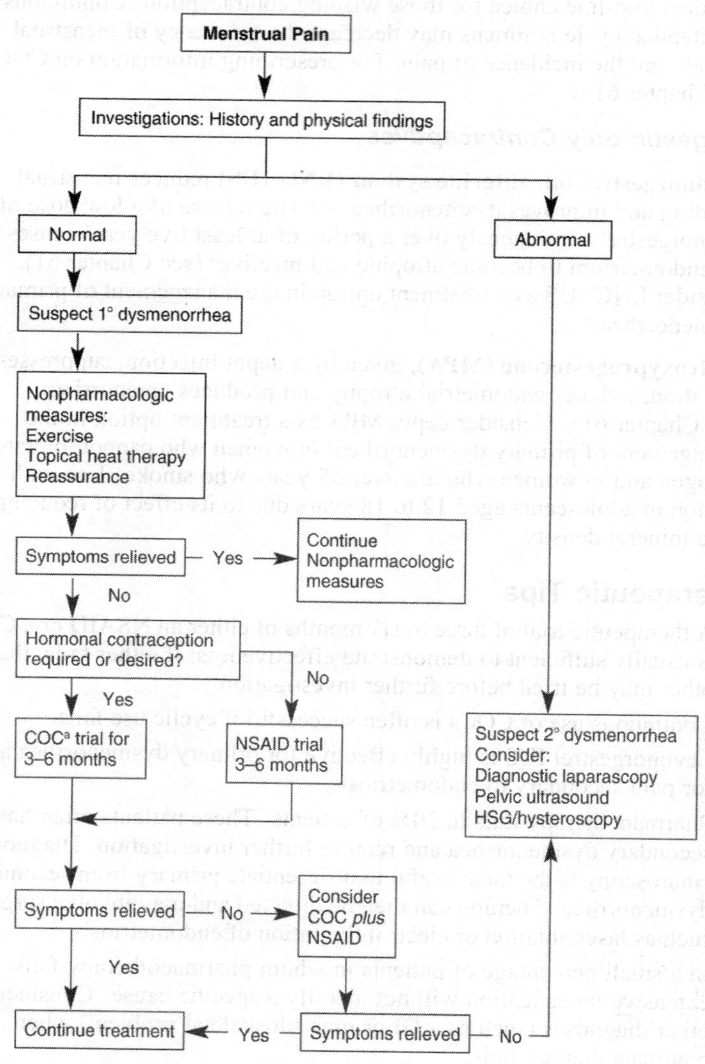

[a] Consider levonorgestrel IUS (Mirena) or depot medroxyprogesterone in certain situations (see text).
Abbreviations: COC = combined oral contraceptive; HSG = hysterosalpingogram

Table 2: **NSAIDs for the Management of Dysmenorrhea**

Class	Drug	Dose	Adverse Effects	Comments	Cost[a]
NSAIDs, acetic acid derivatives	*diclofenac sodium* Voltaren, generics	50–75 mg daily or divided twice daily with food	Very common (> 10%): dyspepsia, nausea/vomiting. Common (5–10%): nonspecific rash, pruritus, dizziness, headache.	First line in the management of dysmenorrhea. Prescribe oral contraceptives if hormonal contraception is required or desired. Can be given in combination if treatment with NSAIDs is inadequate. Contraindications: hypersensitivity to ASA, active pelvic inflammatory bowel disease, existing renal disease, clotting disorders. SSRIs may ↑ risk of gastrointestinal bleeding when used with NSAIDs.	$-$$
	diclofenac potassium Voltaren Rapide, generics	Loading dose of 100 mg then 50 mg Q6–8H with food. Max daily dose: 150 mg	See diclofenac sodium.	See diclofenac sodium.	$$$$
	indomethacin generics	25 mg TID up to six times a day with food. Max daily dose: 200 mg	See diclofenac sodium.	See diclofenac sodium.	$

(cont'd)

Table 2: **NSAIDs for the Management of Dysmenorrhea** *(cont'd)*

Class	Drug	Dose	Adverse Effects	Comments	Cost[a]
NSAIDs, fenamates	*mefenamic acid* generics	Loading dose of 500 mg then 250 mg Q6H with food	See diclofenac sodium.	See diclofenac sodium. Theoretically, the fenamate NSAIDs should be the most effective pain relievers; in addition to inhibiting PG synthesis, they also bind to PG receptors and have an antagonistic effect.	$$
NSAIDs, oxicams	*piroxicam* generics	10–40 mg daily with food	See diclofenac sodium.	See diclofenac sodium.	$-$$
NSAIDs, propionic acid derivatives	*ibuprofen* Advil, Motrin IB, generics	200–600 mg Q6H with food Max daily dose: 2400 mg	See diclofenac sodium.	See diclofenac sodium.	$
	ketoprofen generics	50 mg TID with food	See diclofenac sodium.	See diclofenac sodium.	$
	naproxen Naprosyn, generics	Loading dose of 500 mg then 250 mg Q6–8H or 500 mg BID with food. Max daily dose: 1250 mg	See diclofenac sodium.	See diclofenac sodium.	$
	naproxen sodium Anaprox, generics	275–550 mg BID with food	See diclofenac sodium.	See diclofenac sodium.	$$

[a] Cost of 7-day supply; includes drug cost only.

Dosage adjustment may be required in renal impairment; see Appendix I.

Legend: $ < $5 $-$$ < $5–10 $$ $5–10 $$$ $10–15 $$$$ $15–20

Suggested Readings

Dawood MY. Primary dysmenorrhea: advances in pathogenesis and management. *Obstet Gynecol* 2006; 108(2):428-41.

Emans SJH, Goldstein DP, editors. *Pediatric and adolescent gynecology.* 3rd ed. Boston (MA): Little, Brown; 1990. p.291-9.

Fraser IS. Prostaglandins, prostaglandin inhibitors and their roles in gynaecological disorders. *Baillieres Clin Obstet Gynaecol* 1992;6(4):829-57.

Lefebvre G, Pinsonneault O, Antao V et al. Primary dysmenorrhea consensus guideline. *J Obstet Gynaecol Can* 2005;27(12):1117-46.

Rapkin AJ. Pelvic pain and dysmenorrhea. In: Berek JS, Adashi EY, Hillard PA, editors. *Novak's gynecology.* 12th ed. Baltimore (MD): Williams & Wilkins; 1996. p.399-428.

Speroff L, Glass RH, Kase NG. *Clinical gynecologic endocrinology and infertility.* 6th ed. Baltimore (MD): Lippincott Williams & Wilkins; 1999. p.566-7.

References

1. Dawood MY. Primary dysmenorrhea: advances in pathogenesis and management. *Obstet Gynecol* 2006; 108(2):428-41.
2. Speroff L, Glass RH, Kase NG. *Clinical gynecologic endocrinology and infertility.* 6th ed. Baltimore (MD): Lippincott Williams & Wilkins; 1999.
3. Lefebvre G, Pinsonneault O, Antao V et al. Primary dysmenorrhea consensus guideline. *J Obstet Gynaecol Can* 2005;27(12):1117-46.
4. Marjoribanks J, Proctor ML, Farquhar C. Nonsteroidal anti-inflammatory drugs for primary dysmenorrhoea. *Cochrane Database Syst Rev* 2003;(4):CD001751.
5. Zhang WY, Li Wan Po A. Efficacy of minor analgesics in primary dysmenorrhoea: a systematic review. *Br J Obstet Gynaecol* 1998; 105(7):780-9.
6. Proctor ML, Roberts H, Farquhar CM. Combined oral contraceptive pill (OCP) as treatment for primary dysmenorrhoea. *Cochrane Database Syst Rev* 2001;(4):CD002120.
7. Barrington JW, Bowen-Simpkins P. The levonorgestrel intrauterine system in the management of menorrhagia. *Br J Obstet Gynaecol* 1997;104(5):614-6.
8. Andersson JK, Rybo G. Levonorgestrel-releasing intrauterine device in the treatment of menorrhagia. *Br J Obstet Gynaecol* 1990; 97(8):690-4.
9. Critchley HO, Wang H, Jones RL et al. Morphological and functional features of endometrial decidualization following long-term intrauterine levonorgestrel delivery. *Hum Reprod* 1998;13(5):1218-24.
10. Proctor ML, Smith CA, Farquhar CM et al. Transcutaneous electrical nerve stimulation and acupuncture for primary dysmenorrhoea. *Cochrane Database Syst Rev* 2002;(1):CD002123.
11. Proctor ML, Latthe PM, Farquhar CM et al. Surgical interruption of pelvic nerve pathways for primary and secondary dysmenorrhoea. *Cochrane Database Syst Rev* 2005;(4):CD001896.
12. Wilson ML, Murphy PA. Herbal and dietary therapies for primary and secondary dysmenorrhoea. *Cochrane Database Syst Rev* 2001;(3):CD002124.

CHAPTER 63
Endometriosis

G. Barry Gilliland, MD, FRCSC

Endometriosis, diagnosed by finding tissue that histologically resembles endometrium at sites outside the uterine cavity, can cause pelvic pain, dysmenorrhea and infertility. Histological confirmation requires at least two of the following: endometrial epithelium, endometrial glands, endometrial stroma and hemosiderin-laden macrophages. Although endometriosis is most often classified according to the revised American Fertility Sterility Classification[1] (r-AFS) there is no direct correlation between the volume of endometriotic tissue, i.e., stage of disease, and either pregnancy rates or severity of symptoms.

Recurrent pain from endometriosis occurs frequently. After treatment with gonadotropin-releasing hormone analogues (GnRH-analogues), the rate of recurrent pelvic pain over five years ranges from 37% in patients with mild endometriosis to 74% in those with severe disease.[2] Following surgical ablation/resection of endometriosis, the risk of recurrence of pain is estimated to be as high as 40% at ten years of follow-up.[3]

Endometriosis may be treated with drugs, surgery or both. Individualize treatment according to age, duration of infertility, severity of pelvic pain, response to previous therapies, anticipated side effects and cost.

This chapter focuses on endometriosis-associated pain, endometriosis-associated infertility and recurrent endometriosis.

Goals of Therapy

- Relieve pain
- Treat infertility
- Prevent recurrence

Investigations

Diagnosis of endometriosis is difficult due to its variable presentation. Significant overlap with other conditions, e.g., irritable bowel syndrome, has been observed.[4]

- History
  - history of pelvic pain (cyclical at first, becomes continuous as endometriosis worsens), dysmenorrhea (does not diminish after menstrual day 2), deep dyspareunia or infertility suggests endometriosis
- Physical examination
  - pelvic examination: tenderness, particularly in the uterosacral ligament area, especially around the time of menses, suggests endometriosis

- Objective measurements
  - laparascopy ± biopsy: gold standard. Endometriotic tissue may have a typical or atypical appearance. Focal deposits may have the classic blue or black appearance. They may also appear yellow, brown, white or red—81% of such areas show histological evidence of endometriosis[5]
  - serum CA 125 (a tumor-associated protein) levels: often significantly elevated (> 35 IU/mL) but not always found with endometriosis. Other causes of elevated serum CA 125 levels: pelvic inflammatory disease, epithelial ovarian cancer and pregnancy. Serum CA 125 levels are useful for treatment follow-up and may aid in identifying infertile women with severe endometriosis who could benefit from surgery[6]
  - ultrasound: reliably identify masses with features of endometriomas;[7] however, these features are nonspecific. Sensitivity of ultrasound is poor for the detection of focal implants[8]
  - MRI: useful for identifying deep subperitoneal lesions and for monitoring residual or recurrent disease after surgery

Endometriosis-associated Pain

Therapeutic Choices (Figure 1)

Combined surgery and drug treatment offer the best options to maximize pain relief. Some authors report a 30% placebo response rate and about 20% of patients will have no benefit from surgery.[9] As conservative surgery is considered to be cytoreductive in the higher stages of disease, it is reasonable to use surgery to "reduce" this stage of the disease before initiating drug treatment. Once drug treatment is discontinued, symptoms may recur.

Nonpharmacologic Choices

Surgery (Table 1)

The primary goals in the surgical treatment of endometriosis-associated pain include the removal of typical and atypical endometriotic implants and the restoration of pelvic anatomy.

Definitive therapy of endometriosis-associated pain requires total abdominal hysterectomy and bilateral salpingo-oophorectomy with complete excision or ablation of endometriosis. It is considered 90 to 95% effective for pain relief.[10] Many patients have persistent pain due to other pelvic pathology, notably interstitial cystitis and irritable bowel syndrome or regional sympathetic syndrome. The major indication for definitive therapy is intractable pain in patients who have not responded to more conservative measures or who have completed their families. Estrogen replacement therapy postoperatively is associated with minimal (1 to 3%) risk of disease recurrence.[11]

Conservative surgery for endometriosis is a cytoreductive procedure that is not necessarily curative. Sixty to 100% of patients experience decreased severity of pain after ablative surgery.[12] Recurrence rates range from 13.5 to 40.3% at five years.[13] Conservative surgery can be performed by laparoscopy or laparotomy and both procedures are equally effective.[14]

Potential advantages of laparoscopy include the ability to treat the disease at the time of diagnosis, enhanced removal and ablation of endometriosis, reduced morbidity, shorter hospital stay, rapid recovery and potential decrease in the rate of postoperative adhesion formation.[15] Laser ablation and laparascopic uterosacral nerve ablation (LUNA) effectively relieved pain in 62.5% of treated patients, compared to 22.6% in the control group.[16]

Presacral neurectomy, in conjunction with conservative surgery for endometriosis, may be effective in relieving severe midline dysmenorrhea associated with endometriosis if the surgeon completely resects the presacral nerve plexus.[17] Results of adding this procedure to conservative surgery are mixed.

Table 1: **Surgical Management of Endometriosis-associated Infertility or Pain**

Surgical Approach	Comments
Conservative surgery (laparoscopy or laparotomy)	Used in endometriosis-associated infertility Laparoscopy offers advantage of shorter hospital stay, less postoperative pain and quicker convalescence, but requires surgical expertise and expensive equipment Used in endometriosis-associated pain Cytoreductive procedure that is not necessarily curative 2/3 of patients treated with surgery have pain relief for at least one year
Laparoscopic uterosacral nerve ablation (LUNA)	Used with conservative surgery in women with dysmenorrhea, dyspareunia or pelvic pain to relieve endometriosis-associated pain
Presacral neurectomy (PSN)	Used in conjunction with conservative surgery for relieving severe midline dysmenorrhea associated with endometriosis
Hysterectomy	Limited role in treatment-resistant endometriosis-associated dysmenorrhea in women with endometriosis confined to the uterus if completed bearing children Major indication is intractable pain that has not responded to more conservative measures
Hysterectomy plus bilateral salpingo-oophorectomy	May be offered as definitive therapy for treatment-resistant endometriosis-associated pelvic pain or adnexal masses in women with extensive extra-uterine disease

Pharmacologic Choices (Table 2)

Nonsteroidal Anti-inflammatory Drugs (NSAIDs)

NSAIDs inhibit endometrial prostaglandins, which cause abnormal uterine contractions (see Chapter 62), and are recommended as first-line treatment of mild endometriosis-associated pelvic pain and dysmenorrhea. They are most effective if started at the onset of menstrual symptoms and given throughout the menstrual period. NSAIDs are well tolerated, safe and inexpensive.

Opioids

Opioid analgesics are used but their effect on bowel motility may contribute to pelvic pain. Although long-term use may lead to addiction, use may be appropriate in select patients with intractable chronic pain and no history of drug abuse. Avoid opiates with short half-lives as they are associated with rebound pain. Fentanyl transdermal patches may be a good choice as more consistent serum levels are maintained.[18]

Contraceptives

Combined oral contraceptives (COC) relieve symptoms in 75 to 100% of cases of endometriosis-associated pain, reduce menstrual blood flow and suppress ovulation. The use of a COC, either cyclically or continuously, may delay the onset or recurrence of disease. When used continuously, low-dose monophasic COCs (20–35 µg ethinyl estradiol) produce amenorrhea.[19,20] Pain, associated with estrogen and progestin withdrawal, may be suppressed.[19,20]

Progestin-only contraceptives inhibit ovulation and suppress gonadotropin secretion thereby inducing a hypoestrogenic, acyclic hormonal environment.

Medroxyprogesterone acetate (MPA), 150 mg every 6 to 12 weeks given by a depot injection (Depo-Provera), significantly reduces pain and induces amenorrhea.[21] Do not use MPA in younger women who wish to become pregnant immediately after stopping treatment because resumption of ovulation is delayed following cessation of therapy. As depot MPA may decrease bone mineral density (see Chapter 61),[22,23,24] reserve use for older patients who do not want to conceive and wish to avoid surgery. Continuous oral MPA, 20–40 mg daily, relieves endometriosis-associated pain. Spotting frequently occurs but ovulation resumes promptly after discontinuation. **Levonorgestrel (LNG)** intrauterine system (IUS) provides an alternative route of delivering the drug directly into the uterine cavity at a steady rate of 20 µg/day over a five-year period.[25] An effective hormonal option for the treatment of symptomatic endometriosis (mild to moderate disease), LNG IUS alters the staging of disease[26] and is effective in symptom control for up to three years.[27] Advantages include lower cost, no repeated treatments and fewer side effects. Breakthrough bleeding is common especially in the first three months. Amenorrhea occurs in up to 35% of patients in one year.

Androgen Agonists

Danazol inhibits ovarian estrogen production and causes atrophy of endometrial deposits. It is highly effective in the treatment of endometriosis-associated dysmenorrhea but less effective in the management of chronic pelvic pain.[28] Endometriomas greater than 1 cm in diameter respond poorly to danazol. Doses of 600–800 mg/day for six months effectively alleviate symptoms of endometriosis, particularly in the earlier stages of the disease.[29] Hypoandrogenic side effects such as hirsutism and acne are common with danazol therapy.

Gonadotropin-releasing Hormone Analogues (GnRH-analogues)

Gonadotropin-releasing hormone analogues (GnRH-analogues) inhibit the hypothalamic-pituitary-gonadal axis, reducing the secretion of LH and FSH required for follicular development and resulting in a markedly hypoestrogenic state, which induces atrophy and regression of endometriotic implants.[30] Endometriomas respond poorly to GnRH-analogues.

Use **nafarelin** 200 μg intranasally twice daily, **goserelin** 3.6 mg subcutaneously monthly or **leuprolide** 3.75 mg intramuscularly monthly. There is no advantage of one GnRH-analogue over another. No significant differences in pain relief or clinical symptoms were observed using GnRH-analogue therapy for three or six months.[31] Hypoestrogenic adverse effects are common and include hot flashes, insomnia, mood changes and vaginal atrophy. Decrease in bone mineral density of 1–3% is seen when GnRH-analogue is taken for three to six months.[32] Recurrence of endometriosis symptoms commonly occurs within nine to twelve months after completion of therapy.

Add-back hormone therapy, consisting of continuous estrogen (e.g., oral conjugated estrogens 0.625 mg daily) plus progestin (e.g., oral MPA 2.5 mg daily) improves hypoestrogenic symptoms and prevents bone density loss, which may allow a longer duration of therapy.[33] GnRH-analogue therapy, combined with add-back therapy, is as effective as GnRH-analogue therapy alone for relieving pelvic symptoms.[34] GnRH-analogues are used for six to twelve months with add-back hormone therapy[35] or for six months if no add-back hormones are given. Optimal use of add-back therapy has not been established.

Bisphosphonates can be used in patients who are on GnRH-analogue for longer than six months or who are at a high risk or have evidence of osteoporosis (see Chapter 73). [36]

Aromatase Inhibitors

Patients with endometriosis have a high level of aromatase P450 expression in eutopic and ectopic endometrium. Aromatase P450 inhibitors (**anastrozole, letrozole**) reduce estrogen produced from sources other than the ovary such as the adrenal gland. Aromatase inhibitors are used with oral contraceptives, GnRH-analogues or a progestin to reduce the risk of developing ovarian cysts.[37] Aromatase inhibitors represent a promising new approach to the therapy for endometriosis,[37,38,39] but remain investigational.[40]

Antiprogestins

Mifepristone (RU-486) shows promise in the management of pain in endometriosis but larger controlled clinical trials are needed to establish the role of antiprogestins in the management of endometriosis.[41] Mifepristone is not available in Canada.

Endometriosis-associated Infertility

Therapeutic Choices (Figure 1)

Nonpharmacologic Choices

Surgery (Table 1)

Laparoscopy and laparotomy are equally successful in the surgical treatment of endometriosis-associated infertility.[42,14] Laparoscopy offers the advantage of a shorter hospital stay, less pain and quicker convalescence but requires surgical expertise and expensive equipment.

Laparoscopic resection or ablation of minimal or mild endometriosis enhances fecundity in infertile women.[10] There is no relative advantage to any of the various cytoreductive techniques (coagulation, laser vaporization or excision of endometriosis).

The addition of postsurgical gonadotropin-releasing hormone analogue (GnRH-analogue) therapy offers no advantage over surgery alone in terms of pain relief or increased fertility.[11]

Assisted Reproductive Technologies

The efficacy of in vitro fertilization–embryo transfer (IVF–ET) in treating endometriosis-associated infertility has not been evaluated based on severity of disease or other important prognostic variables such as age and duration of infertility. With improvements in IVF programs, this form of therapy may be considered in milder forms of endometriosis-associated infertility.

Pharmacologic Choices (Table 2, Table 3)

Ovulation Induction

Clomiphene 50 mg daily for five days, administered on days three to seven of the menstrual cycle, is simple and inexpensive. Clomiphene use for ovulation induction with or without intrauterine insemination does not significantly increase pregnancy rates but helps with timing intercourse or intrauterine insemination. **Human chorionic gonadotropin (hCG)**

is sometimes added in a dose of 5000 to 10 000 units im at midcycle, ± intrauterine insemination.

A Cochrane review concluded that administering GnRH-analogues for three to six months prior to IVF or intracytoplasmic sperm injection (ICSI) in women with endometriosis results in a fourfold increase in the odds of clinical pregnancy.[43] Use gonadotropin therapy, referred to as superovulation or controlled ovarian hyperstimulation, together with intrauterine insemination, to treat minimal or mild endometriosis-associated infertility.[44] Live birth rates diminish with successive treatments. Because of its cost, limit gonadotropin therapy to three cycles.

As fecundity significantly decreases and spontaneous abortion rate increases in women > 35 years, these patients may benefit from an aggressive therapeutic plan with superovulation/intrauterine insemination or IVF–ET.[45]

Ovarian Suppression

Ovarian suppression is inappropriate to use for endometriosis-associated infertility as it prevents pregnancy. It may be used as an option if there is severe coexisting endometriosis-associated pain.[46]

Recurrent Endometriosis

Therapeutic Choices (Figure 1)

Nonpharmacologic Choices

Surgery (Table 1)

Conservative surgery may be considered for recurrent disease, if pain relief is required,[47] or a patient declines *definitive* surgery. Between 20 and 40% of patients suffer recurrence five years after conservative surgery.[47] Pregnancy does not influence the average time to recurrence of symptoms.[48]

Hysterectomy, with or without bilateral oophorectomy, is often used as a definitive therapy for the treatment of endometriosis associated with pelvic pain or adnexal masses. A retrospective study of recurrence of symptoms after definitive surgery, with a mean follow-up of 4 years, 10 months, showed that 62% of patients with ovarian conservation had recurrent symptoms and 31% required further surgery. In women with bilateral oophorectomy, 10% had recurrent symptoms and 3.7% required further surgery.[49] The majority of patients who had bilateral oophorectomy had subsequently taken estrogen replacement therapy with no adverse effect on endometriosis. There is no advantage in delaying the introduction of estrogen replacement therapy after surgery.[49]

Pharmacologic Choices (Table 2, Table 3)

Mild Disease

Low-dose **OCs** reduce symptoms of mild disease (suggested by pelvic tenderness, no nodularity). Low-dose OCs can be used for an unlimited time. Use **medroxyprogesterone**, **danazol** or a **GnRH-analogue** if low-dose OC therapy is ineffective.

Advanced Disease

Medroxyprogesterone, danazol or a GnRH-analogue relieve the pain of advanced disease (suggested by an adnexal mass, a fixed uterus or obliteration of the cul-de-sac) but may not affect the disease process. Although these drugs may reduce the size of endometriomas, their use is not necessarily associated with a reduction in surgical time or the eventual outcome of surgery.

Use danazol or a progestin as alternative treatment when there has been marked unrecovered bone loss with GnRH-analogue therapy, bone density is not being evaluated or the patient has other risk factors for osteoporosis.

Use GnRH-analogue treatment, combined with add-back hormonal therapy as an alternative to repeated GnRH monotherapy (see Endometriosis-associated Pain: Gonadotropin-releasing Hormone Analogues). The addition of a bisphosphonate prevents bone loss in a small group of endometriosis patients treated with a GnRH-analogue.[36] Add-back therapy (adding HT to GnRH-analogue) does not increase the recurrence rates of endometriosis. Efficacy of treatment is not reduced, and adverse hypoestrogenic effects are decreased although not abolished.[50]

Therapeutic Tips

- Endometriosis must be diagnosed by laparoscopy ± biopsy.
- Chronic pelvic pain is a diagnosis, in itself, and should be treated as such.
- Drug treatment of endometriosis does not improve fecundity.[45]
- NSAIDs can be used as an adjunct with combined oral contraceptives, progestin-only contraceptives, GnRH-analogues or danazol, if needed.[19]
- Currently, no single add-back hormone therapy has been recommended for all women treated with GnRH-analogues.
- GnRH-analogues are not more effective than COCs or progestins in managing endometriosis-associated pain.
- Hormonal treatment may be used prior to surgery to reduce the size of endometrial implants; however, this strategy does not prolong pain-free interval, decrease recurrence rates or increase pregnancy rates.
- Postsurgery residual disease treated with progestin, danazol or GnRH-analogue in combination with surgery (laparotomy,

laparoscopic conservative, definitive surgical treatment) results in prolonged pain-free interval and delayed recurrence rates.[51]

Figure 1: **Endometriosis Management**

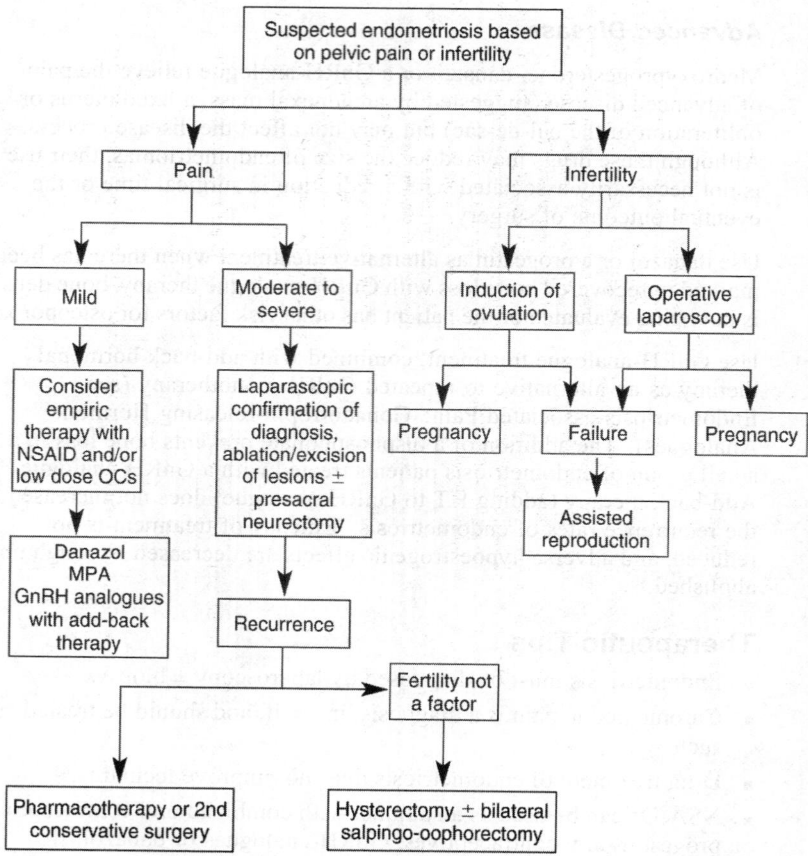

Abbreviations: NSAID = nonsteroidal anti-inflammatory drug; OCs = oral contraceptives; MPA = medroxyprogesterone acetate.

Table 2: Drugs Used for Endometriosis-associated Pain

Class	Drug	Dose	Adverse Effects	Comments	Cost[a]
Contraceptives, oral—combined estrogen (< 50 µg EE) and progestin, monophasic	*EE 35 µg/ norethindrone 1 mg* Brevicon 1/35, Ortho 1/35, Select 1/35	1 tab po daily	Major: thromboembolism (rare), stroke, retinal artery thrombosis, myocardial infarction, benign liver tumour, cholelithiasis, hypertension. Common: breakthrough bleeding/spotting, amenorrhea, nausea/vomiting, bloating, chloasma, breast tenderness, mood changes such as depression, headaches.	Continuous use (no break for period) of COCs produces anovulation and amenorrhea. Cyclic or continuous use of COCs may delay onset or recurrence of disease. If used continuously, may consider short breaks Q3 mo. Watch for danger signals: ACHES—abdominal pain, chest pain, headaches, eye problems, severe leg pain. Advise physician consult. *Absolute contraindications:* history of MI or ischemic heart disease, cerebrovascular disease, complicated valvular heart disease, current or past history VTE, severe cirrhosis, liver tumour, breast cancer, diabetes with microvascular complications, migraines with aura, < 6 wk postpartum if breastfeeding, smoker > 35 y (≥ 15 cigarettes/day), hypertension (SBP ≥ 160 mm Hg or DBP ≥ 100 mm Hg), known coagulation-factor deficiency.	$
	EE 35 µg/ norethindrone 0.5 mg Brevicon 0.5/35, Ortho 0.5/35	1 tab po daily	See EE 35 µg/ norethindrone 1 mg.	See EE 35 µg/ norethindrone 1 mg.	$
	EE 35 µg/ cyproterone 2 mg Diane-35	1 tab po daily	See EE 35 µg/ norethindrone 1 mg.	See EE 35 µg/ norethindrone 1 mg.	$

(cont'd)

Table 2: **Drugs Used for Endometriosis-associated Pain** *(cont'd)*

Class	Drug	Dose	Adverse Effects	Comments	Cost[a]
	EE 35 µg/ norgestimate 0.25 mg Cyclen	1 tab po daily	See EE 35 µg/ norethindrone 1 mg.	See EE 35 µg/ norethindrone 1 mg.	$
	EE 30 µg/ desogestrel 0.15 mg Marvelon, Ortho-Cept	1 tab po daily	See EE 35 µg/ norethindrone 1 mg.	See EE 35 µg/ norethindrone 1 mg.	$
	EE 30 µg/ ethynodiol diacetate 2 mg Demulen 30	1 tab po daily	See EE 35 µg/ norethindrone 1 mg.	See EE 35 µg/ norethindrone 1 mg.	$
	EE 30 µg/ norethindrone acetate 1.5 mg Loestrin 1.5/30	1 tab po daily	See EE 35 µg/ norethindrone 1 mg.	See EE 35 µg/ norethindrone 1 mg.	$
	EE 30 µg/ drospirenone 3 mg Yasmin	1 tab po daily	See EE 35 µg/ norethindrone 1 mg.	See EE 35 µg/ norethindrone 1 mg.	$
	EE 20 µg/ norethindrone acetate 1 mg Minestrin 1/20	1 tab po daily	See EE 35 µg/ norethindrone 1 mg.	See EE 35 µg/ norethindrone 1 mg.	$
	EE 20 µg/ levonorgestrel 0.1 mg Alesse	1 tab po daily	See EE 35 µg/ norethindrone 1 mg.	See EE 35 µg/ norethindrone 1 mg.	$

Class	Drug	Dose	Adverse Effects	Comments	Cost[a]
Contraceptives, progestin-only, injectable	*medroxyprogesterone acetate* Depo-Provera	150 mg im Q6–12 wk	Breast tenderness, insomnia or somnolence, fatigue, mood changes such as depression or irritability, dizziness, headache, skin sensitivity reactions, hyperpyrexia, change in weight, acne. Long-term: ↓ in BMD, delayed return of fertility.	Not recommended for women who wish to become pregnant immediately after stopping treatment as resumption of ovulation is significantly delayed after stopping treatment. Consider other options in women with risk factors for osteoporosis. Reserve for patients who are older and/or who do not want to conceive and wish to avoid surgery.	$$/ 3 months
Contraceptives, progestin-only, intrauterine system (IUS)	*levonorgestrel 20 µg/day* Mirena	Insert every 5 years. Releases levonorgestrel 20 µg/day into uterine cavity	Spotting for first 3 mo after insertion; menstrual changes such as amenorrhea.	Inserted within 7 days of onset of menses. Intrauterine progestogen (levonorgestrel) is effective in symptom control for at least 3 years.[52]	$320/unit
Gonadotropin Inhibitors, pituitary	*danazol* Cyclomen	600–800 mg po daily divided BID–QID without interruption for 3 to 6 mo	Androgenic side effects: voice deepening (irreversible), ↓ breast size, ↑ weight, hirsutism, ↑ LDL. Menopausal symptoms: hot flashes, vaginal dryness.	Avoid in patients with dyslipidemia or liver disease. Use limited by poor tolerability. Effective contraception necessary for duration of treatment.	$450
Gonadotropin-releasing Hormone Analogues (GnRH-analogues)	*buserelin acetate* Suprefact	200 µg into each nostril TID × 6 mo	Bone loss (if used for 6 mo, reversible upon cessation of treatment). Vasomotor symptoms: hot flashes, vaginal dryness, insomnia, loss of libido, emotional lability.	A temporary ↑ in pain upon initiation of therapy may occur. Usually given for 6 mo as long-term use associated with significant ↓ in bone mineral density. Symptoms may recur within 9–12 mo after stopping therapy; *add-back* hormonal therapy can improve hypoestrogenic symptoms and control bone loss.	$$$$

(cont'd)

Table 2: **Drugs Used for Endometriosis-associated Pain** *(cont'd)*

Class	Drug	Dose	Adverse Effects	Comments	Cost[a]
	goserelin acetate Zoladex, Zoladex LA	3.6 mg sc every mo × 6 mo 10.8 mg sc Q12 wk × 6 mo	See buserelin acetate.	See buserelin acetate.	3.6 mg: $400/unit 10.8mg: $1100/unit
	leuprolide acetate Lupron Depot	3.75 mg im every mo × 6 mo 11.25 mg im Q3 mo × 6 mo	See buserelin acetate.	See buserelin acetate.	3.75 mg: $340/unit 11.25mg: $1000/unit
	nafarelin acetate Synarel	1 spray (200 µg) into one nostril a.m. and into the other p.m. × 6 mo Total daily dose: 400 µg	See buserelin acetate.	See buserelin acetate.	$295/unit
	triptorelin pamoate Trelstar	3.75 mg im Q28 days × 6 mo	See buserelin acetate.	See buserelin acetate.	$290
NSAIDs, propionic acid derivatives	*ibuprofen* Advil, Motrin IB, generics	400 mg po Q4–6H Max daily dose: 2400 mg	Very common (> 10%): dyspepsia, nausea/vomiting. Common (5–10%): nonspecific rash, pruritus, dizziness, headache.	First line in the management of mild endometriosis-associated pelvic pain and dysmenorrhea. May start treatment at the onset of symptoms. Do not take on an as-needed basis during this time. Contraindications: hypersensitivity to ASA, active pelvic inflammatory bowel disease, existing renal disease, clotting disorders. SSRIs may ↑ risk of gastrointestinal bleeding when used with NSAIDs.	$

Class	Drug	Dose	Adverse Effects	Comments	Cost[a]
	naproxen (renal symbol) Naprosyn, generics	250 mg po Q6–8H Max daily dose: 1250 mg	See ibuprofen.	See ibuprofen.	$
Progestins, oral	*medroxyprogesterone acetate (MPA)* Provera, generics	20–40 mg po daily	Well tolerated. Breakthrough bleeding, weight gain, fluid retention, mood swings.	Ovulation resumes promptly after stopping oral MPA.	$

[a] Cost of 30-day supply unless otherwise specified; includes drug cost only.
(renal symbol) Dosage adjustment required in renal impairment; see Appendix I.
Legend: $ < $25 $$ $25–50 $$$ $50–100 $$$$ $100–125

Table 3: **Drugs Used for Endometriosis-associated Infertility**

Class	Drug	Dose	Comments	Cost[a]
Ovulation Stimulators	*clomiphene* Clomid, Serophene	50 mg po daily × 5 days. Start on 5th day of menstrual cycle if bleeding occurs. May start at any time if no recent uterine bleeding. Can ↑ dose to 100 mg po daily × 5 days, if ovulation does not occur after initial course within 30 days of previous course.	Repeat regimen for 3 or 4 cycles if conception does not occur with ovulation.	$25

[a] Cost of 5-day supply; includes drug cost only.

Suggested Readings

Crosignani P, Olive D, Bergqvist A et al. Advances in the management of endometriosis: an update for clinicians. *Hum Reprod Update* 2006;12(2):179-89.

Jarrell JF, Vilos GA, Allaire C et al. Consensus guidelines for the management of chronic pelvic pain. *J Obstet Gynaecol Can* 2005;27(8):781-826. Available from: http://sogc.org/guidelines/public/164E-CPG1-August2005.pdf Accessed May 29, 2007.

Jarrell JF, Vilos GA, Allaire C et al. Consensus guidelines for the management of chronic pelvic pain. *J Obstet Gynaecol Can* 2005;27(9):869-87. Available from: http://sogc.org/guidelines/public/164E-CPG2-September2005.pdf Accessed May 29, 2007.

References

1. [No authors listed]. Revised American Fertility Society classification of endometriosis: 1985. *Fertil Steril* 1985;43(3):351-2.
2. Waller KG, Shaw RW. Gonadotropin-releasing hormone analogues for the treatment of endometriosis: long-term follow-up. *Fertil Steril* 1993;59(3):511-5.
3. Wheeler JM, Malinak LR. Recurrent endometriosis: incidence, management, and prognosis. *Am J Obstet Gynecol* 1983;146(3):247-53.
4. Zondervan KT, Yudkin PL, Vessey MP et al. Patterns of diagnosis and referral in women consulting for chronic pelvic pain in UK primary care. *Br J Obstet Gynaecol* 1999;106(11):1156-61.
5. Nisolle M, Paindaveine B, Bourdon A et al. Histologic study of peritoneal endometriosis in infertile women. *Fertil Steril* 1990;53(6):984-8.
6. Mol BW, Bayram N, Lijmer JG et al. The performance of CA-125 measurement in the detection of endometriosis: a meta-analysis. *Fertil Steril* 1998;70(6):1101-8.
7. Guerriero S, Mais V, Ajossa S et al. The role of endovaginal ultrasound in differentiating endometriomas from other ovarian cysts. *Clin Exp Obstet Gynecol* 1995;22(1):20-2.
8. Friedman H, Vogelzang RL, Mendelson EB et al. Endometriosis detection by US with laparoscopic correlation. *Radiology* 1985;157(1):217-20.
9. Hornstein MD, Hemmings R, Yuzpe AA et al. Use of nafarelin versus placebo after reductive laparoscopic surgery for endometriosis. *Fertil Steril* 1997;68(5):860-4.
10. Olive DL, Schwartz LB. Endometriosis. *N Engl J Med* 1993;328(24):1759-69.
11. Malinak LR. Surgical treatment and adjunct therapy of endometriosis. *Int J Gynaecol Obstet* 1993;40(Suppl):S43-7.
12. Lu PY, Ory SJ. Endometriosis: current management. *Mayo Clin Proc* 1995;70(5):453-63.
13. Revelli A, Modotti M, Ansaldi C et al. Recurrent endometriosis: a review of biological and clinical aspects. *Obstet Gynecol Surv* 1995;50(10):747-54.
14. Crosignani PG, Vercellini P, Biffignandi F et al. Laparoscopy versus laparotomy in conservative surgical treatment for severe endometriosis. *Fertil Steril* 1996;66(5):706-11.
15. Cook AS, Rock JA. The role of laparoscopy in the treatment of endometriosis. *Fertil Steril* 1991;55(4):663-80.
16. Sutton CJ, Ewen SP, Whitelaw N et al. Prospective, randomized, double-blind, controlled trial of laser laparoscopy in the treatment of pelvic pain associated with minimal, mild, and moderate endometriosis. *Fertil Steril* 1994;62(4):696-700.
17. Candiani GB, Fedele L, Vercellini P et al. Presacral neurectomy for the treatment of pelvic pain associated with endometriosis: a controlled study. *Am J Obstet Gynecol* 1992;167(1):100-3.
18. Caplin RA et al. Transdermal fentanyl: an overview of clinical progress. In: Estafanous FG, editor. *Opioids in anesthesia II*. Boston (MA): Butterworth-Heinemann; 1991.
19. Jarrell JF, Vilos GA, Allaire C et al. Consensus guidelines for the management of chronic pelvic pain. *J Obstet Gynaecol Can* 2005;27(8):781-826.
20. Vercellini P, De Giorgi O, Mosconi P et al. Cyproterone acetate versus a continuous monophasic oral contraceptive in the treatment of recurrent pelvic pain after conservative surgery for symptomatic endometriosis. *Fertil Steril* 2002;77(1):52-61.
21. Vercellini P, De Giorgi O, Oldani S et al. Depot medroxyprogesterone acetate versus an oral contraceptive combined with very-low-dose danazol for long-term treatment of pelvic pain associated with endometriosis. *Am J Obstet Gynecol* 1996;175(2):396-401.
22. Curtis KM, Chrisman CE, Peterson HB et al. Contraception for women in selected circumstances. *Obstet Gynecol* 2002;99(6):1100-12.

23. Scholes D, LaCroix AZ, Ichikawa LE et al. Change in bone mineral density among adolescent women using and discontinuing depot medroxyprogesterone acetate contraception. *Arch Pediatr Adolesc Med* 2005;159(2):139-44.
24. Cromer BA, Lazebnik R, Rome E et al. Double-blinded randomized controlled trial of estrogen supplementation in adolescent girls who receive depot medroxyprogesterone acetate for contraception. *Am J Obstet Gynecol* 2005;192(1):42-7.
25. Andersson K, Odlind V, Rybo G. Levonorgestrel-releasing and copper-releasing (Nova T) IUDs during five years of use: a randomized comparative trial. *Contraception* 1994;49(1):56-72.
26. Lockhat FB, Emembolu JO, Konje JC. The evaluation of the effectiveness of an intrauterine-administered progestogen (levonorgestrel) in the symptomatic treatment of endometriosis and in the staging of the disease. *Hum Reprod* 2004;19(1):179-84.
27. Lockhat FB, Emembolu JE, Konje JC. Serum and peritoneal fluid levels of levonorgestrel in women with endometriosis who were treated with an intrauterine contraceptive device containing levonorgestrel. *Fertil Steril* 2005;83(2):398-404.
28. Barbieri RL, Evans S, Kistner RW. Danazol in the treatment of endometriosis: analysis of 100 cases with a 4-year follow-up. *Fertil Steril* 1982;37(6):737-46.
29. Dmowski WP. Danazol. A synthetic steroid with diverse biologic effects. *J Reprod Med* 1990;35(1 Suppl):69-74.
30. Bergqvist IA. Hormonal regulation of endometriosis and the rationales and effects of gonadotrophin-releasing hormone agonist treatment: a review. *Hum Reprod* 1995;10(2):446-52.
31. Heinrichs WL, Henzl MR. Human issues and medical economics of endometriosis. Three- vs. six-month GnRH-agonist therapy. *J Reprod Med* 1998;43(3 Suppl):299-308.
32. Dawood MY, Ramos J, Khan-Dawood FS. Depot leuprolide acetate versus danazol for treatment of pelvic endometriosis: changes in vertebral bone mass and serum estradiol and calcitonin. *Fertil Steril* 1995;63(6):1177-83.
33. Friedman AJ, Hornstein MD. Gonadotropin-releasing hormone agonist plus estrogen-progestin "add-back" therapy for endometriosis-related pelvic pain. *Fertil Steril* 1993;60(2):236-41.
34. Surrey ES, Hornstein MD. Prolonged GnRH agonist and add-back therpay for symptomatic endometriosis: long-term follow-up. *Obstet Gynecol* 2002;99(5 Pt 1):709-19.
35. Hornstein MD, Surrey ES, Weisberg GW et al. Leuprolide acetate depot and hormonal add-back in endometriosis: a 12-month study. Lupron Add-Back Study Group. *Obstet Gynecol* 1998;91(1):16-24.
36. Surrey ES, Voigt B, Fournet N et al. Prolonged gonadotropin-releasing hormone agonist treatment of symptomatic endometriosis: the role of cyclic sodium etidronate and low-dose norethindrone "add-back" therapy. *Fertil Steril* 1995;63(4):747-55.
37. Amsterdam LL, Gentry W, Jobanputra S et al. Anastrazole and oral contraceptives: a novel treatment for endometriosis. *Fertil Steril* 2005;84(2):300-4.
38. Soysal S, Soysal ME, Ozer S et al. The effects of post-surgical administration of goserelin plus anastrozole compared to goserelin alone in patients with severe endometriosis: a prospective randomized trial. *Hum Reprod* 2004;19(1):160-7.
39. Ailawadi RK, Jobanputra S, Kataria M et al. Treatment of endometriosis and chronic pelvic pain with letrozole and norethindrone acetate: a pilot study. *Fertil Steril* 2004;81(2):290-6.
40. Attar E, Bulun SE. Aromatase inhibitors: the next generation of therapeutics for endometriosis? *Fertil Steril* 2006;85(5):1307-18.
41. Kettel LM, Murphy AA, Morales AJ et al. Preliminary report on the treatment of endometriosis with low-dose mifepristone (RU 486). *Am J Obstet Gynecol* 1998;178(6):1151-6.
42. Adamson GD, Pasta DJ. Surgical treatment of endometriosis-associated infertility: meta-analysis compared with survival analysis. *Am J Obstet Gynecol* 1994;171(6):1488-504.
43. Sallam HN, Garcia-Velasco JA, Dias S et al. Long-term pituitary down-regulation before in vitro fertilization (IVF) for women with endometriosis. *Cochrane Database Syst Rev* 2006;(1):CD004635.
44. Tummon IS, Asher LJ, Martin JS et al. Randomized controlled trial of superovulation and insemination for infertility associated with minimal or mild endometriosis. *Fertil Steril* 1997;68(1):8-12.
45. Practice Committee of the American Society for Reproductive Medicine. Endometriosis and infertility. *Fertil Steril* 2006;86(5 Suppl):S156-60.
46. Hughes EG, Fedorkow DM, Collins JA. A quantitative overview of controlled trials in endometriosis-associated infertility. *Fertil Steril* 1993;59(5):963-70.
47. Redwine DB. Conservative laparoscopic excision of endometriosis by sharp dissection: life table analysis of reoperation and persistent or recurrent disease. *Fertil Steril* 1991;56(4):628-34.
48. Wheeler JM, Malinak LR. Recurrent endometriosis: incidence, management, and prognosis. *Am J Obstet Gynecol* 1983;146(3):247-53.
49. Namnoum AB, Hickman TN, Goodman SB et al. Incidence of symptom recurrence after hysterectomy for endometriosis. *Fertil Steril* 1995;64(5):898-902.
50. Howell R, Edmonds DK, Dowsett M et al. Gonadotropin-releasing analogue (goserelin) plus hormone replacement therapy for the treatment of endometriosis: a randomized controlled trial. *Fertil Steril* 1995;64(3):474-81.

51. Kennedy S, Bergqvist A, Chapron C et al. ESHRE guideline for the diagnosis and treatment of endometriosis. *Hum Reprod* 2005;20(10):2698-704.

52. Lockhat FB, Emembolu JO, Konje JC. The efficacy, side effects and continuation rates in women with symptomatic endometriosis undergoing treatment with an intra-uterine administered progestogen (levonorgestrel): a 3-year follow-up. *Hum Reprod* 2005;20(3):789-93.

CHAPTER 64
Menopause

Amie J. Cullimore, MD, MSc, FRCSC

Natural menopause is defined as cessation of menses of one year's duration secondary to lack of estrogen production by the ovary. Menopause may also be induced by medical or surgical intervention such as radiation or chemotherapy treatment or removal of the ovaries at time of hysterectomy.

Vasomotor symptoms, commonly known as hot flashes and night sweats, are the most common presenting complaint of menopausal women. The average age of menopause in Canada is 51 and this has been constant throughout the last few centuries.[1] The frequency of bothersome hot flashes appears to commence about two years before the final menstrual period with maximum symptoms occurring within the first two years after the last period. The frequency of hot flashes gradually decreases over six years;[1,2] however, some women experience hot flashes many years after menopause.

Other associated complaints of menopause, including vaginal symptoms such as dryness, itching, vaginitis and dyspareunia generally persist or worsen with aging due to low estrogen levels. Women tend to complain of vaginal symptoms a few years after the last menstrual period. Unlike hot flashes, vaginal atrophy does not improve over time. Some women notice decreasing libido and an alteration in sexual function with the onset of menopause. The cause of this change is multifaceted and has been linked to decreasing testosterone production from the ovary (see Chapter 65).

Mood changes have also been reported in the menopausal transition and may continue into early menopause.

Goals of Therapy

- Reduce symptoms associated with declining estrogen levels including vasomotor instability (hot flashes, hot flushes, night sweats), urogenital atrophy (vaginal dryness, dyspareunia) and mood-related changes (depression, anxiety, sleeplessness)
- Avoid harm that may be increased with the use of estrogen therapies including endometrial and breast carcinoma, myocardial infarction or stroke and venous thromboembolism (VTE).

Investigations

- Confirm cessation of ovarian activity (Figure 1)
  - if cessation of menses is greater than six months, ovarian failure is virtually certain

  - if ovarian function is uncertain, continued elevation of serum follicle stimulating hormone (FSH) in excess of 30 IU/L confirms ovarian failure
- Health maintenance screening
  - initial evaluation should include blood pressure assessment, breast examination and cervical cytology
  - mammography is indicated for all women over 50 years of age. Consider younger women for mammography if at higher risk for breast cancer, e.g., strong family history
  - screen women at high risk for cardiovascular disease or osteoporosis for dyslipidemia or bone mineral density, respectively
- Investigate any unexpected bleeding by means of endometrial sampling to rule out endometrial carcinoma

Therapeutic Choices (Figure 1)

Nonpharmacologic Choices

- Lifestyle modification may positively impact vasomotor symptoms.
  - passive smoke exposure and high body mass index ($\geq$ 27 kg/m^2) are associated with greater prevalence of hot flashes.[3]
  - lowering the ambient temperature may help reduce the intensity of hot flashes.
  - stretching improves flushing in overweight postmenopausal women.[4]
  - practising paced respiration may reduce frequency of flushing.[5]
  - reducing core body temperature, e.g., dressing in layers and getting regular exercise may help manage hot flashes.[6]

Pharmacologic Choices (Table 1, Table 2)

The treatment of vasomotor symptoms, vaginal symptoms and mood changes associated with menopause are addressed.

Vasomotor Symptoms

Vasomotor symptoms have a significant impact on quality of life. Intolerance to heat, flushing and perspiration are uncomfortable and also embarrassing. Flushing or night sweats can lead to sleepless nights, fatigue and decreased productivity at work.[7]

Hormone Therapy

Estrogen is indicated for the short-term relief of vasomotor symptoms to decrease the frequency and severity of hot flashes.[6,8,9,10] Use estrogen at the lowest effective dose that can control menopausal symptoms for the shortest possible time.[11] Beginning with a dose of 0.3 mg of conjugated estrogen (or equivalent) is reasonable and then increase the dose after three weeks if no improvement in menopausal symptoms are noted.

Estrogen preparations may be administered orally, transdermally, vaginally or parenterally. Surrogate outcomes such as increased triglycerides is seen with oral estrogens but not with the transdermal route of administration.[6] However, there is no evidence that route of administration affects the clinical outcomes of greatest interest, such as myocardial infarction or fracture.

The effect of estrogen therapy on vasomotor symptoms is dose related, with substantial relief seen within 4 weeks with standard doses (estradiol 1 mg or equivalent) and 8 to 12 weeks with low doses (conjugated estrogens 0.3 mg or equivalent).[12] Lower doses of estrogen are associated with decreased incidence of irregular bleeding or breast tenderness compared to standard doses.[12]

Estrogen *alone* in women without a uterus should be used continuously through the month to reduce the risk of exacerbation of menopausal symptoms.

Table 1: Absolute Contraindications to Estrogen and Progestin Therapy

Estrogen Therapy	• Undiagnosed vaginal bleeding • Active liver disease • Active thromboembolic disease
The risk of recurrence of breast cancer or thrombosis following estrogen therapy is unknown. Caution is recommended in women with cardiovascular disease. For all women, the risk versus the benefit must be taken into consideration when prescribing estrogen therapy.	
Progestin Therapy	• Undiagnosed vaginal bleeding • Known or suspected carcinoma of the breast • Pregnancy

Progestin is indicated in women using systemic estrogen who have an intact uterus. The dose is the equivalent of 5 mg **medroxyprogesterone acetate (MPA)** for cyclical regimens or 2.5 mg for continuous regimens. Absolute contraindications to estrogen and progestin therapy are listed in Table 1.

Consider progestins such as oral and injectable MPA and **megestrol acetate** as alternative treatments for hot flashes in symptomatic women who cannot or who do not want to use estrogen therapy. Do not recommend progesterone cream because it does not prevent endometrial hyperplasia when used in combination with estrogen therapy in women with an intact uterus.[6] It is currently unknown whether progestin monotherapy increases the risk of breast cancer.[6]

Continuous estrogen with *cyclical* progestin helps reduce the risk of endometrial hyperplasia or carcinoma in women with a uterus. In cyclic regimens, estrogen is taken continuously and progestin is taken from day 1 to 14 of the calendar month. A woman can expect a withdrawal bleed when the progestin is stopped. This regimen is less favoured because of the induced bleeding.

Continuous combined therapy with estrogen and progestin taken daily without a break is the most commonly prescribed regimen. This reduces the risk of bleeding and the risk of endometrial carcinoma. During the first year of use, unexpected spotting or light bleeding may occur.

There is no good evidence to suggest the best way to discontinue hormone therapy. All women should have an annual review of their therapy with their health care provider. Avoid the abrupt discontinuation of therapy by gradually reducing the dose and frequency. If the patient becomes symptomatic with lower doses, continue that dose until the vasomotor symptoms abate.[6]

Prevention of Cardiovascular Disease and Osteoporosis with Estrogen Use

Estrogen is not indicated for the primary or secondary prevention of cardiovascular disease and osteoporosis.[6,13,14,15] Two randomized, controlled trials have shown that estrogen-progestin treatment is ineffective for primary or secondary prevention of coronary artery disease (CAD).[16,17] Prevention of CAD is best achieved by improving health, diet and fitness and, where necessary, risk reduction with drug therapy such as antihypertensives and lipid-lowering agents (see Chapter 32 and Chapter 31).

Current evidence indicates that the prevention of osteoporosis should be achieved by diet, exercise, calcium supplementation and vitamin D, as well as bisphosphonates or selective estrogen receptor modulators (see Chapter 73).

Risks Associated with Estrogen Therapy

In the estrogen-progestin Women's Health Initiative (WHI) study, the risks of breast cancer, MI, stroke and VTE outweighed the benefits of reduced fractures and colorectal cancer frequency after five years of treatment. VTE risk in the first year of use was 3.6-fold higher with estrogen-progestin compared to placebo. Although the risk declined over time, the overall risk over five years remained significantly elevated (Hazard Ratio 2.11, 95% CI 1.26-3.55).[16] Thus, use of estrogen with or without progestin for treatment of menopausal symptoms should be reviewed each year to determine if continued use is expected to result in more benefit than risk.

The risk of breast cancer with estrogen-progestin use mirrors the increased risk with delayed menopause (i.e., the additional risk with each year of estrogen-progestin treatment is similar to the additional risk with each year of delayed menopause).[18] In the WHI study, breast cancer risk was higher among estrogen-progestin users than placebo users, rising to a statistically significant difference after five years. The difference began at four years of use. The absolute risk for individual users, however, is small (38 cases in hormone users compared with 30 in placebo users, per 10 000 women per annum).[3] There was no difference in breast cancer rates, however, among women in the estrogen-alone arm (i.e., women with hysterectomy) and the placebo arm.

Nonhormonal Therapies

Not all women are candidates for hormonal therapy (HT) or care to consider HT as a therapeutic option. A systematic review showed reduced frequency and severity of menopausal hot flashes with **paroxetine**, **venlafaxine**, **clonidine** and **gabapentin** in highly symptomatic women.[19] Their use may be limited by side effects.[19] Venlafaxine, 75 mg and 150 mg, reduced hot flash scores by 61% compared to 27% seen with placebo in postmenopausal women after 4 weeks of treatment.[20] Paroxetine controlled release 12.5 mg decreased daily hot flash composite score by 62.2% compared to 37.8% seen with placebo after 6 weeks of treatment.[21] Consider venlafaxine and paroxetine as first line in women experiencing hot flashes who have significant perimenopausal/menopausal mood and anxiety problems. Gabapentin 900 mg daily reduced hot flash frequency and severity by 54% compared to 31% seen with placebo after 12 weeks of treatment in postmenopausal women experiencing ≥7 hot flashes a day[22]. A phase III clinical trial showed a 50% reduction in hot flash scores with **fluoxetine** compared to 36% with placebo in women with a history of breast cancer experiencing ≥14 hot flashes per week.[23] Clonidine, a centrally acting antihypertensive, and a combination product containing phenobarbital, ergotamine and belladonna (**Bellergal Spacetabs**), are indicated for the relief of hot flashes but are associated with side effects.[6]

Black cohosh and **red clover–derived isoflavones** may have a small effect or no effect on vasomotor symptoms.[19,24,25,26,27,28] Case reports link black cohosh to liver damage.[29,30] **Vitamin E** 800 IU daily has shown a small effect in decreasing hot flashes.[31] Progesterone cream cannot be recommended because it effectively prevents endometrial hyperplasia when used in combination with estrogen therapy.[6]

There is insufficient evidence to support the use of *acupuncture*.[6,24]

Vaginal Symptoms

Estrogens administered intravaginally (creams, vaginal tablets and/or estradiol-releasing ring) are effective for treating the symptoms of vaginal atrophy in postmenopausal women[32] and may be considered in patients experiencing only vaginal symptoms.[6] Vaginal estrogens are preferred over systemically administered estrogens (oral, transdermal) as they elicit lower systemic estradiol levels and therefore reduces endometrial stimulation, uterine bleeding and breast tenderness.[32]

Vaginal moisturizers (Replens) improve vaginal dryness and dyspareunia when used continuously. **Vaginal lubricants** can be used as needed (see Table 2).

Mood Changes

Women progressing through the menopausal transition may notice changes in mood resulting in anxiety and irritability which is often compounded by sleeplessness. Women at greatest risk of development of depression include those with a previous history of depressive disorders, poor physical health and a long perimenopausal transition.[6] Treat mood disorders and anxiety with SSRIs. Add low-dose hormone therapy for those who do not respond to antidepressants alone.[33]

Therapeutic Tips

- Consider the needs and wants of each patient prior to recommending a course of therapy for menopausal symptoms. Each patient has a unique health history and risk profile that affects the relative benefit she will derive from hormone therapy and how she makes decisions about life and health. Unswerving policy applied to all patients is unlikely to meet the individual needs of many.
- Consider lifestyle choices either alone or in combination with hormone therapy, after assessing the individual's risks and benefits.
- Prescribe vaginal estrogen preparations if menopausal symptoms are vaginal only.
- Prescribe hormone therapy for patients who enter menopause prior to age 40, as premature ovarian failure is associated with an early rise in the incidence of cardiovascular disease and osteoporosis. Continue treatment until at least the age of 50, the age when most women reach natural menopause.[34]

Figure 1: **Treatment of Menopausal Symptoms**

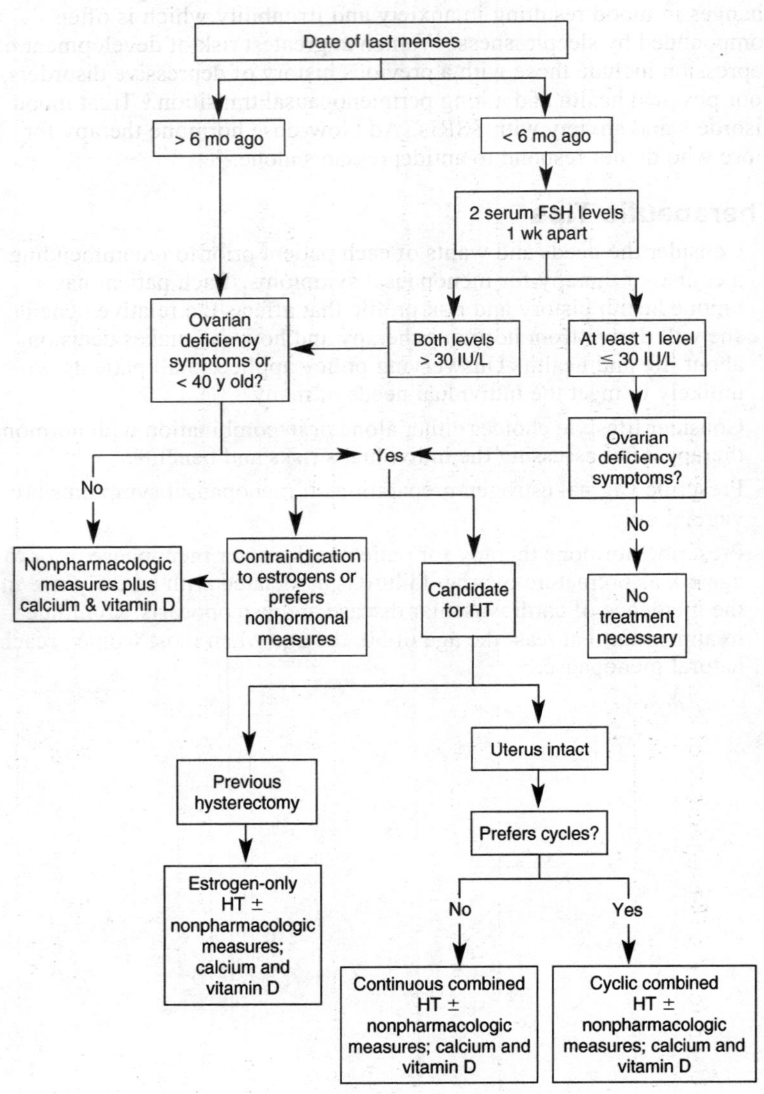

Abbreviations: FSH = follicle stimulating hormone; HT = hormone therapy

Table 2: Drugs Used for the Management of Menopausal Symptoms

Class	Drug	Dose	Adverse Effects	Comments	Cost[a]
Alpha$_2$-adrenergic Agonists	*clonidine* Dixarit, generics	0.05 mg po BID	Dizziness, dry mouth, drowsiness, constipation.	Indicated for the treatment of vasomotor symptoms in patients who do not want to take or cannot take estrogens. Discontinue if no benefit after 2 to 4 wk or side effects. Monitor blood pressure with concomitant use of other antihypertensives.	$
Ergot Combination Products	*ergotamine/belladonna alkaloids/phenobarbital* Bellergal Spacetabs	1 tablet po in the morning and 1 tablet po in the evening Max: 16 tabs/wk	Dizziness, dry mouth, drowsiness, constipation.	Indicated for the treatment of vasomotor symptoms in patients who do not want to take or cannot take estrogens. Avoid in combination with CYP3A4 inhibitors, e.g., erythromycin, clarithromycin, ritonavir, nelfinavir, ketoconazole, itraconazole.	$$$$
Estrogens, oral	*conjugated equine estrogen* Premarin	0.3–1.25 mg po daily given continuously or cyclically	Bloating, headache, nausea, breast tenderness, dose-related bleeding.	Administer with progestin in patients with uteri to prevent endometrial hyperplasia or cancer. Consider vaginal estrogen for patients with vaginal symptoms only.	$
	conjugated estrogen sulfate C.E.S., generics	0.3–1.25 mg po daily given continuously or cyclically	See conjugated equine estrogen.	See conjugated equine estrogen.	$
	estradiol, micronized Estrace	0.5–2 mg po daily given continuously or cyclically	See conjugated equine estrogen.	See conjugated equine estrogen.	$

(cont'd)

Table 2: **Drugs Used for the Management of Menopausal Symptoms** *(cont'd)*

Class	Drug	Dose	Adverse Effects	Comments	Cost[a]
Estrogens, transdermal	*estradiol-17β, patch* Climara, Estraderm, Estradot, Oesclim	Depending on the product: 1 patch applied 1–2 times weekly, delivering 0.025–0.1 mg daily	Redness, skin irritation.	Avoids first-pass effect. May benefit women with malabsorption conditions. Less effect on hepatic sex-hormone binding globulin synthesis than oral estrogens. May benefit women who complain of ↓ sexual desire.	$$
	estradiol-17β, topical gel Estrogel	0.75–1.5 mg (1.25–2.5 g gel) applied to arms daily 1 actuation of metered dose pump is applied to arm. Total dose from 1 actuation is 1.25 g gel or 0.75 mg estradiol	See estradiol-17β, patch.	Less effect on hepatic protein synthesis than oral estrogens; alternate application sites include abdomen or inner thighs.	$$
Estrogens, vaginal	*conjugated equine estrogen (CEE), vaginal cream* Premarin	0.625 mg CEE/g: 0.3–1.25 mg CEE (0.5–2 g) daily or as directed intravaginally or topically depending on the severity of condition	Local burning, irritation, vaginal leakage.	Indicated for the treatment of atrophic vaginitis and dyspareunia. Improves vaginal vascularity and lubrication. Administer cyclically at the lowest dose for short term (e.g., 3 wk on and 1 wk off). Administer with progestin in patients with uteri to prevent endometrial hyperplasia or cancer. Absorbed into systemic circulation with ↑ doses resulting in ↑ systemic estrogen concentrations. Intermittent therapy may also be used.	$$
	estradiol-17β vaginal ring Estring	Insert 1 ring pv Q 3 mo Delivers 7.5 μg estradiol over 24-h period at a sustained rate for up to 12 weeks	Spotting, discharge, genital pruritus.	Indicated for the treatment of atrophic vaginitis and dyspareunia. Improves vaginal vascularity and lubrication.	$$$$/ring

Class	Drug	Dose	Adverse Effects	Comments	Cost[a]
	estradiol-17β, vaginal tablet Vagifem	25 µg/vaginal tablet: insert 1 vaginal tablet daily for 2 weeks then twice weekly with a 3–4 day interval between doses	Vaginal secretion, vaginal discomfort.	See estradiol-17β vaginal ring.	$$$
Gamma Aminobutyric Acid Derivatives	*gabapentin* Neurontin, generics	300 mg po TID	Somnolence, dizziness.	For vasomotor symptoms in patients who do not want to take or cannot take estrogens. Start at 300 mg daily and ↑ to 300 mg TID over 3 to 7 days. Discontinue over a one week period.	$$$
Lubricants, vaginal	*vaginal gels or jelly* K-Y Jelly, Gynemoistrin, Astroglide	Apply when needed		Provides rapid, short term relief. Can be applied to penis and the opening of vagina to decrease discomfort in dyspareunia.	$
Moisturizers, vaginal	*polycarbophil gel* Replens	Apply 2–3 × per week		Provides longer duration of action than vaginal lubricants. Used on a continuous basis. Replens was equivalent to local hormone therapy for improvement of dyspareunia.[35] Provides long-term relief (2–3 days) of vaginal dryness by changing fluid content of epithelium and lowering vaginal pH.	$

(cont'd)

Table 2: **Drugs Used for the Management of Menopausal Symptoms** *(cont'd)*

Class	Drug	Dose	Adverse Effects	Comments	Cost[a]
Progestins, oral	*medroxyprogesterone acetate* Provera, generics	*In combination with estrogen in patients with uterus:* 5–10 mg po daily cyclically *or* 2.5–5 mg po daily continuously *For prevention of hot flashes:* 20 mg po daily[6]	Bloating, irritability, weight gain, mood swings.	Progestins normalize the endometrial response and ↓ breakthrough bleeding; when given continuously, they prevent blood flow.	$
	megestrol acetate Megace, generics	For prevention of hot flashes: 20 mg po daily[6]	See medroxyprogesterone acetate.	See medroxyprogesterone acetate. For symptomatic women who cannot or who do not want to use estrogen therapy.	$
	norethindrone Micronor	0.35–0.7 mg po daily continuously	See medroxyprogesterone acetate.	See medroxyprogesterone acetate.	$
	progesterone, micronized Prometrium	*In combination with estrogen in patients with uterus:* 200–300 mg po HS cyclically *or* 100–200 mg po HS continuously	See medroxyprogesterone acetate.	Contains peanut oil. Lack of evidence of effectiveness for vasomotor symptoms. Better side effect profile and beneficial effect on sleep.	$$–$$$

Class	Drug	Dose	Adverse Effects	Comments	Cost[a]
Progestins, injectable	*medroxyprogesterone* Depo-Provera	150 mg im every 1–3 months	See medroxyprogesterone acetate, oral.	See medroxyprogesterone acetate, oral.	$$/vial
Progestins, intrauterine system	*levonorgestrel* Mirena	52 mg/IUS	To a lesser extent of bloating, irritability, weight gain and mood swings compared to medroxyprogesterone acetate.	See medroxyprogesterone acetate.	$320/IUS
Serotonin-norepinephrine Reuptake Inhibitors	*venlafaxine* Effexor XR, generics	37.5–75 mg daily	Gastrointestinal upset, nervousness, insomnia.	*Not an approved indication for the treatment of vasomotor symptoms.* For vasomotor symptoms in patients who do not want to take or cannot take estrogens. Start with 37.5 mg daily and ↑ to 75 mg daily after 1 week, if necessary. Higher doses are not useful for the treatment of vasomotor symptoms and are associated with side effects.[19] Result may take 2–3 weeks. Taper gradually when stopping.	$$-$$$
Selective Serotonin Reuptake Inhibitors	*paroxetine* Paxil CR	12.5–25 mg po daily	See venlafaxine.	*Not an approved indication for the treatment of vasomotor symptoms.* For vasomotor symptoms in patients who do not want to take or cannot take estrogens. Result may take 2–3 weeks. Taper gradually when stopping. Avoid combination with sibutramine. May ↓ efficacy of tamoxifen.	$$$

(cont'd)

Table 2: **Drugs Used for the Management of Menopausal Symptoms** *(cont'd)*

Class	Drug	Dose	Adverse Effects	Comments	Cost[a]
	fluoxetine Prozac, generics	20 mg po daily	See venlafaxine.	*Not an approved indication for the treatment of vasomotor symptoms.* For vasomotor symptoms in patients who do not want to take or cannot take estrogens. Result may take 2–3 weeks. Avoid combination with sibutramine. May ↓ efficacy of tamoxifen.	$$

[a] Cost of 30-day supply unless otherwise specified; includes drug cost only.

Dosage adjustment may be required in renal impairment; see Appendix I.

Legend: $ < $20 $-$$ < $20–40 $$ $20–40 $$–$$$ $20–60 $$$ $40–60 $$$$ $60–80

Suggested Readings

Brass LM. Estrogens and stroke: use of oral contraceptives and postmenopausal use of estrogen: current recommendations. *Curr Treat Options Neurol* 2004;6(6):459-67.

[No authors listed]. Proceedings from the NIH State-of-the-Science Conference on Management of Menopause-Related Symptoms, March 21-23, 2005, Bethesda, Maryland, USA. *Am J Med* 2005;118(Suppl 12B):S1-171.

SOGC Clinical Practice Guideline. Canadian Consensus Conference on Menopause, 2006 update. *J Obstet Gynaecol Can* 2006;28:S1-S112. Available from: http://www.sogc.org/guidelines/public/171E-CONS-February2006.pdf Accessed April 12, 2007.

References

1. Guthrie JR, Dennerstein L, Taffe JR et al. The menopausal transition: a 9-year prospective population-based study. The Melbourne Women's Midlife Health Project. *Climacteric* 2004;7(4):375-89.
2. Kronenberg F. Hot flashes: epidemiology and physiology. *Ann N Y Acad Sci* 1990;592:52-86.
3. Gold EB, Sternfeld B, Kelsey JL et al. Relation of demographic and lifestyle factors to symptoms in a multi-racial/ethnic population of women 40-55 years of age. *Am J Epidemiol* 2000;152(5):463-73.
4. Aiello EJ, Yasui Y, Tworoger SS et al. Effect of a yearlong, moderate-intensity exercise intervention on the occurrence and severity of menopause symptoms in postmenopausal women. *Menopause* 2004;11(4):382-8.
5. Freedman RR, Woodward S. Behavioral treatment of menopausal hot flushes: evaluation by ambulatory monitoring. *Am J Obstet Gynecol* 1992;167(2):436-9.
6. Belisle S, Blake J, Basson R et al. Canadian consensus conference on menopause, 2006 update. *J Obstet Gynaecol Can* 2006;28(2 Suppl 1):S7-S94.
7. Ohayon MM. Severe hot flashes associated with chronic insomnia. *Arch Intern Med* 2006;166:1262-8.
8. Nelson HD. Commonly used types of postmenopausal estrogen for treatment of hot flashes: scientific review. *JAMA* 2004;291(13):1610-20.
9. Brunner RL, Gass M, Aragaki A et al. Effects of conjugated equine estrogen on health-related quality of life in postmenopausal women with hysterectomy: results from the Women's Health Initiative Randomized Clinical Trial. *Arch Intern Med* 2005;165(17):1976-86.
10. MacLennan AH, Broadbent JL, Lester S et al. Oral oestrogen and combined oestrogen/progestogen therapy versus placebo for hot flushes. *Cochrane Database Syst Rev* 2002;1:CD002978.
11. Stephenson J. FDA orders estrogen safety warnings: agency offers guidance for HRT use. *JAMA* 2003;289(5):537-8.
12. Ettinger B. Vasomotor symptom relief versus unwanted effects: role of estrogen dosage. *Am J Med* 2005;118(Suppl 12B):74-8.
13. Mosca L, Banka CL, Benjamin EJ et al. Evidence-based guidelines for cardiovascular disease prevention in women: 2007 update. *Circulation* 2007;115(11):1481-501.
14. Farquhar CM, Marjoribanks J, Lethaby A et al. Long term hormone therapy for perimenopausal and postmenopausal women. *Cochrane Database Syst Rev* 2005;(3):CD004143.
15. U.S. Preventive Services Task Force. Hormone therapy for the prevention of chronic conditions in postmenopausal women: recommendations from the U.S. Preventive Services Task Force. *Ann Intern Med* 2005;142(10):855-60.
16. Rossouw JE, Anderson GL, Prentice RL et al. Risks and benefits of estrogen plus progestin in healthy postmenopausal women: principal results from the Women's Health Initiative randomized controlled trial. *JAMA* 2002;288(3):321-33.
17. Hulley S, Grady D, Bush T et al. Randomized trial of estrogen plus progestin for secondary prevention of coronary heart disease in postmenopausal women. Heart and Estrogen/progestin Replacement Study (HERS) Research Group. *JAMA* 1998;280(7):605-613.
18. [No authors listed]. Breast cancer and hormone replacement therapy: collaborative reanalysis of data from 51 epidemiological studies of 52,705 women with breast cancer and 108,411 women without breast cancer. Collaborative Group on Hormonal Factors in Breast Cancer. *Lancet* 1997;350(9084):1047-59.
19. Nelson HD, Vesco KK, Haney E et al. Nonhormonal therapies for menopausal hot flashes: systematic review and meta-analysis. *JAMA* 2006;295(17):2057-71.
20. Loprinzi CL, Kugler JW, Sloan JA et al. Venlafaxine in management of hot flashes in survivors of breast cancer: a randomised controlled trial. *Lancet* 2000;356(9247):2059-63.
21. Stearns V, Beebe KL, Iyengar M et al. Paroxetine controlled release in the treatment of menopausal hot flashes: a randomized controlled trial. *JAMA* 2003;289(21):2827-34.

22. Guttuso T, Kurlan R, McDermott MP et al. Gabapentin's effects on hot flashes in postmenopausal women: a randomized controlled trial. *Obstet Gynecol* 2003;101(2):337-45.
23. Loprinzi CL, Sloan JA, Perez EA et al. Phase III evaluation of fluoxetine for treatment of hot flashes. *J Clin Oncol* 2002;20:1578-1583.
24. Nedrow A, Miller J, Walker M et al. Complementary and alternative therapies for the management of menopause-related symptoms: a systematic evidence review. *Arch Intern Med* 2006;166(14):1453-65.
25. Newton KM, Reed SD, LaCroix AZ et al. Treatment of vasomotor symptoms of menopause with black cohosh, multibotanicals, soy, hormone therapy, or placebo: a randomized trial. *Ann Intern Med* 2006;145(12):869-79.
26. Uebelhack R, Blohmer JU, Graubaum HJ et al. Black cohosh and St. John's wort for climacteric complaints: a randomized trial. *Obstet Gynecol* 2006;107(2 Pt 1):247-255.
27. Pockaj BA, Gallagher JG, Loprinzi CL et al. Phase III double-blind, randomized, placebo-controlled crossover trial of black cohosh in the management of hot flashes: NCCTG Trial N01CC1. *J Clin Oncol* 2006;24(18):2836-41.
28. Tice JA, Ettinger B, Ensrud K et al. Phytoestrogen supplements for the treatment of hot flashes: the Isoflavone Clover Extract (ICE) Study: a randomized controlled trial. *JAMA* 2003;290(2):207-14.
29. Lynch CR, Folkers ME, Hutson WR. Fulminant hepatic failure associated with the use of black cohosh: a case report. *Liver Transpl* 2006;12(6):989-92.
30. Cohen SM, O'Connor AM, Hart J et al. Autoimmune hepatitis associated with the use of black cohosh: a case study. *Menopause* 2004;11(5):575-7.
31. Barton DL, Loprinzi CL, Quella SK et al. Prospective evaluation of vitamin E for hot flashes in breast cancer survivors. *J Clin Oncol* 1998; 16(2):495-500.
32. Suckling J, Lethaby A, Kennedy R. Local oestrogen for vaginal atrophy in postmenopausal women. *Cochrane Database Syst Rev* 2006;(4):CD001500.
33. Cohen LS, Soares CN, Joffe H. Diagnosis and management of mood disorders during the menopausal transition. *Am J Med* 2005;118(Suppl12B):93-7.
34. Writing Group for the British Menopause Society. Management of premature menopause. *J Br Menopause Soc* 2007;13(1):44-5.
35. Nachtigall LE. Comparative study: Replens versus local estrogen in menopausal women. *Fertil Steril* 1994;61(1):178-80.

CHAPTER 65
Female Sexual Dysfunction

Rosemary Basson, MD, FRCP(UK)

Ongoing sexual difficulties causing distress affect between 15 and 34% of women.[1,2] Sexual response is a biopsychosocial phenomenon. Adaptation to past and present untoward circumstances may result in dysfunction. Frequently nothing is intrinsically wrong with the sex response system. However, medical conditions, medications, surgery, radiation or aging may contribute to impairment.[3,4,5] In assessing a woman's sexual problems, it may be helpful to interview both partners together and separately.[6]

Interviewing for Female Sexual Dysfunction[6]

- Assess partners together
  - sexual problems in the patient's own words: Clarify with direct questions; give options rather than leading questions
  - duration, consistency, priority: Are problems present in all situations and which is most severe?
  - context of sexual problems: Emotional intimacy with partner, activity/behaviour just prior to sexual activity, privacy, safety, birth control, risk of sexually transmitted infections (STIs), usefulness of sexual stimulation, sexual skills of partner, sexual communication, time of day, cultural context
  - other aspects of each partner's sexual response: Check this currently and prior to the onset of the sexual problems—sexual motivation, subjective arousal, enjoyment, orgasm, pain, erection and ejaculation in a male partner
  - reaction of each partner to sexual problems: How each has reacted emotionally, sexually and behaviourally
  - previous help: Compliance with recommendations and effectiveness
  - determine what precipitated this request for help
- Assess each partner alone
  - partner's own assessment of the situation: Sometimes it is easier to acknowledge symptoms, e.g., total lack of desire, in the partner's absence
  - sex response with self stimulation as well as sexual thoughts and fantasies
  - the following items may be omitted for a recent problem after decades of healthy sexual function
    - past sexual experiences: Positive, negative aspects
    - developmental history: Relationships to others in the home while growing up, losses, traumas, how they coped. Who (if

anyone) was this person close to, shown affection by, felt loved by, respected by? Clarify if some of these themes are playing out in the current sexual relationship

- enquire regarding sexual, emotional and physical abuse: Explain that abuse questions are routine and do not necessarily imply causation of the problems

Women's Sexual Desire/Interest Disorder

Absent or diminished feelings of sexual interest or desire, absent sexual thoughts or fantasies and a lack of responsive desire defines women's sexual desire/interest disorder. Motivations (defined as reasons/incentives) for attempting to become sexually aroused are scarce or absent. The lack of interest is considered to be beyond normal lessening with age and relationship duration.[7]

Goals of Therapy

- Identify psychological, interpersonal and medical factors
- Provide patient and partner with knowledge and understanding of sexual response cycle (Figure 1).[7] Address problematic areas
- Identify need for psychological or psychiatric consultation for deep-seated issues that prevent the woman from responding to sexual stimuli or that result in her experiencing negative emotions such as shame, guilt or disgust with arousal

Investigations

- Sexual history including current and past sexual function of both partners (see Interviewing for Female Sexual Dysfunction[6]). Past sexual function strongly modulates current sexual function[8]
- Medical history including medication (Table 1) and mood
- Relationship details, both past and present, focusing on nonsexual intimacy, trust and respect, safety, birth control, fertility and stressors. Feelings for the partner and for the relationship correlate with women's sexual function[1,9,10]
- Lab investigations only as indicated by medical history. No correlation has been found between androgen levels and sexual function.[11,12] This may, in part, be because about 50% of testosterone is made within cells and not reflected in serum levels.[13] Available assays of testosterone (total, free, bioavailable) are unreliable in the female range[14]

Table 1: **Drugs[a] Associated with Female Sexual Dysfunction[15,16,17,18]**

Alcohol at higher doses	Antiandrogens	Beta blockers
Alkylating agents	Cimetidine	Clonidine
Amphetamines	Spironolactone	Digoxin
Anticholinergics	Antiepileptic drugs	GnRH agonists
Antidepressants	Antihistamines	Ketoconazole
MAOIs	Antipsychotics	Lithium
SNRIs	Aromatase inhibitors	Methadone
SSRIs	Barbiturates	Metoclopramide
TCAs	Benzodiazepines	Oral contraceptives
		Trazodone

[a] This list is not exhaustive. A trial off the drug may help determine whether or not the drug is contributing to the problem.

Abbreviations: GnRH = gonadotropin-releasing hormone; MAOIs = monoamine oxidase inhibitors; SNRIs = serotonin and norepinephrine reuptake inhibitors; SSRIs = selective serotonin reuptake inhibitors; TCAs = tricyclic antidepressants

Therapeutic Choices

Nonpharmacologic Choices

- Counsel or refer the couple when their emotional intimacy is insufficient to motivate her sexually and/or impairs her subjective arousal/pleasure
- Address lack of stimuli, e.g., insufficient nongenital stimuli or nonpenetrative genital stimuli
- Address psychological factors that are inhibiting the effectiveness of sexual stimulation:
  - distractions/nonsexual stressors
  - dysphoric arousal (may indicate previous abuse)
  - constant sexual self-monitoring
  - low self-esteem/poor body image
  - expectation of pain—a past history of dyspareunia can interfere with the processing of sexual stimuli, even if pain is currently absent
  - negative outcome, e.g., partner's sexual dysfunction. In this situation, address the primary problem
- Address biological factors limiting the effectiveness of stimulation:
  - depression
  - medications (Table 1)
  - chronic ill health
  - fatigue, e.g., sleep disorder, shift work, disturbed nights
  - decreased androgen activity (Table 2)
  - irregular or absent menstrual cycles, e.g., hyperprolactinemia
  - hypothyroidism

Table 2: **Theoretical Causes of Androgen Insufficiency**[19]

Premature ovarian failure
Chemotherapy-associated menopause
Hypopituitary states
Primary or secondary hypoadrenal states
Bilateral oophorectomy in a young woman
Chronic cortisone administration
Gonadotropin-releasing hormone (GnRH) therapy
Oral contraceptive use[a], oral estrogen use
Aging with excessive reduction of adrenal precursors of testosterone

[a] All combined estrogen and progestin contraceptives and postmenopausal oral estrogen therapy reduce available testosterone by markedly increasing sex hormone binding globulin, though clinical impact varies in individuals.

The diagnosis of androgen insufficiency is based on clinical symptoms of desire/interest disorder in the presence of one of the conditions listed in Table 2.[19] The lack of ability to trigger desire and to become aroused at any time during the sexual experience is now considered integral to this disorder. Suspect androgen insufficiency when one of the conditions listed in Table 2 exists.

Pharmacologic Choices

There are no approved pharmacologic treatments for women's sexual desire/interest disorder. Although physicians experienced in women's sexual dysfunction are investigating **testosterone** therapy with careful follow-up for women with conditions associated with marked reduction in androgen activity (Table 2), guidelines from the American Endocrine Society recommend against the use of testosterone patches in women until further safety data becomes available.[14]

There are no approved formulations of androgen for women.[14] Treating estrogenized postmenopausal women with a transdermal patch containing testosterone 300 μg has been investigated.[20,21,22,23,24] Such therapy results in testosterone levels at the upper limit of normal for young healthy women. The dose delivered by available patches, intramuscular and oral forms of testosterone causes unwanted supraphysiological testosterone levels[25,26,27] and should not be used.

Women's Sexual Arousal Disorders

A lack of subjective arousal frequently occurs despite a normal genital vasocongestive response.[28] A woman's awareness of the engorgement of the genitalia is often minimal. Her subjective experience is influenced more consistently by concurrent thoughts and emotions than by feedback from the vasocongesting genitalia.[28]

- *Combined genital and subjective sexual arousal disorder* is absence of or markedly diminished feelings of sexual arousal (sexual excitement and sexual pleasure) from any type of sexual stimulation as well as complaints of absent or impaired genital sexual arousal (vulval swelling, lubrication).[7] Both subjective arousal from any type of sexual stimulus and any awareness of genital vasocongestion are absent.

- *Subjective sexual arousal disorder* is the absence of or markedly diminished feelings of sexual arousal (sexual excitement and sexual pleasure) from any type of sexual stimulation. Vaginal lubrication or other signs of physical response still occur.[7] Despite lack of subjective arousal from any type of stimulus, lubrication and/or genital swelling is noted.
- *Genital arousal disorder* is absent or impaired genital sexual arousal, i.e., minimal vulval swelling or vaginal lubrication from any type of sexual stimulation and reduced sexual sensation from caressing the genitalia. Subjective sexual excitement still occurs from a variety of nongenital stimuli but a "genital deadness" is reported.[7]

Goals of Therapy

- Address any lack of required auditory, visual or physical sexual stimuli
- Address psychological factors impairing subjective arousal, e.g., distractions, sexual anxiety, stressors, relationship issues, previous abuse
- Address biological factors impairing subjective arousal, e.g., fatigue, depression, medications (Table 1), androgen insufficiency (Table 2)
- Address biological factors impairing genital vasocongestion, e.g., estrogen deficiency, vaginitis, autonomic nerve damage, medications (Table 1), androgen insufficiency (Table 2)

Investigations

- Sexual history: current and past sexual functioning of both partners (Interviewing for Female Sexual Dysfunction[6])
- Medical history including medication (Table 1) and mood
- Relationship details, both past and present, focusing on nonsexual intimacy, trust, respect, safety, birth control, fertility and stressors
- Genital examination: although physical examination is usually normal, a reported lack of genital response may be the result of vulvovaginal atrophy or conditions such as lichen sclerosus
- Lab investigations only as indicated by medical history

Therapeutic Choices

Nonpharmacologic Choices

- Provide information if there is lack of stimuli or suitable context
- Counsel or refer when the couple's emotional intimacy is insufficient to allow the vulnerability needed for sexual arousal
- Address psychological factors, e.g., nonsexual distractions, feeling sexually substandard or unsafe, expecting a negative outcome, negative

emotions with arousal, suppressed anger and therefore suppressed sexual emotions, learned pattern of feeling emotions minimally

Pharmacologic Choices

There are no approved pharmacologic treatments for absent sexual arousal; however, when decreased androgen activity is clinically present (Table 2), physicians experienced in women's sexual dysfunction are investigating **testosterone** therapy (see Women's Sexual Desire/Interest Disorder, Pharmacologic Choices).

Address medications and other biological factors such as depression.

Use local **estrogen** when lack of genital congestion, loss of pleasure from genital stimulation, loss of lubrication or dyspareunia are associated with estrogen-deficient states (see Chapter 64). Vaginal lubricants (e.g., Gynemoistrin, Astroglide) or moisturizers (i.e., Replens) used regularly improve lubrication.

Genital arousal disorder may continue despite adequate estrogen if there is autonomic nerve damage, e.g., from radical hysterectomy or multiple sclerosis. If there is no contraindication to their use (see Chapter 66), consider the investigational use of PDE5 inhibitors[29,30,31] in women with neurologic disease (in addition to estrogen, local or systemic, in postmenopausal women).

Dyspareunia/Vaginismus

Dyspareunia is persistent or recurrent pain with attempted or complete vaginal entry and/or penile vaginal intercourse.[7]

Vaginismus is the persistent or recurrent difficulty of the woman to allow vaginal entry of a penis, a finger and/or any object, despite the woman's expressed wish to do so. There is often phobic avoidance and anticipation/fear/experience of pain, along with variable and involuntary pelvic muscle contraction.

Goals of Therapy

- Address biological factors:
  - estrogen deficiency
  - increased pelvic muscle tone
  - infection, e.g., chronic vaginitis, chronic pelvic inflammatory disease
  - pelvic pathology, e.g., endometriosis, interstitial cystitis, inflammatory bowel disease
  - rare congenital abnormalities, e.g., vaginal septum
  - reflexive pelvic muscle tightening on introital contact (vaginismus)

  - vulvar vestibulitis (VVS); vulvodynia (ongoing tenderness, burning, irritation around urethral meatus and vestibular area) may also be present
- Address psychosocial factors:
  - fear of pain or being damaged by something entering the vagina, difficulty with relinquishing control
  - ambivalence about being sexual with intercourse (the pain may be solely from *appropriate* tightening of perivaginal muscles)
  - lack of sexual arousal and therefore lack of increased elasticity, lubrication and expansion of proximal vagina
  - a subset of women with VVS show marked psychological distress associated with intense fear of negative evaluation and anxiety
- Address psychological factors:
  - lowered sexual self-confidence and decreased desire to self-stimulate
  - avoiding sexual stimuli or finding stimuli ineffective because of the focus on negative outcome
  - feelings of being extremely abnormal, shame, guilt and fears of permanent infertility especially when intercourse has never been possible
  - partner may be confused, feel unattractive and withdraw emotionally, compounding the woman's low sexual self-image

Investigations

- Determine timing of pain. Pain may occur with:
  - external contact, minimal entry of penis, dildo, finger (compatible with vaginismus)
  - partial entry of penis (compatible with vaginismus, VVS, urogenital atrophy, tears of posterior fourchette)
  - full entry and thrusting (compatible with lack of arousal, VVS, pelvic pathology)
  - penile movement (typical of VVS, urogenital atrophy, infection)
  - postcoital urination, partner's ejaculation (typical of VVS but also compatible with urogenital atrophy and with tears of posterior fourchette)
  - pain continues for hours after intercourse (typical of VVS, endometriosis)
- Gynecologic and medical history
- Physical exam looking for:
  - abdominal tenderness, masses
  - vulvar atrophy (associated with estrogen deficiency)
  - interlabial fissures (associated with estrogen deficiency or candidiasis)

  - signs of past tears of posterior fourchette
  - adhesions between labia minora which preclude penile entry and require surgical division
  - deficient posterior fourchette requiring simple perineoplasty
  - abnormal discharge (vaginal infection or possibly more serious pelvic pathology)
  - erythema of introital margin (consistent with VVS)
  - allodynia (sensation of pain from simple touch) of introital margin (consistent with VVS)
  - lichen sclerosus involving the introitus
  - bimanual exam: pain on palpation of uterus, cervix or adnexae, nodularity along uterosacral ligaments or in the pouch of Douglas, all evidence of possible pelvic pathology; pelvic muscle hypertonicity with "trigger points" in deep levator ani muscles; abnormalities in urethra, bladder or rectum
  - woman unable to be examined: encourage "practising" at home in private for 10 minutes daily. She should recline on couch or bed, or in the bathtub, partially abducting her thighs and learning to tolerate self-touch to the vulva, ultimately to the introitus, spreading the labia so the introitus can be examined. When she is ready for the exam, allow her to be in control, separating her labia, and any touch (e.g., with a Q-tip for VVS) can be done by her. Full examination is preferably delayed to a subsequent visit
- Laboratory investigations as indicated by history and physical examination:
  - KOH whiff test (fishy odour intensified by addition of a few drops of potassium hydroxide 10% to vaginal secretions on speculum or smear) to detect bacterial vaginosis
  - microscopy and pH for bacterial vaginosis, candidiasis, trichomoniasis
  - fasting glucose and HIV status if chronic candidiasis present
  - biopsy of any vulval area with abnormal appearance
  - DNA and/or culture for gonococcus and chlamydia

Therapeutic Choices

Benefit is more likely when psychosexual and medical approaches are combined.[32]

Nonpharmacologic Choices

- Advise couples to focus on nonpenetrative sex and avoid actual intercourse to break cycle of pain
- Address concomitant lack of arousal and desire
- Refer for definitive treatment if pelvic pathology suspected

- Refer if conservative therapy for recurrent tearing of posterior fourchette fails
- Assess pelvic muscle hypertonicity[33]
  - refer to pelvic muscle physiotherapist or teach "reverse Kegel exercises" with use of conical vaginal inserts of gradually increasing diameter
- Explain role of stress in chronic pain, and counsel on management

Pharmacologic Choices

There is no good evidence for the treatment of dyspareunia/vaginismus. The following recommendations are based on the author's experience and a recent international consensus.[34]

Local **estrogen** can be used for vulvovaginal atrophy (see Chapter 64).

For VVS, consider **antiepileptic** drugs, e.g., **topiramate** or **gabapentin**. Begin at the lowest dose and increase slowly as for neuropathic pain syndromes (see Chapter 15). **Venlafaxine** or **tricyclic antidepressants** may also be used. Begin at the lowest dose and increase slowly. Nondepressed patients are very susceptible to side effects.[35] Warn against sudden discontinuation of both antiepileptic drugs and antidepressants.

Topical anti-inflammatory medications for the allodynia of VVS help some women. In a subset of women, **sodium cromoglycate** 2% in glaxal base may be more effective and possibly safer than **hydrocortisone** 1% although there are no head-to-head trials. Medication must be placed on sites of allodynia, preferably with a needleless syringe, under direct vision using a mirror. Predicting which medication is optimal for which woman is currently not possible. Higher potency steroids provide short-term relief but are associated with rebound exacerbations and not recommended.

Treat any STIs that are identified (see Chapter 104).

Topical **estrogen cream** can be used for recurrent posterior fourchette tearing. Topical **testosterone** 2% is also helpful. Apply sparingly daily to the posterior fourchette and review in three months.

Vaginal lubricants and vaginal moisturizers can be helpful (see Chapter 64).

Therapeutic Tips

- Information is often therapeutic, especially for changes in sexual function and needs in both men and women with life cycle changes and aging. Women's desire "normally" lessens with duration of relationships. The need for orgasm with each sexual interaction, "normally" lessens with age in men and women. Gradual loss of spontaneous/initial desire, but the ability to become aroused and trigger desire "once into it" is "normal" for middle-aged and older women.
- Loss of sexual desire is a common symptom of depression. Many antidepressants can cause not only orgasmic dysfunction but loss of

desire. Bupropion, mirtazapine and moclobemide appear to be less likely to cause sexual dysfunction.

- For the woman complaining of low sexual desire or arousal, construct her sex response cycle (Figure 1) to identify the breaks. This logic is therapeutic as she may feel less dysfunctional and become aware of the contextual changes needed to restore her motivation and ability to become sexually aroused.
- Most women complaining of lack of arousal have normal vulval and vaginal congestion. Focus assessment and therapy on the adequacy of stimuli and context and the biological and psychological factors interfering with arousability of her mind.
- When the etiology of desire and arousal disorders appears to stem from deep-seated themes in childhood and adolescence and/or there is a history of abuse (mental, emotional, physical), refer to a psychiatrist or psychologist. When the relevant factors are lack of useful sexual contexts, stimuli, sexual information, needed eroticism and attractive behaviours of partners, consider referral to a sex therapist.

Figure 1: **Model of Female Sexual Response Cycle**

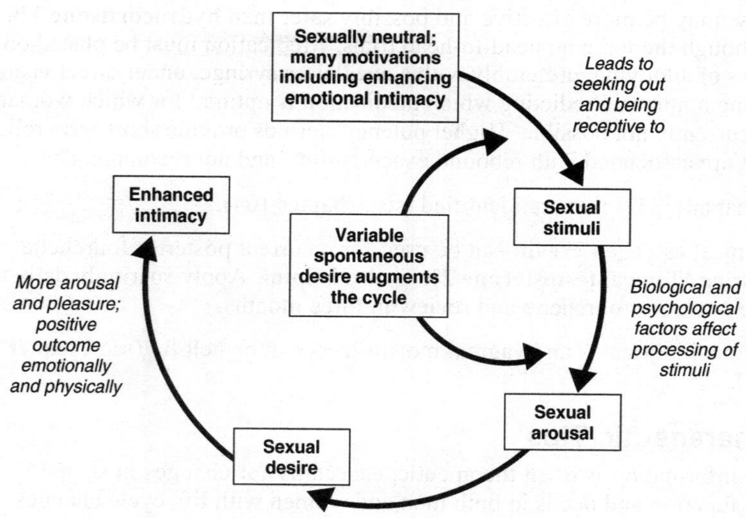

Adapted with permission from Lippincott Williams & Wilkins. R. Basson. Female sexual response: the role of drugs in the management of sexual dysfunction. *Obstet Gynecol* 2001;98(2):350-3.

Suggested Readings

Basson R. Clinical practice. Sexual desire and arousal disorders in women. *N Engl J Med* 2006;354(14):1497-506.

Basson R, Schultz WW. Sexual sequelae of general medical disorders. *Lancet* 2007;369(9559):409-24.

Bhasin S, Enzlin P, Coviello A et al. Sexual dysfunction in men and women with endocrine disorders. *Lancet* 2007;369(9561):597-611.

Rees PM, Fowler CJ, Maas CP. Sexual function in men and women with neurological disorders. *Lancet* 2007;369(9560):512-25.

Women's difficulties with low sexual desire and sexual avoidance. In: Levine SB, editor. *Handbook of clinical sexuality for mental health professionals*. New York (NY): Brunner-Routledge; 2003.

References

1. Fugl-Meyer AR, Sjögren Fugl-Meyer K. Sexual disabilities, problems and satisfaction in 18-74 year old Swedes. *Scand J Sexol* 1999;2(2):79-105.
2. Mercer CH, Fenton KA, Johnson AM et al. Sexual function problems and help seeking behaviour in Britain: national probability sample survey. *BMJ* 2003;327(7412):426-7.
3. Basson R, Schultz WW. Sexual sequelae of general medical disorders. *Lancet* 2007;369(9559):409-24.
4. Rees PM, Fowler CJ, Maas CP. Sexual function in men and women with neurological disorders. *Lancet* 2007;369(9560):512-25.
5. Bhasin S, Enzlin P, Coviello A et al. Sexual dysfunction in men and women with endocrine disorders. *Lancet* 2007;369(9561):597-611.
6. Basson R. Introduction to special issue on women's sexuality and outline of assessment of sexual problems. *Menopause* 2004;11(6 Pt 2):709-13.
7. Basson R, Leiblum S, Brotto L et al. Definitions of women's sexual dysfunction reconsidered: advocating expansion and revision. *J Psychosom Obstet Gynaecol* 2003;24(4):221-9.
8. Dennerstein L, Lehert P. Modeling mid-aged women's sexual functioning: a prospective, population-based study. *J Sex Marital Ther* 2004;30(3):173-83.
9. Bancroft J, Loftus J, Long JS. Distress about sex: a national survey of women in heterosexual relationships. *Arch Sex Behav* 2003;32(3):193-208.
10. Laumann EO, Nicolosi A, Glasser DB et al. Sexual problems among women and men aged 40-80 y: prevalence and correlates identified in the Global Study of Sexual Attitudes and Behaviors. *Int J Impot Res* 2005;17(1):39-57.
11. Davis SR, Guay AT, Shifren JL et al. Endocrine aspects of female sexual dysfunction. *J Sex Med* 2004;1(1):82-6.
12. Santoro N, Torrens J, Crawford S et al. Correlates of circulating androgens in mid-life women: the study of women's health across the nation. *J Clin Endocrinol Metab* 2005;90(8):4836-45.
13. Labrie F, Luu-The V, Labrie C et al. Endocrine and intracrine sources of androgens in women: inhibition of breast cancer and other roles of androgens and their precursor dehydroepiandrosterone. *Endocr Rev* 2003;24(2):152-82.
14. Weirman ME, Basson R, Davis SR et al. Androgen therapy in women: an Endocrine Society Clinical Practice guideline. *J Clin Endocrinol Metab* 2006;91(10):3697-710.
15. Finger WW, Lund M, Slagle MA. Medications that may contribute to sexual disorders. A guide to assessment and treatment in family practice. *J Fam Pract* 1997;44(1):33-43.
16. Gregoria RS, Golden KA, Bahce A et al. Antidepressant-induced sexual dysfunction. *Ann Pharmacother* 2002;36(10):1577-89.
17. Morrell MJ, Flynn KL, Done S et al. Sexual dysfunction, sex steroid hormone abnormalities, and depression in women with epilepsy treated with antiepileptic drugs. *Epilepsy Behav* 2005;6(3):360-5.
18. Sanders SA, Graham CA, Bass JL et al. A prospective study of the effects of oral contraceptives on sexuality and well-being and their relationship to discontinuation. *Contraception* 2001;64(1):51-8.
19. Guay AT. Screening for androgen deficiency in women: methodological and interpretive issues. *Fertil Steril* 2002;77(Suppl 4):S83-8.
20. Braunstein GD, Sundwall DA, Katz M et al. Safety and efficacy of a testosterone patch for the treatment of hypoactive sexual desire disorder in surgically menopausal women: a randomized, placebo-controlled trial. *Arch Intern Med* 2005;165(14):1582-9.
21. Simon J, Braunstein G, Nachtigall L et al. Testosterone patch increases sexual activity and desire in surgically menopausal women with hypoactive sexual desire disorder. *J Clin Endocrinol Metab* 2005;90(9):5226-33.
22. Shifren JL, Davis SR, Moreau M et al. Testosterone patch for the treatment of hypoactive sexual desire in naturally menopausal women: results from the INTIMATE NMI Study. *Menopause* 2006;13(5):770-9.

23. Buster JE, Kingsberg SA, Aguirre O et al. Testosterone patch for low sexual desire in surgically menopausal women: a randomized trial. *Obstet Gynecol* 2005;105(5 Pt 1):944-52.
24. Davis SR, van der Mooren MJ, van Lunsen RH et al. Efficacy and safety of a testosterone patch for the treatment of hypoactive sexual desire disorder in surgically menopausal women: a randomized, placebo-controlled trial. *Menopause* 2006;13(3):387-96.
25. Floter A, Carlstrom K, von Schoultz B et al. Administration of testosterone undecanoate in postmenopausal women: effects on androgens, estradiol, and gonadotrophins. *Menopause* 2000;7(4):251-6.
26. Padero MC, Bhasin S, Friedman TC. Androgen supplementation in older women: too much hype, not enough data. *J Am Geriatr Soc* 2002;50(6):1131-40.
27. Chu MC, Lobo RA. Formulations and use of androgens in women. *Mayo Clin Proc* 2004;79(4 Suppl):S3-7.
28. van Lunsen RH, Laan E. Genital vascular responsiveness and sexual feelings in midlife women: psychophysiologic, brain, and genital imaging studies. *Menopause* 2004;11(6 Pt 2):741-8.
29. Sipski ML, Rosen RC, Alexander CJ et al. Sildenafil effects on sexual and cardiovascular responses in women with spinal cord injury. *Urology* 2000;55(6):812-5.
30. Basson R, Brotto LA. Sexual psychophysiology and effects of sildenafil citrate in oestrogenised women with acquired genital arousal disorder and impaired orgasm: a randomised controlled trial. *BJOG* 2003;110(11):1014-24.
31. Caruso S, Rugolo S, Agnello C et al. Sildenafil improved sexual functioning in premenopausal women with type 1 diabetes who are affected by sexual arousal disorder: a double-blind crossover, placebo-controlled pilot study. *Fertil Steril* 2006;85(5):1496-501.
32. Brotto LA, Basson R, Gehring D. Psychological profiles among women with vulvar vestibulitis syndrome: a chart review. *J Psychosom Obstet Gynaecol* 2003;24(3):195-203.
33. McKay E, Kaufman RH, Doctor U et al. Treating vulvar vestibulitis with electromyographic biofeedback of pelvic floor musculature. *J Reprod Med* 2001;46(4):337-42.
34. Basson R, Althof S, Davis S et al. Summary of the recommendations on sexual dysfunctions in women. *J Sex Med* 2004;1(1):24-34.
35. Reed BD, Haefner HK, Cantor L. Vulvar dysesthesia (vulvodynia). A follow-up study. *J Reprod Med* 2003;48(6):409-16.

CHAPTER 66
Male Sexual Dysfunction

Rosemary Basson, FRCP (UK)

This chapter addresses erectile dysfunction and premature ejaculation.

Erectile Dysfunction

Erectile dysfunction (ED) is the persistent inability to obtain or maintain an erection sufficiently firm for satisfactory sexual activity. Addressing sexual function is an integral part of general medical assessment as impairment can signal serious disease. Of note is the frequency with which vascular erectile dysfunction heralds asymptomatic coronary artery disease.[1]

Goals of Therapy

- Address underlying conditions that present as ED
- Assess the safety of resuming intercourse and orgasm after serious illness
- Correct reversible ED
- Safely prescribe medical enhancement for irreversible ED
- Restore sexual intimacy to allow sexual arousal

Investigations (Figure 1)

- Sexual history (Table 1) with attention to:
  - reversible causes of ED (Table 2)
  - identifying psychological issues underlying or contributing to ED, or that may hinder the efficacy of pharmacotherapy
- Medical history with attention to damage from:
  - reversible factors, e.g., medications (Table 3), depression, decreased testosterone, prostatitis (Table 2)
  - irreversible factors, e.g., hypertension, smoking, elevated cholesterol, neurologic disease, penile structural problems (e.g., Peyronie's disease), diabetes mellitus, pelvic surgery or trauma damaging pelvic autonomic nerves
  - known risks associated with resumption of intercourse and orgasm, e.g., cardiac risk or, less commonly, risk of recurrent cerebral bleed, respiratory or other physical compromise

Table 1: Questions to Clarify Sexual History and Current Sexual Status

- For how long have you had difficulty getting and keeping erections?
- On a scale of 1–10/10 where 1/10 is a flaccid penis, 10/10 is completely firm and erect and 6/10 allows (but only just allows) intercourse, how firm are erections when you have sexual play with your partner, when you attempt intercourse, when you waken from sleep, and when you self-stimulate?
- Despite those changes, are you two still touching each other in sexual ways, and being a sexual couple?
- Your willingness to try and have sex may well be reduced given the disappointments, but do you still have sexual thoughts, sexual fantasies and the desire to self-stimulate, and become aroused mentally if you see or hear something erotic? How sexually excited (in your mind) are you when sexually active with your partner?
- Your experience of orgasm—has that changed?
- Are you reaching ejaculation—and has that changed?
- Does your partner have sexual difficulties? Will I be able to interview your partner? Is your partner in agreement with reinstitution of sexual activity including intercourse?
- What effects have these difficulties had on you, on your relationship and on your partner?

Table 2: Clues to Potentially Reversible Erectile Dysfunction

Clues in Sexual History	Potential Reversible Factor
Sleep-induced and self-stimulated erections are firmer than erections with sexual partner	Psychological factors: intrapersonal (e.g., insecurity, perfectionism, distractions, depression); interpersonal (i.e., difficulties within the relationship)
Decreased sexual desire (fewer sexual thoughts and fantasies)	Depression, ↓ testosterone, ↑ prolactin, medications, psychodynamic issues (likely complex, such as a learned response not to feel emotions generally)
Ejaculation delayed	Drug effect, ↓ testosterone
Ejaculation early and painful	Prostatitis
Decreased orgasm intensity	Drug effect, depression, ↓ testosterone
ED generalized and lifelong	Congenital or past traumatic vascular damage, potentially amenable to microvascular surgery

Table 3: Drugs Associated with Erectile Dysfunction

Acetazolamide	Clonidine	Metoclopramide
Alcohol (acute, chronic)	Digoxin	Phenytoin
Alpha blockers	Finasteride	Propranolol
Atenolol	Ketoconazole	Phenothiazines
Barbiturates	Labetalol	Spironolactone
Carbamazepine	Lithium	SSRIs
Cimetidine	MAOIs	Tricyclic Antidepressants
Clofibrate	Methadone	Thiazides

Abbreviations: MAOIs = monoamine oxidase inhibitors; SSRIs = selective serotonin reuptake inhibitors.

- Personal psychosexual history preferably from each partner individually with attention to:
  - negative thoughts during sexual engagement, e.g., fear of loss of erection, anger, resentment, distractions
  - past sexual experiences both positive and negative
  - childhood experiences that may have affected ability to be intimate, to feel emotions (especially for long-term dysfunction)
- Physical examination with attention to:
  - cardiovascular (CV) signs that may indicate irreversible vascular cause, e.g., bruits, hypertension, fundal changes, poor peripheral pulses, heart failure

    Note: Normal CV exam does not exclude vascular etiology, e.g., endothelial cells lining corpora cavernosal sinusoids cannot be examined
  - CNS signs that may indicate irreversible neurologic damage, e.g., multiple sclerosis, dementia, Parkinson's disease, peripheral neuropathy, spinal cord injury or diabetes mellitus
  - late signs of hypotestosteronism including fine body hair, smooth skin, testicular atrophy, lessening of beard, gynecomastia, hepatomegaly
  - rectal exam to detect signs of prostatic pathology
  - assessment of *cardiovascular risk* (Table 4) associated with sexual activity, using stress testing to four metabolic equivalents (METs), to identify silent or symptomatic cardiac ischemia that could occur with sexual intercourse and orgasm. Two consensus panels have developed similar guidelines for management of ED based on cardiovascular risk.[2,3]

Table 4: **Management Recommendations Based on Graded Cardiovascular (CV) Risk Assessment**

Grade of Risk	Categories of CVD	Management Recommendations
Low risk	• Asymptomatic, < 3 major risk factors for CAD excluding age and gender • Controlled hypertension • Mild, stable angina • Post-successful coronary revascularization • Uncomplicated past MI (> 6–8 wk) • Mild valvular disease • LVD/CHF (NYHA Class I)	• Primary-care management • Consider all first-line therapies • Reassess at regular intervals (6–12 months)

(cont'd)

Table 4: **Management Recommendations Based on Graded Cardiovascular (CV) Risk Assessment** *(cont'd)*

Grade of Risk	Categories of CVD	Management Recommendations
Intermediate Risk	• ≥ 3 major risk factors for CAD, excluding gender • Moderate, stable angina • Recent MI (> 2, < 6 wk) • LVD/CHF (NYHA Class II) • Noncardiac sequelae of atherosclerotic disease (e.g. CVA, peripheral vascular disease)	• Evaluation by a cardiologist prior to initiation of any therapy for erectile dysfunction, due to risk of myocardial ischemia during sexual activity and orgasm • Specialized CV testing, e.g., ETT, Echo • Restratification into high risk or low risk based on the results of CV assessment
High Risk	• Unstable or refractory angina • Uncontrolled hypertension • LVD/CHF (NYHA Class III/IV) • Recent MI (< 2 wk), CVA • High-risk arrhythmias • Hypertrophic obstructive and other cardiomyopathies • Moderate/severe valvular disease	• Priority referral for specialized CV management • Treatment for sexual dysfunction to be deferred until cardiac condition stabilized and dependent on specialist recommendations

Abbreviations: CAD = coronary artery disease; CHF = congestive heart failure; CVA = cerebrovascular accident; CVD = cardiovascular disease; Echo = echocardiogram; ETT = exercise tolerance test; LVD = left ventricular dysfunction; NYHA = New York Heart Association.

- Laboratory investigations:
  - calculated free testosterone or bioavailable testosterone and prolactin levels, if the patient is identified as having a primary decrease in sexual desire, LH, FSH if testosterone low
  - fasting blood glucose, lipid profile, CBC and liver function tests as needed (abnormalities in these parameters may clarify etiology of ED, but correcting them is unlikely to improve it)
  - serum creatinine and calculated GFR

Therapeutic Choices

Nonpharmacologic Choices

Address Sexual Avoidance

- Remind couples who have deliberately avoided sexual intimacy because of dysfunction that reinstating sexual intimacy requires effort:
  - the first priority is to make time to be together, away from responsibilities, to create a context appropriate for reinstituting sex
  - reintroduce sexual/sensual/intimate remarks and behaviours throughout the day to allow each individual to once again view the other as a potential sexual partner
  - address perceived negative consequences of attempting to be sexual together, e.g., performance failure, pregnancy, moral issues, dyspareunia in the woman

Address Lack of Subjective Sexual Arousal

- Address intra- and interpersonal psychological issues identified in history that are contributing to the ED and/or would likely preclude benefit from pharmacologic intervention.
- Address partner sexual dysfunction/lack of enjoyment
- Address lack of useful stimulation/contexts

Vacuum Erection Devices (VEDs)

VEDs, also known as vacuum constrictive devices, create a vacuum and draw venous blood back into the penis. The blood is then trapped by the use of a retaining band around the base of the penis, to attain adequate firmness for intercourse. There is a learning curve with the use of VEDs. Warn patients that the tightness of the retention band is critical and the band must be removed within 30 minutes after being applied. Some men cannot tolerate the degree of tightness required. Any condition that predisposes to priapism (e.g., leukemia, polycythemia, myelofibrosis and sickle cell disease) is a relative contraindication to the use of a VED. VED is contraindicated in patients who are on warfarin or have an increased INR.

Pharmacologic Choices (Table 6)

Phosphodiesterase Type 5 (PDE5) Inhibitors

Sildenafil, **vardenafil** and **tadalafil** are the drugs of first choice for ED, given their safety, efficacy and oral administration.[4,5,6] Safety and efficacy data are more extensive for sildenafil as it has been on the market for a longer time. PDE5 inhibitors can only enhance an erection that is partially developing as a result of effective sexual stimulation and mental sexual arousal.

Duration of action is longest with tadalafil but, contrary to previous information, sildenafil[7] and vardenafil[8] may last up to 8-12 hours. Vardenafil may have an onset of action of as early as 10 minutes.[9] Vardenafil and sildenafil have some affinity for PDE_6 present in the retina accounting for occasional visual side effects. Tadalafil has some affinity for PDE_{11A} which may underlie myalgia associated with this drug. The onset of action of tadalafil and sildenafil appears not to be influenced by food.

Head-to-head studies of these three drugs are just beginning.

Contraindications to the use of PDE5 inhibitors include: concurrent use of nitrates or nonselective alpha-blockers; symptomatic hypotension (these are mildly hypotensive drugs); previous priapism; any condition in which even a slight lowering of systemic pressure would be poorly tolerated, including conditions restricting aortic outflow and volume depletion states; conditions predisposing to priapism, e.g., leukemia, polycythemia, myelofibrosis and sickle cell disease.

Prostaglandin E_1 (PGE_1) Analogues

Alprostadil Intracavernosal Injection[10]

If sufficient corporal erectile tissue is still present, injected alprostadil will cause erections even in the absence of mental sexual arousal.

Because alprostadil directly stimulates nociceptors, the technique, dose and dilution are critical for efficacy and comfort of erection. Proper dilution and measurement of the dose are particularly important in neurogenic ED, which often requires doses of only 1 to 3 µg. Doses up to 40 to 60 µg may be needed for vascular ED.

Contraindications to the use of intracavernosal alprostadil include: anticoagulation; previous priapism; symptomatic thrombocytopenia; conditions predisposing to priapism, e.g., leukemia, polycythemia, myelofibrosis, sickle cell disease and valve lesions with significant risk of subacute bacterial endocarditis.

Alprostadil by Urethral Instillation[11]

Instilling alprostadil in the form of a pellet into the urethra allows the drug to enter the corpus spongiosum. Retrograde venous passage from spongiosum to cavernosa is unpredictable and depends on the individual's venous anatomy. Therefore, a trial of intraurethral alprostadil pellets is necessary to determine efficacy in a particular patient.

By entering the communicating veins between the corpora, the drug is introduced into the systemic circulation, and hypotensive systemic side effects are possible.

Contraindications to the use of intraurethral alprostadil include: previous priapism; symptomatic hypotension; conditions predisposing to priapism (e.g., leukemia, polycythemia, myelofibrosis and sickle cell disease); distal urethral pathology.

Therapeutic Tips

- ED is a couple entity. Interview the partner whenever possible. There may be reasons not to intervene (e.g., the man's desire for intercourse is low but he feels his partner expects/needs intercourse, when in reality she is pleased intercourse is no longer possible, never enjoyed it, has chronic dyspareunia and prefers nonpenetrative sex).
- Sex is a biopsychosocial entity. If a patient's erections with self-stimulation are more firm and erect than with his partner, addressing the couple's interaction is more relevant than drug therapy. Prescribing alprostadil will address only the erectile difficulty. PDE5 inhibitors are unlikely to be effective, given the minimal arousal.
- Plan follow-up, since "drug failures" are usually due to lack of sexual arousal, poor technique with intracavernosal therapy or low desire in the partner.

- Reinforce the contraindications to the use of nitrates and alpha-blockers.
- Assess safety of resumption of sexual activity in cardiac patients prior to initiation of any therapy—this applies, of course, to both partners.

Premature Ejaculation

Ejaculation is described as *premature* or rapid when it occurs with minimal sexual stimulation, before or shortly after penetration, and before the person wishes it.

Goals of Therapy

- Address underlying conditions if premature ejaculation (PE) is acquired (as opposed to lifelong)
- Address psychological factors contributing to PE
- Address possible sequelae of PE in both the patient and his partner (Table 5)
- Provide reassurance that PE can be considered as "very efficient sexual function" rather than a dysfunction and that many couples simply adapt
- Choose therapy appropriate to the man's or couple's circumstances

Table 5: **Sequelae of PE for Both Patient and Partner**

Low sexual self-confidence (which creates more anxiety, compounding PE and possibly provoking ED)
Arousal, desire or orgasmic disorder in partner resulting from rushing on to (brief) intercourse
Intercourse itself never resulting in partner's orgasm
Dyspareunia from premature entry into vagina without woman's arousal

Investigations

- Psychosexual history with attention to:
  - description of current problem and previously tried interventions
  - possible psychological factors predisposing to PE (e.g., anxiety related to: intimacy, lack of sexual skill or attractiveness, losing erection or causing pain to the partner; feelings of guilt or shame associated with sex). Sexual anxiety when with the partner is implied since men with PE typically take longer to ejaculate with self-stimulation
- For acquired PE:
  - genitourinary history and prostate examination to identify underlying causes such as prostatic pathology, urinary tract irritation, e.g., bladder calculus
  - CNS history and exam in context of neurological disease, e.g., MS. However, these conditions more often cause *delayed* ejaculation.

- urinalysis and pelvic ultrasound if infection or bladder calculus suspected. Cystoscopy may be indicated if other underlying pathology is suspected, or ultrasound findings require clarification.

Therapeutic Choices

Nonpharmacologic Choices

The following sex therapy techniques must include suggestions for pleasuring the partner, to avoid feelings of being used. They are not appropriate for couples with poor relationships for whom referral for relationship counselling is the appropriate therapy.

- Adaptation
  - ejaculation stimulated by his partner's hand can be the beginning of a more leisurely sexual experience for the younger man with PE. If the couple then proceeds towards mutual sexual touching and then intercourse, his erection will return, but his orgasmic response will be slower with the "second" erection.

The following 3 techniques emphasize the appreciation of low intensity sexual arousal without a "goal," e.g., of intercourse.

- Stop/start technique
  - the couple has a series of experiences (6 to 12) where low key stimulation, e.g., his partner's hand is used. When he reaches moderate mental sexual arousal, the stimulation is deliberately stopped for one minute. It is then continued, to be stopped and restarted four times before he moves on to ejaculation. These exercises can be used to slow down his self-stimulated response but typically the difficulty occurs when with the partner. The objective is for him to learn to focus and enjoy lower degrees of sexual arousal. Numbing the penile skin with local anesthetic, reinforces the man's inability to recognize lower states of sexual arousal and is generally not used.
- Squeeze technique
  - the stop/start method is modified to include a brief, firm squeeze to the glans with the "stop."[9] This will decrease his excitement more than just discontinuing the stimulus. Most clinicians do not recommend this addition because of the negative/painful intervention.
- Quiet vagina
  - to decrease the immediate excitement (and ejaculation) resulting from vaginal stimulation with movement, the woman sits astride her partner, her vagina containing his penis, but with minimal movement for the first four to five minutes.

Pharmacologic Choices

Medications to slow down the ejaculatory reflex by increasing serotonergic transmission (SSRIs such as **citalopram**,[12] **fluoxetine**,[13]

paroxetine[14] and **sertraline**[14] or tricyclic antidepressants such as **clomipramine**,[15] in the usual initial dose range given either four to six hours prior to sexual activity or daily) are effective, but rarely allow permanent change. (For prescribing information, see Chapter 5). Combining pharmacologic and behavioural techniques is recommended, to prolong benefit and ultimately allow withdrawal of medication.

Sildenafil has been shown to significantly delay ejaculation.[16,17] None of the men had ED and the mechanism underlying this apparent sildenafil-induced delay in ejaculation is unknown.

For more severe refractory PE, intracavernosal therapy may result in erectile persistence after ejaculation, allowing for partner satisfaction.

Therapeutic Tips

- The overall objective of the adaptation and sex therapy techniques (± medication) is to enable the man to focus his attention away from the act of intercourse and concentrate instead on his enjoyment of the total sexual experience, including the pleasure he gives to, and receives from, his sexual partner. The more he can become aware of lower states of arousal, coupled with his ability to enjoy them, the less anxious he will be and the slower his response.

Figure 1: **Assessment and Management of Acquired Erectile Dysfunction**

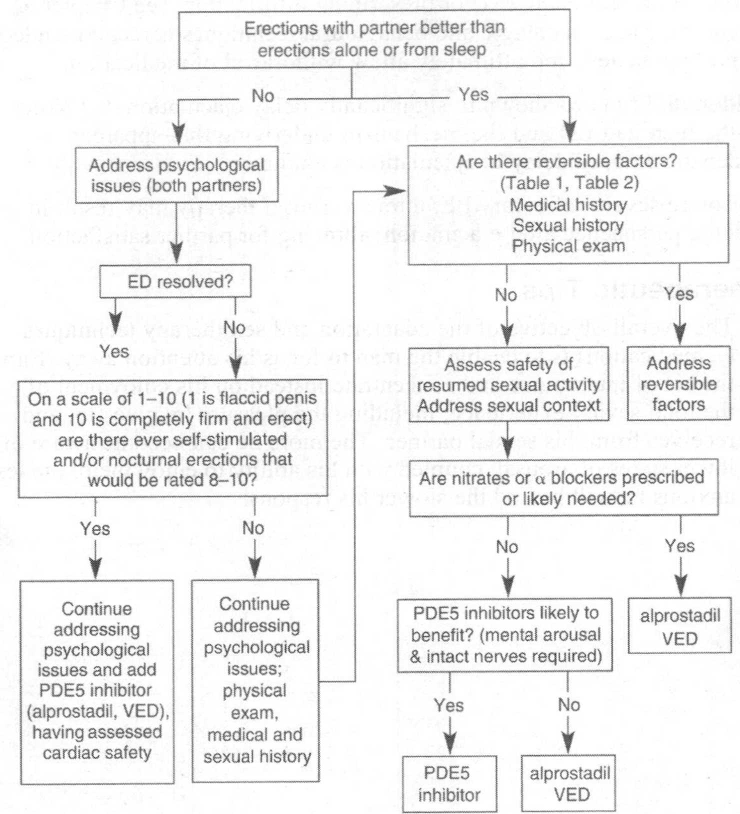

Abbreviations: VED = vacuum erection device; ED = erectile dysfunction; PDE5 inhibitor = phosphodiesterase type 5 inhibitor.

Table 6: **Drug Therapy for Erectile Dysfunction**

Class	Drug	Dose	Adverse Effects	Drug Interactions	Comments	Cost
PDE_5 Inhibitors	*sildenafil* Viagra	50–100 mg 30–60 min before sexual activity. Use only 25 mg in hepatic or renal disease (< 30 mL/min) and in the elderly. May use a smaller dose (e.g., 25 mg) with concomitant use of CYP3A4 inhibitors. Max dose 25 mg every 48 hours with ritonavir.	Headache (15%), flushing (10%), dyspepsia (7–17%), nasal congestion (4%), transient visual disturbances (3–11%), dizziness (2%), skin rash (2%). Rare: priapism, permanent vision loss.	Contraindicated with nitrates (seek emergency care if chest pain present within 24–48 hours of taking PDE5 inhibitor; not to be given for 5 days after stopping long-acting nitrates); contraindicated with nonselective alpha-blockers (hypotension); inhibitors of CYP3A4 (e.g., cimetidine, efavirenz, erythromycin, ketoconazole, itraconazole, ritonavir) can significantly ↓ sildenafil's metabolism. Avoid grapefruit juice.	Efficacy dependent on mental arousal. Duration of effect may be up to 12 hours. Dyspepsia and transient visual disturbances (impaired blue/green discrimination, blurred vision or increased light sensitivity) > 10% with doses of 100 mg. Use with caution in retinitis pigmentosa.	$10–11 per dose
	vardenafil Levitra	5–20 mg, 30–60 min before sexual activity. Use only 5 mg in moderate hepatic impairment or renal disease and in the elderly. Adjust with concomitant use of CYP3A4 inhibitors (2.5 mg/24h with ritonavir, indinavir, ketoconazole or itraconazole 400 mg/day; 5 mg/24h as single dose with ketoconazole or itraconazole, 200 mg/day, erythromycin)	Headache (15%), flushing (11%), dyspepsia (4%), rhinitis (3–9%), sinusitis (3%), transient visual disturbances (1–2%). Slight prolongation of QT interval. Rare: priapism, permanent vision loss.	See sildenafil. Slight prolongation of QT interval. Do not use with quinidine, procainamide, amiodarone or sotalol due to ↑ QT interval.	Efficacy dependent on mental arousal. Duration of effect may be up to 12 hours. Delayed absorption after food if high fat content. Do not use in men with congenital long QT syndrome.	$ 10–11 per dose

(cont'd)

Table 6: **Drug Therapy for Erectile Dysfunction** *(cont'd)*

Class	Drug	Dose	Adverse Effects	Drug Interactions	Comments	Cost
	tadalafil Cialis	2.5–20 mg, at least 60 min before sexual activity. Max: 10 mg/day in mild-to-moderate hepatic impairment. Max: 5 mg daily, or a single daily dose of 10 mg in a 48-h period in moderate renal insufficiency. Max: 5 mg in severe renal insufficiency or hemodialysis. No dose adjustment needed in the elderly.	Headache (11–15%), flushing (2–3%), dyspepsia (4–10%), nasal congestion (2–3%), myalgia (1–3%), back pain (3–6%). Rare: visual disturbances, permanent vision loss.	See sildenafil. Can use tamsulosin with tadalafil.	Efficacy dependent on mental arousal. Duration of effect up to 36 hours. Desirable in couples who want more freedom in timing their sexual activity. No delay in absorption after food. Should take tadalafil no more frequently than every 2nd day. Not recommended in severe hepatic impairment.	$10–11 per dose
PGE_1 Ana-logues	*alpros-tadil (intra-cavernosal injection)* Caverject	Effective dose provides an erection sufficient for intercourse with an erection duration ≤ 1 h. Neurogenic ED: start with 1.25 μg and titrate to response. May ↑ to 2.5 μg then to 5 μg, then by 5 μg increments until effective dose is reached. Vascular, psychogenic or mixed ED: start with 2.5 μg and titrate to response. Severe vascular ED may require up to 40–60 μg. Use 10–30 min prior to sexual	Penile pain (37%), hematoma (3%), ecchymosis (2%), penile fibrosis (3%). Rare: priapism.		Should not be used more than once daily or 3 times/wk, at least 24 hours between each dose. Caution re: needle stick injury and risk of STI transmission. Stress strict sterile technique, especially if known risk of endocarditis. Stress one time use of needle and syringe provided in Caverject kit. The initial dose is determined in the physician's office.	$14–21 per 10–20 μg dose

Class	Drug	Dose	Adverse Effects	Drug Interactions	Comments	Cost
		activity. Max dose is 60 μg once daily.				
	alprostadil (intraurethral pellet) MUSE	250–1000 μg 10–30 min before sexual activity. Dose depends on venous anatomy rather than ED etiology. Onset of effect within 5–10 min.	Penile pain (35%), dizziness (4%). Rare: syncope, priapism.	Additive hypotension with antihypertensives.	Do not use more than once per 24-h period. Monitor BP during in-office titration to detect asymptomatic hypotension.	$21 per dose

Abbreviations: STI = sexually transmitted infection; BP = blood pressure; ED = erectile dysfunction

Suggested Readings

Erectile Dysfunction

Bhasin S, Enzlin P, Coviello A et al. Sexual dysfunction in men and women with endocrine disorders. *Lancet* 2007;369(9561):597-611.

Rees PM, Fowler CJ, Maas CP. Sexual function in men and women with menopause with neurological disorders. *Lancet* 2007;369(9560):512-25.

Seftel AD, Mohammed MA, Althof SE. Erectile dysfunction: etiology, evaluation and treatment options. *Med Clin North Am* 2004;88(2):387-416.

Premature Ejaculation

Basson R, Schultz WW. Sexual sequelae of general medical disorders. *Lancet* 2007;369(9559):409-24.

Leiblum SR, editor. *Principles and practice of sex therapy.* 4th ed. New York (NY): Guilford Press; 2007. p. 212–40.

References

1. Basson R, Schultz WW. Sexual sequelae of general medical disorders. *Lancet* 2007;369(9559):409-24.
2. DeBusk R, Drory Y, Goldstein I et al. Management of sexual dysfunction in patients with cardiovascular disease: recommendations of The Princeton Consensus Panel. *Am J Cardiol* 2000;86(2):175-81.
3. Cheitlin MD, Hutter AM, Brindis RG et al. ACC/AHA expert consensus document. Use of sildenafil (Viagra) in patients with cardiovascular disease. American College of Cardiology/American Heart Association. *J Am Coll Cardiol* 1999;33(1):273-82.
4. Goldstein I, Lue TF, Padma-Nathan H et al. Oral sildenafil in the treatment of erectile dysfunction. Sildenafil Study Group. *N Engl J Med* 1998;338(20):1397-404.
5. Porst H, Rosen R, Padma-Nathan H et al. The efficacy and tolerability of vardenafil, a new, oral, selective phosphodiesterase type 5 inhibitor, in patients with erectile dysfunction: the first at-home clinical trial. *Int J Impot Res* 2001;13(4):192-9.
6. Brock GB, McMahon CG, Chen KK et al. Efficacy and safety of tadalafil for the treatment of erectile dysfunction: results of integrated analyses. *J Urol* 2002;168(4 Pt 1):1332-6.
7. Zinner N. Do food and dose timing affect the efficacy of sildenafil? A randomized placebo-controlled study. *J Sex Med* 2007;4(1):137-44.
8. Padma-Nathan H, Christ G, Adaikan G et al. Pharmacotherapy for erectile dysfunction. *J Sex Med* 2004;1(2):128-40.
9. Montorsi F, Padma-Nathan H, Buvat J et al. Earliest time to onset of action leading to successful intercourse with vardenafil determined in an at-home setting: a randomized, double-blind, placebo-controlled trial. *J Sex Med* 2004;1(2):168-78.
10. Porst H, Buvat J, Meuleman E et al. Intracavernous Alprostadil Alfadex--an effective and well tolerated treatment for erectile dysfunction. Results of a long-term European study. *Int J Impot Res* 1998;10(4):225-31.
11. Porst H. Transurethral alprostadil with MUSE (medicated urethral system for erection) vs intracavernous alprostadil--a comparative study in 103 patients with erectile dysfunction. *Int J Impot Res* 1997;9(4):187-92.
12. Atmaca M, Kuloglu M, Tezcan E et al. The efficacy of citalopram in the treatment of premature ejaculation: a placebo-controlled study. *Int J Impot Res* 2002;14(6)502-5.
13. Haensel SM, Klem TM, Hop WC et al. Fluoxetine and premature ejaculation: a double-blind, crossover, placebo-controlled study. *J Clin Psychopharmacol* 1998;18(1):72-7.
14. Waldinger MD, Zwinderman AH, Olivier B. Antidepressants and ejaculation: a double-blind, randomized, placebo-controlled, fixed-dose study with paroxetine, sertraline, and nefazodone. *J Clin Psychopharmacol* 2001;21(3):293-7.
15. Haensel SM, Rowland DL, Kallan KT. Clomipramine and sexual function in men with premature ejaculation and controls. *J Urol* 1996;156(4):1310-5.
16. Chen J, Greenstein A, Mabjeesh NJ et al. Role of sildenafil in the treatment of premature ejaculation [abstract]. *Int J Impot Res* 2001;13(Suppl 4):S48.
17. Montorsi F, Salonia A, Zanoni M et al. Premature ejaculation: a prospective study comparing paroxetine alone vs paroxetine plus sildenafil. Preliminary results [abstract]. *Int J Impot Res* 2001;13(Suppl 4):S48.

CHAPTER 67

Fibromyalgia

Howard Stein, , MD, , FRCPC

Fibromyalgia is characterized by chronic widespread pain, increased tenderness at specific sites known as "tender points," fatigue, headache and unrefreshing sleep. Fibromyalgia affects 2 to 4% of the general population. Of those affected, 80 to 90% are females. In general, symptom onset occurs between the ages of 30 and 60.

Goals of Therapy

- Reduce pain, fatigue, distress and sleep problems
- Improve physical and emotional well-being, functioning and quality of life
- Address the associated conditions
- Provide education and promote self-management

Investigations (Figure 1, Figure 2)

Therapeutic Choices

Nonpharmacologic Choices

- Empathy and encouragement from health care providers.
- A comprehensive, multidisciplinary program of education, self-management, nonpharmacologic pain reduction techniques, graded aerobic exercises, sleep hygiene, stress management and cognitive behavioural therapy can be effective.[1]
- Supervised aerobic exercise, walking programs, pool exercises and strength training can improve function, symptoms and well-being.[2]
- Nonpharmacologic pain reduction techniques include cold, heat, transcutaneous electrical nerve stimulation (TENS), acupuncture, massage, and relaxation techniques such as biofeedback, meditation and hypnosis.
- Patient education, such as the Arthritis Self-Help Course, can improve pain, sleep, fatigue, quality of life and the 6-minute walk. Improvement can last at least 3 to 12 months.[1]
- Cognitive behavioural strategies performed over 6 to 14 weeks show improvement in tender points, Visual Analogue Scale (VAS) pain scores, pain coping, pain behaviours, depression and physical function.[3]
- Electroacupuncture reduces pain and analgesic requirements.[4]

Pharmacologic Choices (Table 1)

Because the etiology of fibromyalgia remains unknown, drug treatments are largely empiric. Studies have been of short duration and varying quality.

- Low doses of **tricyclic antidepressants** (e.g., amitriptyline) at bedtime can improve sleep and reduce pain somewhat.[5] Only short-term efficacy has been shown. If taken two to three hours before bedtime the effect will start at bedtime, and morning hangover will be lessened.
- The only muscle relaxant that is somewhat effective is **cyclobenzaprine**, perhaps because it too is a tricyclic.[6]
- **Selective serotonin reuptake inhibitors** (SSRIs) are not as helpful as tricyclics but may have a role when used with amitriptyline in depressed patients with fibromyalgia.They are better tolerated than tricyclics. **Fluoxetine** in the morning with evening **amitriptyline** was more effective than either agent alone in a double-blind controlled trial in fibromyalgia sufferers.[7,8]
- Dual-action noradrenaline and serotonin reuptake inhibitors such as **venlafaxine** may help more individuals with fibromyalgia than do tricyclics (60% vs 40%).[9,10]
- Analgesics such as **acetaminophen** and **nonsteroidal anti-inflammatory drugs** (NSAIDs) (especially ibuprofen) deserve a trial but help very few patients. These drugs may not be useful for fibromyalgia because the pain is probably a result of central sensitization rather than peripheral pain or inflammation. However, **tramadol** (with or without acetaminophen) reduces pain and improves health-related quality of life in individuals with fibromyalgia.[11,12] The use of tramadol with antidepressants may cause serotonin syndrome. Other opioids should be avoided because of limited benefit, dependency and side effects.
- Sedatives may benefit those with severe sleep dysfunction but do not provide effective reduction of pain. Dependency and adverse effects are also concerns. **Clonazepam** or **zopiclone** might be useful intermittently but studies are lacking.[13]
- **Human growth hormone** improved symptoms in a placebo-controlled trial, although further investigation is required.[14] It may help only those with low growth hormone levels. Expense and availability limit its use.
- **S-adenosyl-methionine** (SAM-e) improved depression, pain, fatigue, morning stiffness and global disease measures in fibromyalgia.[5]
- Treatment of peripheral pain generators by local injection (e.g., usually **lidocaine** 1% with or without a depot form of **corticosteroid**) to myofascial trigger points may reduce the total pain burden and the perpetuation of central pain sensitization.[15]

Therapeutic Tips

- The treatment of arthritis and other conditions may be complicated by concomitant fibromyalgia.
- Pharmacologic agents work best when combined with nonpharmacologic modalities, ideally as part of a multidisciplinary treatment program.[1]
- It is important to document not only reduced pain but also improved function.
- Because patients with fibromyalgia are unduly sensitive to drug side effects, start medications at low doses and increase slowly by small increments.
- The initial improvement of fibromyalgia with drugs fades with time. Significant and sustained clinical improvement due to drugs occurs only in a minority of patients. However, about 20% of patients experience remission not necessarily related to any specific therapy. Conversely, there are subsets of patients who are intolerant of and/or unresponsive to all pharmacologic therapy.
- Sleep problems may need further study in a sleep disorder clinic.
- Concomitant mood disorders require higher doses of antidepressants than are used for fibromyalgia.

Figure 1: Investigation of Diffuse Aches and Pains

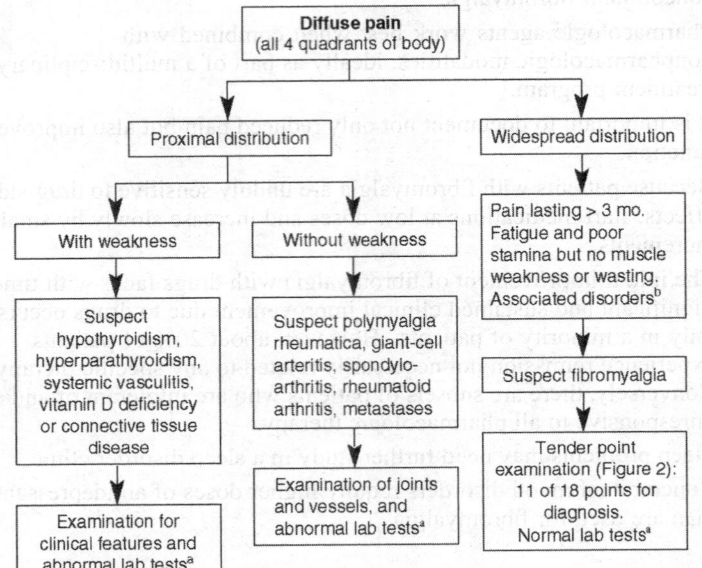

[a] CBC, ESR, creatinine, AST, alkaline phosphatase, calcium, TSH.

[b] Associated disorders include mood disturbances, cognitive dysfunction, irritable bowel syndrome, irritable bladder syndrome, dizziness, cold intolerance, subjective swelling, paresthesiae and temporomandibular joint syndrome.

Abbreviations: CBC = complete blood count; ESR = erythrocyte sedimentation rate; AST = aspartate transaminase; TSH = thyroid-stimulating hormone

Figure 2: **Tender Point Examination**[a]

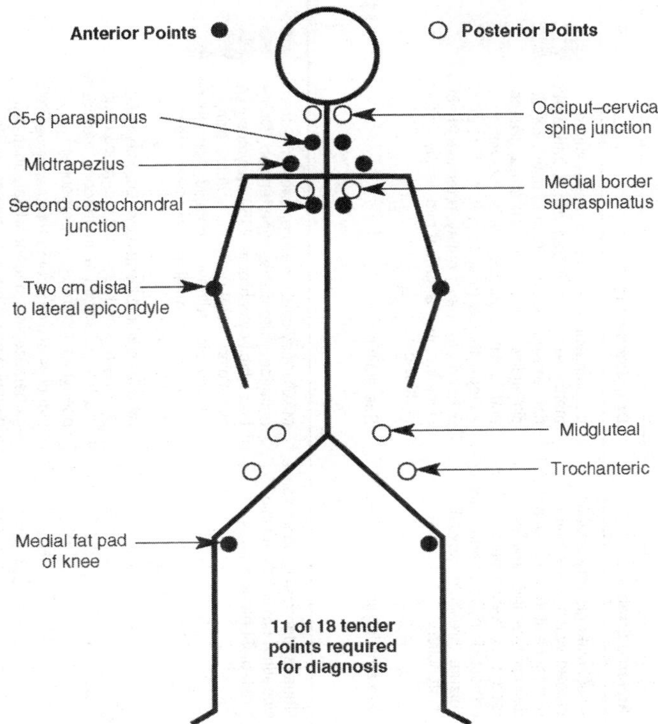

[a] Using thumb pressure sufficient to blanch fingernail.

Table 1: **Drugs Used in Fibromyalgia**

Class	Drug	Dose	Adverse Effects	Drug Interactions	Cost[a]
Tricyclic Agents[b]	*amitriptyline* generics	5–20 mg 2–3 h before bedtime	Anticholinergic (dry mouth, blurred vision, constipation, urinary hesitancy, tachycardia, delirium), antihistaminergic (sedation, weight gain), orthostatic hypotension, lowered seizure threshold; sexual dysfunction.	Combination with MAOIs may result in mania, excitation, hyperpyrexia; barbiturates, carbamazepine and rifampin may ↓ effect; cimetidine and antipsychotics may ↑ effect and toxicity; possible interaction with antiarrhythmics (may lead to ↑ effect of either drug); may ↓ antihypertensive effect of clonidine; may augment hypotensive effect of thiazides.	$
	cyclobenzaprine generics	10–40 mg/day in 2 to 4 divided doses	See amitriptyline.	See amitriptyline.	$-$$$
Selective Serotonin Reuptake Inhibitors[b]	*fluoxetine* Prozac, generics	10–20 mg/day with amitriptyline	Nausea, dry mouth, somnolence, sweating, sexual dysfunction. ↑ risk of GI bleeding.	MAOIs may cause severe reaction — tremor, agitation, hypomania, hypertension. Drugs that inhibit cytochrome P450 enzymes (e.g., cimetidine, clarithromycin, erythromycin, fluconazole, indinavir, isoniazid, itraconazole, ketoconazole, quinidine, ritonavir) may ↑ SSRI levels. All SSRIs inhibit certain cytochrome P450 isoenzymes and can ↓ the clearance of other drugs (e.g., clozapine, methadone, mexiletine, phenytoin, pimozide, propafenone). Inducers of cytochrome P450 enzymes (e.g., carbamazepine, phenobarbital, phenytoin, rifampin) can ↑ the clearance of SSRIs. ↑ risk of GI bleeding with NSAIDs.	$$

Class	Drug	Dose	Adverse Effects	Drug Interactions	Cost[a]
Serotonin-Norepinephrine Reuptake Inhibitors	*venlafaxine* Effexor XR, generic	75 mg/day	Nausea, sweating, somnolence, dry mouth, dizziness, insomnia, hypertension, abnormal ejaculation/orgasm.	Alcohol, warfarin, clozapine, MAOIs, tramadol. Drugs that inhibit cytochrome P450 may ↑ venlafaxine levels.	$$$
Hypnotics[b]	*zopiclone* Imovane, Rhovane, generics	3.75–7.5 mg HS	Bitter taste, drowsiness.	Alcohol, CNS depressants, antidepressants.	$
Analgesics	*acetaminophen* Tylenol, Atasol Preparations, generics[c]	325–1000 mg Q4H Max. 4 g/day	Hepatotoxicity, urticaria, rash.	Excessive alcohol intake may ↑ the risk of hepatotoxicity. Warfarin: ↑ anticoagulant effect with regular use of > 2 g/day.	$
	tramadol / acetaminophen Tramacet	1–2 tablets Q4–6H as needed Max. 8 tabs/day	Somnolence, dizziness, flushing, constipation, nausea, pruritus, seizures, anaphylactoid reactions, dependence, withdrawal syndrome.	See acetaminophen. Possible ↑ risk of seizure with SSRI antidepressants or anorectics, MAOIs, tricyclic antidepressants and other tricyclic compounds, neuroleptics, amphetamines, linezolid, opioids or any drugs that reduce the seizure threshold. Use with SSRIs or MAOIs may also ↑ risk of serotonin syndrome. Use with CNS depressants may ↑ the risk of CNS and respiratory depression. Carbamazepine may ↑ the metabolism of tramadol. Also, tramadol may ↑ the risk of seizures in patients taking anticonvulsants.	$$$$$

(cont'd)

Table 1: **Drugs Used in Fibromyalgia** *(cont'd)*

Class	Drug	Dose	Adverse Effects	Drug Interactions	Cost[a]
Nonsteroidal Anti-inflammatory Drugs[b]	*ibuprofen*◗ Advil, Motrin IB, generics[c]	200–600 mg Q6H	Peptic ulcer, dyspepsia, fluid retention, hypertension, renal impairment, hypersensitivity.	Warfarin: ↑ anticoagulant effect. Antihypertensives: possible ↓ in hypertensive effect; may require additional antihypertensive therapy. Lithium: may interfere with sodium/water balance. Monitor lithium levels when NSAID added. SSRIs may ↑ risk of gi bleeding when used with NSAIDs.	$
Natural Health Products	*S-adenosyl-L-methionine* SAM-e, SAM-e IsoActive[c]	800 mg daily	Flatulence, diarrhea, nausea, vomiting, constipation, headache, anorexia, insomnia, dizziness. SAMe can cause anxiety in depressed patients. It has been associated with a worsening of manic symptoms in patients with bipolar disorder.	Antidepressants: concurrent use may cause an ↑ serotonergic effects including agitation, tremor and tachypnea. Avoid in patients taking MAOIs and for 2 wk after discontinuing the MAOI. Use with dextromethorphan, meperidine, pentazocine or tramamdol could theoretically cause additive serotonergic effects. Levodopa: SAMe methylates levodopa, which may worsen parkinsonian symptoms.	$$$$$

[a] Cost of 30-day supply; includes drug cost only.
[b] Listed drugs are examples of medications in this class.
[c] Available without a prescription.
◗ Dosage adjustment may be required in renal impairment; see Appendix I.
Abbreviations: CNS = central nervous system; MAOIs = monoamine oxidase inhibitors
Legend: $ < $20 $$ $20-40 $-$$$ < $20–60 $$$ $40–60 $$$$ $60–80 $$$$$ > $80

Suggested Readings

Bennett RM. Rational management of fibromyalgia. *Rheum Dis Clin North Am* 2002;28(2):xiii-xv.

Goldenberg MD, Burckhardt C, Crofford L. Management of fibromyalgia syndrome. *JAMA* 2004;292(19):2388-95.

Mease P. Fibromyalgia syndrome: review of clinical presentation, pathogenesis, outcome measures and treatment. *J Rheumatol Suppl* 2005;75:6-21.

Puttick MP. Rheumatology: 11. Evaluation of the patient with pain all over. *CMAJ* 2001;164(2):223-7.

References

1. Bennett RM. Multidisciplinary group programs to treat fibromyalgia patients. *Rheum Dis Clin North Am* 1996;22(2):351-67.
2. Mannerkorpi K. Exercise in fibromyalgia. *Curr Opin Rheumatol* 2005;17(2):190-4.
3. Burckhardt CS. Nonpharmacologic management strategies in fibromyalgia. *Rheum Dis Clin North Am* 2002;28(2):291-304.
4. Deluze C, Bosia L, Zirbs A et al. Electroacupuncture in fibromyalgia: results of a controlled trial. *BMJ* 1992;305(6864):1249-52.
5. Arnold LM, Keck PE, Welge JA. Antidepressant treatment of fibromyalgia. A meta-analysis and review. *Psychosomatics* 2000;41(2):104-13.
6. Tofferi JK, Jackson JL, O'Malley PG. Treatment of fibromyalgia with cyclobenzaprine: a meta-analysis. *Arthritis Rheum* 2004;51(1):9-13.
7. Goldenberg D, Mayskiy M, Mossey C et al. A randomized, double-blind crossover trial of fluoxetine and amitriptyline in the treatment of fibromyalgia. *Arthritis Rheum* 1996;39(11):1852-9.
8. Arnold LM, Hess EV, Hudson JI et al. A randomized, placebo-controlled, double-blind, flexible-dose study of fluoxetine in the treatment of women with fibromyalgia. *Am J Med* 2002;112(3):191-7.
9. Littlejohn GO, Guymer EK. Fibromyalgia syndrome: which antidepressant drug should we choose. *Curr Pharm Des* 2006;12(1):3-9.
10. Sayar K, Aksu G, Ak I et al. Venlafaxine treatment of fibromyalgia. *Ann Pharmacother* 2003;37(11):1561-5.
11. Bennett RM, Kamin M, Karim R et al. Tramadol and acetaminophen combination tablets in the treatment of fibromyalgia pain: a double-blind, randomized, placebo-controlled study. *Am J Med* 2003;114(7):537-45.
12. Bennett RM, Schein J, Kosinski MR et al. Impact of fibromyalgia pain on health-related quality of life before and after treatment with tramadol/acetaminophen. *Arthritis Rheum* 2005;53(4):519-27.
13. Thorpy MJ. New paradigms in the treatment of restless legs syndrome. *Neurology* 2005;64(12 Suppl 3):S28-33.
14. Bennett RM, Clark SC, Walczyk J. A randomized, double-blind, placebo-controlled study of growth hormone in the treatment of fibromyalgia. *Am J Med* 1998;104(3):227-31.
15. Borg-Stein J. Management of peripheral pain generators in fibromyalgia. *Rheum Dis Clin North Am* 2002;28(2):305-17.

CHAPTER 68
Chronic Fatigue Syndrome

Elizabeth Mann, MD, FRCPC

Fatigue, usually short-lived, is common and is often related to some identified cause. Chronic fatigue syndrome (CFS) is a biopsychosocial illness of persistent, prolonged and profound fatigue, which may be disabling. The prevalence is 0.2 to 2.6%, varying somewhat with the population and criteria used.[1] It is found in all ages, races and socio-economic groups. About 50% more women are affected than men. The peak prevalence is ages 40 to 49.[2]

Chronic fatigue syndrome is the subject of significant debate and controversy. No single factor appears etiologic in this illness.[3] Rather it is more likely an individual response to a number of potential stimuli, including infection, major illness or life stress. Twin studies reveal a possible genetic component,[4] suggesting a predisposition requiring an environmental trigger. Approximately 50% of patients will have psychiatric complaints or prior psychiatric history, and many will become depressed after the onset of this prolonged illness. CFS is not felt to be a solely psychologic entity.[3]

There are significant overlaps with other medically undefined syndromes, including fibromyalgia, idiopathic environmental intolerances/multiple chemical sensitivities, and even irritable bowel syndrome.[3] The syndrome tends to improve over time, but even the best treatments available are not a cure.[5]

The development of diagnostic criteria (Table 1) has encouraged research in this area. Results are often conflicting, both for pathophysiology and for treatment. Many studies are unable to document defects in cognitive function despite subjective complaints. There is some evidence of slowed cognitive processing speed in patients who complain of cognitive dysfunction.[6]

Goals of Therapy

- Provide the patient with a supportive treatment environment
- Improve function and well-being and reduce fatigue
- Educate and promote self-management including exercise

Investigations

Diagnostic criteria are presented in Table 1.[7] Although the diagnosis of CFS cannot be seriously entertained before six months of fatigue, investigations should proceed in the interim to medically evaluate the patient for other causes of fatigue. This clinical evaluation (Table 2) must rule out other potentially treatable causes of fatigue.

As well as six months of fatigue, at least four of eight physical symptoms must occur (Table 1). Well-controlled illness, both medical and psychiatric, does not preclude a diagnosis of CFS.[7]

Neither viral titres nor neuro-imaging studies are required or helpful in routine clinical practice. There are no consistent, well-defined abnormalities in neuro-imaging studies. There are no specific findings in muscle or muscle metabolism to explain the fatigue.

Table 1: Diagnostic Criteria for Chronic Fatigue Syndrome[7]

- Clinically evaluated fatigue (history, physical, laboratory investigations) (Table 2)
- Persistent or relapsing fatigue for ≥ 6 months
- New or definite onset
- Not significantly relieved by rest
- Substantial, significant reduction in function (occupation, education, social or personal)

PLUS four or more of the following symptoms — concurrent, recurrent, or persistent:

- Reduced short-term memory or concentration
- Sore throat
- Tender cervical or axillary lymph nodes
- Muscle pain
- Diffuse arthralgia without arthritis
- New headaches
- Unrefreshing sleep
- Post-exercise fatigue lasting more than 24 hours

Adapted with permission from Fukuda K et al. The chronic fatigue syndrome: a comprehensive approach to its definition and study. International Chronic Fatigue Syndrome Study Group. *Ann Intern Med* 1994;121(12):953-9.

Table 2: Clinical Evaluation of Prolonged Fatigue[7]

1. History and physical exam
2. Mental status exam
3. Neurologic and psychiatric exam if indicated
4. Routine laboratory tests (CBC with differential, BUN, creatinine, electrolytes, fasting glucose, calcium, phosphorus, ESR or CRP, urinalysis, TSH, liver enzymes, total protein, albumin, anti-tissue transglutaminase)
5. Any additional tests as indicated from 1–4 above
6. Label chronic fatigue syndrome if above negative or unhelpful AND all diagnostic criteria are met
7. Label idiopathic chronic fatigue if either duration or severity criteria are not met

Adapted with permission from Fukuda K et al. The chronic fatigue syndrome: a comprehensive approach to its definition and study. International Chronic Fatigue Syndrome Study Group. *Ann Intern Med* 1994;121(12):953-9.

Therapeutic Choices

There are no specific treatments for CFS.[1,8] Patients benefit from being given a positive diagnosis with reasonable explanations of their symptoms. Treatment should stress nonpharmacologic approaches, attempts at symptom control, a supportive environment and recognition of suffering.

Nonpharmacologic Choices

Nonpharmacologic therapies should be utilized primarily.

- Healthy diet: No specific diet or nutritional supplements have been proven to benefit this condition. Patients with exaggerated orthostatic hypotension should ingest salt.
- Regular progressive aerobic exercise: Bedrest confers no long-term benefit. Physical deconditioning prolongs disability and prevents recovery. Gradual progressive aerobic exercise programs are of proven benefit (Table 3).[9]
- *Positive Pacing*:
  - lifestyle issues are major. Using the excuse of pacing ("living within my limits") to avoid gradual increases in exercise perpetuates the disability.
  - wide fluctuations in physical activity are self-defeating and perpetuate the notion that exercise is to be avoided. There should be periods of planned activity and a definite sleep routine. Graded increases in activity (Table 3) are mandatory. It is better to be somewhat (and increasingly) active every day, than to do nothing most days and then attempt to walk five miles.
- Psychologic counselling and lifestyle management: Cognitive behavioural therapy (CBT) including counselling regarding belief systems about chronic fatigue and illness, usually in association with progressive exercise therapy, results in best outcomes. Randomized controlled trials of cognitive behavioural therapy have shown improvement in 60 to 75% of patients receiving this treatment, compared with < 30% of patients receiving standard care.[1]

  Inability to access trained psychotherapists can limit formal CBT. Similar results have been obtained using patient education and gradual progressive exercise with appropriate follow-up by family physicians.[10] One trial demonstrates that benefits of CBT are long lasting.[11]

Table 3: **Exercise Guidelines**

- Prescribe exercise
- Choose walking, bicycle, treadmill, swimming, etc; any exercise patient can do
- Gradual progressive aerobic exercise
- Supervised, or independent with follow-up by physician/nurse
- Start where patient is comfortable, e.g., five minutes per day
- Increase weekly by increments, even one to two minutes per session, to 30 minutes per day
- Do not miss any days, as it can delay further progression for a week

Pharmacologic Choices

- Since there are no proven pharmacologic treatments for CFS, treat symptomatically (Table 4). Symptomatic treatment usually includes medication for sleep, most often with low-dose **antidepressants**.

There is no convincing evidence that one agent is superior to another. Short trials of six to eight weeks are sufficient to notice benefit.

- Although several short-term clinical trials have been published using standard replacement dose or low-dose **corticosteroids**, there is no convincing evidence that benefit outweighs risk. Use of combined low-dose steroids and fludrocortisone are of no benefit. Use of intravenous **immunoglobulins** provides mild benefit with severe side effects and risks, and is not standard therapy.[1]
- One short-term trial notes benefit from **methylphenidate** 10 mg twice daily in CFS patients with severe cognitive complaints. This has not yet been confirmed and is not standard therapy.[12]

Therapeutic Tips

- In several referral clinic–based studies, the prognosis for recovery was poor for severely ill patients, who may remain ill for many years. Poor outcome is predicted by rigid beliefs in a physical cause for the illness, and unwillingness to participate in either psychologic therapy or exercise-based treatments.[5,13,14]
- There is *no role* for nystatin, fludrocortisone, rigid diets and/or megavitamin routines.
- Patients experiencing pain can be offered analgesics usually starting with acetaminophen.

Table 4: **Drugs for Symptomatic Management of Chronic Fatigue Syndrome**

Class	Drug	Dose	Adverse Effects	Drug Interactions	Comments	Cost[a]
Tricyclic Antidepressants (TCAs)[b]	*amitriptyline* generics	Initial: 10–25 mg/day Usual: 75 mg/day	Anticholinergic (dry mouth, blurred vision, constipation, urinary hesitancy, tachycardia, delirium), antihistaminergic (sedation, weight gain), orthostatic hypotension, lowered seizure threshold; sexual dysfunction.	Combination with MAOIs may result in mania, excitation, hyperpyrexia. Barbiturates, carbamazepine and rifampin may ↓ effect. Cimetidine and antipsychotics may ↑ effect and toxicity. Possible interaction with antiarrhythmics: may ↑ effect of either drug; may also ↑ risk of cardiac arrhythmias. May ↓ antihypertensive effect of clonidine. May augment hypotensive effect of thiazides.	Use for sleep and mood, especially nonrestorative sleep. No evidence for superiority of any agent. Use side effects (anticholinergic, weight gain) to guide therapy. Should be taken in the evening. Only about 50% respond.	$
	desipramine Norpramin, generics	Initial: 10–25 mg/day Usual: 100 mg/day	See amitriptyline.	See amitriptyline.	See amitriptyline.	$-$$$

Class	Drug	Dose	Adverse Effects	Drug Interactions	Comments	Cost[a]
Selective Serotonin Reuptake Inhibitors (SSRIs)[b]	*fluoxetine* Prozac, generics	Initial: 10–20 mg/day Usual: 20–40 mg/day	Nausea, nervousness, anorexia, insomnia. ↑ risk of GI bleeding	MAOIs may cause severe reaction — tremor, agitation, hypomania, hypertension. Drugs that inhibit cytochrome P450 enzymes (e.g., cimetidine, clarithromycin, erythromycin, fluconazole, indinavir, isoniazid, itraconazole, ketoconazole, quinidine, ritonavir) may ↑ SSRI levels. All SSRIs inhibit certain cytochrome P450 enzymes and can ↓ the clearance of other drugs (e.g., clozapine, methadone, phenytoin, pimozide, propafenone). Inducers of cytochrome P450 enzymes (e.g., carbamazepine, phenobarbital, phenytoin, rifampin) can ↑ the clearance of SSRIs. ↑ risk of GI bleeding with NSAIDs.	Use for sleep and mood. No evidence for superiority of any agent. Can use early in the day for the hypersomnolent. May be better tolerated than TCAs.	$$-$$$$
	sertraline Zoloft, generics	Initial: 25–50 mg/day Usual: 50–100 mg/day	Nausea, tremors, diarrhea, dry mouth. ↑ risk of GI bleeding.	See fluoxetine.	See fluoxetine.	$-$$

(cont'd)

Table 4: **Drugs for Symptomatic Management of Chronic Fatigue Syndrome** *(cont'd)*

Class	Drug	Dose	Adverse Effects	Drug Interactions	Comments	Cost[a]
Serotonin-Norepinephrine Reuptake Inhibitors	*venlafaxine* Effexor XR, generic	Initial: 37.5 mg/day Usual: 112.5–225 mg/day	Nausea, drowsiness, nervousness, dizziness, dry mouth, may increase BP if dose > 300 mg/day.	Avoid combination with or use within 2 wk of discontinuation of MAOIs. Drugs that inhibit cytochrome P450 (e.g., cimetidine) may increase venlafaxine levels. St. John's wort may increase sedative-hypnotic effects.	This may be more helpful for patients with pain/fibromyalgia type complaints.	$$-$$$$$
Antidepressants, miscellaneous	*trazodone* Desyrel, generics	Initial: 50 mg QHS Usual: 50–100 mg QHS	Drowsiness, nausea, vomiting, headache, dry mouth, priapism. Adverse events appear more common with higher doses.	May potentiate effects of other CNS depressants and augment hypotensive effects of antihypertensives.	Useful for sleep. May be combined with SSRI.	$
Analgesics[b]	*acetaminophen* Atasol preparations, Tylenol, generics	325–650 mg TID	May cause hepatotoxicity if taken in excess or by patients with liver diseases.	Excessive alcohol intake may increase the risk of hepatotoxicity. Warfarin: increased anticoagulant effect with regular use of > 2 g/day.		$

Class	Drug	Dose	Adverse Effects	Drug Interactions	Comments	Cost[a]
	ibuprofen Advil, Motrin IB, generics	200–600 mg TID	Peptic ulcers, dyspepsia, fluid retention, hypertension, renal impairment, hypersensitivity. MI, CVA, heart failure all possible. Extent of CV risk still not completely defined.	Warfarin: increased anticoagulant effect. Antihypertensives: possible reduction in hypertensive effect; may require additional antihypertensive therapy. Lithium: may interfere with sodium/water balance. Monitor lithium levels when NSAID added. SSRIs may ↑ risk of GI bleeding when used with NSAIDs.	Other NSAIDs may be used. No evidence for superiority of any agent.	$

[a] Cost of 30-day supply; includes drug cost only.
[b] Listed drugs are examples of medications in this class.
Dosage adjustment may be required in renal impairment; see Appendix I.
Abbreviations: BP = blood pressure; MAOI = monoamine oxidase inhibitor; NSAIDs = nonsteroidal anti-inflammatory drugs; SSRI = selective serotonin reuptake inhibitor; TCA = tricyclic antidepressant
Legend: $ < $20 $-$$ < $20–40 $$ $20–40 $-$$$ < $20–60 $$$ $40–60 $$-$$$$ $20–80 $$$$ $60–80 $$-$$$$$ $20– >80 $$$$$ >$80

Suggested Readings

Centers for Disease Control and Prevention (US). *Chronic fatigue syndrome*. Atlanta (GA): CDC. Available from: www.cdc.gov/cfs/ Accessed December 6, 2006.

Evengard B, Klimas N. Chronic fatigue syndrome: probable pathogenesis and possible treatments. *Drugs* 2002;62(17):2433-46.

Fukuda K, Straus SE, Hickie I et al. The chronic fatigue syndrome: a comprehensive approach to its definition and study. International Chronic Fatigue Study Group. *Ann Intern Med* 1994;121(12):953-9.

Prins JB, van der Meer JW, Bleijenberg G. Chronic fatigue syndrome. *Lancet* 2006;367(9507):346-55.

References

1. Reid S, Chalder T, Cleare A et al. Chronic fatigue syndrome. *BMJ* 2000;320(7230):292-6.
2. Jason LA, Richman JA, Rademaker AW et al. A community-based study of chronic fatigue syndrome. *Arch Intern Med* 1999;159(18):2129-37.
3. Natelson BH. Chronic fatigue syndrome. *JAMA* 2001;285(20):2557-9.
4. Buchwald D, Herrell R, Ashton S et al. A twin study of chronic fatigue. *Psychosom Med* 2001;63(6):936-43.
5. Hill NF, Tiersky LA, Scavalla VR et al. Natural history of severe chronic fatigue syndrome. *Arch Phys Med Rehabil* 1999;80(9):1090-4.
6. Deluca J, Christodoulou C, Diamond BJ et al. Working memory deficits in chronic fatigue syndrome: differentiating between speed and accuracy of information processing. *J Int Neuropsychol Soc* 2004;10(1):101–9.
7. Fukuda K, Straus SE, Hickie I et al. The chronic fatigue syndrome: a comprehensive approach to its definition and study. International Chronic Fatigue Syndrome Study Group. *Ann Intern Med* 1994;121(12):953-9.
8. Whiting P, Bagnall AM, Sowden AJ et al. Interventions for the treatment and management of chronic fatigue syndrome: a systematic review. *JAMA* 2001;286(11):1360-8.
9. Edmonds M, McGuire H, Price J. Exercise therapy for chronic fatigue syndrome. *Cochrane Database Syst Rev* 2004;(3):CD003200.
10. Powell P, Bentall RP, Nye FJ, Edwards RH. Randomized controlled trial of patient education to encourage graded exercise in chronic fatigue syndrome. *BMJ* 2001;322:1–5.
11. Deale A, Husain K, Chalder T et al. Long-term outcome of cognitive behavior therapy versus relaxation therapy for chronic fatigue syndrome: a 5-year follow-up study. *Am J Psychiatry* 2001;158(12):2038-42.
12. Blockmans D, Persoons P, Van Houdenhove B et al. Does methylphenidate reduce the symptoms of chronic fatigue syndrome? *Am J Med* 2006;119(2):167.e23-30.
13. Lawrie SM, Pelosi AJ. Chronic fatigue syndrome: prevalence and outcome. *BMJ* 1994;308(6931):732-3.
14. Bentall RP, Powell P, Nye FJ et al. Predictors of response to treatment for chronic fatigue syndrome. *Br J Psychiatry* 2002;181:248-52.

CHAPTER 69
Polymyalgia Rheumatica and Giant-Cell Arteritis

John G. Hanly, MD, MRCPI, FRCPC

Polymyalgia rheumatica (PMR) and giant-cell arteritis (GCA) are related conditions that affect older individuals and may reflect two ends of a spectrum of the same disease. PMR is characterized by aching and stiffness in the muscle groups of the neck, pectoral and pelvic girdles and thighs. The prevalence approaches 1% of people over the age of 50.[1]

GCA is a chronic vasculitis of large and medium-sized arteries with a predominance for the cranial branches of the arteries originating from the aortic arch. Thus, headache, jaw claudication and visual loss are common presentations. It is less frequent than PMR and affects approximately 0.2% of people 50 years of age and older.[2]

Both conditions are two-fold more frequent in women than in men. There is a clear association between PMR and GCA. Approximately 16 to 21% of patients with PMR will develop GCA concurrently or subsequent to the diagnosis of PMR;[1,3] conversely 40 to 60% of patients with GCA will develop symptoms of PMR. Although the etiology of both conditions is unknown, PMR is characterized pathologically by a low grade synovitis of the proximal joints while the hallmark of GCA is granulomatous inflammation with giant cells of affected arterial walls. Both conditions may be associated with systemic clinical manifestations.

Goals of Therapy

- Eliminate symptoms of musculoskeletal pain and stiffness and associated malaise
- Restore function
- Relieve symptoms due to GCA and prevent permanent visual loss
- Minimize the frequency and severity of corticosteroid toxicity

Investigations

The value of a thorough history and physical examination cannot be overemphasized. PMR and GCA are clinical diagnoses. Other than a positive temporal artery biopsy there are no laboratory tests that are specific for either disease.

The diagnostic approach is outlined in Table 1 and Figure 1.

History

Patients with PMR typically present with the following characteristics:

- Significant proximal muscle discomfort, especially around the shoulders, across the neck, and in the buttocks and thighs. The pain is generally severe and usually interferes with activities of daily living.
- Many patients describe an acute onset and can pinpoint the start of their symptoms to a specific day.
- Musculoskeletal morning stiffness lasting for hours is a prominent feature. Symptoms tend to worsen through the night, and movement during sleep causes discomfort severe enough to wake the patient.
- Systemic symptoms such as fever, malaise, anorexia and fatigue may be present in one-third of patients.[4]

Patients with GCA most frequently present with the following characteristics:

- Headache in the temporal or occipital areas, claudication of the jaw or tongue and partial or complete monocular visual loss which may affect the contralateral eye within two weeks even after starting corticosteroid therapy.
- Additional distinct clinical presentations may occur based upon the pattern of vascular involvement and the degree of systemic symptoms.[5] For example, involvement of the branches of the aortic arch, similar to that seen in Takayasu's arteritis, may occur in up to 15% of cases and is manifested by audible bruits and upper limb claudication.
- Systemic symptoms, including fever, occur in up to 50% of cases.
- A recognized late complication of GCA is a 17-fold increase in thoracic aortic aneurysm.[6]
- Patients who present with PMR should be questioned specifically about symptoms of GCA.

Physical Examination

- The physical findings in PMR are nonspecific and usually reveal a reduction in range of motion of the neck and shoulders.
- Large and small joint synovitis may be present but is unusual in locations distal to the wrist and ankle. Severe swelling with pitting edema over the dorsum of both hands and feet may also occur and forms a distinct clinical subset.[7,8]
- Proximal muscle tenderness may be present but muscle weakness, although difficult to assess due to pain, is not a predominant feature of PMR.
- Diminished or absent temporal artery pulsation and associated scalp tenderness, coupled with an appropriate history, is suggestive of GCA.
- Funduscopic findings related to GCA include optic neuritis with pallor and edema of the optic disc, cotton-wool patches, and small hemorrhages.

Laboratory Tests

- A rapid erythrocyte sedimentation rate (ESR) and elevated levels of C-reactive protein (CRP) are usually present. However, 5 to 6% of patients with PMR and GCA will have a normal ESR[9,10] although in the majority of such cases the CRP is elevated.[9]
- Anemia and/or thrombocytosis may also be found in patients presenting with PMR or GCA.
- Temporal artery biopsy is indicated only if there is a clinical suspicion of GCA and is not routinely recommended in patients who present with isolated PMR. Due to patchy involvement of affected vessels, a normal biopsy does not exclude the diagnosis. Thus, even when up to 5 cm of bilateral temporal arteries are sampled, 9% of suspected cases have normal biopsies.[11,12,13,14] More recent studies have suggested that performing bilateral temporal artery biopsies increases the diagnostic yield by only 1 to 5%.[15] *Corticosteroid therapy should not be withheld* while awaiting the result of a temporal artery biopsy. This biopsy can still show changes of arteritis when performed up to four weeks following the commencement of corticosteroid therapy.[16,17]

The diagnostic approach is outlined in Figure 1. A number of conditions must be considered in the differential diagnosis of PMR (Table 1) although GCA can usually be readily distinguished from other forms of vasculitis.

Table 1: **Differential Diagnosis of Polymyalgia Rheumatica (PMR)**

Diagnosis	Distinguishing Features From PMR
Myositis	Muscle weakness on physical examination ↑ CPK Abnormalities on EMG and muscle biopsy
Fibromyalgia	Usually seen in younger patients Widespread pain and tenderness at a significant number of soft tissue sites not limited to the shoulders and hips Normal ESR and CRP
Rheumatoid Arthritis	Synovitis distal to the wrist and ankle Seropositivity for rheumatoid factor Inadequate response to low dose prednisone therapy Radiographic erosions
Malignancy	As directed by clinical examination, laboratory evaluation (e.g., iron deficiency anemia), and lack of response to conventional therapy. However, the incidence of malignancy is not increased in PMR

Abbreviations: CPK = creatine phosphokinase; EMG = electromyelogram; ESR = erythrocyte sedimentation rate; CRP = C-reactive protein

Therapeutic Choices

Pharmacologic Choices

Corticosteroids

Nonsteroidal anti-inflammatory drugs (NSAIDs) are generally ineffective or provide only partial improvement of symptoms in patients with PMR. Thus, systemic corticosteroids are the cornerstone of therapy. **Prednisone** 10 to 20 mg/day results in rapid and sustained clinical improvement[4] (Table 2). Substantial, if not complete, resolution of symptoms occurs within days. In fact, the diagnosis of PMR should be reconsidered if symptoms fail to improve significantly after one week of corticosteroid therapy.

GCA requires higher doses of corticosteroids, with an initial dose of 40 to 60 mg of prednisone daily. Although the infusion of large doses of methylprednisolone (1000 mg daily for three days) has been used for the treatment of patients with impending visual loss, there is no evidence that this approach is more effective than oral prednisone.[20] The chances of vision loss are reduced by prompt diagnosis and treatment[15] but once vision loss occurs, corticosteroids will not usually reverse it. Most patients require one to two years of therapy, although 30 to 50% will experience exacerbations over this period.[21,22] Some patients require corticosteroids for 5 to 10 years[22,23] or indefinitely.[24]

Prevention of Corticosteroid Toxicity

Since corticosteroids are associated with significant side effects, the lowest dose of corticosteroid needed to control symptoms should be used for the shortest period of time possible in order to minimize toxicity. Treatment with prednisone doses greater than 7.5 mg daily for more than three months has been associated with significant bone loss. Bisphosphonates (e.g., **etidronate** 400 mg daily for two weeks every three months, **alendronate** 5 to 10 mg daily or 70 mg weekly or **risedronate** 5 mg daily or 35 mg weekly) prevent the bone loss associated with corticosteroid use and should be prescribed in patients with PMR or GCA commencing corticosteroid therapy.[25] Weight-bearing exercise, calcium (total daily dose 1500 mg) and vitamin D supplementation (400 to 800 IU daily) also reduce the risk of osteoporosis and should be prescribed in conjunction with bisphosphonates.

Immunosuppressives and Biologic Response Modifiers

Methotrexate and **azathioprine** have been used in the treatment of PMR and GCA primarily to minimize corticosteroid exposure. However, studies have yielded conflicting results.[26,27,28,29,30] Two out of three [28,29,30] placebo-controlled studies of methotrexate did not detect a statistically significant benefit in patients with GCA and only one placebo-controlled study of methotrexate has shown benefit in patients with PMR.[31] These drugs should be considered only in those patients with significant corticosteroid toxicity and/or in those unable to wean below 7.5 mg of prednisone daily.

Preliminary observations with the use of anticytokine therapies such as **infliximab**[32] and **etanercept**[33] in steroid-resistant cases provided encouraging results. However, recent controlled studies of infliximab did not confirm benefit in the treatment of either PMR or GCA.[34,35] Consult a rheumatologist for initiation of an immunosuppressive or anticytokine agent.

Therapeutic Tips

- Prompt diagnosis and initiation of corticosteroid therapy is critical for the prevention of vision loss in patients with giant-cell arteritis. Treatment should not be delayed while awaiting a temporal artery biopsy which can still be positive up to four weeks after the initiation of corticosteroid therapy.
- Patients may report a transient increase in musculoskeletal symptoms after each corticosteroid dose reduction. These symptoms usually subside spontaneously over the ensuing week and do not necessarily represent a disease flare.
- The ESR and CRP usually parallel disease activity in patients with PMR and GCA. These tests can be used to confirm the clinical suspicion of a disease flare but should not be used in isolation to make treatment decisions.
- Reduction in shoulder range of motion may occur in some patients with PMR due to a localized rotator cuff tendonitis or capsulitis. This is more likely to occur when there has been a delay in diagnosis and initiation of therapy. A local corticosteroid injection (e.g., methylprednisolone acetate, triamcinolone hexacetonide) of the subacromial bursa or glenohumeral joint is often helpful.

Figure 1: **Diagnostic Approach in Patients with Suspected Polymyalgia Rheumatica (PMR) and Giant-Cell Arteritis (GCA)**

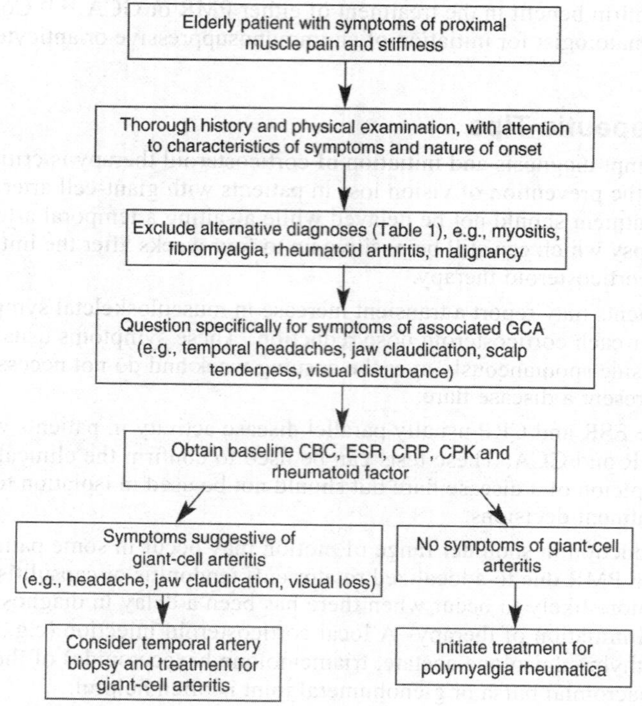

Abbreviations: CBC = complete blood count; ESR = erythrocyte sedimentation rate; CRP = C-reactive protein; CPK = creatine phosphokinase

Table 2: Drug Therapy of Polymyalgia Rheumatica (PMR) and Giant-Cell Arteritis (GCA)

Drug Class	Drug	Dose	Adverse Effects	Drug Interactions	Comments	Cost[a]
Corticosteroids	*prednisone* generics	PMR: 15 mg daily x 2 wk. Taper as follows: 12.5 mg daily x 2 wk, 10 mg daily x 4 wk, then decrease daily prednisone dose by 1 mg/mo until completion GCA: 60 mg daily x 4 wk. Taper as follows: decrease dose by 5 mg/wk until the dose is 10 mg daily. Then taper more gradually by 1 mg/mo until completion.	Acne, glucose intolerance, weight gain, mood alteration, cataracts, myopathy, hypertension, osteoporosis, aseptic necrosis of large joints, adrenal suppression, increased susceptibility to infection.	Barbiturates, phenytoin and rifampin ↓ corticosteroid effect.	Avoid alternate day corticosteroid dosing as it is associated with a higher rate of relapse.[18,19] Ensure regular clinical assessments to look for recurrence of the original symptoms while concurrently checking CBC, ESR and CRP during the prednisone taper. An isolated rise in ESR or CRP is usually not sufficient justification to increase the dose of corticosteroids. If a disease flare does occur, increase the dose of prednisone to the lowest level that was previously effective in controlling the disease. Maintain at that level for one mo, then taper as before. Immunosuppressive agents may be required in some cases.	$

[a] Cost of 1-day supply; includes drug cost only.
Legend: $ < $1

Suggested Readings

Nordborg E, Nordborg C. Giant cell arteritis: strategies in diagnosis and treatment. *Curr Opin Rheumatol* 2004;16(1):25-30.

Salvarani C, Cantini F, Boiardi L et al. Polymyalgia rheumatica and giant-cell arteritis. *N Engl J Med* 2002;347(4):261-71.

Salvarani C, Macchioni P, Boiardi L. Polymyalgia rheumatica. *Lancet* 1997;350(9070):43-7.

Weyland CM, Goronzy JJ. Giant-cell arteritis and polymyalgia rheumatica. *Ann Intern Med* 2003;139(6):505-15.

References

1. Salvarani C, Gabriel SE, O'Fallon WM et al. Epidemiology of polymyalgia rheumatica in Olmsted County, Minnesota, 1970-1991. *Arthritis Rheum* 1995;38(3):369-73.
2. Salvarani C, Gabriel SE, O'Fallon WM et al. The incidence of giant cell arteritis in Olmsted County, Minnesota: apparent fluctuations in a cyclic pattern. *Ann Intern Med* 1995;123(3):192-4.
3. Franzen P, Sutinen S, von Knorring J. Giant cell arteritis and polymyalgia rheumatica in a region of Finland: an epidemiologic, clinical and pathologic study, 1984-1988. *J Rheumatol* 1992;19(2):273-6.
4. Salvarani C, Cantini F, Boiardi L et al. Polymyalgia rheumatica and giant-cell arteritis. *N Engl J Med* 2002;347(4):261-71.
5. Weyand CM, Goronzy JJ. Giant-cell arteritis and polymyalgia rheumatica. *Ann Intern Med* 2003;139(6):505-15.
6. Evans JM, O'Fallon WM, Hunder GG. Increased incidence of aortic aneurysm and dissection in giant cell (temporal) arteritis. A population-based study. *Ann Intern Med* 1995;122(7):502-7.
7. Oide T, Ohara S, Oguchi K et al. Remitting seronegative symmetrical synovitis with pitting edema (RS3PE) syndrome in Nagano, Japan: clinical, radiological, and cytokine studies of 13 patients. *Clin Exp Rheumatol* 2004;22(1):91-8.
8. Queiro R. RS3PE syndrome: a clinical and immunogenetical study. *Rheumatol Int* 2004;24(2):103-5.
9. Cantini F, Salvarani C, Olivieri I et al. Erythrocyte sedimentation rate and C-reactive protein in the evaluation of disease activity and severity in polymyalgia rheumatica: a prospective follow-up study. *Semin Arthritis Rheum* 2000;30(1):17-24.
10. Salvarani C, Hunder GG. Giant cell arteritis with low erythrocyte sedimentation rate: frequency of occurrence in a population-based study. *Arthritis Rheum* 2001;45(2):140-5.
11. Hall S, Persellin S, Lie JT et al. The therapeutic impact of temporal artery biopsy. *Lancet* 1983;2(8361):1217-20.
12. Klein RG, Campbell RJ, Hunder GG et al. Skip lesions in temporal arteritis. *Mayo Clin Proc* 1976;51(8):504-10.
13. Gonzalez-Gay MA, Garcia-Porrua C, Llorca J et al. Biopsy-negative giant cell arteritis: clinical spectrum and predictive factors for positive temporal artery biopsy. *Semin Arthritis Rheum* 2001;30(4):249-56.
14. Hedges TR, Gieger GL, Albert DM. The clinical value of negative temporal artery biopsy specimens. *Arch Ophthalmol* 1983;101(8):1251-4.
15. Nordborg E, Nordborg C. Giant cell arteritis: strategies in diagnosis and treatment. *Curr Opin Rheumatol* 2004;16(1):25-30.
16. Achkar AA, Lie JT, Hunder GG et al. How does previous corticosteroid treatment affect the biopsy findings in giant cell (temporal) arteritis? *Ann Intern Med* 1994;120(12):987-92.
17. Ray-Chaudhuri N, Kine DA, Tijani SO et al. Effect of prior steroid treatment on temporal artery biopsy findings in giant cell arteritis. *Br J Ophthalmol* 2002;86(5):530-2.
18. Bengtsson BA, Malmvall BE. An alternate-day corticosteroid regimen in maintenance therapy of giant cell arteritis. *Acta Med Scand* 1981;209(5):347-50.
19. Hunder GG, Sheps SG, Allen GL et al. Daily and alternate-day corticosteroid regimens in treatment of giant cell arteritis: comparison in a prospective study. *Ann Intern Med* 1975;82(5):613-8.
20. Hayreh SS, Zimmerman B. Management of giant cell arteritis. Our 27-year clinical study: new light on old controversies. *Ophthalmologica* 2003;217(4):239-59.
21. Salvarani C, Macchioni PL, Tartoni PL et al. Polymyalgia rheumatica and giant cell arteritis: a 5-year epidemiologic and clinical study in Reggio Emilia, Italy. *Clin Exp Rheumatol* 1987;5(3):205-15.
22. Andersson R, Malmvall BE, Bengtsson BA. Long-term corticosteroid treatment in giant cell arteritis. *Acta Med Scand* 1986;220(5):465-9.
23. Bengtsson BA, Malmvall BE. Prognosis of giant cell arteritis including temporal arteritis and polymyalgia rheumatica. A follow-up study on ninety patients treated with corticosteroids. *Acta Med Scand* 1981;209(5):337-45.

24. Gonzalez-Gay MA, Blanco R, Rodriguez-Valverde V et al. Permanent visual loss and cerebrovascular accidents in giant cell arteritis: predictors and response to treatment. *Arthritis Rheum* 1998;41(8):1497-504.

25. [No authors listed]. Recommendations for the prevention and treatment of glucocorticoid-induced osteoporosis: 2001 update. American College of Rheumatology Ad Hoc Committee on Glucocorticoid-Induced Osteoporosis. *Arthritis Rheum* 2001;44(7):1496-503.

26. De Silva M, Hazleman BL. Azathioprine in giant cell arteritis/polymyalgia rheumatica: a double-blind study. *Ann Rheum Dis* 1986;45(2):136-8.

27. Ferraccioli G, Salaffi F, De Vita S et al. Methotrexate in polymyalgia rheumatica: preliminary results of an open, randomized study. *J Rheumatol* 1996;23(4):624-8.

28. Hoffman GS, Cid MC, Hellmann DB et al. A multicenter, randomized, double-blind, placebo-controlled trial of adjuvant methotrexate treatment for giant cell arteritis. *Arthritis Rheum* 2002;46(5):1309-18.

29. Spiera RF, Mitnick HJ, Kupersmith M et al. A prospective, double-blind, randomized, placebo controlled trial of methotrexate in the treatment of giant cell arteritis (GCA). *Clin Exp Rheumatol* 2001;19(5):495-501.

30. Jover JA, Hernandez-Garcia C, Morado IC et al. Combined treatment of giant-cell arteritis with methotrexate and prednisone. a randomized, double-blind, placebo-controlled trial. *Ann Intern Med* 2001;134(2):106-14.

31. Caporali R, Cimmino MA, Ferraccioli G et al. Prednisone plus methotrexate for polymyalgia rheumatica: a randomized, double-blind, placebo-controlled trial. *Ann Intern Med* 2004;141(7):493-500.

32. Salvarani C, Cantini F, Niccoli L et al. Treatment of refractory polymyalgia rheumatica with infliximab: a pilot study. *J Rheumatol* 2003;30(4):760-3.

33. Tan AL, Holdsworth J, Pease C et al. Successful treatment of resistant giant cell arteritis with etanercept. *Ann Rheum Dis* 2003;62(4):373-4.

34. Salvarani C, Macchioni P, Manzini C et al. Infliximab plus prednisone or placebo plus prednisone for the initial treatment of polymyalgia rheumatica: a randomized trial. *Ann Intern Med* 2007; 146(9):631-639.

35. Hoffman GS, Cid MC, Rendt-Zagar KE et al. Infliximab for maintenance of glucocorticosteroid-induced remission of giant cell arteritis: a randomized trial. *Ann Intern Med* 2007; 146(9):621-630.

CHAPTER 70
Gout and Hyperuricemia

Suneil Kapur, MD, FRCPC and
Gunnar Kraag, MD, FRCPC

Gout is a disease in which monosodium urate monohydrate (MSU) crystals deposit in joints, soft tissues such as cartilage, tendon and bursa, or in renal tissues such as glomeruli, the interstitium and tubules. This can result in gouty arthritis, tophi, nephropathy or uric acid nephrolithiasis. Gouty arthritis is the most common cause of inflammatory arthritis in men older than 40 years of age. The mean age of onset is the fourth decade in males and the sixth decade in females. It is unusual for an attack to occur before age 30 in males and age 50 in females unless the patient has an inherited enzyme abnormality.

Goals of Therapy

- Terminate the acute attack of arthritis
- Prevent recurrence
- Prevent or reverse complications
- Deal with associated disorders

The four stages of gouty arthritis are asymptomatic hyperuricemia, acute gouty arthritis, intercritical gout and chronic tophaceous gout.

Asymptomatic Hyperuricemia

This refers to elevated serum urate levels without any clinical manifestations. It is defined as a level greater than 360 μmol/L in females and 420 μmol/L in men.[1] During puberty, male serum urate levels increase by 60 to 120 μmol/L to levels of 240 to 360 μmol/L. These values remain sustained. Women develop increased urate levels after menopause, where values approach those of men. In 70% of patients with hyperuricemia, an underlying cause such as drugs or systemic conditions is discovered by history and physical examination (Table 1 and Table 2).[1] Hyperuricemia is not an indication for urate-lowering therapy. Most patients with hyperuricemia remain asymptomatic throughout life. The annual incidence of acute arthritis is 0.1 to 0.5% among patients with a urate level between 420 and 540 μmol/L, and 5% when greater than 540 μmol/L.[2] Similarly, the risk of nephrolithiasis increases with the serum urate level and the 24-hour urinary uric acid excretion. This phase ends with the first attack of gouty arthritis or urolithiasis, typically after 20 years of sustained hyperuricemia.

Table 1: **Drugs That May Cause Hyperuricemia**

Alcohol	Nicotinic acid
Cyclosporine	Pyrazinamide
Diuretics	Salicylates, low-dose
Ethambutol	Theophylline
Levodopa	

Table 2: **Conditions Associated With Hyperuricemia**

Alcohol consumption	Intrinsic renal disease
Atherosclerosis	Ischemic heart disease
Diabetes	Myeloproliferative disorders and some cancers
Hyperlipidemia	Obesity
Hypertension	

Acute Gouty Arthritis

Investigations

- History, physical and laboratory examinations:
  - abrupt onset of excruciating pain and inflammation of joint during the night or early morning
  - patients cannot tolerate even light pressure such as a bed sheet on the affected joint
  - most commonly affects joints of lower limb. There is a higher frequency of upper limb joint involvement in women compared to men[3]
  - about 85% of first attacks are monoarticular; however, elderly patients often have a polyarticular presentation
  - podagra (inflammation of first metatarsophalangeal [MTP] joint) involved in first attack > 50% of time and eventually > 90% of time; other joints involved include, in decreasing order, insteps, ankles, heels, knees, wrists, interphalangeal joints and elbows
  - predilection for damaged joints with osteoarthritis
  - acute gouty bursitis may occur in prepatellar or olecranon bursa
  - attacks often resolve spontaneously over 3 to 10 days
  - precipitants of acute attacks include acute illness, surgery, trauma, alcohol, high purine diet and drugs (Table 1)
  - definitive diagnosis by identification of intracellular monosodium urate crystals in synovial fluid
  - presumptive diagnosis with triad of acute monoarthritis, hyperuricemia and dramatic response to colchicine

Therapeutic Choices (Figure 1)

Pharmacologic Choices (Table 4)

Perhaps because many commonly used therapies for gout were available before the standards for clinical trials were developed, there is a general absence of well-controlled trials and systematic reviews regarding gout therapy.

NSAIDs are the first choice in the treatment of acute gout. NSAIDs are started in full doses, reduced by one-half as soon as improvement is noted and then withdrawn over several more days. Adverse effects are greatest in elderly patients with renal dysfunction. **COXIBs** and/or cytoprotection with **proton pump inhibitor** (PPI) or **misoprostol** may be offered to patients at risk for ulcer complications (e.g., age > 65, previous GI bleed or patients receiving anticoagulants or corticosteroids).

The intra-articular injection of corticosteroids into a single joint at the time of diagnostic arthrocentesis is ideal therapy and usually results in rapid control of inflammation and symptoms. Systemic corticosteroid therapy can be used for refractory attacks, particularly polyarticular gout, or when other agents are contraindicated, e.g., some elderly patients.

Colchicine relieves pain within 24 hours in 90% of patients when treated within the first few hours. However, its role is limited due to its toxicity (Table 4). Gastrointestinal (GI) toxicity may precede clinical response in many patients.[4] Because of severe potential toxicity, the use of i.v. colchicine should be avoided and restricted to hospitalized patients when other options have been exhausted.

Used in acute and prophylactic management of gout, **uricase-PEG20** is a drug that dissolves uric acid, but with potential for immunogenic side effects. It is not yet available in Canada.

Therapeutic Tips

- The earlier therapy is started, the quicker the attack will be resolved.
- Do not start or stop urate-lowering drugs during an acute attack because symptoms may be exacerbated or prolonged.
- Colchicine is not a good choice to treat acute gout because of the severity of side effects and the ready availability of other options.
- If prednisone is the best option, use high doses, e.g., 30 mg daily.

Intercritical Period and Prophylaxis

The intercritical period is asymptomatic. Most patients have a second attack within 6 to 24 months. Subsequent attacks are less explosive but more frequent, severe and enduring. These attacks are often polyarticular with upper extremity involvement and constitutional symptoms. Erosive radiographic changes and tophi may develop during the intercritical period, especially with frequent attacks of gouty arthritis. About 12 to 58% of patients have urate crystals in synovial fluid during this phase.[1]

Therapeutic Choices

Nonpharmacologic Choices

In a large observational study it was found that higher amounts of meat and seafood consumption were associated with an increased risk of gout.[5,6] Total protein intake and total amount of purine-rich vegetable intake were not associated with an increased risk of gout. There was a strong inverse association between consumption of dairy products, especially those with low fat content, and incidence of gout.[5,6] There is also a clear relationship between obesity (body mass index > 30 kg/m^2) and gout. Higher consumption of beer and liquor was associated with an increased risk of gout attacks while wine consumption was not associated with an increased risk.[5,6]

Pharmacologic Choices (Figure 2, Table 4)

When used for three months after attaining a serum urate concentration of < 390 µmol/L, **colchicine** (0.6 mg twice daily) effectively reduces the frequency and severity of acute flares when starting allopurinol for chronic gouty arthritis; it also reduces the likelihood of recurrent flares.[7] If it cannot be used, a low-dose NSAID (e.g., **indomethacin** 25 mg twice daily or **naproxen** 250 mg twice daily) may be substituted. Colchicine and NSAIDs should be used with caution in elderly patients with renal and hepatic insufficiency.

Antihyperuricemic Drugs

The decision of when to initiate urate-lowering therapy remains controversial. One view is that the first attack is a late event in the gouty diathesis; even if further attacks do not occur, it cannot be assumed that renal damage will not.[8] The other view is that, because recurrence may be delayed for many years and chronic tophaceous gout develops only in a minority, therapy can be delayed until recurrence or detection of tophi. The aim of antihyperuricemic therapy is to reduce the serum urate concentration to below 380 µmol/L, the saturation point of monosodium urate in the extracellular fluid.[1] Therapy should be lifelong since acute arthritis occurs within six months and tophi within three years of discontinuation.

Allopurinol, a xanthine oxidase inhibitor, inhibits the production of uric acid. Full doses reduce serum urate concentrations to normal in 80% of patients with gout.[2] To avoid unnecessary risks and costs, reserve allopurinol for select patients (Table 3).[2] The incidence of side effects is about 15%, with rash being the most common. Severe toxicity can occur: a hypersensitivity syndrome occurs in less than 1 in 1000 cases and includes exfoliative dermatitis, vasculitis, bone marrow suppression, liver dysfunction, fever, eosinophilia, acute interstitial nephritis or death.[2]

Patients can be desensitized to allopurinol as long as reactions are not severe.[9] The metabolite of allopurinol, **oxypurinol**, is available in Canada through the Special Access Program. There is 50% cross-reactivity with allopurinol, but it may be safer to desensitize with oxypurinol in patients with mild allergic reactions to allopurinol.[10]

Uricosuric agents such as **probenecid** and **sulfinpyrazone** are good substitutes but are not effective in the presence of renal insufficiency or gross over-production.[2] The combination of allopurinol and a uricosuric may be required to mobilize extensive urate deposits.

Table 3: **Indications for Antihyperuricemic Drugs**

Greater than 2 attacks/year
Presence of tophaceous gout
24-hour urinary uric acid excretion > 1000 mg
Severe and persistent hyperuricemia (> 720 µmol/L)
Hypoxanthine-guanine phosphoribosyl transferase (HGPRT) deficiency or phosphoribosyl pyrophosphate (PRPP) synthetase overactivity (both increase uric acid production)
Nephrolithiasis
Uric acid nephropathy
Chronic gouty arthritis with bony erosions
Prophylaxis of hyperuricemia prior to cytotoxic agents

Therapeutic Tips

- Do not treat asymptomatic hyperuricemia.
- Minimize the risk of acute gout during the intercritical period by protecting with a low-dose NSAID when initiating urate-lowering therapy.
- Adjust allopurinol dosage according to creatinine clearance.
- Improve compliance by explaining the objectives of therapy, e.g., allopurinol does not relieve pain and must be used continuously.

Chronic Tophaceous Gout

This stage typically occurs 12 years from onset with a reported range of 3 to 42 years.[1] Only 2% of patients develop severe crippling disease. The strongest associated risk factor for developing tophi is the serum urate level.[1] Other factors include the frequency of attacks, duration of hyperuricemia and severity of renal disease. Common locations of tophi are the synovium, subchondral bone, digits of the hands and feet, olecranon bursa, Achilles tendon and helix of the ear. They can, however, occur anywhere including the conduction system of the heart. Tophi themselves are painless but they can lead to destruction of joints and deformities. Radiographic changes include paramarginal erosions with sclerotic margins and calcified tophi.[1] The optimal therapy for chronic tophaceous gout is prevention by aggressive management of acute gout and correction of hyperuricemia. The aims of therapy are to control pain and inflammation, typically with NSAIDs, and to decrease serum uric acid levels. After several years of therapy, resorption of urate deposits will eventually lead to disappearance of tophi.

Figure 1: **Treatment of Acute Gout**[a]

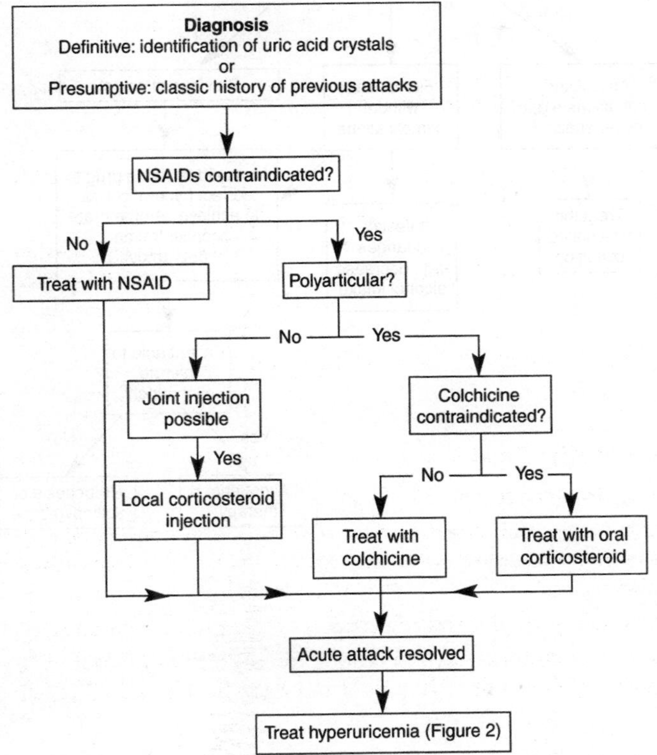

[a]Note: Never alter dose of urate-lowering drug during an attack.

Figure 2: **Treatment of Hyperuricemia**

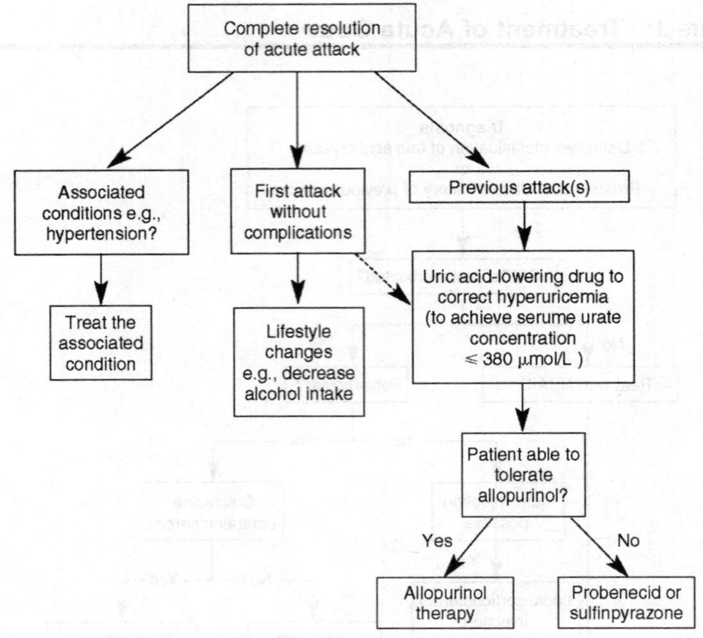

Table 4: **Drug Therapy of Gout**

Class	Drug	Dose	Adverse Effects	Drug Interactions	Comments	Cost[a]
NSAIDs[b]	*indomethacin* generics	Acute attack: 75 mg STAT, then 50 mg Q6H ×2 days then 50 mg Q8H ×1 day then 25 mg Q8H ×1 day Prophylaxis: 25 mg BID	(For all NSAIDs) GI disturbances; other adverse effects uncommon with short-term therapy but include fluid retention, hypertension, renal impairment, hypersensitivity.	Warfarin: ↑ anticoagulant effect. Antihypertensives: Possible ↓ in antihypertensive effect; may require additional antihypertensive therapy. Lithium: May interfere with sodium/water balance. Monitor lithium levels when NSAID added. SSRIs may ↑ risk of GI bleeding when used with NSAIDs.	Indomethacin and naproxen are listed as examples. There is no good evidence to suggest one NSAID is more efficacious than another. Suppositories may be used if oral route inadvisable.	$
	naproxen Naprosyn, generics	Acute attack: 750 mg STAT, then 500 mg BID × 4–5 days Prophylaxis: 250 mg BID	See indomethacin.	See indomethacin.	See indomethacin.	$
Antimitotics	*colchicine* generics	Acute attack: 0.6 mg TID-QID until relief or side effects occur; Usual max: 6 doses Prophylaxis: 0.6–1.8 mg/day; usual: 1 mg/day	Very common: abdominal pain and cramps, diarrhea, nausea and vomiting. Rare: neuropathy, myopathy, bone marrow suppression.	Patients receiving colchicine with erythromycin or clarithromycin should be monitored for colchicine toxicity (fever, GI symptoms, leukopenia).	Low benefit/toxicity ratio in acute gout. May be given iv: consult specialized references. Dosage should be ↓ in elderly and in renal impairment.	$$-$$$

(cont'd)

Table 4: **Drug Therapy of Gout** *(cont'd)*

Class	Drug	Dose	Adverse Effects	Drug Interactions	Comments	Cost[a]
Corticosteroids, intra-articular	*triamcinolone hexacetonide* Aristospan	Acute attack: Large joints: 10–20 mg intra-articular Small joints: 2–6 mg intra-articular	Not usually significant after single intra-articular injection.			$
	methylprednisolone acetate Depo-Medrol, generics	Acute attack: Large joints: 20–80 mg intra-articular Medium joints: 10–40 mg intra-articular Small joints: 4–10 mg intra-articular	Not usually significant after single intra-articular injection.			$
Corticosteroids, systemic	*methylprednisolone sodium succinate* Solu-Medrol, generics	Acute attack: 50–100 mg iv ×1 dose	Not usually significant after single injection.		Use when prednisone cannot be used po.	$$
	prednisone generics	Acute attack: 30 mg daily × 5 days Effective dose range: 20–50 mg/day	Except for GI disturbances and glucose intolerance, not usually significant in short-term use. Long-term effects are numerous.	Barbiturates, phenytoin and rifampin ↓ steroid effect.	Doses < 20 mg/day tend to be ineffective. Simultaneous low-dose colchicine or NSAID helps prevent rebound when steroid stopped.	$
Uricosurics	*probenecid* generics	Starting dose: 250 mg BID; titrate gradually; max: 3 g/day	May precipitate acute attack during initial phase of therapy; renal calculi, hypersensitivity reactions, GI irritation.	Salicylates ↓ effect of probenecid. Probenecid: ↑ levels of dapsone, methotrexate. Heparin activity ↑ by probenecid.	Liberal fluid intake and alkalinizing the urine can help prevent stones. Severe toxicity is rare.	$$-$$$

Class	Drug	Dose	Adverse Effects	Drug Interactions	Comments	Cost[a]
	sulfinpyrazone (renal symbol) generics	Starting dose: 50 mg BID with meals; titrate gradually; max. 800 mg/day	See probenecid.	Salicylates may ↑ bleeding time, ↓ uricosuric effect of sulfinpyrazone. Action of oral hypoglycemics, insulin and anticoagulants ↑ by sulfinpyrazone.	See probenecid.	$
Xanthine Oxidase Inhibitors	*allopurinol* Zyloprim, generics (renal symbol)	Starting dose: 100 mg daily Usual: 300 mg/day titrated to urate levels: max. 800 mg/day ↓ maintenance dose in renal impairment: 100 mg/day if ClCr 10–20 mL/min; 100 mg Q2–3 days if ClCr < 5 mL/min Chemotherapy/irradiation: 600–800 mg/day × 2–3 days before therapy Children with malignancies or enzyme deficiencies: 10 mg/kg/day	Skin rash, GI upset, hepatotoxicity, fever, severe hypersensitivity syndrome, xanthine stones (rare). May precipitate attack during initial phase of therapy.	Half-life of azathioprine and 6-mercaptopurine ↑ by allopurinol. May ↑ toxicity of cyclophosphamide. Allopurinol inhibits hepatic metabolism of warfarin. ↑ incidence of rashes when used with ampicillin or amoxicillin.	May need to ↑ dose or combine with uricosuric agents in chronic tophaceous gout. To prevent acute attacks on initiation of therapy, give prophylactic NSAID or colchicine for 2–3 wk. Desensitization to allopurinol can be achieved in some patients, but sensitivity may recur.	$

[a] Cost of 30-day supply; includes drug cost only
[b] Listed drugs are examples of medications in this class.
(renal symbol) Dosage adjustment may be required in renal impairment; see Appendix I.
Legend: $ < $10 $$ $10–20 $$-$$$ $10–30 $$$ $20–30

Suggested Readings

Choi HK, Mount DB, Reginato AM. Pathogenesis of gout. *Ann Intern Med* 2005;143:499-516.

Rott KT, Agudelo CA. Gout. *JAMA* 2003;289(21):2857-60.

Schlesinger N. Management of acute and chronic gouty arthritis: present state-of-the-art. *Drugs* 2004;64(21):2399-416.

References

1. Wortmann RL et al. Gout and hyperuricemia. In: Ruddy S et al., eds. *Kelley's textbook of rheumatology*. 6th ed. Philadelphia (PA): WB Saunders; 2001.
2. Emmerson BT. The management of gout. *N Engl J Med* 1996;334(7):445-51.
3. De Souza AW, Fernandes V, Ferrari AJ. Female gout: clinical and laboratory features. *J Rheumatol* 2005;32 (11):2186-8.
4. Ahern MJ, Reid C, Gordon TP et al. Does colchicine work? The results of the first controlled study in acute gout. *Aust N Z J Med* 1987;17(3):301-4.
5. Lee SJ, Terkeltaub RA, Kavanaugh A. Recent developments in diet and gout. *Curr Opin Rheumatol* 2006;18(2):193-8.
6. Choi HK, Atkinson K, Karlson EW et al. Purine-rich foods, dairy and protein intake and the risk of gout in men. *N Engl J Med* 2004; 350(11):1093-103.
7. Borstad GC, Bryant LR, Abel MP et al. Colchicine for prophylaxis of acute flares when initiating allopurinol for chronic gout arthritis. *J Rheumatol* 2004;31(12):2429-32.
8. Fam AG. Should patients with interval gout be treated with urate lowering drugs? *J Rheumatol* 1995;22(9):1621-3.
9. Fam AG, Lewtas J, Stein J et al. Desensitization to allopurinol in patients with gout and cutaneous reactions. *Am J Med* 1992;93(3):299-302.
10. Earl JM, Saavedra M. Oxipurinol therapy in allopurinol-allergic patients. *Am Fam Physician* 1983;28(5):147-8.

CHAPTER 71

Osteoarthritis

Paul Davis, MD, FRCP UK, FRCPC and
Angela Juby, MBChB

Osteoarthritis (OA) is the most prevalent of the rheumatic diseases and a leading cause of disability. The condition is divided into primary and secondary forms. Risk factors for primary OA include advancing age, obesity and genetic susceptibility.[1] Secondary OA may occur in younger age groups, usually as a result of previous traumatic or inflammatory damage to peripheral joints. Originally believed to be a simple degenerative process of aging cartilage, OA is now recognized as a highly complex condition associated with biochemical changes within the cartilage matrix. Treatment is usually only initiated at the end stages of the pathologic process when symptoms appear.

Goals of Therapy

- Reduce joint pain
- Improve joint function and mobility
- Maintain normal articular and periarticular structures
- Prevent (and possibly reverse) joint cartilage damage

The first three goals are achievable with currently available modalities, while the goal of cartilage protection and repair is under intense research.

Investigations

OA is largely a clinical diagnosis.

- History:
  - joint pain usually worse after exercise; improves with rest; joint and periarticular muscle stiffness (gelling) usually < 30 minutes
  - absence of obvious underlying inflammatory polyarthritis
  - joint pain in particular distribution (hips, knees, first metatarsophalangeal joint, distal interphalangeal joints, carpal metacarpal joint and axial skeleton)
  - secondary OA possible with history of trauma, prior inflammatory arthropathy, acromegaly
- Physical examination:
  - pain, limitation and stiffness of both passive and active movement of joint
  - possible crepitus, deformity and/or bony swelling
  - later stages may include disruption of joint architecture with ligamentous and capsular laxity and significant disabling deformity
  - varying degrees of mild synovitis possible

- Imaging:
  - radiographic imaging usually only serves to confirm clinical diagnosis and determine extent of damage, but a discrepancy often exists between signs and symptoms of OA and radiographic findings. It is of particular value when surgery is a consideration. Joint space narrowing, osteophyte formation, subchondral cysts (geodes) and bony sclerosis are radiographic hallmarks of uncomplicated OA. Chondrocalcinosis may be seen in patients with underlying metabolic disorders predisposing to secondary OA
  - bone scan, CT scan and MRI are of little value in routine clinical practice
- Lab tests:
  - routine blood work is largely unhelpful in diagnosis
  - joint fluid analysis usually shows relatively minor inflammatory changes except when complicated by crystal-induced synovitis where calcium pyrophosphate may be identified

Therapeutic Choices (Figure 1)

Prevention

Primary prevention consists of appropriate physical activity and weight control. Secondary preventive interventions include avoidance of trauma and inappropriate mechanical stresses on predisposed joints as well as weight loss.

Nonpharmacologic Choices

- Nonpharmacologic options should play a major role in improving quality of life of OA sufferers but are underutilized and undervalued. *Patient education* sessions such as those designed by the Arthritis Society should be initiated.[2] OA patients should be treated by a team including allied health professionals, e.g., occupational therapists, physiotherapists, social workers, pharmacists.
- *Physical therapies* such as transcutaneous electrical nerve stimulation (TENS) and laser therapy may benefit some patients.[3] There is no evidence that ultrasound is of benefit in knee OA.[4] The statistical benefit of acupuncture remains a subject of debate.[5,6]
- *Orthotics* such as wedge insoles may be helpful.[7] *Aids to daily living* including canes and walkers may be suggested for those with hip and knee OA. *Bracing* of affected joints may also assist patients.[8]
- *Exercise*,[9] weight loss, or exercise plus *physiotherapy*[10] provide modest reductions in pain and disability.

Pharmacologic Choices

Oral or Topical Therapy (Table 2, Table 3)

- Oral **analgesics** and, to a lesser extent, topical analgesics are the mainstays of therapy. Compared to **acetaminophen**, NSAIDs are superior in controlling pain in OA but with more GI side effects.[11,12,13] Consequently, acetaminophen should be the initial choice due to its safety and tolerability.[14] Two to three weeks of acetaminophen at doses not exceeding 4 g/day constitutes an appropriate trial. Some clinicians feel acetaminophen is most efficacious in chronic noninflammatory mechanical knee pain.[15] Analgesic/anti-inflammatories such as **ibuprofen** or **naproxen** can be used at low (analgesic) dose if an appropriate trial of acetaminophen has failed.

- In more symptomatically resistant patients, oral narcotics such as **morphine** or **oxycodone** can be considered as an adjunct for one to two weeks;[16] however, narcotic analgesics are not recommended for maintenance therapy[14] and must be used in lower doses in the elderly.
- Topical analgesics can be used adjunctively but evidence supporting their use is limited. They may be offered to those refusing systemic therapy. In a few small studies **capsaicin** was superior to placebo for pain control, but study patients were permitted to use oral analgesics.[17,18] The burning sensation caused by capsaicin is often not well tolerated. A **topical diclofenac** solution has recently been approved for treating the symptoms of OA of the knee. Its place in therapy remains to be determined but was effective in a recent trial.[19]
- For inflammatory pain, many patients require more than simple analgesia with acetaminophen. **Anti-inflammatory medications** such as NSAIDs are recommended second-line after a failure of simple analgesics.[14] Traditional NSAIDs (e.g., naproxen, diclofenac) in low doses (or full doses if necessary) can be used for symptomatic management of OA. Side effects with NSAIDs include GI complications, fluid retention, hypertension and renal effects (Table 2).

  Expert reviews have highlighted the risk of increased cardiovascular events for both the COX-2 inhibitors and nonselective NSAIDs. COX-2 inhibitors appear to be associated with a reduction in endoscopic ulcers compared to nonselective NSAIDs.[20] Currently, individual patients must be assessed for cardiovascular and gastrointestinal risk factors before selecting a therapy.

  If continuous NSAIDs must be used, especially if patients are at risk of GI complications (Table 1), add **misoprostol** or a **proton pump inhibitor** (PPI) (H_2–receptor antagonists are less effective[21]). Bleeding ulcers still may occur in high risk patients receiving a COX-2 inhibitor or traditional NSAID/PPI combination.[22] In patients with symptomatic OA requiring treatment, traditional NSAIDs and COX-2 inhibitors may be offered, providing that patients are screened for potential adverse effects (e.g., GI, cardiovascular) and are monitored for toxicity. Many clinicians prescribe simple analgesics as baseline therapy supplemented by NSAIDs (with gastroprotection if warranted) at times of increased symptomatology or obvious inflammation.
- Based on a systematic review, the alternative therapy **glucosamine** does not appear to have a clinically significant effect on pain or function (depending on the scale used) when taken for two to three

months.[23] In a recent trial, **chondroitin** did not have a clinically important effect on pain in patients with severe arthritis of the knee but may offer a small protective effect on the joint.[24] Concern exists about analysed content of glucosamine and chondroitin in several commercial products; the lack of standardized quality may affect their efficacy in non-trial settings.[25]

Table 1: **Risk Factors for Development of Upper GI Adverse Effects with NSAIDs[14,26]**

Risk factors
Age ≥ 65
Comorbid medical conditions
Anticoagulants or oral glucocorticoids
History of upper GI bleeding
Presence of H. pylori infection

Intra-articular therapies (Table 4)

- Often used to complement traditional treatments, **corticosteroid** joint injections are of particular value in the management of patients with a small number of symptomatic joints associated with clinical evidence of inflammation.
- The injection of hyaluronan and its derivatives has been used as viscosupplementation in the management of mild to moderate OA although results of studies are varied.[27,28] Because of the nature of this material, the knee is the only joint where it can be used on a regular basis. Other intra-articular procedures such as joint lavage and radioactive colloids have not proven to be of major benefit in OA.

Surgery

Arthroplasty is presently advocated for most patients with moderate to severe OA of the knee and hip with unremitting symptomatology despite adherence to a conservative medical program. Use of Silastic implants and spacers for smaller joints of the hands and feet are also effective in appropriately selected patients. Arthroscopic lavage and joint debridement are of questionable value.[29,30]

Therapeutic Tips

- Patients should receive only one NSAID at a time (with the exception of low-dose cardioprotective ASA). It is not yet known to what extent the addition of low-dose ASA added to COX-2 inhibitors decreases the GI benefits afforded by these agents.[20]
- Dyspepsia with NSAIDs does not correlate with endoscopically proven ulcers or with serious upper GI complications. Patients treated with NSAIDs who complain of dyspepsia in the absence of risk factors (Table 1) can be switched to simple analgesics, offered a trial with a different class of NSAID or treated symptomatically.

- Making patients aware of the GI risks involved with NSAID use has been shown to lower the incidence of acute GI bleeding.[31]
- For most patients, a flexible regimen of appropriate simple analgesics supplemented by anti-inflammatory medications together with nonpharmacologic modalities is sufficient to produce adequate relief of symptoms and functional benefit.
- As many OA sufferers are elderly, always consider drug intolerance. Start with low doses, increasing slowly to therapeutic effect. Drug interactions are also a concern because many of these patients are being treated for other conditions.
- Based on available data, experts have concluded that an increased risk of cardiovascular events may be a class effect for NSAIDs. Further evaluation is ongoing.[32]

Figure 1: **Treatment of Osteoarthritis**

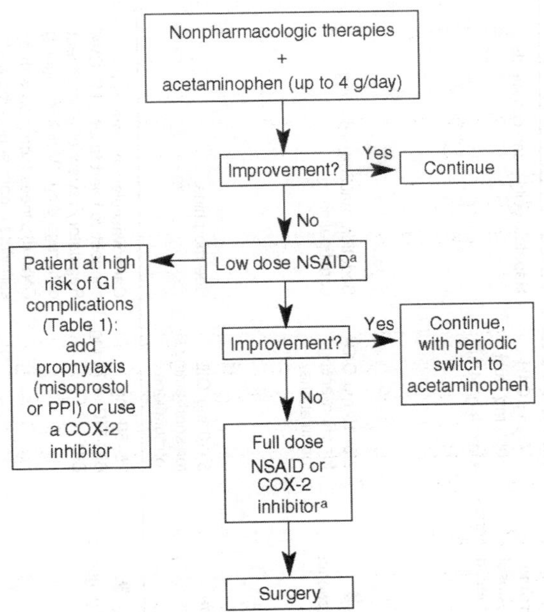

[a] Supplement with topicals, opioids, local injection, alternative therapies.

Table 2: Oral Agents Used in Osteoarthritis

Class	Drug	Dose	Adverse Effects	Drug Interactions	Comments	Cost[a]
Analgesics	*acetaminophen* Tylenol, Atasol Preparations, generics	650 mg Q4H–1000 mg Q6H Max: 4 g/24 h	Hepatotoxicity—see comments.	Alcohol: ↑ risk of hepatotoxicity with excessive alcohol intake (> 3 drinks/day). Warfarin: ↑ anticoagulant effect with regular use of > 2 g/day.	May cause hepatitis if taken in excess or by patients with liver diseases.	$
	morphine MS-IR, generics	2.5–15 mg QID for short-acting formulations	Sedation, nausea, vomiting, constipation.	Concurrent use of other sedating or constipating medications may increase these side effects. Lidocaine: potential enhancement of opioids' effects.	Useful for short-term adjunctive therapy. May be poorly tolerated in the elderly.	$
	oxycodone generics	5–10 mg QID for short-acting formulations	See morphine.	See morphine.	See morphine.	$$$$
NSAIDs, acetic acid derivatives	*diclofenac* Voltaren, generics	25–50 mg BID-TID or 75 mg BID	Cardiovascular: hypertension, congestive heart failure, MI, CVA. Regulatory review of all pertinent data regarding CV risk is ongoing. CNS: dizziness (common with all salicylates, both acetylated and nonacetylated), tinnitus, loss of hearing, disorientation, confusion (tends to occur with all NSAIDs in the elderly), aseptic meningitis (reported with ibuprofen in lupus	Warfarin: ↑ anticoagulant effect. Antihypertensives (diuretics, beta-blockers, ACE inhibitors, alpha-blockers): possible reduction in hypotensive effect; may require additional antihypertensive therapy. Lithium may interfere with sodium/water balance.	All NSAIDs have equivalent efficacy. When possible, avoid NSAIDs, including COX-2 inhibitors, in patients with a history of peptic ulcer disease, risk factors for heart attack or stroke, renal failure, heart failure or asthma.	$$

Class	Drug	Dose	Adverse Effects	Drug Interactions	Comments	Cost[a]
			patients). CNS effects may be dose related and respond to ↓ dosage. Dermatologic: skin rashes, some serious (e.g., erythema multiforme, Stevens-Johnson syndrome). Gastrointestinal: dyspepsia, nausea/vomiting, diarrhea, gastric and duodenal ulcers. Rare: gastric hemorrhage, perforation, small bowel ulceration. Hematologic: antiplatelet effect, agranulocytosis/aplastic anemia (indomethacin), thrombocytopenia. Hepatic: ↑ LFTs, Reye's syndrome in children with chickenpox and flu (primarily ASA), hypersensitivity reaction (hepatitis in adults) with all NSAIDs. Pulmonary: asthma (patients with ASA hypersensitivity). Renal: fluid retention/edema, renal insufficiency (problems more common in elderly patients), hyperkalemia.	Monitor lithium levels when NSAID added. SSRIs may ↑ risk of gi bleeding when used with NSAIDs.		
	etodolac Ultradol, generics	200–300 mg BID	See diclofenac.	See diclofenac.	See diclofenac.	$$$
	indomethacin generics	50–200 mg/day in two to three divided doses	See diclofenac.	See diclofenac.	See diclofenac.	$

(cont'd)

Table 2: **Oral Agents Used in Osteoarthritis** *(cont'd)*

Class	Drug	Dose	Adverse Effects	Drug Interactions	Comments	Cost[a]
	sulindac generics	150–200 mg BID	See diclofenac.	See diclofenac.	See diclofenac.	$$
NSAIDs, oxicams	*piroxicam* generics	10–20 mg daily	See diclofenac.	See diclofenac.	See diclofenac.	$
	tenoxicam generics	20–40 mg daily	See diclofenac.	See diclofenac.	See diclofenac.	$$
	meloxicam Mobicox, generics	7.5–15 mg daily	See diclofenac.	See diclofenac.	See diclofenac.	$
NSAIDs, propionic acid derivatives	*flurbiprofen* Ansaid, Froben, generics	50–100 mg BID-TID	See diclofenac.	See diclofenac.	See diclofenac.	$$
	ibuprofen Advil, Motrin, generics	200–600 mg Q6H-Q8H	See diclofenac.	See diclofenac.	See diclofenac.	$
	ketoprofen Orudis, generics	50–75 mg TID-QID	See diclofenac.	See diclofenac.	See diclofenac.	$
	naproxen Naprosyn, generics	250–500 mg BID	See diclofenac.	See diclofenac.	See diclofenac.	$
	naproxen sodium Anaprox, generics	275–550 mg BID	See diclofenac.	See diclofenac.	See diclofenac.	$$$

Class	Drug	Dose	Adverse Effects	Drug Interactions	Comments	Cost[a]
	oxaprozin Daypro, generics	600–1200 mg/day	See diclofenac.	See diclofenac.	See diclofenac.	$$$
	tiaprofenic acid Surgam, generics	200–300 mg BID	See diclofenac.	See diclofenac.	See diclofenac.	$$
NSAIDs, salicylic acid derivatives	*ASA* Aspirin, Bufferin, Coated Aspirin, generics	325–650 mg Q4H	See diclofenac.	See diclofenac.	See diclofenac.	$
	diflunisal generics	250–500 mg BID	See diclofenac.	See diclofenac.	See diclofenac.	$$
NSAIDs, naphthylalkanone derivatives	*nabumetone* generics	1000–2000 mg daily or in 2 divided doses	See diclofenac.	See diclofenac.	See diclofenac.	$$$$
COX-2 Inhibitors	*celecoxib* Celebrex	100 mg BID or 200 mg once daily	Usual doses do not appear to have antiplatelet effects. Serious skin reactions have been reported. Patients with history of heart attack or stroke, serious heart disease–related chest pain or serious heart disease such as HF should not use COX-2 inhibitors. Assess risk in patients with risk factors for heart attack and stroke. See diclofenac.	See diclofenac.	See diclofenac. Two COX-2 inhibitors, rofecoxib and valdecoxib, were removed from the Canadian market because of safety concerns. Celecoxib contraindicated if sulfonamide allergy.	$$

(cont'd)

Table 2: **Oral Agents Used in Osteoarthritis** *(cont'd)*

Class	Drug	Dose	Adverse Effects	Drug Interactions	Comments	Cost[a]
	lumiracoxib Prexige	100 mg daily	See celecoxib. See diclofenac.	See diclofenac.	See diclofenac. See celecoxib	$$
Alternative Therapies	*chondroitin* various	400 mg TID	None known.	None known.	Lack of product standardization.	$$
	glucosamine various	500 mg TID	Mild GI problems.	None known.	Lack of product standardization.	$

[a] Cost of 1 week's therapy; includes drug cost only.

Dosage adjustment may be required in renal impairment; see Appendix I.

Legend: $ < $5 $$ $5–10 $$$ $10–15 $$$$ > $15

Table 3: Topical Agents Used in Osteoarthritis

Class	Drug	Dose	Adverse Effects	Drug Interactions	Comments	Cost[a]
Topical Agents	*capsaicin* Zostrix, generics	Apply TID-QID	Transient burning on application.		Avoid contact with eyes or open lesions.	$$$
	methyl salicylate Rub A-535, others	Apply TID-QID	Skin irritation.	Warfarin: ↑ anticoagulant effect.	Avoid in ASA allergic patients. Avoid contact with eyes and mucous membranes.	$
	diclofenac, topical Pennsaid	Apply QID	Skin dryness or irritation, hypersensitivity. Serious GI toxicity has not been seen to date in clinical trials.		For external use only. Approved for treatment regimen of not more than 3 months' duration (continuous or intermittent).	$$$$

[a] Cost of 1 week's therapy; includes drug cost only.
Legend: $ < $5 $$ $5–10 $$$ $10–15 $$$$ > $15

Table 4: Intra-articular Agents Used in Osteoarthritis

Class	Drug	Dose	Adverse Effects	Comments	Cost[a]
Corticosteroids, intra-articular	*methylprednisolone acetate* Depo-Medrol	Large joints[b]: 20–80 mg Medium joints[c]: 10–40 mg Small joints[d]: 4–10 mg	No clinically significant systemic effects.	Inexpensive, safe and effective therapy for individual joints (esp. hips/knees) Maximum 3 injections/joint/year Minimize joint activity for 3 days following injection. Benefits last 4-6 wk	$$
	triamcinolone acetonide Kenalog 10 Injection, Kenalog 40 Injection	Large joints[b]: 5–40 mg Small joints[d]: 2.5–10 mg	See methylprednisolone.	See methylprednisolone.	$$
	triamcinolone hexacetonide Aristospan	Large joints[b]: 10–20 mg Small joints[d]: 2–6 mg	See methylprednisolone.	See methylprednisolone.	$$
Viscosupplementation	*hyaluronans* NeoVisc, Synvisc, OrthoVisc, Hyalgan, Durolane	1 injection/wk given once or repeated depending on product	No general systemic effect. Pseudogout. Pseudosepsis has been reported rarely in patients receiving Synvisc.[33,34]	Used in knee joint; sometimes used in shoulder and hip (e.g., Hyalgan).	(>$125)

[a] Cost of one injection; includes drug cost only.
[b] Large joints: hips, knees, shoulders, ankles.
[c] Medium joints: elbows, wrists.
[d] Small joints: metacarpophalangeal, interphalangeal, sternoclavicular, acromioclavicular.
Legend: $ < $5 $$ $5–10

Suggested Readings

Jordan KM, Arden NK, Doherty M et al. EULAR Recommendations 2003: an evidence based approach to the management of knee osteoarthritis: Report of a Task Force of the Standing Committee for International Clinical Studies Including Therapeutic Trials (ESCISIT). *Ann Rheum Dis* 2003;62(12):1145-55.

Ontario Program for Optimal Therapeutics. *Ontario treatment guidelines for osteoarthritis, rheumatoid arthritis and acute musculoskeletal injury.* 1st ed. Toronto (ON): OPOT; 2000.

Recommendations for the medical management of osteoarthritis of the hip and knee: 2000 update. American College of Rheumatology Subcommittee on Osteoarthritis Guidelines. *Arthritis Rheum* 2000;43(9):1905-15.

Rostom A, Dubé C, Jolicoeur E, Boucher M, Joyce J. *Gastroduodenal ulcers associated with the use of non-steroidal anti-inflammatory drugs: a systematic review of preventive pharmacological interventions.* Ottawa (ON): Canadian Coordinating Office for Health Technology Assessment; 2004. Technology Overview No: 12. Available from: http://www.ccohta.ca/publications/pdf/261_gastro_to_e.pdf. Accessed August 16, 2005.

References

1. Creamer P, Hochberg MC. Osteoarthritis. *Lancet* 1997;350(9076):503-8.
2. Superio-Cabuslay E, Ward MM, Lorig KR. Patient education interventions in osteoarthritis and rheumatoid arthritis: a meta-analytic comparison with nonsteroidal antiinflammatory drug treatment. *Arthritis Care Res* 1996;9(4):292-301.
3. Osiri M, Welch V, Brosseau L et al. Transcutaneous electrical nerve stimulation for knee osteoarthritis. *Cochrane Database Syst Rev* 2000;(4):CD002823.
4. Welch V, Brosseau L, Peterson J et al. Therapeutic ultrasound for osteoarthritis of the knee. *Cochrane Database Syst Rev* 2001;(3):CD003132.
5. Vas J, Mendez C, Perea-Milla E et al. Acupuncture as a complementary therapy to the pharmacological treatment of osteoarthritis of the knee: randomised controlled trial. *BMJ* 2004;329(7476):1216.
6. Berman BM, Lao L, Langenberg P et al. Effectiveness of acupuncture as adjunctive therapy in osteoarthritis of the knee: a randomized, controlled trial. *Ann Intern Med* 2004;141(12):901-10.
7. Kerrigan DC, Lelas JL, Goggins J et al. Effectiveness of a lateral-wedge insole on knee varus torque in patients with knee osteoarthritis. *Arch Phys Med Rehabil* 2002;83(7):889-93.
8. Brouwer RW, Jakma TS, Verhagen AP et al. Braces and orthoses for treating osteoarthritis of the knee. *Cochrane Database Syst Rev* 2005;(1):CD004020.
9. van Baar ME, Assendelft WJ, Dekker J et al. Effectiveness of exercise therapy in patients with osteoarthritis of the hip or knee: a systematic review of randomized clinical trials. *Arthritis Rheum* 1999;42(7):1361-9.
10. Deyle GD, Henderson NE, Matekel RL et al. Effectiveness of manual physical therapy and exercise in osteoarthritis of the knee. A randomized, controlled trial. *Ann Intern Med* 2000;132(3):173-81.
11. Lee C, Straus WL, Balshaw et al. A comparison of the efficacy and safety of nonsteroidal antiinflammatory agents versus acetaminophen in the treatment of osteoarthritis: a meta-analysis. *Arthritis Rheum* 2004;51(5):746-54.
12. Zhang W, Jones A, Doherty M. Does paracetamol (acetaminophen) reduce the pain of osteoarthritis? A meta-analysis of randomised controlled trials. *Ann Rheum Dis* 2004;63(8):901-7.
13. Wegman A, van der Windt D, van Tulder M et al. Nonsteroidal antiinflammatory drugs or acetaminophen for osteoarthritis of the hip or knee? A systematic review of evidence and guidelines. *J Rheumatol* 2004;31(2):344-54.
14. Recommendations for the medical management of osteoarthritis of the hip and knee: 2000 update. American College of Rheumatology Subcommittee on Osteoarthritis Guidelines. *Arthritis Rheum* 2000;43(9):1905-15.
15. Miceli-Richard C, Le Bars M, Schmidely N et al. Paracetamol in osteoarthritis of the knee. *Ann Rheum Dis* 2004;63(8):923-30.
16. Sachs CJ. Oral analgesics for acute nonspecific pain. *Am Fam Physician* 2005;71(5):913-8.
17. Altman RD et al. *Semin Arthritis Rheum* 1994;23(6 Suppl 3):25-33.

18. Deal CL, Schnitzer TJ, Lipstein E et al. Treatment of arthritis with topical capsaicin: a double-blind trial. *Clin Ther* 1991;13(3):383-95.
19. Bookman AA, Williams KS, Shainhouse JZ. Effect of a topical diclofenac solution for relieving symptoms of primary osteoarthritis of the knee: a randomized controlled trial. *CMAJ* 2004;171(4):333-8.
20. Rostom A, Dubé C, Jolicoeur E, Boucher M, Joyce J. *Gastroduodenal ulcers associated with the use of non-steroidal anti-inflammatory drugs: a systematic review of preventive pharmacological interventions.* Ottawa (ON): Canadian Coordinating Office for Health Technology Assessment; 2004. Technology Overview No: 12. Available from: http://www.ccohta.ca/publications/pdf/261_gastro_to_e.pdf. Accessed August 16, 2005.
21. Koch M, Dezi A, Ferrario F et al. Prevention of nonsteroidal anti-inflammatory drug-induced gastrointestinal mucosal injury. A meta-analysis of randomized controlled clinical trials. *Arch Intern Med* 1996;156(20):2321-32.
22. Chan FK, Hung LC, Suen BY et al. Celecoxib versus diclofenac and omeprazole in reducing the risk of recurrent ulcer bleeding in patients with arthritis. *N Engl J Med* 2002;347(26):2104-10.
23. Towheed TE, Maxwell L, Anastassiades TP et al. Glucosamine therapy for treating osteoarthritis. *Cochrane Database Syst Rev* 2005;(2):CD002946.
24. Michel BA, Stucki G, Frey D et al. Chondroitins 4 and 6 sulfate in osteoarthritis of the knee: a randomized, controlled trial. *Arthritis Rheum* 2005;52(3):779-86.
25. Adebowale AO, Cox DS, Liang Z et al. Analysis of glucosamine and chondroitin sulfate content in marketed products and caco-2 permeability of chondroitin sulfate raw materials. *J Am Nutraceutical Assoc* 2000;3:37-44.
26. Hunt R, Fallone C, Veldhuyzan van Zanten S et al. Canadian Helicobacter Study Group Consensus Conference: Update on the management of Helicobacter pylori--an evidence-based evaluation of six topics relevant to clinical outcomes in patients evaluated for H pylori infection. *Can J Gastroenterol* 2004;18(9):547-54.
27. Bellamy N, Campbell J, Robinson V et al. Viscosupplementation for the treatment of osteoarthritis of the knee. *Cochrane Database Syst Rev* 2005;(2):CD005321.
28. Arrich J, Piribauer F, Mad P et al. Intra-articular hyaluronic acid for the treatment of osteoarthritis of the knee: systematic review and meta-analysis. *CMAJ* 2005;172(8):1039-43.
29. Moseley JB, O'Malley K, Petersen NJ et al. A controlled trial of arthroscopic surgery for osteoarthritis of the knee. *N Engl J Med* 2002;347(2):81-8.
30. Felson DT, Buckwalter J. Debridement and lavage for osteoarthritis of the knee. *N Engl J Med* 2002;347(2):132-3.
31. Wynne HA, Long A. Patient awareness of the adverse effects of non-steroidal anti-inflammatory drugs (NSAIDs). *Br J Clin Pharmacol* 1996;42(2):253-6.
32. Health Canada. Drugs & Health Products. Report of the Expert Advisory Panel on the safety of Cox-2 selective non-steroidal anti-inflammatory drugs (NSAIDs). Available from: http://www.hc-sc.gc.ca/dhp-mps/prodpharma/activit/sci-consult/cox2/sap_report_gcs_rapport_cox2_e.html. Accessed August 23, 2005.
33. Canadian Adverse Reaction Newsletter. Hyalgan G–F 20 (Synvisc): reported incidents of joint inflammation and pain. 2005;15(2).
34. Altman RD, Status of hyaluronan supplementation therapy in osteoarthritis. *Curr Rheumatol Rep* 2003;5(1):7–14.

Pharmacoeconomic Considerations: Osteoarthritis

Nicole Mittmann, MSc, PhD

Epidemiology	
Country	**Prevalence**
Canada (2000)[1]	16% (range 11.6 –23.3%) of Canadians aged ≥ 15 years (3.9 million)

(cont'd)

Cost of Illness Data		
Country and Year of Estimate	**Direct Costs[a]**	**Indirect Costs[b]**
Canada (1993)[2]	$2.46 billion	Not reported
Canada (1997)[2]	Not reported	$17.6 billion

Commentary

Osteoarthritis (OA) is a disabling condition that places an enormous medical and economic burden on society. In 1998, physician visit rates for arthritis ranged from 146 to 207 per 1000 people for those aged greater than 15 years.[1] It has been reported that 82% of patients seeking medical advice for arthritis and arthritis related conditions made at least one visit to a primary care physician.[1]

Nonsteroidal anti-inflammatory agents (NSAIDs), acetaminophen and cyclooxygenase-2 (COX-2) inhibitors are frequently used to treat OA.[1] COX-2 inhibitors (celecoxib, lumiracoxib and meloxicam) are more expensive than traditional NSAIDs and acetaminophen. COX-2 inhibitors and NSAIDs have similar efficacy but different adverse event profiles; the rate of gastrointestinal bleeding is lower in patients receiving COX-2 inhibitors than NSAIDs.[3]

Acetaminophen is frequently used for OA and is inexpensive. However, as it is an over-the-counter agent it places an economic burden on the patient. Economic evaluations comparing acetaminophen with NSAIDs and COX-2s show a reduction in gastrointestinal adverse events at a low cost in patients at high risk of having gastrointestinal events.[4]

COX-2 inhibitors are generally not economically attractive in patients with "average" risk for gastrointestinal bleeds.[5] Celecoxib is considered to be cost-effective relative to some traditional NSAIDs in patients who are at high risk of gastrointestinal events (i.e., elderly patients or those with a history of gastrointestinal adverse events). In a Canadian economic evaluation, celecoxib was more effective and less expensive than ibuprofen plus a proton pump inhibitor in high-risk patients. In the same study, diclofenac was more effective and less expensive in both average-risk patients treated without a proton pump inhibitor and in high-risk patients with a proton pump inhibitor.[5] Other COX-2 inhibitors have also been shown to be cost-effective in older patients and in patients with risk factors for gastrointestinal adverse events.[6]

[a] Direct costs include those associated with physician services, nursing care, diagnostic procedures, drugs and hospitalization.
[b] Indirect costs include those associated with lost productivity and days off work due to morbidity or premature mortality.

References

1. Health Canada. Arthritis is Canada: An Ongoing Challenge, Ottawa, Health Canada 2005 (http://www.phac-aspc.gc.ca/publicat/ac/ac_2e.html)
2. Institute of Health Economics. *The Burden of osteoarthritis in Canada: a review of current literature.* November 9, 2000.

3. Silverstein FE, Faich G, Goldstein JL et al. Gastrointestinal toxicity with celecoxib vs nonsteroidal anti-inflammatory drugs for osteoarthritis and rheumatoid arthritis: the CLASS study: a randomized controlled trial. Celecoxib Long-term Arthritis Safety Study. *JAMA* 2000;284(10):1247-55.
4. Kamath CC, Kremers HM, Vanness DJ et al. The cost-effectiveness of acetaminophen, NSAIDs, and selective COX-2 inhibitors in the treatment of symptomatic knee osteoarthritis. *Value Health* 2003;6(2):144-157.
5. Maetzel A, Krahn M, Naglie G. The cost-effectiveness of rofecoxib and celecoxib in patients with osteoarthritis or rheumatoid arthritis. *Arthritis Rheum* 2003;49(3):283-92.
6. Moore A, Phillips C, Hunsche E et al. Economic evaluation of etoricoxib versus non-selective NSAIDs in the treatment of osteoarthritis and rheumatoid arthritis patients in the UK. *Pharmacoeconomics* 2004;22(1):643-60.

CHAPTER 72
Rheumatoid Arthritis

Vivian P. Bykerk, MD, FRCPC

Rheumatoid arthritis (RA) is a systemic autoimmune disease manifesting primarily as a symmetric and erosive polyarthritis. It can cause pain, stiffness and fatigue as well as joint destruction resulting in disability and premature mortality and can be associated with systemic manifestations including most internal organs. The incidence is .05% per year and prevalence is 1% of the adult population. Onset can occur at any age, including childhood, but most frequently starts at age 40 to 50. It affects women three times more frequently than men.

Erosions will be seen at the first visit in 20% of patients and will be present in up to 70% of patients at one year if left untreated.[1] Rheumatologists recommend an *early optimal approach to management.*[1]

Goals of Therapy

- To fully control signs and symptoms of the disease and to halt radiographic progression. All patients should reach a low disease activity state at minimum, aiming for remission. Treatment should:
  - alleviate pain, stiffness and fatigue
  - prevent any/further joint damage and destruction
  - maintain function and maximize quality of life

Investigations (Table 1)

Table 1: **Evaluation of Disease Activity and Damage**

Subjective
Degree of joint pain (scored /10 on ascending pain scale)
Duration of morning stiffness (in minutes or hours)
Duration of fatigue (scored /10 on ascending fatigue scale)
Limitation of function
Physical examination
Determine the number of actively inflamed joints
Mechanical joint problems: loss of motion, crepitus, instability, malalignment and/or deformity
Extra-articular manifestations including dry eyes, nodules, pulmonary findings

(cont'd)

Table 1: **Evaluation of Disease Activity and Damage** *(cont'd)*

Laboratory
Erythrocyte sedimentation rate/C-reactive protein level: monitor every 1–2 months
Rheumatoid factor-titre: at baseline
Complete blood cell count monitor during most therapies: every 1–3 months
Creatinine level: monitor at least twice per year
Urinalysis at baseline and during an annual visit
Synovial fluid analysis if available: at baseline to exclude other conditions or sepsis
Other
Fatigue, pain and extent of morning stiffness at each visit
Physician and patient global assessment of disease activity at each visit
Imaging
Radiographs of hands and feet and selected involved joints annually and as indicated
Consider joint ultrasound or, if available, MRI to identify subclinical erosions if radiographs normal in the first year.

Guidelines for the management of rheumatoid arthritis: 2002 update. American College of Rheumatology Subcommittee on Rheumatoid Arthritis Guidelines. *Arthritis Rheum* 2002. Reprinted by permission of Wiley-Liss, Inc., a subsidiary of John Wiley & Sons Inc.

Therapeutic Choices (Figure 1)

Nonpharmacologic Choices

RA is best treated though a *multidisciplinary team approach* that provides patient education, emotional and psychological support and physical rehabilitation. Advise patients regarding energy conservation, appropriate levels of activity and work roles, types of exercise, methods of pain modulation with heat and cold applications,[2] adjustments to activities of daily living and maintenance of joint range of motion and muscle strength. Recent studies show improvement in functional ability with dynamic exercise training, which increases aerobic capacity and muscle strength without increasing disease activity.[3] Periodically evaluate patients for splints, foot orthoses, proper footwear and surgery.

Pharmacologic Choices

Disease-Modifying Antirheumatic Drugs (DMARDs) (Table 2)

The diagnosis of RA should be confirmed by a rheumatologist who will start the patient on DMARD therapy within two to four weeks of disease onset.[4] Reassess patients every three to four months until their RA is in remission, then reduce to every six to 12 months. Adjust treatment if the patient presents with repetitive flares, ongoing disease activity after three months of maximum therapy, progressive joint damage or evidence of drug toxicity.

Severity of illness, prognostic factors,[5] presence of extra-articular features and comorbid conditions, potential adverse events, dosing intervals, routes of administration, monitoring requirements, patient preferences and costs must all be considered before selecting an initial therapy. Most DMARDs reach maximum effect in three to six months.

Frequently Used DMARDs

Methotrexate (MTX) is the reference DMARD and is an anchor drug in the treatment of RA.[6] An adequate trial of MTX consists of a weekly dose of 20 to 25 mg (orally or parenterally) for at least three months. The minor side effects of MTX can be reduced by concurrent use of folic or folinic acid.[7]

Monotherapy with **hydroxychloroquine (HCQ)** or **sulfasalazine (SSZ)** is sometimes used for early, very mild disease defined as < 2 swollen joints in a setting of a negative or low titre rheumatoid factor (RF), normal ESR and CRP and absence of radiographic erosions in the hands or feet. Initial combination of MTX with hydroxychloroquine and/or sulfasalazine is also recommended early for moderate to severe disease (swollen joint count ≥ 3 joints).

There is evidence of efficacy using combination therapy with MTX, HCQ and SSZ ("triple therapy")[8] or **gold salts**[9] or MTX with **leflunomide**,[10] **azathioprine**[11] or **cyclosporine**.[12]

At times rheumatologists recommend adding the DMARD **leflunomide** to MTX. They prefer not to discontinue MTX due to a significant risk of disease flare when MTX is discontinued even if the patient is an incomplete responder to MTX. Leflunomide can be used in place of MTX for patients who have contraindications to MTX. The loading dose of leflunomide often causes significant diarrhea and is thus no longer recommended. There have been concerns that leflunomide may be associated with an increased risk of serious adverse events, including acute liver failure, when compared to MTX.[13] However, the FDA concluded that there is presently insufficient evidence of an increase in the risk of life-threatening events with leflunomide.[14]

Less Frequently Used DMARDs

Oral and parenteral **gold**, **D-penicillamine**, **azathioprine** and **cyclosporine** are now used less frequently and mostly in combination with other DMARDs. They are used in patients who have failed MTX and who do not have access to biologic response modifiers.

Biologic Response Modifiers (Table 3)

Biologic response modifiers block tumor necrosis factor-alpha (TNFα) and interleukin-1 (IL-1), key mediators of inflammatory synovitis and bone and cartilage destruction. These agents improve the signs and symptoms of active RA and reduce the radiologic progression of the disease.[15] They are most effective in combination with MTX.[16,17,18,19] All anti-TNFα agents are thought to have comparable efficacy leading to rapid improvement in signs and symptoms, as well as laboratory parameters of inflammation, usually within 8 to 12 weeks. In patients with a partial response, increasing the dose, decreasing the dosing interval (in the case of infliximab), adding or maximizing the use of MTX or adding other

DMARDs may provide additional improvement. All biologic agents can be added to or substituted for previous DMARDs.

Anti-TNFα agents have all rarely been associated with both serious bacterial and opportunistic infections and reactivation of tuberculosis.[20] If there is a suspicion of latent TB infection, rule out active tuberculosis. Prophylactic treatment with **isoniazid** is warranted. Long-term safety with respect to lymphoproliferative and other malignancies continues to be investigated.[21] Combination therapy with two biologic response modifiers is contraindicated due to increased risk of serious infections and malignancy.[22] The risk of malignancy with the use of TNF antagonists remains low.[23]

Infliximab, a chimeric mouse-human monoclonal antibody to TNFα, has been approved only in combination with MTX in order to reduce the immune reaction to the murine component. In the case of inadequate response to infliximab, it is recommended that methotrexate doses be maximized. If this is ineffective, infliximab should be increased to 3 to 5 mg/kg every 6 to 8 weeks.

Etanercept monotherapy is effective in early RA[24] and more effective when given with MTX in preventing radiographic damage.[25] Etanercept can be given subcutaneously 25 mg twice weekly[24] or 50 mg once weekly.[26]

Adalimumab is another anti-TNFα agent effective in RA.[27] As with other TNF antagonists, it is recommended that it be used after failing DMARDs and that MTX be continued.

Anakinra is a biologic response modifier that blocks the IL-1 receptor. It is indicated in patients who are not candidates for an anti-TNFα agent or who have failed such therapy. It is associated with up to 70% chance of developing injection site reactions which are amnestic but usually resolve within a month. It may result in less symptomatic relief than the anti-TNFα agents and is effective in reducing radiographic damage. Anakinra appears to be associated with fewer significant infections compared to the anti-TNFα agents.

Two new biologic response modifiers with efficacy in RA, **abatacept** and **rituximab**, were recently approved for use in Canada. Abatacept is a fusion protein which includes a natural inhibitor of T cell costimulation called CTLA4. This can bind to a receptor on T cells to block T cell interaction with other antigen presenting cells. It is used in patients who have had an inadequate response to one or more DMARDs and/or to anti-TNFα agents. Rituximab is a chimeric monoclonal antibody which effectively removes B cells, but not plasma cells, from the circulation of patients with RA. It is to be used with MTX in patients who have failed or are intolerant of therapy with an anti-TNFα agent.

Nonsteroidal Anti-Inflammatory Drugs (NSAIDs)

Traditional **NSAIDs** (See Chapter 71, Table 2) are believed to be effective via their inhibition of COX-2. Some adverse reactions of NSAIDs, including gastrointestinal effects, may result from their inhibition of COX-1, whereas an increased risk of cardiovascular adverse events may be linked to the inhibition of COX-2. COX-2 inhibitors were specifically designed to access only the COX-2 enzyme. Their efficacy is similar to nonselective NSAIDs. Patients with heart disease should be on concurrent low-dose ASA, with appropriate gastroprotection if they are at risk of peptic ulcer disease.[28]

Glucocorticoids

Glucocorticoids rapidly reduce inflammation.[29] Some clinicians suggest that chronic low doses of **prednisone** ≤ 10 mg/day may have disease-modifying properties.[30] Prednisone is the preferred oral preparation because of its moderate glucocorticoid potency, intermediate duration of action and low mineralocorticoid potency. Depot preparations are used as bridging therapy.[31] **Triamcinolone** is preferred for deep intra-articular injections because of low systemic absorption and long action. Depot preparations of steroids may cause atrophy after infiltration of superficial subcutaneous soft tissues, thus **methylprednisolone acetate** is recommended for small joints and tendon sheaths.

Glucocorticoids are associated with a number of serious side effects including metabolic abnormalities (e.g., hyperglycemia, hypertension, muscle atrophy, truncal obesity), adrenal suppression, cataracts, infections and avascular necrosis. In combination with NSAIDs, glucocorticoids increase the risk of peptic ulcer disease. Moreover, glucocorticoids will further aggravate osteoporosis and cardiovascular disease, conditions independently associated with RA. Patients on prolonged steroid therapy should be on **calcium** 1500 mg/day and **vitamin D** 800 IU/day supplementation and an antiresorptive agent (e.g., **etidronate** 400 mg daily for two weeks every three months, **alendronate** 5 to 10 mg daily or 70 mg weekly or **risedronate** 5 mg daily or 35 mg weekly) to prevent the bone loss associated with corticosteroid use.[32] They should also be considered for prophylactic gastroprotective therapy and antiplatelet therapy with low-dose ASA.

Analgesia

RA is increasingly recognized as a *chronic pain syndrome*.[33] Many adjunctive medications and alternative therapies are being used. Although controlled trials supporting their effectiveness in RA are not available, some are compatible with the medications used to treat RA and have fewer serious side effects than NSAIDs. Avoid propoxyphene, meperidine and pentazocine because of lack of proven efficacy, risk of accumulation and serious toxicity with prolonged use. Also, up to 10% of the population lacks the enzyme that converts codeine to morphine. Failure to respond to codeine warrants a trial with hydromorphone or morphine, preparations that do not require metabolic activation.

RA Treatment During Pregnancy[34]

Pregnancy itself has a favourable influence on disease activity. Medications can often be reduced or discontinued during pregnancy.

- Glucocorticoids remain the safest therapy during pregnancy and lactation. They pose a small risk of orofacial clefts when used in the first trimester, however, benefits often appear to outweigh risks.[35]
- Data relating to the use of **hydroxychloroquine** in pregnancy is scarce. Existing data do not indicate that the drug poses significant fetal risk.[35] Despite concerns regarding a potential risk of kernicterus, **sulfasalazine** has been used in pregnancy with relative safety.[35] Because sulfasalazine is a folic acid antagonist, folic acid supplementation should be ensured in women of reproductive age. It is still recommended to monitor for hyperbilirubinemia in fetuses exposed to sulfasalazine close to term. Continue other DMARDs when potential benefits outweigh risks.
- **NSAIDs** rarely pose risks in the first and second trimesters but their use in the last month of pregnancy may be of concern. Because of antiprostaglandin effects, NSAIDs can increase risks of fetal and maternal bleeding, premature closure of the ductus arteriosus and also interfere with labour onset or duration.
- Antifolate metabolic effects of **MTX** may cause open neural tube defects and other CNS abnormalities, facial anomalies, growth retardation as well as other problems. It is contraindicated in pregnancy. Women of childbearing age should use reliable contraception while taking MTX. The drug should be stopped in both males and females at least three months before attempting conception. MTX also has abortifacient properties.[35]
- **Leflunomide** is known to be *teratogenic* and is contraindicated in pregnancy. Because of the long half-life of leflunomide, males and females wishing to conceive must stop the medication for one year prior to conceiving or stop for two months and undergo a drug elimination (washout procedure), as follows. Cholestyramine 8 g is administered three times a day for 11 days. Leflunomide plasma levels are then documented on two occasions 14 days apart. (Blood level kits are available from the manufacturer.)
- A number of registries have documented outcomes of patients who became pregnant while receiving **biologic response modifiers** and to date there has been no reported increase in adverse outcomes.[36] However, there are currently insufficient data to recommend the use of any biologic response modifiers in pregnancy or during lactation.
- The anti-TNFα agents are not associated with teratogenicity in animal studies. Although there are no studies in humans, it is recommended these be discontinued if possible during pregnancy. Safety in lactation is unknown.

Therapeutic Tips

- Referral to a rheumatologist and institution of prompt therapy is essential. Early, aggressive treatment is linked to a positive outcome in RA.
- Comorbidities, including infections, cardiovascular disease[37], lymphoma[38] and osteoporosis are common in RA patients. Routine care should include prevention and treatment of these conditions.
- Only 30% of patients have a positive RF at initial presentation. A negative RF does not exclude the possibility of rheumatoid arthritis.

Figure 1: Management of Rheumatoid Arthritis

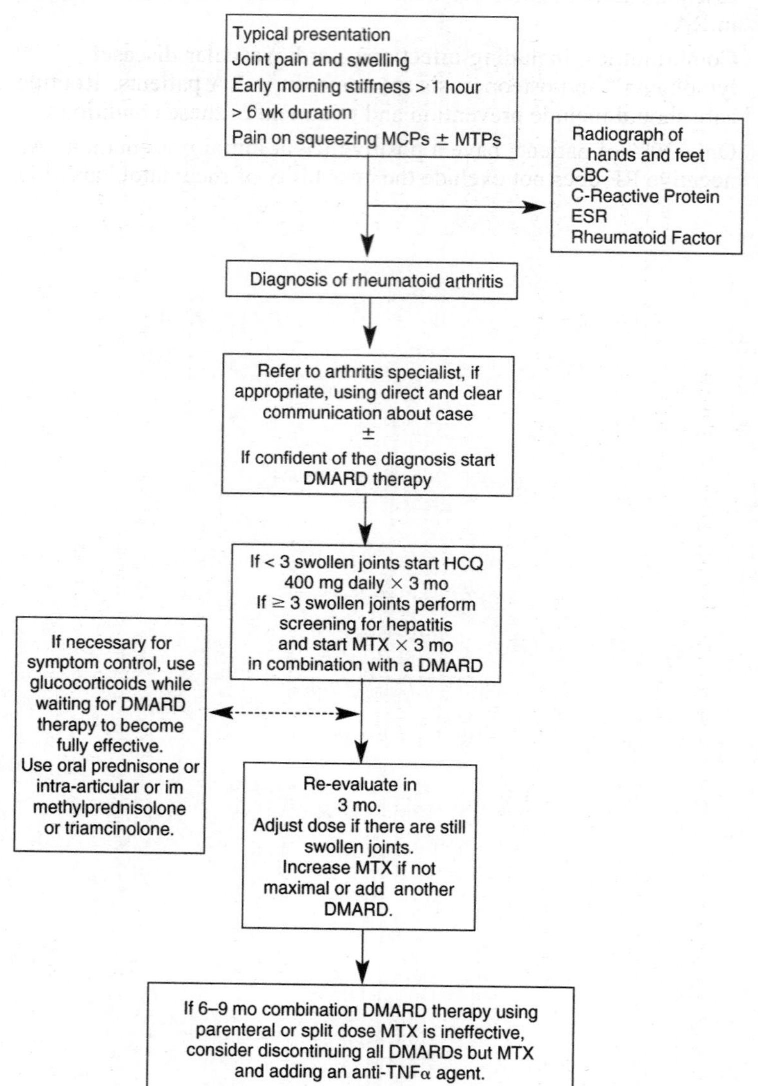

Abbreviations: DMARD=disease-modifying antirheumatic drug; HCQ=hydroxychloroquine; MCD=metacarpal phalangeal; MTP=metatarsal phalangeal; MTX=methotrexate; TNFα=tumor necrosis factorα

Table 2: **Disease-Modifying Antirheumatic Drugs for Rheumatoid Arthritis**

Class	Drug	Dose	Adverse Effects	Monitoring[39]	Drug Interactions	Cost [a]
DMARDs	*methotrexate* Methotrexate, Methotrexate Tablets USP, generics	Initial: 7.5–15 mg po Q wk, increase by 2.5–5 mg Q 1–4 wk Maintenance: 7.5–25 mg po, sc or im Q wk (single dose if tolerated, or divided in 2 doses Q12H) For doses > 15 mg sc, divided dose better absorbed	Nausea, malaise, flu-like aches, headache, oral ulcers, transient loose stools; rarely: bone marrow and liver toxicity, pneumonitis, immunosuppression, malignancy. Not to be used in patients with hepatitis B or C, renal insufficiency or lung disease.	Baseline hepatitis B and C serology and chest x-ray; CBC, LFTs, albumin, creatinine every mo × 6 mo then every 2 mo thereafter.	Alcohol restriction may minimize hepatotoxicity. NSAIDs or ASA may increase MTX serum concentrations minimally but this is not clinically significant; these can be combined at low doses. Penicillins (e.g., amoxicillin, cloxacillin, piperacillin) and sulfonamides (e.g., trimethoprim/sulfamethoxazole) may decrease MTX clearance.	$
	hydroxychloroquine Plaquenil, generics	Initial: 400–600 mg daily Maintenance: 200–400 mg daily. Reduce dose if < 60 kg	Nausea, cramps, diarrhea, rash, nightmares, hyperpigmentation. Rarely, if dosed too high for too long, corneal and retinal deposition can occur.	Ophthalmologic exam Q12–18 mo	Avoid concomitant use of related drugs such as quinine.	$
	sulfasalazine Salazopyrin, generics	Initial: 500 mg po daily or BID, increase 500 mg Q wk to a maintenance dose of 2–3 g po daily (divided in 2 doses)	Rash, marrow toxicity, gastrointestinal intolerance. May cause sun sensitivity. Do not use if sulfa allergy or G6PD deficiency.	CBC, LFTs every 3 mo.	Sulfasalazine may decrease GI absorption of digoxin.	$-$$

(cont'd)

Table 2: **Disease-Modifying Antirheumatic Drugs for Rheumatoid Arthritis** *(cont'd)*

Class	Drug	Dose	Adverse Effects	Monitoring[39]	Drug Interactions	Cost [a]
	leflunomide Arava, generics	10–20 mg po daily	Nausea, diarrhea, anorexia, alopecia, hypertension, rash. May cause hepatic toxicity, cytopenias, profound anorexia and weight loss, pulmonary fibrosis, interstitial lung disease.	Baseline hepatitis B and C serology; CBC, LFTs, creatinine Q2–8 wk, LFTs Q mo if also on MTX.	Avoid alcohol because of possible ↑ risk of hepatotoxicity. Pregnancy is contraindicated while taking this medication. Washout procedure with cholestyramine 8 g TID for 11 days recommended for serious toxicity or imminently planned pregnancy (see RA Treatment During Pregnancy[34]).	$$$$
	azathioprine Imuran, generics	Initial: 50 mg po daily, increase by 25–50 mg Q1–2 wk (dose 2–2.5 mg/kg/day) Maintenance: 50–150 mg (divided in 1–3 doses)	Hepatitis, drug fever, myelosuppression, immunosuppression, unconfirmed risk of malignancy.	CBC, LFTs every 1–3 mo.	Allopurinol may ↑ azathioprine toxicity; dosage adjustment may be necessary (1/4 of regular dose).	$-$$
	cyclosporine Neoral, generics	Initial: 2.5 mg/kg/day, divided in 2 doses, increase every 1–2 wk Maintenance: 2.5–5 mg/kg/day (divided in 2 doses)	Renal toxicity, hypertension, hypertrichosis, cytopenia, gum hyperplasia.	Blood pressure every mo, periodic CBC, LFTs, electrolytes and drug blood levels.	Metabolized by cytochrome P450—many possible drug interactions (e.g., grapefruit, erythromycin, ketoconazole, rifampin).	$$$$
	minocycline Enca, Minocin, generics	100 mg po BID	Hyperpigmentation, autoimmune diseases.	None.		$$$$

Class	Drug	Dose	Adverse Effects	Monitoring[39]	Drug Interactions	Cost [a]
	penicillamine Cuprimine	Initial: 125–250 mg po daily, increase by 125–250 mg q 1–3 mo Maintenance: 250–750 mg po daily (single dose)	Proteinuria, cytopenia, autoimmune diseases.	CBC, urine dipstick Q1–2 mo.	Food: Since the effectiveness of penicillamine may be decreased by food, administer on an empty stomach at least 1 h before or 2 h after meals and at least 1 h apart from any other drug or milk.	$$–$$$
	sodium aurothiomalate ❥ Myochrysine, generics	Initial: 10 mg im 1st wk, 25 mg 2nd wk, then 50 mg Q wk for 20 wk, then reduce to maintenance. Maintenance: 50 mg im Q2–6 wk, usually monthly	Post-dose reactions (arthralgias, flushing, hypotension). Stomatitis, pruritic dermatitis, cytopenia, proteinuria.	CBC, dipstick for urinary protein with every 1–2 injections. Hold if pruritus, mucosal ulcers, or > 1+ proteinuria.		$-$$

[a] Cost of 4-week supply for maintenance dose; includes drug cost only.

❥ Dosage adjustment may be required in renal impairment; see Appendix I

Legend: $ < $25 $-$$ < $25–50 $$ $25–50 $$-$$$ $25–75 $$$ $50–75 $$$$ > $75

Table 3: **Biologic Response Modifiers for Rheumatoid Arthritis**

Class	Drug	Dose	Adverse Effects	Monitoring[39]	Contraindications	Cost[a]
Biologic Response Modifiers	*etanercept* Enbrel	25 mg sc twice weekly or 50 mg sc once weekly	Injection site reactions, infections including tuberculosis and opportunistic organisms, autoimmune phenomena.	History of TB exposure. Baseline PPD and chest x-ray to assess for latent TB.	Demyelinating disease and susceptibility to or presence of serious or recurrent infection; consider CHF a relative contraindication.	$
	infliximab Remicade	3–5 mg/kg iv at 0, 2, 6 wk and Q4–8 wk thereafter Always give with MTX.	Infusion reactions, infections including tuberculosis and opportunistic organisms, autoimmune phenomena.	History of TB exposure. Baseline PPD and chest x-ray to assess for latent TB.	Congestive heart failure if using > 5 mg/kg/infusion, demyelinating disease, susceptibility to or presence of serious and/or recurrent infection; lupus a relative contraindication.	$$
	anakinra Kineret	100 mg sc daily	Injection site reactions (70%).	None recommended.	Susceptibility to infection.	$$$$$
	adalimumab Humira	40 mg sc every other wk	Injection site reactions (17%).	History of TB exposure. Baseline PPD and chest x-ray to assess for latent TB.	Demyelinating disease, susceptibility to or presence of serious and/or recurrent infection; consider lupus and CHF relative contraindications.	$

Class	Drug	Dose	Adverse Effects	Monitoring[39]	Contraindications	Cost[a]
	abatacept Orencia	Dosing based on weight: < 60 kg: 500 mg iv initial infusion; 60–100 kg: 750 mg iv initial infusion; > 100 kg: 1 g iv initial infusion. After baseline dosing administer at 2 wk, 4 wk and then monthly. Indicated in DMARD or anti-TNFα agent failures	Rare minor infusion reactions.	No cases of TB documented to date.	Susceptibility to infection.	$$$
	rituximab Rituxan	1 g iv × 2 doses 2 wk apart. Infusions are given with 100 mg of methylprednisolone; doses can be repeated after 5–6 mo. Indicated in patients who have failed an anti-TNFα agent	Mild to moderate infusion reactions.	CD19 counts can monitor B cell levels.	Susceptibility to infection. Contraindicated in patients with known Type I hypersensitivity or anaphylactic reactions to murine proteins, Chinese Hamster Ovary (CHO) cell proteins or to any component of the product.	$$$$$

[a] Cost of 4–week supply; includes drug cost only.

Dosage adjustment may be required in renal impairment; see Appendix I

Abbreviations: PPD = purified protein derivative

Legend: $ $1000–2000 $$ $2000–4000 $$$ $4000–6000 $$$$ $6000–8000 $$$$$ $8000–10 000

Suggested Readings

American College of Rheumatology Subcommittee on Rheumatoid Arthritis Guidelines. Guidelines for the management of rheumatoid arthritis: 2002 update. *Arthritis Rheum* 2002;46(2):328-46.

Haraoui et al. *Updated position paper on the use of TNF antagonists in rheumatic diseases*. Available from: www.rheum.ca/en

[No authors listed]. Guidelines for monitoring drug therapy in rheumatoid arthritis. American College of Rheumatology Ad Hoc Committee on Clinical Guidelines. *Arthritis Rheum* 1996;39(5):723-31.

Scott DL, Kingsley GH. Tumor necrosis factor inhibitors for rheumatoid arthritis. *N Engl J Med* 2006;355(7):704-12.

Tannenbaum H, Bombardier C, Davis P et al. An evidence-based approach to prescribing nonsteroidal antiinflammatory drugs. Third Canadian Consensus Conference. *J Rheumatol* 2006;33(1):140-57.

References

1. Bykerk VP, Baron M, Boire G et al. Canadian consensus statement on early optimal therapy in early rheumatoid arthritis. *CRAJ* 2004;14(3):11-3. Available from: http://www.stacommunications.com/customcomm/Back-issue_pages/CRAJ/crajPDFs/fall2004e/11.pdf Accessed March 7, 2007.
2. Bykerk VP, Keystone EC. What are the goals and principles of management in the early treatment of rheumatoid arthritis? *Best Pract Res Clin Rheumatol* 2005;19(1):147-61.
3. Hakkinen A. Effectiveness and safety of strength training in rheumatoid arthritis. *Curr Opin Rheumatol* 2004; 6(2):132-7.
4. Alliance for the Canadian Arthritis Program. *Standards of Care Conference, 2007*. Available from: http://www.arthritisalliance.ca/home/index.html
5. Visser H, le Cessie S, Vos K et al. How to diagnose rheumatoid arthritis early: a prediction model for persistent (erosive) arthritis. *Arthritis Rheum* 2002;46(2):357-65.
6. Pincus T, Yazici Y, Sokka T et al. Methotrexate as the "anchor drug" for the treatment of early rheumatoid arthritis. *Clin Exp Rheumatol* 2003; 21(5 Suppl 31):S179-85.
7. Shiroky JB. Folic acid and methotrexate in rheumatoid arthritis. *Ann Intern Med* 1996;124(1 Pt 1):73-4.
8. O'Dell JR, Leff R, Paulsen G et al. Treatment of rheumatoid arthritis with methotrexate and hydroxychloroquine, methotrexate and sulfasalazine, or a combination of the three medications: results of a two-year, randomized, double-blind, placebo-controlled trial. *Arthritis Rheum* 2002;46(5):1164-70.
9. Lehman AJ, Esdaile JM, Klinkhoff AV et al. A 48-week, randomized, double-blind, double-observer, placebo-controlled multicenter trial of combination methotrexate and intramuscular gold therapy in rheumatoid arthritis: results of the METGO study. *Arthritis Rheum* 2005;52(5):1360-70.
10. Kremer JM, Genovese MC, Cannon GW et al. Concomitant leflunomide therapy in patients with active rheumatoid arthritis despite stable doses of methotrexate. A randomized, double-blind, placebo-controlled trial. *Ann Intern Med* 2002;137(9):726-33.
11. Willkens RF, Stablein D. Combination treatment of rheumatoid arthritis using azathioprine and methotrexate: a 48 week controlled clinical trial. *J Rheumatol Suppl* 1996;44:64-8.
12. Stein CM, Pincus T, Yocum D et al. Combination treatment of severe rheumatoid arthritis with cyclosporine and methotrexate for forty-eight weeks: an open-label extension study. The Methotrexate-Cyclosporine Combination Study Group. *Arthritis Rheum* 1997;40(10):1843-51.
13. Public Citizen's Health Research Group letter. 2002.
14. Goldkind L. *Hepatotoxicity: leflunomide*.
15. Furst DE, Breedveld FC, Kalden JR et al. Updated consensus statement on biological agents for the treatment of rheumatoid arthritis and other rheumatic diseases (May 2002). *Ann Rheum Dis* 2002;61(Suppl 2:)ii2-7.
16. van der Heijde D, Klareskog L, Rodriguez-Valverde V et al. Comparison of etanercept and methotrexate, alone and combined, in the treatment of rheumatoid arthritis: two-year clinical and radiographic results from the TEMPO study, a double-blind, randomized trial. *Arthritis Rheum* 2006;54(4):1063-74.
17. Maini R, St Clair EW, Breedveld F et al. Infliximab (chimeric anti-tumour necrosis factor alpha monoclonal antibody) versus placebo in rheumatoid arthritis patients receiving concomitant methotrexate: a randomised phase III trial. ATTRACT Study Group. *Lancet* 1999;354(9194):1932-39.

18. St Clair EW, van der Heijde DM, Smolen JS et al. Combination of infliximab and methotrexate therapy for early rheumatoid arthritis: a randomized, controlled trial. *Arthritis Rheum* 2004;50(11):3432-43.
19. Weinblatt ME, Keystone EC, Furst DE et al. Adalimumab, a fully human anti-tumor necrosis factor alpha monoclonal antibody, for the treatment of rheumatoid arthritis in patients taking concomitant methotrexate: the ARMADA trial. *Arthritis Rheum* 2003;48(1):35-45.
20. Gardam MA, Keystone EC, Menzies R et al. Anti-tumour necrosis factor agents and tuberculosis risk: mechanisms of action and clinical management. *Lancet Infect Dis* 2003;3(3):148-55.
21. Askling J, Fored CM, Baecklund E et al. Haematopoietic malignancies in rheumatoid arthritis: lymphoma risk and characteristics after exposure to tumour necrosis factor antagonists. *Ann Rheum Dis* 2005;64(10):1414-20.
22. Weinblatt M, Schiff M, Goldman A et al. Selective costimulation modulation using abatacept in patients with active rheumatoid arthritis while receiving etanercept: a randomised clinical trial. *Ann Rheum Dis* 2007;66(2):228-34.
23. Askling J, Fored CM, Brandt L et al. Risks of solid cancers in patients with rheumatoid arthritis and after treatment with tumour necrosis factor antagonists. *Ann Rheum Dis* 2005;64(10):1421-6.
24. Bathon JM, Martin RW, Fleischmann RM et al. A comparison of etanercept and methotrexate in patients with early rheumatoid arthritis. *N Engl J Med* 2000;343(22):1586-93.
25. Klareskog L, van der Heijde D, de Jager JP et al. Therapeutic effect of the combination of etanercept and methotrexate compared with each treatment alone in patients with rheumatoid arthritis: double-blind randomised controlled trial. *Lancet* 2004;363(9410):675-81.
26. Keystone EC, Schiff MH, Kremer JM et al. Once-weekly administration of 50 mg etanercept in patients with active rheumatoid arthritis: results of a multicenter, randomized, double-blind, placebo-controlled trial. *Arthritis Rheum* 2004;50(2):353-63.
27. Keystone EC, Kavanaugh AF, Sharp JT et al. Radiographic, clinical, and functional outcomes of treatment with adalimumab (a human anti-tumor necrosis factor monoclonal antibody) in patients with active rheumatoid arthritis receiving concomitant methotrexate therapy: a randomized, placebo-controlled, 52-week trial. *Arthritis Rheum* 2004;50(5):1400-11.
28. Tannenbaum H, Bombardier C, Davis P et al. An evidence-based approach to prescribing nonsteroidal antiinflammatory drugs. Third Canadian Consensus Conference. *J Rheumatol* 2006;33(1):140-57.
29. Goekoop-Ruiterman YP, de Vries-Bouwstra JK, Allaart CF et al. Clinical and radiographic outcomes of four different treatment strategies in patients with early rheumatoid arthritis (the BeSt study): a randomized, controlled trial. *Arthritis Rheum* 2005;52(11):3381-90.
30. Kirwan JR. The effect of glucocorticoids on joint destruction in rheumatoid arthritis. The Arthritis and Rheumatism Council Low-Dose Glucocorticoid Study Group. *N Engl J Med* 1995;333(3):142-6.
31. Grigor C, Capell H, Stirling A et al. Effect of a treatment strategy of tight control for rheumatoid arthritis (the TICORA study): a single-blind randomised controlled trial. *Lancet* 2004;364(9430):263-9.
32. Brown JP, Fortier M, Frame H et al. Canadian consensus conference on osteoporosis, 2006 update. *J Obstet Gynaecol Can* 2006;28(2 Suppl 1):S95-S112.
33. American Pain Society. *Guideline for the management of pain in osteoarthritis, rheumatoid arthritis and juvenile chronic arthritis*. 2nd edition. Glenview (IL): American Pain Society; 2002.
34. Janssen NM, Genta MS. The effects of immunosuppressive and anti-inflammatory medications on fertility, pregnancy, and lactation.*Arch Intern Med* 2000;160(5):610-9.
35. Briggs GG, Freeman RK, Yaffe SJ, editors. *Drugs in pregnancy and lactation: a reference guide to fetal and neonatal risk.* 7th ed. Philadelphia (PA): Lippincott Williams & Wilkins; 2005.
36. British Society of Rheumatology. *British Society of Rheumatology Biologics Registry*. 2007.
37. Gabriel S. Heart disease in rheumatoid arthritis: changing the paradigm of systemic inflammatory disorders. *J Rheumatol* 2007;34(1):220-3.
38. Baecklund E, Iliadou A, Askling J et al. Association of chronic inflammation, not its treatment, with increased lymphoma risk in rheumatoid arthritis. *Arthritis Rheum* 2006;54(3):692-701.
39. American College of Rheumatology Subcommittee on Rheumatoid Arthritis Guidelines. Guidelines for the management of rheumatoid arthritis: 2002 update. *Arthritis Rheum* 2002;46(2):328-46.

Pharmacoeconomic Considerations: Rheumatoid Arthritis

Nicole Mittman, MSc, PhD

Epidemiology	
Country (Year)	**Prevalence (%)**
Canada (2000)[1]	4.6% to 6.8% of adults aged ≥ 55 years
Cost of Illness Data	
Country and Year of Estimate	**Indirect Costs[a]**
Finland (2002)[2]	€ 7217 per patient–year of lost productivity
Commentary	

Rheumatoid arthritis (RA) has a significant impact on both direct and indirect costs and health-related quality of life. Poor functioning is correlated with high costs.[3,4]

The main driver for overall costs of RA is lost productivity.[3,5,6] Work disability is the most costly consequence of rheumatoid arthritis.[7,8] Patients enrolled in a randomized trial reported taking 17 days of sick leave per year and 3 days of disability leave per year.[9] Predictors of work loss in patients with RA include old age disability level, severity of RA and education level.[10]

Disease-modifying antirheumatic drugs (DMARDs) may reduce work disability,[10,11] however, disease progression still occurs. Biologic agents (adalimumab, etanercept, infliximab) are expensive and have significantly increased the cost of care. These agents improve symptoms and slow the radiological progression of disease, but only limited data are available on long-term outcomes. Several economic analyses, most of which were sponsored by pharmaceutical manufacturers, have examined the use of biologic agents given after DMARDs.[12,13] The results of these analyses suggest that the high cost of biologics is offset by improved functioning in patients with moderate to severe RA.[13,14]

A comprehensive pharmacoeconomic analysis in the UK concluded that the most cost-effective approach to using biologic agents is to use them as last line therapy in patients who do not have a satisfactory response to methotrexate.[15] First-line use of these agents reduces their cost-effectiveness considerably. The cost of biologics would be beyond the means of most patients; therefore it is essential to confirm insurance coverage before prescribing these agents.

[a] Indirect costs include costs associated with lost productivity and days off work due to morbidity or premature mortality.

References

1. Badley EM, Wang PP. The contribution of arthritis and arthritis disability to nonparticipation in the labor force: a Canadian example. *J Rheumatol* 2001;28(5):1077-82.

2. Puolakka K, Kautiainen H, Pekurinen M et al. Monetary value of lost productivity over a five year follow up in early rheumatoid arthritis estimated on the basis of official register data on patients' sickness absence and gross income: experience from the FIN-RACo trial. *Ann Rheum Dis* 2006;65(7):899-904.
3. Kobelt G, Eberhardt K, Jonsson L et al. Economic consequences of the progression of rheumatoid arthritis in Sweden. *Arthritis Rheum* 1999;42(2):347-56.
4. Kobelt G, Jonsson L, Lindgren P et al. Modeling the progression of rheumatoid arthritis: a two-country model to estimate costs and consequences of rheumatoid arthritis. *Arthritis Rheum* 2002;46(9):2310-9.
5. McIntosh E. The cost of rheumatoid arthritis. *Br J Rheumatol* 1996;35(8):781-90.
6. Yelin E, Wanke LA. An assessment of the annual and long-term direct costs of rheumatoid arthritis: the impact of poor function and functional decline. *Arthritis Rheum* 1999;42(6):1209-18.
7. Ruof J, Hulsemann JL, Mittendorf T et al. Costs of rheumatoid arthritis in Germany: a micro-costing approach based on healthcare payer's data sources. *Ann Rheum Dis* 2003;62(6):544-9.
8. Pugner KM, Scott DI, Holmes JW et al. The costs of rheumatoid arthritis: an international long-term view. *Semin Arthritis Rheum* 2000;29(5):305-20.
9. Merkesdal S, Ruof J, Huelsemann JL et al. Indirect cost assessment in patients with rheumatoid arthritis (RA): comparison of data from the health economic patient questionnaire HEQ-RA and insurance claims data. *Arthritis Rheum* 2005;53(2):234-40.
10. Puolakka K, Kautiainen H, Mottonen T et al. Predictors of productivity loss in early rheumatoid arthritis: a 5 year follow up study. *Ann Rheum Dis* 2005;64(1):130-3.
11. Puolakka K, Kautiainen H, Mottonen T et al. Impact of initial aggressive drug treatment with a combination of disease-modifying antirheumatic drugs on the development of work disability in early rheumatoid arthritis: a five-year randomized followup trial. *Arthritis Rheum* 2004;50(1):55-62.
12. Kobelt G, Lindgren P, Singh A et al. Cost effectiveness of etanercept (Enbrel) in combination with methotrexate in the treatment of active rheumatoid arthritis based on the TEMPO trial. *Ann Rheum Dis* 2005;64(8):1174-9.
13. Bansback NJ, Brennan A, Ghatnekar O. Cost effectiveness of adalimumab in the treatment of patients with moderate to severe rheumatoid arthritis in Sweden. *Ann Rheum Dis* 2005;64(7):995-1002.
14. Kobelt G, Eberhardt K, Geborek P. TNF inhibitors in the treatment of rheumatoid arthritis in clinical practice: costs and outcomes in a follow up study of patients with RA treated with etanercept or infliximab in southern Sweden. *Ann Rheum Dis* 2004;63(1):4-10.
15. Chen YF, Jobanputra P, Barton P et al. A systematic review of the effectiveness of adalimumab, etanercept and infliximab for the treatment of rheumatoid arthritis in adults and an economic evaluation of their cost-effectiveness. *Health Technol Assess* 2006;10(42):iii-xiii, 1-229.

CHAPTER 73
Osteoporosis

David A. Hanley, MD, FRCPC

Goals of Therapy

- Prevent fractures, disability and loss of independence
- Preserve or enhance bone mass

Investigations

Evidence-based clinical practice guidelines identify four key predictors of osteoporosis-related fracture: age, history of previous fragility fracture, low bone mineral density and family history of osteoporotic fracture, especially maternal hip fracture.[1]

Table 1 lists risk factors used to select candidates for bone density testing. After age 50 or menopause, one major or two minor factors should qualify an individual for a bone density test.[1]

Table 1: **Risk Factors Prompting Assessment for Osteoporosis**

Major Risk Factors	Minor Risk Factors
Age > 65 y	Rheumatoid arthritis
Vertebral compression fracture	Past history of clinical hyperthyroidism
Fragility fracture after age 40	Chronic anticonvulsant therapy
Family history of osteoporotic fracture (especially maternal hip fracture)	Low dietary calcium intake
Systemic glucocorticoid therapy of > 3 mo duration	Smoker
Malabsorption syndrome	Excessive alcohol intake
Primary hyperparathyroidism	Excessive caffeine intake
Propensity to fall	Weight < 57 kg
Osteopenia apparent on x-ray film	Weight loss > 10% of weight at age 25
Hypogonadism	Chronic heparin therapy
Early menopause (before age 45)	

"2002 clinical practice guidelines for the diagnosis and management of osteoporosis in Canada" – Reprinted from *CMAJ* 12 November 2002;167 (10 Suppl) by permission of the publisher © 2002 Canadian Medical Association.

- *History:*
  - peak height as a young adult (4 cm greater than current *measured* height)
  - chronic or acute back pain
  - endocrine diseases: hyperthyroidism, hyperparathyroidism, hypogonadism, Cushing's syndrome; renal diseases, organ transplantation, gastrointestinal disease: gastric surgery, malabsorption; chemotherapy for malignancy

- medications recently associated with fractures: proton pump inhibitors, SSRIs. High doses of vitamin A are associated with increased risk of hip fracture. Advise patients not to take double doses of multivitamins to obtain higher doses of vitamin D[2]
- See Table 1 for other risk factors

- *Physical examination*
  - kyphosis
  - factors increasing risk of falling: muscle weakness (inability to rise from a chair), impaired visual acuity, poor balance or disability causing a tendency to fall
- *Laboratory investigations*
  - all should be normal: CBC, calcium, alkaline phosphatase (may be elevated in acute recovery from fracture), creatinine. Consider serum 25-OH vitamin D if the patient has an apparent increased risk of deficiency (e.g., malabsorption syndromes, housebound); measure TSH if there is a clinical suspicion of thyroid disease; serum protein electrophoresis can be performed if there is a suspicion of secondary causes of osteoporosis.
  - other more specific markers of calcium or bone metabolism are not routinely available or appropriate[1]
- *Diagnostic imaging*
  - x-rays are mainly used for detecting fractures.[1] If x-ray shows osteopenia (decreased bone mineral), confirm with a bone density measurement.[1]
  - bone scans can identify new fracture activity in patients with back pain and no obvious new fracture on x-ray
- *Bone density measurements*
  - bone mineral density (BMD) of the spine and hip by dual-energy x-ray absorptiometry (DXA) is the preferred method of assessing bone mass and fracture risk, as well as monitoring response to therapy.[1] Other methods (e.g., heel ultrasound) are acceptable for assessing fracture risk if DXA is not available.[3]
  - recommendations for reporting DXA that combine age, BMD and epidemiologic data yield an estimated 10-year risk of osteoporotic fracture (Figure 1), which is reported as "low" (≤ 10%), intermediate (11–19%) or high (≥ 20%).[4] This risk stratification is borrowed from the Framingham-based cardiovascular risk assessment strategy, and has not yet been validated as an osteoporosis management strategy. Nevertheless, an individual in the "low risk" category is not likely to receive clinically meaningful fracture prevention benefit from pharmacologic therapy. Glucocorticoid therapy or a fragility fracture moves a patient to a higher risk category than that indicated by BMD and age.

Therapeutic Choices

Osteoporosis therapy may be subdivided into *prevention* and *treatment* of established osteoporosis (Figure 2). Chronic glucocorticoid therapy requires special attention for preventive intervention.[1]

Nonpharmacologic Choices

- Regular exercise (especially impact type).
- Reduce risk of falling: minimize hazards for falling in the home, assess drugs implicated in falls such as benzodiazepines and other psychotropics; improve strength and balance.
- Adequate protein, calcium and vitamin D intake (Table 2).
- Facilitate smoking cessation; encourage avoidance of excessive alcohol (> 2 drinks/day) and caffeine intake (> 4 cups of coffee per day or equivalent).

Pharmacologic Choices (Table 2)

Therapies for osteoporosis manipulate the normal process of bone remodelling, either by reducing bone resorption (antiresorptive or anticatabolic agents) or stimulating bone formation (anabolic).[5] Most approved drugs are primarily *antiresorptive*. By acting to reduce both the depth and rate of bone resorption while bone formation proceeds normally, these agents cause an initial increase in bone mass. This increase eventually plateaus, as bone formation slows to match the reduced rate of resorption.[5]

Anticatabolic Agents

Bisphosphonates

Alendronate, risedronate and cyclical etidronate are approved for prevention and treatment of postmenopausal bone loss, treatment of established osteoporosis and glucocorticoid-induced osteoporosis. All bisphosphonates have very poor intestinal absorption, e.g., alendronate < 1%. They must be taken on an empty stomach and only with water, as other medications or food will prevent absorption. Strict adherence to dosing instructions is mandatory.

The main side effects of bisphosphonates are minor gastrointestinal upset and allergic reactions. An important rare side effect of alendronate and risedronate is esophageal ulceration.

Etidronate taken for two weeks every three months increases bone density and prevents vertebral fractures.[6] Safety and efficacy for up to seven years of cyclical etidronate therapy has been demonstrated.[7] The dose schedule of etidronate (only two weeks every three months) and its lower cost are attractive to some patients.

Didrocal provides 14 days of etidronate 400 mg followed by 76 days of elemental calcium 500 mg as calcium carbonate. Additional calcium supplements may be used as needed.

Alendronate increases bone mass throughout the skeleton and reduces the risk of all fractures (including hip).[8,9,10]

Risedronate, like alendronate, is associated with a reduced risk of all osteoporosis-associated fractures.[11,12]

Gains in spinal bone density appear to be greater with alendronate and risedronate than with etidronate; a meta-analysis places these agents ahead of etidronate in preventing vertebral and nonvertebral fractures.[13] Guidelines recognize alendronate and risedronate as first-line therapies for osteoporosis.[1]

There have been no well-designed, direct comparison trials of bisphosphonates that have been powered to look at fracture prevention. A recent randomized trial showed alendronate had a greater effect on BMD and biochemical markers of bone turnover than risedronate, but fracture prevention was no different.[14] However, an observational study suggests earlier and greater fracture prevention with risedronate than alendronate.[15]

Although not approved in Canada for the treatment of osteoporosis, *intravenous bisphosphonates* have become more commonly used for patients who cannot tolerate oral bisphosphonates. **Pamidronate** 30 or 60 mg iv over two to three hours *every three months* causes a similar improvement in BMD to that seen with the oral bisphosphonates, and a small study suggests fracture prevention.[16,17] A recent placebo-controlled large clinical trial of **zoledronate** 5 mg iv infusion *once yearly* shows improved BMD and reduction in all osteoporotic fractures, including hip fractures.[18]

Selective Estrogen Receptor Modulators

Raloxifene prevents postmenopausal bone loss,[19] increasing bone density by approximately 3% and reducing new vertebral fractures by 30 to 40%.[20] It is an estrogen antagonist in breast and uterine tissue, but has estrogen-like activity in bone and lipid metabolism. Like estrogen, there is a modestly increased risk of deep vein thrombosis and pulmonary embolism in postmenopausal women.[20] It also significantly reduces the relative risk of diagnosis of estrogen receptor–positive breast cancer by 76%.[21] Raloxifene is not associated with increased cardiovascular risk.[22]

Estrogen and Progesterone

Postmenopausal estrogen or estrogen/progesterone therapy (ET or EPT) is no longer a first choice for treatment of osteoporosis.[1,23] However, to prevent osteoporosis in women experiencing an early menopause (i.e., before age 45), it is recommended that hormone therapy (HT) be taken until normal age of menopause.[1] For women entering menopause at the usual age, Canadian guidelines suggest HT *only* for relief of menopausal symptoms.[1] For the treatment of established osteoporosis in older postmenopausal women, HT is now considered second-line,[1] because the reduction in hip and other fractures is offset by increased risk of breast cancer and heart disease, according to the Women's Health Initiative (WHI) studies.[23] It should be noted, however, that women participating in the WHI were at low risk for osteoporosis but had a high incidence of obesity and hypertension, increasing their risk for breast cancer and cardiovascular disease. The risk/benefit ratio may be different for postmenopausal women with osteoporosis.

Calcitonin

Salmon calcitonin nasal spray has been shown to prevent vertebral fractures, but because of weaker clinical trial data, calcitonin is a second-line therapy.[1,24] Calcitonin reduces pain associated with acute vertebral fractures. The effective dose of injectable calcitonin has not been standardized.

Anabolic Agents

Teriparatide

Teriparatide, a parathyroid hormone (PTH) analogue, is an anabolic agent that causes a steady gain in bone density and a reduction in osteoporotic fractures by more than 50%.[25]

The major clinical trials of teriparatide were stopped at a median of 19 months of therapy because of occurrence of osteogenic sarcoma in teratogenicity studies in rats given lifelong treatment with very high doses. This finding is not likely to be relevant to its use in humans at a lower dose for a much shorter relative duration of therapy. Teriparatide has been approved for 18 months' lifetime exposure in Canada (and two years in the United States).

Human Parathyroid Hormone

In a large placebo-controlled, 18-month clinical trial in patients at low risk of fracture, recombinant **human PTH** 100 µg sc daily significantly increased BMD and reduced the incidence of vertebral fractures.[26] This drug is approved for osteoporosis therapy in Europe, and is under review in North America.

After PTH or teriparatide therapy is completed, treatment with a bisphosphonate or other anticatabolic agent is advised, as much of the increase in BMD is lost during the first year after stopping the drug, unless an anticatabolic is started.[27]

Strontium Ranelate

Strontium replaces calcium in bone matrix and also appears to uncouple bone remodelling, causing a modest reduction in bone resorption in conjunction with a similarly modest increase in bone formation.[28] The dramatic increases in bone density are partly explained by strontium having a higher atomic weight than calcium, and partly by the positive bone balance.

Clinical trials of strontium ranelate have shown similar fracture prevention to that seen with bisphosphonates.[28] Strontium ranelate 2 g orally is taken as powder mixed with water, once per day. Side effects appear to be minimal.

Combination Therapy

Combining a bisphosphonate with other anticatabolic agents, estrogen or raloxifene, has additive or synergistic effects on BMD, but no fracture benefit has yet been demonstrated.[29,30]

Combining anticatabolic with anabolic therapy may seem an attractive approach, but mixed results have been reported. Giving a bisphosphonate concurrently with PTH or teriparatide may actually blunt the anabolic response. However, combining teriparatide with either estrogen or raloxifene therapy does not interfere with the anabolic action, and may even enhance it.[31]

After PTH or teriparatide therapy is completed, treatment with a bisphosphonate or other anticatabolic agent is advised, to preserve and consolidate the gains achieved with the anabolic agent.[27]

Therapeutic Tips

- A person over the age of 50 with a vertebral compression fracture, wrist fracture or hip fracture should be considered to have osteoporosis until proven otherwise. Test these individuals with bone densitometry. These patients are still candidates for therapy if bone densitometry is not available.
- In all age groups, adequate **calcium** and **vitamin D** preserves or enhances bone mass and prevents fractures in the elderly.[32] Ensure adequate intake of both of these nutrients when prescribing pharmacologic therapy for osteoporosis. Vitamin D insufficiency is a common problem in Canada,[33] and many experts believe even the current recommendation for vitamin D supplements of 800 IU per day is too low.
- For the prevention of osteoporosis in early postmenopause, if estrogen deficiency symptoms also require treatment, estrogen or estrogen/progesterone remains a reasonable choice. If menopausal symptoms are not a problem, raloxifene is an alternative, with the potential added benefit of reducing breast cancer risk.
- For patients with established osteoporosis (e.g., a fragility fracture and bone density in the osteoporosis range), bisphosphonates are recommended first-line therapy. Raloxifene is also ranked as first-line therapy but in the absence of hip fracture prevention data, it would be considered after bisphosphonate therapy for individuals at high risk of hip fracture (age > 70 years with a prior fragility fracture history). Consider teriparatide for severe cases characterized by more than one fragility fracture and a very low BMD.[34]

- For the prevention and treatment of *glucocorticoid-induced osteoporosis*, bisphosphonates are the agents of choice.[1]
- In the absence of fracture prevention data, calcitriol, androgens and sodium fluoride are no longer considered appropriate alternative therapies.
- Osteoporosis is often ignored in men, but men are affected by this disorder almost as frequently as women.[35]

Figure 1: **Use of Bone Density and Age to Predict Fragility Fracture Risk in Women**

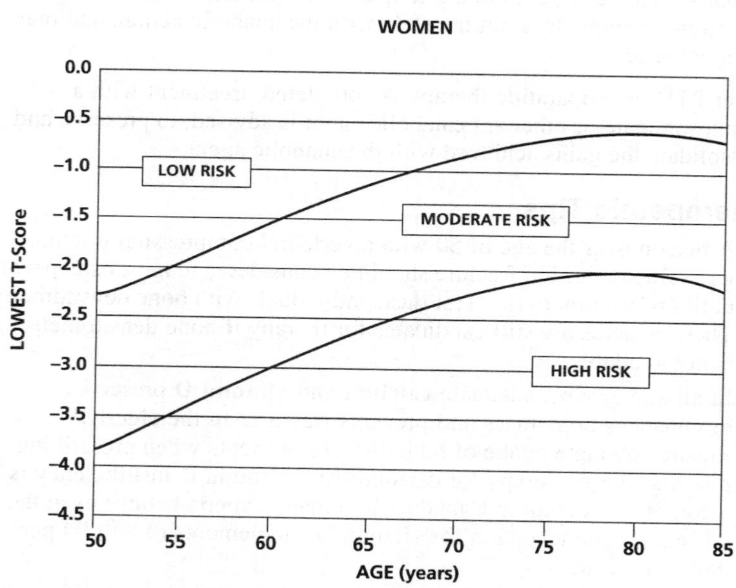

Calculated 10-year absolute risk of typical osteoporotic fracture (hip, forearm, proximal humerus and symptomatic vertebral compression) for women over age 50 who have not received osteoporosis therapy. Most therapies reduce relative risk of fracture by 40 to 50%. Reprinted from *Can Assoc Radiol J* 2005;56(3):182 by permission of the publisher © 2005 Canadian Association of Radiologists.

Figure 2: **Use of Bone Density and Risk Factors in Osteoporosis Management**

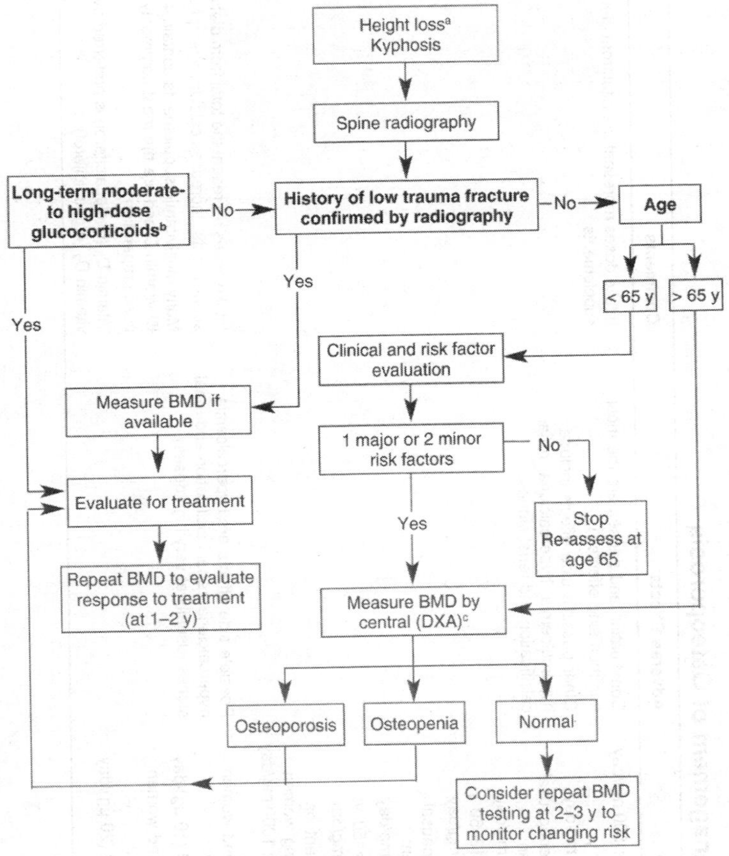

[a] 4 cm historical height loss; 2 cm prospective height loss.
[b] Low to moderate: 2.5–7.5 mg prednisone/day; moderate to high: > 7.5 mg prednisone/day.
[c] Central DXA = spine and hip.
Abbreviations: BMD = bone mineral density; DXA = dual-energy x-ray absorptiometry
"2002 clinical practice guidelines for the diagnosis and management of osteoporosis in Canada". Reprinted from *CMAJ* 12 November 2002;167(10 Suppl):S7 by permission of the publisher © 2002 Canadian Medical Association.

Table 2: **Drugs Used for the Management of Osteoporosis**

Class	Drug	Dose	Adverse Effects	Comments	Cost[a]
Nutritional Supplements	*calcium* Caltrate 600, Os-Cal, Tums, generics	4–8 y: 800 mg/day 9–18 y: 1300 mg/day Premenopausal women: 1000 mg/day Men 18–50 y: 1000 mg/day Menopausal women: 1500 mg/day Men > 50 y: 1500 mg/day Pregnant or lactating women > 18 y: 1000 mg/day	Constipation and nausea are the most common side effects. Other possible side effects include hypercalcemia, hypercalciuria, renal calcification and renal stones.	Intake doses represent the total from diet and supplements.	$
	vitamin D Drisdol, generics	Men and women < 50 y: 400 IU (10 μg)/day Men and women > 50 y: 800 IU (20 μg)/day	Possible side effects are hypercalcemia, hypercalciuria, renal calcification and renal stones (usually at very high doses).	Intake doses represent the total from diet and supplements. Increases calcium absorption. Many multivitamin supplements contain 400 IU vitamin D and are the most commonly used preparation. Vitamin D_3 (cholecalciferol) is preferred over vitamin D_2 (ergocalciferol).	$

Class	Drug	Dose	Adverse Effects	Comments	Cost[a]
Bisphosphonates	*etidronate* Didronel, generics Didrocal (packaged with calcium in 3 month kit)	Cyclic: 400 mg/day × 14 days Q3 mo, then calcium alone	Side effects are usually minimal: GI symptoms, altered taste, nighttime leg cramps. Rarely reported: acute-phase reactions involving fever and lymphopenia, joint or muscle pain, skin reactions, ocular effects. Safety in impaired renal function (ClCr < 35 mL/min) is unknown. Osteonecrosis of the jaw (ONJ) has been reported rarely in patients receiving bisphosphonates in doses used for osteoporosis; it is not known whether the incidence is any different from the general population. If possible, patients are advised to have elective dental work done before starting bisphosphonates.[36]	Etidronate should be taken on an empty stomach with a full glass of water. To aid compliance, it is recommended that patients take the therapy at bedtime, at least 2 h before or after eating. Calcium supplements should be separated by at least 2 h before or after.	$$ Didrocal: $$/3 months
	alendronate Fosamax, generic	Prevention: 5 mg/day Treatment: 10 mg/day or 70 mg once weekly	See etidronate. Esophageal ulceration is a rare side effect of bisphosphonates and appears to be more common with aminobisphosphonates; patient must take it with a full glass of water and not lie down for 30 min after taking the pill.	Must be taken at least 30 min before the first food, beverage, or medication with plain water only. Retrospective analysis suggests alendronate prevents fractures within the first year of therapy.	$$
	risedronate Actonel	5 mg/day or 35 mg once weekly	See alendronate.	Risedronate should be taken on an empty stomach at least 30 min before consuming the first food, drink (other than plain water) and/or any other medication. Patients should not lie down for at least 30 min after taking the medication. Risedronate has been shown to prevent fractures within the first year of therapy.	$$$

(cont'd)

Table 2: **Drugs Used for the Management of Osteoporosis** *(cont'd)*

Class	Drug	Dose	Adverse Effects	Comments	Cost[a]
Bisphosphonate/Nutritional Supplement Combinations	*alendronate/ vitamin D* Fosavance	alendronate 70 mg plus vitamin D 2800 IU once weekly	See alendronate.	See alendronate.	$$$
	risedronate/ calcium Actonel Plus Calcium	35 mg/week (day 1 of the 7–day cycle)plus calcium (as carbonate) 500 mg (days 2–7)	See alendronate.	See risedronate.	$$$
Selective Estrogen Receptor Modulators	*raloxifene* Evista	60 mg/day	Leg cramps, hot flashes especially in younger postmenopausal women. Venous thromboembolism risk similar to estrogen.	May aggravate hot flushes; should not be started until menopause is established.	$$$
Hormone Therapy (See Chapter 64)					
Calcitonin Peptides	*calcitonin salmon, intranasal* Miacalcin NS	200 IU/day intranasally	Local effects such as rhinitis, nasal dryness with crusting, nonsevere epistaxis and sinusitis. Rarely associated with systemic effects such as nausea, vomiting, dizziness, flushing accompanied by a sensation of heat and, uncommonly, polyuria and chills.		$$$

Class	Drug	Dose	Adverse Effects	Comments	Cost[a]
	calcitonin salmon, subcutaneous Calcimar, Caltine	50–100 IU sc/day or Q 2nd day or 5 days/wk	See intranasal salmon calcitonin. Pain at site of injection, nausea, facial flushing, metallic taste, hypersensitivity (rare).	Not approved for osteoporosis; restrict to patients who fail conventional therapy. Dose is not standardized.	\$\$\$\$\$
Anabolic Agents	*teriparatide* Forteo	20 µg sc/day for 18 months	Nausea, dizziness, leg cramps. Not to be prescribed to patients with an increased baseline risk of osteosarcoma. Patients should be in a supine or sitting position for administration because of the risk of orthostatic hypotension.	Limited data available concerning use in renal or hepatic impairment.	Ap-prox: \$750

[a] Cost of 30-day supply unless otherwise specified, includes drug cost only.

Dosage adjustment may be required in renal impairment; see Appendix I.

Legend: \$ < \$20 \$\$ \$20–40 \$\$\$ \$40–60 \$\$\$\$ \$60–80 \$\$\$\$\$ > \$80

Suggested Readings

Brown JP, Josse RG; Scientific Advisory Council of the Osteoporosis Society of Canada. 2002 clinical practice guidelines for the diagnosis and management of osteoporosis in Canada. *CMAJ* 2002;167(10 Suppl):S1-34.

Brown JP, Fortier M, Frame H et al. Canadian consensus conference on osteoporosis, 2006 update. *J Obstet Gynaecol Can* 2006;28(2 Suppl 1):S95-S112.

Cranney A, Guyatt G, Griffith L et al. Meta-analyses of therapies for postmenopausal osteoporosis. IX: Summary of meta-analyses of therapies for postmenopausal osteoporosis. *Endocr Rev* 2002;23(4):570-8.

Siminoski K, Leslie WD, Frame H et al. Recommendations for bone mineral density reporting in Canada. *Can Assoc Radiol J* 2005;56(3):178-88.

References

1. Brown JP, Josse RG; Scientific Advisory Council of the Osteoporosis Society of Canada. 2002 clinical practice guidelines for the diagnosis and management of osteoporosis in Canada. *CMAJ* 2002;167(10 Suppl):S1-34.
2. Feskanich D, Singh V, Willett WC et al. Vitamin A intake and hip fractures among postmenopausal women. *JAMA* 2002;287(1):47-54.
3. Bauer DC, Gluer CC, Cauley JA et al. Broadband ultrasound attenuation predicts fractures strongly and independently of densitometry in older women. A prospective study. Study of Osteoporotic Fractures Research Group. *Arch Intern Med* 1997;157(6):629-34.
4. Siminoski K, Leslie WD, Frame H et al. Recommendations for bone mineral density reporting in Canada. *Can Assoc Radiol J* 2005;56(3):178-88.
5. Riggs BL, Melton LJ. The prevention and treatment of osteoporosis. *N Engl J Med* 1992;327(9):620-7.
6. Storm T, Thamsborg G, Steiniche T et al. Effect of intermittent cyclical etidronate therapy on bone mass and fracture rate in women with postmenopausal osteoporosis. *N Engl J Med* 1990;322(18):1265-71.
7. Miller PD, Watts NB, Licata AA et al. Cyclical etidronate in the treatment of postmenopausal osteoporosis: efficacy and safety after seven years of treatment. *Am J Med* 1997;103(6):468-76.
8. Black DM, Cummings SR, Karpf DB et al. Randomised trial of effect of alendronate on risk of fracture in women with existing vertebral fractures. Fracture Intervention Trial Research Group. *Lancet* 1996;348(9041):1535-41.
9. Black DM, Thompson DE, Bauer DC et al. Fracture risk reduction with alendronate in women with osteoporosis: the Fracture Intervention Trial. FIT Research Group. *J Clin Endocrinol Metab* 2000;85(11):4118-24.
10. Pols HA, Felsenberg D, Hanley DA et al. Multinational, placebo-controlled, randomized trial of the effects of alendronate on bone density and fracture risk in postmenopausal women with low bone mass: results of the FOSIT study. Fosamax International Trial Study Group. *Osteoporos Int* 1999;9(5):461-8.
11. Harris ST, Watts NB, Genant HK et al. Effects of risedronate treatment on vertebral and nonvertebral fractures in women with postmenopausal osteoporosis: a randomized controlled trial. Vertebral Efficacy With Risedronate Therapy (VERT) Study Group. *JAMA* 1999;282(14):1344-52.
12. McClung MR, Geusens P, Miller PD et al. Effect of risedronate on the risk of hip fracture in elderly women. Hip Intervention Program Study Group. *N Engl J Med* 2001;344(5):333-40.
13. Cranney A, Guyatt G, Griffith L et al. Meta-analyses of therapies for postmenopausal osteoporosis. IX: Summary of meta-analyses of therapies for postmenopausal osteoporosis. *Endocr Rev* 2002;23(4):570-8.
14. Rosen CJ, Hochberg MC, Bonnick SL et al. Treatment with once-weekly alendronate 70 mg compared with once-weekly risedronate 35 mg in women with postmenopausal osteoporosis: a randomized double-blind study. *J Bone Miner Res* 2005;20(1):141-51.
15. Silverman SL, Watts NB, Delmas PD et al. Effectiveness of bisphosphonates on nonvertebral and hip fractures in the first year of therapy: the risedronate and alendronate (REAL) cohort study. *Osteoporos Int* 2007;18(1):25-34.
16. Kim SH, Lim SK, Hahn JS. Effect of pamidronate on new vertebral fractures and bone mineral density in patients with malignant lymphoma receiving chemotherapy. *Am J Med* 2004;116(8):524-8.

17. Vis M, Bultink IE, Dijkmans BA et al. The effect of intravenous pamidronate versus oral alendronate on bone mineral density in patients with osteoporosis. *Osteoporos Int* 2005;16(11):1432-5.
18. Black DM, Delmas PD, Eastell R et al. Once-yearly zoledronic acid for treatment of postmenopausal osteoporosis. *N Engl J Med* 2007;356(18):1809-22.
19. Delmas PD, Bjarnason NH, Mitlak BH et al. Effects of raloxifene on bone mineral density, serum cholesterol concentrations, and uterine endometrium in postmenopausal women. *N Engl J Med* 1997;337(23):1641-7.
20. Ettinger B, Black DM, Mitlak BH et al. Reduction of vertebral fracture risk in postmenopausal women with osteoporosis treated with raloxifene: results from a 3-year randomized clinical trial. Multiple Outcomes of Raloxifene Evaluation (MORE) Investigators. *JAMA* 1999;282(7):637-45.
21. Cummings SR, Eckert S, Krueger KA et al. The effect of raloxifene on risk of breast cancer in postmenopausal women: results from the MORE randomized trial. Multiple Outcomes of Raloxifene Evaluation. *JAMA* 1999;281(23):2189-97.
22. Barrett-Connor E, Mosca L, Collins P et al. Effects of raloxifene on cardiovascular events and breast cancer in postmenopausal women. *N Engl J Med* 2006;355(2):125-37.
23. Rossouw JE, Anderson GL, Prentice RL et al. Risks and benefits of estrogen plus progestin in healthy postmenopausal women: principal results From the Women's Health Initiative randomized controlled trial. *JAMA* 2002;288(3):321-33.
24. Cranney A, Tugwell P, Zytaruk N et al. Meta-analyses of therapies for postmenopausal osteoporosis. VI. Meta-analysis of calcitonin for the treatment of postmenopausal osteoporosis. *Endocr Rev* 2002;23(4):540-51.
25. Neer RM, Arnaud CD, Zanchetta JR et al. Effect of parathyroid hormone (1-34) on fractures and bone mineral density in postmenopausal women with osteoporosis. *N Engl J Med* 2001;344(19):1434-41.
26. Greenspan SL, Bone HG, Ettinger MP et al. Effect of recombinant human parathyroid hormone (1-84) on vertebral fracture and bone mineral density in postmenopausal women with osteoporosis: a randomized trial. *Ann Intern Med* 2007;146(5):326-39.
27. Black DM, Bilezikian JP, Ensrud KE et al. One year of alendronate after one year of parathyroid hormone (1-84) for osteoporosis. *N Engl J Med* 2005;353(6):555-65.
28. Reginster JY, Seeman E, De Vernejoul MC et al. Strontium ranelate reduces the risk of nonvertebral fractures in postmenopausal women with osteoporosis: Treatment of Peripheral Osteoporosis (TROPOS) study. *J Clin Endocrinol Metab* 2005;90(5):2816-22.
29. Lindsay R, Cosman F, Lobo RA et al. Addition of alendronate to ongoing hormone replacement therapy in the treatment of osteoporosis: a randomized, controlled clinical trial. *J Clin Endocrinol Metab* 1999;84(9):3076-81.
30. Wimalawansa SJ. A four-year randomized controlled trial of hormone replacement and bisphosphonate, alone or in combination, in women with postmenopausal osteoporosis. *Am J Med* 1998;104(3):219-26.
31. Deal C, Omizo M, Schwartz EN et al. Combination teriparatide and raloxifene therapy for postmenopausal osteoporosis: results from a 6-month double-blind placebo-controlled trial. *J Bone Miner Res* 2005;20(11):1905-11.
32. Chapuy MC, Arlot ME, Duboeuf F et al. Vitamin D3 and calcium to prevent hip fractures in the elderly women. *N Engl J Med* 1992;327(23):1637-42.
33. Hanley DA, Davison KS. Vitamin D insufficiency in North America. *J Nutr* 2005;135(2):332-7.
34. Hodsman A; Scientific Advisory Council of Osteoporosis Canada; Papaioannou A et al. Clinical practice guidelines for the use of parathyroid hormone in the treatment of osteoporosis. *CMAJ* 2006;175(1):48.
35. Khan AA, Hodsman AB, Papaioannou A et al. Management of osteoporosis in men: an update and case example. *CMAJ* 2007;176(3):345-8.
36. Shane E, Goldring S, Christakos S et al. Osteonecrosis of the jaw: more research needed. *J Bone Miner Res* 2006;21(10):1503-5.

Pharmacoeconomic Considerations: Osteoporosis

Nicole Mittmann, MSc, PhD

Epidemiology	
Country (Year)	**Prevalence**
Canada (2003)[1]	1.0–1.4 million 1 : 4 male : female sex ratio
Cost of Illness Data	
Country and Year of Estimate	**Direct Costs[a]**
Canada (1995-96)[2]	$650 million annually
Commentary	

Complications of osteoporosis, namely vertebral and nonvertebral fractures, are associated with a large economic burden. Death is a real complication of both vertebral and nonvertebral fractures. Hospitalization, rehabilitation, rehospitalization, chronic care and long-term care significantly drive the direct medical costs of treatment and management of osteoporosis.[2] Inpatient length of stay increases exponentially with age, thereby increasing the costs of management.[3] Personal care and nursing care are also considerable.[4]

Lost productivity associated with fractures is also a consideration. Intangible costs, including pain and suffering associated with fractures, can be substantial, but have not been quantified.

A number of drugs are available to prevent fractures and reduce vertebral and nonvertebral fractures including bisphosphonates, selective estrogen receptor modulators and teriparatide.

In general, economic studies for all bisphosphonates have reported good clinical outcomes and economic benefit in terms of reducing complications (i.e., hip fracture) and mortality when compared with no treatment, indicating that these drugs are cost-effective.[5,6,7]

Raloxifene, an oral selective estrogen receptor modulator used in the prevention of osteoporosis, is expensive but reduces fracture rates when used for both primary and secondary prevention.[8] The cost-effectiveness ratios are high for the reduction in fracture rates achieved with raloxifene.[7,9] Raloxifene has been associated with a reduction in coronary heart disease and cancer in postmenopausal women when compared with no therapy,[7,8] which may make the drug more cost-effective.[7]

(cont'd)

Commentary

Teriparatide, a recombinant form of parathyroid hormone, is more expensive than the bisphosphonates but decreases vertebral fractures in older individuals and reduces the incidence of moderate to severe fractures.[10] There is controversy about the cost-effectiveness of teriparatide. Some studies have reported that teriparatide is not cost-effective when compared with alendronate,[11] and others show favourable cost-effectiveness ratios when patients are treated early and include consideration of reductions in mortality and fracture rates.[12] Differences in these analyses can be attributed to study design, patient characteristics and outcomes considered.

[a] Direct costs include those associated with physician services, nursing care, diagnostic procedures, drugs and hospitalization.

References

1. Osteoporosis Society of Canada. Osteoporosis update: a practical guide for Canadian physicians. *Osteoporosis Update* 2003;7(1):1-19. Available from: http://www.osteoporosis.ca/local/files/health_professionals/pdfs/osteoupdate_special_e.pdf Accessed June 28, 2007.
2. Wiktorowicz ME, Goeree R, Papaioannou A et al. Economic implications of hip fracture: health service use, institutional care and cost in Canada. *Osteoporos Int* 2001;12(4):271-8.
3. Papadimitropoulos EA, Coyte PC, Josse RG et al. Current and projected rates of hip fracture in Canada. *CMAJ* 1997;157(10):1357-63.
4. Brecht JG, Schadlich PK. Burden of illness imposed by osteoporosis in Germany. *Health Economics in Prevention and Care* 2000;1(1):26-32.
5. Grima DT, Burge RT, Becker DL et al. Short-term cost-effectiveness of bisphosphonate therapies for postmenopausal osteoporotic women at high risk of fracture. *P&T* 2002;27(9):448-51. Available from: http://www.ptcommunity.com/ptjournal/fulltext/27/9/PTJ2709448.pdf Accessed June 28, 2007.
6. Kennedy CC, Papaioannou A, Adachi JD. Treating osteoporosis: economic aspects of bisphosphonate therapy. *Expert Opin Pharmacother* 2006;7(11):1457-67.
7. Goeree R, Blackhouse G, Adachi J. Cost-effectiveness of alternative treatments for women with osteoporosis in Canada. *Curr Med Res Opin* 2006;22(7):1425-36.
8. Meadows ES, Klein R, Rousculp MD et al. Cost-effectiveness of preventative therapies for postmenopausal women with osteopenia. *BMC Womens Health* 2007;7:6.
9. Brecht JG, Kruse HP, Mohrke W et al. Health-economic comparison of three recommended drugs for the treatment of osteoporosis. *Int J Clin Pharmacol Res* 2004;24(1):1-10.
10. Dobnig H. A review of teriparatide and its clinical efficacy in the treatment of osteoporosis. *Expert Opin Pharmacother* 2004;5(5):1153-62.
11. Liu H, Michaud K, Nayak S et al. The cost-effectiveness of therapy with teriparatide and alendronate in women with severe osteoporosis. *Arch Intern Med* 2006;166(11):1209-17.
12. Lundkvist J, Johnell O, Cooper C et al. Economic evaluation of parathyroid hormone (PTH) in the treatment of osteoporosis in postmenopausal women. *Osteoporos Int* 2006;17(2):201-11.

CHAPTER 74

Neck Pain and Whiplash

Eldon Tunks, MD, FRCPC

Goals of Therapy

Acute phase

- Reduce distress
- Identify patients in need of urgent surgical intervention

1 to 4 weeks

- Promote therapy to restore function
- Return to normal activities as soon as possible

Subacute period (4 to 12 weeks)

- Interrupt progress to chronicity
- Promote active therapy while encouraging return to work

Chronic pain (6 months or more)

- Multimodal therapy aimed at management of chronic pain/disability, with emphasis on restoring function and independence

Acute Phase to 30 Days

Investigations

Acute Phase (days 1 to 7)

- History and physical examination. Assess for "red flags" (Table 1) and, based on history, physical and laboratory findings, classify according to WAD (Whiplash-Associated Disorders) criteria (Table 2, Figure 1).
- Decision to x-ray is based on history of severe trauma, impaired consciousness and neurological signs and symptoms. However, neurological findings may not be present or prominent with cervical fracture, so clinical judgment/experience and imaging are necessary when fracture is suspected.[1]

Table 1: **Possible Red Flags Associated with Neck Pain[1]**

History of severe trauma	Sensory or motor deficits
Impaired consciousness	Lower body sensory changes
Loss of reflexes	Loss of bowel or bladder function

Table 2: **WAD Classification**[1]

WAD-I: neck pain, stiffness or tenderness, but no physical signs/limitations
WAD-II: pain and tenderness and reduced range
WAD-III: pain and neurological signs; sensory or motor or reflex changes without fracture/instability
WAD-IV: fracture or dislocation

Therapeutic Choices

Nonpharmacologic Choices

WAD-I to WAD-III: Provide symptomatic relief as indicated, reassure, and counsel to resume normal activity as soon as possible. Avoid immobilization or passive therapy. WAD-IV: Urgent referral and surgical management.[1]

There is considerable agreement among opinion leaders that initial management is most effective if patients are counselled to maintain activity or return to activity as soon as tolerated, avoiding collars, bedrest or immobilization and limiting or avoiding work absence. This results in improved range of motion in the short term and favourable symptomatic improvement in the longer term.[1,2]

If progress is not occurring as expected within the first month or by the end of the first month, consider the possibility of psychosocial barriers or complications. Active exercise combined with psychosocial intervention results in reduced pain in the short term and accelerates return to work.[1,2]

Pharmacologic Choices (Chapter 75, Table 3)

A short course of an analgesic or **NSAID** combined with other interventions is effective for back pain (and presumably also for neck pain).[1] In the first month, NSAIDs are more effective for symptom relief than placebo, but there is no evidence that any one NSAID is more effective for reducing pain.[3] However, given the risks associated with use of NSAIDs, **acetaminophen** and/or an **opioid** are appropriate alternatives in the acute phase although available literature is inadequate.

There is an absence of adequate evidence regarding efficacy of muscle relaxants in neck pain. In acute low back pain, all types of muscle relaxants are more effective than placebo but adverse effects are also more common.[4]

During Second and Third Month (Subacute Period)

Order plain radiographs for neck pain lasting more than a few weeks, or if there is nerve root or spinal cord involvement or history of such injury.[5] For those not making progress in function, or suffering unexpected prolongation of pain, review to identify potential psychological risk factors (Table 3).

By this time, combined therapy is preferable: psychosocial, patient education and active exercise. Promote work re-entry if there has been delay.

Table 3: **Identification of Psychological Risk Factors**[6,7]

Obvious psychological distress
Severe pain beyond what is expected
History of prior significant pain recurrences
Higher than expected functional impairment
Unexplained widespread pain
Pain and limitation not consistent with objective findings

There is a lack of quality evidence for the efficacy of passive and palliative physical therapy modalities or medications for symptom relief, but they may be used in conjunction with active measures if they appear to promote patient comfort and adherence to the active treatments.[2]

The role of manual therapies, e.g., manipulation or mobilization of the spine, is still controversial, partly due to a very small but real risk of catastrophic complications with manipulation and partly due to lack of evidence that manual therapy alone is adequate treatment for neck problems.[1,8] Manipulation should be performed only by an expert therapist with certified skills in manual therapy and with appropriate clinical screening to exclude patients with risk factors for complications. There is limited evidence that exercise combined with manual therapy is efficacious.[8,9]

By Three Months

If functional improvement and return to work/activity has not happened by this point, there is an increasing risk of chronic pain and poor function. Identify psychosocial and related risk factors that may impair progress. If work return (with or without modifications) is not successful, refer to multidisciplinary rehabilitation, in liaison with stakeholders, with the goal of return to work and function.

By Six Months or More (Chronic Neck Pain)

Therapeutic Choices

With time there is increasing probability of associated psychological comorbidity.[6] Assess and treat comorbid depression, anxiety or adjustment problems. If necessary, refer to an appropriate specialist.

Nonpharmacologic Choices

For chronic musculoskeletal pain in general, there is limited evidence that intensive multimodal/multidisciplinary treatment programs (cognitive-behavioural therapy with active exercise and psychosocial intervention, work hardening and planning for work re-entry) are effective for improving function and sense of well-being.[10,11] This will be more effective if the program involves other stakeholders and the workplace.[10] For chronic neck and shoulder pain in particular, there is insufficient evidence to judge the efficacy of multidisciplinary biopsychosocial therapy.[12]

In the chronic stage, individual supervised active exercises (but not group exercise classes) can improve pain and function.[13]

There is limited evidence for the efficacy of radiofrequency denervation of the dorsal root ganglion for cervicobrachial pain and of the primary dorsal rami for cervical zygapophyseal pain.[14]

Pharmacologic Choices

There is limited evidence for the efficacy of **NSAIDs** or **opioids** for chronic pain,[3,11] but there is increasing clinical acceptance of the use of the latter.[11]

Although amitriptyline is widely used for soft tissue pain, **tricyclic antidepressants** have not been proven effective for mixed musculoskeletal and soft tissue pain relief.[11] They may nevertheless be helpful for neuralgias, headache, insomnia and comorbid depression, and use should be governed by patient clinical response, absence of contraindications and tolerability.

Several poor-quality studies suggest that local infiltration of anesthetic to trigger/tender points may be beneficial.[11,15] Support is lacking for the use of injection therapy alone for management of persistent neck pain/whiplash, and rehabilitation is recommended in addition to pain relief methods.

Therapeutic Tips

- The strongest predictors of chronicity in neck pain problems include self-reported, severe pain levels and a history of previous occurrences of whiplash/neck pain.

Figure 1: **Early Management of Whiplash Disorder**

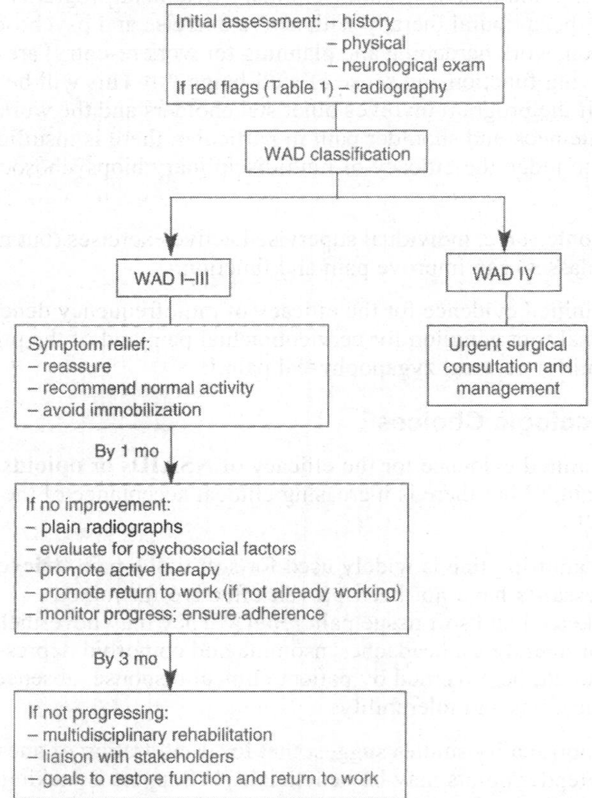

Abbreviations: WAD = whiplash-associated disorders.

Suggested Readings

Binder A. Clinical Evidence Concise: Neck pain. *Am Fam Physician* 2005;71(1). Available from: http://www.aafp.org/afp/20050101/bmjx.html Accessed March 2, 2006.

College of Physicians and Surgeons of Ontario. *Evidence-based recommendations for medical management of chronic non-malignant pain: reference guide for clinicians*. Toronto (ON): CPSO; 2000. Available from: http://www.cpso.on.ca/publications/pain.PDF Accessed March 1, 2006.

Devereaux MW. Neck pain. *Prim Care* 2004;31(1):19-31.

References

1. Spitzer WO, Skovron ML, Salmi LR et al. Scientific monograph of the Quebec Task Force on Whiplash-Associated Disorders: redefining "whiplash" and its management. *Spine* 1995;20(8 Suppl):1S-73S.
2. Verhagen AP, Scholten-Peeters GG, de Bie RA et al. Conservative treatments for whiplash. *Cochrane Database Syst Rev* 2004;(1):CD003338.
3. van Tulder MW, Scholten RJ, Koes BW et al. Non-steroidal anti-inflammatory drugs for low back pain. *Cochrane Database Syst Rev* 2000;(2):CD000396.
4. van Tulder MW, Touray T, Furlan AD et al. Muscle relaxants for non-specific low-back pain. *Cochrane Database Syst Rev* 2003;(2):CD004252.
5. Tsang I. Rheumatology: 12. Pain in the neck. *CMAJ* 2001;164(8):1182-7.
6. Tunks E et al. Natural history and efficacy of treatment of chronic pain arising from musculoskeletal injury. In: Sullivan T, editor. *Injury and the new world of work.* Vancouver (BC): UBC Press; 2000.
7. Borghouts JA, Koes BW, Bouter LM. The clinical course and prognostic factors of non-specific neck pain: a systematic review. *Pain* 1998;77(1):1-13.
8. Gross AR, Hoving JL, Haines TA et al. Manipulation and mobilisation for mechanical neck disorders. *Cochrane Database Syst Rev* 2004;(1):CD004249.
9. Kay TM, Gross A, Goldsmith C et al. Exercises for mechanical neck disorders. *Cochrane Database Syst Rev* 2005;(3):CD004250.
10. Loisel P, Abenhaim L, Durand P et al. A population-based, randomized clinical trial on back pain management. *Spine* 1997;22(24):2911-8.
11. College of Physicians and Surgeons of Ontario. *Evidence-based recommendations for medical management of chronic non-malignant pain: reference guide for clinicians.* Toronto (ON): CPSO; 2000. Available from: http://www.cpso.on.ca/publications/pain.PDF Accessed March 1, 2006.
12. Karjalainen K, Malmivaara A, van Tulder M et al. Multidisciplinary biopsychosocial rehabilitation for neck and shoulder pain among working age adults. *Cochrane Database Syst Rev* 2003;(2):CD002194.
13. Philadelphia Panel. Philadelphia Panel evidence-based clinical practice guidelines on selected rehabilitation interventions for neck pain. *Phys Ther* 2001;81(10):1701-17.
14. Niemisto L, Kalso E, Malmivaara A et al. Radiofrequency denervation for neck and back pain. A systematic review of randomized controlled trials. *Cochrane Database Syst Rev* 2003;(1):CD004058.
15. Nelemans PJ, de Bie RA, de Vet HC et al. Injection therapy for subacute and chronic benign low back pain. *Cochrane Database Syst Rev* 2000;(2):CD001824.

CHAPTER 75
Low Back Pain

Eldon Tunks, MD, FRCPC

This chapter summarizes the nonsurgical management of low back pain (LBP).

Goals of Therapy

Acute LBP

- Promote rapid recovery and reduce distress

Subacute/recurrent LBP

- Assess appropriately and prevent chronicity
- Prevent or minimize work absence

Chronic LBP

- Promote or restore healthy behaviour, fitness and appropriate role functions by defining and treating medical and psychological factors associated with persistent/recurrent pain, according to evidence-based principles

Acute LBP (0–30 days) (Figure 1)

Investigations

Clinical history, relevant physical examination and neurological assessment. Identify "red flags" (Table 1).[1,2] When red flags are present, further investigation and/or referral for consultation are indicated. Arrange diagnostic imaging and laboratory tests consistent with bedside examination findings.

Therapeutic Choices

Nonpharmacologic Choices

0 to 30 days: Promoting earlier recovery

For acute or recurrent back pain of less than three weeks, provide symptomatic relief, encourage the patient to continue or resume activity and work as soon as tolerated and educate the patient to expect early recovery. Avoid unnecessary bedrest for uncomplicated back pain as well as premature physical therapy. This approach results in the shortest duration of sick leave and pain.[1,2,3,4,5,6]

Acute back pain with sciatica: physiotherapy offers slightly better functional status at four weeks' follow-up compared to bedrest, with no difference in outcomes for pain. There is no advantage to bedrest in acute back pain with sciatica.[3]

Pharmacologic Choices (Table 3)

For acute uncomplicated low back pain, **NSAIDs** are effective for pain relief, particularly during the first few weeks, but there is no evidence that one NSAID is more effective than another.[7] When selecting an NSAID, consider tolerability and cost.

There is conflicting evidence that NSAIDs are more effective than acetaminophen for back pain.[7] Given the greater safety profile compared to NSAIDs, a trial of **acetaminophen with codeine** is a reasonable option in acute uncomplicated back pain.

During the acute phase of low back pain, **muscle relaxants** (benzodiazepines, nonbenzodiazepines such as cyclobenzaprine, or antispasticity drugs) may be effective for short-term use,[2] but consider potential adverse effects such as drowsiness and dizziness.[8]

Strong **opioids** such as morphine may be indicated in more severe acute pain, especially if NSAIDs or acetaminophen provide insufficient relief, or in the presence of NSAID intolerance or contraindications.

Table 1: **"Red Flag" Symptoms/Signs in Assessment of Low Back Pain[1]**

Herniated Nucleus Pulposus	Cancer	Spinal Osteomyelitis	Compression Fracture	Cauda Equina Syndrome
Positive SLR (leg pain at < 60°) Weak dorsiflexion of ankle (L4-5), or great toe (L5-S1 or L4-5) Reduced ankle reflex (L5-S1) Reduced light touch in L4, L5 or S1 dermatomes of foot/leg	Age > 50 Nighttime pain, or bedrest does not relieve pain Failure to improve after > 1 mo therapy Previous cancer history Unexplained weight loss	Intravenous drug abuse Sources of infection (e.g., skin, teeth, urinary tract, or indwelling catheter) Fever Vertebral tenderness	Age > 70 Osteoporosis Corticosteroid use History of a fall/trauma, especially if osteoporotic or with history of bone disease	Acute urinary retention or overflow incontinence Loss of anal sphincter tone/fecal incontinence Perineal numbness Change in sexual function Weakness of legs
Investigation: MRI of lumbar spine	Investigation: positive laboratory tests and imaging	Investigation: positive laboratory tests and imaging	Investigation: positive laboratory tests including plain x-rays	Investigation: emergency laboratory assessment and imaging

Abbreviations: MRI = magnetic resonance imaging; SLR = straight leg raising

Subacute LBP (4 to 12 weeks) and recurrent LBP (up to 6 months) (Figure 2)

Investigations

When there is persistent or recurrent pain and interference with vocational function, re-evaluate the patient.[1,2] When red flags are present (Table 1), imaging and consultation are recommended. After the first four to six weeks, in addition to imaging, electromyogram may be helpful if there are clinical findings suggestive of nerve root involvement.

One of the strongest predictors of satisfactory adjustment is vocational status, and delay in work return significantly reduces the likelihood of ever returning.

Table 2: **Factors Adversely Affecting Prognosis of LBP**

Psychosocial Factors	Mental Status Indicators of Significant Anxiety or Depression
Duration of work absence	Insomnia or nightmares
High levels of self-reported functional disability	Irritability
Self-report of extreme pain and constant pain in multiple body areas	Withdrawal
History of prolonged sick-listing after previous injuries	Panic episodes or anxiety during the day or night
Prior history of absenteeism	Persistent tearfulness
Delays/obstacles in work re-entry process	Poor concentration
Patients who believe that they will never return to work	Inability to enjoy (anhedonia)
Adversarial attitude toward employer	Poor appetite/weight loss
Longstanding history of psychiatric distress or maladjustment	Poor libido
	Thoughts that "life is not worth living"

For recurrent back pain or persistent back pain of three to six months, reassessment is advised. This should include screening for psychosocial complications (Table 2).[2,6,9] Although compensation or litigation alone has an indefinite effect on prognosis, where compensation levels are high or when the employee is in conflict, compensation and litigation may significantly impair prognosis.[9]

Therapeutic Choices

Nonpharmacologic Choices

If the pain and sick-listing are not resolved *after the first month*, early active treatment aimed at return to productive function has the greatest efficacy with regard to resolving pain, restoring functional ability and successful work return.[10] Setting a treatment timeline and projected date for return to work is essential for management. Workplace-based interventions that avoid the patient having to cease work for treatment have the greatest efficacy.[4,5,6,11]

Patient education at this stage should stress that low back pain usually has a favourable outcome if it is managed by active exercise and timely return to function and occupation, rather than expecting the pain to completely resolve first. Screen for and treat psychosocial factors or refer when necessary.[6,9,12]

There are many potential modalities of symptomatic physical therapy, e.g., ice, heat, laser, ultrasound, massage, manipulation, acupuncture, transcutaneous electrical nerve stimulation (TENS). Evidence for efficacy of any individual modality is presently inadequate, with the exception that active exercise and avoidance of unnecessary bedrest improves outcomes.[3,4,11,13]

At approximately three to six months, the focus is on interrupting progress toward chronic pain (Figure 2). If there is marked functional disability associated with pain that is recurrent or persisting for three months or more, establish a coordinated program between the primary care provider, patient, employer and compensation agency. If the coordinated program is unsuccessful, consider timely referral to a multidisciplinary chronic pain management clinic for intensive treatment.[1,2,9]

Pharmacologic Choices (Table 3)

Acetaminophen with codeine, or opioid analgesics, are effective in some cases of chronic pain in general. Evidence of efficacy is limited, but strong enough to recommend a trial.[12]

There is insufficient evidence to recommend for or against muscle relaxants, NSAIDs or antidepressants for relief of subacute back pain.

Chronic LBP (persistent pain after 6 months or more) (Figure 2)

Investigations

Be aware of co-existing psychological and social complications which at this time are the strongest obstacles to improvement or recovery (Table 2).

Therapeutic Choices

Nonpharmacologic Choices

"Back school" or patient education alone tends to be ineffective at this point unless there is an active exercise and/or functional restoration focus tied closely with the workplace for work re-entry.[1,11] Patients must be engaged in goal-setting and monitoring progress.[6,9] Cognitive-behavioural therapy or relaxation therapy are effective for pain and for behavioural outcomes in chronic low back pain,[14] but efficacy for work return is associated with conducting therapy in the context of a planned work re-entry.[11] The focus should include multidisciplinary rehabilitation, cognitive-behaviour therapy, active exercise, functional restoration, patient education and vocational counselling toward work re-entry, and may also include psychosocial intervention and training in coping skills.[1,2,9,12,15,16]

There is a lack of evidence whether patients who have failed treatment in a multidisciplinary rehabilitation program (or chronic pain management program) will benefit from a second attempt. After treatment failure, barriers that interfered with progress must be identified and addressed. These might include, for example, an Axis I disorder (especially major depression, anxiety disorder or dysthymia), an attitude problem such as unwillingness to set goals for change, a substance or medication abuse problem, a previously undetected medical/surgical problem, or obstacles to work re-entry or lack of cooperation within the job environment.

Pharmacologic Choices (Table 3)

Some patients with persistent low back pain respond to **opioid analgesics**. If opioids are to be used in more than small doses and for a longer period of time, sustained-release preparations are preferable. Consider opioid analgesics when pain is a significant barrier to function, an unremitting source of distress and if there are otherwise no significant psychological or medical contraindications. If in doubt, obtain a consultation.[12]

Injection therapies for chronic low back pain have not had statistically significant efficacy; however, there is a tendency toward positive results with only minor side effects. This applies to facet joint, epidural and local injection therapy. At the moment there is no justification for abandoning injection therapy in patients with low back pain, provided it is well tolerated and accompanied by patient improvement. Also, consider the duration of improvement.[17]

Therapeutic Tips

- A significant minority of chronic pain sufferers have comorbid depression, anxiety or dysthymia (chronic depression/anxiety), often masked by the pain presentation. Key symptoms (Table 2) can reveal the underlying mood disorder. Comorbid mood disorders often respond to antidepressants, which can improve coping with pain.
- For back pain and chronic soft tissue pain, **tricyclic** or other types of **antidepressants** have equivocal efficacy, but may be useful for their antidepressant effect.[9]

Figure 1: **Management of Acute Low Back Pain**

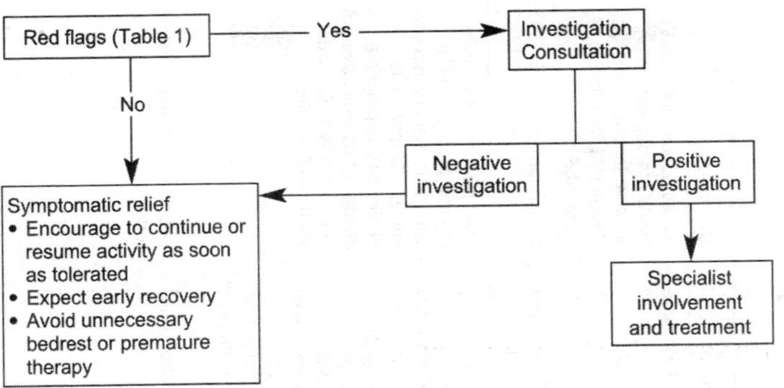

Figure 2: **Management of Persistent Low Back Pain**

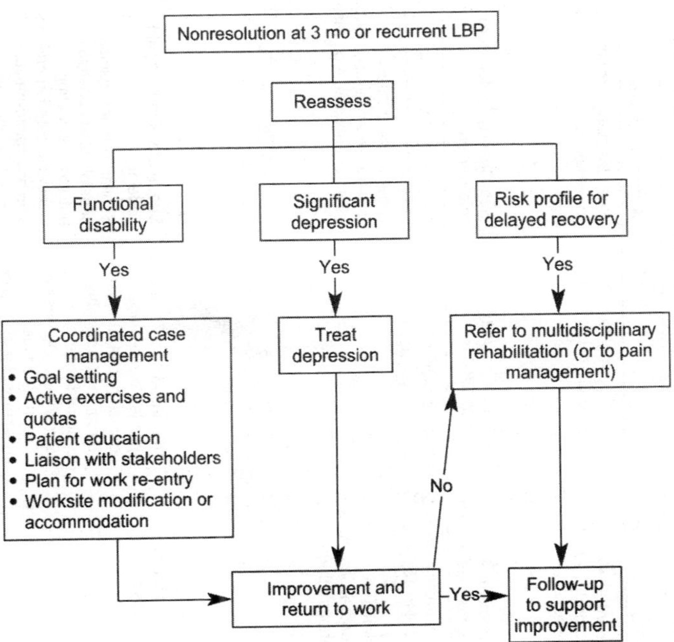

Reprinted from *Rheum Dis Clin North Am*, 22(3), Pain Clinics, 599-611, 1996, with permission from Elsevier.

Table 3: **Drugs Used in the Treatment of Back and Neck Pain**

Class	Drug	Dosage	Adverse Effects	Drug Interactions	Comments	Cost[a]
NSAIDs[b]	*ibuprofen* Motrin IB, Advil, generics	600–1200 mg/day po divided Q6-8H.	See Chapter 71 for more information.	See Chapter 71 for more information.	No evidence that one NSAID is superior to another for back pain. See Chapter 71 for a listing of other NSAIDs.	$
	naproxen Naprosyn, generics	500–1000 mg/day po divided Q8-12H.	See Chapter 71 for more information.	See Chapter 71 for more information.	See ibuprofen.	$-$$
Opioids	*acetaminophen with codeine 15, 30 or 60 mg* Tylenol with codeine preparations, Atasol, various others	1–2 tabs QID max: 8 tabs/day.	Nausea and vomiting, constipation, sedation or drowsiness, confusion, urinary retention, dry mouth, allergic reactions, e.g., rash.	CNS depressants including sedatives, tranquilizers, alcohol may increase CNS depression. Avoid use with MAO inhibitors because of enhanced CNS depressant effects. Avoid use of opioid antagonists. Be cautious of drugs that may precipitate withdrawal reactions.	Start low. Titrate dosage against pain gradually enough to manage adverse effects. Upper limits of clinically appropriate dosage of opioids have not been identified. Consider addition of laxative.	$
	fentanyl patch Duragesic	After initiating with oral opioids, to morphine equivalence of at least 40 mg/day (preferably to equivalence of 60 mg/day). Duragesic 25 µg/hr can be substituted for oral opioid.	See acetaminophen with codeine. Similar to other opioids, possibly less constipation but more sweating. Contraindicated in patients who are opioid-naïve.	See acetaminophen with codeine.	See acetaminophen with codeine.	$$$$$

Class	Drug	Dosage	Adverse Effects	Drug Interactions	Comments	Cost[a]
	hydromorphone sustained-release Hydromorph Contin	Initial: 3 mg Q12H po for sustained-release products.	See acetaminophen with codeine.	See acetaminophen with codeine.	See acetaminophen with codeine.	$$
	morphine sustained-release M-Eslon, MS Contin, generics	Initial: 15 mg Q12H po for sustained-release products.	See acetaminophen with codeine.	See acetaminophen with codeine.	See acetaminophen with codeine. MS Contin has been tested in randomized controlled trials for back pain.	$$
	oxycodone sustained-release OxyContin	Initial: 10 mg Q12H po for sustained-release products.	See acetaminophen with codeine.	See acetaminophen with codeine.	See acetaminophen with codeine.	$$$
Muscle Relaxants	*cyclobenzaprine* generics	5–10 mg po TID.	Drowsiness, dry mouth, dizziness, fatigue, nausea, constipation.	See amitriptyline. Combination with opiates or other CNS depressants may ↑ risk of CNS depression.	Can be given as one pm dose.	$-$$
	methocarbamol Robaxin	1 g po QID.	See cyclobenzaprine.	Combination with opiates or other CNS depressants may ↑ risk of CNS depression.		$$
	orphenadrine Norflex, generics	100–200 mg/day po divided BID.	See cyclobenzaprine.	Use with propoxyphene may ↑ CNS effects.	Can be given as one pm dose.	$-$$
Benzodi-azepines	*diazepam* generics	2–5 mg BID to QID po for acute pain.	Drowsiness, cognitive impairment, drug dependence, falls, accumulation in the elderly and in presence of pulmonary, liver or kidney disease.	Potentiation of cognitive impairment when used with opioids. Potentiation of alcohol intoxication.	In acute pain, short-term use as muscle relaxant. Not recommended in the elderly.	$

(cont'd)

Table 3: **Drugs Used in the Treatment of Back and Neck Pain** *(cont'd)*

Class	Drug	Dosage	Adverse Effects	Drug Interactions	Comments	Cost[a]
Tricyclic Antidepressants	*amitriptyline* generics	Initial: 10–25 mg QHS, increase by 10–25 mg QHS weekly until effect.	Anticholinergic (dry mouth, blurred vision, constipation, urinary hesitancy, tachycardia, delirium), antihistaminergic (sedation, weight gain), orthostatic hypotension, lowered seizure threshold; sexual dysfunction.	Do not use with MAOIs; SSRIs ↑ serum levels of TCAs; carbamazepine and rifampin may ↓ effect; cimetidine and antipsychotics may ↑ effect and toxicity; possible interaction with antiarrhythmics (may lead to ↑ effect of either drug); may ↓ antihypertensive effect of clonidine; may augment hypotensive effect of thiazides.	May be helpful for comorbid chronic headache or neuralgia or for depression/anxiety, but inadequate evidence for use in fibromyalgia or musculoskeletal and soft tissue pain.	$
	desipramine Norpramin, generics	Initial: 10 mg QAM or QHS, increase to 25–75 mg/day.	See amitriptyline.	See amitriptyline.	See amitriptyline.	$

[a] Cost of 30-day supply, includes drug cost only
[b] Listed drugs are examples of medications in this class.
Dosage adjustment may be required in renal impairment; see Appendix I
Legend: $ <$20 $-$$ <$20–40 $$ $20–40 $$$ $40–60 $$$$ $60-80 $$$$$ > $80

Suggested Readings

College of Physicians and Surgeons of Ontario. *Evidence-based recommendations for medical management of chronic non-malignant pain: reference guide for clinicians*. Toronto (ON): CPSO; 2000. Available from: http://www.cpso.on.ca/publications/pain.PDF Accessed March 1, 2006.

Harwood MI, Smith BJ. Low back pain: a primary care approach. *Clinics in Family Practice* 2005;7(2):279-303.

References

1. Bigos S et al. *Acute low back problems in adults. Clinical Practice Guideline No. 14.* AHCPR Publication No. 95-0642. Rockville (MD): Agency for Health Care Policy and Research, Public Health Service, U.S. Department of Health and Human Services; December 1994.
2. Scientific approach to the assessment and management of activity-related spinal disorders. A monograph for clinicians. Report of the Quebec Task Force on Spinal Disorders. *Spine* 1987;12(7 Suppl):S1-59.
3. Hagen KB, Hilde G, Jamtvedt G, Winnem M. Bed rest for acute low-back pain and sciatica. *Cochrane Database Syst Rev* 2004;(4):CD001254.
4. Philadelphia Panel. Philadelphia Panel evidence-based clinical practice guidelines on selected rehabilitation interventions for low back pain. *Phys Ther* 2001;81(10):1641-74.
5. NHS Centre for Reviews and Dissemination, University of York. Acute and chronic low back pain. *Eff Health Care* 2000;6(5):1-8. Available from: http://www.york.ac.uk/inst/crd/ehc65.pdf Accessed March 1, 2006.
6. Carter JT, Birrell LN, editors. *Occupational health guidelines for the management of low back pain at work: principal recommendations.* London (UK): Faculty of Occupational Medicine of the Royal College of Physicians; 2000.
7. van Tulder MW, Scholten RJ, Koes BW, Deyo RA. Non-steroidal anti-inflammatory drugs for low back pain. *Cochrane Database Syst Rev* 2000;(2):CD000396.
8. van Tulder MW, Touray T, Furlan AD, Solway S, Bouter LM. Muscle relaxants for non-specific low back pain. *Cochrane Database Syst Rev* 2003;(2):CD004252.
9. Tunks E et al. Natural history and efficacy of treatment of chronic pain arising from musculoskeletal injury. In: Sullivan T, editor. *Injury and the New World of Work.* Vancouver (BC): UBC Press; 2000.
10. Karjalainen K, Malmivaara A, van Tulder M et al. Multidisciplinary biopsychosocial rehabilitation for subacute low back pain among working age adults. *Cochrane Database Syst Rev* 2003;(2):CD002193.
11. Loisel P, Abenhaim L, Durand P et al. A population-based, randomized clinical trial on back pain management. *Spine* 1997;22(24):2911-8.
12. College of Physicians and Surgeons of Ontario. *Evidence-based recommendations for medical management of chronic non-malignant pain: reference guide for clinicians.* Toronto (ON): CPSO; 2000. Available from: http://www.cpso.on.ca/publications/pain.PDF Accessed March 1, 2006.
13. Assendelft WJ, Morton SC, Yu EI et al. Spinal manipulative therapy for low back pain. *Cochrane Database Syst Rev* 2004;(1):CD000447.
14. Ostelo RW, van Tulder MW, Vlaeyen JW et al. Behavioural treatment for chronic low-back pain. *Cochrane Database Syst Rev* 2005;(1):CD002014.
15. Schonstein E, Kenny DT, Keating J, Koes BW. Work conditioning, work hardening and functional restoration for workers with back and neck pain. *Cochrane Database Syst Rev* 2003;(1):CD001822.
16. Guzman J, Esmail R, Karjalainen K et al. Multidisciplinary bio-psycho-social rehabilitation for chronic low back pain. *Cochrane Database Syst Rev* 2002;(1):CD000963.
17. Nelemans PJ, de Bie RA, de Vet HC, Sturmans F. Injection therapy for subacute and chronic benign low back pain. *Cochrane Database Syst Rev* 2000;(2):CD001824.

CHAPTER 76
Sports Injuries

James Kissick, MD, CCFP, Dip Sport Med

The majority of sports injuries encountered by physicians involve the soft tissues: strains, sprains and contusions.

Goals of Therapy

- To reduce acute symptoms (pain, inflammation) and recurrences
- To correct contributing factors, e.g., malalignment, muscle weakness
- To return the athlete's weight-bearing capability, flexibility, range of motion, strength and proprioception to normal
- To enable the athlete to participate comfortably, safely and fully in all pre-injury activities

Therapeutic Choices

For management of specific injuries, see Table 1.

Nonpharmacologic Choices

Acute treatment is best summarized by the RICE protocol:

- **R**est the injured part.
- **I**ce: Wrap an ice bag, cold pack or package of frozen peas in a damp, thin cloth and apply to the injured area for 15 to 20 minutes at a time, at least QID for the first 48 hours (or longer if swelling continues).
- **C**ompress with an elastic bandage if there is swelling such as in an ankle sprain.
- **E**levation: Try to elevate the injured part above the heart.

Initial rehabilitation is directed toward allowing the injured tissues to heal. Aggravation of the injury must be avoided, but alternative activities should be encouraged (e.g., the runner with a stress fracture of the fibula should not run but can swim or run in deep water). The next phase is directed toward restoring and improving range of motion, strength, endurance and proprioception. A progression toward full activity is then undertaken. Before the patient resumes activity, any factors that may have contributed to the injury (improper shoes, poor protective equipment) should be corrected, and sport-specific skills regained.

Pharmacologic Choices

NSAIDs or **ASA** (if not contraindicated) can decrease swelling and discomfort but should be used for short periods only.

Table 1: **Management of Specific Sports Injuries**

Injury	Investigations	Therapeutic Choices
Rotator Cuff Disorders Degenerative tears (tendonosis), acute tears (partial or full thickness), less commonly overuse inflammation (tendonitis) of the rotator cuff muscles of the shoulder. These muscles act as movers (rotation, initial abduction) and stabilizers of the humeral head in the glenoid. Often results in subacromial impingement of supraspinatus (cuff muscle) and subacromial bursa.	**History:** Sudden pain if traumatic onset (e.g., fall), gradual onset of pain if tendonosis. Pain noted with shoulder movement (can vary with location of injury), especially over-shoulder level. Often sore at night, hard to find comfortable sleep position. Weakness if complete or significant partial tear. **Physical Exam:** Wasting may be noted posteriorly over scapula if full thickness tear, disuse. Pain on active, passive, and resisted tests depending on injury type and location. Weakness if more significant tear. If subacromial impingement, often get "painful arc" in flexion or abduction, pain with Hawkins' test (pain when shoulder placed at 90° of flexion and internally rotated) and Neer's test (pain with pronated arm brought into full overhead elevation). If significant supraspinatus tear, get positive "drop arm" test (unable to hold arm in flexion or abduction above 90°). Test for instability. **Imaging:** X-ray if concern re: bony injury (acute trauma), or osteoarthritis. Ultrasound good at detecting rotator cuff tears. MRI good at detecting cuff tears, other shoulder pathology (usually need MRI arthrogram if concern re: labral tear).	Rest from aggravating activities. Ice may help if acute injury. Nonsteroidal anti-inflammatory medication for acute pain. May need analgesic medication for nighttime. Physiotherapy: strengthening of scapular stabilizers, correction of impaired scapulohumeral rhythm, addressing soft tissue tightness followed by rotator cuff strengthening. Persistent impingement symptoms and signs often benefit from subacromial corticosteroid injection (e.g., triamcinolone acetonide 40 mg mixed with 3–4 mL lidocaine 1%) followed by resumption of exercise program. Surgery if full thickness tear in younger, active person (repair cuff); also if persistent pain and/or impingement despite above measures: debridement, acromioplasty; limited repair; repair.

(cont'd)

Table 1: **Management of Specific Sports Injuries** *(cont'd)*

Injury	Investigations	Therapeutic Choices
Lateral Epicondylitis ("Tennis Elbow") **Medial Epicondylitis ("Golfer's Elbow")** Lateral epicondylitis: Tendonosis of the common extensor tendon at its origin at the lateral epicondyle of the humerus. Medial epicondylitis: Tendonosis of the common flexor/pronator tendon at its origin at the medial epicondyle.	**History** of pain at the lateral elbow or medial elbow usually due to overuse and/or faulty mechanics. **Physical examination:** tenderness just distal to the lateral or medial epicondyle, painful resisted wrist extension (lateral elbow), wrist flexion (medial elbow). **X-ray** rarely required (only if any concern about bony pathology).	Rest from aggravating activities. Tennis elbow "counter-force" brace. Ice, ice massage with "ice cup." Physiotherapy:[1] acupuncture, mobilizations, soft tissue techniques, stretching. Strengthening exercises as improvement occurs. **Correction of predisposing factors:** in tennis—correct poor strokes, especially backhand (leading with the elbow), correct grip size, string tension to maximum 50–55 lbs, lighter racquet, avoid heavy duty or wet balls. Suggest consultation with teaching professional. Work activities important (e.g., ergonomic factors). Gradual return to activity. If above is unsuccessful, consider corticosteroid injection (e.g., triamcinolone acetonide 20 mg) to common extensor origin area at lateral epicondyle or common flexor origin at medial epicondyle. Maximum 3 injections, at least 1 mo apart. If still unsuccessful, consider surgery.

Injury	Investigations	Therapeutic Choices
Patellofemoral Syndrome Anterior knee pain resulting from patellofemoral articulation dysfunction (also known as patellofemoral pain syndrome or anterior knee pain syndrome).	**History** of anterior knee pain, worse with prolonged flexion, running, stairs (down). **Physical examination:** malalignment, pain with patellar pressure, painful quads setting, poor flexibility, medial quadricep weakness, lateral patellar tracking, pain with squat, stairs. **X-rays** (including skyline view of patella) if trauma or bony pathology is a concern.	**Relief of acute symptoms:** Rest from aggravating activities (emphasize alternative activities); ice, both PRN and postactivity; physiotherapy, NSAIDs, taping. **Correction of contributing factors:** *Foot overpronation*: appropriate shoes with straight to slightly curved last, good medial arch and support. If severe, may require custom foot orthotic. *Muscle factors*: VMO (vastus medialis obliquus) strengthening (e.g., closed kinetic chain exercises such as quarter squats, step ups and downs). Hip abductor and external rotator strengthening. Electrical muscle stimulation and/or biofeedback can assist. *Improve flexibility*: quadriceps, hamstrings, gastrocnemius, ilio-tibial band stretches may help (no firm evidence). *Taping techniques*:[2] to correct patellar malposition. *Correction of training errors*: in runners, more gradual distance increases, fewer hills. Decrease jumping, squats; avoid resisted leg extensions to ≥ 90° flexion. *Patellar stabilizing brace*: with supporting buttress and/or straps. Use with activities or more regularly if subluxation. *Surgery*: e.g., lateral release of tight retinacula, patellar tendon transfer is rarely required and should be a last resort.

(cont'd)

Table 1: **Management of Specific Sports Injuries** *(cont'd)*

Injury	Investigations	Therapeutic Choices
Lower Leg Pain **"Shin Splints"** (Tibial periostitis, medial tibial stress syndrome) Inflammation of the tibialis posterior at its origin or of the tibial periosteum.	**History** of diffuse shin pain, usually in inexperienced and/or inadequately stretched or strengthened athletes. **Physical examination:** tenderness, usually diffuse, at medial border of tibia and adjacent muscle. If localized bony tenderness, rule out stress fracture. If normal exam at rest, rule out exertional compartment syndrome. **X-rays** normal; may need bone scan to differentiate from stress fracture.	Rest from aggravating activities (e.g., running). Alternative activities: cycling, swimming, pool running (running in deep water with flotation belt). Ice. Muscle stretching and strengthening. Correction of predisposing anatomic factors (e.g., with foot orthotics) and training errors. Gradual return to running or activity.
Stress fractures of the tibia/fibula Failure of bone due to repetitive overload, resulting in microfractures.	**History** of well-localized shin pain with pounding activities. **Physical examination:** localized bony tenderness. **X-rays** usually negative until at least 2 wk after onset; may see periosteal thickening. Bone scan will show discrete increased uptake at stress fracture site. Note: Beware of anterior midshaft tibial stress fractures ("the dreaded black line"). On x-ray, they appear as a horizontal fissure extending into the cortex of the tibia. These are slow to heal and often go on to nonunion.	No pounding activities until pain-free and nontender (usually 6–8 wk). Alternative activities: cycling, swimming, pool running. Flexibility and strength work. Long Air Cast-type brace often provides more comfort and possibly earlier return to pounding activities (if pain-free in Air Cast). Correction of anatomic factors, training errors. Gradual return to running when pain-free on walking and nontender. One example is: Wk 1: Run every other d, 1/2 usual distance, 1 min off usual mile pace Wk 2: Usual run frequency, 3/4 usual distance, 1 min off mile pace Wk 3: Usual frequency, 3/4 distance, 30 s off mile pace Wk 4: Usual frequency, full distance, 30 s off mile pace[3] Anterior midshaft tibial stress fractures should be assessed by orthopedic surgeon; may need immobilization.

Injury	Investigations	Therapeutic Choices
Ankle Sprain Partial or complete tear to ankle-stabilizing ligaments, most commonly lateral (anterior and posterior talofibular, calcaneofibular). **Grade I:** No laxity, bears weight without pain, minimal swelling **Grade II:** Swelling, painful weight bearing, possible slight laxity **Grade III:** Unstable, significant laxity, complete disruption of at least 2 ligaments	**History** of acute inversion (eversion less common). **Physical examination:** tenderness (most marked over injured ligament), swelling, pain with passive inversion and plantar flexion, positive drawer test in Grade III sprains. **X-rays**: clinical decision rules for the use of x-rays in acute ankle sprains are outlined in the Ottawa Ankle Rules.[4]	**Grade I & II Sprains** Initial RICE protocol. Gradual ↑ weight bearing; may use tape/brace as support. Begin as soon as pain and stability allow (facilitates healing and proprioception). Early range of motion exercises. Stretching in dorsiflexion and plantar flexion. Strengthening: dorsiflexors, plantar flexors, then invertors and evertors. Proprioceptive retraining Progressive ↑ activities: walk → jog → run → run backward → curves → zig-zags. **Grade III Sprains** Removable cast brace for 3–6 wk (allows icing, physiotherapy); then stirrup-type ankle brace. Once stable, follow protocol for Grade I and II sprains. Refer for orthopedic consultation if not improved after 6 weeks conservative therapy, recurrent pain or instability. Note: Don't forget to check for associated injury more proximally in the leg.

(cont'd)

Table 1: **Management of Specific Sports Injuries** *(cont'd)*

Injury	Investigations	Therapeutic Choices
Achilles Tendonitis Inflammation (tendonitis) or degenerative micro-tears (tendonosis) of Achilles tendon mainly occurring at insertion or distal part of tendon. In tendonitis, paratenon may also be inflamed.	**History:** Pain, often swelling, of distal Achilles tendon. May be acute—usually caused by rapid increase in training/activity (e.g., running, jumping), or chronic (usually in those over 30, usually tendonosis). Aggravated by running, jumping, walking. Sore first few steps in morning. Beware history of sudden acute pain (and occasionally feeling of "pop"), which may indicate tear of tendon. **Physical Exam:** Occasionally swelling distal Achilles. When chronic, may have nodule. Tender to squeeze over tendon. Pain with passive ankle dorsiflexion and resisted plantar flexion (especially in weight bearing). May have pes planus or cavus. Thompson test (squeeze of calf should produce ankle plantar flexion against gravity) normal. If test not normal (no plantar flexion), suspect complete tear. **Imaging:** If concern re: possible tear, or if swelling, ultrasound helpful.	Rest from aggravating activities (try bike as alternate). Ice. Heel lift (approx. 1/4"). Nonsteroidal anti-inflammatory medication if inflamed/swollen. Night splint (prevents plantar flexion of ankle while sleeping). Physiotherapy. Progressive strengthening exercises as improves (start with eccentric work first[5]). Stretching with improvement. Orthotics/arch supports if overpronates. Extracorporeal shock wave therapy (conflicting evidence).[6] Surgery rarely required for chronic tendonosis. If concern re: complete tear, immediate orthopedic referral.
Plantar fasciitis Microtears of the plantar fascia and inflammation of the periosteum at its calcaneal origin (heel bone).	**History** of pain at plantar aspect of calcaneus, worse upon arising in the morning, getting up after a prolonged sit, and with running or prolonged walking. **Physical examination:** Tender at plantar fascial origin at the heel; pes planus or cavus, overpronation with walking. **X-ray** not usually needed, may show "spur" as a result of more chronic fasciitis.	Rest from aggravating activities (e.g., bike instead of run). Limit overpronation, cushion heel. Footwear important; running shoe best. Should wear for all weight bearing. Arch supports, heel pads or cups may be necessary. Custom foot orthotics needed in some cases. Ice or ice massage. Roll foot on soup can before weight bearing in morning. Stretches: gastrocnemius, soleus, plantar fascia,[7] foot intrinsics. Night splint to prevent ankle plantar flexion while sleeping; decreases fascial shortening and morning pain.[8]

Injury	Investigations	Therapeutic Choices
		Corticosteroid injection if not improving with above (e.g., triamcinolone acetonide 20 mg mixed with 0.5 mL xylocaine 1% to tender area). Extracorporeal shock wave therapy (conflicting evidence).[9] Surgery rarely required.

Suggested Readings

Brukner P, Khan K. *Clinical sports medicine*. 3rd ed. New York (NY): McGraw-Hill ; 2007.

Crossley K, Bennell K, Green S et al. A systematic review of physical interventions for patellofemoral pain syndrome. *Clin J Sport Med* 2001;11(2):103-10.

Hershman EB, Mailly T. Stress fractures. *Clin Sports Med* 1990;9(1):183-214.

Kibler WB. Shoulder rehabilitation: principles and practice. *Med Sci Sports Exerc* 1998;30(4 Suppl):S40-50.

Press JM, Kibler WB, editors. *Functional rehabilitation of sports and musculoskeletal injuries*. Gaithersburg (MD): Aspen; 1998.

References

1. Bisset L, Beller E, Jull G et al. Mobilisation with movement and exercise, corticosteroid injection, or wait and see for tennis elbow: randomized trial. *BMJ* 2006;333(7575):939.
2. McConnell J. The management of chondromalacia patellae: a long term solution. *Aust J Physiother* 1986;32(4):215-23.
3. Mellion MB. *The team physician's handbook* . 3rd ed. Philadelphia (PA): Hanley & Belfus; 2002.
4. Stiell IG, Greenberg GH, McKnight RD et al. Decision rules for the use of radiography in acute ankle injuries. Refinement and prospective validation. *JAMA* 1993;269(9):1127-32.
5. Wallmann H. Achilles tendinitis: eccentric exercise prescription. *ACSM's Health & Fitness Journal* 2000;4(1):7-16.
6. Costa ML, Shepstone L, Donell ST et al. Shock wave therapy for chronic Achilles tendon pain: a randomized placebo-controlled trial. *Clin Orthop Relat Res* 2005;440:199-204.
7. DiGiovanni BF, Nawoczenski DA, Lintal ME et al. Tissue-specific plantar fascia-stretching exercise enhances outcomes in patients with chronic heel pain. A prospective, randomized study. *J Bone Joint Surg Am.* 2003;85-A(7):1270-7.
8. Batt ME, Tanji JL, Skattum N. Plantar fasciitis: a prospective randomized clinical trial of the tension night splint. *Clin J Sport Med* 1996;6(3):158-62.
9. Crawford F, Thomson C. Interventions for treating plantar heel pain. *Cochrane Database Syst Rev* 2003;(3):CD000416.

CHAPTER 77

Acne

Duane Lichtenwald, MD, FRCPC

Acne vulgaris is the most common skin disorder, typically starting at puberty, increasing in severity until the late teens then slowly abating. There is a great degree of variability in the age of onset, distribution, severity and age of resolution. It often results in disfigurement, scarring and/or emotional stress. Even mild acne can cause major and sometimes permanent psychological disturbance.[1] Fortunately acne can be safely and effectively treated.

Acne vulgaris is usually classified by the number, type and distribution of acne lesions. Comedones are sebaceous glands that have developed a keratin plug. If the plug is high in the duct, the keratin becomes oxidized, recognized as a blackhead or open comedone. When the blockage is deeper, a flesh-coloured papule or closed comedone develops. As these lesions become overgrown with bacteria, cytokines are released, which cause transformation into an inflammatory papule which may eventually develop a central pustule. If this inflammatory lesion ruptures below the dermis, an inflammatory cyst ensues. These are the lesions most likely to trigger scarring.

Goals of Therapy

- Clear existing lesions
- Prevent new lesions
- Minimize scarring

Investigations

- Usually not required
  - the diagnosis is a clinical one
- Culture and sensitivity of pustules
  - *Propionibacterium acnes*, a gram-positive anaerobe, is the prevalent organism
  - when patients are resistant to antibiotic therapy, perform cultures to identify gram-negative folliculitis and guide further therapy
- Hormonal investigations are indicated if there are other signs of hyperandrogenism such as:
  - hirsutism
  - infertility
  - infrequent menses
  - insulin-resistant diabetes
  - middle-age onset in women

Therapeutic Choices

Nonpharmacologic Choices

The management of acne is primarily pharmacologic. There are no controlled trials that support restriction of specific foods or food groups.[2] Acne is not the result of improper or lack of cleansing.[3] Modifying skin care regimens has a minimal preventative effect. Sunlight and other sources of ultraviolet light can help but are rarely recommended in view of the risks of photo damage and carcinogenic effects. Various lasers, intense pulsed light, microdermabrasion, chemical peels and photodynamic therapy are all helpful in certain situations but are expensive, rarely insured, often painful and must be administered on an ongoing basis. They are rarely required for effective acne management. Laser treatments have a greater role in acne scar therapy.

Pharmacologic Choices (Figure 1)

There are numerous pharmacologic agents that can have some positive effect on acne. The most useful agents are as follows:

Topical Agents (Table 1)

Benzoyl peroxide is antibacterial and mildly comedolytic. It has the ability to prevent or eliminate *P. acnes*.[4] It is a mild skin irritant and rare cause of allergy. Formulations can bleach clothing. Over-the-counter 5% gel is as effective as prescription 10% gel.[5]

Topical retinoids are the most powerful comedolytic agents yet still take months to be effective. **Tretinoin** is the most cost effective but also the most photosensitizing. **Adapalene** is the least irritating. **Tazarotene** is the most potent.[6]

Of the topical antibiotics, **clindamycin** and **erythromycin** are the most useful. Use in combination with benzoyl peroxide reduces the chance of bacterial resistance developing. They are mainly used in papulopustular acne to decrease skin colonization with *P. acnes*.

Glycolic acid (alpha hydroxy acid) is mildly comedolytic. It can be used when topical retinoids are not tolerated. At higher concentrations it is used for chemical peels which are a rapid but highly irritating method of clearing comedones.

Systemic Agents (Table 2)

The **tetracyclines**, **erythromycin** and **trimethoprim** alone or in combination with **sulfamethoxazole**, are the most useful systemic antibiotics. Bacterial resistance is an increasing problem and can be reduced by using oral antibiotics in combination with benzoyl peroxide gel. Limit duration of therapy when possible.[7]

Oral contraceptives with a progestational agent that has minimal androgenic effects are useful, especially in women with other signs of androgen excess (Table 2). **Cyproterone acetate** and **spironolactone** are anti-androgens with good efficacy in acne management. Cyproterone acetate with ethinyl estradiol taken cyclically appears to be associated with the same risk of thromboembolic events as other oral contraceptives.[8]

Isotretinoin is a systemic retinoid. It remains the most powerful anti-acne agent with reliable clearing and sustained remission of even the most severe cases. It is a well-documented and potent teratogen. Baseline and monthly pregnancy tests should be performed by women of childbearing age. As well, women should use two reliable methods of birth control or remain abstinent during therapy. Risk of adverse effects limits its use to severe or recalcitrant cases. Increased risk of depression and suicide secondary to isotretinoin remain unsubstantiated.[9,10] It is still prudent to warn patients that these remain potential side effects. In the case of acne relapse, eight weeks should pass before starting a second course of isotretinoin therapy.

Table 1: **Topical Acne Preparations**

Class	Drug	Dosage form/Dose
Peroxides	*benzoyl peroxide 2.5%–10%* Benzagel, Desquam-X , Proactive, Solugel, others	Cream, lotion, gel; concentrations ≤ 5% available without a prescription
Retinoids	*tretinoin 0.01%, 0.025%, 0.05%, 0.1%* Retin-A, Retin-A Micro, Stieva-A, Vitamin A Acid	Cream, gel; apply HS to limit photosensitivity
	tazarotene 0.05%, 0.1% Tazorac Cream, Tazorac Gel	Cream, gel; apply HS to limit photosensitivity
Retinoid Analogues	*adapalene 0.1%* Differin	Cream, gel; least irritating and photosensitizing
Antibiotics	*erythromycin 2%* Erysol	Gel; apply BID
	clindamycin 1% Dalacin T solution, Clindasol cream, Clindets (plegets)	Apply BID
Combination Products	*benzoyl peroxide 5%/erythromycin 3%* Benzamycin	Gel; apply BID
	benzoyl peroxide 5%/clindamycin 1% Clindoxyl, Benzaclin	Gel
	tretinoin 0.01%, 0.025% or 0.05%/ erythromycin 4% Stievamycin Mild, Regular, Forte	Gel; apply HS
Alpha-hydroxy Acids	*glycolic acid 2% – 15%* Reversa, Neostrata, others	Gel, lotion, cream; available without prescription

Therapeutic Tips

- Topical acne therapies should be applied to the affected zone to prevent new lesions rather than to the lesions alone.
- As many acne treatments are irritating, the skin care regimen should be gentle, avoiding astringents and abrasives.
- It can take several weeks for treatments to be effective. Each time an agent is added or changed, give adequate time to note effectiveness.
- Acne is a disease that usually lasts years. Once control has been achieved, the treatment regimen may be simplified but some suppressive therapy will be required. The exception to this is **isotretinoin**, which can produce prolonged remission.

Figure 1: **Management of Acne**

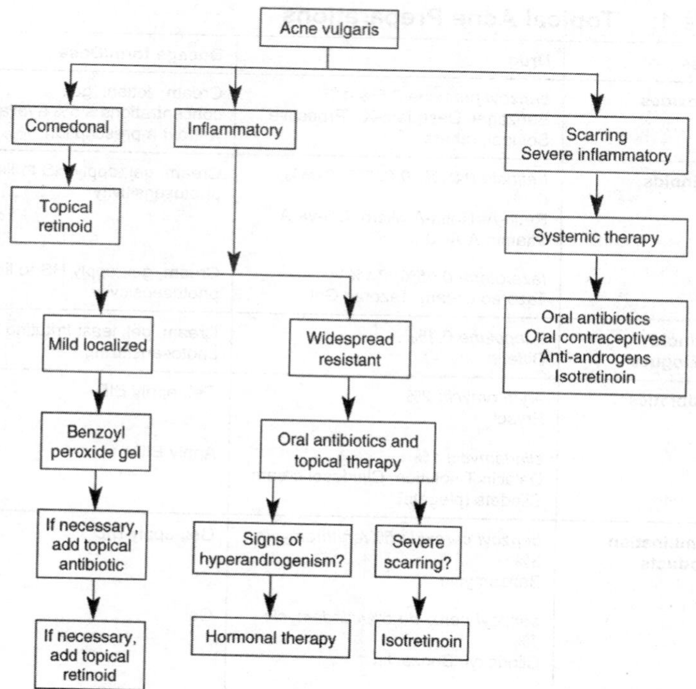

Table 2: Systemic Drugs Used for Acne Therapy

Class	Drug	Dose	Adverse Effects	Drug Interactions	Cost[a]
Tetracyclines	*tetracycline* generics	Initial: 500 mg BID Maintenance: 250–1000 mg/day	GI effects; fungal overgrowth; photosensitivity; pseudotumor cerebri; contraindicated in children < 8 y and pregnant women.	GI absorption impaired by iron, bismuth, aluminum and magnesium in drugs and foods. Separate doses by 2 h.	$
	minocycline Minocin, generics	Initial: 100 mg/day Maintenance: 50–200 mg/day	See tetracycline. Also dizziness; vertigo; cutaneous pigmentation; rarely LE-like syndrome; hepatic dysfunction.	See tetracycline.	$$
	doxycycline Vibra-Tabs, generics	Initial: 100 mg/day Maintenance: 100–200 mg/day	See tetracycline. Photosensitivity may occur.	See tetracycline.	$
Macrolides	*erythromycin* Eryc, PCE, others	Initial: 500 mg BID Maintenance: 250–1000 mg/day	GI effects: nausea, vomiting, epigastric distress, diarrhea.	May ↑ blood levels of theophylline, cyclosporine, carbamazepine, warfarin, digitalis, ergotamine.	1 g/day base: $ EC caps: $$
Diaminopyrimidines	*trimethoprim* generics	100–200 mg/day	GI upset, very rare agranulocytosis or toxic epidermal necrolysis.	↑ phenytoin levels; ↑ myelosuppression with methotrexate.	$
Sulfonamide Combinations	*trimethoprim/ sulfamethoxazole* generics	2–4 regular strength tabs/day divided BID	GI upset, very rare agranulocytosis, toxic epidermal necrolysis or sulfa hypersensitivity syndrome.	↑ phenytoin levels, ↑ INR with warfarin, hypoglycemia with sulfonylureas, ↑ nephrotoxicity with cyclosporine.	$

(cont'd)

Table 2: **Systemic Drugs Used for Acne Therapy** *(cont'd)*

Class	Drug	Dose	Adverse Effects	Drug Interactions	Cost[a]
Retinoids	*isotretinoin* Accutane, Clarus	0.5–2.0 mg/kg/day for 12–16 wk	Teratogenicity. Common: mucocutaneous dryness, myalgia, arthralgia, headache, photosensitivity. Uncommon–Rare: hypertriglyceridemia, mood disorder, possibly suicide ideation, pseudotumor cerebri.	Tetracyclines: rare cases of benign intracranial hypertension (pseudotumor cerebri).	$$$
Contraceptives, Oral	*EE 0.035 mg/ cyproterone 2 mg* Diane-35	1 tab/day × 21 days, off for 7 days and repeat cycle	Major: rare thromboembolism, stroke, retinal artery thrombosis, myocardial infarction, benign liver tumor, cholelithiasis, hypertension. Common: breakthrough bleeding/spotting, amenorrhea, nausea/vomiting, weight gain, bloating, chloasma, breast tenderness, depression, headaches. Discontinue 3–4 cycles after acne resolved.	Antibiotics: there is controversy as to whether a barrier method of birth control should also be used when women are using antibiotics and oral contraceptives. Patients with diarrhea or breakthrough bleeding may be at higher risk. Rifampin is the only antibiotic consistently shown to reduce estrogen levels.	$$
	EE 0.02 mg/ levonorgestrel 0.1 mg Alesse	1 tab/day × 21 days, off for 7 days and repeat cycle	See EE/cyproterone.	See EE/cyproterone.	$
	EE 0.035 mg/ norgestimate 0.18 mg × 7 days, 0.255 mg × 7 days, 0.25 mg × 7 days Tri-Cyclen	1 tab/day × 21 days, off 7 days and repeat cycle	See EE/cyproterone.	See EE/cyproterone.	$

Class	Drug	Dose	Adverse Effects	Drug Interactions	Cost[a]
	EE 0.03 mg/ drospirenone 3 mg Yasmin	1 tab/day × 21 days, off 7 days and repeat cycle	See EE/cyproterone.	See EE/cyproterone.	$
Androgen Receptor Antagonists	*spironolactone* [renal] Aldactone, generics	25–200 mg/day	Hyperkalemia, irregular menses, breast tenderness, nausea, headache.	ACE inhibitors, digoxin.	$

[a] Cost of 30-day supply based on 70 kg body weight; includes drug cost only.
[renal] Dosage adjustment may be required in renal impairment; see Appendix I.
Abbreviations: EE = ethinyl estradiol
Legend: $ < $20 $$ $20–50 $$$ $50–100

Suggested Readings

James WD. Acne *N Engl J Med* 2005;352:1463–72.

Purdy S, de Berker D. Acne. *BMJ* 2006;333(7275):949-53.

Strauss JS, Krowchuk DP, Leyden JJ et al. Guidelines of care for acne vulgaris management. *J Am Acad Dermatol* 2007;56(4):651-63.

References

1. Magin P, Adams J, Heading G et al. Psychological sequelae of acne vulgaris: results of a qualitative study. *Can Fam Physician* 2006;52:978-9.
2. Yan AC. Current concepts in acne management. *Adolesc Med Clin* 2006;17(3):613-37.
3. Leyden JJ. Therapy for acne vulgaris. *N Engl J Med* 1997;336(16):1156-62.
4. Burkhart CG, Burkhart CN. Antibacterial properties of benzoyl peroxide in aerobic and anaerobic conditions. *Int J Dermatol* 2006;45(11):1373-4.
5. Mills OH, Kligman AM, Pochi P et al. Comparing 2.5%, 5% and 10% benzoyl peroxide on inflammatory acne vulgaris. *Int J Dermatol* 1986;25(10):664-7.
6. Kalita L. Tazarotene versus tretinoin or adapalene in the treatment of acne vulgaris. *J Am Acad Dermatol* 2000;43(2 Pt 3):S51-4.
7. Strauss JS, Krowchuk DP, Leyden JJ et al. Guidelines of care for acne vulgaris management. *J Am Acad Dermatol* 2007;56(4):651-63.
8. Lidegaard O. Absolute and attributable risk of venous thromboembolism in women on combined cyproterone acetate and ethinylestradiol. *J Obstet Gynaecol Can* 2003;25(7):575-7.
9. Jick SS, Kremers HM, Vasilakis C et al. Isotretinoin use and risk of depression, psychotic symptoms, suicide, and attempted suicide. *Arch Dermatol* 2000;136(10):1231-6.
10. Chia CY, Lane W, Chibnall J et al. Isotretinoin therapy and mood changes in adolescents with moderate to severe acne: a cohort study. *Arch Dermatol* 2005;141(5)557-60.

CHAPTER 78
Rosacea

W. Stuart Maddin, MD, FRCPC

Rosacea is the fifth most common diagnosis made by dermatologists and is estimated to affect 10% of the population, more commonly Celts and North Europeans with fair skin.[1] It is seen in women two to three times more often than in men.

The release of proinflammatory mediators from neutrophils seems to be the underlying cause. Damage to dermal connective tissue such as that caused by sun exposure may initiate the problem. It is a chronic and progressive cutaneous vascular disorder and is often misdiagnosed as adult acne. More than 50% of patients with rosacea suffer eye involvement characterized by irritation, dryness, blepharitis and conjunctivitis. See Table 1 for classification of rosacea.

Table 1: **Classification of Rosacea**

Classification
Erythematotelangiectatic 1. mild: flushing, faint erythema and occasionally telangiectatic 2. moderate: frequent flushing, moderate persistent erythema, distinct telangiectasia 3. severe: frequent severe flushing, pronounced and persistent erythema, many prominent telangiectasias
Papulopustular 1. mild: few papules or pustules, mild erythema 2. moderate: scattered papules or pustules, moderate erythema 3. severe: many papules or pustules, pronounced erythema, plaques or edema may be present
Phymatous 1. mild: slight puffiness of nose, patulous follicular orifices 2. moderate: bulbous nasal swelling, dilated patulous follicular orifices, hypertrophy of sebaceous glands and change in nasal contour 3. severe: marked nasal swelling, large dilated follicles, distortion of nasal contour with nodular component
Ocular 1. mild: mild itch, dryness, fine scaling and erythema of lid margins and conjunctival injection 2. moderate: burning, stinging, crusting of lid margins with erythema/edema, conjunctival hyperemia, chalazion 3. severe: pain, photosensitivity or blurred vision, loss of lashes, severe conjunctival injection corneal changes with potential loss of vision

Adapted from Wilkin J, Dahl M, Detmar M et al. Standard classification of rosacea: report of the National Rosacea Society Expert Committee on the Classification and Staging of Rosacea. *J Am Acad Dermatol* 2002;46(4):584-7 and Powell FC. Clinical practice. Rosacea. *N Engl J Med* 2005;352(8):793-803.

Goals of Therapy

- Increase awareness of events that can trigger outbreaks of cutaneous rosacea, and how to avoid these triggers

- Make the patient aware of signs and symptoms of ocular rosacea and how they can be managed
- Reduce the number and severity of recurrences of cutaneous and ocular rosacea
- Prevent the development of rhinophyma (nose enlargement) with aggressive early treatment

Investigations

- Establish the diagnosis:
  - family history
  - later onset than acne (late 20s to 40s)
  - history of recurrent bouts of papules and pustules, inappropriate flushing and/or persistent redness of the face
  - history of eye irritation, blepharitis, dry eyes or recurrent styes
  - flare-up of rosacea following sun exposure
- Physical examination:
  - presence of papules or pustules along with erythema of the central face; absence of comedones
  - existence of telangiectasia
  - evidence of conjunctivitis, blepharitis, stye formation or complaint of dry eyes
  - rhinophyma (not common)
- Differential diagnosis:
  - acne vulgaris, perioral dermatitis, seborrheic dermatitis, photosensitivity reactions or discoid lupus erythematosus

Therapeutic Choices (Figure 1)

Nonpharmacologic Choices

- Advise patients how to avoid triggers that can worsen rosacea (Table 2).
- Protect from the sun with the use of proper clothing, hat and regular use of an effective sunscreen (Chapter 79). The sun and other climatic influences, such as intense cold or harsh winds may cause an exacerbation.
- Avoid hot beverages, soups, spices, vinegar and undiluted liquor. Dietary factors may precipitate flushing.
- *Scalpel, electrosurgery* or *laser therapy* — telangiectasia and persistent erythema may significantly improve after one to three laser treatments. For rhinophyma, the use of a scalpel to shave the nose or an electric loop or carbon dioxide laser to sculpt the nose to more normal proportions are worthwhile options.

Table 2: **Triggers That Can Worsen Rosacea**

Sunlight
Heat
Hot beverages
Spicy foods, vinegar
Alcohol
Application of topical corticosteroids to the face
Use of astringents
Emotional stress

Pharmacologic Choices (Table 3, Table 4, Table 5)

Table 3: **Treatment of Rosacea**

	Topical	Systemic	Physical
Erythematotelang-iectatic	Metronidazole Azelaic acid	Tetracycline, minocycline or doxycycline Erythromycin Isotretinoin	Lasers Intense pulsed light
Papulopustular		Tetracycline, minocycline or doxycycline	
Phymatous		To combat lymphedema: prednisone, isotretinoin	To combat rhinophyma: shave or debulk
Ocular	Fusidic acid 1% eye drops		Cosmetic camouflage Lasers Intense pulsed light

Start with **topical metronidazole** or **azelaic acid**. Azelaic acid is not available in Canada as a commercial product but can be compounded.

For severe and persistent rosacea, stress avoidance of triggers and do not hesitate to use oral antibiotics such as **tetracycline**, **doxycycline**, **minocycline** or **erythromycin** in full dosage for up to six months.

The use of low-dose **isotretinoin** is an effective and useful option for the management of patients with treatment-resistant rosacea.[2] Isotretinoin can also be used to treat persistent facial edema (Morbihan's disease), which may accompany rosacea.[3]

If there is clinical evidence of ocular involvement, it is critical to initiate treatment with tetracycline or doxycycline as well as **fusidic acid** 1% eye drops twice daily.

Therapeutic Tips

- Sun protection is very important.

- For female patients, recommend the use of a green-tinted foundation which works well at camouflaging the erythema of rosacea.
- Avoid topical corticosteroids; they can precipitate or worsen rosacea by adding to the dermal dystrophy that characterizes the disorder.
- When evaluating patients with cutaneous rosacea, inquire about ocular symptoms and examine the eyelids. This is especially important in patients with mild disease who are more likely to be treated with topical treatment alone.
- Counsel patients with particularly intense erythema that following successful treatment, posterythema-revealed telangiectasia (PERT) may become apparent. This preempts subsequent worries that the antibiotic therapy "produced" the telangiectasia.
- Pulsed dye laser and other laser systems (e.g., variable pulse width laser) can be very effective for telangiectasia. These procedures should be performed by skilled practitioners.

Figure 1: **Treatment of Rosacea**

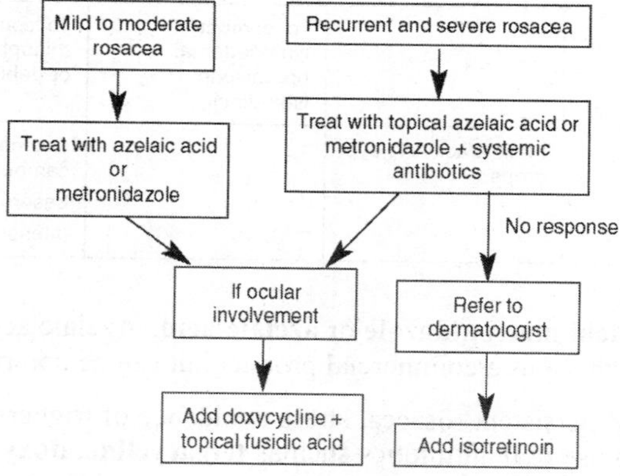

Table 4: Topical Treatment of Rosacea

Class	Drug	Dose	Adverse Effects	Comments	Cost[a]
Fusidane	*fusidic acid* 1% eye drops Fucithalmic	One drop in each eye twice per day	Rare: irritation.	Provides worthwhile benefit over a period of weeks.	$
Nitroimidazole	*metronidazole* 0.75%: MetroCream, MetroGel, MetroLotion 1%: Noritate, Rosasol (with SPF 15)	0.75% gel or cream, or 1% cream applied as thin film daily or BID × 9 wk, then as needed	Local irritation.	Treatment of choice. If discontinued, relapse can occur. May need up to 12 wk therapy to show pronounced improvement. Can be used in combination with oral tetracyclines. Inclusion of sunscreen provides sun protection and reduces dryness and irritation.[4]	$$$

[a] Cost of smallest available pack size; includes drug cost only.
Legend: $ < $10 $$ $10–20 $$$ $20–40

Table 5: Oral Drugs for the Treatment of Rosacea

Class	Drug	Dose	Adverse Effects	Drug Interactions	Comments	Cost[a]
Macrolides	*erythromycin* Eryc, PCE, others	0.5–1 g/day divided BID × 6–8 wk	GI effects; hepatotoxicity, especially with the estolate; candidiasis.	May ↑ blood levels of theophylline, cyclosporine, carbamazepine, warfarin, digitalis, ergotamine, methylprednisolone.	May be taken with food.	$
Retinoids	*isotretinoin* Accutane, Clarus	0.5–1 mg/kg/day for 4–5 mo	Teratogenicity (major concern); cheilitis, dry skin; mucocutaneous effects, myalgia; psychiatric events.	NB: No adverse interaction known between retinoids and oral contraceptives.	For recalcitrant cases.[5] Provides worthwhile benefit, but not as consistent. Requires at least **2 types** of contraception when used in females of childbearing age.	$$$$
Tetracyclines	*tetracycline* generics	500 mg BID × 2 wk, then 500 mg daily until rosacea controlled. Then 250 mg daily × 3–4 wk	GI effects; fungal overgrowth; photosensitivity; may ↑ azotemia; pseudotumor cerebri; contraindicated in pregnant women.	GI absorption of tetracycline may be impaired by iron, bismuth, aluminum, calcium, magnesium, in drugs and foods (e.g., dairy products). Separate doses by 2 h.	Lowest in cost; used in combination with topical metronidazole. Not to be taken with milk or milk products. Recurrences of rosacea do occur after treatment is discontinued.	$

Class	Drug	Dose	Adverse Effects	Drug Interactions	Comments	Cost[a]
	minocycline Enca, Minocin, generics	50–100 mg daily × 6–8 wk	See tetracycline. Also dizziness; vertigo; abnormal cutaneous pigmentation; rarely LE-like syndrome; hepatic dysfunction.		Can be tried if tetracycline fails after compliant 4–6 wk trial. No food restriction required. Recurrences of rosacea do occur after treatment is discontinued.	$$-$$$
	doxycycline Vibra-Tabs, generics	100 mg daily × 12 wk	See tetracycline. Photosensitivity may occur.	Serum concentrations of doxycycline may be reduced by carbamazepine, chronic alcohol ingestion, phenobarbital and phenytoin. Methotrexate concentrations may be increased by doxycycline.	Given once daily. No food restriction required. Useful for improving ocular rosacea. Recurrences of rosacea do occur after treatment is discontinued.	$$

[a] Cost of 30-day supply; includes drug cost only.

Dosage adjustment may be required in renal impairment; see Appendix I.

Legend: $ < $10 $$ $10–20 $$-$$$ $10–30 $$$ $20–30 $$$$ > $30

Suggested Readings

Baldwin HE. Oral therapy for rosacea. *J Drug Dermatol* 2006;5(1):16–21.

Baldwin HE. Systemic therapy for rosacea. *Skin Therapy Letter* 2007;12(2):1-5, 9.

Nally JB, Berson DS. Topical therapies for rosacea. *J Drugs Dermatol* 2006;5(1):23–6.

Powell FC. Rosacea. *N Engl J Med* 2005;352:793–803.

van Zuuren EJ, Graber MA, Hollis S et al. Interventions for rosacea. *The Cochrane Database of Systematic Reviews* 2005(3): CD003262.

References

1. Crawford GH, Pelle MT, James WD. Rosacea: I. Etiology, pathogenesis and subtype classification. *J Am Acad Dermatol* 2004;51(3):327-41.
2. Erdogan FG, Yurtsever P, Aksoy D et al. Efficacy of low-dose isotretinoin in patients with treatment-resistant rosacea. *Arch Dermatol* 1998;134(7):884-5.
3. Mazzatenta C, Giorgino G, Rubegni P et al. Solid persistent facial oedema (Morbihan's disease) following rosacea, successfully treated with isotretinoin and ketotifen. *Br J Dermatol* 1997;137(6):1020-1.
4. Tan JK. A new formulation containing sunscreen (SPF 15) and 1% metronidazole (ROSASOL Cream) in the treatment of rosacea. *Skin Therapy Lett* 2001;6(8)1-2.
5. Ortonne JP. Oral isotretinoin treatment policy. Do we all agree? *Dermatology* 1997;195(Suppl 1):34-7.

CHAPTER 79
Sunburn

Lyn Guenther, MD, FRCPC

Sunburn is caused by acute excessive exposure to ultraviolet (UV) radiation. It is characterized by *erythema*, with onset two to six hours after exposure to a threshold dose of UV radiation; it peaks at 15 to 36 hours and regresses by 72 to 120 hours. Erythema resulting from sun bed UVA exposure starts immediately, peaks at 8 hours and regresses by 24 to 48 hours. *Edema*, *pain* and *pruritus* may be present. *Blistering* in severe cases may take a week or more to resolve. Nausea, abdominal cramping, fever, chills, weakness, malaise and headache may also occur. *Desquamation* with resolution results from cellular injury and death.

Sun exposure in children is approximately thrice that of adults.[1] According to a national survey, the highest prevalence of sunburn was in the 15 to 24 age group. Men experienced more sunburns and used fewer sun protective measures.[2] Any person, even black, will burn with large doses of UV radiation. Blue- or green-eyed, lighter-skinned individuals who tan poorly and freckle burn more readily. The trunk, neck and head burn at a lower dose of UV radiation than the upper limbs, which burn more readily than the lower limbs. This may be due to the regional differences in thickness of the epidermis and/or stratum corneum.[3]

Sunburns are common in tanning salons. Sunburns are more common in sun bed users than non-users.[4]

Characteristics of Ultraviolet Radiation

- UV radiation (UVR) accounts for approximately 5% of terrestrial solar radiation. UV light that causes skin injury is classified by wavelength. UVA is responsible for phototoxicity, photoaging, immunosuppression and skin cancer. It also accounts for ~ 95% of radiation found in artificial tanning beds. It penetrates the skin more deeply than UVB and is responsible for most phototoxic reactions to drugs.
- UVB is the primary cause of sunburn from sunlight. It can also cause immunosuppression and skin cancer.

A 1% decrease in ozone results in a 1.5% increase in UVB, leading to a 2 to 6% increase in basal and squamous cell cancers and a 0.3 to 2% increase in melanomas.[5] Radiation effects are enhanced by reflective surfaces (e.g., sand, snow, cement and water). Up to 80% of UV radiation penetrates clouds. Increased humidity decreases the threshold for erythema from UV radiation. The UV index forecasts the intensity of UV rays (Table 1).

Table 1: **UV Index and Risk of Sunburn**

UV index	Risk	Estimated time for fair-skinned person to burn
0–2	minimal	1 h
3–4	low	< 20 min
5–6	moderate	< 15 min
7–9	high	< 10 min
≥10	extreme	< 5 min

Prevention of Sunburn

Prevention is critical since repeated sun exposure and sunburns are associated with skin cancer and premature skin aging. UV exposure has been linked to 90% of nonmelanoma skin cancers and 65% of melanomas.[6] Two blistering sunburns during childhood can double the risk of melanoma later in life.[6] UV radiation can also suppress the immune system and habitual exposure can cause cataracts.

Nonpharmacologic Choices

- Cosmetic tanning should be avoided. Pigmentation does not occur without damage and death of epidermal cells.
- Tanning salons should be avoided.
- Outdoor activities at peak UV irradiance times (10 a.m. to 4 p.m. when your shadow is shorter than you; when the UV index is high or extreme) should be avoided.
- Outdoor activities should be in the shade if possible.
- Umbrellas may reduce UV radiation by about 70%; however, they do not protect against reflected radiation.
- Protective clothing (pants, long-sleeved shirts, gloves) and sunglasses should be worn. Loosely woven, white or wet clothing offers less protection. Women's hosiery provides minimal protection.
- Wide-brimmed hats (at least 7.5 cm) of tightly woven fabric (not straw) should be worn to protect the face, ears and neck. Regular use could decrease the lifetime risk of skin cancer by 40%.[7]
- Sun exposure should be minimized while one is taking phototoxic medications or using certain local agents (Table 2), which can interact with UV/visible light to cause a dose-related sunburn.

Table 2: **Medications That May Cause Phototoxic Reactions**[a]

Amiodarone	Psoralens
Antimicrobials	Methoxsalen
Ceftazidime	Trioxsalen
Griseofulvin	Psychiatric medications
Quinolones	Alprazolam
Ciprofloxacin	Chlordiazepoxide
Nalidixic acid	Chlorpromazine
Norfloxacin	Desipramine
Ofloxacin	Imipramine
Sulfonamides	Perphenazine
Tetracyclines	Prochlorperazine
Demeclocycline	Thioridazine
Doxycycline	Trifluoperazine
Tetracycline	Quinidine
Trimethoprim	Quinine
Antineoplastics	Retinoids, systemic
Dacarbazine	Acitretin
5-fluorouracil	Isotretinoin
Vinblastine	Retinoids, topical[b]
Clofibrate	Adapalene
Coal tar derivatives, topical	Tazarotene
Diuretics	Tretinoin
Furosemide	Sulfites
Hydrochlorothiazide	Sulfonylureas
Hematoporphyrin	Tolbutamide
NSAIDs	
Diclofenac	
Ibuprofen	
Indomethacin	
Ketoprofen	
Naproxen	
Piroxicam	
Sulindac	
Tiaprofenic acid	

[a] Radiation in the UVA range causes most drug-related phototoxic reactions.
[b] After continued use due to thinning of the stratum corneum.

Pharmacologic Choices

No sunscreen offers complete protection from the sun. Sunscreens should be adjunctive rather than the primary means of protection. It is estimated that regular sunscreen use for the first 18 years could decrease the lifetime risk of skin cancer by about 80%.[8] Daily sunscreen use for 4.5 years decreased the incidence of squamous cell cancer.[9] Sunscreens can also prevent UV-induced immunosuppression.[10]

Topical Sunscreens

Sunscreens should be used to protect the skin and not to prolong sun exposure. They should provide protection against both UVB and UVA and have an SPF of at least 30, where SPF is defined as: least amount of UVB energy to produce erythema with sunscreen divided by the least amount of UVB energy to produce erythema without sunscreen. The FDA rates sunscreens with an SPF of 2 to 11 as providing minimum protection, 12 to 29 moderate and ≥ 30 high. The SPF of sunscreens is measured under ideal laboratory conditions and may be considerably less when applied thinly and used outdoors. There is no internationally accepted UVA standard testing procedure, making it difficult for the consumer to determine the degree of UVA protection afforded by commercially available sunscreens. Topical sunscreens should be applied generously (2 mg/cm^2) to all exposed surfaces including lips, tops of ears and tops of feet. Approximately 30 mL is needed for full coverage. Most people only apply a quarter to half the tested amount, effectively reducing the SPF. A second application shortly after the first increases the amount of sunscreen applied and may result in an SPF closer to that stated on the sunscreen product.

Reapplication of sunscreen 15 to 30 minutes after sun exposure begins improves coverage and may increase photoprotection.[11] Sunscreens should also be reapplied after swimming, towelling off or sweating. Waterproof sunscreens maintain their efficacy after 80 minutes of water immersion, water-resistant sunscreens after 40 minutes of water immersion, and sweat-resistant after 30 minutes of continuous heavy sweating. Reapplication does not extend the period of protection. A person who burns in 10 minutes will burn in 300 minutes using a sunscreen with an SPF of 30, no matter how many times it is applied. This person will develop erythema in < 300 minutes if the sunscreen is not reapplied after swimming, towelling off or sweating. Although sunscreens can prevent sunburn, many biological effects (e.g., immunosuppression, carcinogenicity) can occur before the UV erythema threshold is reached. Outdoor workers and fair-skinned individuals should be encouraged to apply sunscreens as part of their daily cosmetic regimen.

Chemical Sunscreens (Table 3)

Commercial products usually contain more than one active ingredient. They should be applied 15 to 60 minutes before UV exposure to allow active ingredients to bind to the skin. They can be used in children older than six months of age. Chronic sunscreen use has not been associated with vitamin D deficiency.[12] Only a few minutes of sun daily, to the back of one hand, results in sufficient vitamin D production. In addition, adequate amounts of vitamin D can be absorbed from cereal, dairy products and fish.

Table 3: **Chemical Sunscreens**[a]

Class	Active Ingredient	Comments
UVB Absorbers Para-aminobenzoic acid (PABA) esters	*padimate O (octyl dimethyl PABA)*	Adhere well to skin. May cause contact/photocontact dermatitis. May cross-react with sulfonamides, thiazides, sulfonylurea hypoglycemics, ester anesthetics.
UVB Absorbers Salicylates	*homosalate (homomenthyl salicylate)*	Does not adhere well to skin; easily removed by perspiration or swimming. Rarely causes contact dermatitis.
	octyl salicylate	See homosalate.
	triethanolamine salicylate	See homosalate.
UVB Absorbers Cinnamates	*octyl methoxycinnamate (Parsol MCX)*	Does not adhere well to skin; easily removed by sweating and swimming. May cross-react with balsam of Peru, cocoa leaves, benzyl and methyl cinnamate, cinnamic alcohol, cinnamic aldehyde, cinnamon oil. Photostabilizes dibenzoylmethanes.
	2-ethoxyethyl p-methoxycinnamate (Cinoxate)	See octyl methoxycinnamate.
	octocrylene	See octyl methoxycinnamate.
UVB Absorbers Benzylidene camphor derivative	*4-methylbenzylidene camphor*	Maximum absorption at 300 nm. Photostabilizes dibenzoylmethanes.
UVA Absorbers Benzophenones	*oxybenzone (benzophenone-3)*	Broad-spectrum UVA/UVB protection. May cause contact/photocontact dermatitis.
	dioxybenzone (benzophenone-8)	May cause contact urticaria/contact dermatitis.
UVA Absorbers Anthranilates	*menthyl anthranilate*	Incomplete UVA protection. Rarely causes sensitization.
UVA Absorbers Dibenzoylmethanes	*avobenzone or t-butylmethoxy-dibenzoylmethane (Parsol 1789)*	Broad UVA absorption. Better protection against UVA than benzophenones, anthranilates and Mexoryl SX. Photodegradable. May cause contact and photocontact dermatitis.
UVA Absorbers Benzylidene camphor derivative	*terephthalylidene dicamphor sulfonic acid (Mexoryl SX)*	Maximum absorption at 345 nm. Good photostability.

[a] For a listing of Canadian Dermatology Association-recognized sunscreens, see http://www.dermatology.ca/patients_public/info_patients/sun_safety/recognized_sunscreens.html

Physical Sunscreens

Titanium dioxide, zinc oxide, kaolin, talc (magnesium silicate), ferric chloride and melanin protect against UVA and UVB and can be used in people of all ages including infants. They reflect and scatter UV and visible light. Titanium dioxide and zinc oxide can also absorb UVA wavelengths up to 400 nm. Physical sunscreens are generally thicker, less cosmetically elegant and may rub off easily or melt with the sun's heat. Although they pose less risk of sensitization, their occlusive effect may cause miliaria and folliculitis. Micronized titanium dioxide and zinc oxide are relatively transparent to visible light but scatter UV light well.

Oral Sunscreens

There is no effective oral sunscreen. Oral beta-carotene, antimalarials, vitamin A, vitamin E and oral PABA *do not* provide effective protection against sunburn. Combined systemic vitamin C 2 g/day and vitamin E 1000 IU/day provide minimal protection (SPF 1.4).[13] Vitamin C or E in a topical sunscreen may enhance photoprotection.[14]

Treatment of Sunburn

Mild sunburn does not usually require any specific treatment; however, it provides an opportunity for education about the associated risks and use of photoprotection. The following may provide relief if given at the time of sunburn or shortly after.

Nonpharmacologic Choices

Cool baths or **wet compresses** with tap water or saline for 20 minutes four to six times a day provide some relief. **Moisturizers** help with dryness and peeling. **Fluids** should be replenished with nonalcoholic beverages.

Pharmacologic Choices

Topical vitamin E (alpha-tocopherol) applied two minutes after UV exposure may decrease erythema and edema. The effect is diminished if applied later post-irradiation and is probably insignificant if applied after five hours.[15]

Celecoxib 200 mg twice daily suppressed erythema in approximately 50% of treated individuals.[16]

Indomethacin 25 mg or **ibuprofen** 400 mg Q6H for four doses or topical 1% indomethacin, starting at time of insult, may decrease erythema and reduce the degree of epidermal injury.

Diclofenac gel applied six and ten hours after irradiation may decrease pain, erythema and edema.[17]

Potent topical corticosteroids transiently decrease erythema by causing vasoconstriction but do not reduce epidermal damage. They may soothe stinging and itching. Their effect is additive when used with indomethacin or ibuprofen.[18]

Glycolic acid 8% cream applied once daily for one week starting within 24 hours of excessive sun exposure may accelerate resolution of the erythema.[19]

Pramoxine lotion, **calamine** and **colloidal oatmeal** may be soothing.

Acetaminophen may relieve pain.

Therapeutic Tips

- Systemic corticosteroids have little effect in treating sunburn and may increase the risk of secondary infection.
- Topical anesthetic sprays are associated with a risk of sensitization and should be avoided.
- After a sunburn, the skin should not be exposed to the sun for at least a week.
- Blisters should not be unroofed since the overlying skin protects against secondary infection.
- Blistering sunburns may require treatment in a burn unit if there is extensive denudation of skin and fluid and electrolyte loss.
- Scarring rarely occurs unless there is secondary infection.

Suggested Readings

Bissonnette R, Claveau J, Gupta AK. Ultraviolet A radiation and the need for protection. *J Cutan Med Surg* 2006;10(Suppl 1):1-7.

Driscoll MS, Wagner RF. Clinical management of the acute sunburn reaction. *Cutis* 2000;66(1):53-8.

[No authors listed]. Prevention and treatment of sunburn. *Med Lett Drugs Ther* 2004;46(1184):45-6.

Provost N, Landells I, Maddin S. Sunscreens: past, present, and future. *J Cutan Med Surg* 2006;10(Suppl 1):14-21.

Rivers JK, Bang B, Marcoux D. Ultraviolet radiation exposure: public health concerns. *J Cutan Med Surg* 2006;10(Suppl 1):8-13.

References

1. Stern RS. Proportion of lifetime UV dose received by age 18, what Stern et al actually said in 1986. *J Invest Dermatol* 2005;124(5):1079-80.
2. Lovato C, Shoveller J, Rivers J. *National survey on sun & protective behaviours. Final report.* Vancouver (BC): Institute of Health Promotion Research, UBC; 1998.
3. Waterston K, Naysmith L, Rees JL. Variation in skin thickness may explain some of the within-person variation in ultraviolet radiation-induced erythema at different body sites. *J Invest Dermatol* 2005;124(5):1078.
4. Thieden E, Philipsen PA, Sandby-Moller J et al. Sunburn related to UV radiation exposure, age, sex, occupation, and sun bed use based on time-stamped personal dosimetry and sun behavior diaries. *Arch Dermatol* 2005;141(4):482-8.
5. Coldiron BM. Thinning of the ozone layer: facts and consequences. *J Am Acad Dermatol* 1992;27(5 Pt 1):653-62.
6. Geller AC, Cantor M, Miller DR et al. The Environmental Protection Agency's National SunWise School Program: sun protection education in US schools (1999-2000). *J Am Acad Dermatol* 2002;46(5):683-9.
7. Marks R. Photoprotection and prevention of melanoma. *Eur J Dermatol* 1999;9(5):406-12.

8. Stern RS, Weinstein MC, Baker SG. Risk reduction for nonmelanoma skin cancer with childhood sunscreen use. *Arch Dermatol* 1986;122(5):537-45.
9. Green A, Williams G, Neale R et al. Daily sunscreen application and betacarotene supplementation in prevention of basal-cell and squamous-cell carcinomas of the skin: a randomised controlled trial. *Lancet* 1999;354(9180):723-9.
10. Baron ED, Stevens SR. Sunscreens and immune protection. *Br J Dermatol* 2002;146(6):933-7.
11. Diffey BL. When should sunscreen be reapplied? *J Am Acad Dermatol* 2001;45(6):882-5.
12. Marks R, Foley PA, Jolley D et al. The effect of regular sunscreen use on vitamin D levels in an Australian population. Results of a randomized controlled trial. *Arch Dermatol* 1995;131(4):415-21.
13. Eberlein-Konig B, Placzek M, Przybilla B. Protective effect against sunburn of combined systemic ascorbic acid (vitamin C) and d-alpha-tocopherol (vitamin E). *J Am Acad Dermatol* 1998;38(1):45-8.
14. Darr D, Dunston S, Faust H et al. Effectiveness of antioxidants (vitamin C and E) with and without sunscreens as topical photoprotectants. *Acta Derm Venereol* 1996;76(4):264-8.
15. Trevithick JR. Vitamin E prevention of ultraviolet-induced skin damage. In: Fuchs J, Packer L, editors. *Oxidative stress in dermatology*. New York (NY): Dekker; 1993.
16. Rodriguez-Burford C, Tu JH, Mercurio M et al. Selective cyclooxygenase-2 inhibition produces heterogeneous erythema response to ultraviolet irradiation. *J Invest Dermatol* 2005;125(6):1317-20.
17. Kienzler JL, Magnette J, Queille-Roussel C et al. Diclofenac-Na gel is effective in reducing the pain and inflammation associated with exposure to ultraviolet light - results of two clinical studies. *Skin Pharmacol Physiol* 2005;18(3):144-52.
18. Hughes GS, Francom SF, Means LK et al. Synergistic effects of oral nonsteroidal drugs and topical corticosteroids in the therapy of sunburn in humans. *Dermatology* 1992;184(1):54-8.
19. Perricone NV, DiNardo JC. Photoprotective and antiinflammatory effects of topical glycolic acid. *Dermatol Surg* 1996;22(5):435-7.

CHAPTER 80
Burns

David Warren, MD, FRCPC

Goals of Therapy

- Provide early management of serious burns to reduce associated morbidity and mortality
- Optimize cosmetic results and minimize functional morbidity of burns
- Provide appropriate analgesia, burn wound management and follow-up

Investigations

- A thorough history of the burn injury with special attention to:
  - burning agent and its temperature and duration of exposure
  - fire in open or enclosed space, explosion, fall, electrical or chemical exposure
  - past medical history, medications and tetanus status
- Physical examination:
  - general physical examination with attention initially to airway, breathing and circulation
  - head to toe examination to assess for other systemic or musculoskeletal injuries
  - presence of headache, irritability, nausea, confusion, agitation and uncoordination, which may indicate *carbon monoxide poisoning*
  - assess for *pulmonary complications*. Upper airway edema may occur from direct thermal injury, especially with steam. Smoke inhalation doubles the mortality risk of a burn from systemic and direct toxicant effects to the airway. Indicators include fire in an enclosed space, inhalation of noxious fumes, facial burns, pharyngeal burns, carbonaceous sputum, hoarseness, elevated carboxyhemoglobin > 5% and abnormal pulmonary function. Pulmonary edema may be an early or late finding
  - assess *depth of wound* (Table 1)
  - triage patients for inpatient, referral and outpatient care
  - assess the *extent of the burn* quantified as the percentage of total body surface area (BSA). The palm size of the victim is approximately 1% BSA, or estimate following the rule of nines (Figure 1)
  - some burns, due to their extent or potential morbidity, should be considered for *referral to a burn centre* or specialized care (Table 2). Transfer should be facilitated by contact between physicians. All pertinent documentation, tests, flow sheets and transfer records should accompany the patient

- Laboratory tests in moderate and severe burns:
  - CBC, electrolytes, glucose, BUN, creatinine, blood type and clotting studies
  - ethanol and drug toxicology if warranted
  - carboxyhemoglobin level and other toxins in suspected inhalation injuries
  - urinalysis and, if blood positive or > 30% BSA burn, urine myoglobin
  - arterial blood gas and chest radiograph, often normal early with findings 6 to 24 hours later

Table 1: **Burn Depth Classification**[1]

Degree	Class	Description	Example	Healing Time
1st	Superficial	Involves epidermis: skin red and painful	Sunburn	7 days
2nd	Superficial partial thickness	Epidermis and upper dermis: blisters, underlying skin red and moist, very painful	Scald with water	10–21 days
	Deep partial thickness	Epidermis and deep dermis: some hair follicle and sweat gland damage, blisters to charring	Flame, oil	> 14 days, some scarring
3rd	Full thickness	Epidermis through dermis to subcutaneous fat: skin pale, painless, leathery	Flame, hot metal	scars — will not heal; surgery ± grafts

Therapeutic Choices

Nonpharmacologic Choices

Initial First Aid Management

- Remove the victim from the source of injury, taking care to limit risk to rescuers in electrical and chemical burn injuries.
- Remove any burning clothing or hot material.
- Assess airway, breathing and circulation (ABC).
- In chemical exposures, copiously irrigate burn region with lukewarm water until testing demonstrates a normal tissue pH, often prolonged with alkali burns.
- Cover the exposed area with a clean cloth soaked in cool water. Avoid hypothermia in young infants and in extensive burns. Avoid putting ice or home remedies on burn.
- Cover with clean dry cloth on transport to hospital.

Table 2: **Criteria for Referral or Transfer to a Burn Centre**[2]

- Partial thickness burn > 10% BSA if patient < 10 y or > 50 y of age
- Partial thickness burns > 20% BSA in other age groups
- Partial and full thickness burns involving the face, eyes, ears, hands, feet, perineum or overlying major joints
- Full thickness burns > 5% BSA
- Significant chemical or electrical burns
- Inhalation injuries
- Patients with pre-existing illness likely to complicate recovery
- Patients with concomitant trauma should be initially treated in an appropriate trauma setting and subsequently transferred to a burn centre
- Children should be treated in facilities with appropriate capabilities and equipment
- Patients with special psychosocial needs and/or rehabilitative support (child abuse, mental health needs, drug addiction)

Initial Medical Management

- Initially assess ABC.
- Consider the need for early *intubation* if any airway or breathing compromise.
- Use humidified oxygen if any suspicion of inhalation injury.
- Employ *oxygen* 100% if known carbon monoxide exposure or fire in an enclosed space. This will drop the half-life of carboxyhemoglobin from 330 to 90 minutes.
- Establish iv access for any burn > 10% BSA, in noninvolved areas of the upper body if possible.
- Major burns will always require significant *fluid resuscitation*. The Parkland formula, 4 mL × (total burn surface area [%]) × (body weight [kg]) is a good initial estimate of fluid requirements. Half should be given in the first 8 hours and the remainder over subsequent 16 hours postburn. Adjustments may be required as clinical assessment and urinary output indicate.
- Children should receive maintenance fluid in addition, at an hourly rate of:
  - 4 mL/kg for the first 10 kg of body weight plus
  - 2 mL/kg for second 10 kg of body weight plus
  - 1 mL/kg for > 20 kg of body weight[3]
- *Nasogastric tube* drainage for ileus is likely in any major burn.
- *Bladder catheterization* to monitor appropriate urinary output, minimum 0.5 mL/kg/h (children < 25 kg, 1 mL/kg/h).[4]
- Elevate any encircling limb burn and closely assess for neurovascular status. Assess chest burns for restriction of normal excursion and pulmonary compromise. Consider surgical escharotomy as required.
- Ensure adequate *tetanus prophylaxis*; 0.5 mL **tetanus toxoid** in previously immunized patient with additional 250 units **tetanus immune globulin** if previously unimmunized.

Burn Wound Management

- Remove any attached clothing and loose tissue.
- Gently wash the burn surface with sterile water or normal saline.
- Débride open blisters and loose tissue.
- Use petroleum-based ointments such as **neomycin/bacitracin/polymyxin B** to act as emulsifying agents to remove tar.[5]
- The application of **topical antibiotic** agents will lower the incidence of wound infections.[4] Often not used with superficial burns, they have a more significant role with deeper, more extensive injuries (Table 4). Apply topical antibiotics using sterile technique to approximately 2 mm twice daily or as required if rubbed off. Cleanse the wound prior to reapplication.

Dressings (Table 3)

Most commonly used are *semi-closed dressings* which permit ambulatory management while maintaining hygiene, limiting mobilization and preventing tampering with the wound. They consist of:

- an innermost dressing layer of porous mesh gauze impregnated with nonpetroleum-based water-soluble lubricant or antibiotic;
- a second layer of bulky, fluffed coarse mesh gauze to absorb exudate and protect the wound;
- an outer layer of semi-elastic coarse mesh, which provides moderate pressure to keep the dressing in place but should not be constrictive.

Dressing changes for semi-closed dressings should be every other day, daily or twice daily depending on the wound, antibiotic use and the patient.

An alternative for superficial partial thickness wounds are *semisynthetic occlusive dressings* (e.g., Biobrane, DuoDerm, Tegaderm) used in flat partial thickness burns. Dressing changes: removal, cleansing and redressing is required if fluid collects beneath, otherwise removal at 7 to 10 days.

Open therapy is often used on the head, neck and perineum, which are areas that are difficult to dress and prone to maceration.

Moisture retentive dressings are designed to lock exudates away from the wound, reducing maceration.[6,7] They can be used in mild and moderate thickness burns. These dressings offer an antimicrobial barrier to the wound; impregnated silver provides prolonged antimicrobial activity. Central gels and fewer dressing changes assist pain relief. To use:

- Cleanse and débride wound, moisten as directed if dry.
- Cover wound with dressing sheets, extending dressing beyond wound edges; trim as required.
- Cover dressing with sterile gauze.

- Cover may be removed periodically to inspect wound, but leave dressing in place for 3 to 14 days as per product directions.
- Trim dressing as it detaches; inspect frequently if any signs of infection.

Table 3: **Wound Dressings Used for the Treatment of Burns**

Dressing	Type of Burn Wound	Characteristics of Dressing
silver antimicrobial moisture retentive Aquacel, Acticoat	Superficial, exudative and deep partial thickness wounds.	Moisten dressing as directed if wound dry. Antimicrobial coverage for 3-14 days.
semisynthetic Duoderm, Tegaderm Hydrocolloid	Superficial, minimal exudate, partial thickness wounds.	No antimicrobial coverage. Easy application.
biosynthetic Biobrane, Curasorb	Large, mid-partial thickness burns and donor sites.	Permeable to topical antibiotics. Limits evaporative water losses.

Pharmacologic Choices

- Avoid prophylactic oral and parenteral antibiotics in all but exceptional circumstances to avoid development of resistant infections.
- **Topical antibiotics:** various agents have been used with specific indications and limitations (Table 4).

Pain Management

- **NSAIDs** manage pain in minor burns and suppress the inflammatory response in major burns. Standard doses for soft tissue injury given on a regular basis can be used (e.g., **ibuprofen** 400 mg every four to six hours).
- Potent analgesia with small aliquots of **morphine** (0.1 to 0.15 mg/kg iv) or **fentanyl** (0.5 to 1.0 μg/kg iv), titrated to effect, are often required initially to manage pain.[8]
- Take care not to suppress the signs of other injuries initially with analgesia.
- Children especially require analgesia to manage their burns.
- Longer term and outpatient analgesia can be achieved with oral **codeine**.

Therapeutic Tips

- Avoid contamination of the wound; infection is the major threat to burn outcome.
- Advise patients regarding signs of infection; any evidence of infection should be reviewed quickly and treatment altered as appropriate.

- Outpatient follow-up schedule may be daily initially and extended as dressing requirements and healing progress.
- Electrical burns often have more extensive damage below the surface than is initially identified and should be followed appropriately.
- Moisturize healed burns and protect them from sun exposure with clothing or sunscreen.

Figure 1: **Rule of Nines Estimation of Body Surface Area for Child and Adult**

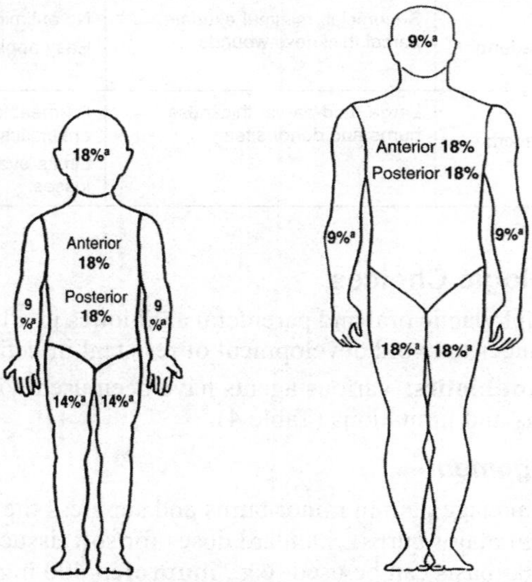

[a] Includes both anterior and posterior aspects.

Table 4: Topical Anti-infectives for the Treatment of Burns

Class	Drug	Application[a]	Limitations	Comments	Cost[b]
Antibiotics, topical	*bacitracin* Baciguent, generics	Daily, BID open or semi-closed	Poor eschar penetration, moderate antibacterial spectrum.	Transparent, easy to apply, cosmetically acceptable.	$
	framycetin 1% Sofra-Tulle	Daily, semi-closed	Poor penetration, moderate antibacterial action.	Easy to use.	$
	fusidic acid 2% Fucidin Cream	Daily to QID open or semi-closed	Moderate antibacterial spectrum.	Development of resistance.	$$–$$$$
	mupirocin 2% Bactroban Cream, Bactroban Ointment, generics	TID, open	Limited antimicrobial coverage.	Gram-positive coverage.	$$
	silver sulfadiazine 1% Dermazin, Flamazine, SSD	BID–QID open or semi-closed	Only fair penetration, sulfonamide sensitivity (rash), leukopenia.	Broad antibacterial spectrum, painless, washable.	$–$$
Antiseptics	*povidone/iodine 1%* Betadine, Proviodine	BID open or semi-closed	Poor penetration, tissue staining, painful, iodine absorption.	Broad antibacterial action.	$$

[a] Approximately 5 g per 1% BSA burn per application.
[b] Cost of 7-day supply based on 1% BSA burn; includes drug cost only.
Legend: $ < $10 $-$$ < $10–25 $$ $10–25 $$$ $25–50 $$-$$$$ $10– >50 $$$$ > $50

Suggested Readings

American College of Surgeons. Injuries due to burns and cold. In: *Advanced trauma life support*. 7th ed. Chicago (IL): American College of Surgeons; 2004. p.231-42.

Benson A, Dickson WA, Boyce DE. Burns. *BMJ* 2006;332(7542):649-52.

Husspith J, Rayatt S. First aid treatment of minor burns. *BMJ* 2004;328(7454):1487-9.

Papini R. Management of burn injuries of various depths. *BMJ* 2004;329(7458):158-60.

Reed J, Pomerantz WJ. Emergency management of pediatric burns. *Pediatr Emerg Care* 2005;21(2):118-29.

References

1. [No authors listed]. Appendix B to hospital resources document. Guidelines for service standards and severity classifications in the treatment of burn injury. American Burn Association. *Bull Am Coll Surg* 1984;69(10):24-8.
2. [No authors listed]. Hospital and prehospital resources for optimal care of patients with burn injury: guidelines for development and operation of burn centers. American Burn Association. *J Burn Care Rehabil* 1990;11(2):98-104.
3. Hettiaratchy S, Papini R. Initial management of a major burn: II--assessment and resuscitation. *BMJ* 2004;329(7457):101-3.
4. Monafo WW. Initial management of burns. *N Engl J Med* 1996;335(21):1581-6.
5. Edlich RF et al. Thermal burns. In: Marx JA et al., editors. *Rosen's emergency medicine: concepts and clinical practice*. 5th ed. St. Louis (MO): Mosby; 2002.
6. Tredget EE, Shankowsky HA, Groeneveld A et al. A matched-pair, randomized study evaluating the efficacy and safety of Acticoat silver-coated dressing for the treatment of burn wounds. *J Burn Care Rehabil* 1998;19(6):531-7.
7. Bowler PG, Jones SA, Walker M et al. Microbicidal properties of a silver-containing hydrofiber dressing against a variety of burn wound pathogens. *J Burn Care Rehabil* 2004;25(2):192-6.
8. Henry DB, Foster RL. Burn pain management in children. *Pediatr Clin North Am* 2000;47(3):681-98, ix-x.

CHAPTER 81
Pressure Ulcers

Stephen R. Tan, MD, FRCPC

Goals of Therapy

- Recognize and modify risk factors for pressure ulcer formation
- Improve existing lesions with the ability to heal
- Recognize and manage the complications of pressure ulcers
- Prevent recurrences in at-risk patients

Staging of Pressure Ulcers

Table 1: Staging of Pressure Ulcers[1]

Stage I	Non-blanchable erythema of intact skin. In darker skin types, discolouration, warmth, edema or induration may be indicators.
Stage II	Partial-thickness skin loss involving the epidermis, dermis, or both. Clinically, this presents as an abrasion, blister or shallow crater.
Stage III	Full-thickness skin loss with damage to subcutaneous tissue which extends down to, but not through, underlying fascia. Clinically, this presents as a deep crater that may have undermining of adjacent tissue.
Stage IV	Full-thickness skin loss with extensive destruction, tissue necrosis, or damage to muscle, bone, or supporting structures such as tendon or joint capsule. Undermining and sinus tracts may be present.

When eschar is present, a pressure ulcer cannot be accurately assessed until the eschar is removed.

Pressure ulcers do not necessarily progress in order, nor do they heal by reverse staging.

Investigations

- Complete history, including:
  - risk factors for pressure ulcer formation (Table 2)
  - concurrent medical problems that may impair wound healing, including peripheral vascular disease, diabetes mellitus, immune deficiencies, collagen vascular diseases, malignancy, malnutrition, psychosis and depression[1,2]
  - medications, especially steroids or immunosuppressives that impair wound healing. Also, drugs that can decrease the level of consciousness/sensory perception, e.g., sedatives, analgesics
- Physical examination:
  - assess the pressure ulcer for location, depth, size, sinus tracts, undermining, tunneling, exudate, necrotic tissue and the presence or absence of granulation tissue and epithelialization (Table 1)[1,3,4]

- Laboratory tests:
  - prealbumin[4] or albumin

Table 2: **Select Risk/Causative Factors for Pressure Ulcers[3,5]**

Local	Systemic
Dry skin	Circulatory disturbance
Excessive moisture	Malnutrition
Friction	Prolonged immobilization, e.g., fractures, spinal cord injury
Pressure, especially overlying bony prominences	Sensory deficit
Shearing forces	Smoking

Therapeutic Choices (Figure 1)

Strategies for the management of pressure ulcers include risk/causative factor modification and local ulcer care.

Risk/Causative Factor Modification

Healing of pressure ulcers is unlikely unless the underlying causative factors are corrected.

Pressure: External pressure is concentrated over bony prominences and will rapidly lead to tissue necrosis. If pressure is intermittently relieved, minimal skin changes occur.[3] Less pressure is required to create tissue ischemia in patients with impaired circulation secondary to disease process or injury, in patients receiving vasopressors and in patients with conditions resulting in impaired oxygenation or perfusion.[4] Pressure relief is the cornerstone of both prevention and treatment[6] and may be accomplished by:

- not placing patients on the pressure ulcer. If possible, raise the ulcer off the support surface. If the ulcer is on a sitting surface, the patient should not be placed in a sitting position. Avoid using ring cushions (donuts), as these cause venous congestion and edema and are more likely to cause pressure ulcers than to prevent them.[1]
- encouraging patients with enough mobility to shift position every 15 to 30 minutes.[7]
- turning bedridden patients every two hours and repositioning sitting individuals without adequate mobility every hour.[1] Implement a written repositioning schedule to protect intact skin.[4]
- avoiding the placement of patients directly on bony prominences.[1] Positioning the patient in the 30° lateral side-lying position instead of directly over the trochanter allows for reduced pressure and improved circulation to the skin overlying the trochanters.[4]
- using soft pillows between bony prominences.[1]
- using commercially available pressure-reducing surfaces.[3,6] Pressure-reducing surfaces may be static or dynamic. Static surfaces

include mattresses or mattress overlays, which are filled with air, water, gel, foam or a combination of these. Dynamic support surfaces include alternating-pressure mattresses, low-air-loss beds and air-fluidized mattresses.[8] There is no compelling evidence that one support surface, static or dynamic, consistently performs better than all others under all circumstances.[1,8] However, specially designed products are generally more effective than standard mattresses for preventing and healing pressure ulcers.[8,9]

Shearing forces: Shearing forces diminish circulation, and damage both tissue and blood vessel integrity.[4] When the head of a supine patient is raised more than 30°, shearing forces occur in the sacral and coccygeal areas.[3] Maintain the head of the bed at the lowest degree of elevation consistent with concurrent medical conditions and other restrictions.[1]

Friction: Friction ulcers often occur over elbows and heels in bedridden patients as they use their elbows and heels to aid in movement.[4] Friction can be minimized by lifting rather than dragging a bedridden patient across bed sheets, by keeping the bed free of particulate matter such as crumbs, and by keeping sheets loose to avoid restricting movement.

Excessive moisture: A long-term moist environment may result from perspiration or fecal or urinary incontinence. Cleanse the skin and remove moisture at the time of soiling.[1] Moisture barrier creams and incontinence briefs may be used for incontinence.[10] A bowel routine and intermittent or permanent catheterization may be considered.

Dry skin: There is an association between pressure ulcers and dry, flaky, scaling skin.[5,8] Well-moisturized skin retains its barrier properties and helps to prevent skin breakdown.

Malnutrition: Although a causal relationship has not been established, nutritional parameters have been correlated with the development of pressure ulcers. There is suggestive evidence that improving nutritional status can help with pressure ulcer prevention and healing.[8,11] Prealbumin is a more sensitive indicator of nutritional status than albumin. Albumin may be affected by hydration status and has a 21-day half-life, whereas prealbumin has a 2-day half-life and is more reflective of current nutritional status.[4] Encourage dietary intake or supplementation if an individual with a pressure ulcer is malnourished. Malnourished patients with a high protein diet have a higher frequency of ulcer healing and a greater decrease in ulcer size than patients with a low protein diet.[12,13] Give vitamin and mineral supplements if deficiencies are suspected or confirmed.[1] A dietary consultation may be warranted.

Immobilization: Early mobilization is encouraged. A physiotherapy consultation may be valuable.

Sensory and circulatory compromise: Optimization of the treatment of contributing medical problems, such as diabetes, will assist in the healing of existing pressure ulcers and the prevention of new ones.

Smoking: Excessive smoking may cause anorexia, contributing to malnutrition.[14] Smoking also causes vasoconstriction and relative tissue hypoxia, which may impair wound healing.

Local Ulcer Care

- The ulcer should be monitored at every dressing change and reassessed at least once per week.[1,2]
- Tracings or colour photos may be helpful for record keeping.[3]
- Local ulcer care involves wound débridement, wound cleansing and appropriate dressing choices.[1]

Wound Débridement

Removal of devitalized tissue and inflammatory agents is necessary to allow granulation tissue formation and subsequent re-epithelialization.[3,15] Wound débridement may be accomplished in four ways:

- *Sharp débridement* with scissors or scalpel is indicated for thick adherent eschars, extensive devitalized tissue or urgent débridement in infected ulcers.[3] Use sterile instruments.[1] If there is bleeding during débridement, pressure should be applied with gauze until the bleeding is controlled. Electrocautery may also be used for hemostasis. A clean, dry dressing may be used for 6 to 24 hours, after which a moist dressing may be reinstated.[1,16] Algosteril, an absorptive dressing from the xerogels category, also functions as a procoagulant and can be used to obtain hemostasis in oozing wounds.[17]
- *Autolytic débridement* involves synthetic dressings, especially hydrocolloids and hydrogels, to cover a wound and allow devitalized tissue to self-digest with wound fluid enzymes. Autolytic débridement may be appropriate for patients who cannot tolerate other methods and have uninfected wounds.[1,3] Wounds must be frequently and effectively cleansed to wash out partially degraded tissue fragments at each dressing change.[15] If wound fluid remains in prolonged contact with intact skin, maceration and further skin impairment may occur. Periwound skin protection is vital, and skin sealants or barrier ointments should be used to protect the surrounding intact skin.[4]
- *Mechanical débridement* may be performed in several ways, including wet-to-dry dressings, hydrotherapy or wound irrigation at moderate pressures. Wet-to-dry dressings adhere to eschar and remove the eschar when the dry dressing is removed.[1] They should be used only for débridement and then immediately discontinued.[3] Hydrotherapy and wound irrigation are useful for softening and mechanically removing eschar and debris.[1] Proper irrigation pressure may be obtained using a 35 mL syringe with a 19-gauge angiocatheter.[3]
- *Enzymatic débridement* is performed by applying enzyme-impregnated dressings to wounds.[17] This method may be used in long-term care facilities and in home care on uninfected ulcers.[1]

Wound Cleansing

- Wounds should be cleansed at initial examination and at each dressing change.
- Irrigation with normal saline may be used to clean most ulcers. Following irrigation, the surrounding skin should be gently patted dry to facilitate optimal adherence of the dressing.[1,16] Care must be taken to avoid maceration and to avoid spreading bacteria to other skin sites.
- To avoid traumatizing the wound, minimal mechanical force should be used when cleansing with gauze, cloth or sponges.[1] Use the smoothest and softest device possible.[6] Antiseptic agents, hydrogen peroxide and skin cleansers are toxic to wound tissue and should not be used.[1,16]
- Whirlpool treatment may be helpful for ulcers with thick exudate, slough and necrotic tissue, but is inappropriate for clean wounds.[1,2] Discontinue whirlpool treatment when the ulcer is clean.[1]

Choice of Dressings

The categories of wound dressings are shown in Table 3. Wound dressing choices for ulcer stages are outlined in Figure 2.

- The goals are to choose a dressing that will:
  - keep the ulcer bed continuously moist but not macerated[18]
  - be absorbent enough to control exudate without desiccating the ulcer bed[1,18]
  - keep the surrounding skin intact and dry[1]
  - protect the wound[3]
- Hydrocolloid dressings are more efficacious than conventional dressings when treating pressure ulcers, with increased healing rates and reduced healing times.[19] Comparisons between advanced dressings do not demonstrate significant differences in healing rates.[19] One trial suggests that sequential treatment with calcium alginate dressings for four weeks for débridement, followed by hydrocolloid dressings for four weeks to promote tissue granulation, will accelerate the healing of grade III and IV pressure ulcers.[20]
- As wounds heal, the dressing needs may change and the wound care plan should be re-evaluated.
- When applying the dressing:
  - dead space should be eliminated by loosely filling all cavities. Tissue must not be overpacked, as this may increase intra-wound pressure and cause additional tissue damage[1,3]
  - optimal secondary dressings should cover about 3 cm of intact, dry skin around the ulcer[16]
  - dressings should not exert tension on the skin, as the resulting shearing forces increase the risk of further tissue breakdown[16]
  - change dressing when drainage has seeped out from beneath it, indicating that the bacterial barrier has been compromised[16]

- frequency of dressing changes must be individually determined. For uncomplicated wounds, change occlusive dressings every three to seven days, as this minimally disturbs healing tissue between dressing changes. If there are other factors, such as an underlying infection or excessive exudate, the dressing changes should be more frequent

Negative pressure wound therapy (NPWT) is a newer technology that promotes wound healing by draining and removing infectious material or other fluids through continuous and/or intermittent (five minutes on/two minutes off) negative pressure.[21]

- NPWT applies subatmospheric pressure to the wound bed via a computerized therapy unit attached to a reticulated foam dressing placed in the wound and secured with an adhesive drape.[21,22]
- This application causes mechanical stress on tissue and the wound is drawn closed. While the degree of pressure to the wounded tissue is small, all areas of the wound work together in an effort to close towards the centre point. NPWT results in quicker closure and resolution of wounds.[21]
- NPWT is best used for Stage III or IV pressure ulcers.[21]
- The wound should be large enough for adequate contact between the foam dressing and the wound bed, and for safe removal of the foam.[21]
- NPWT should be considered if the wound has inadequate or poor granulation tissue and heavy exudate.[21]
- Overall nursing time may be reduced, as fewer dressing changes are required.[22]

Complications

Infection: All stage II to IV ulcers are colonized with bacteria. In most cases, adequate cleansing and débridement prevent colonization from progressing to clinical infection, and healing will still occur.[1]

Inapparent infection may occur, with increased bacterial burden and the usual signs of infection absent. Consider a two-week trial of **topical antibiotics** for clean pressure ulcers that are not healing or are continuing to produce excessive exudate after two to four weeks of optimal patient care.[1,3] Contact dermatitis, bacterial resistance and systemic absorption may occur with topical antibiotics.

Infected pressure ulcers may lead to cellulitis, bacteremia, sepsis or osteomyelitis.[1] Surrounding erythema or swelling greater than 2 cm may indicate cellulitis. If a sterile probe can be inserted to bone, the patient should be considered to have osteomyelitis until proven otherwise,[23] and appropriate **systemic antibiotic therapy** instituted.[1,3] Quantification of bacterial levels in wound tissue may be accomplished by culture swab, tissue biopsy or needle aspiration. When performing a swab culture, proper technique is imperative. Thoroughly cleanse the wound with normal saline, superficially débride to access the deepest wound compartment and swab the culturette in the part of the wound with the most visible signs of infection.[4] Consider an internal medicine or infectious disease consult.

Malignancy: Squamous cell carcinoma has been reported in pressure ulcers, and malignancy should be considered in nonhealing ulcers.[1] If suspected, obtain a dermatology or plastic surgery consultation.

Sinus tracts: Sinus tracts may occur even in superficial pressure ulcers and may contribute to abscess formation or osteomyelitis.[1] If suspected, consider a plastic surgery consultation.

Pain: Patients should be assessed regularly for pain related to the pressure ulcer. Pain relief may be appropriate at certain times, such as before dressing changes.[24] If necessary, administer analgesics prior to wound examination or manipulation.[4,24] Potential topical medications include the **lidocaine** 5% patch or the **eutectic mixture of local anesthetics (EMLA)** consisting of lidocaine 2.5% and prilocaine 2.5%.[24] If pain continues to be an issue, consider the pain-reducing properties of various dressings. Hydrogels and hydrocolloids are both associated with decreased pain.[4]

Therapeutic Tips

- Stage I and II pressure ulcers should show evidence of healing within one to two weeks, and stage III and IV pressure ulcers should show evidence of healing within two to four weeks. If no progress is seen, consider the presence of complications and re-evaluate the treatment plan.[1,2]
- In general, stage I, II and III pressure ulcers are more likely to heal with local therapy. Stage IV pressure ulcers, especially over ischial tuberosities, often require surgical intervention.[14]
- Patients should be continually assessed for adequate pain management throughout the treatment of the pressure ulcer. Nonmedicinal methods to reduce pain at dressing changes include identifying what the patient recognizes as pain triggers and as pain-alleviating factors. Involve the patient in the dressing change, if possible, including allowing the patient to remove the dressing themselves. Encourage slow, rhythmic breathing throughout the procedure, and offer the patient the option of a "time-out" during the dressing change.[24]
- When using NPWT, patients may experience pain during dressing changes. Unless medically contraindicated, 1% lidocaine solution may be introduced down the tubing or injected into the foam dressing before a dressing change. The pump must be set no higher than 50 mm Hg during this procedure. Wait 15 to 20 minutes before removing the dressing.[21]
- Caregiver time and associated labour costs are a significant component of the total cost of caring for a pressure ulcer and should be considered when selecting a dressing. Caregiver labour costs can exceed the cost of supplies in wound management. For example, continuously moistened saline gauze is inexpensive, but can consume up to 10 times

more nursing time than more expensive occlusive dressings such as hydrocolloids or transparent film.[18]

- The early recognition and correction of risk factors will expedite the healing of existing pressure ulcers and may prevent the formation of new pressure ulcers. Specialized support surfaces and dressings do not replace the need for vigilant nursing care. Consider incorporating pressure ulcer risk factor monitoring and prevention into regular nursing procedures to cue nurses to implement preventive measures.[4]

Table 3: **Classification of Wound Dressings**[1,10,17]

Dressing	Characteristics	Wound
Transparent film dressings Biocclusive, Opsite, TegaDerm	Semi-permeable, highly flexible dressings that reduce evaporative water loss, provide good antibacterial barriers, and reduce shearing forces.	Superficial wounds, abrasions and partial-thickness wounds.
Gauze dressings Adherent: 4 × 4 Gauze Non-adherent: Telfa, N-Terface	Débrides, but painful upon removal unless moistened first. Must be secured in place.	Partial- or full-thickness wounds with necrotic debris or covered with antibiotic ointment.
Hydrocolloid dressings DuoDerm, Restore, Comfeel	Available as composite sheets with a hydrophilic polymer and a water-impermeable vapor-transmitting backing or in paste form. They are occlusive and provide an excellent barrier. Wound exudate is absorbed and a gel is formed that expands into the wound cavity. Promotes autolytic débridement. Usually requires less frequent changes.	Both partial- and full-thickness wounds, especially superficial wounds.
Hydrogel dressings Intrasite gel, Vigilon, Nu-Gel, Clearsite, Duoderm gel	Three-dimensional networks of hydrophilic polymers made from gelatin and polysaccharides. Absorbs exudate with medium capacity and provides cooling and pain relief. Promotes autolytic débridement and granulation. Can both absorb fluid and hydrate desiccated eschars.	Full-thickness wounds with or without undermining.

(cont'd)

Table 3: **Classification of Wound Dressings**[1,10,17] *(cont'd)*

Dressing	Characteristics	Wound
Xerogel dressings Kaltostat, Algosteril, Sorbsan, Debrisan, Aquacel	Dry dressings with high absorptive capacity that change into a gel-like substance upon contacting wound exudate. After the exudate is absorbed, xerogels act similarly to hydrogels in facilitating moist wound healing. Alginates (xerogels with hemostatic properties) are also procoagulants and can be used to obtain hemostasis in oozing wounds.	Full-thickness wounds with slough, with or without undermining.
Foam dressings Lyofoam, Epilock, Hydrosorb, Allevyn	Polymeric dressings that maximize absorbency and vapour permeability to provide optimal exudate handling. May be combined with a water-impermeable but vapour-transmitting backing to allow vapour loss. When the exudate contacts the backing, evaporative loss facilitates exudate control. Expansion of the foam as it absorbs exudate creates gentle pressure on the wound, possibly reducing wound edema.	Full-thickness wounds with exudate. Can be used around wound drains and tubes or over incisions.
Enzymatic dressings Collagenase	Enzymatic dressings apply topical débriding agents to devitalized tissue on the wound surface. A clean moist dressing should be applied over the ulcer after enzyme application.	Wounds with eschar.

Figure 1: **Pressure Ulcer Therapy**

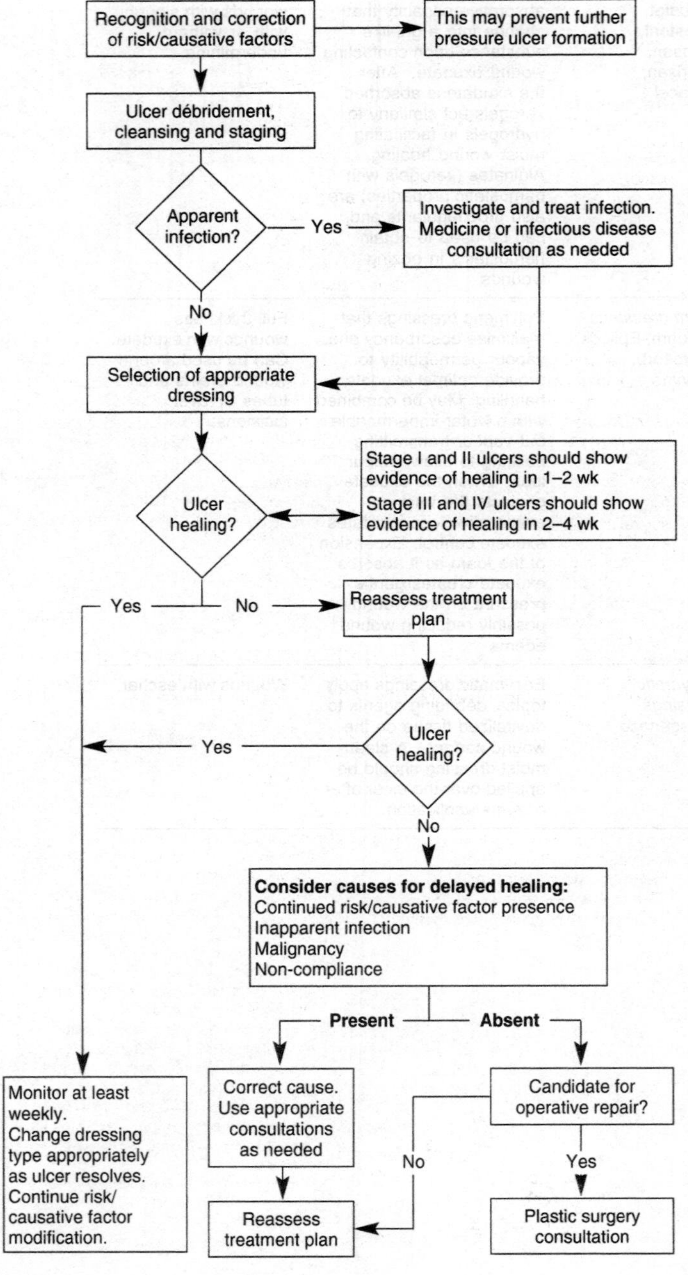

Figure 2: **Dressing Choices for Pressure Ulcers**

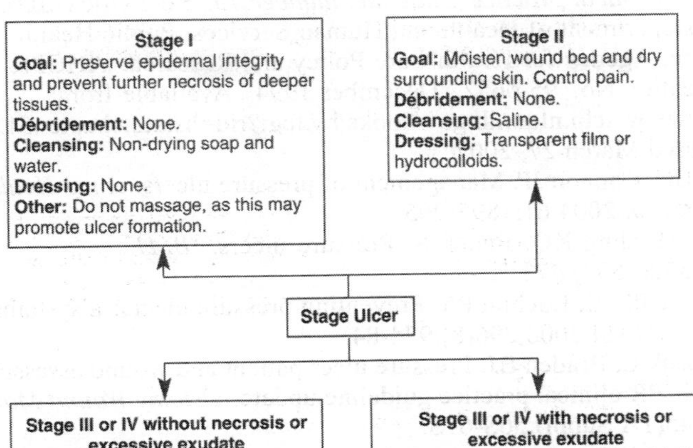

Stage III or IV without necrosis or excessive exudate

Goal: Moisten wound bed and dry surrounding skin.
Débridement: Autolytic with occlusive dressings.
Cleansing: Saline irrigation (35 cc syringe with 19-gauge angiocatheter).
Dressing:

1. If very shallow, use hydrocolloids or hydrogel wafers.
2. If dead space present, lightly fill with hydrogels.

Apply hydrocolloid dressing over wound filler.

3. If no signs of healing are seen after several weeks of appropriate care, consider referral for negative pressure wound therapy.

Stage III or IV with necrosis or excessive exudate

Goal: Débride necrotic material, minimize damage to granulating tissue, keep surrounding skin intact and dry.
Débridement:

1. Infection (advancing cellulitis, bacteremia or sepsis) — sharp débridement.
2. Eschars — soften with an occlusive dressing then use sharp débridement.
3. Slough — use mechanical wet-to-dry saline dressings, enzymatic, or autolytic débridement. Switch once slough resolved. Whirlpool baths may be used.

Cleansing: Saline irrigation (35 cc syringe with 19-gauge angiocatheter).
Dressing:

1. If mechanical débridement is appropriate, use wet-to-dry saline-soaked gauze.

Loosely fill dead space and undermined area.
Do not moisten before removal.

2. After sharp débridement with bleeding, dry dressing or alginate for 6-24 h.

Moisten any dry dressings before removal.

3. If excessive exudate, use xerogels or foams. Protect surrounding skin with barrier ointment.
4. If malodorous or purulent exudate, topical antibacterial agents. If cellulitis, use systemic antibiotics.
5. If no signs of healing are seen after several weeks of appropriate care, consider referral for negative pressure wound therapy.
6. Once necrosis is no longer present, stop débridement and refer to **Stage III and IV without necrosis or excessive exudate.**

At all stages: Search for and correct risk/causative factors. Especially relieve local pressure and optimize systemic condition.

Suggested Readings

Bergstrom N, Allman RM, Alvarez OM et al. *Treatment of pressure ulcers. Clinical practice guideline, number 15.* Rockville (MD): U.S. Department of Health and Human Services, Public Health Service, Agency for Health Care Policy and Research. AHCPR Publication No. 95-0652. December 1994. Available from: http://www.ncbi.nlm.nih.gov/books/bv.fcgi?rid=hstat2.chapter.5124 Accessed March 27, 2007.

Cannon BC, Cannon JP. Management of pressure ulcers. *Am J Health Syst Pharm* 2004;61:1895-905.

Grey JE, Harding KG, Enoch S. Pressure ulcers. *BMJ* 2006;332(7539):472-5.

Reddy M, Gill SS, Rochon PA. Preventing pressure ulcers: a systematic review. *JAMA* 2006;296(8):974-84.

van Rijswijk L, Braden BJ. Pressure ulcer patient and wound assessment: an AHCPR clinical practice guideline update. *Ostomy Wound Manage* 1999;45(1A Suppl):56S-67S.

References

1. Bergstrom N, Allman RM, Alvarez OM et al. *Treatment of pressure ulcers. Clinical practice guideline, number 15.* Rockville (MD): U.S. Department of Health and Human Services, Public Health Service, Agency for Health Care Policy and Research. AHCPR Publication No. 95-0652. December 1994. Available from: http://www.ncbi.nlm.nih.gov/books/bv.fcgi?rid=hstat2.chapter.5124 Accessed March 27, 2007.
2. van Rijswijk L, Braden BJ. Pressure ulcer patient and wound assessment: an AHCPR clinical practice guideline update. *Ostomy Wound Manage* 1999;45(1A Suppl):56S-67S.
3. Kanj LF, Wilking SV, Phillips TJ. Pressure ulcers. *J Am Acad Dermatol* 1998;38(4):517-36.
4. Arnold MC. Pressure ulcer prevention and management: the current evidence for care. *AACN Clin Issues* 2003;14(4):411-28.
5. Guralnik JM, Harris TB, White LR et al. Occurrence and predictors of pressure sores in the National Health and Nutrition Examination survey follow-up. *J Am Geriatr Soc* 1988;36(9):807-12.
6. Wysocki AB. Decubitus ulcers. In: Freedberg IM et al, editors. *Fitzpatrick's dermatology in general medicine.* 5th ed. New York (NY): McGraw-Hill; 1999.
7. Grey JE, Harding KG, Enoch S. Pressure ulcers. *BMJ* 2006;332(7539):472-5.
8. Reddy M, Gill SS, Rochon PA. Preventing pressure ulcers: a systematic review. *JAMA* 2006;296(8):974-84.
9. Cullum N, Nelson EA, Flemming K et al. Systematic reviews of wound care management: (5) beds; (6) compression; (7) laser therapy, therapeutic ultrasound, electrotherapy and electromagnetic therapy. *Health Technol Assess* 2001;5(9):1-221.
10. Bergstrom NI. Strategies for preventing pressure ulcers. *Clin Geriatr Med* 1997;13(3):437-54.
11. Thomas DR. Improving outcome of pressure ulcers with nutritional interventions: a review of the evidence. *Nutrition* 2001;17(2):121-5.
12. Cannon BC, Cannon JP. Management of pressure ulcers. *Am J Health Syst Pharm* 2004;61(18):1895-905.
13. Lyder CH. Pressure ulcer prevention and management. *Annu Rev Nurs Res* 2002;20:35-61.
14. Staas WE, LaMantia JG. Decubitus ulcers and rehabilitation medicine. *Int J Dermatol* 1982;21(8):437-44.
15. Rodeheaver GT. Pressure ulcer debridement and cleansing: a review of current literature. *Ostomy Wound Manage* 1999;45(1A Suppl):80S-85S.
16. Goode PS, Thomas DR. Pressure ulcers. Local wound care. *Clin Geriatr Med* 1997;13(3):543-52.
17. Ladin DA. Understanding dressings. *Clin Plast Surg* 1998;25(3):433-41.
18. Ovington LG. Dressings and ajunctive therapies: AHCPR guidelines revisited. *Ostomy Wound Manage* 1999;45(1A Suppl):94S-106S.
19. Bouza C, Saz Z, Munoz A et al. Efficacy of advanced dressings in the treatment of pressure ulcers: a systematic review. *J Wound Care* 2005;14(5):193-9.
20. Belmin J, Meaume S, Rabus MT et al. Sequential treatment with calcium alginate dressings and hydrocolloid dressings accelerates pressure ulcer healing in older subjects: a multicenter randomized trial of sequential versus nonsequential treatment with hydrocolloid dressings alone. *J Am Geriatr Soc* 2002;50(2):269-74.

21. Gupta S, Baharestani M, Baranoski S et al. Guidelines for managing pressure ulcers with negative pressure wound therapy. *Adv Skin Wound Care* 2004;17(Suppl 2):1-16.
22. Banwell PE, Teot L. Topical negative pressure (TNP): the evolution of a novel wound therapy. *J Wound Care* 2003;12(1):22-8.
23. Grayson ML, Gibbons GW, Balogh K et al. Probing to bone in infected pedal ulcers. A clinical sign of underlying osteomyelitis in diabetic patients. *JAMA* 1995;273(9):721-3.
24. [No authors listed]. Local approaches to the pain of pressure ulcers. *Ostomy Wound Manage* 2005;51(1):20, 22.

CHAPTER 82
Psoriasis

Jean-Pierre DesGroseilliers, MD, MSc, FRCPC

Psoriasis is a chronic skin disease with markedly increased epidermal cellular turnover. Activation of T cells also plays a role in the etiology of psoriasis. Before making therapeutic choices, it is essential that other conditions that affect the same areas of the body be ruled out and the correct diagnosis be established. A regional approach is provided since patients often present with a skin problem affecting their scalp, face, hands and feet, body, fold areas or nails.

Goals of Therapy

- Improve the physical signs of psoriasis and the patient's quality of life
- Facilitate the patient's acceptance of this chronic disease coupled with realistic expectations
- Provide psoriasis control for the longest periods possible

The management of psoriasis affecting all areas of the body is illustrated in Figure 1.

Scalp

Seborrheic dermatitis most often mimics psoriasis. However, the psoriatic scale is thicker and more adherent than that seen in seborrheic dermatitis. As well, there are often signs of psoriasis on the knees, elbows or sacral area.

Pharmacologic Choices (Table 3)

Removal of the scales is essential. This can be done with oil-based products with or without **salicylic acid**, **calcipotriol scalp solution**, and/or a medium-strength **corticosteroid** such as **betamethasone** left on the scalp overnight. For more resistant cases, **tar-based shampoos** can be used in the morning to wash off the oil and scales. Results depend on the frequency of application so it is better to apply tar shampoo every two to three nights than not at all.

Face

On the face, the nature of the scale helps to differentiate.

- Psoriasis—sharply demarcated, silvery scale
- Seborrheic dermatitis—greasy, brownish-yellow scale
- Discoid lupus erythematosus—adherent, carpet-tack scale
- Tinea of face—little or no scale except at the margins

Pharmacologic Choices (Table 3)

Hydrocortisone 1% cream is often sufficient to control psoriasis of the face as long as it is applied regularly. At first, applications should be in the morning and at bedtime. As improvement occurs, decrease the frequency of application to bedtime only and eventually every two to three nights. Avoid long-term use of medium- or higher-strength corticosteroids on the face as these products have been associated with skin thinning, striae, telangiectasias, purpura and acne.

Topical **calcineurin inhibitors** such as **tacrolimus** and **pimecrolimus** are indicated for the treatment of atopic dermatitis. These agents have also been used in patients with facial psoriasis since they are not associated with cutaneous atrophy or acneiform eruptions. The long-term risk of malignancy related to the use of calcineurin inhibitors is controversial, but currently there are insufficient data to support a strong association. Use the minimum amount of these medications for the shortest time necessary.[4,5,6]

Hands and Feet

Psoriasis of palms and soles is one of the most difficult dermatologic conditions to treat. Correct diagnosis is important, as each condition requires very different treatment (see Table 1). The time spent in making the correct diagnosis is worthwhile. Trauma to these areas should be minimized.

Table 1: **Differential Diagnosis for Psoriasis of the Hands and Feet**

	Psoriasis	Tinea	Eczema
Lesion	Well-defined scaling, hyperkeratosis and/or pustules	Scaling and vesicles	Poorly defined scaling, vesicles, pustules
	Maceration between all toes	Maceration between 4th and 5th toes	Maceration between all toes
Site	Weight-bearing areas of soles	Instep area	Weight-bearing area
	Bilateral hands and feet	Asymmetrical	Symmetrical
	Pits of nails	Asymmetrical nail changes	Nonspecific nail changes
	Psoriasis elsewhere	Tinea cruris	Eczema elsewhere
Response to topicals			
Tar	++	–	+

(cont'd)

Table 1: **Differential Diagnosis for Psoriasis of the Hands and Feet** *(cont'd)*

	Psoriasis	Tinea	Eczema
Topical steroids	+	–/+	++
Antifungals	–	++	–

Pharmacologic Choices

Topical Therapy (Table 3)

One choice is frequent lubrication with **petrolatum** and medium- to high-potency **corticosteroid ointment** with or without added salicylic acid. Ointments are the most effective delivery system since they increase permeability in areas that are dry and scaly. Lotions can be used in thinner-skinned areas. Creams are cosmetically more acceptable and can be used in areas involved in movement.

Agents such as **tazarotene** (vitamin A derivative) and **calcipotriol** (vitamin D derivative) alone or combined with betamethasone dipropionate can be used with ultraviolet light (UV).[3]

Phototherapy[8]

Phototherapy includes UVB with tar, anthralin, calcipotriol or tazarotene, or UVA with **psoralen** (PUVA) applied topically as a soak for 10 minutes prior to UVA exposure (20 mg psoralen dissolved in 2 L of water). This treatment is best guided by a dermatologist. Some centres have added Narrow-Band UVB (NBUVB–311 to 313 nm) to their phototherapy modalities. These newer lamps obviate the need for topical or systemic treatments. Phototherapy is also advancing with the use of excimer laser (308 nm) for resistant localized psoriatic plaques as well as topical 5-aminolevulinic acid cream followed by broadband visible light exposure.[1,3,8]

Systemic Therapy (Table 4)

Acitretin, an oral retinoid, 25 to 75 mg daily, **methotrexate** 7.5 to 22.5 mg once a week or **cyclosporine** for short periods at a starting dose of 2 mg/kg/day have been used in the treatment of moderate to severe psoriasis.

Body and Extremities

Classic psoriasis with nonpruritic, silvery scaling plaques affecting the elbows, knees and sacral areas is usually easy to diagnose. Tinea versicolor has a fine orange-brown scale and is limited to the upper thorax. Pityriasis rosea has oval, pink lesions with a fine collarette of central scale and rarely affects elbows and knees. Eczematous dermatitis is itchy and often crusty, lichenified and excoriated. Tinea corporis has an active periphery with a clear centre and a positive potassium hydroxide (KOH) examination for fungal elements.

Pharmacologic Choices (Table 3 and Table 4)

Choosing the appropriate therapy from a number of effective topical and systemic pharmacologic agents is difficult. The tars used with UVB are either 2% **crude coal tar** or 10% **coal tar distillate** with or without **salicylic acid**. For PUVA bath, the patient soaks in a psoralen solution for 10 minutes prior to UVA exposure (100 mg psoralen dissolved in 75 L of water.) For systemic PUVA, the dose of methoxsalen is 0.5 to 0.8 mg/kg body weight given two hours prior to UVA radiation.

As a rule, phototherapy is used only if common local treatments with corticosteroids, calcipotriol, tazarotene, tars or anthralin are ineffective on their own. If required, consult a dermatologist who is familiar with phototherapy and the various systemic therapies (see Table 4).

Fold Areas

In these areas, the diagnosis can be difficult to make (see Table 2), but the treatment will usually include a topical corticosteroid.

Table 2: **Differential Diagnosis for Psoriasis in Fold Areas**

Psoriasis	Tinea	Eczema	Moniliasis
Bright red, well-defined	Scaling at edge	Very itchy	Satellite papules and pustules
KOH -ve	KOH +ve	KOH -ve	KOH +ve
Psoriasis elsewhere	Maceration between 4th and 5th toes	Eczema elsewhere	Affects fold areas mainly

Abbreviations: KOH = potassium hydroxide stain, which is diagnostic for fungi.

Pharmacologic Choices (Table 3)

In most cases, daily to twice daily applications of **hydrocortisone 1% cream** with or without an antimonilial/antifungal agent, such as **ketoconazole**, will dramatically improve the eruption with little or no adverse effects.

Nails

Psoriatic nail changes can be difficult to differentiate from fungal infection of the nails. Both cause yellowish-white discolouration of the distal nail plate but psoriasis produces small "ice pick" pits of the nail.

Pharmacologic Choices (Table 4)

Most topical therapeutic measures are unsatisfactory. Systemic therapy is often required for patients with psoriatic nail changes. It is advisable to keep the nails short to decrease the risk of nail separation caused by trauma. Discourage aggressive manicures.

Therapeutic Tips

- Customize the treatment to the patient. A number of factors need to be considered when opting for one treatment versus another, and the patient must be an equal partner in the decision process.
  - Consider affordability of prescribed medication. This may be especially important when considering the use of a biologic agent.
  - Topicals can be problematic as tar has an odour and anthralin stains.
  - Phototherapy sessions require considerable patient commitment (three to five sessions per week).
  - Side effects of systemic therapies can be severe and must be understood by the patient.
  - Question the diagnosis if there is no relief of disease within one month of optimal therapy.
- Combining oral retinoids and phototherapy gives better results in severe psoriasis than using each treatment separately. The use of biologics with UV is currently under investigation.
- Biologic therapies are alternatives for patients with moderate to severe psoriasis.[9] **Alefacept**, **efalizumab** and **etanercept** are approved in Canada for the treatment of psoriasis.
- Intralesional steroid injections (e.g., triamcinolone every three to six weeks to a maximum of 20 mg) are used occasionally for very resistant psoriatic plaques.
- Length of remission is longer with phototherapy but there still is no definitive cure for psoriasis.
- The continued care of the patient by the family physician should be the foundation on which occasional evaluations by the dermatologist can be added as needed.

Figure 1: **Management of Psoriasis**[1,2,3]

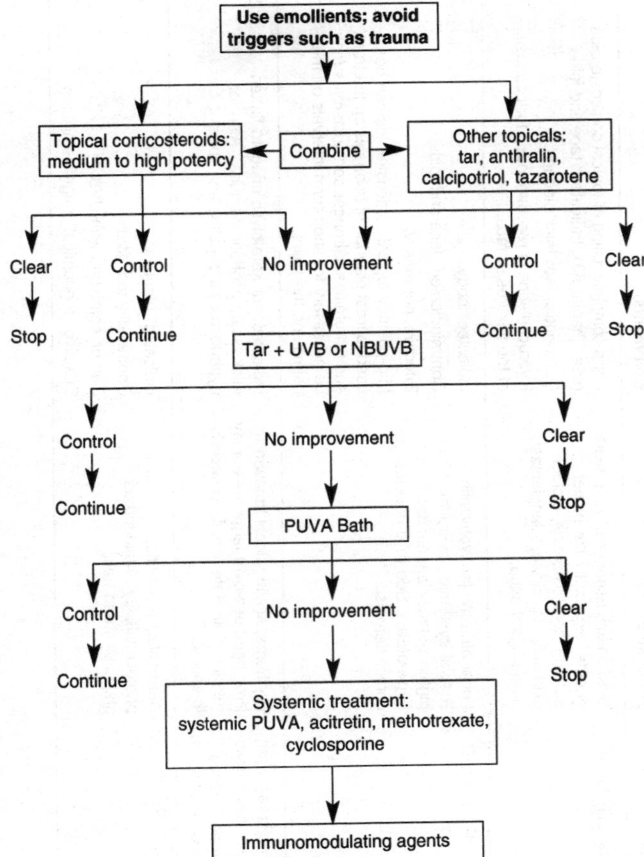

Abbreviations: UVB = ultraviolet-B; NBUVB = narrow-band ultraviolet-B; PUVA = psoraien ultraviolet light

Table 3: Topical Psoriasis Therapies

Class	Drug	Dose	Adverse Effects	Comments	Cost[a]
Corticosteroids, mild potency[b]	*hydrocortisone 1% cream* Emo-Cort, Prevex HC, Sarna HC, generics	Once daily to BID	Side effects associated with these agents, especially the higher potency corticosteroids, include skin thinning, striae, telangiectasis, purpura and acne.	For a complete listing of topical corticosteroids (see Chapter 83). Indicated: face and folds. Contraindicated: thick plaques. Hydrocortisone is recommended for psoriasis of the flexures or face.	$-$$
Corticosteroids, mid- to high-potency[b]	*betamethasone valerate* Betaderm, Valisone Scalp Lotion, generics	Once daily to BID	Local atrophy, tachyphylaxis. Risk of systemic absorption with higher potency agents used over large areas. See mild potency corticosteroids.	Indicated: body. Contraindicated: face and folds. Effective, not messy. Mid-potency topical corticosteroids can be used to treat plaques of psoriasis on the trunk and extremities. Stronger corticosteroids may be necessary for short-term intervals on the palms and the soles.	$-$$
Keratolytic Agents	*salicylic acid*[c] 3-10%	Lotion, cream, gel: once or twice daily Shampoo: Once or twice weekly	Erythema, scaling, local irritation. Prolonged use over large areas may result in salicylate toxicity especially in children.	Indicated: for keratolytic effect to flatten thick, scaly psoriatic plaques. Also for hyperkeratosis of palms and soles.	$$
Tars	*coal tar* Balnetar, Liquor Carbonis Detergens, Targel, others	Once daily	Dermatitis, folliculitis, photosensitivity. Malodorous, stains skin and hair.	Indicated: plaques. Contraindicated: folds. Can be combined with UVB. Effective, economical, longer remission.	$

Class	Drug	Dose	Adverse Effects	Comments	Cost[a]
Anthracene Derivatives	*anthralin* Anthraforte, Anthranol, Micanol, others	Once daily	Irritating to surrounding normal skin. Stains skin and fabrics.	Indicated: plaques. Contraindicated: folds. Can be combined with UVB. Effective, economical, longer remission.	$$
Retinoids	*tazarotene* *0.05%, 0.1%* Tazorac Cream, Tazorac Gel	Once daily	Skin irritation.	Indicated: body. Contraindicated: face and folds. Longer remission.	$$$$
Vitamin D Derivatives	*calcipotriol* Dovonex	Dovonex: BID	Skin irritation.	Indicated: body. Contraindicated: face and folds. Longer remission.	$$$
	calcipotriol/ betamethasone Dovobet	Dovobet: once daily	Skin irritation.	See calcipotriol.	$$$$

[a] Cost of 50 g or 50 mL for topical products or 30-day supply; includes drug cost only.
[b] Listed drugs are examples of medications in this class.
[c] Extemporaneously compounded preparations can be used.
Legend: $ < $10 $-$$ < $10–25 $$ $10–25 $$$ $25–50 $$$$ $50–100

Table 4: Systemic Psoriasis Therapies

Class	Drug	Dose	Adverse Effects	Drug Interactions	Comments	Cost[a]
Psoralens with UVA (PUVA)	*methoxsalen* Oxsoralen, Ultramop	Bath: 100 mg/75 L bath water. Soak in aqueous solution for 10 min before UVA exposure. Oral: 0.5–0.8 mg/kg 2 h before UVA exposure 3 ×/wk	Photosensitivity, exaggerated sunburn. Nausea, pruritus, cataracts.		Indicated: total area. Use 3 ×/wk. Longest remission. Increased risk of skin cancer with long-term PUVA.	Bath:$$$$ Oral: $$$ (40 mg/dose)
Cytotoxics	*methotrexate* Methotrexate, Methotrexate Tablets, generics	7.5–22.5 mg/wk po	Bone marrow suppression, hepatotoxicity, gastrointestinal effects, pulmonary toxicity, blood dyscrasias.	Ethanol and acitretin may increase the risk of MTX-induced liver injury. Cholestyramine and colestipol may bind MTX in the gut. Trimethoprim may increase bone marrow suppression.	Indicated: total area. Contraindicated: liver disease. Use in conjunction with folic acid.	$$-$$$
Retinoids	*acitretin* Soriatane	25–75 mg/day po	Arthralgia, myalgia, alopecia, dry lips and mucosa, hyperlipidemia, hepatotoxicity.	Women should abstain from alcohol during treatment and for ≥ 2 months after stopping acitretin because of its conversion to etretinate (major teratogen). Risk of MTX-induced liver injury may be ↑ with acitretin.	Indicated: hands and feet. Teratogen, contraindicated in pregnancy.	$$$$-$$$$$

Class	Drug	Dose	Adverse Effects	Drug Interactions	Comments	Cost[a]
				"Minipill" progestin-only contraceptives may not be effective in patients taking acitretin. Avoid this combination.		
Biologic Response Modifiers	*alefacept* Amevive	15 mg im weekly for 12 weeks	Dose-dependent reduction of CD4+ counts, infections, malignancy. Mild injection site reactions, chills.	No formal drug interaction studies completed. Avoid use in patients receiving other immunosuppressant drugs. Safety and efficacy of live or attenuated vaccines have not been evaluated.	Indicated: moderate to severe psoriasis. CD4+ counts should be monitored every 2 weeks. Treatment withheld if count less than 250 cells/μL.	Approx. $15,000 for 12 wk
	efalizumab Raptiva	Initial: 0.7 mg/kg then 1 mg/kg weekly sc (maximum single dose of 200 mg)	Infection, immune-mediated hemolytic anemia and thrombocytopenia, malignancies, first-dose reaction (e.g., fever, chills, headache, myalgia).	No formal drug interaction studies completed. Immunosuppressants: concurrent use may increase risk of infection. Immunizations: acellular, live, and live-attenuated vaccines should not be administered during therapy.	Indicated: moderate to severe plaque psoriasis. Monitor platelet counts monthly at start of treatment and every 3 months as therapy continues.	Approx. $20,000 for 1 year
	etanercept Enbrel	Initial: 50 mg sc twice weekly for 3 months. Maintenance: 50 mg sc weekly	Injection site reactions, infections, autoimmune phenomena, worsening HF. Not to be used in patients with demyelinating disease. May ↑ risk of malignancy.	Live vaccines should not be administered during therapy. Anakinra: increased risk of serious infections when used concurrently. Sulfasalazine: decrease in mean white blood cell counts.	Indicated: chronic moderate to severe plaque psoriasis.	Approx. $20,000 for 1 year

[a] includes drug cost only

Dosage adjustment may be required in renal impairment; see Appendix I.

Legend: $ < $10 $$ $10–25 $$-$$$ $10–50 $$$ $25–50 $$$$ $50–100 $$$$-$$$$$ $50– >100 $$$$$ > $100

Suggested Readings

Guenther L, Langley RG, Shear NH et al. Integrating biologic agents into management of moderate-to-severe psoriasis: a consensus of the Canadian Psoriasis Expert Panel. *J Cutan Med Surg* 2004;8(5):321-37.

Kipnis CD, Myers WA, Opeola M, Gottlieb AB. Biologic treatments for psoriasis. *J Am Acad Dermatol* 2005;52(4):671-82.

Lui H. Phototherapy of psoriasis: update with practical pearls. *J Cutan Med Surg* 2002;6(3 Suppl):17-21.

Schon MP, Boehncke WH. Psoriasis. *N Engl J Med* 2005;352(18):1899-912.

Tremblay JF, Bissonnette R. Topical agents for the treatment of psoriasis, past, present and future. *J Cutan Med Surg* 2002;6(3 Suppl):8-11.

References

1. Lebwohl M, Ali S. Treatment of psoriasis. Part 1. Topical therapy and phototherapy. *J Am Acad Dermatol* 2001;45(4):487-98.
2. Lebwohl M, Ali S. Treatment of psoriasis. Part 2. Systemic therapies. *J Am Acad Dermatol* 2001;45(5):649-61.
3. Tremblay JF, Bissonnette R. Topical agents for the treatment of psoriasis, past, present and future. *J Cutan Med Surg* 2002;6(3 Suppl):8-11.
4. Health Canada. *Advisory: Safety information about Elidel cream and Protopic ointment*. Ottawa (ON): Health Canada; April 27, 2005. Available from: http://www.hc-sc.gc.ca/ahc-asc/media/advisories-avis/2005/2005_31_e.html Accessed March 28, 2006.
5. Food and Drug Administration. Pediatric Advisory Committee. *Briefing information*. Rockville (MD): FDA; February 15,2005. Available from: http://www.fda.gov/ohrms/dockets/ac/05/briefing/2005-4089b2.htm Accessed March 28, 2006.
6. Ormerod AD. Topical tacrolimus and pimecrolimus and the risk of cancer: how much cause for concern? *Br J Dermatol* 2005;153(4):701-5.
7. Fonacier L, Spergel J, Charlesworth EN et al. Report of the Topical Calcineurin Inhibitor Task Force of the American College of Allergy, Asthma and Immunology and the American Academy of Allergy, Asthma and Immunology. *J Allergy Clin Immunol* 2005;115(6):1249-53.
8. Lui H. Phototherapy of psoriasis: update with practical pearls. *J Cutan Med Surg* 2002;6 (3 Suppl):17-21.
9. Kipnis CD, Myers WA, Opeola M, Gottlieb AB. Biologic treatments for psoriasis. *J Am Acad Dermatol* 2005;52(4):671-82.

CHAPTER 83
Atopic Dermatitis

Miriam Weinstein, MD, FRCPC

Atopic dermatitis (AD) is an inflammatory disorder of the skin with an onset in early childhood. Patients typically have flares of dermatitis that are ill-defined patches of erythema, scale and excoriations. Significant pruritus and generalized xerosis are usually prominent features. Atopic dermatitis may be associated with other atopic conditions such as asthma, allergic rhinoconjunctivitis and food allergies.

Goals of Therapy

Atopic dermatitis is a chronic, recurring condition without a cure, so the major focus is control of dermatitis, pruritus and xerosis. Goals of therapy are:

- Relieve generalized xerosis and pruritus particularly when it interferes with activities of daily living
- Treat patches of dermatitis to reduce inflammation, pruritus and reduce risk of secondary infection
- Prevent flare-ups caused by environmental irritants
- Promptly treat complications of atopic dermatitis such as secondary bacterial or viral infection

Investigations

Physical exam may show one of three typical morphologic patterns:

- facial and extensor dermatitis in infants
- flexural and fold dermatitis in older children
- prominence of facial and hand dermatitis in adults

Investigations are rarely required for the work-up of classic atopic dermatitis. Bacterial swabs showing moderate or heavy growth of organisms may suggest secondary bacterial infections in resistant patches of dermatitis. However, many patients with atopic dermatitis are colonized with *S. aureus* so swabs with minimal growth may be difficult to interpret.

Therapeutic Choices (Figure 1)
Nonpharmacologic Choices

Reducing environmental irritants is very useful: use nonirritating soaps, double rinse clothing and avoid fabric softeners, perfumed products, wool and synthetic fibers, dry grass and leaves.

Patients with AD have abnormal barrier function so they cannot maintain adequate hydration. Frequent use of lubricating skin emollients such as petrolatum helps seal in moisture. Emollients are first-line therapy for prevention of flares and treatment of minimal irritation and itch. Even when medication is required, emollients should be used at least twice daily. After bathing, apply emollients within three minutes of light drying. Remind patients to apply medicated treatments directly against the skin, not over top of emollients. Emollients should contain no fragrances, few or no preservatives and no irritants (e.g., salicylic acid). Plain petrolatum jelly, while greasy, is highly effective, nonirritating and inexpensive.

Pharmacologic Choices

There are two classes of topical anti-inflammatory agents: **corticosteroids** and **calcineurin inhibitors**. Corticosteroids affect several inflammatory pathways in the skin and carry a risk of skin atrophy, telangiectasia, striae and purpura. Corticosteroids work quickly, are available in a wide variety of potencies and vehicles and their side effects are well known.

The actual clinical potency of topical corticosteroids depends on the molecular structure and vehicle as well as the thickness and integrity of the skin. There is no formula to calculate the precise relationship between these factors.[1] Some principles, however, can guide appropriate treatment selection (see Table 1, Table 2 and Table 3). A systematic review of once-daily versus more frequent use of potent topical corticosteroids in atopic dermatitis found little difference between regimens with respect to clinical outcomes and adverse events.[2] Use the fewest daily doses that will achieve control.

The calcineurin inhibitors (also referred to as topical immune modulators) are a newer class of medications designed to specifically block calcineurin. Calcineurin inhibitors provide a targeted, specific anti-inflammatory mechanism in contrast to the wide-ranging effects of corticosteroids. **Tacrolimus** and **pimecrolimus** are available in Canada. These products work slower than corticosteroids and generally require twice-daily dosing. Short-term safety data for these products are good.[3]

Concerns have been raised about the long-term safety of the calcineurin-inhibitors, in particular, the long-term risk of malignancy.[3] Currently, insufficient data exist to adequately support or refute this claim.[3,4,5] These agents can be useful adjuncts to the therapy of atopic dermatitis but should be used only as indicated: in patients over two years of age, as second-line therapy and on an intermittent basis. Both pimecrolimus and tacrolimus significantly reduce eczema severity scores compared to placebo.[6] Tacrolimus has demonstrated better efficacy than a mild corticosteroid and tacrolimus 0.1% has shown no difference compared to a mid-potency corticosteroid.[7,8] Pimecrolimus was not as effective as betamethasone valerate in patients with eczema of at least moderate severity although it is indicated for patients with mild to moderate eczema.[9]

Other systemic agents such as cyclosporine, methotrexate, azathioprine and UV therapy have been used in patients with extensive dermatitis, patients who have not responded to topical treatment or those who are unable to tolerate topical therapy. Referral to a dermatologist is recommended.

Table 1: **Selection of Topical Therapy by Vehicle**

Vehicle	Advantages	Disadvantages
Cream	Cosmetically elegant	Less absorption; additives can irritate
Lotion	Evaporates well, good for large areas, good for hairy areas	Alcohol base will sting/irritate open areas of eczema
Gel	Good for hairy areas, oily skin	Alcohol base will sting/irritate open areas of eczema
Ointment	Excellent penetration, offers emollient effect, little or no irritation	Cosmetically less acceptable, thick, greasy

Table 2: **Selection of Topical Corticosteroid by Body Area**

Body Area	Skin Properties	Steroid Type
Face, intertriginous folds	Thin skin, more absorption	Low potency
Body and scalp	Medium thickness	Medium potency
Palms, soles	Thick skin	High potency

Therapeutic Tips

- Ointments are less irritating and penetrate better than creams or lotions. They are an excellent choice for atopic dermatitis but cosmetic acceptability and adherence is lower. Generally the same corticosteroid molecule will be more potent in the ointment form than in cream or lotion.
- Education is a key part of therapy. Patients have to understand they have a chronic, recurring condition that can be controlled not cured.
- Sweating, stress and overheating can all increase itching.
- Patches of dermatitis that are resistant to treatment despite compliance may require a short course of a more potent corticosteroid.
- Pruritus in atopic dermatitis is not histamine-mediated and therefore does not respond well to histamine blockade. Nonsedating antihistamines are of little use in the pruritus of atopic dermatitis but may help associated allergic symptoms (e.g., allergic conjunctivitis). Potent sedating antihistamines (e.g., diphenhydramine, hydroxyzine) taken 30 to 60 minutes prior to bedtime may provide some relief possibly through central sedation.

Figure 1: **Management of Atopic Dermatitis**

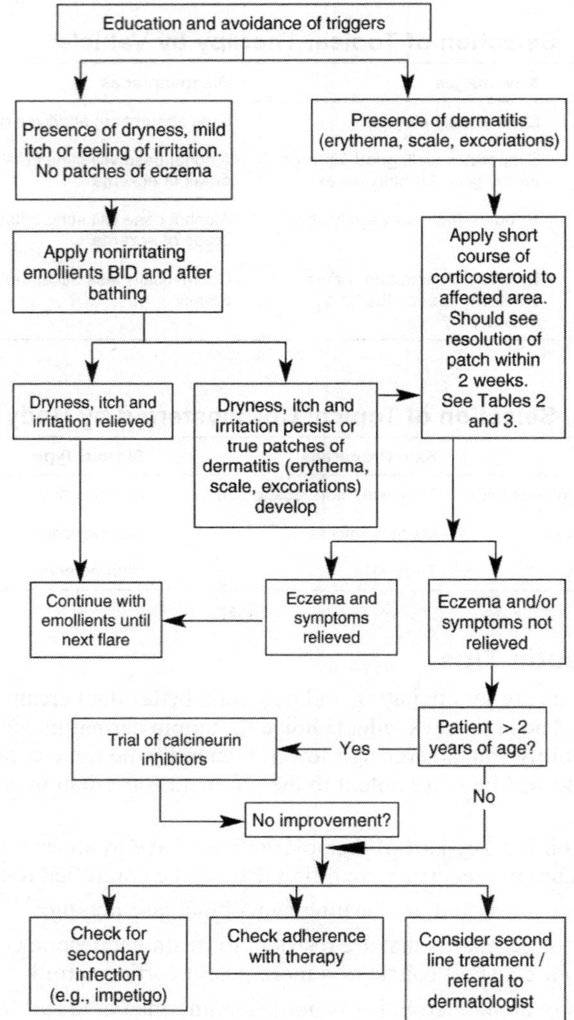

Table 3: **Topical Treatments for Atopic Dermatitis**

Class	Drug	Dose	Adverse Effects	Comments	Cost[a]
Corticosteroids, low potency	*desonide* Desocort, generics	BID-TID	Striae, telangiectasia, atrophy, purpura. When used around the eye for longer periods of time there can be ocular side effects. Systemic effects include suppression of HPA axis, growth suppression and increased risk of glaucoma.	Good for face, intertriginous areas. Safe and effective when used appropriately.	$
	hydrocortisone 1% Emo-Cort, Prevex HC, Sarna HC, generics	BID-TID	See desonide.	See desonide.	$
	hydrocortisone 2.5% Emo-Cort	BID-TID	See desonide.	See desonide.	$
Corticosteroids, medium potency	*betamethasone valerate* Betaderm, Prevex B, generics	Daily-BID	See desonide.	Good for body areas. Safe and effective when used appropriately.	$
	clobetasone butyrate Eumovate	BID-TID	See desonide.	See betamethasone valerate.	$$
	diflucortolone valerate Nerisone	Daily-BID	See desonide.	See betamethasone valerate.	$$
	fluticasone propionate Cutivate	Daily-BID	See desonide.	See betamethasone valerate.	$$

(cont'd)

Table 3: **Topical Treatments for Atopic Dermatitis** *(cont'd)*

Class	Drug	Dose	Adverse Effects	Comments	Cost[a]
	hydrocortisone valerate Hydroval, Westcort	BID-TID	See desonide.	See betamethasone valerate.	$
	mometasone furoate Elocom, generics	Daily	See desonide.	See betamethasone valerate.	$$
	prednicarbate Dermatop	BID	See desonide.	See betamethasone valerate.	$$
	triamcinolone acetonide Aristocort Topicals, generics	BID	See desonide.	See betamethasone valerate.	$
Corticosteroids, high potency	*amcinonide* Cyclocort, generics	BID-TID	See desonide.	Good for thick lichenified plaques. Safe and effective when used appropriately.	$-$$
	desoximetasone Topicort	BID	See desonide.	See amcinonide.	$$
	fluocinolone acetonide Fluoderm, Synalar	BID-TID	See desonide.	See amcinonide.	$
	fluocinonide Lyderm, Tiamol	BID-TID	See desonide.	See amcinonide.	$-$$
	halcinonide Halog	BID-TID	See desonide.	See amcinonide.	$$
Corticosteroids, ultra potent	*betamethasone dipropionate* Diprosone, generics	BID	See desonide.	Good for palms and soles. Safe and effective when used appropriately.	$

Class	Drug	Dose	Adverse Effects	Comments	Cost[a]
	clobetasol propionate Clobex Lotion, Dermovate, generics	BID	See desonide.	See betamethasone dipropionate.	$-$$
	halobetasol propionate Ultravate	BID	See desonide.	See betamethasone dipropionate.	$$$
Antibiotic + Corticosteroid	*fusidic acid/hydrocortisone* Fucidin H	TID	See desonide.	For use in dermatitis with associated *S. aureus.*	$$$
Calcineurin Inhibitors	*pimecrolimus cream* Elidel	BID	Transient burning sensations, skin tingling, pruritus at site of application.	For use as a second-line agent until skin clears. Not for use in children < 2 years of age or in patients who are immunocompromised. Apply in a thin layer and avoid unnecessary UV exposure. Indicated for patients with mild to moderate atopic dermatitis.	$$$$
	tacrolimus 0.03% and 0.1% ointment Protopic	Pediatric (> 2 years of age): 0.03% ointment BID Adult (age 16 and over): 0.03% or 0.1% ointment BID	See pimecrolimus.	See pimecrolimus. Indicated for patients with moderate to severe atopic dermatitis.	$$$$$

[a] Cost of 30 g or 30 mL for topical products; includes drug cost only.
Legend: $ < $10 $-$$ < $10–20 $$ $10–20 $$$ $20–50 $$$$ $50–60 $$$$$ $60–70

Suggested Readings

Ashcroft DM, Dimmock P, Garside R et al. Efficacy and tolerability of topical pimecrolimus and tacrolimus in the treatment of atopic dermatitis: meta-analysis of randomized controlled trials. *BMJ* 2005;330(7490):516.

Eichenfield LF, Hanafin JM, Luger TA et al. Consensus conference on pediatric atopic dermatitis. *J Am Acad Dermatol* 2003;49(6):1088-95.

Ellis C, Luger T, Abeck D et al. International Consensus Conference on Atopic Dermatitis II (ICCAD II): clinical update and current treatment strategies. *Br J Dermatol* 2003;148(suppl.63):3-10.

Hengge UR, Ruzicka T, Schwartz RA, Cork MJ. Adverse effects of topical glucocorticosteroids. *J Am Acad Dermatol* 2006;54(1):1-15.

Williams HC. Clinical practice. Atopic dermatitis. *N Engl J Med* 2005;352(22):2314-24.

References

1. Wolverton SE, editor. *Comprehensive dermatologic drug therapy*. Philadelphia (PA): WB Saunders; 2001.
2. Green C, Colquitt JL, Kirby J, Davidson P. Topical corticosteroids for atopic eczema: clinical and cost effectiveness of once-daily vs. more frequent use. *Br J Dermatol* 2005;152(1):130-41.
3. Food and Drug Administration Pediatric Advisory Committee. February 15, 2005, Briefing information. http://www.fda.gov/ohrms/dockets/ac/05/briefing/2005-4089b2.htm.
4. Ormerod AD. Topical tacrolimus and pimecrolimus and the risk of cancer: how much cause for concern? *Br J Dermatol* 2005;153(4):701-5.
5. Fonacier L, Spergel J, Charlesworth EN et al. Report of the Topical Calcineurin Inhibitor Task Force of the American College of Allergy, Asthma and Immunology and the American Academy of Allergy, Asthma and Immunology. *J Allergy Clin Immunol* 2005;115(6):1249-53.
6. Iskedjian M, Piwko C, Shear NH et al. Topical calcineurin inhibitors in the treatment of atopic dermatitis: a meta-analysis of current evidence. *Am J Clin Dermatol* 2004;5(4):267-79.
7. Reitamo S, Harper J, Bos JD et al. 0.03% Tacrolimus ointment applied once or twice daily is more efficacious than 1% hydrocortisone acetate in children with moderate to severe atopic dermatitis: results of a randomized double-blind controlled trial. *Br J Dermatol* 2004;150(3):554-62.
8. Reitamo S, Rustin M, Ruzicka T et al. Efficacy and safety of tacrolimus ointment compared with that of hydrocortisone butyrate ointment in adult patients with atopic dermatitis. *J Allergy Clin Immunol* 2002;109(3):547-55.
9. Luger T, Van Leent EJ, Graeber M et al. SDZ ASM 981: an emerging safe and effective treatment for atopic dermatitis. *Br J Dermatol*. 2001(144):788–94.

CHAPTER 84
Pruritus

Laura A. Finlayson, MD, FRCPC

Goals of Therapy

- Determine etiology of pruritus in each patient (commonly a skin disease). See Table 1
- Rule out underlying systemic disease (found in about 20% of pruritic patients without skin disorders)[1]
- Decrease or abolish the itching sensation

Investigations

- A complete history including:
  - nature, location, duration, severity of pruritus
  - skin rash or dryness
  - past history or symptoms to suggest renal, hepatic, hematopoietic, lymphoreticular or endocrine disease
  - hygiene practices, topical contacts to the skin
  - weight loss or night sweats
  - prescription, OTC and illicit drug use, particularly opiates
- Physical examination with assessment for presence of skin rash or dryness, excoriations, dermatographism, uremic pigmentation, jaundice, plethora, lymphadenopathy, hepatosplenomegaly
- Laboratory investigations are indicated only if a primary dermatologic cause for the pruritus has been excluded and include CBC with differential, fasting serum glucose, liver function tests, renal function tests, chest x-ray, HIV testing
- Depending on the index of suspicion, further investigations may be required to identify underlying systemic disease (Figure 1)

Therapeutic Choices (Figure 1)

Nonpharmacologic Choices

- *Skin hydration:* Dry skin frequently causes or exacerbates pruritus. Avoid very hot water, harsh soaps and bubble bath preparations that dry and irritate the skin. Ensure adequate indoor humidity, especially during cold weather.

  Bathing is therapeutic for dry skin if water from the bath can be trapped within the skin. A daily tepid bath or shower for 5 to 10 minutes, using mild unscented soap mainly on intertriginous areas, face and feet, can be taken to hydrate skin. Colloidal oatmeal bath preparations or four tablespoons of baking soda in the bath can be soothing. An unscented bath oil, baby oil or mineral oil may be applied to the skin shortly before bathing is finished. Skin is then patted with a towel. Unscented moisture cream or white petrolatum should be applied while the skin is still slightly damp to retard water evaporation.

- *Avoid agents that can enhance histamine release* (e.g., ASA, opiates, shellfish, strawberries and red wine).

Table 1: **Pruritic Skin Diseases**

Morphology	Skin Disease	Treatment
Urticarial	Urticaria	Avoid precipitants; antihistamines
	Dermatographism	Avoid precipitants; antihistamines
	Pruritic urticarial papules and plaques of pregnancy	Symptomatic; deliver baby
	Drug eruption	Discontinue drug; symptomatic
Dermatitic	Atopic dermatitis	Mild topical corticosteroids; hydrate skin
	Xerosis	Hydrate skin
	Contact dermatitis	Avoid precipitants; topical corticosteroids
Dermatitic with burrows	Scabies	Topical permethrin Treat household contacts (see Chapter 85).
Papular	Drug eruption	Discontinue drug; symptomatic
	Swimmer's itch	Symptomatic, topical corticosteroids
	Viral exanthem	Symptomatic
Papulosquamous	Lichen planus	Topical or oral corticosteroids
	Lichen simplex chronicus	Cover to prevent scratching; topical corticosteroids
Pustular	Folliculitis	Minimize friction to hair follicles; topical antibiotics
	Miliaria (heat rash)	Keep skin cool; talcum powder
	Insect bites	Prevention; topical antipruritics
Nodular	Nodular scabies	Topical permethrin; treat household contacts (see Chapter 85).
	Prurigo nodularis	Cover to prevent scratching; topical corticosteroids
Vesiculobullous	Dermatitis herpetiformis	Dapsone; gluten-free diet
	Bullous pemphigoid	Oral corticosteroids, immunosuppressive agents

Table 1: **Pruritic Skin Diseases** *(cont'd)*

Morphology	Skin Disease	Treatment
	Varicella	Symptomatic; acyclovir or other antivirals
Pigmented macules	Urticaria pigmentosa (mastocytosis)	Antihistamines; avoid ASA, opiates, rubbing skin

- *Minimize friction and irritation to the skin.* Clothing should be soft and loose. Wool and synthetic clothing should be avoided as well as rough, exposed seams or interfacing. Washing detergent should be rinsed well from clothing, and antistatic agents in the dryer not be used. Avoid fragranced products.
- *Minimize scratching.* Generalized pruritus produces a powerful, almost uncontrollable stimulus to scratch the skin. The scratch-itch cycle is self-perpetuating. Fingernails should be kept short. Cool tap water compresses applied for 20 minutes four to six times daily can be applied for acute localized itch. A covering of light clothing over the itchy area decreases nonintentional scratching.
- *Avoid vasodilatory stimuli* (e.g., excessive exercise, high environmental temperature and humidity, hot or prolonged showers or baths, spicy foods, caffeine and alcohol).
- *Ensure adequate sleep.* Pruritus is frequently worse at night, mostly because lack of distracting stimuli allows one to focus on the itch. Scratching at night perpetuates the scratch-itch cycle. Antipruritic topical lotion, applied just before bedtime, use of light bedclothes, and a sedative or sedating antihistamine may be helpful.

Pharmacologic Choices

Topical Antipruritics

Menthol 0.25 to 0.5%, **camphor** 0.25 to 0.5% in a light nonperfumed lotion applied TID or PRN, is soothing. **Pramoxine hydrochloride** 1% is a topical anesthetic with low sensitizing potential that may provide short-term relief. Avoid topical benzocaine and other "caine" topical anesthetics, topical diphenhydramine and phenol because they can sensitize the skin. Phenol is also contraindicated in pregnancy. **Crotamiton,** a scabicide, may also be used for its nonspecific antipruritic properties. **Calamine** is useful for acute conditions such as contact dermatitis but will dry the skin excessively with long-term use. Preparations containing topical mast cell stabilizers are presently being evaluated for potential relief of pruritus.

Topical corticosteroids and **topical immune modulators** are only useful and appropriate if the pruritus is caused by an inflammatory skin condition. The strength of topical steroid chosen is based on many factors including location and extent of the eruption, severity and type of inflammation, age of the patient and anticipated duration of use (see Chapter 83). A topical immune modulator such as **tacrolimus** or **pimecrolimus** may be useful in specific conditions such as atopic dermatitis.

Antihistamines (Table 2)

Histamine is directly involved in many, but not all cases of pruritus; therefore, antihistamines may have a variable effect, providing profound to minimal relief. They are most effective in urticaria. Histamine$_1$ (H_1) blockers are the agents of choice because H_2 receptors are not directly involved in itch.[2]

First-generation (classic) antihistamines have effects on adrenergic, serotonergic and cholinergic receptors in addition to histamine receptors. They are more likely to cause central sedative and anticholinergic adverse effects such as dry mouth, blurred vision and urinary retention. Second-generation antihistamines are less lipid soluble and cross the blood-brain barrier poorly, causing fewer CNS effects, and are more selective for the H_1 site resulting in fewer anticholinergic effects.[3] Several second-generation antihistamines occasionally caused cardiotoxicity and drug interactions that led to them being taken off the market and replaced with their active metabolites or enantiomers, which have not demonstrated these problems.

Choosing an antihistamine: Patient responses to these agents vary. Consider precautions and contraindications, adverse effect profile, individual patient factors, occupation, underlying condition and response to initial treatment.

Precautions and contraindications: Antihistamines must be used with caution in patients with glaucoma, stenosing peptic ulcer, urinary retention and those taking MAOIs. Avoid antihistamines in epileptic patients unless the benefits outweigh the possible risks. Especially for these patients, nonpharmacologic measures should be tried first.

Adverse effect profile: Consider the risk and implications of the various side effects (particularly drowsiness and anticholinergic effects) for each patient (Table 2).

Individual patient factors: Antihistamines, particularly the sedating ones, are more likely to cause drowsiness, confusion, hypotension, syncope and dizziness in the *elderly*.[4] *Children* may show paradoxical excitation rather than sedation. Studies have shown, however, that children do not show decreased school performance with either the older or newer antihistamines.[5] **Chlorpheniramine** has been used in pregnant patients who are not controlled with nonpharmacologic or topical measures.

Allergies to antihistamines are uncommon but if a patient is *allergic to or intolerant of* an antihistamine, consider them to also be sensitive to other drugs in the same class.

Occupation: Working adults and school children can function more safely with *nonsedating antihistamines*, e.g., **loratadine, desloratadine** or **fexofenadine** during the day. With **cetirizine**, drowsiness occurs in about 10% of patients; however, the incidence and severity of sedation is less than with classic antihistamines. First-generation antihistamines, e.g., diphenhydramine, clemastine and some second-generation antihistamines may significantly impair driving performance but fexofenadine does not appear to impair driving abilities.[6] Desloratidine and fexofenadine have mild stimulating effects on tasks involving high levels of performance.[7]

Underlying condition: The H_1 antihistamines have proven effectiveness in treatment of urticaria, but have not been proven to treat pruritus from other skin diseases or systemic conditions. However, they are still often used as first-line treatment for pruritus, whatever the cause.[8] Acute or severe pruritus and skin conditions other than urticaria often respond better to the older antihistamines as the sedative properties may contribute directly to relief of the pruritus. Antihistamines are more effective at preventing histamine release than combating the effects of previously released histamine. Therefore, in chronic pruritic conditions antihistamines should be administered regularly for at least a week rather than intermittently when itch is most severe.[9]

Response to initial treatment: Antihistamines are classified by chemical structure (Table 2). If a patient does not respond to an antihistamine from one class, change to an agent from another class. At times, prescribing two antihistamines from different classes at the same time is useful, but it is rarely necessary to prescribe more than two.[3]

Other Systemic Pharmacologic Treatments

Doxepin, an antidepressant with potent antihistaminic properties, is useful in some cases of chronic urticaria (Table 2). It has anticholinergic effects and is contraindicated in patients with congestive heart failure and in those taking MAOIs.

Ketotifen, a selective H_1 antihistamine that also stabilizes mast cells and inhibits mediator release, is used primarily in asthma prophylaxis but can be useful in urticaria and mastocytosis (Table 2).

Patients who scratch uncontrollably at night may benefit from a small dose of **diazepam, chlordiazepoxide** or **lorazepam** at bedtime. Avoid large doses of sedating antihistamines administered at the same time.

Cholestyramine and **colestipol resins** are effective for pruritus related to cholestatic liver disease (Chapter 51). These agents have also been used successfully in uremic pruritus and polycythemia rubra vera.[2]

Opiate antagonists (e.g., **naltrexone**) can significantly reduce the pruritus associated with cholestatic liver disease, renal disease and opioid-induced pruritus.

Serotonin antagonists (e.g., **ondansetron**) are useful in some cases of pruritus of renal or hepatic origin. Although case reports support their use,[10] further studies are required to clarify efficacy and dosing recommendations for both opiate antagonists and serotonin antagonists in the treatment of pruritus.

Phototherapy

Phototherapy with ultraviolet B (UVB) wavelength (290–320 nm) is an effective treatment for uremic pruritus. Eight to 10 treatments usually result in symptomatic improvement. Maintenance therapy may be administered as required. UVB phototherapy is often effective for pruritus of other etiology, particularly primary dermatoses.

Therapeutic Tips

- Dry skin causes or exacerbates pruritus so frequently that ensuring adequate skin hydration is worthwhile general treatment for all itchy patients.
- Do not use histamine$_2$ antagonists (e.g., cimetidine) unless the H_1 receptors are blocked with an H_1 antihistamine. H_2 antagonists alone can exacerbate pruritus by interfering with a negative feedback mechanism.
- Avoid topical steroids and immune modulators in the absence of clinically evident skin disease.
- Test for dermatographism or pressure sensitivity (urticarial lesion appears in site of superficial scratch on skin) because symptomatic dermatographism or subclinical urticaria is a common cause of pruritus that can be suppressed with antihistamines.
- Careful follow-up is required. The itching of scabies, urticaria and drug eruptions may precede onset of skin manifestations. Likewise, symptoms of a systemic disease may eventually develop in a patient with apparent idiopathic pruritus.
- Topical agents may be kept in a refrigerator because the physical cooling enhances their antipruritic effect.
- Antihistamines requiring a single daily dose (e.g., cetirizine, loratadine, desloratadine) are more effective if given in the evening than the morning.

Figure 1: **Management of Pruritus**

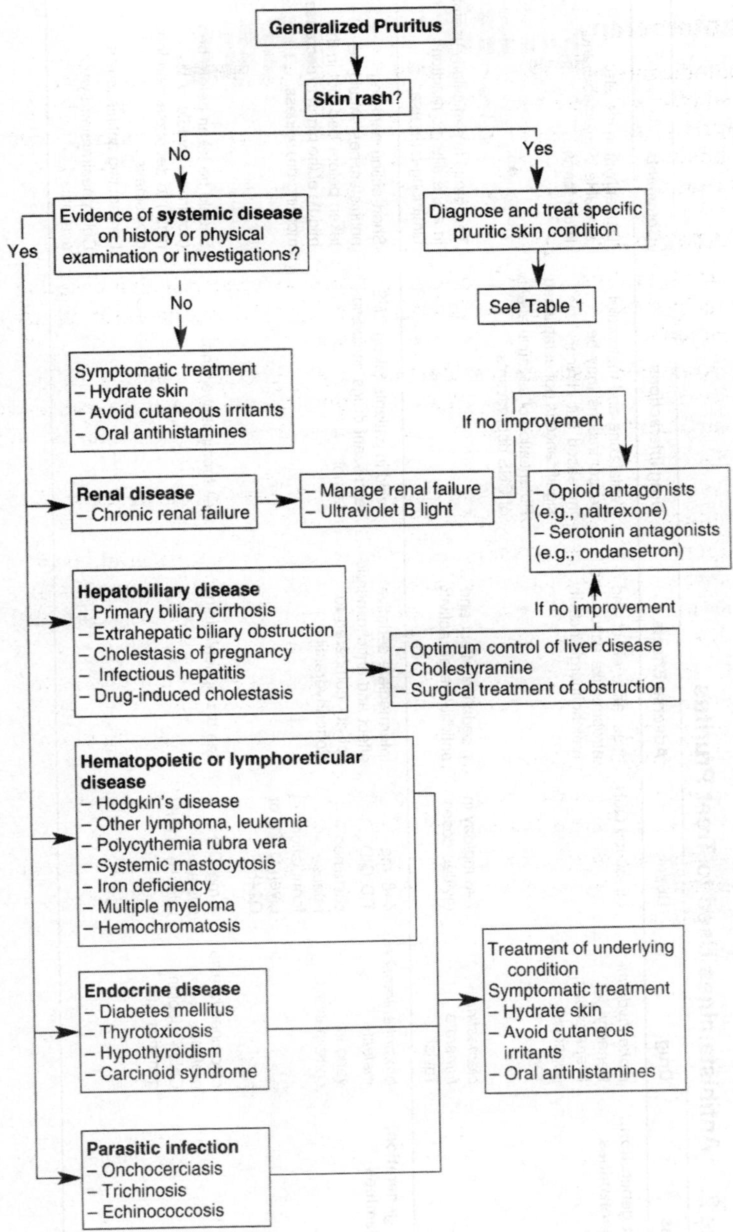

Table 2: Antihistamines Used to Treat Pruritus

Class	Drug	Dose	Adverse Effects	Drug Interactions	Comments	Cost[a]
First generation, ethanolamines	*diphenhydramine* Benadryl Preparations, generics	25–50 mg Q6H	↑ sedative effect and atropine-like action and anticholinergic activity.	Venlafaxine and metoprolol concentrations may be increased but clinical significance is not established. Potentiation of sedative effects of CNS depressants.	Diphenhydramine also available in injectable and liquid forms.	$-$$
	clemastine fumarate Tavist	2–6 mg/day in divided doses	↑ sedative effect and anticholinergic activity.		This group is particularly useful in acute allergic reactions. Limit long-term use.	$$–$$$
First generation, alkylamines	*brompheniramine maleate* various combinations	4–8 mg TID-QID sustained release formulations given Q12H or Q24H	Intermediate sedative effect and anticholinergic activity compared to diphenhydramine.	Avoid in patients taking CNS depressant drugs, including alcohol.	Short-acting sedating antihistamines should be taken before bed (not in the middle of the night) to decrease morning drowsiness.	$$–$$$
	chlorpheniramine maleate Chlor-Tripolon, generics	4 mg Q6H; sustained release Q12H	See brompheniramine.	See brompheniramine.	Should be taken before bed (not in the middle of the night) to decrease morning drowsiness. Long-acting antihistamine. Chlorpheniramine syrup available.	$–$$

Class	Drug	Dose	Adverse Effects	Drug Interactions	Comments	Cost[a]
First generation, piperazines	*hydroxyzine* Atarax, generics	25–75 mg TID–QID	Occasionally may cause paradoxical excitation in children. ↑ sedative effects. Intermediate anticholinergic activity compared to diphenhydramine.	Be aware that hydroxyzine may inhibit the antipsychotic response to neuroleptics.	Hydroxyzine useful in both acute and chronic allergic conditions. Some anxiolytic and antiemetic properties. Liquid form available.	$-$$
First generation, piperidines	*azatadine maleate* Optimine	1–2 mg BID	↑ sedative effects and anticholinergic activity.	MAO inhibitors prolong effect. Effect of oral anticoagulants may be reduced. Additive effect with CNS depressants.	Azatadine and cyproheptadine may stimulate appetite. Caution in glaucoma, bladder neck obstruction.	$$–$$$
	cyproheptadine[b] generics	4–8 mg TID	Intermediate sedative effects compared to diphenhydramine. ↑ anticholinergic activity.	Monitor for reduced antidepressant response to fluoxetine (and possibly other SSRIs) when cyproheptadine started.	See azatadine.	$$
First generation, phenothiazines	*promethazine* generics	12.5 mg QID or 25 mg QHS	↑ sedative effect and anticholinergic activity. Extrapyramidal symptoms, photosensitivity.	Potentiation of sedative effects of CNS depressants.	Promethazine syrup available.	$
	trimeprazine tartrate Panectyl	2.5–5 mg TID	↑ sedative effect and anticholinergic activity. Extrapyramidal symptoms.	See promethazine. May reverse pressor effect of epinephrine.	Best taken after meals. Antiemetic.	$$

(cont'd)

Table 2: **Antihistamines Used to Treat Pruritus** *(cont'd)*

Class	Drug	Dose	Adverse Effects	Drug Interactions	Comments	Cost[a]
Second generation, piperidines	*loratadine*[b] Claritin, generics	10 mg/day	Little sedative effect or anticholinergic activity.	Does not share the drug interactions of previously available nonsedating antihistamines. Cimetidine, erythromycin and ketoconazole may increase plasma concentrations of loratadine; clinical effect minimal.	Long-acting, nonsedating antihistamine. Unchanged loratadine does not appear to be cardiotoxic. Loratadine available as liquid and rapid dissolve tablet.	$$
	fexofenadine Allegra 12 Hour	60 mg BID	Little sedative effect or anticholinergic activity.	Does not share drug interactions of terfenadine (parent compound). ↓ AUC and plasma concentration of fexofenadine with concomitant administration of antacids containing aluminum and magnesium. Erythromycin and ketoconazole may increase plasma concentrations of fexofenadine; clinical effect probably minimal.	Long-acting, nonsedating antihistamine. Metabolite of terfenadine lacking the cardiotoxic effects of the parent compound. Has some anti-inflammatory properties (inhibits COX-2).	$$
Second generation, piperazines	*cetirizine HCl* Reactine, generics	10–20 mg/day	Headache and fatigue in up to 10% of patients. Sedative effects in 10% of patients; little anticholinergic activity.		Metabolite of hydroxyzine. Long-acting and inhibits the late phase reaction of allergy. Liquid form available.	$-$$

Class	Drug	Dose	Adverse Effects	Drug Interactions	Comments	Cost[a]
Third generation, piperidines	*desloratadine* (renal symbol) Aerius	5 mg/day	Little to no sedative effect or anticholinergic activity; some antimuscarinic effects.	Potential kinetic interaction when used with drugs affecting hepatic microsomal enzymes. No ECG changes reported.	Nonsedating antihistamine. Also inhibits many inflammatory mediators in addition to histamine. Liquid form available.	$$
Antihistamines, other	*doxepin* Sinequan, generics	10 mg po TID	Anticholinergic activity; sedation.	Combination with MAOIs may result in mania, excitation, hyperpyrexia; barbiturates, carbamazepine and rifampin may ↓ effect; cimetidine and antipsychotics may ↑ effect and toxicity; possible interaction with antiarrhythmics (may lead to ↑ effect of either drug); may ↓ antihypertensive effect of clonidine; may augment hypotensive effect of thiazides.	Tricyclic antidepressant with potent antihistaminic properties. Used in some cases of chronic urticaria.	$
	ketotifen (renal symbol) Zaditen, generics	1 mg po BID	Sedation, dizziness, headache, rash, nausea, weight gain.	Oral antihyperglycemics: thrombocytopenia rarely seen in patients concomitantly receiving ketotifen. May potentiate sedative effects of alcohol, hypnotics, sedatives or antihistamines.	Used in urticaria and mastocytosis.	$$

[a] Cost of 7-day supply; includes drug cost only.
[b] Dosage adjustment may be required in hepatic impairment.
(renal symbol) Dosage adjustment may be required in renal impairment; see Appendix I.
Abbreviations: AUC = area under the concentration curve
Legend: $ < $5 $–$$ < $5–10 $$ $5–10 $$–$$$ $5–15 $$$ $10–15

Suggested Readings

Charlesworth EN, Beltrani VS. Pruritic dermatoses: overview of etiology and therapy. *Am J Med* 2002;113(Suppl 9A):25S-33S.

Etter L, Myers SA. Pruritus in systemic disease: mechanisms and management. *Dermatol Clin* 2002;20(3):459-72.

Moses S. Pruritus. *Am Fam Physician* 2003;68(6)1135-42.

Walsh GM. Emerging safety issues regarding long-term usage of H(1) receptor antagonists. *Expert Opin Drug Saf* 2002;1(3) :225-35.

References

1. Kantor GR, Lookingbill DP. Generalized pruritus and systemic disease. *J Am Acad Dermatol* 1983;9(3):375-82.
2. Denman ST. A review of pruritus. *J Am Acad Dermatol* 1986;14(3):375-92.
3. Fisher AA. The antihistamines. *J Am Acad Dermatol* 1980;3(3):303-6.
4. Gengo FM. Reduction of the central nervous system adverse effects associated with antihistamines in the management of allergic disorders: strategies and progress. *J Allergy Clin Immunol* 1996;98 (6 Pt 3):S319-25.
5. Bender BG, McCormick DR, Milgrom H. Children's school performance is not impaired by short-term administration of diphenhydramine or loratadine. *J Pediatr* 2001;138(5):656-60.
6. Verster JC, Volkerts ER. Antihistamines and driving ability: evidence from on-the-road driving studies during normal traffic. *Ann Allergy Asthma Immunol* 2004;92(3):294-303.
7. Theunissen EL, Vermeeren A, Vuurman EF et al. Stimulating effects of H1-antagonists. *Curr Pharm Des* 2006;12(20):2501-9.
8. O'Donoghue M, Tharp MD. Antihistamines and their role as antipruritics. *Dermatol Ther* 2005;18(4):333-40.
9. Mattila MJ, Paakkari I. Variations among non-sedating antihistamines: are there real differences? *Eur J Clin Pharmacol* 1999;55(2):85-93.
10. Frigon C, Desparmet J. Ondansetron treatment in a child presenting with chronic intractable pruritus. *Pain Res Manag* 2006;11(4):245-7.

CHAPTER 85
Scabies and Pediculosis

Sandra Knowles, BScPhm and
Neil H. Shear, MD, FRCPC

Scabies and pediculosis are common infestations that cause significant discomfort and are associated with large outbreaks in institutions (e.g., long-term care facilities, schools).

Goals of Therapy

- Eradicate causative organisms and eggs
- Control symptoms (pruritus) and prevent complications (secondary bacterial infection)
- Prevent spread to contacts

Investigations (Table 1)

- History of exposure and itching
- Physical examination for identification of organisms (or evidence of organisms such as eggs or nits)[1]

Therapeutic Choices (Figure 1)

Nonpharmacologic Choices

- Although time-consuming and tedious, *lice* and *nits* should be mechanically removed after pharmacologic treatment.[1,2] Because of increased resistance to various pharmacologic treatments, nit removal is becoming increasingly important.[3] However, wet combing, which involves combing wet hair with a specially designed comb every three to four days, alone produces poor results. There are a variety of different louse or nit combs available (e.g., LiceMeister developed by the National Pediculosis Association).
- Other methods of nit removal include vinegar (wrapping hair in vinegar-soaked towel for 30 to 60 minutes) or formic acid 8% (Step 2).[2] An uncontrolled study showed that Cetaphil cleanser ("Nuvo" lotion) was effective in treatment of lice; the lotion, which is applied to the scalp and allowed to dry in place, suffocates the lice.[4] Other unconventional treatments include hot air,[5] hair styling gels and isopropyl myristate (Resultz).
- *Treatment of room*: wash and dry (with heat) pillowcases, sheets, nightclothes, towels, personal articles (e.g., hats, shared helmets, headphones) and stuffed animals. Alternatively, items that cannot be washed can be dry cleaned or sealed in a plastic bag for two weeks. Vacuum the patient's room. Head lice usually do not exist for more than 48 hours when separated from a person.[2] Treatment of clothing

and bed linen (washing at 65°C or putting in a hermetically sealed bag for several days) is recommended for patients with crusted scabies.[6]

- *Combs and brushes*: soak in a disinfectant solution (e.g., 2% Lysol for one hour) or in hot water (65°C for 5 to 10 minutes).
- Identify and examine *potential human contacts* to prevent a cycle of reinfection. For head lice, only those contacts with live lice or nits within 1 cm of the scalp should be treated.[3] Pets do not transmit human lice and should not be treated for pediculosis. *All* contacts of scabies, even if asymptomatic, require treatment.[7] This includes sexual and close personal or household contacts within the preceding month.

Pharmacologic Choices (Table 2 and Table 3)

- No product is considered reliably ovicidal and many patients are not fully compliant with application; therefore retreatment in 1 week to 10 days is recommended.[8,9]
- In patients with head lice, treatment may fail if hair is not thoroughly soaked with **permethrin**. Two bottles are often needed for thick or long hair.
- *Treatment failure for head lice* may be due to resistance to topical agents.[10] Switching to a different pharmacologic class may be helpful, although resistance to permethrin may cross over to pyrethrins and other pyrethroids.[8] The following have been advocated: permethrin 5% cream applied to scalp and left on for several hours or overnight;[1] oral **sulfamethoxazole-trimethoprim** in combination with permethrin 1%;[7] or oral **ivermectin** 200 μg/kg (available through the Special Access Programme, Health Canada), repeated in 10 days.[8]
- In patients with *pubic lice*, **permethrin** 5% cream,[8] **lindane** 1% shampoo or **pyrethins with piperonyl butoxide** is recommended. Pediculicides are generally unnecessary for patients with body lice, although oral ivermectin (12 mg x 3 doses administered weekly) is effective.[11] Nonpharmacologic treatment measures, such as bathing and laundering of infested clothing and linens in hot water, are usually sufficient.
- Insufficient treatment of itch and fear of infestation may cause patients with scabies to overuse scabicides, resulting in skin irritation and unnecessary repeated therapy.
- In patients with scabies, itching can persist for weeks after mites are eradicated. Medium-potency **topical corticosteroids** (e.g., betamethasone valerate 0.1% cream) and intensive use of emollients are helpful.[7] (See Chapter 84).
- *Crusted scabies* can be treated with oral **ivermectin** 200 μg/kg and repeated in two weeks.[6]

Therapeutic Tips

- Various alternative therapies including acetomicellar complex (SH-206) and naturally occurring substances (e.g., tea tree oil, other essential oils, herbal remedies) have been advocated for the treatment of head lice. However, there is no published evidence to suggest that any of these are consistently effective.[8,12]

- **White petrolatum** (e.g., Vaseline) can be applied to *eyelashes* two to four times daily for 10 days.[8] Removal of lice and nits with forceps or tweezers prior to application is recommended.

Figure 1: Management of Scabies or Lice

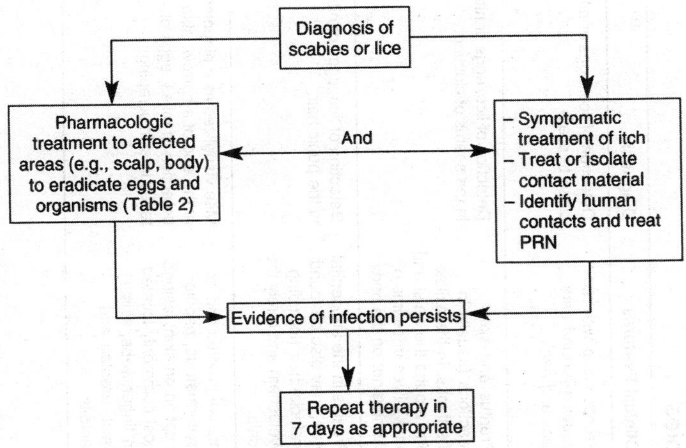

Table 1: Clinical Features of Pediculosis and Scabies

Type	Organism	Mode of Transmission	Clinical Features	Diagnosis	Differential Diagnosis
Pediculosis capitis (head lice)	*Pediculus humanus capitis*	Head-to-head contact; sharing personal items such as combs, brushes, hats.	Pruritic scalp with red papules around ears, face and neck.	Detection of lice, eggs or nits close to scalp.	Dandruff, hair casts, hairspray droplets.
Pediculosis corporis (body lice)	*Pediculus humanus corporis*	Via clothing and bedding; poor hygiene.	Pruritus and skin reactions (usually in the flanks, in the axillae and around the waist and neck); lives in seams of clothing not on the body.	Detection of lice, eggs or nits in the seams of clothing.	Seborrheic dermatitis, flea or insect bites, eczema, folliculitis.
Pediculosis pubis (pubic lice)	*Phthirus pubis*	Sexual contact; may be associated with other sexually transmitted diseases.	Pruritus in the anogenital area; may also be found on facial hair (including eyelashes) and rarely the scalp.	Detection of lice, eggs or nits in the pubic hair.	Seborrheic dermatitis, folliculitis, dermatophytosis.
Scabies	*Sarcoptes scabiei*	Skin-to-skin contact (also via bedding, furniture).	Intense pruritus and an erythematous, papular eruption on skin; lesions most commonly located on finger webs, wrists, waist, areolae and genitals.	Mite visualized as a pinpoint at the end of a burrow; also detection of mites, eggs or feces in skin scrapings.	Impetigo, seborrheic dermatitis, atopic dermatitis.

Table 2: Drugs Used for Pediculosis

Class	Drug	Directions	Adverse Effects	Comments	Cost[a]
Pediculicides	*permethrin 1%* Nix Creme Rinse, Kwellada-P Creme Rinse	Head lice: Wash hair with conditioner-free shampoo, rinse with water and towel dry. Apply permethrin to saturate the hair and scalp (1/2–1 bottle for adults and children with long hair); leave on for 10 min then rinse. May repeat after 7 days if live lice are observed.	May temporarily exacerbate the pruritus, erythema and scalp edema of lice infestation. Burning/stinging, tingling, numbness or scalp discomfort are usually mild and transient.	Drug of choice for most patients. Contraindicated in patients with chrysanthemum allergy. Permethrin resistance may result in treatment failure.	$
	pyrethrins/piperonyl butoxide R&C Shampoo, R&C II Spray, Pronto Lice Killing Shampoo	Shampoo: Apply to thoroughly saturate dry hair and massage scalp; leave on for 10 min. Add a little water; work the shampoo into the hair and skin to form a lather. Rinse thoroughly. Repeat treatment in 7 days. Aerosol: Saturate area (5–10 squirts); wash off after 30 min.	Few adverse effects, although contact dermatitis and eye irritation have been reported.	Contraindicated in patients allergic to ragweed, chrysanthemums or other pyrethrin products.	$

(cont'd)

Table 2: **Drugs Used for Pediculosis** *(cont'd)*

Class	Drug	Directions	Adverse Effects	Comments	Cost[a]
	lindane 1% (gamma benzene hexachloride) Shampoo: Hexit Shampoo, generics Lotion (for pubic lice): Hexit Lotion, generics	Shampoo: Apply enough to dry hair to soak hair and skin. Massage for 4 min; add water a little at a time to produce lather; massage again for 4 min then rinse. Lotion: Apply to affected area, then dress in clean clothes. Leave on for 8–12 h, then thoroughly wash off.	Neurotoxicity (e.g., nausea, vomiting, headache, irritability, insomnia, seizures) has been reported after oral ingestion, repeated application, excessive doses or prolonged treatment or in high-risk populations (e.g., young children, elderly, patients with extensive skin disease).	Not first-line treatment. Avoid contact with eyes, nose, mouth, mucous membranes. Contraindicated in neonates, young children (< 2 y), pregnant women and nursing mothers. Use with caution in any patient weighing < 50 kg.	$

[a] Cost of 1 unit (tube or bottle) of product; includes drug cost only. NB: All products are available without prescription; retail mark-ups may vary.
Legend: $ < $10

Table 3: Drugs Used for Scabies

Class	Drug	Directions	Adverse Effects	Comments	Cost[a]
Scabicides	*permethrin 5%*[b] Nix Dermal Cream, Kwellada-P Lotion	Massage into all skin areas, from the neck down to the soles of the feet; every bit of skin must be treated, including the fingernails, waist and genitalia; leave on for 8–14 h without interruption, then wash off (shower may be the best way).	Pruritus, edema and erythema.	Drug of choice for scabies.[6] Contraindicated in patients allergic to chrysanthemums. Second administration 1 wk after first often routinely prescribed.[7]	Cream:$$ Lotion: $$$
	lindane 1% (lotion recommended; not shampoo) Hexit Lotion, generics	Apply to all skin areas[c] (once); should be left on for 8–12 h and then washed off.	Neurotoxicity (e.g., nausea, vomiting, headache, irritability, insomnia, seizures) has been reported after oral ingestion, repeated application, excessive doses or prolonged treatment or in high-risk populations (e.g., young children, elderly, patients with extensive skin disease).	Used when permethrin has been ineffective or is contraindicated. Not first-line treatment. Avoid contact with eyes, nose, mouth, mucous membranes. Contraindicated in neonates, young children (< 2 y), pregnant women and nursing mothers.	$

(cont'd)

Table 3: Drugs Used for Scabies *(cont'd)*

Class	Drug	Directions	Adverse Effects	Comments	Cost[a]
	crotamiton 10% Eurax cream	Apply to all skin areas[c] daily for 2–5 days; wash off 48 h after last application.	Local irritation.	Less effective than permethrin. Not recommended for patients with exudative or vesicular dermatitis.	$$
	sulfur 5–10%[d]	Apply to all skin areas[c] at bedtime daily for 5–7 days.	Local irritation or dermatitis with repeated applications.	Not popular because it is malodorous, requires multiple applications and stains clothing. Limited study data to support use. Extemporaneously compounded. May be used for small children and pregnant women.	$

[a] Cost of 1 unit (tube or bottle) of product; includes drug cost only. NB: All products are available without prescription; retail mark-ups may vary.
[b] Lower strengths are not effective as scabicides.
[c] As described for permethrin.
[d] Extemporaneously compounded preparations can be used.
Legend: $ < $10 $$ $10–20 $$$ $20–30

Suggested Readings

Burgess I. Head lice. *Clin Evid* 2006;15:1-9.

Chosidow O. Clinical practices. Scabies. *N Engl J Med* 2006;354(16):1718-27.

Ko CJ, Elston DM. Pediculosis. *J Am Acad Dermatol* 2004;50(1):1-12.

Pollack RJ. *Head lice: information and frequently asked questions*. Boston (MA): Harvard School of Public Health, Laboratory of Public Health Entomology, Department of Immunology and Infectious Diseases; 2000. Available from: http://www.hsph.harvard.edu/headlice.html Accessed March 8, 2007.

References

1. Hill N, Moor G, Cameron M, et al. Single-blind, randomised, comparative study of the Bug Buster kit and over the counter pediculicide treatments against head lice in the United Kingdom. *BMJ* 2005;331(7513):384-7.
2. Frankowski BL, Weiner LB; Committee on School Health the Committee on Infectious Diseases. American Academy of Pediatrics. Head lice. *Pediatrics* 2002;110(3):638-43.
3. Elston DM. Controversies concerning the treatment of lice and scabies. *J Am Acad Dermatol* 2002;46(5):794-6.
4. Pearlman DL. A simple treatment for head lice: dry-on, suffocation-based pediculicide. *Pediatrics* 2004;114(3):e275-9.
5. Goates B, Atkin J, Wilding K et al. An effective nonchemical treatment for head lice: a lot of hot air. *Pediatrics* 2006;118(5):1962-70.
6. Heukelbach J, Feldmeier H. Scabies. *Lancet* 2006;367(9524):1767-74.
7. Chosidow O. Clinical practices. Scabies. *N Engl J Med* 2006;354(16):1718-27.
8. Ko CJ, Elston DM. Pediculosis. *J Am Acad Dermatol* 2004;50(1):1-12.
9. Burgess I. Head lice. *Clin Evid* 2006;15:1-9.
10. Meinking TL, Serrano L, Hard B et al. Comparative in vitro pediculicidal efficacy of treatments in a resistant head lice population in the United States. *Arch Dermatol* 2002;138(2):220-4.
11. Foucault C, Ranque S, Badiaga S et al. Oral ivermectin in the treatment of body lice. *J Infect Dis* 2006;193(3):474-6.
12. Roberts RJ. Clinical practice. Head lice. *N Engl J Med* 2002;346(21):1645-50.

CHAPTER 86
Bacterial Skin Infections

Peter Green, MD, FRCPC

This chapter addresses the following bacterial skin infections.

Impetigo: Superficial infection of skin primarily caused by *S. aureus* most often affecting young children. Two clinical forms include crusted or nonbullous (*S. aureus* and/or *S. pyogenes*) and bullous (*S. aureus*-mediated toxin).

Impetiginized: Term describing significant secondary infection of a primary dermatitis, e.g., atopic dermatitis, allergic contact dermatitis resulting from epidermal inflammation severe enough to interfere with normal barrier function; most often related to *S. aureus*.

Folliculitis: Infection of skin and hair follicle to variable depths producing papules and pustules. Infectious causes include *S. aureus* (most common) and *P. aeruginosa*. Noninfectious causes may be termed "*pseudofolliculitis*" and are induced by friction and/or occlusion.

Furuncle (boil): *S. aureus*-mediated infection of hair follicle with extension of suppurative material into dermis and subcutaneous tissue. Interconnecting, multiple furuncles are termed *carbuncles*.

Cutaneous abscess: Deep cutaneous infection harbouring collections of pus that may be polymicrobial or *S. aureus* in origin and located independently of follicular structures.

Cellulitis: Acute onset infection of skin and subcutaneous tissue characterized by poorly circumscribed livid erythema, edema, warmth and tenderness.

Erysipelas: Acute onset infection of skin occurring most commonly on face and lower extremities. Distinguished from cellulitis by more superficial cutaneous involvement, pathogen (most commonly *S. pyogenes*), sharply delineated margins and location.

Necrotizing fasciitis: Limb and life-threatening mono- or polymicrobial infection involving skin, subcutaneous tissue, fascia and muscle.

Therapeutic Choices (Figure 1, Figure 2, Figure 3, Figure 4, Figure 5)

Nonpharmacologic Choices

- For primary impetigo or secondarily impetiginized skin, use normal saline compresses 10–15 minutes two to three times per day to expedite removal of crusts and promote healing.

- Address factors contributing to folliculitis in intertriginous areas by eliminating tight-fitting clothing and reducing friction, moisture and heat.
- Ruptured or inflamed epidermal inclusion cysts, which are sometimes incorrectly called sebaceous cysts, often appear infected or may resemble an abscess given significant erythema and tenderness. Incision with drainage of cystic contents combined with saline compresses is usually sufficient management. Oral antibiotics are reserved for patients with clear signs and symptoms of secondary cellulitis.
- Graduated compression stockings should be considered after cellulitis or erysipelas affecting lower extremities as nearly all will have significant lymphedema. Reducing edema is felt to reduce recurrences of infection.[1]
- If necrotizing infection is suspected, urgent surgical consultation with view to débridement must take place.

Pharmacologic Choices

Systemic Agents (Table 1)

- **Penicillinase-resistant penicillins** are commonly used for uncomplicated bacterial skin infections because of their proven efficacy, familiarity and low cost. **First-generation cephalosporins** are also an excellent choice for uncomplicated skin and soft tissue bacterial infections caused by gram-positive organisms.

  Penicillin monotherapy should not be used for cellulitis or other infections where *S. aureus* is suspected given its resistance to penicillin. Where *S. pyogenes* is the suspected cause of an infection (e.g., erysipelas), penicillin is the treatment of choice.

  A history of minor exanthem (i.e., delayed-onset widespread erythema) from penicillin should be documented but does not exclude patients from cephalosporin use. If there is a history of anaphylaxis or if the nature of the reaction is unknown, avoid cephalosporins in these patients.

  The combination **amoxicillin-clavulanate** should be considered for soft-tissue infections invoked by *animal bites* (e.g., cat, dog) given the presence of *Pasteurella multocida*; resistance of this organism to penicillinase-resistant penicillins (but not penicillin), cephalosporins and clindamycin is documented.[1]
- Macrolide antibiotics (e.g., **erythromycin**) are indicated for gram-positive bacterial skin infections and are frequently used as alternatives to penicillin when patients are penicillin-allergic. Avoid erythromycin if cellulitis is suspected with *H. influenzae* given resistance. Emerging resistance of *S. pyogenes* to erythromycin has also been reported.[1]

Newer macrolide antibiotics (e.g., **azithromycin, clarithromycin**) offer more convenient dosing schedules but use is limited by their cost. Both azithromycin and clarithromycin have better bioavailability than erythromycin and provide coverage for *H. influenzae*.

- **Clindamycin** is a reasonable agent to treat serious skin and soft tissue infections in penicillin-allergic patients, keeping in mind the increased risk for *C. difficile* and pseudomembranous colitis.

  Consider clindamycin when treating patients with community-acquired methicillin-resistant *S. aureus* (MRSA) infections as these strains are often susceptible to non-beta-lactam antibiotics.[1] Consider clindamycin in particularly aggressive or necrotizing skin and soft tissue infections related to group A streptococcus as it offers broader coverage, and in vitro studies have demonstrated toxin suppression and cytokine modulation.[1]
- **Fluoroquinolones** play little role in treating common bacterial skin infections unless gram-negative organisms are suspected. They may play a role in treatment of community-acquired MRSA infections, depending on susceptibility patterns. **Ciprofloxacin** can be used to treat Pseudomonas or so called "hot-tub" folliculitis in select patients with extensive or symptomatic involvement, keeping in mind the typically self-limited course in untreated patients.

Topical Agents (Table 2)

Mupirocin's mechanism of action is not shared by other topical antibiotics and thus resistance has not been an issue to date with the exception of mupirocin-resistant MRSA strains.[2] It is considered particularly useful for localized impetigo and folliculitis caused by *S. aureus*. Applied intranasally, it can be used to eradicate *S. aureus* nasal carriage.[2]

Fusidic acid, like mupirocin, can be used to treat localized skin infections where oral therapy is not indicated. There are reports of increasing resistance of *S. aureus* to fusidic acid; therefore, it should only be used for appropriate indications and for brief, defined treatment courses.[3]

Numerous over-the-counter proprietary preparations containing antibiotics with both gram-positive and gram-negative coverage are available (e.g., **bacitracin, gramicidin, polymyxin B**). These agents have limited efficacy for bacterial skin infections and are best used for prevention of infection and/or wound healing in minor cuts or abrasions.[2]

Framycetin and **silver sulfadiazine** both play a role in reducing microbes in wounds and burns, respectively, but should not be used as monotherapy for established skin and soft tissue infection.

Therapeutic Tips

- When assessing patients with atopic dermatitis, determine whether significant secondary infection due to *S. aureus* is present. This will manifest as crusting, weeping, painful fissured eczema or nonhealing erosions and crusts. Treating the secondary impetiginization is vital for providing symptom relief and control of the eczema.

- If a patient presents with symptoms and signs of a lower extremity cellulitis that is complicated by significant fluid-filled blisters, consider bullous erysipelas and ensure adequate coverage of *S. pyogenes*.
- Any limb cellulitis or serious soft tissue infection that manifests with blisters and/or necrosis, "dusky gray" appearance, severe pain, gas in soft tissue, numbness, exceptionally rapid spread or systemic toxicity should prompt urgent consideration and investigation for *necrotizing fasciitis*.
- In patients with recurrent painful, sterile abscesses and scarring in the axillae and groin, consider *hidradenitis suppurativa* and refer for appropriate specialist care, e.g., dermatology or plastic surgery.
- Avoid prolonged use of topical antibacterials (> 2 weeks) to prevent development of bacterial resistance.
- Given increasing reports of community-acquired MRSA, patients with recurrent impetigo or furuncles should have swabs to rule out MRSA, particularly if risk factors (Figure 2) are identified.[1]
- In patients with refractory folliculitis on upper back and chest accompanied by scale and pigmentary changes (hyper- or hypopigmentation), consider *pityrosporum folliculitis*. This is a deeper, follicular manifestion of pityriasis versicolor infection.
- Avoid routine topical antibiotics in the management of chronic wounds such as *venous stasis ulcers*. Overuse may lead to resistance and possible allergic contact dermatitis.

Figure 1: Management of Impetigo[a]

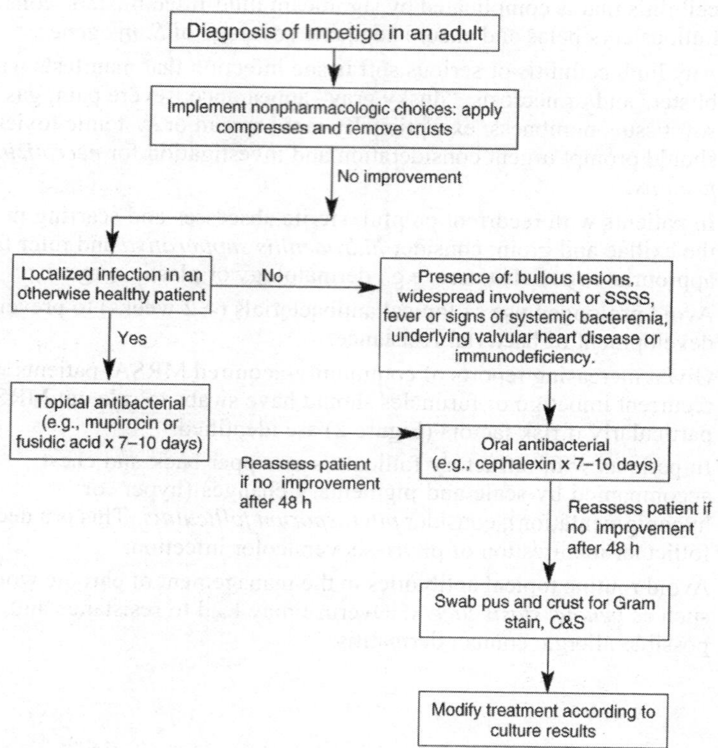

[a] If recurrent impetigo, consider nasal *S. aureus* carriage. Obtain nasal swab and eradicate with mupirocin or fucidin TID intranasally for 3 days.

Abbreviations: SSSS = Staphylococcal scalded skin syndrome; C&S = culture and sensitivity

Figure 2: Management of Folliculitis

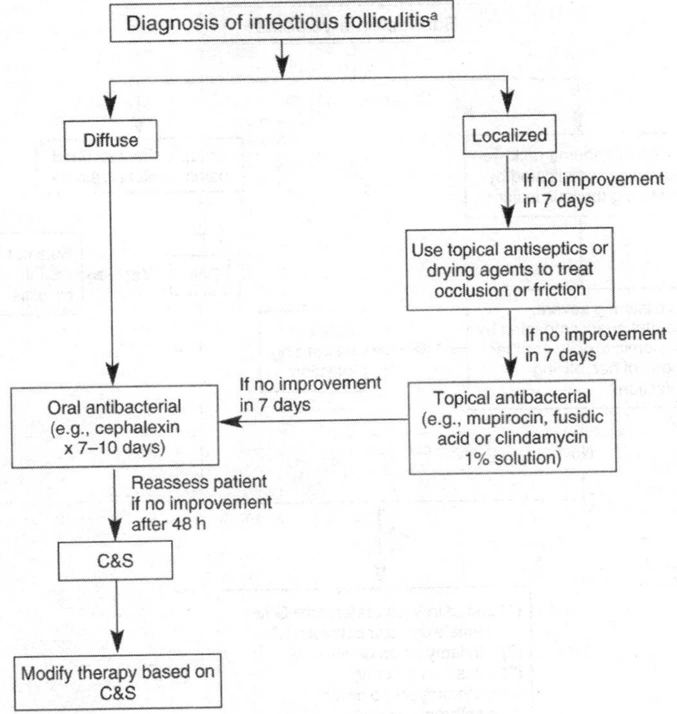

[a] Given the increasing prevalence of community-acquired MRSA skin infections, patients with risk factors who present with recurrent or persistent impetigo and furuncles should have cultures performed to determine antibiotic susceptibilities.[1] Risk factors reported for community-acquired MRSA infection are: incarcerated prisoners, iv drug users, Native Americans, homosexual men, participants in contact sports and children.[1]

Abbreviations: C&S = culture and sensitivity

Figure 3: **Management of Erysipelas**

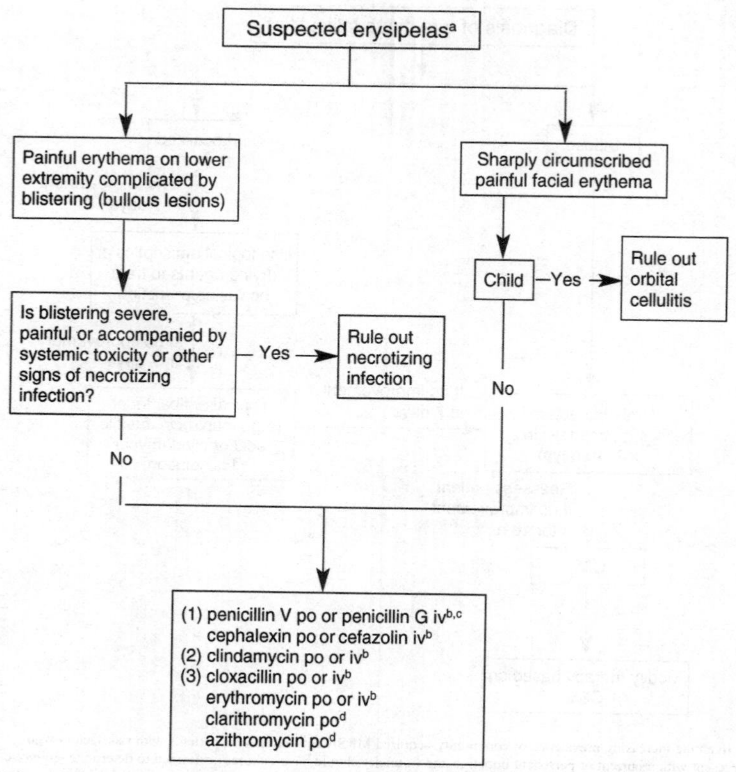

[a] Duration of treatment with erysipelas is usually longer than cellulitis given lymphatic involvement and higher rate of recurrence; consider up to 2 weeks of therapy and may need to extend to 4 to 6 weeks depending on severity of infection.
[b] IV route to be used in severe cases.
[c] Vancomycin iv is recommended in patients who are beta-lactam allergic or who do not respond to therapy.
[d] Organisms resistant to erythromycin will be resistant to clindamycin, clarithromycin and azithromycin also.
Abbreviations: (1) = first line; (2) = second line; (3) = third line

Figure 4: Management of Cellulitis

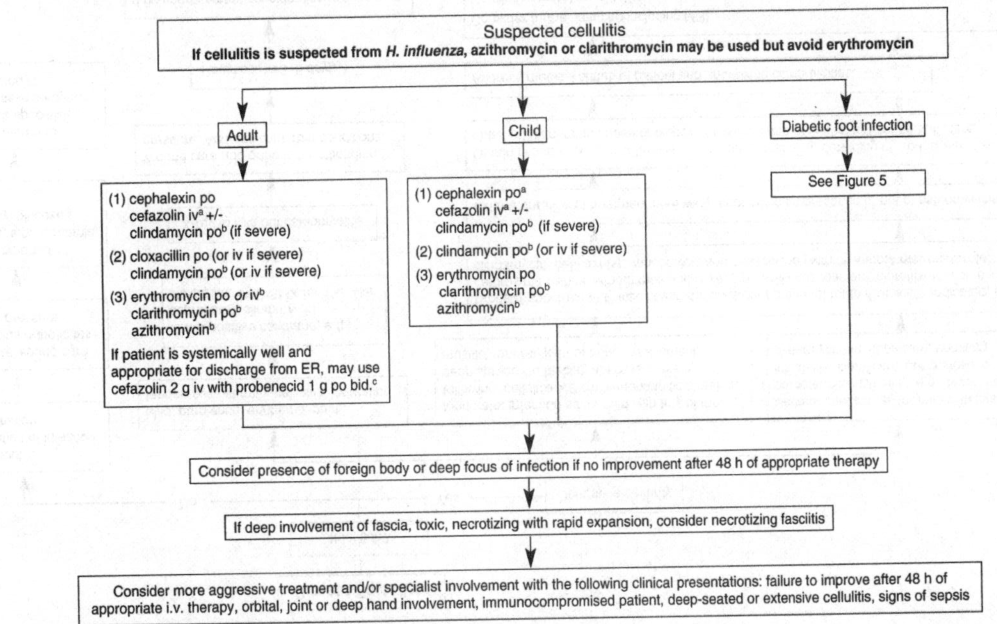

[a] Vancomycin iv is recommended in patients who are beta-lactam allergic or who do not respond to therapy.
[b] Organisms resistant to erythromycin will be resistant to clindamycin, clarithromycin and azithromycin also.
[c] Give probenecid 30 min po PRIOR to cefazolin. May use regimen daily but consider increasing frequency to BID if not improving or worse after 48 h.
Abbreviations: (1) = first line; (2) = second line; (3) = third line

Figure 5: **Management of Diabetic Foot Ulcer**[4]

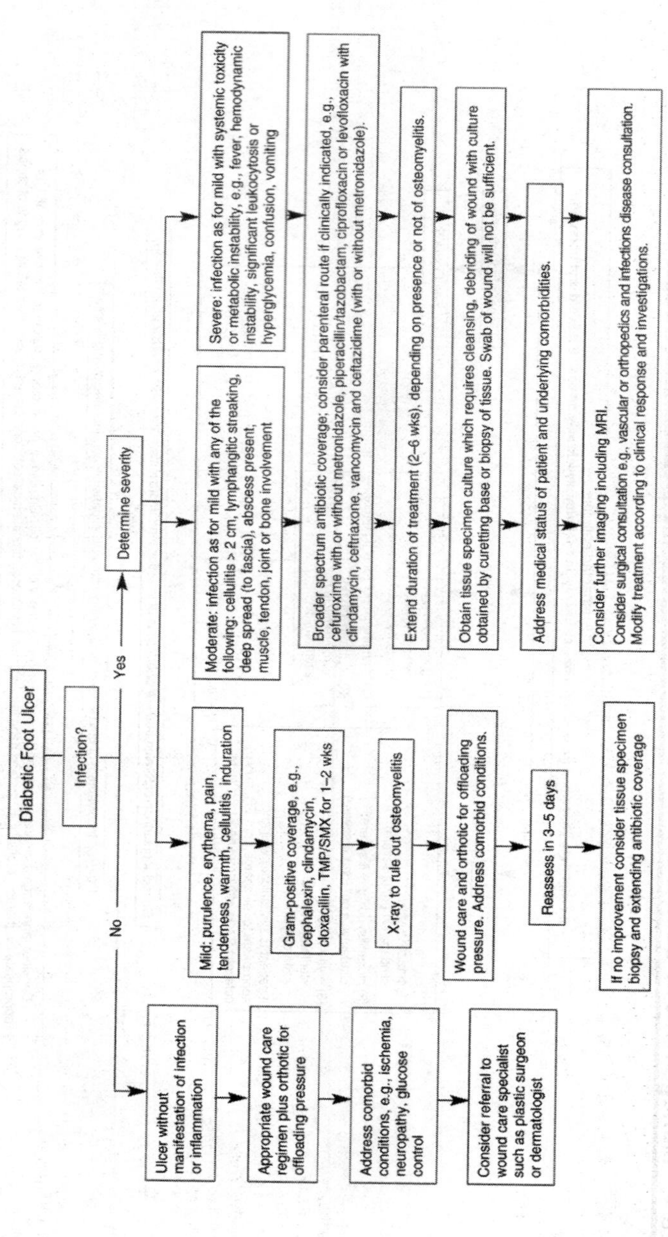

Table 1: Antibiotics Used to Treat Bacterial Skin Infections

Class	Drug	Dose[a]	Adverse Effects[b]	Drug Interactions[b]	Cost[c]
Penicillins	*penicillin V* generics	Adults: 300 mg po Q6H Children: 25–50 mg/kg/day po divided Q6–8H	Rash, drug fever.		$
	penicillin G Crystapen, generics	Adults: 2 million units iv Q4–6H	Electrolyte imbalance possible with high-dose penicillin G Na^+ or K^+ (> 10 million IU/day). See penicillin V.		$$$$$
Penicillinase-resistant Penicillins	*cloxacillin* generics	Adults: 250–500 mg po Q6H Children: 25–50 mg/kg/day po divided Q6H	Hypersensitivity reactions (ranging from minor rashes to anaphylactic shock).		$
Penicillin, Beta-lactamase Inhibitor Combinations	*amoxicillin/clavulanate* Clavulin, generics	Adults: 250–500 mg po Q8H Children: 40 mg/kg/day of amoxicillin po divided Q8H	Nausea, vomiting, diarrhea, rash, eosinophilia. See cloxacillin.		$$
	piperacillin/ tazobactam Tazocin	Adults: 3 g/0.375 g iv Q6H	Hypersensitivity reactions, rash, nausea, vomiting, pseudomembranous colitis, interstitial nephritis.		$$$$$
Cephalosporins	*cephalexin* generics	Adults: 250–500 mg po Q6H Children: 25–50 mg/kg/day po divided Q6H	Hypersensitivity reactions (some cross-reactivity with penicillins).		$
	cefadroxil Duricef, generics	Adults: 1 g po daily	See cephalexin.		$$

(cont'd)

Table 1: **Antibiotics Used to Treat Bacterial Skin Infections** *(cont'd)*

Class	Drug	Dose[a]	Adverse Effects[b]	Drug Interactions[b]	Cost[c]
	cefazolin generics	Adults: 1 g iv Q8H Children: 50–100 mg/kg/day iv divided Q8H	Rash, ↑ AST and ALP, phlebitis. See cephalexin.		$$$$$
	cefuroxime sodium Kefurox, Zinacef, generics	Children: 100–150 mg/kg/day iv divided Q8H to max 750 mg iv Q8H	Eosinophilia, anemia, phlebitis, LFTs. See cephalexin.		$$$$$
Macrolides	*erythromycin* EES, Eryc, generics	Adults: 250 mg po Q6H 500 mg iv Q6H Children: 30–50 mg/kg/day po divided Q6H	GI irritation (common), nausea and vomiting. Cholestatic jaundice with erythromycin estolate (rare).	Inhibits cytochrome P450 enzyme system.[d]	$
	clarithromycin Biaxin	Adults: 250–500 mg po Q12H Children: 15 mg/kg/day po divided Q12H	See erythromycin.	See erythromycin.	Adult: $$$–$$$$$ Children: $$$$
	azithromycin Zithromax, generics	Adults: 500 mg po on day 1, then 250 mg on days 2–5 (total 1.5 g) Children: 10 mg/kg/day po on first day then 5 mg/kg × 4 days	See erythromycin.	Appears less likely to cause interactions than other macrolides.	Adult: $$ Children: $$$
Carbapenems	*imipenem/cilastatin* Primaxin, generics	500 mg iv Q6H	Imipenem has been associated with seizures at doses of 1 g Q6H. Diarrhea, rash, hypersensitivity reactions: interstitial nephritis, neutropenia, hemolytic anemia; thrombocytopenia.		$$$$$

Class	Drug	Dose[a]	Adverse Effects[b]	Drug Interactions[b]	Cost[c]
Glycopeptides	*vancomycin* Vancocin, Vancomycin, generics	Adults: 1 g iv Q12H Children: 40 mg/kg/day iv divided Q6H	Hypotension, flushing, red man syndrome, chills, drug fever, eosinophilia.	↑ toxicity with other nephrotoxic or ototoxic drugs.	$$$$$
Lincosamides	*clindamycin* Dalacin C, Dalacin C Flavored Granules, Dalacin-C Phosphate Sterile Solution, generics	Adults: 150–300 mg po Q6H or 450–600 mg iv Q8H Children: (> 1 mo) 10–30 mg/kg/day po divided Q6H	Diarrhea, pseudomembranous colitis.[e]		Adult po:$$–$$$ Adult iv: $$$$$ Children: $$$
Fluoroquinolones	*ciprofloxacin* Cipro, generics	Adults: 500–750 mg po BID	Nausea, vomiting, diarrhea, abdominal pain.	Multivalent metallic cations, antacids and sucralfate ↓ absorption of ciprofloxacin. Inhibits cytochrome P450 enzyme system.[d]	$$$–$$$$$
Sulfonamide Combinations	*sulfamethoxazole/trimethoprim (cotrimoxazole)* generics	Adults: 800 mg/160 mg daily (2 tabs BID or 1 DS tab BID)	Nausea, vomiting, diarrhea, rash, neutropenia, thrombocytopenia, anemia.	↑ phenytoin levels. ↑ INR with warfarin. Hypoglycemia with sulfonylureas.	$

(cont'd)

Table 1: **Antibiotics Used to Treat Bacterial Skin Infections** *(cont'd)*

Class	Drug	Dose[a]	Adverse Effects[b]	Drug Interactions[b]	Cost[c]
Nitroimidazoles	*metronidazole* Flagyl, generics	Adults: 500 mg po BID Children: 30–50 mg/kg/day po divided TID	Nausea, vomiting, diarrhea, metallic taste, headache, dark urine, neutropenia.	Disulfiram reaction with alcohol. ↑ INR with warfarin. ↓ phenytoin clearance. Phenobarb, phenytoin ↓ effectiveness of metronidazole.	Adult: $ Children: $$

[a] Pediatric dose should not exceed recommended adult dose.
[b] Only select adverse effects/drug interactions are listed; consult product monograph for complete list.
[c] Cost of 7-day supply based on 20 kg body weight for cost of children's dose.; includes drug cost only.
[d] Potential ↑ effect/toxicity of carbamazepine, corticosteroids, cyclosporine, digoxin, theophylline and warfarin.
[e] Commonly associated with clindamycin but any antibiotic may cause this complication.
Dosage adjustment may be required in renal impairment; see Appendix I.
Legend: $ < $10 $$ $10–20 $$-$$$ $10–30 $$$ $20–30 $$$$ $30–40 $$$-$$$$$ $20– > 40 $$$$$ > $40

Table 2: Topical Antibacterials Used in Superficial Bacterial Skin Infections

Class	Drug	Dose	Antibacterial Spectrum	Adverse Effects	Cost[a]
Aminoglycosides	*framycetin* Sofra-Tulle dressing	BID–TID	*S. aureus*, streptococcus, gram-negatives.	Allergic contact dermatitis, cross-reaction with neomycin.	$$$ (10 × 10 cm dressing, 10s)
	gentamicin Garamycin Topical Preparations, generics	BID–TID	*S. aureus*, streptococcus, gram-negatives.	Allergic contact dermatitis.	$$
Antibacterial Combinations	*neomycin with polymyxin B and bacitracin* Neosporin (with polymyxin B and bacitracin), generics	BID–TID	*S. aureus*, streptococcus, gram-negatives.	Allergic contact dermatitis, especially when applied to eczematous skin.	$$[b]
	polymyxin B with gramicidin or bacitracin Polysporin cream or ointment, generics	BID–TID	Gram-negatives.	Nephrotoxicity when used extensively, allergic contact dermatitis.	$[b]
Miscellaneous Antibacterials	*bacitracin* Baciguent, Bacitracin, generics	BID–TID	Gram-positives.	Allergic contact dermatitis, anaphylactic reactions following topical application (rare).	$[b]
	fusidic acid Fucidin Cream	BID–TID	Gram-positives.	Allergic contact dermatitis (rare).	$$

(cont'd)

Table 2: **Topical Antibacterials Used in Superficial Bacterial Skin Infections** *(cont'd)*

Class	Drug	Dose	Antibacterial Spectrum	Adverse Effects	Cost[a]
	mupirocin Bactroban Ointment, generics	BID–TID	Gram-positives.	Stinging, allergic contact dermatitis (rare).	$$[b]
Sulfonamides	*silver sulfadiazine* Dermazin, Flamazine, SSD	BID–TID	*S. aureus*, gram-negatives, *Pseudomonas.*	Allergic contact dermatitis, leukopenia when applied to large area of burned skin.	$

[a] Cost of 15 g tube; includes drug cost only.
[b] Available without prescription; retail mark-up not included.
Legend: $ < $5 $$ $5–10 $$$ $10–15

Suggested Readings

Blume J, Levine E, Heymann W. Bacterial diseases. In: Bolognia J, Jorizzo JL, Rapini RP, editors. *Dermatology*. New York (NY): Mosby; 2003. p. 1117-44.

Lee P, Zipoli M, Weinberg AN et al. Pyodermas: Staphylococcus aureus, streptococcus and other gram-positive bacteria. In: Fitzpatrick TB, Freedberg IM, editors. *Fitzpatrick's dermatology in general medicine*. 6th ed. New York (NY): McGraw-Hill; 2003. p.1856-77.

Stevens DL, Bisno AL, Chambers HF et al. Practice guidelines for the diagnosis and management of skin and soft-tissue infections. *Clin Infect Dis* 2005;41(10):1373-406.

References

1. Stevens DL, Bisno AL, Chambers HF et al. Practice guidelines for the diagnosis and management of skin and soft-tissue infections. *Clin Infect Dis* 2005;41(10):1373-406.
2. Hsu S, Quan LT. Topical antibacterial agents. In: Wolverton SE, editor. *Comprehensive dermatologic drug therapy*. 1st ed. Philadelphia (PA): Saunders; 2001. p.472-96.
3. Dobie D, Gray J. Fusidic acid resistance in Staphylococcus aureus. *Arch Dis Child* 2004;89(1):74-7.
4. Lipsky BA, Berendt AR, Deery HG et.al. Diagnosis and treatment of diabetic foot infections. *Clin Infect Dis* 2004;39(7):885-910.

CHAPTER 87
Common Anemias

S. Rutledge Harding, MD, FRCPC

Anemia is typically defined as a hemoglobin (Hgb) value that is two standard deviations below the mean, according to sex, age and, sometimes, race. This defines the lower limit of the normal range provided by most clinical laboratories with their patient reports. Recently, arguments have been advanced to establish optimal rather than statistical lower limits of Hgb, especially in older adults, based on morbidity and mortality data.[1] Optimal Hgb concentrations were found to be 130 g/L in elderly women and 140 g/L in elderly men.

Goals of Therapy

- Alleviate the signs and symptoms of anemia
- Determine and address the underlying cause(s) of the anemia
- Restore normal or adequate Hgb level
  - improve quality of life[2]
  - possibly prolong survival[3]
- Avoid allogeneic red cell transfusion

Investigations

- Signs and symptoms of anemia occur when the oxygen-carrying capacity of the blood is unable to meet the oxygen requirements of body tissues (Figure 1).[1]
- Identify the underlying cause of anemia. Underlying cause(s) may include medications (cytotoxic agents, antiretrovirals, ribavirin, folate antagonists, etc.), alcohol use, diet (vegans are at particular risk for vitamin B_{12} deficiency), gastrointestinal complaints (blood loss, malabsorption, gastric or terminal ileal surgery), menorrhagia history, cancer, impaired kidney/liver/thyroid function and chronic inflammation. Seek signs and symptoms that point to the etiology of the anemia (e.g., glossitis and koilonychia in iron deficiency, paresthesia in B_{12} deficiency).
- Diagnostic algorithms are given as guidelines in Figure 2, Figure 3 and Figure 4, based on the traditional classification of anemia according to red cell size, as reflected in the mean cell volume (MCV).[4]
- The serum folate level is prone to short-term fluctuations and may be misleading. The red blood cell (RBC) folate level reflects time-averaged folate availability and is a more reliable indicator of tissue folate adequacy.[5]
- There is significant intra- and inter-individual variation in serum cobalamin levels, so patients with macrocytosis and borderline (as defined by the local laboratory) cobalamin levels need further

assessment.[6] Cobalamin levels drop during pregnancy without other evidence of deficiency.[7]

Iron-deficiency Anemia

Nonpharmacologic Choices

Dietary iron, especially from foods rich in heme iron (i.e., liver; lean red meats; seafood such as oyster, clams, tuna, salmon, sardines and shrimp), can contribute to the treatment of iron deficiency anemia, but works more slowly than pharmacologic replacement therapy,[8] and may not be sufficient in the face of more severe or persistent causes of iron deficiency.

Vitamin C enhances the absorption of iron but the effect is small. Consumption of foods that are good sources of vitamin C has a minimal impact on the therapy of iron deficiency anemia.

Pharmacologic Choices (Table 1)

- Simple **oral iron salts** are the mainstay of iron supplementation therapy in most circumstances of iron deficiency anemia.
  - a variety of salts are available, with differing amounts of elemental iron per tablet; however, the gut is limited in its ability to absorb iron and such differences have little effect on the outcome of replacement therapy
  - the usual target dose is 105-200 mg/day of elemental iron, in divided doses
- **Parenteral iron** is reserved for patients with malabsorption or true intolerance to oral iron therapy, or where ongoing losses exceed the capacity of the gut to absorb oral iron. Although newer formulations are somewhat safer and better tolerated than older preparations, anaphylaxis remains a risk.[9]
  - in those who can tolerate and absorb oral iron salts, the use of parenteral iron does not lead to a more rapid resolution of anemia

Therapeutic Tips

- Search for the cause of iron deficiency, including very careful consideration of occult gastrointestinal bleeding (see Suggested Readings). Menorrhagia must be convincing before it is accepted as the sole cause of iron deficiency.[10] This may be an opportunity for early recognition of a gastrointestinal malignancy—don't miss it!
- A reticulocyte response should be evident within one week of beginning iron therapy, with subsequent improvement in the Hgb of about 10 g/L every 7–10 days.
- If the Hgb fails to respond as anticipated, consider that there may be:
  - ongoing blood loss
  - use of other medications that impair iron absorption (Table 1)

  - a different or concurrent cause of anemia and/or an impaired erythropoietic response
  - compliance issues
- Gastrointestinal side effects are the most common reasons for non-compliance:
  - use a graduated approach to dosing. Begin with a single tablet taken after a meal. On a weekly basis, as tolerance permits, add another tablet until the patient is taking one dose with each meal. Thereafter, gradually shift the timing of the doses to the beginning of meals
  - small oral doses may be adequate in patients that are susceptible to gastrointestinal upset.

    In the elderly, daily doses of elemental iron as low as 15 to 50 mg are effective in the treatment of iron deficiency anemia[9]

    In pregnant women, 20 mg/day of elemental iron, started at 20 weeks' gestation, is sufficient to prevent iron deficiency[11]
  - iron contained in enteric-coated tablets is poorly absorbed. These products should be avoided
- Some physicians replenish iron stores while others prefer to stop therapy when the Hgb normalizes, so that further blood loss will not be masked by robust iron stores. As a compromise:
  - completely replenish iron stores when the cause of iron deficiency has been identified and corrected
  - do not replenish iron stores when investigation has failed to identify the cause of the iron deficiency. Recurrence of anemia flags the need and provides the opportunity for further investigation.

Megaloblastic Anemia

Megaloblastic anemias arise because of impaired DNA synthesis from deficiencies of cobalamin (vitamin B_{12}) or folic acid (folate). Other causes of impaired DNA and RNA metabolism (i.e., drugs, myelodysplasia) produce similar hematologic findings.

Cobalamin deficiency may also lead to subacute combined degeneration of the spinal cord. Folate may partially alleviate and mask the hematologic effects of cobalamin deficiency, but does nothing to slow the progression of the neurologic lesion.

Systemic symptoms of megaloblastosis may be subtle in older adults and may precede the development of anemia. A high index of suspicion is warranted.[12]

Cobalamin (Vitamin B_{12}) Deficiency

- Meat and dairy products are the only dietary sources of cobalamin. The typical Canadian diet exceeds the daily requirement, provided that absorption is normal.

- Cobalamin stores are usually sufficient to last several years.
- Strict vegans are at risk of deficiency unless they take cobalamin supplements. Vegetarians may be at risk of deficiency during times of high demand, such as pregnancy.
- The most common cause of cobalamin deficiency is malabsorption due to pernicious anemia, gastrectomy, gastritis, ileal resection, Crohn's disease, blind loops, pancreatic insufficiency and certain drugs (i.e., neomycin, metformin, proton pump inhibitors). Some patients have trouble absorbing cobalamin from food but are able to absorb pharmaceutical cobalamin.

Folic Acid Deficiency

- Dietary deficiency and alcoholism are the most common causes of folate deficiency.
- Although folate is plentiful in a variety of foods (i.e., leafy green vegetables, liver, legumes) it is labile and easily destroyed by exposure to light and during cooking.
- Alcohol inhibits folate absorption and interferes with its enterohepatic cycle.
- Folate deficiency can develop within a few months of adopting a folate-deficient diet and even more quickly in the setting of increased alcohol intake.
- Increased folate requirements are seen in pregnancy, hemolytic anemia and therapy with certain drugs (i.e., methotrexate, phenytoin, trimethoprim).

Nonpharmacologic Choices

Restoring normal dietary intake of cobalamin and folate may be sufficient to completely reverse megaloblastosis. However, patients with neurologic deficits due to cobalamin deficiency should be treated pharmacologically to maximize the likelihood of full neurologic recovery.

Abstinence from alcohol may be necessary.

Pharmacologic Choices (Table 1)

Cobalamin (Vitamin B_{12})

- Cobalamin deficiency is treated with either **cyanocobalamin** or **hydroxocobalamin (hydroxycobalamin)**. The daily requirement is 6–9 µg. Doses greater than 100 µg/day exceed the physiologic binding capacity, but the excess is not toxic and is readily excreted by the kidneys. For this reason there is a tendency to give more rather than less cobalamin, especially in patients with neurologic deficits.
- Cobalamin has traditionally been given parenterally because deficiency is most often due to malabsorption, and most cases of malabsorption are attributable to pernicious anemia with its lack of intrinsic factor.

- High-dose oral cobalamin therapy is effective,[13] feasible[14,15] and cost-effective,[16] but concerns about patient compliance and the need for more attentive monitoring[17] limit adoption of this approach in North America.
- As a compromise:
  - administer parenteral cobalamin until all neurologic and hematologic findings resolve
  - provide maintenance therapy by the route that best fits the patient's circumstances.
- Where dietary deficiency is clearly the cause of the cobalamin deficiency and the patient has no neurologic deficits, oral supplementation is adequate.

Folic Acid

- Prophylaxis with **folate** before and during pregnancy is strongly recommended for the prevention of neural tube defects. (See Chapter 29 for specific dosing recommendations.)
- Otherwise, folate should be given only for confirmed folate deficiency or in situations of increased demand, such as hemolysis.
- The oral route is sufficient to correct folate deficiency, even in patients with malabsorption syndromes.

Therapeutic Tips

- A reticulocyte response should be evident within three to four days of beginning therapy, with improvement in the Hgb level by about day ten. Full resolution of the anemia should occur within about two months.
- The rapid production of new hematopoietic cells leads to a potentially dramatic shift of potassium from extracellular to intracellular compartments, which may cause profound hypokalemia.
  - monitor potassium carefully in the first few days of therapy; consider early and generous potassium supplementation
  - older patients on diuretic therapy for heart failure are at particular risk
- If the Hgb fails to respond as anticipated, consider that there may be:
  - a different or concurrent cause of anemia and/or an impaired erythropoietic response
    - concomitant iron deficiency may show itself with an MCV that shifts from the macrocytic to the microcytic range
  - compliance issues, particularly in patients using oral supplements
- Neurologic deficits may take six months or more to resolve; if severe, some deficits may persist.

Anemias Responsive to Pharmacologic Stimulation of Erythropoiesis

Most patients with nutritional anemias, hemolysis or bleeding have elevated levels of endogenous erythropoietin. There are, however, a number of situations in which pharmacologic stimulation of red cell production is beneficial including:

- Chronic renal failure
- HIV-infected patients receiving antiretroviral therapy[18]
- Chronic hepatitis C patients receiving ribavirin[19]
- Patients receiving chemotherapy for non-hematologic cancers[20,21]
- Surgery patients[20]
- Low-risk myelodysplasia[22]

Other clinical applications are beyond the scope of this discussion.[23,24]

Investigations

Selection of patients is determined in part by baseline endogenous erythropoietin levels (approximately 3–30 IU/L in healthy individuals).

For example:

- A zidovudine-treated HIV patient is unlikely to respond if the baseline erythropoietin level is > 500 IU/L
- A chemotherapy-treated cancer patient is unlikely to respond if the baseline erythropoietin level is > 200 IU/L

It is important to ensure an adequate iron supply in conjunction with erythropoietic stimulation.

Pharmacologic Choices (Table 2)

The choice of agent and dosage regimen varies according to the clinical situation. Both available agents may be given by intravenous or subcutaneous injection. **Epoetin alfa** is a recombinant human erythropoietin with a relatively short half-life that is typically given at least three times per week; daily in some circumstances. **Darbepoetin alfa** is a synthetic erythropoietin analogue with a longer half-life that is typically given weekly or biweekly, and monthly in some patients.

Therapeutic Tips

- These agents have significant potential for toxicity and adverse consequences. They are for judicious use in patients who would otherwise require transfusion support.
- Doses are titrated to achieve a gradual improvement in anemia, without overshooting the target Hgb.
  - in patients with renal failure, higher Hgb targets are not associated with better outcomes[25,26,27]

  - survival was worse in patients treated to higher Hgb targets (> 120 g/L) with erythropoietin as compared with placebo in patients with head and neck cancer[28] and those with breast cancer[29]
- Rapid and/or excessive correction of anemia may provoke hypertension and seizures in susceptible individuals; erythrocytosis may predispose patients to thrombotic complications. Monitor blood pressure three times per week initially, and after each dose thereafter.
- These agents have been associated with the development of pure red cell aplasia (PRCA), a potentially devastating complication in which neutralizing antibodies to the exogenous protein cross-react with endogenous erythropoietin, resulting in profound anemia. Changes in the formulation and handling of these proteins have greatly reduced the risk of PRCA.[3] Nevertheless, PRCA should be considered if a patient becomes refractory to therapy.

Figure 1: **Evaluation of Anemia**

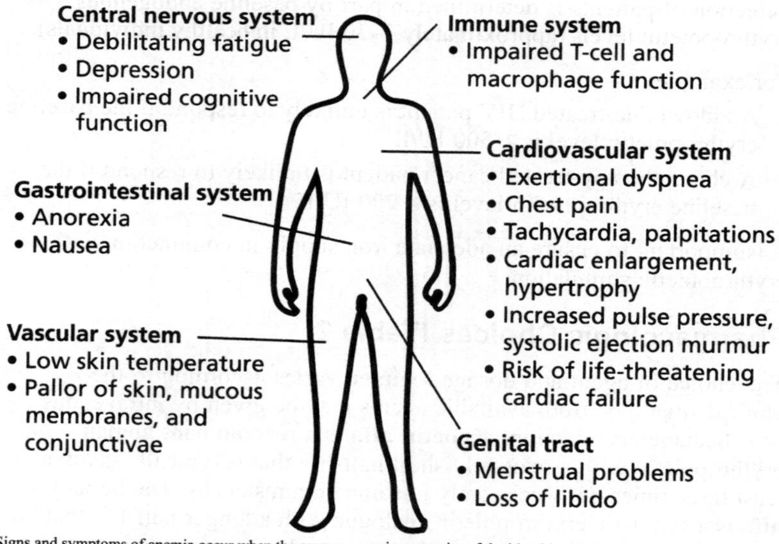

Signs and symptoms of anemia occur when the oxygen-carrying capacity of the blood is unable to meet the oxygen requirements of body tissues. Modified from *Semin Oncol*, Volume 25 (Suppl 7), Ludwig H, Fritz, E. Anemia in cancer patients, pages 2–6, Copyright 1998, with permission from Elsevier Inc.

Figure 2: **Diagnostic Algorithm for Microcytic Anemia**

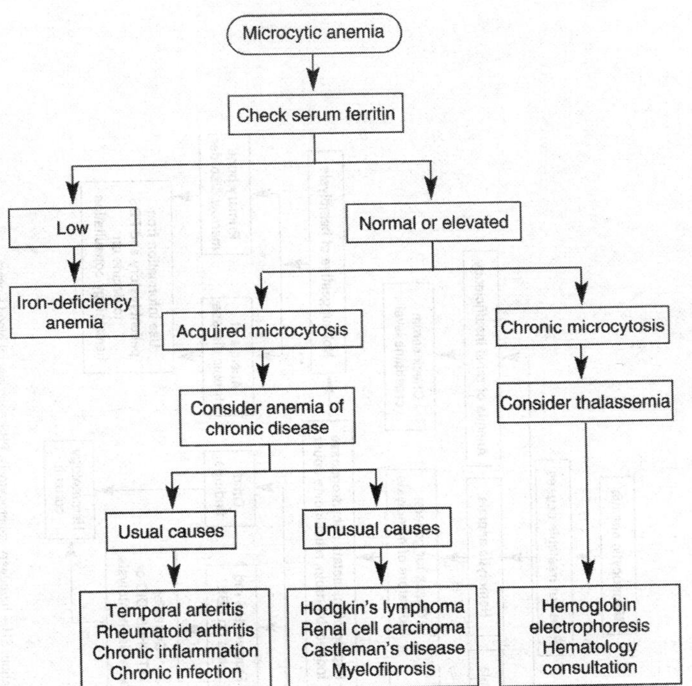

Adapted with permission from: Tefferi A, Hanson DA, Inwards DJ. How to interpret and pursue an abnormal complete blood cell count in adults. *Mayo Clin Proc*. 2005;80:923-936

Figure 3: Diagnostic Algorithm for Normocytic Anemia

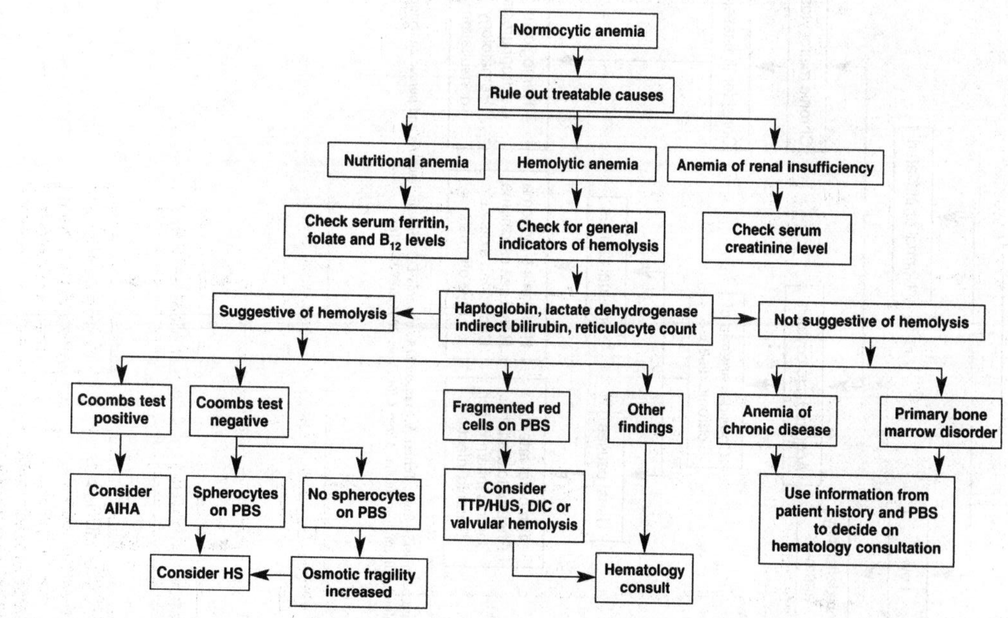

Abbreviations: AIHA = autoimmune hemolytic anemia; DIC = disseminated intravascular coagulation; SH = hereditary spherocytosis; PBS = peripheral blood smear; TTP/HUS = thrombotic thrombocytopenic purpura/hemolytic uremic syndrome

Adapted with permission from: Tefferi A, Hanson DA, Inwards DJ. How to interpret and pursue an abnormal complete blood cell count in adults. *Mayo Clin Proc.* 2005;80:923-936

Figure 4: **Diagnostic Algorithm for Macrocytic Anemia**

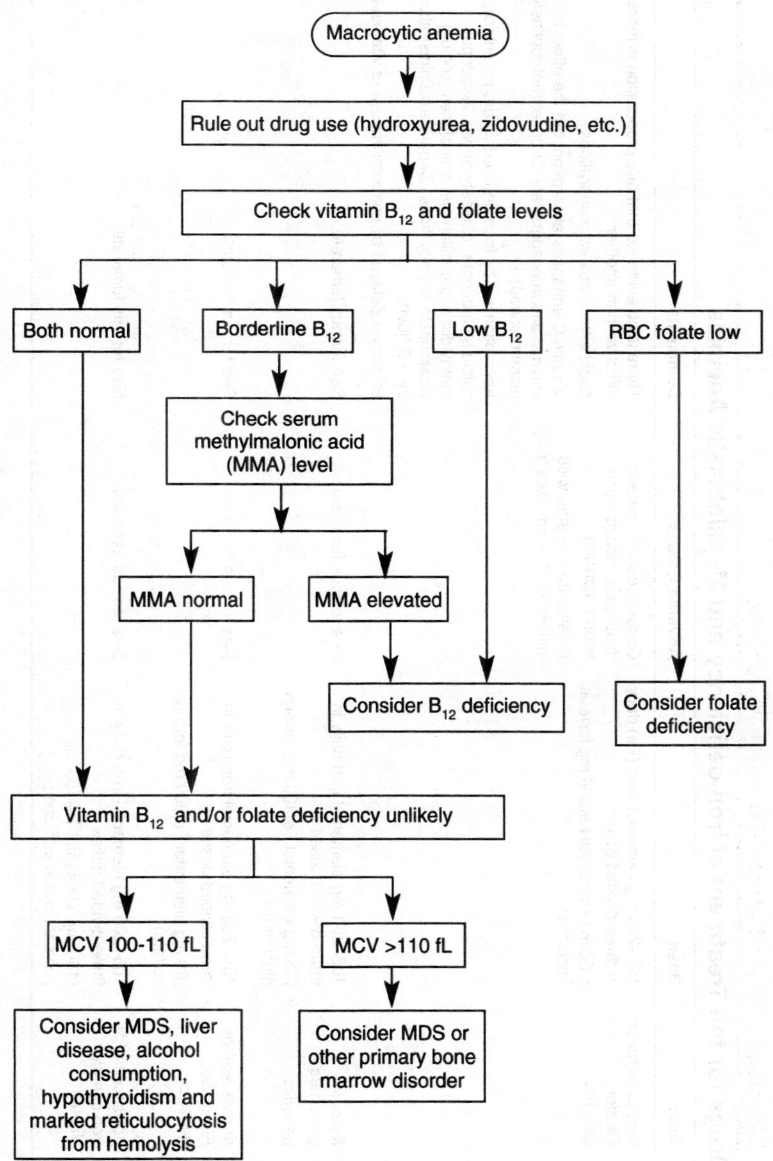

Abbreviations: MCV = mean cell volume; MDS = myelodysplastic syndrome

Adapted with permission from: Tefferi A, Hanson DA, Inwards DJ. How to interpret and pursue an abnormal complete blood cell count in adults. *Mayo Clin Proc.* 2005;80:923-936

Table 1: **Drugs for the Treatment of Iron-deficiency and Megaloblastic Anemias**

Class	Drug	Dose	Adverse Effects	Comments	Cost[a]
Iron Supplements, oral	*ferrous fumarate* Palafer, generics	105–200 mg elemental iron (Fe) daily in three divided doses (100 mg elemental Fe/300 mg ferrous fumarate)	Gastrointestinal: nausea, dyspepsia, constipation and/or diarrhea. Ameliorated by step-wise initiation of therapy (see text).	There is no evidence that one preparation is more effective than another. Avoid enteric-coated preparations. Vitamin C enhances absorption, but the effect is minimal and may aggravate GI upset (not routinely recommended). Absorption is ↓ by food and certain drugs: antacids, calcium carbonate, cholestyramine, levodopa, methyldopa, penicillamine, quinolones, sodium bicarbonate, tetracyclines. Separate administration by ~ 2 hours. Efficacy is delayed by concomitant use of vitamin E.	$
	ferrous gluconate generics	105–200 mg elemental iron daily in three divided doses (35 mg elemental Fe/300 mg ferrous gluconate)	See ferrous fumarate.	See ferrous fumarate.	$
	ferrous sulfate Fer-In-Sol, generics	105–200 mg elemental iron daily in three divided doses (60 mg elemental Fe/300 mg ferrous sulfate)	See ferrous fumarate.	See ferrous fumarate.	$
	polysaccharide-iron complex Niferex	105–200 mg elemental iron daily in three divided doses (150 mg elemental Fe/150 mg polysaccharide iron complex)	See ferrous fumarate.	See ferrous fumarate.	$$

Class	Drug	Dose	Adverse Effects	Comments	Cost[a]
Iron Supplements, parenteral	*iron dextran* Dexlron, Infufer	Total dose infusion: iv dose calculated to restore iron deficit in red cell mass and iron stores. In chronic dialysis patients: 100 mg iv 1–3 ×/wk for 10 doses or until replete; adjust as able to maintain adequate iron availability	Anaphylaxis (rare). Anaphylactoid reactions, hypotension (avoid rapid iv infusion). Fever, chills, headache, myalgia, arthralgia, urticaria, dizziness. May have delayed onset, 24–48 hours after iv infusion and 3–4 days after im administration.	Consult prescribing information for dose calculation, dilution and administration details. 0.9% NaCl is the preferred vehicle. D5W causes more local irritation and phlebitis. Give a 25 mg test dose one h before the initial dose, with epinephrine available. Side effects are more common with larger doses and in underweight patients.	$$$$
	sodium ferric gluconate Ferrlecit	Chronic dialysis patients: 125 mg iv 1–3 ×/wk × 8 doses; adjust as able to maintain adequate iron availability	See iron dextran.	Test doses are no longer recommended by the manufacturer. Incidence of life-threatening adverse effects is lower than with iron dextran.	$$$$
	iron sucrose Venofer	Chronic dialysis patients: 100 mg iv 1–3 ×/wk until replete; adjust as able to maintain adequate iron availability	See iron dextran.	Test doses are not recommended by the manufacturer. Lowest incidence of life-threatening adverse effects among iv iron preparations.	$$$$
Vitamins	*cobalamin (vitamin B_{12})*	Pernicious anemia/other chronic malabsorption disorders: 100 µg sc/im daily × 1 wk; 200 µg sc/im/wk until Hgb normalizes Life-long maintenance: 200 µg sc/im monthly **or** 1000–2000 µg po daily	Occasional peripheral vascular thrombosis, rash, pruritus, headache, nausea and vomiting, diarrhea. Occasional heart failure. Possibility of profound hypokalemia due to intracellular potassium shift.	Oral absorption is ↓ by anticonvulsants, colchicine, metformin, neomycin and omeprazole. Consider generous potassium supplementation with initiation of therapy. Folate supplementation may mask hematologic findings of B_{12} deficiency, without halting progression of the neurologic deficits.	$

(cont'd)

Table 1: **Drugs for the Treatment of Iron-deficiency and Megaloblastic Anemias** *(cont'd)*

Class	Drug	Dose	Adverse Effects	Comments	Cost[a]
	cyanocobalamin generics	Pernicious anemia/other chronic malabsorption disorders: 100 μg sc/im daily × 1 wk; 200 μg sc/im/wk until Hgb normalizes Life-long maintenance: 200 μg sc/im monthly **or** 1000–2000 μg po daily	See Cobalamin (vitamin B_{12}).	See Cobalamin (vitamin B_{12}). Cobalamin has traditionally been given parenterally because deficiency is most often due to malabsorption, and most cases of malabsorption are attributable to pernicious anemia with its lack of intrinsic factor. High-dose oral cobalamin therapy is effective, feasible and cost-effective, but concerns about patient compliance and the need for more attentive monitoring limit adoption of this approach in North America.	$
	hydroxocobalamin generics	Pernicious anemia/other chronic malabsorption disorders: 100 μg sc/im daily × 1 wk; 200 μg sc/im/wk until Hgb normalizes Life-long maintenance: 200 μg sc/im monthly 1000–2000 μg po daily	See Cobalamin (vitamin B_{12}).	See Cobalamin (vitamin B_{12}).	$
	folic acid (folate) generics	1 mg po daily	Occasional allergic reactions—rash, pruritus, flushing, bronchospasm.	Available for iv use in patients who are fasting.	$

[a] Cost of 30-day supply; includes drug cost only.
Legend: $ < $10 $$ $10–20 $$$ $20–250 $$$$ > $250

Table 2: Erythropoiesis-Stimulating Drugs

Class	Drug	Dose	Adverse Effects	Comments	Cost
Erythropoietics	*epoetin alfa*[a] Eprex	**Chronic renal failure** Initial: 50–100 IU/kg sc/iv 3×/wk, then: ↑ 25% Q4–8 wk to max 300 IU/kg/dose to achieve Hgb of 120 g/L As Hgb approaches 120 g/L, ↓ dose by 25% **HIV, on antiretrovirals (endogenous erythropoietin level ≤ 500 IU/L)** Initial: 100 IU/kg sc/iv 3×/wk, then: ↑ by 50 IU/kg/dose Q4–8wk to max 300 IU/kg/dose. **Cancer chemotherapy (endogenous erythropoietin level ≤ 200 IU/L)** Initial: 50 IU/kg sc/iv 3×/wk, or 40 000 IU sc/iv Qwk, then: ↑ by 50 IU/kg/dose Q8wk to max 300 IU/kg/dose. **Chronic hepatitis C, on ribavirin** 40 000 IU sc/iv weekly **Surgery** 600 IU/kg sc/iv 21, 14 and 7 days before surgery and then on the day of surgery	Hypertension, headache, seizures, thrombosis, nausea, vomiting, diarrhea, arthralgia, chest pain, edema, cough. Increases risk of deep venous thrombosis and other thrombotic complications in spine surgery patients. Pure red cell aplasia (rare)	Usually given by sc injection. May be given iv if access already established. Do not exceed target Hgb. If no response to the maximum dose after 8 wk, discontinue. If Hgb ↑ by more than 10 g/L/2 wk, ↓ dose by 25%. Target Hgb ≤ 120 g/L. If no response to the maximum dose after 8 wk, discontinue. In patients with renal failure, achievement of higher Hgb targets is not associated with better outcomes. Survival was worse in patients treated to higher Hgb targets (> 120 g/L) with erythropoietin as compared with placebo in patients with head and neck cancer and in those with breast cancer.	$150/ 10 000 IU
	darbepoetin alfa[a] Aranesp	**Chronic renal failure** 0.45 µg/kg sc/iv Qwk, then: ↑ by 25% monthly if no response. ↓ by 25% as Hgb approaches 120 g/L	Hypertension, hypotension, headache, thrombosis, nausea, vomiting, diarrhea, constipation, arthralgia, myalgia, chest pain,	May be able to shift to biweekly or monthly dosing in some patients. Target Hgb ≤ 120 g/L with ↑ limited to 10 g/L per 2 wk.	$283/ 100 µg

(cont'd)

Table 2: **Erythropoiesis-Stimulating Drugs** *(cont'd)*

Class	Drug	Dose	Adverse Effects	Comments	Cost
		Cancer chemotherapy (endogenous erythropoietin level ≤ 200 IU/L) 2.25 µg/kg sc/iv Qwk If inadequate response after 6 wk, ↑ to 4.5 µg/kg sc/iv Qwk.	arrhythmia, edema, dyspnea, cough.	If excessive response, ↓ dose by 40%. If still excessive, hold dose until Hgb falls.	

[a] Use the lowest dose that will gradually increase the Hgb concentration to the lowest level sufficient to avoid blood transfusions (FDA update, Mar 9, 2007). Dosing recommendations are to be reassessed by the FDA Oncologic Drugs Advisory committee.

Suggested Readings

Kwong JC, Carr D, Dhalla IA et al. Oral vitamin B12 therapy in the primary care setting: a qualitative and quantitative study of patient perspectives. *BMC Fam Pract* 2005;6(1):8.

Macdougall IC, Eckardt KU. Novel strategies for stimulating erythropoiesis and potential new treatments for anaemia. *Lancet* 2006;368(9539):947-53.

Manning-Dimmitt LL, Dimmitt SG, Wilson GR. Diagnosis of gastrointestinal bleeding in adults. *Am Fam Physician* 2005;71(7):1339-46.

Nilsson M, Norberg B, Hultdin J et al. Medical intelligence in Sweden. Vitamin B12: oral compared with parenteral? *Postgrad Med J* 2005;81(953):191-3.

Tefferi A, Hanson CA, Inwards DJ. How to interpret and pursue an abnormal complete blood cell count in adults. *Mayo Clin Proc* 2005;80(7):923-36.

References

1. Culleton BF, Manns BJ, Zhang J et al. Impact of anemia on hospitalization and mortality in older adults. *Blood* 2006;107(10):3841-6.
2. Ross SD, Fahrbach K, Frame D et al. The effect of anemia treatment on selected health-related quality-of-life domains: a systematic review. *Clin Ther* 2003;25(6):1786-805.
3. Macdougall IC, Eckardt KU. Novel strategies for stimulating erythropoiesis and potential new treatments for anaemia. *Lancet* 2006;368(9539):947-53.
4. Tefferi A, Hanson CA, Inwards DJ. How to interpret and pursue an abnormal complete blood cell count in adults. *Mayo Clin Proc* 2005;80(7):923-36.
5. Galloway M, Rushworth L. Red cell or serum folate? Results from the National Pathology Alliance benchmarking review. *J Clin Pathol* 2003;56(12):924-6.
6. Solomon LR. Cobalamin-responsive disorders in the ambulatory care setting: unreliability of cobalamin, methylmalonic acid, and homocysteine testing. *Blood* 2005;105(3):978-85.
7. Metz J, McGrath K, Bennett M et al. Biochemical indices of vitamin B12 nutrition in pregnant patients with subnormal serum vitamin B12 levels. *Am J Hematol* 1995;48(4):251-5.
8. Patterson AJ, Brown WJ, Roberts DC et al. Dietary treatment of iron deficiency in women of childbearing age. *Am J Clin Nutr* 2001;74(5):650-6.
9. Rimon E, Kagansky N, Kagansky M et al. Are we giving too much iron? Low-dose iron therapy is effective in octogenarians. *Am J Med* 2005;118(10):1142-7.
10. Green BT, Rockey DC. Gastrointestinal endoscopic evaluation of premenopausal women with iron deficiency anemia. *J Clin Gastroenterol* 2004;38(2):104-9.
11. Makrides M, Crowther CA, Gibson RA et al. Efficacy and tolerability of low-dose iron supplements during pregnancy: a randomized controlled trial. *Am J Clin Nutr* 2003;78(1):145-53.
12. Dharmarajan TS, Adiga GU, Norkus EP. Vitamin B12 deficiency. Recognizing subtle symptoms in older adults. *Geriatrics* 2003;58(3):30-4,37-8.
13. Vidal-Alaball J, Butler CC, Cannings-John R et al. Oral vitamin B12 versus intramuscular vitamin B12 for vitamin B12 deficiency. *Cochrane Database Syst Rev* 2005;(3):CD004655.
14. Kwong JC, Carr D, Dhalla IA et al. Oral vitamin B12 therapy in the primary care setting: a qualitative and quantitative study of patient perspectives. *BMC Fam Pract* 2005;6(1):8.
15. Nilsson M, Norberg B, Hultdin J et al. Medical intelligence in Sweden. Vitamin B12: oral compared with parenteral? *Postgrad Med J* 2005;81(953):191-3.
16. van Walraven C, Austin P, Naylor CD. Vitamin B12 injections versus oral supplements. How much money could be saved by switching from injections to pills? *Can Fam Physician* 2001;47:79-86.
17. Solomon LR. Oral vitamin B12 therapy: a cautionary note. *Blood* 2004;103(7):2863.
18. Henry DH, Volberding PA, Leitz G. Epoetin alfa for treatment of anemia in HIV-infected patients: past, present, and future. *J Acquir Immune Defic Syndr* 2004;37(2):1221-7.
19. Sherman M, Cohen L, Cooper MA et al. Clinical recommendations for the use of recombinant human erythropoietin in patients with hepatitis C virus being treated with ribavirin. *Can J Gastroenterol* 2006;20(7):479-85.
20. [No authors listed]. Epoetins and darbepoetin alfa in malignant disease. *Drug Ther Bull* 2004;42(3):21-3.
21. Bokemeyer C, Oechsle K, Hartmann JT. Anaemia in cancer patients: pathophysiology, incidence and treatment. *Eur J Clin Invest* 2005;35(Suppl 3):26-31.

22. Rizzo JD, Lichtin AE, Woolf SH et al. Use of epoetin in patients with cancer: evidence-based clinical practice guidelines of the American Society of Clinical Oncology and the American Society of Hematology. *Blood* 2002;100(7):2303-20.
23. Corwin HL. The role of erythropoietin therapy in the critically ill. *Transfus Med Rev* 2006;20(1):27-33.
24. Henry DH, Bowers P, Romano MT et al. Epoetin alfa. Clinical evolution of a pleiotropic cytokine. *Arch Intern Med* 2004;164(3):262-76.
25. Drueke TB, Locatelli F, Clyne N et al. Normalization of hemoglobin level in patients with chronic kidney disease and anemia. *N Engl J Med* 2006;355(20):2071-84.
26. Phrommintikul A, Haas SJ, Elsik M et al. Mortality and target haemoglobin concentrations in anaemic patients with chronic kidney disease treated with erythropoietin: a meta-analysis. *Lancet* 2007;369(9559):381-8.
27. Singh AK, Szczech L, Tang KL et al. Correction of anemia with epoetin alfa in chronic kidney disease. *N Engl J Med* 2006;355(20):2085-98.
28. Henke M, Laszig R, Rube C et al. Erythropoietin to treat head and neck cancer patients with anaemia undergoing radiotherapy: randomised, double-blind, placebo-controlled trial. *Lancet* 2003;362(9392):1255-60.
29. Leyland-Jones B, Semiglazov V, Pawlicki M et al. Maintaining normal hemoglobin levels with epoetin alfa in mainly nonanemic patients with metastatic breast cancer receiving first-line chemotherapy: a survival study. *J Clin Oncol* 2005;23(25):5960-72.
30. Ludwig H, Fritz E. Anemia in cancer patients. *Semin Oncol* 1998;25(3 Suppl 7):2-6.

CHAPTER 88
Dehydration in Children

Gary I. Joubert, MD, FRCPC

Goals of Therapy

- Treat shock/impending shock
- Treat dehydration using an appropriate fluid and route
- Treat electrolyte imbalances
- Prevent complications (seizures or edema)

Fluids in Infants and Children

Newborn and young children have a much higher water content than adolescents and adults (Table 1) and are more prone to both water and salt (sodium [Na^+] and potassium [K^+]) loss during illness.

Table 1: **Age vs Percentage of Body Water**

Age	% Body Water
Newborn	75–80
Child ≤ 1 y	70–75
Child 1–12 y	60–70
Adolescent/adult	55–60

Investigations

- Thorough history with attention to:
  - underlying cause(s): vomiting and/or diarrhea or other excessive fluid loss
  - frequency and amount of loss
  - frequency and amount of urinary output
- Physical examination including a full set of vital signs to assess clinical manifestations and degree of dehydration[1]
- Laboratory tests: electrolytes, BUN, creatinine, glucose, serum bicarbonate (HCO_3), blood gases and urinalysis as indicated clinically

The *assessment of dehydration* in infants and children is challenging (Table 2). This difficulty is related to a child's ability to maintain adequate blood pressure in the face of moderate to severe dehydration.

Table 2: **Estimation of Dehydration**

Extent of Dehydration	Mild	Moderate	Severe
Weight loss–Infants (under 1 y)	5%	10%	15%
Weight loss–Children (over 1 y)	3–4%	6–8%	10%
History	decreased intake decreased urine output normal activity inquire about frequency of vomiting and diarrhea	decreased intake marked decreased urine output listless, weight loss inquire about frequency of vomiting and diarrhea	very decreased intake anuria obtunded inquire about frequency of vomiting and diarrhea longer duration of illness
Pulse	normal	slightly increased	rapid
Blood pressure	normal	normal to orthostatic, > 10 mm Hg change	orthostatic to shock
Behaviour	normal	irritable	hyperirritable to lethargic
Thirst	slight	moderate	intense
Mucous membranes[a]	normal	dry	parched
Tears	present	decreased	absent, sunken eyes
Anterior fontanelle	normal	normal to sunken	sunken
External jugular vein	visible when supine	not visible except with supraclavicular pressure	not visible even with supraclavicular pressure
Skin[a] (less useful in children > 2 y)	capillary refill < 2 sec	slowed capillary refill (2–4 sec), decreased turgor	significant delayed capillary refill (> 4 sec) and tenting; skin cool, acrocyanotic or mottled[a]
Urine specific gravity (SG)	> 1.020	> 1.020, oliguria	oliguria or anuria
Lab values	normal BUN/creatinine	increased BUN/creatinine	increased+++ BUN/creatinine, increased Hgb, low glucose

[a] These signs are less prominent in patients who have hypernatremia.

Therapeutic Choices

Treatment of dehydration involves replacing fluid deficits, then maintaining normal hydration.

Shock must be treated aggressively using isotonic saline (0.9% NaCl).

The calculation of the *fluid deficit* for a given degree of dehydration can be based on historical or objective information (e.g., predehydrational and present dehydrated weight). When the predehydrational weight is known:

Deficit litres (L) = predehydrational weight (kg) – present weight (kg).

Predehydrational body weight can be estimated by:

Body weight (kg) = 3(age) + 7. This gives an estimated weight at or about the 50th percentile for age and can be used for children up to 10 years of age.[2]

Maintenance fluid (Table 4) is the amount of fluid required to maintain normal hydration. Maintenance fluids are linked to caloric requirements and take into account insensible losses.

Dehydration is classified into three types depending on serum Na^+ concentration (Table 3).

Table 3: **Types of Dehydration**

Type of Dehydration (frequency)	Serum Na^+ (mmol/L)	Serum Osmolality (mOsm/kg)
Isonatremic (80%)	130–150	Normal: 280–295 mOsm/kg Equal water and salt loss
Hypernatremic (15%)	> 150	Elevated: 295 mOsm/kg Water loss > salt loss
Hyponatremic (5%)	< 130	↓ or normal or ↑ serum osmolality Must determine subgroup (see text)

Isonatremic dehydration (Figure 1) is the most common form of dehydration, with loss of both K^+ and Na^+. K^+ can be added to the iv mixture following establishment of urinary output. K^+ administration should not exceed 4 mmol/kg/day.[3] Higher K^+ concentrations can be used in life-threatening hypokalemia.

Hypernatremic dehydration usually develops slowly and is corrected slowly to prevent cerebral edema and seizures. Shock is treated aggressively by administering iv 0.9% NaCl until urinary output is re-established, then 0.45% NaCl + D5W is used to correct dehydration states and restore Na^+ to normal levels.

The goal of therapy is to reduce serum Na^+ by 10 to 15 mmol/L/day and to restore hydration to normal in no less than 48 hours. If the serum concentration drops rapidly (i.e., > 10 to 15 mmol/day or >1 mmol every two hours), change the iv solution to 0.9% NaCl + D5W.

Hyponatremic dehydration is classified into three subgroups:

- excessive water
- Na^+ depletion
- fictitious lowering of serum Na^+ concentration due to increased glucose, electrolytes, lipids and proteins

Symptomatic hyponatremia is usually related to the degree of serum Na^+ depletion. Children with serum Na^+ > 120 mmol/L rarely demonstrate any clinical manifestations. When serum Na^+ drops below 120 mmol/L, neurologic manifestations (e.g., seizures) are common. Children who are symptomatic require aggressive replacement using hypertonic saline (3% NaCl) to achieve a serum Na^+ > 125 mmol/L.

Serum Na^+ deficit can be calculated as follows:

$[Na^+]$ deficit = ($[Na^+]$ desired – $[Na^+]$ actual) × body weight (kg) × total body water (L/kg)

After initial elevation of Na^+ to > 125 mmol/L, the remaining deficit can be replaced over 24 to 48 hours.

Remember that children who are dehydrated and continue to have ongoing fluid losses need to have those fluid losses replaced. Those replacements need to be considered in addition to their estimated deficit plus maintenance fluids. The replacement of ongoing fluid losses usually occurs in a ratio of 1 mL of replacement to each 1 mL of fluid lost.[4] Fluid loss replacement is in excess of the usual sensible and insensible losses (i.e., secondary to high urinary output in a diabetic, nasogastric losses, or excessive ongoing vomiting and/or diarrhea). Adjust fluid for electrolyte losses as well.[5]

Table 4: **Maintenance Fluid and Electrolyte Requirements in Children**

Weight (kg)	Daily Fluid Requirement	Hourly Rate	Daily Electrolytes
0–10	100 mL/kg	4 mL/kg	Na^+: 2.5–3 mmol/ 100 mL fluid/day K^+: 2–2.5 mmol/ 100 mL fluid/day
11–20	1000 mL + (50 mL/kg × each kg > 10)	40 mL/h + (2 mL/kg × each kg > 10)	
> 20	1500 mL + (20 mL/kg × each kg > 20)	60 mL/h + (1 mL/kg × each kg > 20)	

Table 5: **Calculation of Maintenance Fluid Requirements**

Using information from Table 4: *Example:* For a 15 kg child use information for 11–20 kg.		
Fluids	**Daily Fluid Rate**	**Hourly Fluid Rate** (quick calculation)
For the first 10 kg	10 kg × 100 mL/kg = 1000 mL	10 kg × 4 mL/kg = 40 mL
For the next 5 kg	5 kg × 50 mL/kg = 250 mL	5 kg × 2 mL/kg = 10 mL
	Total 1250 mL or 52 mL/h	**Total 50 mL/h**
Electrolytes:	**Na^+**	**K^+**
	1250 mL × 3 mmol/100 mL = 37.5 mmol (37.5 mmol/1250 mL or 30 mmol/L)	1250 mL × 2 mmol/100 mL = 25 mmol (25 mmol/1250 mL or 20 mmol/L)
Suggested commercially available solution best meeting the needs would be 0.2% NaCl/D5W + 20 mmol KCl/L.		

Table 6: **Calculation of Fluid Deficit and Replacement for Isonatremic Dehydration**

Example: For a 15 kg child who has 10% isonatremic dehydration **Fluids:** Total fluid replacement equals *deficit* replacement plus *maintenance*. Fluid deficit in 10% dehydration is 100 mL/kg; in 5% dehydration 50 mL/kg
(i) Deficit replacement calculation = 15 kg × 10% (100 mL/kg) or 1500 mL Need to replace 50% or 750 mL over first 8 h at a rate of *94 mL/h*
(ii) Maintenance = 52 mL/h (using calculation from Table 5)
(iii) Total = *146 mL/h* (94 mL/h + 52 mL/h) for first 8 h, then reduce to 100 mL/h for next 16 h (replace remaining deficit of 750 mL + maintenance over 16 h [47 mL/h + 52 mL/h ≈ 100 mL/h]) **Electrolytes:** Na^+ loss would be approximately 120 mmol (8–10 mmol/kg/day) and K^+ loss would be approximately 120 mmol (8–10 mmol/kg/day).[a]

[a] Using a rehydration solution of 0.45% NaCl + D5W at the above rate will replace 115 mmol of Na^+. K^+ 40 mmol/L (not to exceed 4 mmol/kg/day) will replace 60 mmol of total loss. Replacement of K^+ will make up losses over the next 2 days.

Oral Rehydration Therapy (ORT)

Oral rehydration is the treatment of choice in children with mild to moderate dehydration. It can be used in all types of dehydration provided that hypo- and hypernatremic dehydration are not at the extremes of the spectrum.

The fluid deficit is calculated and the rate of replacement is based upon the degree of dehydration.

In the child who is mildly to moderately dehydrated, the rate of replacement is 50 mL/kg over the first 4 hours; for the child who is moderately to severely dehydrated, the rate of replacement is 100 mL/kg over the first 4 hours. The rehydration phase may last from 4 to 12 hours depending upon the degree of dehydration as well as the ability of the child to tolerate oral rehydration. After the first 4 hours, replace the remainder of the deficit over the next 6 to 8 hours.

The fluid should be a balanced electrolyte solution acceptable to the gastrointestinal tract and should facilitate Na^+ transport. Ideal solutions for ORT contain Na^+ 45 to 75 mmol/L, K^+ 20 mmol/L and glucose 20 to 24 g/L; 100 to 150 mL/kg/day is given to the child. Remember in infants less than six months of age, after the oral rehydration phase is completed, restart the child on breast milk or half-strength formula.[6]

Table 7: **Oral Replacement Solutions**

Product	Composition				Cost[a]
	Dextrose g/L	K^+ mmol/L	Na^+ mmol/L	Cl^- mmol/L	
Gastrolyte	17.8	20	60	60	$
Pedialyte	25	20	45	35	$$
Pediatric Electrolyte	20	20	45	35	$$

[a] Cost per litre; includes drug cost only
Legend: $ < $5 $$ $5–10

Commercially available preparations (Table 7) may be used to rehydrate the child with observation in an ambulatory/emergency room setting or at home.

Children who have been started on iv replacement therapy can be switched to ORT at any point. It is important to ensure that no contraindications (shock or impending shock, high diarrheal purge rates, intractable vomiting, altered sensorium) are present.

Another option in the child failing ORT secondary to vomiting is to place an NG tube and use the fluid regimen per hour as described above.

Therapeutic Tips

- Absolute indications for admission to hospital are:
  - shock
  - hypo/hypernatremia
  - intractable vomiting/diarrhea
- Possible indications for admission to hospital are:
  - serum $HCO_3 < 15$ mmol/L at onset of therapy
  - poor response to ORT and ongoing requirement for iv therapy
- Clinical signs of dehydration are often not present until at least 5% of a child's body weight is lost.
- Serum electrolytes should be measured before, at the time of and after starting iv fluids.

Figure 1: Management of Isonatremic Dehydration

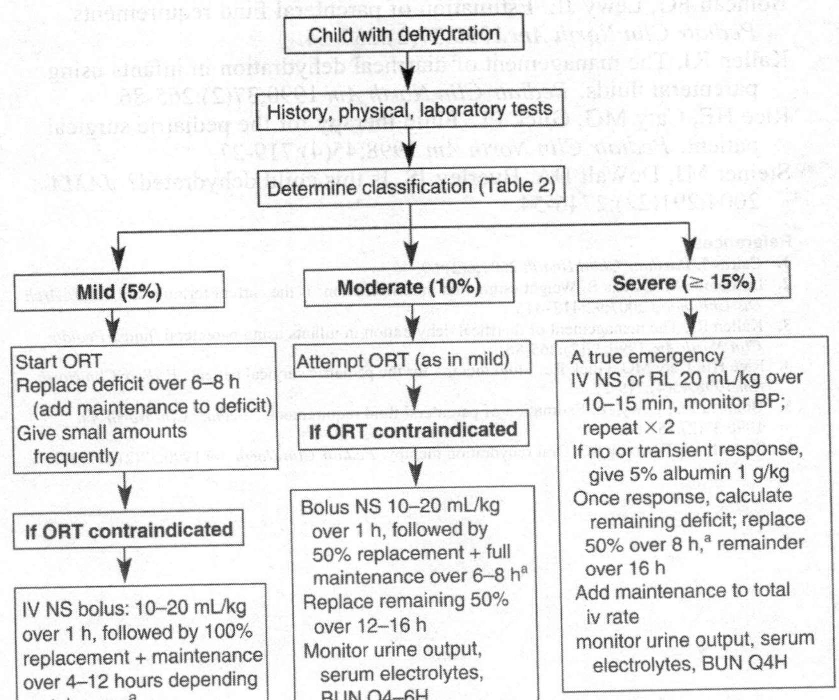

[a] Replacement therapy after bolus should contain 50–60 mmol/L Na^+ plus a source of glucose (e.g., D5W) plus appropriate K^+. An ideal solution is 0.33% NaCl (Na^+ 51.3 mmol/L) + D3.3W (3.3 g glucose/100 mL) + appropriate K^+. K^+ should not exceed 4 mmol/kg/day and replenishment should be done gradually over 2 days. **No urine output, no K^+.**

Abbreviations: BP = blood pressure; NS = normal saline, 0.9% NaCl; ORT = oral replacement therapy; RL = Ringer's lactate

Suggested Readings

Boineau FG, Lewy JE. Estimation of parenteral fluid requirements. *Pediatr Clin North Am* 1990;37(2):257-64.

Kallen RJ. The management of diarrheal dehydration in infants using parenteral fluids. *Pediatr Clin North Am* 1990;37(2):265-86.

Rice HE, Caty MG, Glick PL. Fluid therapy for the pediatric surgical patient. *Pediatr Clin North Am* 1998;45(4):719-27.

Steiner MJ, DeWalt DA, Byerley JS. Is this child dehydrated? *JAMA* 2004;291(22):2746-54.

References

1. Cairns J. *Paediatr Child Health* 2001;6(2):69.
2. Luscombe M, Owens B. Weight estimation in resuscitation: is the current formula still valid? *Arch Dis Childhood* 2007;92:412–415.
3. Kallen RJ. The management of diarrheal dehydration in infants using parenteral fluids. *Pediatr Clin North Am* 1990;37(2):265-86.
4. Rice HE, Caty MG, Glick PL. Fluid therapy for the pediatric surgical patient. *Pediatr Clin North Am* 1998;45(4):719-27.
5. Boineau FG, Lewy JE. Estimation of parenteral fluid requirements. *Pediatr Clin North Am* 1990;37(2):257-64.
6. Casteel HB, Fiedorek SC. Oral rehydration therapy. *Pediatr Clin North Am* 1990;37(2):295-311.

CHAPTER 89
Hypovolemia

Peter J. McLeod, MD, FRCPC, FACP

Hypovolemia is a generic term encompassing volume depletion and dehydration.[1] Volume depletion is the loss of salt and water from the intravascular space. It is more frequently associated with hypotension and tachycardia than is dehydration. Dehydration, such as from excess sweating, implies loss of water from both extracellular (intravascular and interstitial) and intracellular spaces and leads to elevated plasma sodium and osmolality.

Goals of Therapy

- Restore normal volume to relieve symptoms and prevent organ damage

Investigations

- History:
  - symptoms of hypovolemia include thirst, fatigue and postural lightheadedness
  - causes of hypovolemia include: hemorrhage; volume losses from GI tract, kidneys, skin, respiratory tract; fluid sequestration or third-space losses
- Physical exam:
  - determine the presence and severity of hypovolemia
  - pulse: heart rate (HR) increase of more than 30 beats/min after 1 minute of standing from recumbent position is the most accurate sign of volume depletion.[1] The pulse should be counted for 30 seconds and doubled to determine the number of beats per minute. Supine tachycardia is insensitive
  - blood pressure: postural decline of systolic pressure of more than 20 mm Hg suggests volume depletion[1]
  - low jugular venous pressure (JVP) is suggestive of volume depletion. Dry axillae support the diagnosis of hypovolemia.[1] Moist mucous membranes and axillae argue against hypovolemia. Skin turgor, capillary refill time and eyeball tension are late signs and are insensitive in adults[2]
- Laboratory tests:
  - blood: in hypovolemia, hematocrit and albumin concentrations increase and urea increases disproportionately to creatinine. Sodium concentration may be normal, low or high and is dependent on the type and amount of fluid consumed by the patient in response to thirst.

- urine: hypovolemia is suggested if urine volume is < 0.5 mL/kg/h, if Na^+ is < 20 mmol/L or if osmolality is > 450 mOsm/kg.[3] Urine specific gravity (SG) is less accurate but SG > 1.015 suggests concentrated urine and may indicate hypovolemia

Therapeutic Choices (Figure 1, Table 1)

Therapy is designed to restore volume while replacing ongoing losses. Concurrent fluid and electrolyte disorders will influence choice of fluid used.

- *Hypovolemia suspected but uncertain*: consider an IV fluid challenge of 250 to 500 mL of normal saline over 30 minutes. Closely monitor HR and BP to determine if low cardiac output is due to hypovolemia.
- *Mild hypovolemia* (< 5% of body weight): oral therapy is usually adequate. Water, juices, soft drinks or soup broth with extra salt or a commercially available electrolyte solution (see Chapter 88) may be used.[4] Rice-based oral solutions have proven effective for diarrheal conditions in developing countries.
- *Moderate* (5 to 10% of body weight) *or severe* (> 10% of body weight) *hypovolemia* or inability to ingest oral fluids: IV therapy is required and four types of solutions are used:
  - **dextrose 5% in water** (D5W) distributes throughout total body water and is useful for intracellular volume loss (dehydration). It is a poor plasma volume expander as very little remains in the intravascular space and therefore it is not useful for managing acute hypotension or tachycardia.
  - **sodium chloride 0.9%** (normal saline or NS) is the fluid of choice for initial treatment of acute hypotension and tachycardia associated with volume depletion. Like other crystalloid solutions, it distributes to extracellular fluid. For every litre infused, about 250 mL remains in the intravascular space and the remainder goes to the interstitial space.[4]
  - **colloid solutions**, including albumin, gelatins (not available in Canada) and starch compounds, are better intravascular volume expanders than NS because they remain in the intravascular space longer than crystalloids. Their cost is high, and the duration of benefit is relatively short; their use as the primary fluid is not justified in most hypovolemic states.
  - **blood** is an excellent intravascular expander. Packed red blood cells with normal saline is indicated for hemorrhagic hypovolemia.

Determining Fluid Requirements

There is no precise formula since disease, age, source and rate of fluid loss influence needs. In severe and less severe hypovolemia with obvious hemodynamic compromise, give at least 1 L of NS over 30 minutes and a second litre over the next hour. Closely monitor HR, BP and JVP, watching for improvement or fluid overload. In less severe hypovolemia, give 250 to 500 mL/hour of NS. A recent randomized controlled trial has demonstrated the safety and efficacy of 30 mL/kg of normal saline given over 30 minutes to patients with suspected sepsis and a systolic blood pressure of < 90 mm Hg.[5]

Colloid solutions may be needed if NS is ineffective but there are no data indicating that colloid use will provide better outcomes in critically ill patients.[6,7] Fluid resuscitation with 4% albumin or normal saline resulted in similar outcomes, including 28-day mortality, in ICU patients.[8] Maintenance fluids must be added to those given to correct the deficit. In adults, maintenance is possible with approximately 30 mL/kg/day or 2000 to 2500 mL/day containing 75 mmol of Na^+ and 50 mmol of K^+ in a 24-hour period.

Other commercially available crystalloid solutions are more costly and, aside from dextrose 3.3% with sodium chloride 0.3% (2/3–1/3) or dextrose 5% with sodium chloride 0.45% (D5–1/2 NS), they play very little role in managing volume depletion. Users of other crystalloids must be aware of their contents. For example, Ringer's lactate contains calcium, potassium and lactate in addition to sodium and may not be suitable for some patients, e.g., those with renal dysfunction.

Therapeutic Tips

- If presence of hypovolemia is uncertain, consider a fluid challenge.
- Normal saline is the fluid of first choice for patients with hypotension and tachycardia associated with volume depletion. Dextrose in water is a poor plasma volume expander.
- Additional potassium may be required for fluid loss associated with diarrhea, vomiting or over-diuresis with diuretics.
- Colloid solutions are usually reserved as second-line plasma volume expanders; burns and other volume losses containing protein may require additional colloid.
- Bicarbonate may be required in severe metabolic acidosis if the bicarbonate concentration in plasma is < 4 mmol/L. The bicarbonate concentration need only be raised to ≥ 8 mmol/L.

Figure 1: **Management of Suspected Hypovolemia**

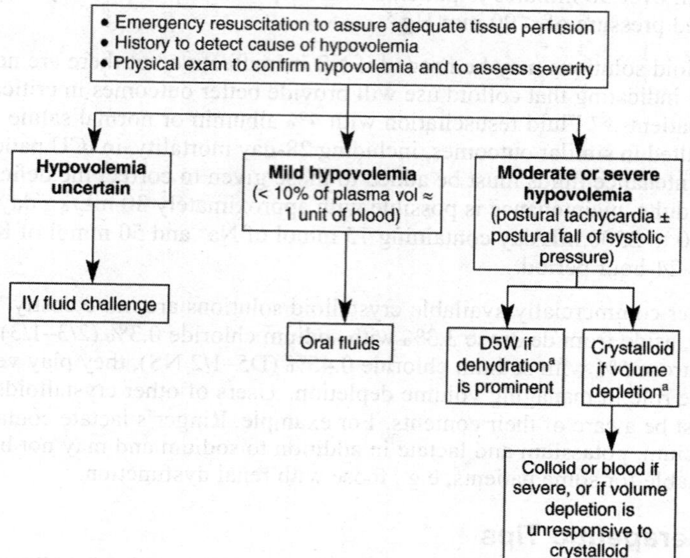

[a] Dehydration refers to loss of intracellular water leading to elevated plasma sodium and osmolality. Patients with dehydration may or may not have hypotension and tachycardia. Volume depletion results from loss of salt and water from the extracellular space. Volume depleted patients exhibit circulatory instability.

Table 1: **Intravenous Solutions for Hypovolemia**

Class	Drug	Use	Adverse Effects	Comments
Crystalloids	*sodium chloride 0.9%, normal saline or NS (Na⁺ 154 mmol/L)* Sodium Chloride Injection USP, generics	Initial treatment of hypovolemia.	Fluid overload; peripheral edema. Dilutional coagulopathy. Hyperchloremic metabolic acidosis with infusion of large amounts of NS (usually >3 L). Hypernatremia.	IV solutions with Na^+ concentrations that approximate normal serum Na^+ cause more intravascular and interstitial expansion than do D5W solutions.
	Ringer's lactate (Na⁺ 130 mmol/L) Lactated Ringer's Injection, generics	Initial treatment of hypovolemia.	Fluid overload; peripheral edema. Dilutional coagulopathy. Hyponatremia. May aggravate pre-existing hyperkalemia.	Contains 1.4 mmol/L Ca^{++}, 4 mEq K^+/L; 109 mEq Cl^-/L; 28 mEq lactate/L.
	dextrose 5% with sodium chloride 0.9%, D5W-NS (Na⁺ 154 mmol/L) generics	Hypovolemia and dehydration.	See sodium chloride 0.9%.	See sodium chloride 0.9%. Compared to NS or Ringer's lactate, D5W results in comparatively small changes in plasma volume because it distributes throughout the total body water space, including the intracellular space.
	dextrose 5% in water, D5W generics	Dehydration; poor plasma volume expander.		Water is distributed to both intracellular fluid and extracellular fluid after dextrose metabolism.

(cont'd)

Table 1: **Intravenous Solutions for Hypovolemia** *(cont'd)*

Class	Drug	Use	Adverse Effects	Comments
	sodium chloride 0.45%, half-normal saline or 1/2 NS (Na⁺ 77 mmol/L) Sodium Chloride Injection USP, generics	Maintenance fluids.	See sodium chloride 0.9%.	See sodium chloride 0.9%.
	dextrose 3.3% with sodium chloride 0.3%, 2/3-1/3 (Na⁺ 51 mmol/L) generics	Maintenance fluids.	See sodium chloride 0.9%.	See sodium chloride 0.9%.
	dextrose 5% with sodium chloride 0.45%, D5-1/2NS (Na⁺ 77 mmol/L) generics	Maintenance fluids.	See sodium chloride 0.9%.	See sodium chloride 0.9%.
Colloids	*albumin* Plasbumin-5, Plasbumin-25, generics	Volume expander, useful for hypoproteinemic hypovolemia. Used to replace or in conjunction with crystalloids. Volume remains within the extracellular compartment. Contraindicated in patients at risk of circulatory overload such as those with history of CHF, renal insufficiency or stabilized chronic anemia.	Rare: anaphylactoid/anaphylaxis. Fluid overload.	Albumin 5% is iso-oncotic (does not pull fluid into the intravascular space) with normal plasma; IV infusion will expand circulating blood volume by an amount approximately equal to the amount infused; does not aggravate tissue dehydration; concomitant use of crystalloids may be necessary to maintain fluid balance. Albumin 25% is used in situations of oncotic deficit, e.g., blood loss due to surgery or trauma; may be used when treatment of shock has been delayed. IV infusion will expand plasma volume 3-4 times the volume infused. May be used in patients with clinical evidence of both edema and hypovolemia, i.e., is normally hydrated or interstitial edema is present. May be used in combination with crystalloids.

Class	Drug	Use	Adverse Effects	Comments
	hetastarch 6% in lactated electrolyte Hextend	Volume expander, alternative to blood.	Bleeding. Macroamylase formation may lead to incorrect diagnosis of pancreatitis because of possibility of increase in blood amylase. Fluid overload.	Hetastarch exhibits comparable plasma expansion with respect to 5% albumin solution. Contraindicated in patients at risk of circulatory overload such as those with history of CHF, renal insufficiency or stabilized chronic anemia.
	pentastarch 10% in normal saline Pentaspan	Volume expander.	May produce coagulopathy if > 28 mL/kg is given over a 24-hour period though this is extremely rare and usually not clinically significant. Hyperchloremic acidosis.	Commonly used in crystalloid refractory patients in critical care areas but there is no evidence of clinical superiority compared to crystalloids.
	dextrans Gentran 70, Gentran 40	Volume expander.	Aggravation of bleeding; interfere with blood coagulation. Anaphylaxis with higher molecular weight solutions.	Not used as plasma expanders as frequently as albumin and starch compounds.
	blood	Packed cells with saline indicated for hemorrhage.	Fluid overload.	Replaces or increases oxygen-carrying capacity but only if not stored for > 3-5 days.

Suggested Readings

Brenner BM, Rector FC, editors. *Brenner and Rector's the kidney*. 6th ed. Philadelphia (PA): W.B. Saunders; 2000.

Halperin ML, Goldstein MB. *Fluid, electrolyte, and acid-base physiology a problem-based approach*. 2nd ed. Philadelphia (PA): W.B. Saunders; 1994.

Maxwell MH, Kleeman CR, Narins RG. *Maxwell & Kleeman's clinical disorders of fluid and electrolyte metabolism*. 5th ed. New York (NY): McGraw-Hill, Health Professions Division; 1994.

McGee S, Abernethy WB, Simel DL. The rational clinical examination. Is this patient hypovolemic? *JAMA* 1999;281(11):1022-9.

References

1. McGee S, Abernethy WB, Simel DL. The rational clinical examination. Is this patient hypovolemic? *JAMA* 1999;281(11):1022-9.
2. Webb AR. Recognizing hypovolaemia.*Minerva Anesthesiol* 2001;67(4):185-9.
3. Sterns RH. Renal function and disorders of water and sodium balance. In: *Scientific American Medicine*. New York (NY): WebMD Professional Publishing; 2002.
4. Boldt J. Volume replacement in the surgical patient--does the type of solution make a difference? *Br J Anaesth* 2000;84(6):783-93.
5. Rivers E, Nguyen B, Havstad S et al. Early goal-directed therapy in the treatment of severe sepsis and septic shock. *N Engl J Med* 2001;345(19):1368-77.
6. Webb AR. The appropriate role of colloids in managing fluid imbalance: a critical review of recent meta-analytic findings.*Crit Care* 2000;4(Suppl 2):S26-S32.
7. Alderson P, Schierhout G, Roberts I et al. Colloids versus crystalloids for fluid resuscitation in critically ill patients. *Cochrane Database Syst Rev* 2000;(2):CD000567.
8. Finfer S, Bellomo R, Boyce N et al. A comparison of albumin and saline for fluid resuscitation in the intensive care unit. *N Engl J Med* 2004;350(22):2247-56.

CHAPTER 90
Edema

Tammy M. Keough-Ryan, MD, MSc, FRCPC

Edema is a sign of an underlying disorder that should be identified and treated prior to initiation of therapy. It results from altered sodium homeostasis that leads to increased extracellular fluid volume (ECFV). Therapy must be individualized.

Peripheral edema is swelling in a dependent area that is palpable on physical examination. *Anasarca* is gross, generalized edema.

Common conditions that are associated with edema include congestive heart failure (CHF), cirrhosis, renal failure, nephrotic syndrome and pregnancy. The main focus of this chapter is peripheral edema. For edema associated with specific conditions, see Chapter 36 and Chapter 51.

Goals of Therapy

- Determine the cause of edema
- Decrease symptomatic fluid overload
- Manage diuretic resistance

Investigations

- History:
  - conditions associated with pitting edema: renal failure, nephrotic syndrome, CHF, hepatic cirrhosis, pregnancy
  - salt intake
  - drugs that may cause or exacerbate edema, e.g., NSAIDs, calcium channel blockers, corticosteroids or drugs that may interact with diuretic agents
- Physical exam:
  - localized or generalized edema, pitting or nonpitting edema

    If lower limb edema is asymmetric, consider lymphedema from lymphatic obstruction, deep vein thrombosis (DVT) or infection.

    If edema is nonpitting, consider lymphatic obstruction or myxedema
  - distribution (symmetric or asymmetric)
  - location of edema: legs if ambulatory or sacrum if recumbent
  - weight, blood pressure, heart rate, respiratory rate
  - signs of fluid overload: jugular venous distention, pulmonary edema, ascites
- Laboratory investigations:
  - electrolytes (including Na^+, K^+, Cl^-, HCO_3^-, Ca^{++}, Mg^{++}), uric acid, urea, creatinine

- urinalysis
- liver function tests
- chest x-ray
- other: TSH, glucose and lipids, albumin, 24-hour urine collection to quantify proteinuria if symptoms/signs are suggestive of primary renal disorder

Therapeutic Choices (Figure 1)

Nonpharmacologic Choices

- Decrease sodium intake to < 100 mmol/day (2.4 g Na^+ or 6 g NaCl).[1,2]
- Decrease fluid intake to 1 L/day.[2]
- Posture: supine position improves cardiac output; elevate legs.
- Consider supportive compression stockings.
- Paracentesis for ascites under direction of a specialist.

Pharmacologic Choices

Consider if nonpharmacologic actions do not significantly reduce the symptoms related to edema and treatment of underlying disorder has been implemented.

Diuretic Therapy (Table 1)

Peripheral edema, in the absence of respiratory/cardiac effect, is not life threatening and fluid removal must be slow. The maximum recommended rate of weight loss is 1 kg/day.[3] Diuretics are not effective if lymphatic or venous drainage obstruction is the underlying problem. Diuretics should not be prescribed in pregnancy; refer pregnant patients to a specialist.

Diuretics decrease sodium reabsorption at various sites in the nephron by interfering with carrier proteins or channels. Diuretics increase sodium and water losses; this decreases ECFV and improves the edema. Closely monitor for electrolyte imbalances (K^+, Cl^-, Ca^{++}, Mg^{++}, HCO_3^-) and prerenal azotemia (urea, creatinine) to avoid significant alterations.

Loop Diuretics

The loop diuretics, **furosemide**, **ethacrynic acid** and **bumetanide**, are potent diuretic agents that act in the loop of Henle in the nephron. The onset and duration of action are short. Loop diuretics are particularly useful in the presence of moderate to severe renal insufficiency (ClCr ≤ 50 mL/min). If there is no response with the maximum dose, switching to an alternate loop diuretic will not be effective.

Bumetanide has no advantage over furosemide. Ethacrynic acid is reserved for use in patients with sulfa allergy that contraindicates the use of furosemide. There are reports of ototoxicity with ethacrynic acid.[4,5]

Potassium-sparing Diuretics

Spironolactone is an aldosterone receptor antagonist. It is the first-line agent in hepatic disease because of the secondary hyperaldosteronism that leads to sodium and water retention.[3] Spironolactone can also be effective adjunctive therapy for edema of NYHA Class III or IV CHF (see Chapter 36) associated with high aldosterone levels.

Amiloride and **triamterene** are other effective potassium-sparing diuretics that are useful in combination therapy with loop diuretics in resistant edema or if hypokalemia complicates the initial diuretic therapy used.

Thiazides

Thiazide diuretics are useful first-line agents if the creatinine clearance is > 50 mL/min.[3,6] Thiazides work in the distal convoluted tube of the nephron and are effective antihypertensive agents. Thiazides have a longer duration of action than the loop diuretics. Alternate thiazides have no advantage over **hydrochlorothiazide**.[1] Thiazides are useful adjunctive agents to loop diuretic therapy for resistant edema. Hyponatremia, as a complication of diuretic therapy, is more common with thiazide diuretics.[2]

Management of Resistant Edema

- Sodium restriction
  - emphasize adherence to 100 mmol/day (2.4 g Na^+ or 6 g NaCl)
  - check 24-hour urine sodium to assess compliance
- Fluid restriction (especially with hyponatremia)
  - emphasize adherence to 1 L/day[2]
- Bedrest
  - supine position and leg elevation can increase glomerular filtration rate by 40%[1]
- Dosing of furosemide
  - increase the dose incrementally until diuresis is achieved by doubling the dose every two to three days.
  - secretion of the diuretic into the tubular lumen of the nephron can be impaired in severe hypoalbuminemia or decreased renal perfusion states such as renal failure or CHF, resulting in ineffective diuresis with initial doses
  - if unable to maintain an acceptable duration of effective diuresis, increase the frequency of dosing to two to three times per day
  - double the dose if switching from intravenous dose to oral dose[1]
  - consider intravenous dosing if the gastrointestinal tract is edematous, as this leads to impaired absorption of oral drug
  - monitor clinical status carefully, including weight, to ensure daily weight loss does not exceed 1 kg
  - monitor for electrolyte disturbances and prerenal azotemia

Combination Diuretic Therapy

- A **thiazide** added to a **loop diuretic** blocks a second site of sodium reabsorption to improve diuresis. If the thiazide is given orally with intravenous furosemide, administer 30–60 minutes prior to the loop diuretic. If both diuretics are taken orally, administer at the same time.
- **Potassium-sparing agents** can be added to further block sodium reabsorption, particularly if the patient is hypokalemic. As life-threatening hyperkalemia can result, exercise caution and monitor electrolytes frequently if the patient has renal failure, diabetes mellitus or is taking any of the following medications: cyclosporine, tacrolimus, ACE inhibitor, angiotensin receptor blocker, pentamidine, trimethoprim, NSAIDs or beta-blockers.
- **Spironolactone** is an effective adjunctive agent in the presence of neurohumoral activation, e.g., hepatic disease, CHF or nephrotic syndrome.
- **Carbonic anhydrase inhibitors** such as **acetazolamide** may occasionally be added on the advice of a specialist if diuresis is ineffective using a combination of other diuretic agents or if diuresis is complicated by metabolic alkalosis.
- If all above measures fail, a specialist may consider other options such as ultrafiltration in renal failure or liver transplantation in cirrhosis.

Idiopathic Edema

This condition occurs most often in postpubertal, young to middle-aged, obese females. It is a diagnosis of exclusion when physical exam and laboratory investigations fail to define an underlying cause for edema. In 80% of cases, the edema is orthostatic, that is, the edema develops in the standing position and is more evident at the end of the day. The edema usually presents in the lower extremities but can also present in the face, hands and breasts, particularly in the morning. This can be demonstrated by weight gains of 0.7 to 1 kg/day from morning to evening weight.[7] An altered homeostatic response to an upright position promotes the retention of sodium and water.

- Consider discontinuation of diuretic therapy.
- Consider nonpharmacologic measures such as restriction of sodium and fluid intake, recumbent position, avoidance of prolonged periods of standing and use of supportive compression stockings.
- Consider intermittent daily diuretic use only when nonpharmacologic measures fail.
- Reassess fluid-restricted diet if rebound edema occurs when diuretics are stopped.

Therapeutic Tips

- Investigate unilateral edema for venous obstruction or infection.
- Refer pregnant patients to a specialist.

- Monitor electrolytes and renal function closely when initiating diuretic therapy, increasing the dose, using combination therapy or the patient is clinically unwell.
- Avoid prescribing potassium-sparing agents for patients with renal failure as these agents may cause life-threatening hyperkalemia.
- Avoid using combination products as dosing is more difficult to titrate or decrease if changes in volume status occur.
- Identify overdiuresis in patients by monitoring for clinical signs of weakness, hypotension and laboratory evidence of prerenal azotemia, hypokalemia and metabolic alkalosis. Rehydrate and refer these patients to a specialist.

Figure 1: **Management of Edema**

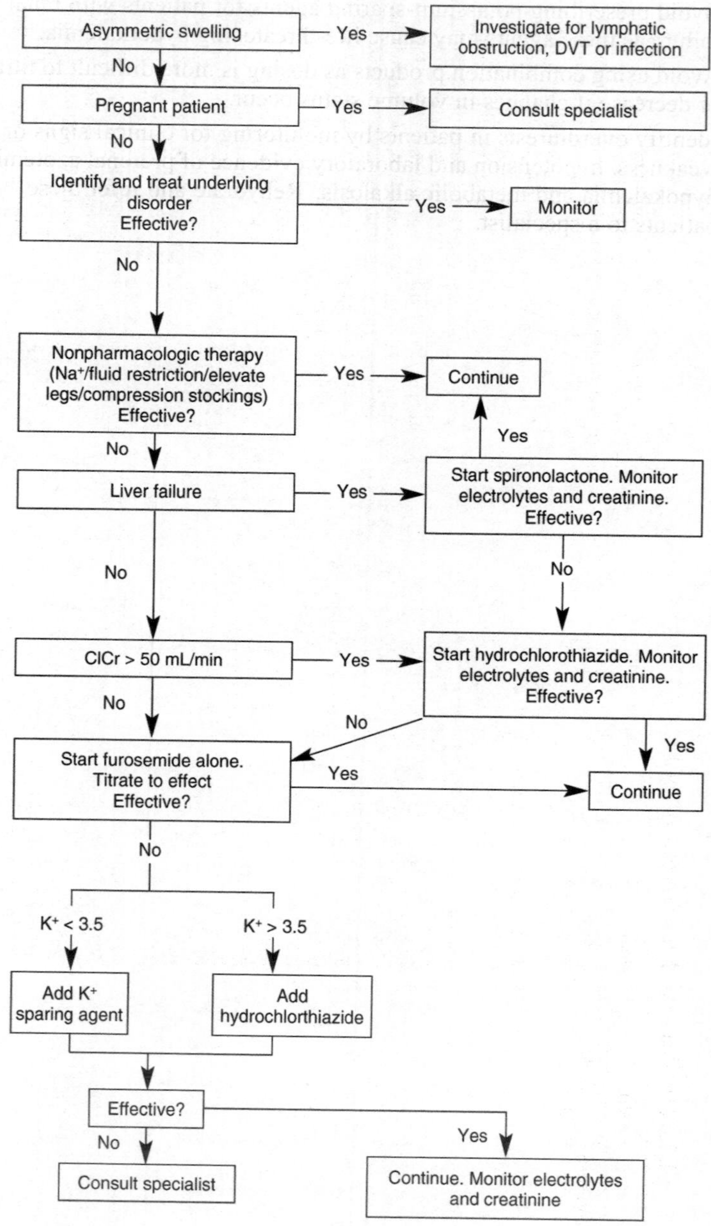

Table 1: Diuretic Agents for Treatment of Edema[1,2,4,6,8,9,10,11,12]

Class	Drug	Dose	Adverse Effects	Drug Interactions	Comments	Cost[a]
Loop Diuretics	*bumetanide* Burinex	Individualize dose according to patient response 0.5–2 mg po as a single dose; max daily dose 10 mg If diuretic response is not adequate with 1 mg, a 2nd and 3rd dose may be given at a 4–5 h interval May dose BID. Evening dose appears to have a greater diuretic effect than morning dose Maintenance: lowest effective daily dose Impaired hepatic function: use minimum effective dose; max daily dose 5 mg	Volume depletion. Electrolyte disturbances: hypochloremia, hypokalemia (evident during first 1–2 wk), hyponatremia, hyperuricemia (usually asymptomatic). Azotemia, increase in serum creatinine. Hyperglycemia. Dizziness, hypotension. Acute interstitial nephritis. Ototoxicity. Myalgias (common with high doses of bumetanide). Allergy (sulfa).	Aminoglycosides, cisplatin: ↑ ototoxicity. Thiazide diuretics: ↑ diuresis and electrolyte abnormalities; monitor for dehydration and electrolyte abnormalities when used in combination. Digoxin: hypokalemia and hypomagnesemia may lead to arrhythmias Lithium: reduced renal clearance of lithium resulting in lithium toxicity; monitor lithium levels and adjust dose as needed. NSAIDs: ↑ risk of renal failure development secondary to ↓ renal blood flow resulting from prostaglandin inhibition; monitor for ↓ diuretic and natriuretic response.	Diuresis within 30–60 min following oral administration. Monitor electrolytes, BUN, creatinine and daily weight. Bumetanide 1 mg produces a diuretic response similar to furosemide 40 mg in healthy patients; in renal failure, bumetanide 2 mg produces a diuretic response similar to furosemide 40 mg. Caution in patients with sulfa allergy. Contraindications: hepatic coma, states of severe electrolyte depletion.	$-$$$
	ethacrynic acid Edecrin	Individualize dose according to patient response Initial: 50 mg as single dose after a meal	See bumetanide. May be associated with severe ototoxicity. Can be used in sulfa-allergic patients.	See bumetanide.	May be considered in individuals with sulfonamide hypersensitivity or in cases of severe, refractory edema. Onset of diuresis: po 30 min; iv 5 min.	$–$$$

(cont'd)

Table 1: Diuretic Agents for Treatment of Edema[1,2,4,6,8,9,10,11,12] (cont'd)

Class	Drug	Dose	Adverse Effects	Drug Interactions	Comments	Cost[a]
		Titrate up gradually in increments of 25–50 mg daily until desired response; may require up to 200 mg BID in severe, refractory cases of edema Maintenance: lowest effective daily dose When adding to another diuretic, start low (i.e., 25 mg daily) and titrate up as necessary			Duration of action: po 6–8 h; iv 2 h. Monitor electrolytes, BUN, creatinine and daily weight. Similar in potency to furosemide. IV route used when oral intake is not viable or in urgent situations such as pulmonary edema.	
	furosemide Lasix, Lasix Special, generics	Individualize dose according to patient response Initial: 20–80 mg po as a single dose preferably in a.m. If desired response has not been achieved, ↑ by 20–40 mg Q6–8H; max single dose dependent on disease state and renal function; ↑ dose if initial dose fails to produce adequate increase in urinary output within 4–6 h of dose	See bumetanide.	See bumetanide.	Half-life: 1.5–2h and prolonged in kidney insufficiency. Extent and rate of absorption varies between patients depending on concomitant disease states. Effectiveness diminishes in the presence of gut wall edema Onset of diuresis: po 30–60 min; iv 5 min. Duration of action: po 4–8 h, iv 2 h.	$–$$

Class	Drug	Dose	Adverse Effects	Drug Interactions	Comments	Cost[a]
		IV dose: 20–40 mg as a single injection, may repeat Q2H. If no response, may ↑ dose in 20 mg increments Continuous infusion: 3–20 mg/h titrated to patient's response Maintenance: lowest effective dose taken daily, BID or intermittently on alternate days Severe edema: can use 250–500 mg tablet po			Monitor electrolytes, BUN, creatinine and daily weight. Furosemide 500 mg tablet: for patients with GFR 5–20 mL/min who have not responded to conventional doses. May use in combination with thiazides for synergy. Caution in patients with sulfa allergy.	
Thiazide Diuretics	*chlorthalidone* generics	Individualize dose according to patient response 50–100 mg once daily; can be given every other day Maintain on lowest effective dose Ineffective as monotherapy in patients with GFR < 50 mL/min When adding to another diuretic, start low and titrate up as necessary	Usually well tolerated. Orthostatic hypotension. Electrolyte abnormalities: hyperuricemia (usually asymptomatic), hyponatremia (common), hypochloremia, hypokalemia (evident during first 1–2 wk). Headache, vertigo, dizziness, asthenia, muscle cramps. Volume depletion. Acute interstitial nephritis.	Loop diuretics: ↑ diuresis and electrolyte abnormalities; monitor for dehydration and electrolyte abnormalities when used in combination. Digoxin: hypokalemia and hypomagnesemia may lead to arrhythmias. Antidiabetic medications: thiazides may ↑ blood sugar—seen at higher doses. Monitor blood glucose and adjust dose of antidiabetic medications as necessary.	Half-life: 24–55 h. Onset: 2–6 h, persists for 24–72 h. Contraindications: severe renal or hepatic failure, hypercalcemia, refractory hypokalemia or hyponatremia, symptomatic hyperuricemia.	$

(cont'd)

Table 1: **Diuretic Agents for Treatment of Edema**[1,2,4,6,8,9,10,11,12] *(cont'd)*

Class	Drug	Dose	Adverse Effects	Drug Interactions	Comments	Cost[a]
			Thiazides can exacerbate gout.	Lithium: ↓ renal clearance of lithium resulting in toxicity; monitor lithium levels and adjust dose as needed. NSAIDs: may negate the diuretic effect and ↑ risk of NSAID-induced renal dysfunction.		
	hydrochloro-thiazide generics	Individualize dose according to patient response Initial: 25–100 mg daily or divided BID or TID Can also be given on alternate days Ineffective as monotherapy in patients with GFR < 50 mL/min When adding to a loop diuretic, start low and titrate up as necessary	See chlorthalidone. ↑ fasting blood glucose may be dose-related as not seen with doses < 12.5 mg.	See chlorthalidone.	Half-life: 2.5 h, prolonged in renal insufficiency. Onset: 2 h with duration of 6–12 h. Used in combination with furosemide for synergistic effect.	$
	indapamide Lozide, generics	Individualize dose according to patient response Initial: 2.5 mg once daily; may ↑ to 5 mg daily if no response within 1 wk	See chlorthalidone.	See chlorthalidone.	Half-life: 15–25 h. Take with food or milk to decrease GI side effects. Monitor electrolytes in patients who may be at increased risk of hypokalemia,	$

Class	Drug	Dose	Adverse Effects	Drug Interactions	Comments	Cost[a]
		When adding to a loop diuretic, start low and titrate up as necessary Ineffective as monotherapy in patients with GFR < 50 mL/min			e.g., patients on digoxin, patients with cardiac arrhythmias. Contraindications: progressive and severe oliguria, hepatic coma.	
	metolazone Zaroxolyn	Individualize dose according to patient response Single daily dose is recommended; start low and titrate up 2.5–20 mg Q24H Ineffective as monotherapy in patients with GFR < 50 mL/min	See chlorthalidone.	See chlorthalidone.	Diuresis and saluresis begin within 1 h and persist for 12–24 h, depending on dose. May be given for a limited time period initially. May be given indefinitely to patients who remain volume-expanded, based on target weight. Contraindications: hepatic coma, sulfa allergy	$-$$
Potassium-sparing Diuretics	*amiloride* Midamor, generics	Individualize dose according to patient response Initial: 5 mg daily; ↑ to 10 mg daily if necessary If persistent hypokalemia is present, may ↑ to 15 mg, then 20 mg daily with careful monitoring of electrolytes	Hyperkalemia – common if used as monotherapy; incidence greater in patients with renal impairment, elderly and in diabetes. Headache, impotence. Hyponatremia, hypochloremia when	ACEI and ARBs: ↑ K^+ levels; monitor renal function and potassium levels when used in combination, especially in patients with renal impairment and type 2 diabetes mellitus; adjust dose as needed. Potassium preparations: ↑ K^+; avoid combination unless documented hypokalemia; monitor K^+ levels.	Contraindications: significant renal function impairment, hyperkalemia.	$–$$

(cont'd)

Table 1: **Diuretic Agents for Treatment of Edema**[1,2,4,6,8,9,10,11,12] *(cont'd)*

Class	Drug	Dose	Adverse Effects	Drug Interactions	Comments	Cost[a]
		ClCr 10–50 mL/min: administer 50% of normal dose	used in combination with other diuretics.	Tacrolimus, cyclosporine: ↑ K^+ levels. NSAIDs: may negate the diuretic effect and ↑ risk of NSAID-induced renal dysfunction.		
	spironolactone Aldactone, generics	Individualize dose according to patient response; 25–200 mg daily ↑ 25–50 mg Q 5 days Continue initial dose for ≥ 5 d, then titrate accordingly If adequate diuresis has not occurred, add a 2nd diuretic which acts proximally in nephron for additive effects ClCr 10–50 mL/min: administer Q12–24H ClCr < 10 mL/min: avoid	See amiloride. Gynecomastia.	See amiloride. Digoxin: ↑ plasma levels due to ↓ in renal tubular secretion; spironolactone may interfere with digoxin radioimmunoassay, resulting in falsely ↑ digoxin levels. Salicylates: may result in sodium retention; monitor sodium levels and blood pressure. Mitotane: antagonism of mitotane activity; avoid combination.	See amiloride.	$

[a] Cost of 30-day supply; includes drug cost only.

Dosage adjustment may be required in renal impairment; see Appendix I

Abbreviations: ACEI = ACE inhibitor; ARB = angiotensin receptor blocker; NSAID = nonsteroidal anti-inflammatory drug

Legend: $ < $20 $-$$ < $20–40 $$ $20-40 $-$$$ < $20– >40 $$$ > $40

Suggested Readings

Andreoli TE. Edematous states: an overview. *Kidney Int Suppl* 1997;59:S2-10.

Brater DC. Diuretic therapy. *N Engl J Med* 1998;339(6):387-95.

Brater DC. Pharmacology of diuretics. *Am J Med Sci* 2000;319(1):38-50.

Morrison RT. Edema and principles of diuretic use. *Med Clin North Am* 1997;81(3):689-704.

O'Brien JG, Chennubhotla SA, Chennubhotla RV. Treatment of edema. *Am Fam Physician* 2005;71(11):2111-7.

Streeten DH. Idiopathic edema. Pathogenesis, clinical features, and treatment. *Endocrinol Metab Clin North Am* 1995;24(3):531-47.

Wilcox CS. Metabolic and adverse effects of diuretics. *Semin Nephrol* 1999;19(6):557-68.

References

1. Rose BD. Diuretics. *Kidney Int* 1991;39(2):336-52.
2. Wilcox CS. Metabolic and adverse effects of diuretics. *Semin Nephrol* 1999;19(6):557-68.
3. Rasool A, Palevsky PM. Treatment of edematous disorders with diuretics. *Am J Med Sci* 2000;319(1):25-37.
4. Greenberg A. Diuretic complications. *Am J Med Sci* 2000;319(1):10-24.
5. Ellison DH. Diuretic resistance: physiology and therapeutics. *Semin Nephrol* 1999;19(6):581-97.
6. Brater DC. Diuretic therapy. *N Engl J Med* 1998;339(6):387-95.
7. Streeten DH. Idiopathic edema. Pathogenesis, clinical features, and treatment. *Endocrinol Metab Clin North Am* 1995;24(3):531-47.
8. Bleich M, Greger R. Mechanism of action of diuretics. *Kidney Int Suppl* 1997;59:S11-5.
9. Brater DC. Pharmacology of diuretics. *Am J Med Sci* 2000;319(1):38-50.
10. Andreucci M, Russo D, Fuiano G et al. Diuretics in renal failure. *Miner Electrolyte Metab* 1999;25(1-2):32-8.
11. Capasso G, Pica A, Saviano C et al. Clinical complications of diuretic therapy. *Kidney Int Suppl* 1997;59:S16-20.
12. Dormans TP, Gerlag PG, Russel FG et al. Combination diuretic therapy in severe congestive heart failure. *Drugs* 1998;55(2):165-72.

CHAPTER 91
Hypercalcemia

Walter Watral, BScPharm, PharmD

Goals of Therapy

- Normalize serum calcium levels
  - correct extracellular fluid (ECF) volume contraction and dehydration
  - enhance renal excretion of calcium
  - inhibit accelerated bone resorption
- Alleviate signs and symptoms of hypercalcemia, e.g., depressed level of consciousness, thirst, polyuria
- Diagnose and treat underlying disorder

Investigations

- Initiating treatment immediately will not interfere with diagnostic tests (see Pharmacologic Choices: General Measures)
- History and physical examination,[1,2] with special attention to:
  - onset and duration of symptoms (anorexia, nausea, vomiting, constipation, altered mental status, malaise, drowsiness, bone pain, polydipsia, polyuria are usually symptoms associated with acute hypercalcemia)
  - chronic hypercalcemia is usually asymptomatic
- Laboratory evaluation:[2,3]
  - ionized calcium (preferred where available) or serum calcium and albumin (see Table 1 to calculate calcium corrected for low albumin)
  - 24-hour urine creatinine and calcium (if familial hypocalciuric hypercalcemia or milk-alkali syndrome is suspected), serum phosphate, serum creatinine and BUN
  - alkaline phosphatase
  - serum intact parathyroid hormone
  - specialists may order other tests (e.g., skeletal survey, bone scan) based on history or physical findings of hypercalcemia-associated conditions, as required
  - consider referral to endocrinologist for a complete endocrine assessment to evaluate the possibility of multiple endocrine neoplasia (MEN) syndrome
  - if hypercalcemia is acute or chronic and PTH is high, consider hyperparathyroidism
  - if hypercalcemia is acute and PTH is low, consider malignancy. Perform a more complete clinical evaluation

- if hypercalcemia is chronic and PTH is low, consider granulamatous diseases, familial disorders, milk-alkali syndrome, drug-induced (e.g., lithium, thiazide diuretics, excess vitamin A or D, derivatives and analogues of vitamin A, estrogens, antiestrogens, progestins, androgens, parental nutrition, ingestion of > 3 g elemental calcium per day), adrenal insufficiency, hyperthyroidism

Therapeutic Choices (Figure 1)

- Aggressiveness of initial interventions depends on the rapidity of onset and severity of the hypercalcemia.
- Definitive therapy for long-term control of hypercalcemia requires diagnosis and treatment of the underlying condition.

Table 1: **Serum Calcium Correction (mmol/L) for Low Serum Albumin**[a]

Albumin (g/L)	Correction (add to measured Ca^{++})	Albumin (g/L)	Correction (add to measured Ca^{++})
10	0.6	23	0.34
11	0.58	24	0.32
12	0.56	25	0.3
13	0.54	26	0.28
14	0.52	27	0.26
15	0.5	28	0.24
16	0.48	29	0.22
17	0.46	30	0.2
18	0.44	31	0.18
19	0.42	32	0.16
20	0.4	33	0.14
21	0.38	34	0.12
22	0.36	35	0.1

[a] corrected Ca^{++} value = (40 – measured albumin) (0.02) + measured Ca^{++}

Nonpharmacologic Choices

Mobilize[2,3,4]

Hypercalcemia is exacerbated by immobilization. Ambulation helps to reduce bone resorption and normalize serum calcium.

Diet[2,3,4]

Dietary changes rarely correct hypercalcemia. Patients with vitamin D-mediated hypercalcemia may benefit from dietary calcium restriction. Excessive use of vitamin D supplements, calcium supplements or calcium-containing antacids should be curtailed in all patients.

Hemodialysis[2,4,5]

If available and able to be instituted promptly, hemodialysis (zero or low calcium bath) provides rapid correction of severe hypercalcemia. It is of particular value in those with severe hypercalcemia and severe renal impairment.

Pharmacologic Choices

General Measures

Stop Offending Agents

If possible, discontinue offending agents (see Investigations) and replace with agents that do not exacerbate hypercalcemia.

Hydrate

Patients with hypercalcemia are often dehydrated as a result of a renal water-concentrating defect induced by hypercalcemia and by decreased fluid intake resulting from nausea and vomiting. Expansion of intravascular volume enhances renal calcium clearance. Hydration alone usually reduces serum calcium by ≤ 0.6 mmol/L. This effect is present only during hydration.[2,3,4] Serum magnesium and potassium may also decrease and should be monitored and replaced as needed.

Patients with mild to moderate asymptomatic hypercalcemia should drink 3 L per day of noncaffeinated beverages to achieve and maintain euvolemia. Patients with moderate to severe symptomatic hypercalcemia should receive **normal saline** (0.9% NaCl) intravenously, typically at 250–500 mL/hour, if safe to do so, until euvolemic, and then the infusion rate should be reduced to maintain normal intravascular volume. Volume correction may require 2 to 3 L of fluid within the first eight hours. Patients with a significant volume deficit may need 3 to 5 L of fluid in the first 24 hours and 2 to 3 L per 24 hours thereafter until a good urine output (≥ 0.5–1 mL/kg/hour) has been established.[5,6,7,8,9] Renal dysfunction is common among hypercalcemic patients. Careful monitoring of hydration is essential, especially in elderly patients and those with preexisting renal insufficiency or left ventricular systolic dysfunction. Refer to Figure 1 for further information on the management of mild, moderate and severe hypercalcemia.

Use a loop diuretic (i.e., **furosemide**, **ethacrynic acid**) to prevent fluid overload and heart failure, as needed, but only after volume contraction is corrected. Thiazide diuretics are contraindicated because they impair calcium excretion.[10,11]

Normalize Serum Phosphate

Hypophosphatemia, seen mostly in primary hyperparathyroidism and malignancy-associated hypercalcemia, exacerbates hypercalcemia by increasing renal synthesis of 1,25-dihydroxyvitamin D, which consequently reduces bone formation, increases bone resorption and increases intestinal absorption of dietary calcium. Oral **phosphates** (1 to 2 g elemental phosphate per day) can be given safely in all patients, except those with renal insufficiency, to increase serum phosphate to the low normal range (0.8 to 1 mmol/L). Though rare, calcium phosphate can precipitate and cause serious organ damage (heart, kidney, lungs, blood vessels) if phosphate levels are increased to > 1 mmol/L or if iv phosphate is administered.[2]

Specific Measures (Table 2)

Primary Hyperparathyroidism

Surgery remains arguably the first-line measure for control of primary hyperparathyroidism in all patients.[1,6,9,12,13,14] Medical management is used for patients who refuse surgery, who are not candidates for surgery or who have had an unsuccessful parathyroid surgery.[3] Oral phosphate therapy can also be used if the dose is titrated to normalize serum calcium, and appropriate monitoring is provided.[8,9] **Bisphosphonate** therapy is usually reserved for patients with moderate to severe hypercalcemia.[13]

Cinacalcet is the first available calcimetic and is indicated for treatment of secondary hyperparathyroidism in patients with chronic kidney disease on dialysis. Its role in treatment of primary hyperparathyroidism is being investigated.[16,17]

Malignancy

Antineoplastic therapy aimed at the underlying malignancy is the key to long-term calcium control, although not all patients are candidates. **Bisphosphonates** are first-line drugs if effective antineoplastic therapy is not available or appropriate, if the patient has severe hypercalcemia (> 3.5 mmol/L with or without symptoms) or if the patient has multiple myeloma. For acute management, parenteral **pamidronate**, **clodronate** or **zoledronic acid** may be used.[18,19] Two hour iv infusion of pamidronate and clodronate is convenient for outpatient therapy (Table 2). Additionally, clodronate can be administered by a subcutaneous infusion, useful in the palliative setting.[20] Zoledronic acid can be infused over 15 minutes in most patients.[21] Response to treatment with an iv bisphosphonate is generally seen within 24 to 48 hours. For patients who respond, serum calcium levels can be maintained at acceptable levels for up to five weeks before re-treatment is required.[19,22,23] Patients with multiple myeloma benefit from reduced bone pain, decreased skeletal morbidity and prevention of hypercalcemia recurrence with prolonged therapy.[18] There is insufficient information about the use of other bisphosphonates (e.g., alendronate, risedronate) for serum calcium control.[24] **Calcitonin** rapidly reduces serum calcium levels in severe hypercalcemia, however, the response tends to abate within 48 hours.[20]

Granulomatous Diseases

Excess production of 1,25-dihydroxyvitamin D is characteristic of granulomatous diseases (e.g., sarcoidosis). Therapy includes restricting vitamin D and calcium intake and avoiding excessive exposure to sunlight. Corticosteroids may be used in acutely ill patients.[8,13]

Therapeutic Tips

- Overly aggressive use of loop diuretics can aggravate hypercalcemia by depleting extracellular fluid volume. Routine prescription of a loop diuretic with hydration therapy is discouraged.
- To reduce serum calcium rapidly, i.e., within 6 to 12 hours in severe hypercalcemia of malignancy, use calcitonin plus hydration. Serum calcium usually declines 0.8 mmol/L at 12 to 24 hours following combined therapy. To augment and prolong serum calcium control, use definitive therapy, e.g., antineoplastic therapy, for the underlying cause. If antineoplastic therapy is not an option, use a bisphosphonate when dehydration is corrected and adequate urine output is achieved—preferably within 24 hours of hypercalcemia diagnosis.
- Premedication with acetaminophen 650 mg can prevent bisphosphonate-induced fever in patients with hypercalcemia of malignancy.
- Adjunctive glucocorticoid therapy, e.g., prednisone 40 to 100 mg/day or equivalent for up to one week, is useful in patients with lymphoma, myeloma, lymphoid leukemia and breast cancer in situations where hypercalcemic flares are caused by hormonal treatment.

Figure 1: **Management of Hypercalcemia**

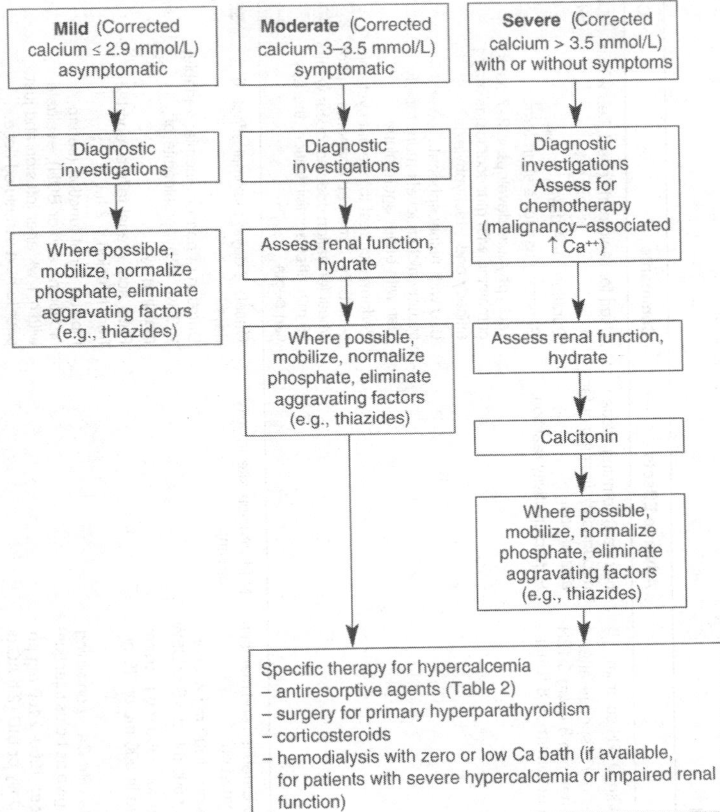

Table 2: **Treatment of Hypercalcemia**

Class	Drug	Dose	Adverse Effects	Comments	Cost[a]
Antiparathyroid Hormone	*calcitonin salmon* Calcimar, Caltine, generics	Initial: 4 IU/kg Q12H sc or im If unsatisfactory response after 1–2 days, may ↑ to 8 IU/kg Q12H. May ↑ to a maximum of 8 IU/kg Q6H	Nausea, vomiting (dose dependent), flushing of face and hands. Hypersensitivity reaction.	Used for rapid early effect, i.e., within 6 h. Duration: 1–4 days. Generally use for a short term. Tachyphylaxis develops in 2–7 days; combining with glucocorticoids may ↑ efficacy and ↓ tachyphylaxis. Use with bisphosphonate lowers serum calcium levels more rapidly than with either agent alone. Perform skin test to rule out systemic sensitivity; if marked erythema and/or wheal formation does not occur within 15 min after administration, therapy can begin.	$46/ 400 IU vial
Bisphosphonates	*clodronate, IV* Bonefos	**Treatment:** Establish and maintain adequate hydration Single infusion: 1500 mg iv over 4 h diluted in 500 mL of NS or D5W Multiple infusion: 300 mg iv over 2–6 h diluted in 500 mL of NS or D5W Do not dilute with Ca^{++}-containing solutions or give as bolus injections **Maintenance:** 1600–2400 mg po given once daily or BID (2 h AC or 2 h PC)	Mild infusion site toxicity, vomiting.	Onset: 2 days; maximal effect: 6 days. Duration of normocalcemia: variable, 2–3 wk in hypercalcemia of malignancy. Fatal acute renal failure reported from infusion < 2 h. Monitor renal function (serum creatinine and/or BUN), evaluate within 1 wk after infusion and just prior to next scheduled dose.	$65/ 300 mg vial

Class	Drug	Dose	Adverse Effects	Comments	Cost[a]
		Maximum daily dose is 3200 mg. Ensure adequate fluid rehydration			
	clodronate, oral Bonefos, Clasteon, Ostac	**Maintenance:** 1600–2400 mg po given once daily or BID (2 h AC or 2 h PC) Maximum daily dose is 3200 mg. Ensure adequate fluid rehydration	Nausea, vomiting, anorexia, diarrhea, muscle cramps	Concomitant intake of oral iron, calcium, magnesium, aluminum, e.g., antacids, may prevent absorption of oral clodronate. Do not take with or within 1 h before or after food or milk. Reintroduce iv clodronate if elevated serum calcium present during oral clodronate treatment.	$1.50/ 400 mg capsule
	pamidronate Aredia, Pamidronate Disodium for Injection, generics	**Tumor-induced hypercalcemia:** Adequate hydration with normal saline necessary before treatment Not to exceed 90 mg in 500 mL over 4 h; infusion rate not to exceed 22.5 mg/h. Consult product monograph for dosing for serum Ca^{++} > 3 mmol/L Total dose can be given as a single infusion or multiple infusions spread over 2–4 consecutive days. Maximum dose is 90 mg per treatment. Do not dilute with Ca^{++}-containing solutions or give as bolus injections	Local infusion site reactions, febrile reaction within 24–48 h of infusion—may be accompanied by malaise, rigor, fatigue, flushes, osteonecrosis of the jaw[25] Rare: posterior uveitis.[26]	Onset: 4–72 h; decrease in calcium levels seen in 24–48 h; maximum lowering occurs in 3–7days. Duration: 3–4 wk. Repeat infusion if calcium level does not decrease within 2 days or if hypercalcemia recurs. Monitor renal function (serum creatinine and/or BUN), evaluate within 1 wk after infusion and just prior to next scheduled dose. Case reports of safe and effective use, without dosage modification, in patients on hemodialysis. Osteonecrosis of the jaw: regular dental exam, especially prior to	$475/ 90 mg vial

(cont'd)

Table 2: **Treatment of Hypercalcemia** *(cont'd)*

Class	Drug	Dose	Adverse Effects	Comments	Cost[a]
				therapy or within 3 months if possible, as well as good oral hygiene.	
	zoledronic acid Zometa Concentrate	**Tumor-induced hypercalcemia:** Establish and maintain adequate hydration 4 mg in patients with albumin-corrected serum calcium ≥ 3.0 mmol/L given as a single dose iv infusion over 15 min[19] Retreatment: 8 mg as a single dose over 15 minutes. In patients demonstrating complete or partial response without normalization of Ca^{++} levels. Only for patients who can tolerate standard rehydration procedures (3–5 L fluids and > 400 mEq of NaCl per day) Do not dilute with Ca^{++}-containing solutions or give as bolus injections	Febrile reactions, nausea, vomiting, flu-like syndrome, local infusion site reactions, mild hypomagnesemia, hypokalemia and hypophosphatemia, osteonecrosis of the jaw[25]	Onset: 24–48 h. Duration: 4–5 wk. Monitor renal function, evaluate within 1 wk after infusion and just prior to next scheduled dose. More potent than pamidronate. Renal function deterioration reported with infusion < 15 min. Osteonecrosis of the jaw: regular dental exam, especially prior to therapy or within 3 months if possible, as well as good oral hygiene.	$550/ 4mg vial
Corticosteroids, systemic	*hydrocortisone sodium succinate* Solu-Cortef, generics	200–300 mg iv daily for 3–5 days		Slow onset. Potential for diabetes mellitus, osteoporosis, increased susceptibility to infection.	$36/ 500 mg vial
	prednisone generics	40–60 mg daily for 5–10 days		See hydrocortisone.	$8/ 20 mg vial

Class	Drug	Dose	Adverse Effects	Comments	Cost[a]
Calcimetics	*cinacalcet* Sensipar	Starting: 30 mg once daily; titrate every 2–4 wk to a maximum dose of 180 mg once daily to achieve a target parathyroid hormone (PTH) level No dosage adjustment required in renal impairment	Nausea, vomiting, diarrhea, myalgia, hypocalcemia.	Inhibits CYP2D6; dose adjustments may be required for concomitant CYP2D6-metabolized drugs with narrow therapeutic index, e.g., TCAs, flecainide. Increases the sensitivity of the calcium-sensing receptor to circulating serum calcium, thereby decreasing the secretion of PTH. Onset: PTH level decreases within 2–6 h after a dose. Food increases bioavailability. Monitor serum calcium, serum phosphate and PTH.	$23/ 60 mg tablet
Crystalloids	*sodium chloride 0.9% (normal saline, NS)* Sodium Chloride Injection USP	Initial: 200–300 mL/h Dependent on concomitant disease states and extent of hypercalcemia		Onset: 24–48 h. Can be given ± other electrolytes. Contraindications: renal insufficiency, congestive heart failure.	$7/ 500 mL bag
Diuretics, loop	*furosemide* generics	Initial: 40–80 mg iv Q1–4H after volume expansion	Electrolyte abnormalities, e.g., hypokalemia, orthostatic hypotension.	Given following aggressive rehydration restoring intravascular volume. Prevents fluid overload and inhibits calcium reabsorption in the distal renal tubule.	$30/ 40 mg vial

[a] Drug cost only.

Dosage adjustment may be required in renal impairment; see Appendix I

Suggested Readings

Bilezikian JP and Silverberg SJ. Asymptomatic primary hyperparathyroidism.*N Engl J Med* 2004;350(17):174651.

Jacob TP and Bilezikian JP. Clinical Review: Rare causes of hypercalcemia. *J Clin Endocrinol Metab* 2005;90:631622.

Ariyan CE and Sosa JA. Assessment and management of patients with abnormal calcium. *Crit Care Med* 2004;32 (Suppl): S14654.

Bushinsky DA, Monk RD. Electrolyte quintet: calcium. *Lancet* 1998;352(9124):306-11.

Stewart AF. Clinical practice. Hypercalcemia associated with cancer. *N Engl J Med* 2005;352(4):373-9.

References

1. Carroll MF, Schade DS. A practical approach to hypercalcemia. *Am Fam Physician* 2003;67(9):1959-66.
2. Stewart AF. Clinical practice. Hypercalcemia associated with cancer. *N Engl J Med* 2005;352(4):373-9.
3. Kaye TB. Hypercalcemia. How to pinpoint the cause and customize treatment. *Postgrad Med* 1995;97(1):153-5, 159-60.
4. Deftos LJ. Hypercalcemia: mechanisms, differential diagnosis, and remedies. *Postgrad Med* 1996;100(6):119-21,125-6.
5. Nakashima L. Guidelines for the treatment of hypercalcemia associated with malignancy. *J Oncol Pharm Practice* 1997;3:31-7.
6. Ralston SH, Coleman R, Fraser WD et al. Medical management of hypercalcemia. *Calcif Tissue Int* 2004;74(1):1-11.
7. Chisholm MA, Mulloy AL, Taylor AT. Acute management of cancer-related hypercalcemia. *Ann Pharmacother* 1996;30(5):507-13.
8. Davis KD, Attie MF. Management of severe hypercalcemia. *Crit Care Clin* 1991;7(1):175-90.
9. Bilezikian JP. Clinical review 51: Management of hypercalcemia. *J Clin Endocrinol Metab* 1993;77(6):1445-9.
10. Potts JT. Hyperparathyroidism and other hypercalcemic disorders. *Adv Intern Med* 1996;41:165-212.
11. Strong P, Jewell S, Rinker J. Thiazide therapy and severe hypercalcemia in a patient with hyperparathyroidism. *West J Med* 1991;154(3):338-40.
12. [No authors listed]. NIH conference. Diagnosis and management of asymptomatic primary hyperparathyroidism: consensus development conference statement. *Ann Intern Med* 1991;114(7):593-7.
13. Bushinsky DA, Monk RD. Electrolyte quintet: calcium. *Lancet* 1998;352(9124):306-11.
14. Levine MA. Primary hyperparathyroidism: 7,000 years of progress. *Cleve Clin J Med* 2005;72(12):1084-5, 1088, 1091-2.
15. Grey AB, Stapleton JP, Evans MC et al. Effect of hormone replacement therapy on bone mineral density in postmenopausal women with mild primary hyperparathyroidism. A randomized, controlled trial. *Ann Intern Med* 1996;125(5):360-8.
16. Shoback DM, Bilezikian JP, Turner SA et al. The calcimimetic cinacalcet normalizes serum calcium in subjects with primary hyperparathyroidism. *J Clin Endocrinol Metab* 2003;88(12):5644-9.
17. Peacock M, Bilezikian JP, Klassen PS et al. Cinacalcet hydrochloride maintains long-term normocalcemia in patients with primary hyperparathyroidism. *J Clin Endocrinol Metab* 2005;90(1):135-41.
18. Lacy MQ, Dispenzieri A, Gertz MA. Mayo Clinic consensus statement for the use of bisphosphonates in multiple myeloma. *Mayo Clinic Proceedings* 2006;81(3):1047–53.
19. Major P, Lortholary A, Hon J et al. Zoledronic acid is superior to pamidronate in the treatment of hypercalcemia of malignancy: a pooled analysis of two randomized, controlled clinical trials. *J Clin Oncol* 2001;19(2):558-67.
20. Berenson JR. Treatment of hypercalcemia of malignancy with bisphosphonates. *Semin Oncol* 2002;29(6 Suppl 21):12-8.
21. Berenson J, Hirschberg R. Safety and convenience of a 15-minute infusion of zoledronic acid. *Oncologist* 2004;9(3):319-29.
22. Watters J, Gerrand G, Dodwell D. The management of malignant hypercalcaemia. *Drugs* 1996;52(6):837-48.
23. Perry CM, Figgitt DP. Zoledronic acid: a review of its use in patients with advanced cancer. *Drugs* 2004;64(11):1197-211.
24. Lteif AN, Zimmerman D. Bisphosphonates for treatment of childhood hypercalcemia. *Pediatrics* 1998;102(4 Pt 1):990-3.

25. Woo SB, Hellstein JW, Kalmar JR. Narrative [corrected] review: bisphosphonates and osteonecrosis of the jaws. *Ann Intern Med* 2006 May 16;144(10):753-61.
26. Haverbeke G, Pertile G, Claes C et al. Posterior uveitis: an under-recognized adverse effect of pamidronate: 2 case reports. *Bull Soc Belge Ophtalmol* 2003;(290):71-6.

CHAPTER 92
Potassium Disturbances

Jean Éthier, MD, FRCPC

Potassium, the major intracellular cation in the human body, is found in abundance in fruits (e.g., tomatoes, cucumbers), vegetables (e.g., leafy greens) and meats. The average dietary daily intake is 100 mEq. Normal potassium concentration is 3.5–5.0 mmol/L.

Hypokalemia, defined as a plasma potassium concentration of less than 3.5 mmol/L, can be mild (3–3.5 mmol/L), moderate (2.5–3 mmol/L) or severe (< 2.5 mmol/L). *Hyperkalemia*, defined as a plasma concentration of greater than 5.0 mmol/L, can be mild (5.5–6 mmol/L), moderate (6.1-6.9 mmol/L) or severe (> 7 mmol/L). Hypokalemia and hyperkalemia are associated with potentially fatal cardiac arrhythmias.

Goals of Therapy

- Prevent life-threatening cardiac arrhythmias and improve neuromuscular conductivity
- Re-establish normal body stores of potassium (K^+) and prevent undue losses or accumulations
- Identify and correct underlying causes

Investigations

- History with attention to possible etiology (see Table 1)
- Physical examination to assess cardiac rhythm, paresis, muscle weakness, paresthesias, blood pressure (in suspected hypokalemia)
- ECG when clinically necessary
- Laboratory tests may be useful in assessing hypokalemia or hyperkalemia, if not already evident:
  - urea, creatinine, Na^+, K^+, Cl^-, glucose
  - arterial or venous blood gases or total CO_2
  - spot urine for Na^+, K^+, Cl^- and osmolality to calculate the transtubular K^+ concentration gradient (TTKG) and the potassium-creatinine ratio and, in select cases, 24-hour urine collection for Na^+, K^+ and creatinine
  - renin, aldosterone, cortisol, screening tests for renovascular disease in select cases
  - magnesium in refractory hypokalemia, especially when patient is at risk for hypomagnesemia, e.g., taking diuretics or cisplatin, diarrhea
  - rule out pseudohyperkalemia (possible with thrombocytosis, severe leukocytosis, in vitro hemolysis or forearm contraction)[1]

Table 1: **Causes of Potassium Disturbances**

Hyperkalemia	Hypokalemia
Drug-induced: K^+ supplements, NSAIDs, ACE inhibitors, angiotensin II receptor blockers (ARBs), K^+-sparing diuretics, digoxin overdose, cyclosporine, penicillin G potassium, tacrolimus, trimethoprim or TMP/SMX (high-dose or in susceptible patients, i.e., elderly, renal failure), heparin, aminocaproic acid, beta-blockers, pentamidine, succinylcholine, some herbal and nutritional supplements (e.g., alfalfa, nettle) especially in the presence of renal failure	Diarrhea, vomiting
Renal failure, diabetes, adrenal insufficiency, hyporeninemic hypoaldosteronism	Inadequate dietary intake
Familial history of hyperkalemia	Drug-induced: loop and thiazide diuretics, laxatives, amphotericin B, aminoglycosides, long-term corticosteroid therapy, antipseudomonal penicillins, tocolytic agents, $beta_2$-agonists, carbenoxolone, licorice, insulin, foscarnet, theophylline, caffeine
Acidosis	Familial history (Bartter's or Gitelman's syndrome)
Crush injury, trauma, hemolysis, tumor lysis	Mineralocorticoid excess (e.g., primary aldosteronism)
	Renovascular disease
	Metabolic alkalosis
	Osmotic diuresis (diabetes)
	Hypomagnesemia
	Increased sweat loss
	Dialysis/Plasmapheresis

Abbreviations: ACE = angiotensin converting enzyme; TMP/SMX = trimethoprim/sulfamethoxazole

Hyperkalemia

Therapeutic Choices (Figure 1)

Nonpharmacologic Choices

- Stop K^+ supplements and/or drugs inducing hyperkalemia (see Table 1). If K^+ supplements are strongly indicated, a reduction in dosage may be sufficient.
- Reduce dietary K^+ intake to ≤ 60 mmol/day.

In mild hyperkalemia (plasma $K^+ = 5.5–6$ mmol/L) these measures are usually sufficient. Increasing K^+, ongoing K^+ load or renal failure require further measures, e.g., hemodialysis.

Pharmacologic Choices (Table 2)

Do not rely only on the plasma K^+ or ECG to determine the urgency of treatment. Cardiac toxicity depends not only on the level of plasma K^+ but also on the rate of increase, chronicity of hyperkalemia, levels of other electrolytes (hypocalcemia, hyponatremia and acidosis increase cardiotoxicity) and cardiac irritability. Consider all these factors.

In *severe hyperkalemia* ($K^+ > 6.5–7$ mmol/L) or when significant or advanced ECG changes are present (loss of P waves or widening of QRS complexes), *continuous cardiac monitoring* should accompany treatment. Give **iv calcium** promptly and begin **insulin**. Initiate K^+ removal simultaneously (Figure 1, Table 2).

In less severe situations, K^+ removal with or without redistribution agents may be sufficient. Estimate renal function and ongoing gain of K^+ in extracellular fluid. Initiate treatment early and more aggressively when renal failure is present or there is rapid and severe input of K^+ (e.g., rhabdomyolysis, tumor lysis syndrome) than when there is slow or no input (e.g., hyperkalemia induced by K^+-sparing diuretics).

Membrane Antagonists

Calcium gluconate or **calcium chloride** antagonizes the adverse cardiac effects of potassium and should be used in the presence of ECG changes since it is fast acting. Calcium iv has a rapid onset but relatively short duration of action and should be administered simultaneously with other treatments.

Redistribution Agents

These agents act for a longer period than membrane antagonists as they facilitate reuptake of potassium into cells.

Insulin must be administered iv.[2] **Glucose** (40 to 50 g per 10 units insulin) is given to avoid hypoglycemia, but avoid bolus administration because an acute increase in plasma tonicity can induce a rise in plasma K^+. Expect a 1.0–1.5 mmol/L fall in potassium in 60 minutes.

Sodium bicarbonate ($NaHCO_3$) is usually reserved for hyperkalemia associated with significant metabolic acidosis. It has a synergistic effect with insulin in the presence of mild acidosis.[3] In the absence of low serum bicarbonate concentration or pH, sodium bicarbonate has a smaller effect.[4] To avoid an acute increase in K^+, hypertonic $NaHCO_3$ solutions should not be used. The correction of acidosis in hypocalcemic patients may induce tetany. Insulin administration is faster, more reliable and more effective than sodium bicarbonate.[2]

The beta$_2$-agonist **salbutamol** is effective in lowering plasma K^+. Its effect is similar to insulin, but the mechanism is different; concurrent administration of insulin and salbutamol has a synergistic effect.[5] High doses of nebulized salbutamol have a similar effect to iv salbutamol; however, up to 50% of renal failure patients are resistant to this therapy.[6] Reserve salbutamol for young patients or life-threatening situations when other therapies have failed, because it is arrhythmogenic and has the potential to exacerbate angina.

Potassium Removal

Cation-exchange resins (i.e., sodium polystyrene sulfonate, calcium polystyrene sulfonate) promote the exchange of Na^+ and Ca^{++} for K^+, respectively, in the bowel; they also bind calcium and magnesium. Despite their theoretical value and their widespread clinical use with apparent efficacy, the K^+-lowering effect of single-dose resin-cathartic therapy is questionable.[7,8] The addition of resins does not seem to increase bowel K^+ removal above the effect of the diarrhea induced by the simultaneous administration of osmotic or secretory cathartics.[9] Because cation-exchange resins are constipating, they must be given with a laxative, usually sorbitol.

Resins have serious side effects. The Na^+ released in exchange for K^+ (2 mmol of Na^+ per mmol of K^+) may lead to volume overload. Rectal ulceration or colonic necrosis has been described when sodium polystyrene sulfonate mixed in sorbitol is given orally or by enema postoperatively.[10] Necrosis may be caused by sorbitol rather than by resins.[11,12] The duration of drug contact with the mucosa may be a risk factor. A cleansing enema (sodium-free) is recommended to reduce this risk. Avoid using sorbitol when the resin is administered by enema, especially in postoperative patients.

The administration of **loop diuretics** in patients with sufficient renal function can significantly increase renal K^+ excretion.

If large amounts of K^+must be removed rapidly, hemodialysis is the technique of choice. Because time is required to prepare the equipment and to insert a catheter, other treatments must be initiated while preparing for dialysis. Peritoneal dialysis is far less efficient in acutely reducing plasma K^+.

Therapeutic Tips

- Focus the treatment of chronic hyperkalemia on the cause or pathophysiological mechanism (Table 1). The treatments are similar to those used in acute hyperkalemia ($NaHCO_3$, diuretics, resins).
- The mineralocorticoid 9-alpha-**fludrocortisone** may be used in patients with hypoaldosteronism.
- Closely monitor potassium after introducing or changing the dose of any medication that could induce hyperkalemia such as ACE inhibitors, ARB, K^+-sparing diuretics, in particular in patients at risk of hyperkalemia, e.g., renal failure, elderly, cardiac insufficiency. Monitoring is even more important when a combination of these medications is prescribed (ACE + ARB + spironolactone). Measure potassium one week after the introduction of these medications and after any change in the dose.[13]

Hypokalemia

Therapeutic Choices

Nonpharmacologic Choices

- If clinically appropriate reduce or stop medication leading to K^+ loss.
- Determine and treat the etiology (Table 1).
- If the deficit is slight (plasma K^+ = 3.0–3.5 mmol/L) and there are no ongoing losses or clinical conditions warranting prompt treatment, dietary intake of potassium-rich foods should be adequate. If there

are still unusual losses, K^+ supplements or K^+-sparing diuretics will be needed.

Pharmacologic Choices (Table 3, Table 4)

The appropriate pharmacologic approach is determined by:

- Relative urgency for treatment.
- The *estimated total body deficit* for an adult with plasma K^+ of 3 mmol/L is approximately 200–400 mmol and for plasma K^+ of 2 mmol/L, approximately 500–700 mmol. *Note:* The true deficit will be larger with an extracellular shift of potassium (e.g., acidosis or insulin deficit) and smaller with an intracellular shift of potassium, (e.g., periodic paralysis or hyperadrenergic state).
- *Ongoing losses* must be added to the deficit when replacement therapy is planned. Renal losses can be estimated based on urine K^+ levels and the volume excreted per hour.
- In the presence of renal failure the treatment should be more cautious.

Potassium Salts (Table 3)

In most cases **potassium chloride** (KCl) is the salt of choice, and *oral administration* is the preferred route. If there is no paralytic ileus or suspected absorption problem, oral administration of KCl can rapidly increase plasma K^+ (40–60 mmol of a liquid preparation will increase plasma K^+ by 1.0–1.5 mmol/L).

Reserve **potassium bicarbonate** or **potassium citrate** for hypokalemic patients with metabolic acidosis (e.g., renal tubular acidosis, diarrhea). **Potassium phosphate** is used when severe hypophosphatemia is present.

Reserve iv administration of potassium for patients requiring urgent treatment (e.g., respiratory muscle weakness, cardiac arrhythmias especially if digitalis is present, hepatic encephalopathy) or those unable to take oral supplements (e.g., postsurgery, paralytic ileus). To avoid sclerosis, iv potassium should be administered via a large peripheral vein at a maximum concentration of 40–60 mmol/L. Administer higher concentrations via a central line with the catheter positioned away from the right atrium or ventricle. In patients with severe hypokalemia, administer K^+ in a dextrose-free solution to avoid stimulating insulin secretion and subsequent intracellular K^+ shift.[14] Administering potassium iv rather than po is more likely to result in hyperkalemia. Thrombophlebitis and pain at site of injection are other risks.

The *rate of administration* depends on the urgency to treat (Table 3).

Potassium-sparing Diuretics (Table 4)

If renal K^+ losses are involved in the pathogenesis of hypokalemia (e.g., hyperaldosteronism, concomitant use of other diuretics), K^+-sparing diuretics may be used to decrease these losses; they also prevent or decrease magnesium losses. **Triamterene, amiloride** and **spironolactone** are equally effective but differ in side effects. Use spironolactone in patients with primary or secondary hyperaldosteronism. The most frequent and serious side effect is hyperkalemia.

Avoid K^+-sparing diuretics in patients with renal or adrenal insufficiency, the elderly, patients with diabetes and patients taking other drugs that may increase plasma K^+ (Table 1).

Therapeutic Tips

- Avoid the use of K^+ supplements and K^+-sparing diuretics together as the risk of hyperkalemia is greatly increased. Combined use may be required temporarily at the beginning of replacement therapy if renal K^+ losses are very high; however, frequent monitoring of plasma K^+ is mandatory, and one of the drugs should be stopped when plasma K^+ reaches 3.0–3.5 mmol/L.
- Treat hypomagnesemia if present.

Figure 1: **Management of Hyperkalemia**

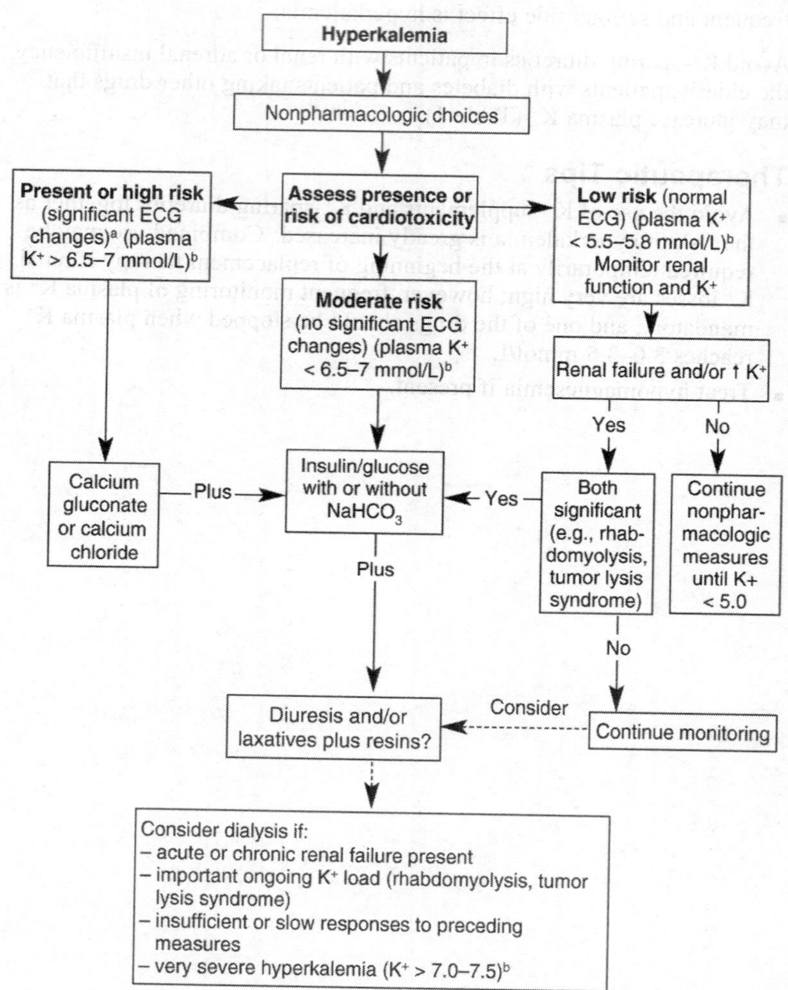

[a] Loss of P waves, widening of QRS complexes or more severe changes are considered significant. Isolated peaked T waves may not be significant.

[b] Plasma potassium level is given only as indicative; **therapy should not rely only on the plasma level.**

Table 2: **Drugs for Treatment of Hyperkalemia**

Class	Drug	Dose	Comments
Beta$_2$-adrenergic Agonists	*salbutamol* Ventolin Nebules P.F., generics	10–20 mg by nebulizer Onset: 30 min Duration of action: 2–4 h	Reserved for life-threatening cases when other treatments have failed; risk of arrhythmia or angina; variable response.
Cation-exchange esins	*sodium polystyrene sulfonate* Kayexalate, generics	**Oral:** 15–60 g in 50–100 mL of 20% sorbitol Q4–6H PRN; usual dose: 30 g Do not mix with orange juice or other fruit juices with high potassium content Onset: 1–2 h **Rectal:** 30–50 g in 100–200 mL of water or 10% dextrose Q4–6H PRN; retain at least 30–60 min. Onset: 30–60 min Duration of action: 4–6 h	Effectiveness seriously questioned. Constipating; watch for Na^+ overload; risk of colonic ulceration or necrosis with hypertonic enema. Cleansing enema before pr use recommended. Cleansing enema after pr use to be given after evacuation of the resins or after retention for 1–6 h. Available as powder and rectal suspension.
	calcium polystyrene sulfonate Resonium Calcium	**Oral:** 15 g 3 or 4 times a day. May mix resin into a paste with sweetened vehicle. Do not mix with orange juice or other fruit juices with high potassium content **Rectal:** 30 g in 100 mL of 2% methylcellulose and 100 mL of water as a daily retention enema; if possible, enema should be retained for 9 h	See sodium polystyrene sulfonate. Avoid concomitant administration of sorbitol with calcium polystyrene sulfonate as use has been associated with colonic necrosis and intestinal obstruction.
Diuretics	*furosemide* Lasix, generics	40–250 mg po/iv depending on renal function Onset: 30–60 min Duration of action: to end of increased diuresis (about 4–6 h)	Risk of volume depletion; transient ototoxicity with high-dose furosemide.

(cont'd)

Table 2: **Drugs for Treatment of Hyperkalemia** *(cont'd)*

Class	Drug	Dose	Comments
Electrolytes	*calcium gluconate 10%* Calcium Gluconate Injection USP, generics	10 mL iv over 2–5 min; may repeat once after 5 min (depending on ECG) Onset: 1–3 min Duration of action: 30–60 min	Continuous ECG monitoring required; infuse more slowly in patients on digoxin because of risk of ↑ digoxin toxicity; incompatible with $NaHCO_3$-containing solutions (precipitation). 1 g calcium gluconate = 93 mg elemental calcium = 4.6 mEq elemental calcium = 2.3 mmol elemental calcium.
	calcium chloride generics	5–10 mL iv over 2–5 min; may repeat once after 5 min (depending on ECG) Onset: 1–3 min Duration of action: 30–60 min	See calcium gluconate. Recommended in cardiac arrest in the presence of hyperkalemia or hypocalcemia or magnesium toxicity. May cause tissue necrosis if extravasation occurs. 1 g calcium chloride = 270 mg elemental calcium = 14 mEq elemental calcium = 7 mmol elemental calcium.
	sodium bicarbonate ($NaHCO_3$)	50–100 mmol iv over 5 min; repeat Q10–15 min (depending on ECG) Onset: variable, within 1 h Duration of action: 2 h	Variable response; risk of tetany if hypocalcemia present (give calcium first); watch for Na^+ overload. Can induce bicarbonaturia with an ↑ in renal K^+ excretion. Hypertonic $NaHCO_3$ solutions should not be used.
Insulin	*insulin with glucose*	Bolus: 5–10 units iv with 25–50 g of dextrose over 5 min. If less urgent, infuse 10 units insulin in 500 mL of 10% dextrose at the rate of 50–100 mL/h Onset: 30 min Duration of action: 4–6 h	The most reliable medication for redistribution of K^+. Risk of hypoglycemia. Avoid bolus administration of glucose because acute increase in plasma tonicity can induce ↑ K^+ in plasma.

Dosage adjustment may be required in renal impairment; see Appendix I.

Table 3: Potassium Supplements Used in the Management of Hypokalemia

Class	Drug	Indication	Dose	Adverse Effects	Comments	Cost[a]
Potassium Supplements, intravenous	*potassium salts, intravenous* Potassium Chloride for Injection Concentrate USP (2 mEq K^+/mL)	*Urgent (immediate treatment required):* Severe hypokalemia (plasma $K^+ < 2.5$ mmol/L) Symptomatic hypokalemia (respiratory muscle weakness or paresis, paralysis) Cardiac arrhythmia or conduction disturbances *Less urgent (prompt treatment required):* Plasma $K^+ = 2.5–3.0$ mmol/L Hypokalemia with digitalis toxicity, myocardial infarction or ischemia Hypokalemia with diabetic ketoacidosis (risk of insulin-induced life-threatening hypokalemia) Hypokalemia with hepatic insufficiency (risk of hepatic encephalopathy)	*Urgent (immediate treatment required):* 20–40 mmol in the first hour with continuous ECG monitoring and frequent serum K^+ measurements to adjust further rate of administration. When plasma $K^+ = 3.0$ mmol/L, correct the remaining deficit more slowly. *Less urgent (prompt treatment required):* 10–20 mmol over one hour (↑ serum K^+ by 0.25–0.5 mmol/L)[15,16] with ECG monitoring if > 10 mmol/h. Should be repeated according to resulting serum K^+. Correct the remaining deficit more slowly.	Sclerosis: Administer via a large peripheral vein at a maximum concentration of 40–60 mmol/L.	Doses > 40 mmol/h have been given in life-threatening hypokalemia.[17] Potassium (20–40 mmol) could be diluted in 100 ml of NaCl 0.9% if administered via a central vein. A maximum concentration of 10 mmol in 100 ml of NaCl 0.9% could be administered in a large peripheral vein; however, it could induce pain and sclerosis of the vein. Serum K+ should be measured frequently when large dose is administered. Measure each time after the administration of 20 to 40 mmol.	$$

(cont'd)

Table 3: **Potassium Supplements Used in the Management of Hypokalemia** *(cont'd)*

Class	Drug	Indication	Dose	Adverse Effects	Comments	Cost[a]
Potassium Supplements, oral	*potassium chloride, oral liquid or powder* K-10 (20 mEq K^+ /15 mL), K-Lor (20 mEq K^+/packet), K-Lyte/Cl (25 mEq K^+/packet)	*Not urgent:* Plasma K^+ > 3.0–3.5 mmol/L	Initially, 40–60 mmol/day (divided 2–4 times daily), is usually sufficient Salt of choice, especially in alkalotic patients. Rapid absorption, good bioavailability.	Unpleasant taste, aftertaste, nausea, heartburn.	Avoid use with potassium-sparing diuretics because of ↑ risk of severe hyperkalemia. If combination therapy is required, frequent monitoring (at least every day) of plasma K^+ is mandatory; discontinue one of the drugs when plasma K^+ reaches 3.0–3.5 mmol/L. Salt substitutes also contain potassium chloride.	$-$$
	potassium chloride, oral wax matrix tablet Apo-K (8 mEq K^+/tab); Slow-K (8 mEq K^+/tab)	*Not urgent:* Plasma K^+ > 3.0–3.5 mmol/L	Initially, 40–60 mmol/day (divided doses), is usually sufficient	GI symptoms, though less frequent than with liquid, GI ulceration (rare).	See potassium chloride, oral liquid or powder. Avoid in patients with delayed GI transit or impaired esophageal or intestinal motility. Empty wax matrix may appear in stool.	$
	potassium chloride, oral micro-encapsulated capsule K-Dur (20 mEq K^+/cap), Micro-K Extencaps (8 mEq K^+/capsule)	*Not urgent:* Plasma K^+ > 3.0–3.5 mmol/L	Initially, 40–60 mmol/day (divided doses), is usually sufficient	May be less ulceration than with wax matrix.	See potassium chloride, oral liquid or powder. Avoid in patients with delayed GI transit or impaired esophageal or intestinal motility.	$

Class	Drug	Indication	Dose	Adverse Effects	Comments	Cost[a]
	potassium citrate, oral effervescent tablets K-Lyte (25 mEq K^+/tablet)	*Not urgent:* Plasma K^+ > 3.0–3.5 mmol/L	Initially, 40–60 mmol/day (divided doses), is usually sufficient	See potassium chloride, oral liquid or powder.	Avoid use with potassium-sparing diuretics because of ↑ risk of severe hyperkalemia. If combination therapy is required, frequent monitoring of plasma K^+ is mandatory; discontinue one of the drugs when plasma K^+ reaches 3.0–3.5 mmol/L. Useful for patients with metabolic acidosis. More convenient for transport. Useful for hypokalemia secondary to thiazides given for kidney stones. ↑ urinary citrate excretion.	$$
	potassium citrate, oral crystals or liquid Polycitra-K (10 mEq K^+/5 mL oral solution)	*Not urgent:* Plasma K^+ > 3.0–3.5 mmol/L	Initially, 40–60 mmol/day (divided doses), is usually sufficient	See potassium chloride, oral liquid or powder.	See potassium citrate, oral effervescent tablets. Also contains 10 mEq of bicarbonate per 5 mL of oral solution.	$
	potassium gluconate, oral liquid generics	*Not urgent:* Plasma K^+ > 3.0–3.5 mmol/L	Initially, 40–60 mmol/day (divided doses), is usually sufficient	See potassium chloride, oral liquid or powder.	See potassium chloride, oral liquid or powder. Useful in patients with acidosis.	$

[a] Cost of 30-day supply of a 20 mmol/day dose; includes drug cost only.
Legend: $ < $10 $-$$ < $10–20 $$ $10–20

Table 4: **Potassium-sparing Diuretics Used in the Management of Hypokalemia**

Class	Drug	Dose	Adverse Effects	Drug Interactions	Cost[a]
Diuretics, potassium-sparing	*spironolactone* [renal] Aldactone, generics	25–200 mg/day (in single or divided doses). Up to 400 mg/day in patients with hyperaldosteronism	Hyperkalemia, gynecomastia, androgen-like side effects, breast tenderness, gastrointestinal symptoms.	Avoid NSAIDs, ACE inhibitors, angiotensin II receptor blockers, potassium supplements: may cause severe hyperkalemia.	$
	amiloride [renal] Midamor, generics	5–20 mg/day	Hyperkalemia, muscle cramps, headaches, gastrointestinal symptoms (rare).	See spironolactone.	$–$$

[a] Cost of 30-day supply; includes drug cost only.
[renal] Dosage adjustment may be required in renal impairment; see Appendix I.
Abbreviations: NSAIDs = nonsteroidal anti-inflammatory agents; ACE = angiotensin converting enzyme
Legend: $ < $20 $-$$ < $20–40 $$ $20–40

Suggested Readings

Allon M. Treatment and prevention of hyperkalemia in end-stage renal disease. *Kidney Int* 1993;43(6):1197-209.

Cohn JN, Kowey PR, Whelton PK et al. New guidelines for potassium replacement in clinical practice: a contemporary review by the National Council on Potassium in Clinical Practice. *Arch Intern Med* 2000;160(16):2429-36.

Gennari FJ. Hypokalemia. *N Engl J Med* 1998;339(7):451-8.

Halperin ML, Kamel KS. Potassium. *Lancet* 1998;352(9122):135-40.

Perazella MA. Drug-induced hyperkalemia: old culprits and new offenders. *Am J Med* 2000;109(4):307-14.

Rastegar A, Soleimani M. Hypokalaemia and hyperkalaemia. *Postgrad Med J* 2001;77(914):759-64.

References

1. Smellie WS. Spurious hyperkalaemia. *BMJ* 2007;334(7595):693-5
2. Blumberg A, Weidmann P, Shaw S et al. Effect of various therapeutic approaches on plasma potassium and major regulating factors in terminal renal failure. *Am J Med* 1988;85(4):507-12.
3. Kim HJ. Combined effect of bicarbonate and insulin with glucose in acute therapy of hyperkalemia in end-stage renal disease patients. *Nephron* 1996;72(3):476-82.
4. Blumberg A, Weidmann P, Ferrari P. Effect of prolonged bicarbonate administration on plasma potassium in terminal renal failure. *Kidney Int* 1992;41(2):369-74.
5. Allon M, Copkney C. Albuterol and insulin for treatment of hyperkalemia in hemodialysis patients. *Kidney Int* 1990;38(5):869-72.
6. Allon M, Dunlay R, Copkney C. Nebulized albuterol for acute hyperkalemia in patients on hemodialysis. *Ann Intern Med* 1989;110(6):426-9.
7. Kamel KS, Wei C. Controversial issues in the treatment of hyperkalaemia. *Nephrol Dial Transplant* 2003;18(11):2215-8.
8. Mahoney BA, Smith WA, Lo DS et al. Emergency interventions for hyperkalaemia. *Cochrane Database Syst Rev* 2005;(2):CD003235.
9. Gruy-Kapral C, Emmett M, Santa Ana CA et al. Effect of single dose resin-cathartic therapy on serum potassium concentration in patients with end-stage renal disease. *J Am Soc Nephrol* 1998;9(10):1924-30.
10. Wootton FT, Rhodes DF, Lee WM et al. Colonic necrosis with Kayexalate-sorbitol enemas after renal transplantation. *Ann Intern Med* 1989;111(11):947-9.
11. Lillemoe KD, Romolo JL, Hamilton SR et al. Intestinal necrosis due to sodium polystyrene (Kayexalate) in sorbitol enemas: clinical and experimental support for the hypothesis. *Surgery* 1987;101(3):267-72.
12. Romolo JL, Williams GM. Effect of kayexalate and sorbitol on colon of normal and uremic rats. *Surg Forum* 1979;30:369-70.
13. Palmer BF. Managing hyperkalemia caused by inhibitors of the renin-angiotensin-aldosterone system. *N Engl J Med* 2004;351(6):585-92.
14. Kunin AS, Surawicz B, Sims EA. Decrease in serum potassium concentrations and appearance of cardiac arrhythmias during infusion of potassium with glucose in potassium-depleted patients. *N Engl J Med* 1962;266:228-33.
15. Hamill RJ, Robinson LM, Wexler HR et al. Efficacy and safety of potassium infusion therapy in hypokalemic critically ill patients. *Crit Care Med* 1991;19(5):694-9.
16. Kruse JA, Carlson RW. Rapid correction of hypokalemia using concentrated intravenous potassium chloride infusions. *Arch Intern Med* 1990;150(3):613-7.
17. Gennari FJ. Hypokalemia. *N Engl J Med* 1998;339(7):451-8.

CHAPTER 93
Acute Otitis Media in Childhood

Joseph V. Vayalumkal, MD, FRCPC

One of the most frequently encountered situations in primary care is the irritable child with a history of two to three days of fever, runny nose and cough. Most children with this clinical presentation have viral infections that do not require antibiotics; however, some will have signs of acute otitis media (AOM) evident on physical examination and may benefit from antibiotic therapy.

AOM can be caused by both viral and bacterial pathogens.[1] It is often preceded by a viral upper respiratory tract infection which may alter respiratory tract defences by disturbing the epithelium and impairing mucociliary clearance. This may subsequently lead to eustachian tube dysfunction.[2,3] The combination of events allows bacterial pathogens colonizing the nasopharynx to invade the middle ear and cause acute infection. A recent investigation of the microbiology of acute otitis media reported that bacteria were isolated in 92% of middle ear effusions while viruses were isolated in 70%. Co-infection was noted in 66% of patients.[4]

A number of prevention strategies for AOM have been assessed. Most strategies involve vaccination against AOM pathogens but risk factor modification has also been studied.[5,6,7,8,9] Exposure to tobacco smoke and exposure to other children (e.g., daycare) are associated with higher risk of AOM in childhood.[6,8,9] Breastfeeding is protective against respiratory tract colonization and is associated with lower rates of acute otitis media in childhood.[7]

Goals of Therapy

- Relieve symptoms (fever, irritability, pain)
- Sterilize the middle ear
- Prevent complications, e.g., mastoiditis, intracranial infection, facial paralysis
- Avoid inappropriate therapy which may lead to the emergence of resistant pathogens and adverse drug effects such as antibiotic-associated diarrhea

Investigations (Figure 1)

- History
  - fever
  - nonspecific symptoms of viral upper respiratory tract infection such as cough and coryza

- otalgia is a common manifestation and may be the best clue to the diagnosis; however, ear pain is not always easily communicated by infants and toddlers (disturbed sleep, irritability, tugging the ear or rubbing the head may suggest otalgia in young children)

- Physical examination
  - focus on the head and neck region to rule out other causes of pain referred to the ear such as mastoiditis or dental abscess
  - proper visual inspection of the tympanic membrane may require the following: child to be restrained by parents, proper lighting, removal of cerumen obscuring proper view of the tympanic membrane
  - assess for signs of middle ear effusion and middle ear inflammation
  - four key features of the tympanic membrane should be evaluated: *colour*, *position*, *translucency* and *mobility*. A red, displaced/bulging, opaque and immobile tympanic membrane indicates acute otitis media

- Referral
  - for treatment failures or recurrences unresponsive to therapy, consider referral to an ENT specialist who can obtain middle ear fluid for culture to identify the pathogen involved and its antibiotic susceptibility profile
  - children who have frequent, recurrent episodes (> 3 episodes in 6 months or > 4 episodes in 12 months) should be referred to an ENT specialist for consideration of myringotomy and tympanostomy tubes
  - children with recurrent episodes of AOM should also have audiology assessment to determine any conductive hearing loss

Therapeutic Choices

Nonpharmacologic Choices

The strategy of watchful waiting has been recommended for clinical situations in which the child is over 2 years of age, illness is mild and uncomplicated and a parent/caregiver can easily access the physician for communication/re-evaluation.[10] Watchful waiting in these circumstances has been accepted and is evident in clinical practice guidelines published in Canada, the United States and some European countries.[10,11,12,13,14]

Pharmacologic Choices

Analgesics

Provide adequate analgesia in the early stages of infection. In most cases, **acetaminophen** 10–15 mg/kg or **ibuprofen** 10 mg/kg every 4–6 hours is sufficient to control the ear pain. If the pain is severe and not responding to usual pain medication, 1–2 doses of **codeine** in the first 24 hours may help but narcotic analgesics have more adverse effects than acetaminophen or ibuprofen.

Antibiotics (Table 1, Table 2)

The primary bacterial pathogens involved in acute otitis media are *Streptococcus pneumoniae*, *Haemophilus influenzae* and *Moraxella catarrhalis*. Clinical observations suggest that spontaneous resolution rates of acute otitis media caused by these three pathogens are 20%, 50% and 75%, respectively.[21] Therefore, a wait and see approach has been proposed for a subset of patients[10] which may lead to reduced number of antibiotic prescriptions.[22,23] Furthermore, with the introduction of pneumococcal conjugate vaccine (Prevnar) the epidemiology of acute otitis media is likely to change, and treatment recommendations may be modified in the future.[24,25,26,27]

Antibiotic resistance is common among these three pathogens; therefore, choosing appropriate therapy depends on understanding the mechanisms of resistance involved. *S. pneumoniae* resistance to penicillin is a result of alteration of penicillin-binding cell wall proteins leading to decreased drug affinity. Doubling the dose of amoxicillin raises the drug concentration in the middle ear to allow effective killing of penicillin-resistant strains. For *H. influenzae* and *M. catarrhalis,* beta-lactamase production confers resistance to amoxicillin and therefore adding a beta-lactamase inhibitor, such as clavulanate, will allow the antibiotic to work effectively.

Standard-dose **amoxicillin** is used in patients without risk factors for antibiotic resistance (recent antibiotic use, daycare attendance, recent episode of acute otitis media, treatment failure or early recurrence). Amoxicillin is most active against *S. pneumoniae*, less effective for penicillin-resistant strains and is not effective against beta-lactamase-producing strains of *H. influenzae* and *M. catarrhalis*.

High-dose **amoxicillin** is used in patients with risk factors for antibiotic resistance; it is effective against most penicillin-resistant strains of *S. pneumoniae*.

Amoxicillin/clavulanate (with high-dose amoxicillin) possesses the added benefit of stability against beta-lactamases, produced by some strains of *H. influenzae* and most strains of *M. catarrhalis*. Amoxicillin/clavulanate is effective against most penicillin-resistant *S. pneumoniae*.

All other treatment options for acute otitis media are less favourable than amoxicillin or amoxicillin/clavulanate. Rates of resistance to other antibiotic classes such as cephalosporins and macrolides are on the rise.[28,29,30] However, in situations of treatment failures and penicillin allergy these antibiotic classes are alternatives.[10,11,12,13,31,32] It is important to differentiate between those patients who have true type I hypersensitivity (anaphylactic) reactions and those who experience a nonspecific adverse effect to the antibiotic. In general, parents and patients overestimate the true frequency of allergic reactions.[33,34] Cephalosporins can be used for patients who have previously experienced a non–type I hypersensitivity reaction to penicillins.

Cefuroxime axetil and **cefprozil** are second-generation cephalosporins with reasonable activity against *H. influenzae* and *M. catarrhalis* because they are less susceptible to the action of beta-lactamases than amoxicillin. However, cephalosporins are less effective than amoxicillin against penicillin-resistant strains of *S. pneumoniae*. They can be used as second-line agents.

Ceftriaxone is the most effective of the cephalosporins against otitis media pathogens but is not used routinely because it is given intravenously or intramuscularly daily for three days.[35]

Reserve **azithromycin** and **clarithromycin** for patients with type I hypersensitivity reactions to beta-lactam antibiotics.

Avoid clindamycin because it does not cover *H. influenzae* or *M. catarrhalis*.

Therapeutic Tips

- Use of vaccines for influenza and *S. pneumoniae* may have a beneficial impact on the incidence of acute otitis media and therefore should be encouraged for eligible patients.[5,15,16,17,18] (See Table 3.)
- Most children will have middle ear effusions after completion of therapy. There is no need to treat an abnormal-appearing tympanic membrane in an asymptomatic child. If middle ear effusion persists over three months, arrange an audiology assessment to assess hearing.
- Nasal and oral decongestants alone or in combination with an antihistamine have not shown efficacy in clinical trials and are not recommended.[1,36]

Figure 1: **Management of Acute Otitis Media**

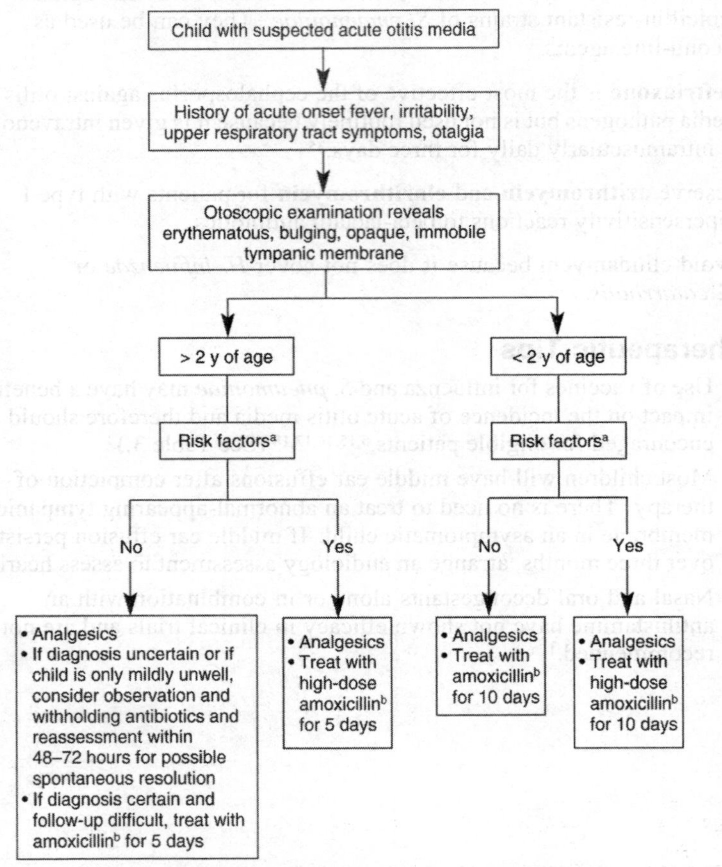

[a] Risk factors: recent antibiotic use, daycare attendance, recent episode of AOM, treatment failure or early recurrence.

[b] If treatment failure or recurrence within one month, consider alternative agents and repeated course of treatment or referral for tympanocentesis.

Table 1: **Antibiotic Treatment Recommendations for AOM[10]**

Characteristics	Therapeutic Tips	First Choice	Treatment Failure Noted on Day 3	Treatment Failure Noted on Day 10–28
Age < 1 mo	Investigate for bacteremia; acute otitis media often due to gram-negative bacteria	Refer to nearest emergency department for further assessment; symptoms such as fever may be related to sepsis in this age group.	n/a	n/a
Age < 2 y No risk factors (no antibiotics in prior 3 months, no daycare attendance)	Treat most cases of acute otitis media with antibiotic for 10 days	Standard-dose amoxicillin: 40–45 mg/kg/day divided TID *or* high-dose amoxicillin[a]: 80–90 mg/kg/day divided BID or TID	High-dose amoxicillin/ clavulanate *or* cefprozil *or* cefuroxime axetil *or* ceftriaxone im for 3 days	High-dose amoxicillin/ clavulanate *or* cefprozil *or* cefuroxime axetil *or* ceftriaxone im for 3 days
Age < 2 y With risk factors (received antibiotics in prior 3 months or daycare attendance)	Treat most cases of acute otitis media with antibiotic for 10 days	High-dose amoxicillin[a]: 80–90 mg/kg/day divided BID or TID	High-dose amoxicillin/ clavulanate or cefprozil 30 mg/kg/day *or* cefuroxime axetil 30 mg/kg/day *or* ceftriaxone im for 3 days Consider tympanocentesis	High-dose amoxicillin/ clavulanate *or* cefprozil 30 mg/kg/day *or* cefuroxime axetil 30 mg/kg/day *or* ceftriaxone im for 3 days Consider tympanocentesis
Age > 2 y No risk factors (no frequent bouts AOM and no antibiotics in prior 3 months)	Consider deferring treatment to see if acute otitis media resolves in 48–72 h only if follow-up can be ensured and if antibacterial therapy can be initiated if symptoms worsen Treat for 5 days[10]	High-dose amoxicillin[a]: 80 mg/kg/day divided BID or TID	High-dose amoxicillin /clavulanate *or* cefprozil 30 mg/kg/day *or* cefuroxime axetil 30 mg/kg/day *or* ceftriaxone im for 3 days	High-dose amoxicillin/ clavulanate *or* cefprozil 30 mg/kg/day *or* cefuroxime axetil 30 mg/kg/day *or* ceftriaxone im for 3 days Consider tympanocentesis

(cont'd)

Table 1: **Antibiotic Treatment Recommendations for AOM**[10] *(cont'd)*

Characteristics	Therapeutic Tips	First Choice	Treatment Failure Noted on Day 3	Treatment Failure Noted on Day 10–28
Age > 2 y With risk factors (received antibiotics in prior 3 months)	Consider deferring treatment to see if acute otitis media resolves in 48–72 h only if follow-up can be ensured and if antibacterial therapy can be initiated if symptoms worsen. Treat for 5 days[10]	High-dose amoxicillin[a]/clavulanate	High-dose amoxicillin /clavulanate *or* cefprozil 30 mg/kg/day *or* cefuroxime axetil 30 mg/kg/day *or* ceftriaxone im for 3 days. Consider tympanocentesis	High-dose amoxicillin/clavulanate *or* cefprozil 30 mg/kg/day *or* cefuroxime axetil 30 mg/kg/day *or* ceftriaxone im for 3 days. Consider tympanocentesis
Any age Frequent bouts of acute otitis media	Verify acute otitis media. Treat acute otitis media episode for ≥ 10 days. Consider Prevnar if age < 5 y. Give influenza vaccine every year, all ages	High-dose amoxicillin[a]/clavulanate	Ceftriaxone im for 3 days. Consider tympanocentesis	High-dose amoxicillin/clavulanate *or* cefprozil *or* cefuroxime axetil *or* ceftriaxone im for 3 days
Allergic to penicillin	Verify true anaphylactic-type allergy: hives; swollen lip, mouth, or throat; wheezing; ↓ BP	Clarithromycin 15 mg/kg/day *or* azithromycin	Tympanocentesis	Clarithromycin 15 mg/kg/day *or* azithromycin. Consider tympanocentesis

[a] High-dose amoxicillin: a) amoxicillin 40 mg/kg/day plus amoxicillin/clavulanate liquid (Clavulin-200 or Clavulin-400) 40 mg/kg/day of the amoxicillin component or b) amoxicillin/clavulanate liquid (Clavulin-200 or Clavulin-400) can be given at a dose of 80 mg/kg/day of the amoxicillin component (may cause diarrhea). May be given TID rather than BID to minimize gastrointestinal side effects.

Abbreviations: BP = blood pressure; n/a = not applicable

Table 2: **Antibiotics for Acute Otitis Media**

Class	Drug	Dose[a]	Adverse Effects	Comments	Cost[b]
Penicillins	*amoxicillin* generics	*Standard dose:* 40 mg/kg/day divided BID-TID. *High dose:* 80–90 mg/kg/day divided BID-TID Reserve standard-dose amoxicillin for the limited number of children at low risk of being infected with drug-resistant bacteria, i.e., no daycare, no antibiotic in the prior three-month period	Excellent safety profile. Occasionally causes mild diarrhea. Maculopapular rash occurs uncommonly but is difficult to distinguish from a concomitant viral exanthem.	Most active agent against pneumococci with ↓ susceptibility to penicillins and cephalosporins. For pneumococci with ↓ susceptibility to penicillins and cephalosporins, amoxicillin is more active than cephalosporins.	$
	amoxicillin/ clavulanate Clavulin, generics	80–90 mg/kg/day amoxicillin divided BID-TID Best given as two simultaneous prescriptions to minimize the risk of diarrhea: One prescription of amoxicillin 40 mg/kg/day *plus* one prescription of new formulation amoxicillin/clavulanate liquid (Clavulin-200 or Clavulin-400) 40 mg/kg/day of the amoxicillin component Alternatively, one of the new formulations of amoxicillin/clavulanate liquid (Clavulin-200 or Clavulin-400) can be given at a dose of 80 mg/kg/day of the amoxicillin component, but may cause diarrhea. Some patients will tolerate these high-dose regimens better if doses are given three times daily rather than twice daily	Excellent safety profile. Diarrhea occurs frequently.	Do not use the original formulations of amoxicillin/clavulanate (Clavulin-125F and Clavulin-250F) in the high-dose protocol because they have so much clavulanate in them that they are almost certain to cause diarrhea. To avoid confusion when prescribing high-dose regimens, confirm intention on the prescription (e.g., write "**high dose amoxicillin intended**" at the bottom). Active against most bacteria likely to cause acute otitis media.	$$

(cont'd)

Table 2: **Antibiotics for Acute Otitis Media** *(cont'd)*

Class	Drug	Dose[a]	Adverse Effects	Comments	Cost[b]
Cephalosporins	*cefprozil* Cefzil	30 mg/kg/day divided BID	Low incidence of diarrhea or GI upset.	Most children like the taste of the liquid formulation and it is well absorbed.	$$$$
	ceftriaxone Rocephin	50 mg/kg (max 1 g) im Q24H for 3 days	Pain at injection site can be minimized with use of 1% plain lidocaine as diluent.	Second- or third-line agent.	$$$$$
	cefuroxime axetil Ceftin, generics	30 mg/kg/day divided BID	See cefprozil.	Available as suspension.	$$$$$
Macrolides	*azithromycin* Zithromax, generics	Day 1: 10 mg/kg Days 2–5: 5 mg/kg Administer once daily at bedtime	Low incidence of diarrhea or GI upset.	Most children like the taste of the suspension. Pneumococci with ↓ susceptibility to penicillins and cephalosporins are sometimes resistant to azithromycin. Short course may improve compliance. Use if true anaphylactic-type β-lactam allergy.	$$$$$
	clarithromycin Biaxin	15 mg/kg/day divided BID Because it sometimes has a bitter aftertaste, the suspension should be taken with food and/or juice	Diarrhea or vomiting (15%).	Pneumococci with ↓ susceptibility to penicillins and cephalosporins are sometimes resistant to clarithromycin. Use if true anaphylactic-type β-lactam allergy.	$$$

[a] Duration of treatment is 5 days for children over 2 years and 10 days if under 2 years; exceptions are ceftriaxone and azithromycin.
[b] Cost of 10-day supply based on 20 kg body weight, except 5-day supply for azithromycin, 3-day supply for ceftriaxone; includes drug cost only.
Dosage adjustment may be required in renal impairment; see Appendix I.
Legend: $ < $10 $$ $10–20 $$$ $20–30 $$$$ $30–40 $$$$$ > $40

Table 3: **Vaccines for Prevention of Acute Otitis Media**

Class	Drug	Dose[19]	Comments	Cost[a]
Vaccines, viral	*influenza vaccine, inactivated* Fluviral S/F, Fluzone, Influvac, Vaxigrip	Children 6 mo–8 y who have not previously received influenza vaccine should receive a second dose ≥ 1 mo after the first dose. *6–35 mo:* 0.25 mL im *36 mo–8 y:* 0.5 mL im *≥ 9 y:* 0.5 mL im	Pretreatment with acetaminophen may help minimize soreness and mild flu-like symptoms. Contraindicated in persons with history of anaphylactic reaction to a previous dose or eggs.	$
Vaccines, bacterial	*pneumococcal vaccine, 7-valent conjugate* Prevnar	2–6 mo: 4 doses im: 2, 4, 6 and 12–15 mo 7–11 mo: 2 doses im given 4 wk apart *plus* a booster after 12 mo 12–23 mo: 2 doses im given 2 mo apart 24–59 mo: 1 dose im	Pretreatment with acetaminophen may help minimize soreness at injection site.	$$$

[a] Cost of 1 dose; includes drug cost only.
$ < $10 $$ $10–80 $$$ $80–90

Suggested Readings

American Academy of Pediatrics Subcommittee on Management of Acute Otitis Media. Diagnosis and management of acute otitis media. *Pediatrics* 2004;113(5):1451-65.

Neff MJ; American Academy of Pediatrics; American Academy of Family Physicians. AAP, AAFP release guideline on diagnosis and management of acute otitis media. *Am Fam Physician* 2004;69(11):2713-5.

Rovers MM, Glasziou P, Appelman CL et al. Antibiotics for acute otitis media: a meta-analysis with individual patient data. *Lancet* 2006;368(9545):1429-35.

Rovers MM, Glasziou P, Appelman CL et al. Predictors of pain and/or fever at 3 to 7 days for children with acute otitis media not treated initially with antibiotics: a meta-analysis of individual patient data. *Pediatrics* 2007;199(3):579-85.

References

1. Chonmaitree T. Acute otitis media is not a pure bacterial disease. *Clin Infect Dis* 2006;43(11):1423-5.
2. Faden H, Stanievich J, Brodsky L et al. Changes in nasopharyngeal flora during otitis media of childhood. *Pediatr Infect Dis J* 1990;9(9):623-6.
3. Sanyal MA, Henderson FW, Stempel EC et al. Effect of upper respiratory tract infection on eustachian tube ventilatory function in the preschool child. *J Pediatr* 1980;97(1):11-5.
4. Ruohola A, Meurman O, Nikkari S et al. Microbiology of acute otitis media in children with tympanostomy tubes: prevalences of bacteria and viruses. *Clin Infect Dis* 2006;43(11):1417-22.
5. Klein JO, Chonmaitree T, Loosmore S et al. Otitis media: a preventable disease? Proceedings of an international symposium organized by the Marcel Merieux Foundation, Veyrier-du-Lac, France, February 13 to 16, 2000. *Pediatr Infect Dis J* 2001;20(5):473-81.
6. Adair-Bischoff CE, Sauve RS. Environmental tobacco smoke and middle ear disease in preschool-age children. *Arch Pediatr Adolesc Med* 1998;152(2):127-33.
7. Duffy LC, Faden H, Wasielewski R et al. Exclusive breastfeeding protects against bacterial colonization and day care exposure to otitis media. *Pediatrics* 1997;100(4):E7.
8. Paradise JL, Rockette HE, Colborn DK et al. Otitis media in 2253 Pittsburgh-area infants: prevalence and risk factors during the first two years of life. *Pediatrics* 1997;99(3):318-33.
9. Greenberg D, Givon-Lavi N, Broides A et al. The contribution of smoking and exposure to tobacco smoke to Streptococcus pneumoniae and Haemophilus influenzae carriage in children and their mothers. *Clin Infect Dis* 2006;42(7):897-903.
10. American Academy of Pediatrics Subcommittee on Management of Acute Otitis Media. Diagnosis and management of acute otitis media. *Pediatrics* 2004;113(5):1451-65.
11. Alberta Medical Association. *Guideline for the diagnosis and treatment of acute otitis media in children.* Edmonton (AB): Toward Optimized Practice, Alberta Medical Association; 2007. Available from: http://www.topalbertadoctors.org/NR/rdonlyres/F78DD01F-1577-4AE3-BA3A-B3603B6915F6/0/AOM_guideline.pdf Accessed May 3, 2007.
12. Ontario Guidelines Advisory Committee. *Otitis media: antibiotic therapy.* Toronto (ON): Ontario Guidelines Advisory Committee; 2004. Available from: http://www.gacguidelines.ca/index.cfm?ACT=topics&Summary_ID=50&Topic_ID=32 Accessed May 3, 2007.
13. British Columbia Medial Association, Guidelines and Protocols Advisory Committee. *Acute otitis media (AOM).* Victoria (BC): British Columbia Medical Association; 2004. Available from: http://www.health.gov.bc.ca/gpac/pdf/otitaom.pdf Accessed May 3, 2007.
14. Hoberman A, Marchant CD, Kaplan SL et al. Treatment of acute otitis media consensus recommendations. *Clin Pediatr (Phila)* 2002;41(6):373-90.
15. Eskola J, Kilpi T, Palmu A et al. Efficacy of a pneumococcal conjugate vaccine against acute otitis media. *N Engl J Med* 2001;344(6):403-9.
16. Jenson HB, Baltimore RS. Impact of pneumococcal and influenza vaccines on otitis media. *Curr Opin Pediatr* 2004;16(1):58-60.
17. Ozgur SK, Beyazova U, Kemaloglu YK et al. Effectiveness of inactivated influenza vaccine for prevention of otitis media in children. *Pediatr Infect Dis J* 2006;25(5):401-4.
18. Clements DA, Langdon L, Bland C et al. Influenza A vaccine decreases the incidence of otitis media in 6- to 30-month-old children in day care. *Arch Pediatr Adolesc Med* 1995;149(10):1113-7.
19. National Advisory Committee on Immunization. Canadian Immunization Guide. 7th ed. Ottawa, Ontario: Public Health Agency of Canada 2006.

20. Hoberman A, Paradise JL, Reynolds EA et al. Efficacy of Auralgan for treating ear pain in children with acute otitis media. *Arch Pediatr Adolesc Med* 1997;151(7):675-8.
21. Klein JO. Microbiologic efficacy of antibacterial drugs for acute otitis media. *Pediatr Infect Dis J* 1993;12(12):973-5.
22. Rovers MM, Glasziou P, Appelman CL et al. Antibiotics for acute otitis media: a meta-analysis with individual patient data. *Lancet* 2006;368(9545):1429-35.
23. Spiro DM, Tay KY, Arnold DH et al. Wait-and-see prescription for the treatment of acute otitis media: a randomized controlled trial. *JAMA* 2006;296(10):1235-41.
24. Casey JR, Pichichero ME. Changes in frequency and pathogens causing acute otitis media in 1995-2003. *Pediatr Infect Dis J* 2004;23(9):824-8.
25. Garbutt J, St Geme JW, May A et al. Developing community-specific recommendations for first-line treatment of acute otitis media: is high-dose amoxicillin necessary? *Pediatrics* 2004;114(2):342-7.
26. Garbutt J, Rosenbloom I, Wu J et al. Empiric first-line antibiotic treatment of acute otitis in the era of the heptavalent pneumococcal conjugate vaccine. *Pediatrics* 2006;117(6):e1087-94.
27. Leibovitz E, Jacobs MR, Dagan R. Haemophilus influenzae: a significant pathogen in acute otitis media. *Pediatr Infect Dis J* 2004;23(12):1142-52.
28. Doern GV, Pfaller MA, Kugler K et al. Prevalence of antimicrobial resistance among respiratory tract isolates of Streptococcus pneumoniae in North America: 1997 results from the SENTRY antimicrobial surveillance program. *Clin Infect Dis* 1998; 27(4):764-70.
29. Jacobs MR, Bajaksouzian S, Zilles A et al. Susceptibilities of Streptococcus pneumoniae and Haemophilus influenzae to 10 oral antimicrobial agents based on pharmacodynamic parameters: 1997 U.S. Surveillance study. *Antimicrob Agents Chemother* 1999;43(8):1901-8.
30. Jacobs MR. Increasing antibiotic resistance among otitis media pathogens and their susceptibility to oral agents based on pharmacodynamic parameters. *Pediatr Infect Dis* J 2000;19(5 Suppl):S47-55.
31. Brook I. Use of oral cephalosporins in the treatment of acute otitis media in children. *Int J Antimicrob Agents* 2004;24(1):18-23.
32. Dunne MW, Latiolais T, Lewis B et al. Randomized, double-blind study of the clinical efficacy of 3 days of azithromycin compared with co-amoxiclav for the treatment of acute otitis media. *J Antimicrob Chemother* 2003;52(3):469-72.
33. Langley JM, Halperin SA, Bortolussi R. History of penicillin allergy and referral for skin testing: evaluation of a pediatric penicillin allergy testing program. *Clin Invest Med* 2002;25(5):181-4.
34. Langley JM, Halperin S. Allergy to antibiotics in children: perception versus reality. *Paediatr Child Health* 2002;7(4): 233-7. Available from: http://www.pulsus.com/Paeds/07_04/Pdf/lang_ed.pdf Accessed May 3, 2007.
35. Leibovitz E, Piglansky L, Raiz S et al. Bacteriologic and clinical efficacy of one day vs. three day intramuscular ceftriaxone for treatment of nonresponsive acute otitis media in children. *Pediatr Infect Dis J* 2000;19(11):1040-5.
36. Flynn CA, Griffin GH, Schultz JK. Decongestants and antihistamines for acute otitis media in children. *Cochrane Database Syst Rev* 2004;(3):CD001727.

CHAPTER 94
Streptococcal Sore Throat

David P. Speert, MD

Goals of Therapy

- Provide symptomatic relief
- Prevent suppurative complications, e.g., mastoiditis, cervical lymphadenitis
- Prevent nonsuppurative complications, e.g., acute rheumatic fever
- Prevent spread of group A streptococci to contacts

Investigations

The probability of culturing group A streptococci is greatest in a child with an acute sore throat who is > 3 years old, lacks signs of a viral upper respiratory infection and has signs and symptoms as listed below.[1] However, the diagnosis of streptococcal pharyngitis (strep throat) should be considered seriously in any child presenting with an acute sore throat, with or without "classic" signs and symptoms.

- Clinical diagnosis of streptococcal infection: adenitis and positive throat cultures are the only predictive features[1]
- Although not diagnostic, signs and symptoms include:
  - signs: tender cervical adenopathy, erythematous pharynx and tonsils, pharyngeal exudate, excoriated nares, scarlatiniform rash
  - symptoms: sore throat (in general of sudden onset), pain on swallowing, headache, abdominal pain, nausea, vomiting, fever (see Chapter 116)
- Laboratory diagnosis:
  - throat culture is "gold standard" (results available in 24 to 48 hours). Viral throat culture rarely influences therapy (results available in days to weeks). A partial list of etiologic agents for acute sore throat is presented in Table 1
  - repeat cultures are not necessary at the end of therapy or from asymptomatic family contacts
  - antigen screen of throat secretions (rapid test): results available in 7 to 70 minutes but sensitivity (< 90%) too low to rule out streptococcal infection in children or adolescents[2]. If the rapid antigen detection test is unavailable or is negative, obtain a culture and withhold antibiotics for 24 to 48 hours until the results are available. If positive, recall and treat patients for group A streptococci. This approach does not increase the risk of acute rheumatic fever[3] but avoids the unnecessary use of antibiotics
  - streptococcal serology (antistreptolysin O or ASO, others): useful retrospectively in patients who have possible complications of

streptococcal infection (e.g., rheumatic fever)[4] but are not useful in the diagnosis of acute streptococcal pharyngitis

Table 1: **Selected Pathogens of Acute Pharyngitis**

Viruses (adenoviruses, enteroviruses, cytomegalovirus, Epstein-Barr, influenza, herpes simplex virus, and parainfluenza viruses)
Group A β-hemolytic streptococci (children: 15–30%; adults: 5–10%)[2]
Groups C and G β-hemolytic streptococci
Neisseria gonorrhoeae (consider sexual abuse if recovered from child's throat)
Mycoplasma pneumoniae[a]
Chlamydia trachomatis[a]
Chlamydophila pneumoniae[a,b]
Corynebacterium diphtheriae
Arcanobacterium hemolyticum[a]

[a] Role in acute pharyngitis is controversial.
[b] Previously *Chlamydia pneumoniae*.

Therapeutic Choices (Figure 1)

Nonpharmacologic Choices

- Strict hand-washing to prevent spread of infection.
- Exclude from school or daycare for 24 hours after antimicrobial therapy is begun.

Pharmacologic Choices (Table 2)

Analgesics

Acetaminophen or **ibuprofen** may be given for fever and pain. Lozenges and gargles may be indicated for symptomatic treatment of sore throat.

Antibiotics

Antibiotic therapy for group A streptococcal pharyngitis can shorten the course of the acute illness and prevent both suppurative and nonsuppurative complications if started early in the course of illness.[4]

Penicillin is the drug of choice.[2] Although **cephalosporins** are effective, they should *not* replace penicillin as the drug of choice.[5] **Amoxicillin** is often used in children requiring liquid medication due to the poor palatability of penicillin V suspension.[5] **Erythromycin** is the preferred alternative in patients allergic to penicillin.

Therapeutic Tips

- Early institution of antibiotic therapy shortens the duration of fever, cervical adenitis and pharyngeal infection and hastens the overall clinical improvement.[6] Early treatment can hasten the return of children to school or daycare and minimize work time lost by their parents.
- Since there is no efficient way to differentiate between the acutely infected child and the carrier of group A streptococci,[1] all symptomatic

patients with positive cultures should receive antistreptococcal therapy. A large percentage of cases of acute rheumatic fever develop after mild or subclinical streptococcal infections.[7]

- It is impossible to reliably differentiate between acute streptococcal infection and chronic carriage; a means of eradicating chronic carriage is therefore desirable. Unfortunately, penicillin, the drug of choice for treating acute streptococcal sore throat, often fails to eradicate *pharyngeal streptococcal carriage*. Some advocate the use of **clindamycin** (20 mg/kg/day divided TID for 10 days; maximum 600 mg/day) or the addition of **rifampin** (20 mg/kg/day divided BID; maximum 600 mg/day) for the final four days of penicillin therapy to attempt to interrupt chronic pharyngeal carriage of group A streptococci.[8]

Figure 1: **Management of Acute Sore Throat**

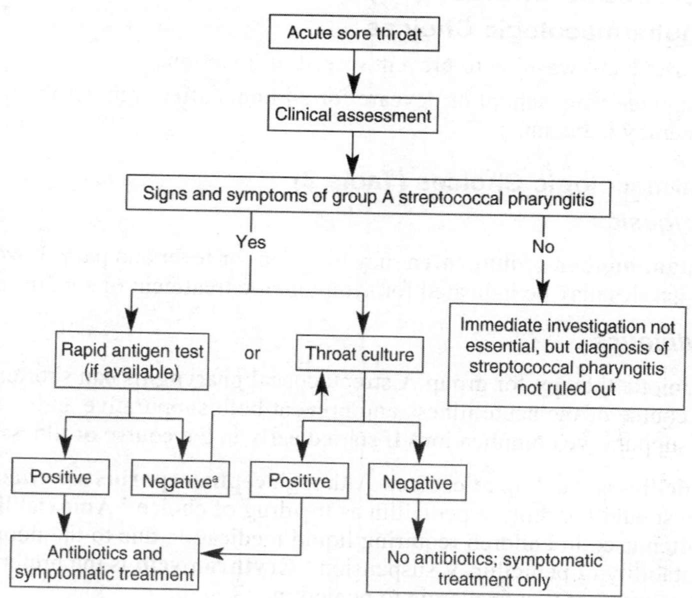

[a] Antibiotic therapy may be safely withheld from an adult based on a negative rapid antigen test.

Table 2: **Drugs for Treatment of Group A Streptococcal Pharyngitis**

Class	Drug	Dose[9]	Adverse Effects	Comments	Cost[a]
Cephalosporins	*cefadroxil* Duricef, generics	Adults: 1 g po daily as a single dose or divided BID × 10 days	Hypersensitivity (some cross-reactivity with penicillins).	**Use if treatment failure with penicillin.**	$$$
	cefixime Suprax	Adults and children > 12 y: 400 mg po daily × 10 days Children 6 mo–12 y: 8 mg/kg po daily × 10 days	See cefadroxil.	**Use if treatment failure with penicillin.** Available as suspension.	$$$$
	cefprozil Cefzil	Adults and children ≥ 13 y: 500 mg po daily × 10 days Children 6 mo–12 y: 15 mg/kg po daily divided Q12H × 10 days; max 1 g/day	See cefadroxil.	**Use if treatment failure with penicillin.** Available as suspension.	$$$$
	cefuroxime axetil Ceftin, generics	Adults and children ≥ 12 y: 250 mg po BID × 10 days Children 3 mo–12 y: 20 mg/kg daily po divided BID × 10 days; max 500 mg/day	See cefadroxil.	**Use if treatment failure with penicillin.** Available as a suspension. Prior to administration, may add dose to milk, fruit juice or lemonade.	$$
	cephalexin generics	Adults: 250 mg po QID × 10 days Children: 25–50 mg/kg po daily divided QID × 10 days; max 1 g/day	See cefadroxil.	**Use if treatment failure with penicillin.** Available as suspension.	$

(cont'd)

Table 2: **Drugs for Treatment of Group A Streptococcal Pharyngitis** *(cont'd)*

Class	Drug	Dose[9]	Adverse Effects	Comments	Cost[a]
Ketolides	*telithromycin* Ketek	Adults: 800 mg po daily × 5 days	Diarrhea, nausea, vomiting, elevated liver enzymes, hepatotoxicity.[10]	**Consider in treatment failures with β-lactam antibiotics.** ↑ telithromycin levels: atorvastatin, lovastatin, simvastatin, itraconazole, ketoconazole. ↑ digoxin levels: monitor digoxin levels and side effects upon initiation and discontinuation of telithromycin. Coadministration with ergot alkaloids, pimozide and disopyramide is contraindicated. Reports of exacerbation of myasthenia gravis with telithromycin.[11]	$$$$
Lincosamides	*clindamycin* Dalacin C, Dalacin C Flavored Granules, generics	Adults:[2] 600 mg po daily divided BID-QID × 10 days Children:[2] 20–30 mg/kg po daily divided TID × 10 days	*C. difficile* colitis, diarrhea (common).	An alternative for patients with erythromycin-resistant strain of group A Streptococcus and who cannot tolerate β-lactam antibiotics. May be used for treatment in symptomatic patients with multiple, recurrent episodes of pharyngitis.[2] Available as suspension.	$$$$

Class	Drug	Dose[9]	Adverse Effects	Comments	Cost[a]
Macrolides	*azithromycin* Z-Pak, Zithromax, generics	Adults: 500 mg po × 1 day, then 250 mg po daily × 4 days Children: 12 mg/kg po daily × 5 days; max 500 mg/day	Lower frequency of GI effects than erythromycin.	A 5-day course is effective. Available as suspension. Less likely than other macrolides to interact with other drugs.	$$
	clarithromycin Biaxin	Adult: 250 mg po BID × 10 days Children: 15 mg/kg po daily divided BID × 10 days	Lower frequency of GI effects than erythromycin.	Available as suspension. ↑ levels of atorvastatin, carbamazepine, digoxin, lovastatin, prednisone, simvastatin, theophylline.	$$
	erythromycin PCE, Erybid, generics	Adults: 1 g po daily divided BID-QID × 10 days Administer 1 hour before meals to prevent acid inactivation	Nausea, vomiting, epigastric distress, diarrhea, elevated liver enzymes, cholestatic jaundice.	**An alternative for penicillin-allergic patients.** ↑ levels of atorvastatin, carbamazepine, digoxin, lovastatin, prednisone, simvastatin, theophylline.	$$
	erythromycin estolate generics	Adults: 1 g po daily divided BID-QID × 10 days Children: 20–40 mg/kg po daily divided BID-TID × 10 days; max 1 g/day	See erythromycin.	Contraindicated in pregnancy. Incidence of cholestatic hepatitis greater in pregnancy. **An alternative for penicillin-allergic patients** Available as suspension. ↑ levels of atorvastatin, carbamazepine, digoxin, lovastatin, prednisone, simvastatin, theophylline.	$$

(cont'd)

Table 2: **Drugs for Treatment of Group A Streptococcal Pharyngitis** *(cont'd)*

Class	Drug	Dose[9]	Adverse Effects	Comments	Cost[a]
	erythromycin ethylsuccinate EES, generics	Adults: 1 g po daily divided BID-QID × 10 days Children: 40–50 mg/kg po daily divided BID-QID × 10 days; max 1 g/day	See erythromycin.	**An alternative for penicillin-allergic patients.** Available as suspension. ↑ levels of atorvastatin, carbamazepine, digoxin, lovastatin, prednisone, simvastatin, theophylline.	$$
Penicillins	*amoxicillin* generics	40 mg/kg po daily divided BID-TID × 10 days	Usually well tolerated. Rash, anaphylaxis (rare).	Available as chewable tablets and suspension.	$$ [b]
	penicillin V potassium generics	Adults: 300 mg po TID or 600 mg po BID × 10 days Children: 25–50 mg/kg po daily divided BID	Anaphylaxis, gastrointestinal upset, diarrhea.	**Drug of choice.** Oral route for penicillin preferred.	$
	pivampicillin Pondocillin	25–60 mg/kg po daily divided BID × 10 days	Rash, anaphylaxis (rare).	Available as suspension.	$$$$ [b]
Penicillinase-resistant Penicillins	*amoxicillin/clavulanate* Clavulin, generics	Adults:[2] 500 mg po BID × 10 days Children:[2] 40 mg/kg po daily divided TID × 10 days; max dose of amoxicillin: 750 mg/day	Diarrhea, gastrointestinal upset, anaphylaxis (rare).	May be used for treatment in symptomatic patients with multiple, recurrent episodes of pharyngitis.[2] Available as suspension.	$$

[a] Cost of 10-day supply of tablets for adult dosage (except 5 days for azithromycin and telithromycin); includes drug cost only.
[b] Cost based on 70 kg body weight.
Dosage adjustment may be required in renal impairment; see Appendix I.
Legend: $ < $5 $$ $5–15 $$$ $15–25 $$$$ $25–35

Suggested Readings

Bisno AL, Gerber MA, Gwaltney JM et al. Practice guidelines for the diagnosis and management of group A streptococcal pharyngitis. Infectious Diseases Society of America. *Clin Infect Dis* 2002;35(2):113-25.

Dajani A, Taubert K, Ferrieri P et al. Treatment of acute streptococcal pharyngitis and prevention of rheumatic fever: a statement for health professionals. Committee on Rheumatic Fever, Endocarditis, and Kawasaki Disease of the Council on Cardiovascular Disease in the Young, the American Heart Association. *Pediatrics* 1995;96(4 Pt 1):758-64.

Gerber MA. Diagnosis and treatment of pharyngitis in children. *Pediatr Clin North Am* 2005;52(3):729-47,vi.

Linder JA, Bates DW, Lee GM et al. Antibiotic treatment of children with sore throat. *JAMA* 2005;294(18):2315-22.

Martin JM, Green M. Group A streptococcus. *Semin Pediatr Infect Dis* 2006;17(3):140-8.

References

1. Wannamaker LW. Perplexity and precision in the diagnosis of streptococcal pharyngitis. *Am J Dis Child* 1972;124(3):352-8.
2. Bisno AL, Gerber MA, Gwaltney JM et al. Practice guidelines for the diagnosis and management of group A streptococcal pharyngitis. Infectious Diseases Society of America. *Clin Infect Dis* 2002;35(2):113-25.
3. Catanzaro FJ, Stetson CA, Morris AJ et al. The role of the streptococcus in the pathogenesis of rheumatic fever. *Am J Med* 1954;17(6):749-56.
4. Bisno AL. Group A streptococcal infections and acute rheumatic fever. *N Engl J Med* 1991;325(11):783-93.
5. Gerber MA. Diagnosis and treatment of pharyngitis in children. *Pediatr Clin North Am* 2005;52(3):729-47, vi.
6. Randolph MF, Gerber MA, DeMeo KK et al. Effect of antibiotic therapy on the clinical course of streptococcal pharyngitis. *J Pediatr* 1985;106(6):870-5.
7. Carapetis JR, McDonald M, Wilson NJ. Acute rheumatic fever. *Lancet* 2005;366(9480):155-68.
8. Tanz RR, Poncher JR, Corydon KE et al. Clindamycin treatment of chronic pharyngeal carriage of group A streptococci. *J Pediatr* 1991;119(1 Pt 1):123-8.
9. Rosser W, Pennie R, Pilla N; Anti-infective Review Panel. *Anti-infective guidelines for community-acquired infections*. Toronto (ON): MUMS Guideline Clearinghouse; 2005.
10. Clay KD, Hanson JS, Pope SD et al. Brief communication: severe hepatotoxicity of telithromycin: three case reports and literature review. *Ann Intern Med* 2006;144(6):415-20.
11. Perrot X, Bernard N, Vial C et al. Myasthenia gravis exacerbation or unmasking associated with telithromycin treatment. *Neurology* 2006;67(12):2256-8.

CHAPTER 95
Sinusitis

Susan R. Fryters, BScPharm, ACPR and
Edith M. Blondel-Hill, MD, FRCPC

Sinusitis is defined as inflammation and/or mucosal thickening of one or more of the paranasal sinus cavities, the cause of which may be allergic, viral, bacterial or (rarely) fungal.[1] *Acute sinusitis* refers to sinusitis lasting four weeks or less, while recurrent sinusitis is defined as four or more episodes of acute sinusitis per year, each lasting 10 days or more, with an absence of symptoms between episodes.[2,10,31] *Chronic sinusitis* refers to infections lasting 12 weeks or more with or without treatment.[1,10,31,30] Acute sinusitis can also be superimposed on chronic sinusitis.[2] Rhinitis and rhinosinusitis, most commonly associated with a viral or allergic etiology, are often misdiagnosed and treated as bacterial sinusitis.

Many similarities exist between sinusitis and otitis media, including histology, pathogenesis, etiologic agents and risk factors. In children, the two diseases frequently coexist.[2]

The paranasal sinuses are normally sterile. Acute sinusitis is most often secondary to viral respiratory infections. Viral upper respiratory tract infections (URTIs) are complicated by bacterial sinusitis in only 0.2 to 2% of cases.[3,4,5,6,7]

This chapter addresses bacterial sinusitis in children and adults. Bacteria commonly implicated in bacterial sinusitis in children and adults are listed in Table 2 and Table 3, respectively. The most common bacterial pathogens in acute sinusitis are *Streptococcus pneumoniae* and unencapsulated strains of *Haemophilus influenzae*. *Moraxella catarrhalis* is more common in children.[1] Up to 10% of cases of acute sinusitis in adults may be due to mixtures of anaerobic bacteria; these are often associated with concurrent dental disease. The etiology of chronic sinusitis is less clear, although anaerobes and *Staphylococcus aureus* are more common than in acute sinusitis.[8]

Goals of Therapy

- Optimize the symptomatic management of sinusitis, especially drainage of congested sinuses
- Eradicate infection
- Prevent recurrences and complications
- Reduce antibiotic use in ill-defined URTI to avoid the development of antibiotic resistance

Investigations

The diagnosis of acute bacterial sinusitis relies on history and physical examination. Differentiation of bacterial sinusitis from viral URTI is determined by the duration and severity of the symptoms described below.[6]

Symptoms

- Adults: Persistent symptoms of URTI without improvement after 10 to 14 days, or worsening after 5 days, with both nasal congestion/purulent nasal discharge and facial pain, with or without fever, maxillary toothache or facial swelling. Nonspecific concurrent symptoms include headache, halitosis, hyposmia/anosmia, ear pain/pressure, fatigue and cough.[1,2,9,10]
- Children: Symptoms of acute bacterial sinusitis are similar in children but often also include irritability, lethargy, prolonged cough and vomiting that occurs in association with gagging on mucus.[1,2,10]
- Chronic: Patients with chronic sinusitis typically complain of purulent nasal discharge, postnasal drip and nasal obstruction accompanied by facial pain. Symptoms can mimic the pain of atypical and typical migraine, dental disease and tension headaches.[11]

Physical Examination

- Physical findings of swelling and/or erythema over the symptomatic area, tenderness on palpation/percussion of paranasal sinuses, periorbital swelling, erythema/swelling of nasal mucosa, postnasal drip.
- In addition:
  - assess patient for changes in extraocular movements and visual acuity to look for orbital complications
  - look for associated dental infection by checking the maxillary teeth for tenderness

Objective measurements

- Transillumination of the sinuses has limited value in adults and no diagnostic value in children as findings are not specific for bacterial infection, and in children, the sinuses are not yet fully formed.
- Nasal/nasopharyngeal cultures are *not* recommended due to poor correlation with sinus pathogens.
- Plain sinus x-rays and CT scans are not routinely recommended in the diagnosis of sinusitis, as they will not distinguish between sinus abnormalities associated with viral URTI and bacterial sinusitis.
- MRI is not routinely recommended due to poor bone definition.
- CT scans may be useful for:
  - complications of acute sinusitis (e.g., periorbital edema, subperiosteal abscess)[2]
  - chronic sinusitis unresponsive to treatment[10]

- chronic progressive nasal obstruction without identified cause[2]
- severe presentations where diagnosis is suspected but not clear[2,10]
- patients in whom surgery is being considered[2,12]

Consider underlying risk factors, especially in recurrent and/or chronic sinusitis:

- gastroesophageal reflux disease
- allergic rhinitis
- structural abnormalities
- cystic fibrosis (chronic sinusitis, children with nasal polyps)
- immunodeficiency (chronic, recurrent sinusitis)
- eosinophilic nonallergic rhinitis[2]

Therapeutic Choices

Prevention of Sinusitis[2,10]

- Limit the spread of viral infections. Handwashing is the most effective way to prevent the spread of infection.
- Avoid environmental tobacco exposure.
- Reduce environmental allergen exposure.

Nonpharmacologic Choices

- Local treatment with steam inhalation, cool mist humidifiers and/or saline irrigation/sprays may be of benefit in both acute and chronic sinusitis to liquefy and soften crusting of nasal secretions to facilitate their removal, and to moisturize dry, inflamed nasal mucosa.[13,14]
- Although there are no scientific data on efficacy, the following comfort measures may be helpful in relieving symptoms in some patients:[2]
  - adequate rest and hydration
  - warm facial packs/compresses
  - sleeping with the head of the bed elevated
  - adding pine oil or menthol preparations to steam treatments.
- Surgical drainage for chronic sinusitis may be necessary, especially when it is unresponsive to medical therapy.[15]

Pharmacologic Choices

Principles of Therapy in Sinusitis

Preferred initial strategy for managing symptoms in sinusitis is the use of analgesics/antipyretics and decongestants when needed. Approximately 70% of cases of acute sinusitis will resolve without antibiotic treatment.[16,17,18,19,20,21,22,23] However, if symptoms continue for longer than 10 days, consider antibiotic therapy.

Symptomatic Management

Analgesics/antipyretics, such as **acetaminophen** or **ibuprofen**, can be used for control of pain and/or fever.

Nasal and oral **decongestants** may be beneficial in both acute and chronic infections.[13] Oral decongestants should be used with caution in patients with uncontrolled hypertension, cardiovascular disease, hyperthyroidism, diabetes, angle-closure glaucoma, urinary retention or in conjunction with monoamine oxidase inhibitors. Topical decongestant sprays should be used with caution as extended use (> 3 to 5 days) may result in rhinitis medicamentosa (rebound congestion/hyperemia), which may be refractory to subsequent decongestant therapy.[2]

The efficacy and safety of nasal/oral decongestants has not been well studied in pediatric patients; therefore, these agents are not recommended in children less than 12 years old.[12,24] Overdosage of cough and cold preparations, specifically **pseudoephedrine**, has been associated with deaths in several infants.[25] As a result, the FDA has issued a warning that caregivers should not give cough and cold medications to children < 2 years old without first consulting their health care provider. Clinicians should carefully weigh the risks and benefits of these medications before prescribing and should ask whether other cough and cold preparations are being used so as to avoid overdose from multiple medications that contain the same ingredients, including analgesic medications.

Avoid antihistamines in acute sinusitis because of their tendency to cause excessive dryness with thickening of secretions and crusting.[26] The **second-generation antihistamines** may, however, have a role in chronic sinusitis where a clear allergic component is demonstrated.[13]

The use of nasal **corticosteroid** sprays in acute sinusitis is controversial.[27] They may offer some benefit in patients with recurrent and/or allergic rhinosinusitis.[1] Nasal corticosteroids may also be beneficial in chronic sinusitis due to their ability to decrease nasal edema and inflammation and thus promote drainage.[2]

There is no evidence that **mucolytics**, such as guaifenesin, are useful adjuncts in acute sinusitis.[2]

Antibiotic Therapy (Table 2, Table 3, Table 4, Table 5)

Multiple clinical trials and two meta-analyses have shown that ~70% of cases of acute sinusitis will resolve without antibiotic treatment.[16,17,18,19,20,21,22,23] Antibiotic therapy should be reserved for those patients with bacterial sinusitis as defined by history and physical examination. There are no clinically significant differences in outcomes between first-line and second-line broader spectrum antibiotics.[21,22,23,28,29,30]

Amoxicillin remains the antibiotic of choice for acute bacterial sinusitis for the following reasons:[1,2,10,15,31]

- Adequate coverage for organisms involved in acute sinusitis
- Best activity of all oral beta-lactam agents against *S. pneumoniae*, including strains with intermediate susceptibility to penicillin when high-dose amoxicillin is used
- No other antibiotic has been proven superior to amoxicillin in clinical trials
- Lower potential to induce resistance
- Relatively few adverse effects
- Relatively inexpensive

Failure of First-line Therapy

Amoxicillin-clavulanate offers the most appropriate spectrum of activity and is the agent of choice when first-line antibiotic therapy fails.[10,23,31]

Antibiotic therapy (especially with macrolides or fluoroquinolones) within the previous three months may be a risk factor for multidrug resistant *S. pneumoniae*. If this is the case, use an antibiotic from a different class.

Table 1: Antibiotics *Not* Recommended as Empiric Therapy for Acute Bacterial Sinusitis[2,10,31]

Antibiotic	Comments
Cephalexin	Poor activity against penicillin intermediate/resistant *S. pneumoniae*. No activity against *Haemophilus* or *Moraxella* spp.
Cefaclor	No activity against penicillin intermediate/resistant *S. pneumoniae*. Marginal activity against *H. influenzae*.
Cefixime	No activity against penicillin intermediate/resistant *S. pneumoniae*. Excellent activity against *Haemophilus* spp.
Ceftriaxone	Routine use of this agent is not recommended in acute bacterial sinusitis due to potential for increased resistance to third-generation cephalosporins. May be an option in patients with severe acute bacterial sinusitis who have failed therapy. Three days of im/iv therapy is recommended, as a single dose is not as effective in eradicating penicillin-resistant *S. pneumoniae*.
Clindamycin	Not recommended for acute bacterial sinusitis as no activity against *Haemophilus* or *Moraxella* spp. Clindamycin can be used as an alternative to amoxicillin-clavulanate in chronic sinusitis.
Erythromycin	Poor activity against *H. influenzae/Moraxella* spp. Significant macrolide resistance in *S. pneumoniae*.
Ciprofloxacin	Suboptimal coverage of *S. pneumoniae*.

Duration of Therapy

Duration of antibiotic therapy in acute bacterial sinusitis is not well defined. Empirically, a 10- to 14-day course of therapy is recommended.[1,2] Some physicians continue antibiotic therapy until the patient is free of symptoms and then for an additional 7 days to ensure eradication of bacteria and to prevent relapse.[2,15] However, short-course optimal dose therapy has been shown, with several different antibiotics, to be effective in acute bacterial sinusitis (e.g., azithromycin[32] or sulfamethoxazole/trimethoprim for 3 days,[33] respiratory quinolones[34] or telithromycin for 5 days[35,36,37]) and has advantages in terms of less development of resistance, better adherence, faster symptom resolution and lower costs.[38] Further study is needed, however, before short course therapy can be extrapolated to all antimicrobials used in the treatment of acute bacterial sinusitis.

Therapeutic Tips

- If patient shows no improvement after 72 hours of symptomatic therapy plus first-line antibiotic, change to a second-line antibiotic.[1,2,9,10,31]
- Inform patients that complete resolution of symptoms may take up to 14 days.[31]
- If the patient deteriorates at any time, reassess for acute complications, other diagnoses and/or adherence to treatment.
- Routine follow-up on completion of therapy in asymptomatic patients is not required.
- If a patient has received antibiotics (especially macrolides or fluoroquinolones) within the past three months, choose an antibiotic from a different class to treat acute bacterial sinusitis as there is a higher risk of multidrug resistant *S. pneumoniae*.
- The presence of tenacious, thick, brown nasal secretions should heighten the suspicion of a fungal infection.
- Refer to ENT specialist if a patient:[10]
  - fails second-line therapy[1]
  - experiences four or more episodes of bacterial sinusitis per year
  - has chronic sinusitis that is not responding to medical therapy (symptomatic and antibiotic)
  - has anatomic anomalies
  - develops complications

Table 2: Recommended Empiric Therapy for Bacterial Sinusitis in Children[10,31]

Infection	Usual Pathogens	Recommended Empiric Therapy	Comments
Acute Sinusitis (symptoms < 4 wk *and* ≤ 3 episodes/y	*S. pneumoniae* *M. catarrhalis* *H. influenzae* Occasionally *S. aureus*, *S. pyogenes*, anaerobes	Standard-dose amoxicillin × 10 days *or* High-dose amoxicillin × 10 days β-lactam allergy: sulfamethoxazole/trimethoprim (SMX/TMP) × 10 days	Refer to ENT specialist if ≥ 4 episodes/y. High-dose amoxicillin should be used in children at high-risk of penicillin-resistant *S. pneumoniae*: recent (< 3 mo) antibiotic exposure and/or daycare centre attendance (extrapolated from acute otitis media data). *S. pneumoniae* resistance to SMX/TMP is increasing. If patient is at high risk of bacterial resistance (see above) and has ß-lactam allergy, use azithromycin or clarithromycin.
Failure of First-line Agents: (No improvement or clinical deterioration after 72 h of antibiotic therapy *or* recurrence within 3 mo)	*S. pneumoniae* *M. catarrhalis* *H. influenzae* Occasionally *S. aureus*, *S. pyogenes*, anaerobes	Amoxicillin/clavulanate (7:1) × 10 days + amoxicillin[a] × 10 days *or* cefuroxime axetil × 10 days β-lactam allergy: azithromycin × 3-5 days[b] *or* clarithromycin × 10 days Severe presentation: iv cefuroxime sodium × 10 days	Consider resistant organisms, especially penicillin-resistant *S. pneumoniae* and ß-lactamase producing *H. influenzae*. If cefuroxime suspension or tablets is not tolerated, cefprozil can be considered. It tastes better than cefuroxime but has inferior coverage of *H. influenzae* and penicillin-intermediate *S. pneumoniae*. Azithromycin and clarithromycin use should be restricted (Table 4).
Chronic Sinusitis (symptoms ≥ 12 wk)	Anaerobes Occasionally *S. aureus*, *S. pneumoniae*, *H. influenzae*, *M. catarrhalis*, *S. pyogenes*, Enterobacteriaceae	Amoxicillin/clavulanate × 3 wk *or* clindamycin × 3 wk	Longer duration of therapy may be required in exceptional circumstances.

[a] If patient has failed high-dose amoxicillin therapy, amoxicillin/clavulanate alone is adequate to cover ß-lactamase producing organisms.

[b] Shorter durations of therapy have been shown to be effective in acute bacterial sinusitis but are not well studied in patients who have failed first-line therapy. Use short-course therapy with caution in this patient population.[32,34] If using azithromycin, consider using 20 mg/kg/day x 3 days.[39,40]

Abbreviations: ENT = ear, nose, throat

Table 3: Recommended Empiric Therapy for Bacterial Sinusitis in Adults[10,31]

Infection	Usual Pathogens	Recommended Empiric Therapy	Comments
Acute Sinusitis (symptoms < 4 wk *and* ≤ 3 episodes/y)	*S. pneumoniae* *H. influenzae* *M. catarrhalis* Occasionally *S. aureus*, *S. pyogenes*, anaerobes	Amoxicillin × 10 days β-lactam allergy: doxycycline × 10 days *or* sulfamethoxazole/trimethoprim (SMX/TMP) × 10 days	Refer to ENT specialist if ≥ 4 episodes/y. *S. pneumoniae* resistance to SMX/TMP is increasing. If ß-lactam allergy and previous antimicrobial exposure, use azithromycin, clarithromycin, levofloxacin or moxifloxacin. Advise patients that symptoms are likely to last up to 14 days. Studies have demonstrated efficacy with shorter courses of therapy.[32,34]
Failure of First-line Agents: (Clinical deterioration after 72 h of antibiotic therapy *or* no improvement post therapy)	*S. pneumoniae* *M. catarrhalis* *H. influenzae* Occasionally *S. aureus*, *S. pyogenes*, anaerobes	Amoxicillin/clavulanate × 10 days *or* cefuroxime axetil × 10 days β-lactam allergy: azithromycin × 3–5 days[a] *or* clarithromycin × 10 days *or* levofloxacin × 5–10 days[a] *or* moxifloxacin × 5–10 days[a]	Consider resistant organisms, especially penicillin-resistant *S. pneumoniae* and β-lactamase producing *H. influenzae*. Cefuroxime axetil provides best coverage of all oral cephalosporins against penicillin-intermediate strains of *S. pneumoniae* and provides good coverage of *H. influenzae*, *M. catarrhalis* and *S. aureus*. Macrolide and quinolone use should be restricted (Table 5).
Chronic Sinusitis (symptoms ≥ 12 wk)	Anaerobes Occasionally *S. aureus*, *S. pneumoniae*, *H. influenzae*, *M. catarrhalis*, *S. pyogenes*, Enterobacteriaceae	Amoxicillin/clavulanate × 3 wk β-lactam allergy: clindamycin × 3 wk	A single prolonged (3 wk) course of antibiotic may be of value in chronic sinusitis. Repeated courses of antibiotics are not recommended. Refer to ENT specialist if not responding.

[a] Shorter durations of therapy have been shown to be effective in acute bacterial sinusitis but not well studied in patients who have failed first-line therapy. Use short-course therapy with caution in this patient population.[32,34]

Abbreviations: ENT = ear, nose, throat

Table 4: Antibiotics for Bacterial Sinusitis in Children

Class	Drug	Pediatric Dose	Adverse Effects	Drug Interactions	Comments	Cost[a]
Cephalosporins	*cefprozil* Cefzil	30 mg/kg/day po divided BID; max 1 g/day	Nausea, vomiting, diarrhea,[b] hypersensitivity reactions (cross-reactivity with penicillins < 2%).		Alternative to cefuroxime if suspension or tablets not tolerated. Cefprozil has a better taste than cefuroxime but inferior coverage of *H. influenzae* and penicillin-intermediate *S. pneumoniae*.	$$$
	cefuroxime axetil Ceftin, generics	30 mg/kg/day po divided BID; max 1 g/day	See cefprozil.		If cefuroxime suspension/tablets not tolerated, consider using cefprozil.	$$$
	cefuroxime sodium Zinacef, generic	100–150 mg/kg/day iv divided Q8H; max 4.5 g/day	See cefprozil.		Use if severe presentation of acute sinusitis.	$$$$$
Lincosamides	*clindamycin* Dalacin C, Dalacin C Flavored Granules, generics	30 mg/kg/day po divided TID or QID; max 1.2–1.8 g/day	Diarrhea.[b]		Not active against *H. influenzae* or *M. catarrhalis*. Alternative to amoxicillin/clavulanate in chronic sinusitis.	capsules: $$$ granules: $$$$
Macrolides	*azithromycin* Zithromax, generics	10 mg/kg (max 500 mg) po first day, then 5 mg/kg (max 250 mg) po daily × 4 days (5 days total) or 10 mg/kg (max 500 mg) po × 3 days	GI irritation, nausea, vomiting, diarrhea,[b] rash.	May ↑ warfarin effect (clarithromycin > azithromycin).	Use of azithromycin and clarithromycin should be restricted because *S. pneumoniae* resistance to macrolides is increasing and macrolides have been shown (in acute otitis media) to be less efficacious than amoxicillin/clavulanate.	$$

Class	Drug	Pediatric Dose	Adverse Effects	Drug Interactions	Comments	Cost[a]
		or 30 mg/kg/day po × 1 day (max 1500 mg)			If using azithromycin **in patients who have failed first-line therapy**, consider using 20 mg/kg/day x 3 days.[39,40]	
	clarithromycin Biaxin	15 mg/kg/day po divided BID; max 1 g/day	See azithromycin.	See azithromycin. Coadministration with pimozide contraindicated. Rifampin and efavirenz ↓ clarithromycin concentrations. Clarithromycin may ↑ levels of some benzodiazepines, buspirone, carbamazepine, cyclosporine, digoxin, ergot alkaloids, statins, tacrolimus, theophyllines.	See azithromycin.	$$$
Penicillins	*amoxicillin* generics	Standard dose: 40 mg/kg/day po divided TID; max 1500 mg/day High dose: 90 mg/kg/day po divided TID; max 2–3 g/day	Usually well tolerated. Nausea, vomiting, diarrhea,[b] hypersensitivity reactions.		First-line treatment for bacterial sinusitis in children. High-dose amoxicillin should be used in children at high risk of resistant *S. pneumoniae*: recent (< 3 months) antibiotic exposure *and/or* daycare centre attendance.	$

(cont'd)

Table 4: **Antibiotics for Bacterial Sinusitis in Children** *(cont'd)*

Class	Drug	Pediatric Dose	Adverse Effects	Drug Interactions	Comments	Cost[a]
	amoxicillin/ clavulanate (7:1) ± *additional amoxicillin* Clavulin, generics	amoxicillin/clavulanate 45 mg/kg/day (amoxicillin component) po divided BID-TID + *additional* amoxicillin 45 mg/kg/day po divided BID-TID	Nausea, vomiting, hypersensitivity reactions. Diarrhea[b] more common with amoxicillin/clavulanate than with amoxicillin alone.		If patient has failed standard-dose amoxicillin, amoxicillin/clavulanate should be combined with amoxicillin to increase the total dose of amoxicillin while minimizing diarrhea due to the clavulanate. If patient has failed high-dose amoxicillin therapy, amoxicillin/clavulanate alone is adequate to cover ß-lactamase producing organisms.	$$
Sulfonamide Combinations	*sulfamethoxazole/ trimethoprim (SMX/TMP)* generics	6–12 mg/kg/day (TMP component) po divided BID; max 320 mg/day (TMP component)	Nausea, vomiting, diarrhea, rash.	May ↑ warfarin effect and phenytoin levels. Enhanced bone marrow suppression with methotrexate.	*S. pneumoniae* resistance to SMX/TMP is increasing.	$

[a] Costs are given for a 10-day course of treatment based on 20 kg body weight, except for azithromycin (1, 3, 5 days) and clindamycin (3 weeks); includes drug cost only.
[b] Antibiotic-associated diarrhea/colitis is commonly associated with clindamycin and ß-lactams, but any antibiotic can cause this condition.
Dosage adjustment may be required in renal impairment; see Appendix I.
Abbreviations: TMP = trimethoprim
Legend: $ < $10 $$ $10–25 $$$ $25–50 $$$$ $50–100 $$$$$ > $100

Table 5: **Antibiotics for Bacterial Sinusitis in Adults**

Class	Drug	Dose	Adverse Effects	Drug Interactions	Comments	Cost[a]
Cephalosporins	*cefuroxime axetil* Ceftin, generics	500 mg po BID	Nausea, vomiting, diarrhea,[b] hypersensitivity reactions (cross-reactivity with penicillins < 2%).		Cefuroxime axetil provides best coverage of all oral cephalosporins against penicillin-intermediate strains of *S. pneumoniae* and provides good coverage of *H. influenzae*, *M. catarrhalis* and *S. aureus*.	$$$$
Macrolides	*azithromycin* Zithromax, generics	500 mg po daily × 3 days or 500 mg po on day 1, then 250 mg po daily × 4 days (5 days total)	GI irritation, nausea, vomiting, diarrhea, rash.	May ↑ warfarin effect (clarithromycin > azithromycin).	Macrolide use should be restricted as *S. pneumoniae* resistance to macrolides is increasing and macrolides have been shown (in acute otitis media) to be less efficacious than amoxicillin/ clavulanate.	$$
	clarithromycin Biaxin, Biaxin XL	Regular: 500 mg po BID or extended release (XL): 1 g po daily	See azithromycin.	See azithromycin. Coadministration with pimozide contraindicated. Rifampin and efavirenz ↓ clarithromycin concentrations. Clarithromycin may ↑ levels of some benzodiazepines, buspirone, carbamazepine, cyclosporine, digoxin, ergot alkaloids, statins, tacrolimus, theophyllines.	See azithromycin.	$$$$

(cont'd)

Table 5: **Antibiotics for Bacterial Sinusitis in Adults** *(cont'd)*

Class	Drug	Dose	Adverse Effects	Drug Interactions	Comments	Cost[a]
Fluoro-quinolones	*levofloxacin* Levaquin, generics	750 mg po daily × 5 days or 500 mg po daily	Usually well tolerated. Headache, dizziness may occur. Rare: tendon rupture.	Antacids, sucralfate, metal cations, didanosine chewable/buffered tablets or pediatric powder, dairy products ↓ levofloxacin absorption. Avoid in patients on Class Ia or III antiarrhythmics. May ↑ warfarin effect. NSAIDs may ↑ risk of CNS stimulation/seizures.	Due to broad spectrum and potential for increased resistance, quinolones should be reserved for patients with ß-lactam allergy or those who have failed previous antibiotic therapy.	$$$$
	moxifloxacin Avelox	400 mg po daily	See levofloxacin.	See levofloxacin. No interaction with calcium.	See levofloxacin.	$$$$
Lincosamides	*clindamycin* Dalacin C, generics	300 mg po QID	Diarrhea.[b]		Not active against *H. influenzae* or *M. catarrhalis*. Alternative to amoxicillin/clavulanate in chronic sinusitis.	$$$$
Penicillins	*amoxicillin* generics	500 mg po TID	Usually well tolerated. Nausea, vomiting, diarrhea,[b] hypersensitivity reactions.		First-line treatment for bacterial sinusitis in adults.	$
	amoxicillin/ clavulanate Clavulin, generics	875 mg po BID or 500 mg po TID	Nausea, vomiting, hypersensitivity reactions. Diarrhea[b] more common than with amoxicillin alone.			$$$

Class	Drug	Dose	Adverse Effects	Drug Interactions	Comments	Cost[a]
Sulfonamide Combinations	*sulfamethoxazole/ trimethoprim* (renal adjustment symbol) generics	800/160 mg (1 DS tablet) po BID	Nausea, vomiting, diarrhea, rash.	May ↑ warfarin effect and phenytoin levels. Enhanced bone marrow suppression with methotrexate. May ↑ risk of hypoglycemia with coadministration of rosiglitazone.	*S. pneumoniae* resistance to SMX/TMP is increasing.	$
Tetracyclines	*doxycycline* Vibra-Tabs, generics	200 mg po once, then 100 mg po BID	Nausea, vomiting, diarrhea, rash, photosensitivity.	May ↑ warfarin effect. May ↑ digoxin levels. Doxycyline seems to be minimally affected by food and dairy products as compared to demeclocycline and tetracycline. Aluminum, bismuth, iron and magnesium ↓ absorption. Alcohol, carbamazepine, phenytoin and phenobarbital may ↓ doxycycline concentrations.	Excellent activity against sinusitis pathogens, including ß-lactamase producing *H. influenzae* and *M. catarrhalis*; *S. pneumoniae*, including penicillin-intermediate strains. ~ 50% less doxycycline resistance than macrolide resistance in *S. pneumoniae*. Has not been associated with causing an increase in penicillin resistance among *S. pneumoniae* (macrolides have). Excellent pharmacokinetics/dynamics (high serum levels, concentration-dependent killing).	$

[a] Costs are given for a 10-day course of treatment except for azithromycin (3-5 days) and clindamycin (3 weeks); includes drug cost only.
[b] Antibiotic-associated diarrhea/colitis is commonly associated with clindamycin and ß-lactams, but any antibiotic can cause this condition.
(renal adjustment symbol) Dosage adjustment may be required in renal impairment; see Appendix I.
Legend: $ < $10 $$ $10–25 $$$ $25–50 $$$$ $50–100

Suggested Readings

Desrosiers M, Frenkiel S, Hamid QA et al. Acute bacterial sinusitis in adults: management in the primary care setting. *J Otolaryngol* 2002;31(Suppl 2):2S2-2S14.

Gwaltney JM. Sinusitis. In: Mandell GL, Bennett JE, Dolin R, editors. *Mandell, Douglas and Bennett's principles and practice of infectious diseases*. 6th ed. Philadelphia (PA): Churchill Livingstone; 2005.

Slavin RG, Spector SL, Bernstein IL et al. The diagnosis and management of sinusitis: a practice parameter update. *J Allergy Clin Immunol* 2005;116(6 Suppl):S13-47.

References

1. Desrosiers M, Frenkiel S, Hamid QA et al. Acute bacterial sinusitis in adults: management in the primary care setting. *J Otolaryngol* 2002;31(Suppl 2):2S2-2S14.
2. Slavin RG, Spector SL, Bernstein IL et al. The diagnosis and management of sinusitis: a practice parameter update. *J Allergy Clin Immunol* 2005;116(6 Suppl):S13-47.
3. Hickner JM, Bartlett JG, Besser RE et al. Principles of appropriate antibiotic use for acute rhinosinusitis in adults: background. *Ann Intern Med* 2001;134(6):498-505.
4. O'Brien KL, Dowell SF, Schwartz B et al. Acute sinusitis: principles of judicious use of antimicrobial agents. *Pediatrics* 1998;101(1 Suppl):174-7.
5. Wald ER, Chiponis D, Ledesma-Medina J. Comparative effectiveness of amoxicillin and amoxicillin-clavulanate potassium in acute paranasal sinus infections in children: a double-blind, placebo-controlled trial. *Pediatrics* 1986;77(6):795-800.
6. Druce HM. Diagnosis of sinusitis in adults: history, physical examination, nasal cytology, echo, and rhinoscope. *J Allergy Clin Immunol* 1992;90(3 Pt 2):436-41.
7. Fireman P. Diagnosis of sinusitis in children: emphasis on the history and physical examination. *J Allergy Clin Immunol* 1992;90(3 Pt 2):433-6.
8. Benninger MS, Anon J, Mabry RL. The medical management of rhinosinusitis. *Otolaryngol Head Neck Surg* 1997;117(3 Pt 2):S41-9.
9. Anon JB, Jacobs MR, Poole MD et al. Antimicrobial treatment guidelines for acute bacterial rhinosinusitis. *Otolaryngol Head Neck Surg* 2004;130 (1 Suppl):1-45.
10. Alberta Medical Association. *Diagnosis and management of acute bacterial sinusitis*. Edmonton (AB): Toward Optimized Practice; 2006. Available from: http://www.topalbertadoctors.org/TOP/CPG/AcuteSinusitis/AcuteSinusitis.htm Accessed May 22, 2007.
11. Richards W, Roth RM, Church JA. Underdiagnosis and undertreatment of chronic sinusitis in children. *Clin Pediatr (Phila)* 1991;30(2):88-92.
12. American Academy of Pediatrics. Subcommittee on Management of Sinusitis and Committee on Quality Improvement. Clinical practice guideline: management of sinusitis. *Pediatrics* 2001;108(3):798-808.
13. Poole MD. A focus on acute sinusitis in adults: changes in disease management. *Am J Med* 1999;106(5A):38S-47S.
14. Racicot J. *Pharm Pract* 2002;18:CE1-8.
15. Brook I. Microbiology and antimicrobial management of sinusitis. *J Laryngol Otol* 2005;119(4):251-8.
16. Lindbaek M, Hjortdahl P, Johnsen UL. Randomised, double blind, placebo controlled trial of penicillin V and amoxycillin in treatment of acute sinus infections in adults. *BMJ* 1996;313(7053):325-9.
17. Axelsson A, Chidekel N, Grebelius N et al. Treatment of acute maxillary sinusitis. A comparison of four different methods. *Acta Otolaryngol* 1970;70(1):71-6.
18. Gananca M, Trabulsi LR. The therapeutic effects of cyclacillin in acute sinusitis: in vitro and in vivo correlations in a placebo-controlled study. *Curr Med Res Opin* 1973;1(6):362-8.
19. Stalman W, van Essen GA, van der Graaf Y et al. The end of antibiotic treatment in adults with acute sinusitis-like complaints in general practice? A placebo-controlled double-blind randomized doxycycline trial. *Br J Gen Pract* 1997;47(425):794-9.
20. van Buchem FL, Knottnerus JA, Schrijnemaekers VJ et al. Primary-care-based randomised placebo-controlled trial of antibiotic treatment in acute maxillary sinusitis. *Lancet* 1997;349(9053):683-7.
21. Garbutt JM, Goldstein M, Gellman E et al. A randomized, placebo-controlled trial of antimicrobial treatment for children with clinically diagnosed acute sinusitis. *Pediatrics* 2001;107(4):619-25.
22. Williams JW, Aguilar C, Cornell J et al. Antibiotics for acute maxillary sinusitis. *Cochrane Database Syst Rev* 2003;(2):CD000243.

23. Ip S, Fu L, Balk E et al. *Update on acute bacterial rhinosinusitis*. Evidence Report/Technology Assessment No. 124 AHRQ Publication No. 05-E020-1. Rockville (MD): Agency for Healthcare Research and Quality; 2005. Available from: http://www.ahrq.gov/downloads/pub/evidence/pdf/rhinoupdate/rhinoup.pdf Accessed May 22, 2007.
24. Taverner D, Latte J. Nasal decongestants for the common cold. *Cochrane Database Syst Rev* 2007;(1):CD001953.
25. Infant Deaths Associated with Cough and Cold Medications—Two States, 2005. *MMWR* 2007;56(1): 1-4.
26. Stafford CT. The clinician's view of sinusitis. *Otolaryngol Head Neck Surg* 1990;103(5 Pt 2):870-4.
27. Meltzer EO, Charous BL, Busse WW et al. Added relief in the treatment of acute recurrent sinusitis with adjunctive mometasone furoate nasal spray. The Nasonex Sinusitis Group. *J Allergy Clin Immunol* 2000;106(4):630-7.
28. de Bock GH, Dekker FW, Stolk J et al. Antimicrobial treatment in acute maxillary sinusitis: a meta-analysis. *J Clin Epidemiol* 1997;50(8):881-90.
29. Piccirillo JF, Mager DE, Frisse ME et al. Impact of first-line vs second-line antibiotics for the treatment of acute uncomplicated sinusitis. *JAMA* 2001;286(15):1849-56.
30. Morris P, Leach A. Antibiotics for persistent nasal discharge (rhinosinusitis) in children. *Cochrane Database Syst Rev* 2002;(4):CD001094.
31. Blondel-Hill E, Fryters S. *Bugs and drugs 2006*. Edmonton (AB): Capital Health; 2006.
32. Henry DC, Riffer E, Sokol WN et al. Randomized double-blind study comparing 3- and 6-day regimens of azithromycin with a 10-day amoxicillin-clavulanate regimen for treatment of acute bacterial sinusitis. *Antimicrob Agents Chemother* 2003;47(9):2770-4.
33. Williams JW, Holleman DR, Samsa GP et al. Randomized controlled trial of 3 vs 10 days of trimethoprim/sulfamethoxazole for acute maxillary sinusitis. *JAMA* 1995;273(13):1015-21.
34. Sher LD, McAdoo MA, Bettis RB et al. A multicenter, randomized, investigator-blinded study of 5- and 10-day gatifloxacin versus 10-day amoxicillin/clavulanate in patients with acute bacterial sinusitis. *Clin Ther* 2002;24(2):269-81.
35. Buchanan PP, Stephens TA, Leroy B. A comparison of the efficacy of telithromycin versus cefuroxime axetil in the treatment of acute bacterial maxillary sinusitis. *Am J Rhinol* 2003;17(6):369-77.
36. Luterman M, Tellier G, Lasko B et al. Efficacy and tolerability of telithromycin for 5 or 10 days vs amoxicillin/clavulanic acid for 10 days in acute maxillary sinusitis. *Ear Nose Throat J* 2003;82(8):576-86.
37. Ferguson BJ, Guzzetta RV, Spector SL et al. Efficacy and safety of oral telithromycin once daily for 5 days versus moxifloxacin once daily for 10 days in the treatment of acute bacterial rhinosinusitis. *Otolaryngol Head Neck Surg* 2004;131(3):207-14.
38. Poole MD, Portugal LG. Treatment of rhinosinusitis in the outpatient setting. *Am J Med* 2005;118(Suppl 7A):45S-50S.
39. Arrieta A, Arguedas A, Fernandez P et al. High-Dose Azithromycin versus high-dose amoxicillin-clavulanate for treatment of children with recurrent or persistent acute otitis media. *Antimicrob Agents Chemother* 2003;47(10):3179-86.
40. Arrieta A, Singh J. Management of recurrent and persistent acute otitis media: new options with familiar antibiotics. *Pediatr Infect Dis J* 2004;23:S115-124.

CHAPTER 96

Acute Bronchitis

Cindy Marshall, MD, CCFP, FCFP and
Wayne Putnam, MD, FCFP

Cough is one of the most common presenting symptoms in family practice. When present for less than three weeks, with or without sputum production, it is consistent with the diagnosis of acute bronchitis.[1] Acute bronchitis should be differentiated from the common cold, acute exacerbation of chronic bronchitis, asthma and community-acquired pneumonia.[2] A nonbacterial cause is present in more than 90% of uncomplicated acute bronchitis (Table 1).[3] Acute bronchitis is not a life-threatening illness. It is generally self-limited and symptoms usually resolve in 10 to 14 days.[1]

This chapter focuses on the treatment of acute bronchitis in the otherwise healthy immunocompetent adult.

Table 1: **Etiologic Agents in Acute Bronchitis**[2,4,5,6]

Etiology of Bronchitis	Frequency of Causation	Comments
Viral	> 90 %	Most common viral isolates in acute bronchitis based on age (in order of prevalence): < 1 y—RSV, parainfluenza, coronavirus 1–10 y—parainfluenza, enterovirus, RSV > 10 y—influenza, RSV, parainfluenza (less commonly adenovirus, coronavirus, rhinovirus)
Noninfectious	Not well studied	Includes chemical and fume inhalational exposures
Bacterial	5–10%	The only isolates shown to cause acute bacterial bronchitis are *Chlamydophila pneumoniae*, *Mycoplasma pneumoniae*, *Bordetella pertussis*, and *Bordetella parapertussis*. There is no evidence that *Streptococcus pneumoniae*, *Haemophilus influenzae* or *Moraxella catarrhalis* cause acute bronchitis in adults in the absence of underlying lung disease

Abbreviations: RSV = respiratory syncytial virus.

Goals of Therapy

- "First do no harm"
- Rule out serious illness, e.g., pneumonia
- Minimize symptoms
- Limit the unnecessary use of antibiotics

Investigations (Figure 1)

- History:

  Symptoms:

  - primarily cough, may or may not be productive. Prolonged cough (> 3 weeks) can occur in up to 50% of cases due to viral infections.[5]
  - in children, the infection of the tracheobronchial tree may result in prolonged cough; consider diagnosis of reactive airways, not acute bronchitis (see Chapter 48). Consider a diagnosis of pertussis, especially in children, when the history of spasmodic cough is elicited or a known outbreak exists in the area.[3]
  - other symptoms may include wheezing, tachypnea, respiratory distress and hypoxemia.
  - green sputum production is a function of peroxidase release from leukocytes, hence it implies only inflammation, not necessarily infection.[5,6]
  - consider alternative diagnoses if symptoms persist longer than three weeks.[1,2,5]

  Obtain vaccination history, travel history, use of cigarettes.
- Physical exam is key to diagnosis:
  - absence of tachycardia (heart rate > 100 beats/min), tachypnea (> 24 breaths/min), fever (oral temperature of > 38°C) and localized chest findings suggest acute bronchitis.[7]
- Objective measurements:
  - no role for routine chest x-ray, viral culture, serologic assay, sputum culture or Gram stain or pulmonary function testing/spirometry.[2,5,6,7]

Therapeutic Choices (Figure 1)

Nonpharmacologic Choices

The nonpharmacologic approach is the mainstay of management.

- Limit risk of inoculation and transmission by employing strict hand-washing techniques.[5]
- Increased fluids and humidity may help reduce cough.[5]

Pharmacologic Choices (Table 2)

Analgesics

Antipyretics or analgesics, such as **acetaminophen** or **ibuprofen**, may be used for symptomatic relief.[1,6]

Antitussives

Antitussives (**codeine, dextromethorphan, hydrocodone**) may provide short-term symptom relief but do not shorten the duration of illness.[1,7]

Bronchodilators

Studies in the pediatric population do not support the use of beta$_2$-agonists (**salbutamol, terbutaline**) in the absence of airflow obstruction.[4,8,9] In adults, beta$_2$-agonists may decrease symptoms, such as cough; however, the potential benefit, which is not supported by evidence, must be weighed against potential adverse effects.[8] Adults experiencing cough with wheezing may benefit from treatment.[7]

Antibiotics

Routine antibiotic treatment in uncomplicated acute bronchitis is not recommended.[1,2,3,4,5,7] Antibiotic treatment does not have a consistent impact on the duration or severity of illness or in prevention of potential complications (e.g., pneumonia, otitis media) either in adult[1,5] or pediatric populations.[10]

A Cochrane systematic review assessed nine trials involving more than 750 patients from the age of 8 to over 65 years.[11] Overall, patients taking antibiotics showed a modest benefit compared to placebo. The evidence suggests antibiotics may reduce the duration of cough by half a day.[11] The magnitude of this benefit, however, is offset by the potential for adverse reactions to antibiotics and an increase in antibiotic resistance for treatment of a self-limited illness.[1,11] Current evidence reveals no statistical difference in the amount of sputum production, purulence of sputum, limitation of work activities or reduction in the incidence of lower respiratory tract infections in the six months following antibiotic treatment.[11]

Therapeutic Tips

- Treatment is only supportive in the vast majority of cases of acute bronchitis.
- Patient satisfaction does not depend on receiving an antibiotic; it is related to the quality of the physician–patient communication.[1,3,6,12]
- Educate patients regarding the lack of evidence for the use of antibiotics in most circumstances. It is helpful to review the concerns of increased antibiotic resistance, possible side effects of antibiotic use and the cost of unnecessary treatment.[13] Providing a related patient information handout may also reduce antibiotic use.
- There is no evidence to support the use of inhaled/oral corticosteroids in the management of acute bronchitis.[5]
- In a documented influenza outbreak, consider neuraminidase inhibitors, which are active against both influenza A and B. Initiate within 48 hours of onset of symptoms (see Chapter 97).
- Set the patient's expectations of a 10- to 14-day duration of cough.[3] Most patients feel much better within the first week.[10]
- Mucolytic and expectorant preparations have failed to show any significant benefit in the management of acute bronchitis.[2]

- If the patient has unresolved symptoms in 2–3 weeks from onset of symptoms, consider follow-up.
- Annual influenza vaccine is recommended.

Figure 1: **Management of Acute Bronchitis**

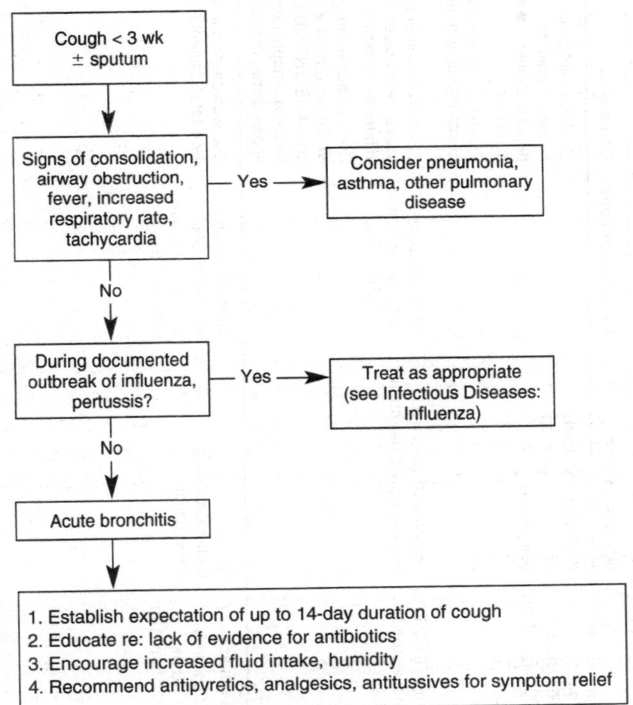

Table 2: **Drugs for the Symptomatic Management of Acute Bronchitis in Adults**

Class	Drug	Dose	Adverse Effects	Drug Interactions	Comments	Cost[a]
Analgesics	*acetaminophen* Atasol, Tempra, Tylenol, generics	325–650 mg Q4–6H PRN (do not exceed 4000 mg/24 h)	Well tolerated (rare GI upset, less than salicylates).		Use with caution in patients with hepatic impairment. Severe hepatic damage can occur with overdose. Preferred agent in children due to experience with this agent.	$[b]
	ibuprofen Advil, Motrin (Children's), Motrin IB, generics	300–400 mg TID-QID PRN (do not exceed 2400 mg/day)	Primarily GI (nausea, epigastric pain, heartburn).	ASA/anticoagulants may increase risk of bleeding.	Contraindicated in patients with active peptic ulcer disease or inflammatory bowel disease. Contraindicated in patients who have a history of or are at risk of ASA/NSAID intolerance (asthma, anaphylaxis, urticaria, angioedema, rhinitis).	$[b]
Antitussives	*codeine* (many products contain additional ingredients): Benylin 2 Cold and Flu with Codeine, CoActifed, Dimetapp-C, Dimetane Expectorant-C, Robitussin AC, generics	Immediate-release: Adults and children > 12 y: 10–20 mg Q4–6H PRN; max 120 mg	Sedation, nausea/vomiting, constipation.	Additive sedation with other CNS depressants; use with caution.	Use with caution in elderly or debilitated patients.	$[b]

Class	Drug	Dose	Adverse Effects	Drug Interactions	Comments	Cost[a]
	dextromethorphan Benylin DM, Robitussin Preparations, generics	30 mg Q6–8H PRN	Rare but can cause nausea, drowsiness, dizziness.	Caution with CNS depressants (can potentiate effects). Do not use with monoamine oxidase inhibitor (MAOI) or for 2 wk after stopping MAOI.	Not recommended in patients with asthma.	$[b]
	hydrocodone Hycodan, generics	5 mg Q4–6H; may ↑ to 10 mg/dose	Lightheadedness, dizziness, sedation, nausea and vomiting, constipation.	Additive sedation with other CNS depressants; use with caution.	Caution in the elderly and debilitated.	$
Inhaled Beta$_2$-adrenergic Agonists, short-acting	*salbutamol* Airomir, Ventolin Diskus, Ventolin HFA, generics	Diskus (200 µg/puff): 1 puff TID-QID; max 800 µg/day MDI: 1–2 puffs (100 to 200 µg) QID PRN; max 800 µg/day	Tremor, restlessness, palpitations, dizziness, headache, nausea.	Caution with other sympathomimetic agents.	Contraindicated in patients with arrhythmias or hypertrophic obstructive cardiomyopathy. Caution with ischemic heart disease, vascular disease and hypertension.	Diskus:$$$ MDI:$$
	terbutaline Bricanyl Turbuhaler	1–2 puffs TID-QID PRN; max 6 puffs/day	See salbutamol.	See salbutamol.	See salbutamol.	$$$

[a] Costs are per day for oral medications and per unit for inhaled medications; includes drug cost only.
[b] Available without prescription; retail mark-up may vary.
Dosage adjustment may be required in renal impairment; see Appendix I.
Legend: $ < $5 $$ $5–10 $$$ $10–15

Suggested Readings

Alberta Clinical Practice Guidelines Working Group. *Guideline for the management of acute bronchitis, 2006 update.* Edmonton (AB): Toward Optimized Practice (TOP) Program, Alberta Medical Association; 2005. Available from: http://www.topalbertadoctors.org/NR/rdonlyres/D3699AF6-7E5C-4C43-9C9C-A04669FCF2B1/0/bronchitis_guideline.pdf Accessed March 8, 2007.

Irwin RS, Baumann MH, Bolser DC et al. Diagnosis and management of cough: ACCP evidence-based clinical practice guidelines. *Chest* 2006;129(1 Suppl):1S-292S.

Wenzel RP, Fowler AA. Clinical practice: acute bronchitis. *N Engl J Med* 2006;355(20):2125-30.

References

1. Snow V, Mottur-Pilson C, Gonzales R et al. Principles of appropriate antibiotic use for treatment of acute bronchitis in adults. *Ann Intern Med* 2001;134(6):518-20.
2. Irwin RS, Baumann MH, Bolser DC et al. Diagnosis and management of cough executive summary: ACCP evidence-based clinical practice guidelines. *Chest* 2006;129(1 Suppl):1S-23S.
3. Alberta Clinical Practice Guidelines Working Group. *Guideline for the management of acute bronchitis, 2006 update.* Edmonton (AB): Toward Optimized Practice (TOP) Program, Alberta Medical Association; 2005. Available from: http://www.topalbertadoctors.org/NR/rdonlyres/D3699AF6-7E5C-4C43-9C9C-A04669FCF2B1/0/bronchitis_guideline.pdf Accessed March 8, 2007.
4. Anish EJ. Lower respiratory tract infection in outpatient adults. *Clinics in Family Practice* 2004;6(1):75-99.
5. Gonzales R, Bartlett JG, Besser RE et al. Principles of appropriate antibiotic use for treatment of uncomplicated acute bronchitis: background. *Ann Emerg Med* 2001;37(6):720-7.
6. Knutson D, Braun C. Diagnosis and management of acute bronchitis. *Am Fam Physician* 2002;65(10):2039-44.
7. Braman SS. Chronic cough due to acute bronchitis: ACCP evidence-based clinical practice guidelines. *Chest* 2006;129(1 Suppl):95S-103S.
8. Smucny J, Becker L, Glazier R. Beta2-agonists for acute bronchitis. *Cochrane Database Syst Rev* 2006;(4):CD001726.
9. Smucny JJ, Flynn CA, Becker LA et al. Are beta2-agonists effective treatment for acute bronchitis or acute cough in patients without underlying pulmonary disease? A systematic review. *J Fam Pract* 2001;50(11):945-51.
10. Snow V, Mottur-Pilson C, Gonzales R et al. Principles of appropriate antibiotic use for treatment of nonspecific upper respiratory tract infections in adults. *Ann Intern Med* 2001;134(6):487-9.
11. Smucny J, Fahey T, Becker L et al. Antibiotics for acute bronchitis. *Cochrane Database Syst Rev* 2004;(4):CD000245.
12. Phillips TG, Hickner J. Calling acute bronchitis a chest cold may improve patient satisfaction with appropriate antibiotic use. *J Am Board Fam Pract* 2005;18(6):459-63.
13. Colgan R, Powers JH. Appropriate antimicrobial prescribing: approaches that limit antibiotic resistance. *Am Fam Physician* 2001;64(6):999-1004.

CHAPTER 97
Influenza

Susan K. Bowles, PharmD and
Robert Strang, MD, MHSc, FRCPC

Influenza is an acute viral illness of the respiratory tract caused by influenza A or influenza B viruses. A typical influenza season in Canada runs from mid-October to the end of April.

Influenza-like illness (ILI) is a term often used in public health surveillance programs for influenza, which refers to any acute illness having symptoms typical of influenza. Adenovirus, parainfluenza or respiratory syncytial virus may cause similar symptoms.

Influenza-like illness[1] is defined as an acute onset of respiratory illness with fever, cough and one or more of: sore throat, arthralgia, myalgia or prostration. Gastrointestinal symptoms may be present in children < 5 years. Fever may not be prominent in children < 5 years or adults ≥ 65 years.

This chapter addresses the prevention and treatment of influenza.

Investigations

- History with particular attention to symptoms and onset of symptoms, the key to appropriate use of antiviral agents:
  - healthy adolescents and adults: when influenza is known to be circulating in the community, abrupt onset of fever of 38.5°C or greater and dry cough is likely to be influenza.[2,3] The predictive value of these symptoms is considerably less in the very young or the elderly
  - young children: can present with either a nonspecific febrile illness or with a respiratory illness resembling croup, bronchitis and occasionally bronchiolitis.[4] GI symptoms (nausea, vomiting, diarrhea) may also be present in children < 5 years
  - older adults: fever may not be prominent.[4,5] When influenza is known to be circulating in the community, have a high index of suspicion for influenza if older patients present with ≥ 2 symptoms of sore throat, arthralgia, myalgia or prostration;[5] this is particularly true of elderly residents of long-term care facilities
- Laboratory testing:
  - beyond formal surveillance programs, widespread laboratory testing in the community is not necessary or practical, but it is important to differentiate between influenza and other respiratory viruses in the event of an outbreak of ILI in the long-term care setting
  - as a general guideline, nasopharyngeal swabs from ill long-term care residents should be sent for laboratory testing in the event of

≥ 2 cases of ILI within a 72-hour period.[6] Obtain swabs from the initial cases as well as the next three to five individuals presenting with ILI. Public health officials should also be notified
- contact the lab to obtain instructions on specimen collection, storage and transport. Some labs may offer rapid tests, which tend to be less sensitive than traditional viral culture, especially in adults
- to decrease the potential for a false negative result, swabs are best obtained within 24 hours of symptom onset and should not be taken more than 48 hours after onset of symptoms

Prevention

Goals of Therapy

- Prevent influenza illness from occurring, especially in individuals at high risk of developing serious influenza-related complications, e.g., pneumonia, exacerbation of cardiac or respiratory disease, death
- Decrease influenza-related hospitalizations and deaths

Therapeutic Choices

Nonpharmacologic Choices

General measures to prevent acquisition of influenza include:

- wash hands often; use hand sanitizer if water and soap are not available.
- cough/sneeze into tissues (or into a sleeve if tissues are not available) and throw all used tissues into the garbage.
- if flu symptoms are present, stay home from work or school and do not visit hospitals, nursing homes or individuals at high risk of influenza-related complications.

In the event of a cluster of ILI in the long-term care setting, implement the following to reduce the potential of influenza spreading from ill to well residents (Figure 1):

- promote and enhance proper hand washing by staff, ambulatory residents and visitors.
- confine ill residents to their rooms until their acute symptoms have resolved.
- enhance environmental controls, e.g., more frequent cleaning.
- if possible, ill residents should be cared for only by staff who have received their annual influenza immunization.
- if possible, ill residents should be cared for by separate staff members who are not looking after well residents. If this is not possible, provide care for well individuals first, with strict hand washing between each patient.
- limit gatherings or activities where residents from different areas of the facility come into contact with each other.

- limit visitors when possible and exclude visits from all individuals with ILI.
- staff with symptoms of ILI should not work until their acute symptoms have resolved.

Pharmacologic Choices (Table 3)

Influenza Vaccine[7]

October to mid-November is the usual recommended time for influenza immunization; however, clinicians should work with their local Public Health Departments to determine the best time for immunization at the local level.

Table 1: **Recommended Recipients of Annual Influenza Immunization**[7]

Persons at high risk for influenza-related complications

- adults and children ≥ 6 mo of age with chronic cardiac or respiratory disorders (includes asthma, bronchopulmonary dysplasia, cystic fibrosis and COPD) requiring regular medical follow-up
- all residents of nursing homes and other long-term care facilities
- all persons ≥ 65 y of age
- adults and children ≥ 6 mo of age with any of the following chronic disorders:
    - diabetes mellitus or other metabolic disorder
    - cancer
    - immunodeficiency
    - immunosuppression (due to underlying disease or treatment)
    - renal disease
    - anemia
    - hemoglobinopathies
- children and adolescents (6 mo to 18 y of age) requiring chronic ASA therapy

Persons capable of transmitting influenza to those at high risk of influenza-related complications

- health care workers and other personnel (e.g., volunteers, housekeeping staff) who have significant contact with those in the above-mentioned high-risk groups, regardless of the practice setting
- adults and children ≥ 6 mo of age who are household contacts of those at high risk of influenza-related complications. This includes household contacts of children < 6 mo old who are at high risk of complications from influenza but for whom there is no currently licensed vaccine. Pregnant women should be immunized if they are expected to deliver during influenza season; they will become household contacts of their newborn.
- those providing regular child care to children age 0 to 23 mo, whether in or out of the home

Other

- people who provide essential community services, e.g., police officers and fire fighters

Annual influenza vaccination of individuals at high risk of influenza-related complications (Table 1) is, and remains, the primary strategy for the reduction of influenza-related morbidity and mortality, in both community and long-term care settings.

Annual vaccination of individuals who have significant contact with individuals at high risk of influenza-related complications (Table 1) or who provide essential community services is also recommended. Encourage healthy individuals aged 2 to 64 years to receive influenza vaccine annually, even if they are not in the aforementioned priority groups.

Travellers may find themselves in areas with high transmission during other months of the year, e.g., Asia, the southern hemisphere and cruise ships. Detailed recommendations for the prevention of influenza related to travel are outlined in the 2005 Committee to Advise on Tropical Medicine and Travel Statement on Travel, Influenza and Prevention—Update (www.phac-aspc.gc.ca/publicat/ccdr-rmtc/05vol31/asc-dcc-11/index.html).

Antiviral Agents

Antiviral agents can be used to prevent influenza in high-risk individuals under several circumstances (Table 2). Their greatest utility is in the long-term care setting (see Figure 1).

When an influenza outbreak is identified in a long-term care setting, give antiviral prophylaxis as soon as possible to all residents who are not yet ill, regardless of their vaccination status, as well as to nonimmunized health care providers.

Table 2: **Criteria for Prophylactic Use of Antivirals**[7]

- Administer to all residents of a long-term care facility who are not already ill, regardless of vaccination status as soon as an influenza outbreak is identified. Duration of prophylaxis is until 8 days after onset of symptoms of last case (covers one infectious period and one incubation period)
- Administer antiviral prophylaxis for the duration of the outbreak to LTC providers who refuse immunization
- Continue prophylaxis for the duration of influenza activity in the community in non-institutionalized people at high risk during outbreak situations when vaccine is not available, contraindicated or unlikely to be effective due to poor match between vaccine and strain circulating in the community and as a supplement to vaccination of those at high risk expected to have an impaired immune response to vaccine.
- Continue prophylaxis for 2 weeks after vaccination (approximately the time required to mount a protective immune response to vaccine) as an adjunct to late vaccination of those at high risk or health care workers caring for those at high risk.

Amantadine has been effective for prophylaxis against influenza A;[7] however, recent data demonstrates high levels of amantadine resistance nationally and internationally.[9,10] If influenza A is sensitive to amantadine, simultaneous use of amantadine for prophylaxis and treatment within a facility is *not* advised due to the increased risk of developing resistance. Future use of amantadine will depend upon resistance patterns. Amantadine dose should be based on renal function to minimize adverse effects (see Appendix I).

Neuraminidase inhibitors, **oseltamivir** and **zanamivir**, are effective for prophylaxis against influenza A and B. Oseltamivir is the first-line agent during outbreaks of influenza A or B, given the current observed amantadine resistance for influenza A and amantadine's lack of activity against influenza B. Zanamivir is not currently recommended in the long-term care setting due to the potential risk of bronchospasm in persons with pre-existing respiratory disease and difficulty in using the inhaler device by some frail elderly. Oseltamivir should be used for prophylaxis in individuals who have experienced an adverse reaction on past exposure to amantadine or in those at high risk of experiencing an adverse reaction to amantadine.

In a long-term care setting, continue surveillance for new cases of ILI to establish effectiveness of antiviral prophylaxis in controlling an influenza outbreak once post-exposure prophylaxis is initiated in a facility. If amantadine is used, reports of amantadine-resistant strains of influenza A during outbreak situations demand change in therapy.

If cases of laboratory-confirmed influenza continue to occur more than 96 hours after initiation of antiviral prophylaxis, consider antiviral prophylaxis failure.[11] Contact the local Medical Officer of Health for assistance.

Treatment

Goals of Therapy

- Relieve influenza symptoms
- Reduce duration of influenza infection
- Reduce the potential for influenza-related complications
- Decrease influenza-related hospitalizations and deaths

Therapeutic Choices

Pharmacologic Choices

Analgesics/Antipyretic agents

Use **acetaminophen** or **ibuprofen** for relief of fever, headache and myalgias. To avoid overdose, caution patients about the concurrent use of cough and cold products that contain acetaminophen or ibuprofen.[12] Cough and cold products contain other ingredients such as antihistamines, which may not be needed.

Children and adolescents less than 18 years of age should *not* take ASA due to the associated risk of Reye's syndrome.

Antiviral Agents

Consider antiviral agents for treatment of influenza, when it is either laboratory confirmed or strongly suspected based on symptoms and known local circulation. The use of antiviral agents for treatment of influenza in the community setting is illustrated in Figure 2.

Studies in otherwise healthy adults taking a **neuraminidase inhibitor**[13] show a reduced duration of illness of 24 to 60 hours compared to placebo in otherwise healthy adults.[14,15,16,17,18,19,20] Early treatment with **oseltamivir** may reduce influenza complications (need for antibiotics, hospitalizations, asthma exacerbations).[21,22,23]

Amantadine is not currently recommended for treatment for influenza A due to increased resistance. When influenza A is sensitive to amantadine, simultaneous use of amantadine for prophylaxis and treatment within a facility, i.e. long-term care or nursing home, is not advised due to the increased risk of developing amantadine resistance.

Do not initiate treatment with any antiviral agent more than 48 hours after the onset of symptoms. The earlier antiviral treatment is started, the better the response.[14]

Do not continue treatment for more than five days. Five days is an adequate treatment period and it minimizes the risk of resistance, a particular concern with amantadine.

Therapeutic Tips

- Antivirals are not substitutes for the influenza vaccine for prevention of influenza.
- Influenza surveillance information can be obtained from the FluWatch program from the Public Health Agency of Canada (http://www.phac-aspc.gc.ca/fluwatch/index.html). Contact local Public Health authorities to determine if influenza is circulating in a specific community and if so, whether it is influenza A or B.
- Rapid identification of influenza in the long-term care setting allows timely implementation of control measures, thereby reducing influenza-related morbidity and mortality. Therefore, each facility should have a surveillance program in place to identify ILI, and policies and procedures regarding laboratory testing for ill residents. Staff should be familiar with the case definition of ILI.
- Consider another antiviral if there is a history of a severe adverse effect (e.g., hallucinations, seizures) with previous use of amantadine.

Figure 1: **Prevention and Control of Influenza in the Long-term Care Setting**

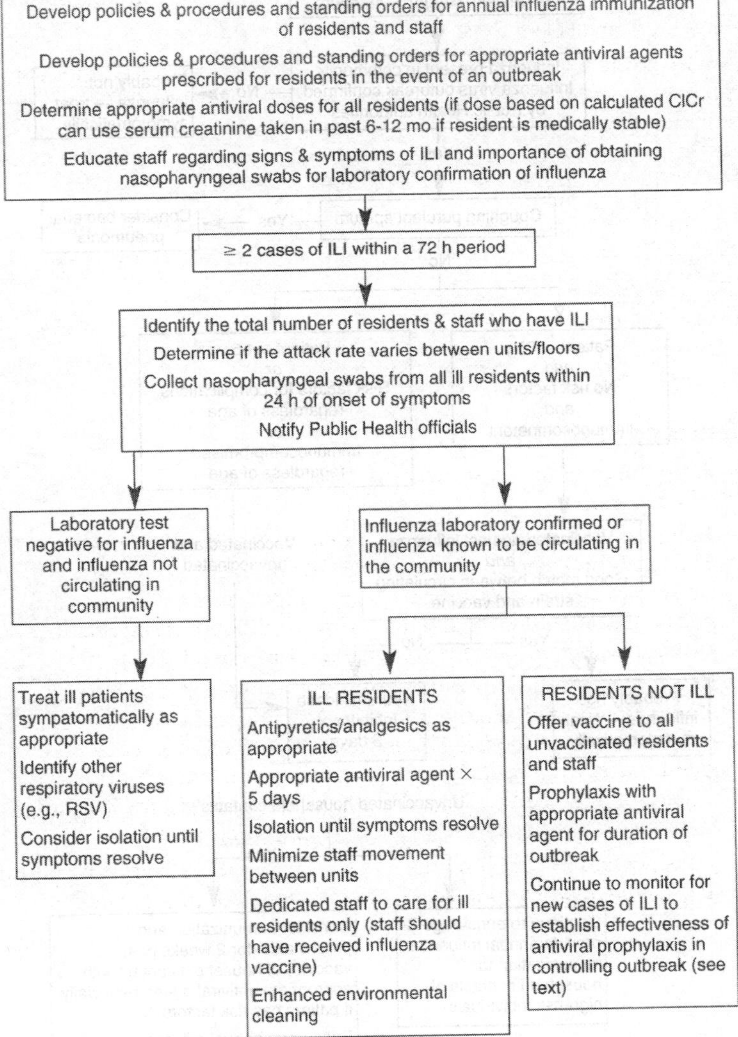

Adapted with permission from Gomolin IH, Kathpalia RK. Influenza. How to prevent and control nursing home outbreaks. *Geriatrics* 2002;57(1):30. Geriatrics is a copyrighted publication of Advanstar Communications Inc. All rights reserved.

Figure 2: **Treatment of Influenza-like Illness in the Community**

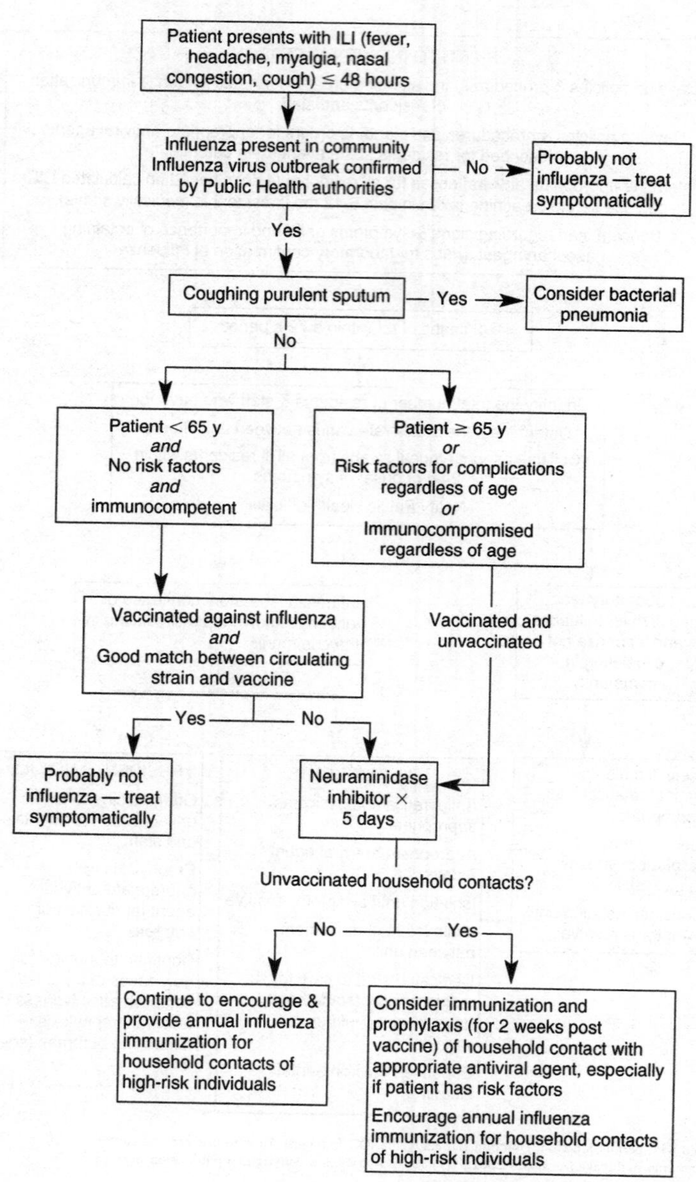

Permission granted by Myra Rudakewich – Adapted with permission from Stiver G. The treatment of influenza with antiviral drugs. *CMAJ* 2003;168(1):49-56.

Table 3: **Drugs Used for the Prevention and Treatment of Influenza**[7]

Class	Drug	Dose	Adverse Effects	Comments	Cost[a]
Antivirals, adamantane derivatives	*amantadine* Endantadine, Symmetrel, generics	Dose is based on age and renal function and is the same for treatment or prophylaxis. Duration of therapy for treatment is 5 days but is variable for prevention. *Treatment/Prevention:* 1–9 y: 5 mg/kg once daily or divided BID; max 150 mg/day 10–64 y: 200 mg once daily or divided BID. If < 40 kg, use dose as listed under 1–9 y. ↓ dose to 100 mg once daily in patients with seizure disorders. ≥ 65 y: 100 mg once daily When dosed according to renal function, the overall rate of adverse effects in elderly nursing home residents is 5–10%, with only 2% requiring discontinuation[7]	Confusion, nausea, vomiting, loss of appetite, ataxia, insomnia, seizures (most likely in those with pre-existing disorder).	Not recommended as treatment or prevention for influenza in the 2006–2007 season due to resistance.[7,8] Consider oseltamivir or zanamivir. Contraindicated if poorly controlled seizure disorders or past history of neuroleptic malignant syndrome. Consider another antiviral if history of severe adverse effects (hallucinations, seizures) with amantadine use. Simultaneous use of amantadine for prophylaxis and treatment within a LTC facility is not advised due to the increased risk of developing resistance. ↑ risk of CNS side effects: anticholinergic therapy. ↑ amantadine concentrations: triamterene, quinidine and quinine. Bupropion may ↑ risk of CNS toxicity and seizures. Consider use of another antiviral agent.	$

(cont'd)

Table 3: **Drugs Used for the Prevention and Treatment of Influenza**[7] *(cont'd)*

Class	Drug	Dose	Adverse Effects	Comments	Cost[a]
Antivirals, neuraminidase inhibitors	*oseltamivir* ◗ Tamiflu	*Treatment:* Adults: 75 mg BID × 5 days. If ClCr 10–30 mL/min: 75 mg once daily × 5 days *Treatment:* Children:[27, 28, b] ≤ 15 kg: 30 mg BID × 5 days > 15–23 kg: 45 mg BID × 5 days > 23–40 kg: 60 mg BID × 5 days > 40 kg: 75 mg BID × 5 days *Prevention:* Adults and children ≥ 13 y: 75 mg once daily. If ClCr 10–30 mL/min: 75 mg every other day *Prevention:* Children:[7] ≤ 15 kg: 30 mg once daily × 5 days > 15–23 kg: 45 mg once daily × 5 days > 23–40 kg: 60 mg once daily × 5 days > 40 kg: 75 mg once daily × 5 days Duration of prophylaxis is variable and is used for the duration of the outbreak	Nausea, vomiting, headache.	Effective for treatment and prevention against influenza A and B. Initiate treatment within 48 hours of exposure after close contact with an infected individual (> 48 hours if significantly immunocompromised with progressive respiratory infection).[29] Do not use if ClCr is < 10 mL/min.	$$-$$$

Class	Drug	Dose	Adverse Effects	Comments	Cost[a]
	zanamivir Relenza	*Treatment:* 10 mg (2 inhalations) BID × 5 days *Prevention* for ≥ 7 y: Household setting: 10 mg (2 inhalations) daily × 10 days Community outbreaks: 10 mg (2 inhalations) daily × 28 days	Bronchospasm has been reported, especially in patients with respiratory disease. Headache, dizziness, gastrointestinal upset, cough.	Effective for treatment and prophylaxis against influenza A and B. Initiate treatment within 48 hours of exposure after close contact with an infected individual (> 48 hours if significantly immunocompromised with progressive respiratory infection).[29] Do not use in patients with asthma or COPD due to risk of serious bronchospasm.	$$$
Vaccines, viral	*influenza vaccine, inactivated* Fluviral S/F, Fluzone, Influvac, Vaxigrip	Children 6 mo–8 y who have not previously received influenza vaccine should receive a second dose ≥ 1 mo after the first dose. *6–35 mo:* 0.25 mL im *36 mo–8 y:* 0.5 mL[b] im ≥ *9 y:* 0.5 mL im	Common: soreness at injection. Mild flu-like symptoms (myalgias, malaise, low-grade fever). Oculorespiratory syndrome (ORS; bilateral red eyes, breathing symptoms or facial swelling): not considered an allergic reaction. People who had mild or moderate cases of ORS, or severe ORS with non–lower respiratory symptoms can be re-immunized.[7,9] Consult the local Medical Officer of Health for advice on more severe reactions.	Pretreatment with acetaminophen may help minimize soreness and mild flu-like symptoms. Contraindicated in persons with history of anaphylactic reaction to a previous dose or eggs. Delay vaccination in adults with an acute febrile illness. Vaccine can be given to those with mild upper respiratory tract illness. Can be used in pregnant and nursing women.[7] Case reports of elevated theophylline blood levels following immunization and increased INR in patients taking warfarin. Monitor following vaccination.	$

[a] Cost of course of adult treatment; includes drug cost only.
[b] Reconstitute into oral suspension of 12 mg/mL.
Dosage adjustment may be required in renal dysfunction; see Appendix I.
Abbreviations: ClCr = creatinine clearance; LTC = long-term care; NACI = National Advisory Committee on Immunization
Legend: $ < $15 $$ $15–30 $$-$$$ $15–45 $$$ $30–45

Suggested Readings

Harper SA, Fukuda K, Uyeki TM et al. Prevention and control of influenza. Recommendations of the Advisory Committee on Immunization Practices (ACIP). *MMWR Recomm Rep* 2005;54(RR-8):1-40.

Moscona A. Neuraminidase inhibitors for influenza. *N Engl J Med* 2005;353(13):1363-73.

National Advisory Committee on Immunization (NACI). Statement on influenza vaccination for the 2006-2007 season. An Advisory Committee Statement (ACS). *Can Commun Dis Rep* 2006;32(ACS-7):1-27.

Stiver G. The treatment of influenza with antiviral drugs. *CMAJ* 2003;168(1):49-56

References

1. Public Health Agency of Canada. *FluWatch. Definitions for the 2006-2007 season.* Ottawa (ON): Public Health Agency of Canada; 2007. Available from: http://www.phac-aspc.gc.ca/fluwatch/06-07/def06-07_e.html Accessed April 5, 2007.
2. Boivin G, Hardy I, Tellier G et al. Predicting influenza infections during epidemics with use of a clinical case definition. *Clin Infect Dis* 2000;31(5):1166-9.
3. Monto AS, Gravenstein S, Elliott M et al. Clinical signs and symptoms predicting influenza infection. *Arch Intern Med* 2000;160(21):3243-7.
4. Cox NJ, Subbarao K. Influenza.*Lancet* 1999;354(9186):1277-82.
5. Govaert TM, Dinant GJ, Aretz K et al. The predictive value of influenza symptomatology in elderly people. *Fam Pract* 1998;15(1):16-22.
6. Gomolin IH, Leib HB, Arden NH et al. Control of influenza outbreaks in the nursing home: guidelines for diagnosis and management. *J Am Geriatr Soc* 1995;43(1):71-4.
7. National Advisory Committee on Immunization (NACI). Statement on influenza vaccination for the 2006-2007 season. An Advisory Committee Statement (ACS). *Can Commun Dis Rep* 2006;32(ACS-7):1-27.
8. Public Health Agency of Canada. *Recommendation for use of Amantadine for treatment and prevention of influenza.* Ottawa (ON): Public Health Agency of Canada; 2006. Available from: http://www.phac-aspc.gc.ca/media/nr-rp/2006/20061101-amantadine_e.htm Accessed April 5, 2007
9. [No authors listed]. Oculo-respiratory syndrome following influenza vaccination: review of post-marketing surveillance through four influenza seasons in Canada. *Can Commun Dis Rep* 2005;31(21):217-25.
10. Bright RA, Medina MJ, Xu X et al. Incidence of adamantane resistance among influenza A (H3N2) viruses isolated worldwide from 1994 to 2005: a cause for concern. *Lancet* 2005;366(9492):1175-81.
11. Bright RA, Shay DK, Shu B et al. Adamantane resistance among influenza A viruses isolated early during the 2005-2006 influenza season in the United States. *JAMA* 2006;295(8):891-4.
12. Bowles SK, Lee W, Simor AE et al. Use of oseltamivir during influenza outbreaks in Ontario nursing homes, 1999-2000. *J Am Geriatr Soc* 2002;50(4):608-16.
13. Carman WF, Elder AG, Wallace LA et al. Effects of influenza vaccination of health-care workers on mortality of elderly people in long-term care: a randomised controlled trial. *Lancet* 2000;355(9198):93-7.
14. Stiver G. The treatment of influenza with antiviral drugs. *CMAJ* 2003;168(1):49-56.
15. Aoki FY, Macleod MD, Paggiaro P et al. Early administration of oral oseltamivir increases the benefits of influenza treatment. *J Antimicrob Chemother* 2003;51(1):123-9.
16. Hayden FG, Osterhaus AD, Treanor JJ et al. Efficacy and safety of the neuraminidase inhibitor zanamivir in the treatment of influenzavirus infections. GG167 Influenza Study Group. *N Engl J Med* 1997; 337(13):874-80.
17. Lalezari J, Campion K, Keene O et al. Zanamivir for the treatment of influenza A and B infection in high-risk patients: a pooled analysis of randomized controlled trials. *Arch Intern Med* 2001;161(2):212-7.
18. Makela MJ, Pauksens K, Rostila T et al. Clinical efficacy and safety of the orally inhaled neuraminidase inhibitor zanamivir in the treatment of influenza: a randomized, double-blind, placebo-controlled European study. *J Infect* 2000;40(1):42-8.
19. Monto AS, Fleming DM, Henry D et al. Efficacy and safety of the neuraminidase inhibitor zanamivirin the treatment of influenza A and B virus infections. *J Infect Dis* 1999;180(2):254-61.

20. Nicholson KG, Aoki FY, Osterhaus AD et al. Efficacy and safety of oseltamivir in treatment of acute influenza: a randomised controlled trial. Neuraminidase Inhibitor Flu Treatment Investigator Group. *Lancet* 2000;355(9218):1845-50.
21. Treanor JJ, Hayden FG, Vrooman PS et al. Efficacy and safety of the oral neuraminidase inhibitor oseltamivir in treating acute influenza: a randomized controlled trial. US Oral Neuraminidase Study Group. *JAMA* 2000;283(8):1016-24.
22. Kaiser L, Wat C, Mills T et al. Impact of oseltamivir treatment on influenza-related lower respiratory tract complications and hospitalizations. *Arch Intern Med* 2003;163(14):1667-72.
23. Machado CM, Boas LS, Mendes AV et al. Use of oseltamivir to control influenza complications after bone marrow transplantation. *Bone Marrow Transplant* 2004;34(2):111-4.
24. Johnston SL, Ferrero F, Garcia ML et al. Oral oseltamivir improves pulmonary function and reduces exacerbation frequency for influenza-infected children with asthma. *Pediatr Infect Dis J* 2005;24(3):225-32.
25. Togo Y, Hornick RB, Felitti VJ et al. Evaluation of therapeutic efficacy of amantadine in patients with naturally occurring A2 influenza. *JAMA* 1970;211(7):1149-56.
26. Wingfield WL, Pollack D, Grunert RR. Therapeutic efficacy of amantadine HCl and rimantadine HCl in naturally occurring influenza A2 respiratory illness in man. *N Engl J Med* 1969;281(11):579-84.
27. Oo C, Barrett J, Hill G et al. Pharmacokinetics and dosage recommendations for an oseltamivir oral suspension for the treatment of influenza in children. *Paediatr Drugs* 2001;3(3):229-36.
28. Oo C, Hill G, Dorr A, Liu B, Boellner S, Ward P. Pharmacokinetics of anti-influenza prodrug oseltamivir in children aged 1-5 years. *Eur J Clin Pharmacol* 2003;59(5-6):411-5.
29. Allen UD, Aoki FY, Stiver HG. The use of antiviral drugs for influenza: recommended guidelines for practitioners. *Can J Infect Dis Med Microbiol* 2006;17(5):273-84. Available from: http://www.pulsus.com/Infdis/17_05/Pdf/Allen.pdf Accessed April 5, 2007.

CHAPTER 98
Community-acquired Pneumonia

Thomas J. Marrie, MD, FRCPC

Community-acquired pneumonia (CAP) is a common and a serious illness. While most (about 80%) cases are treated at home, the mortality rate among those requiring hospitalization is 8–10% and up to 40% for those requiring treatment in an intensive care unit.[1] In general, the clinical presentation of CAP does not allow for an etiologic diagnosis. Many microorganisms can cause CAP (Table 1).

Table 1: Common Pathogens in Community-acquired Pneumonia[2,a]

Pneumonia treated on an ambulatory basis
Streptococcus pneumoniae *Mycoplasma pneumoniae* *Haemophilus influenzae* *Chlamydophila pneumoniae* Respiratory viruses[b] *Moraxella catarrhalis*
Pneumonia requiring admission to hospital ward
Streptococcus pneumoniae *Chlamydophila pneumoniae* *Haemophilus pneumoniae* *Legionella* spp. Aspiration Gram-negative bacilli, e.g., *Escherichia coli*, *Klebsiella* spp., *Enterobacter* spp., *Serratia* spp., *Pseudomonas aeruginosa* Mixed or polymicrobial etiology, e.g., viral *plus* bacterial Respiratory viruses[b] *Mycoplasma pneumoniae*
Pneumonia requiring admission to hospital ICU
Streptococcus pneumoniae *Staphylococcus aureus* *Legionella* spp. Gram-negative bacilli (e.g., *Escherichia coli*, *Klebsiella* spp., *Enterobacter* spp., *Serratia* spp., *Pseudomonas aeruginosa*) *Haemophilus influenzae*

[a] Stratification for severity of illness based on ambulatory or hospital site of care. Pathogens within each stratification are listed in decreasing order of frequency of occurrence.
[b] Influenza A and B, adenovirus, parainfluenza, respiratory syncytial virus.
Abbreviations: ICU = intensive care unit
Adapted from Mandell LA, Wunderink RG, Anzueto A et al. Infectious Diseases Society of America/American Thoracic Society consensus guidelines on the management of community-acquired pneumonia in adults. *Clin Infect Dis* 2007;44(Suppl 2):S27-72.

Each microbe can result in an illness that spans the spectrum from mild to life-threatening disease. *Streptococcus pneumoniae* accounts for about 50% of all cases of CAP that require hospital admission.[1]

This chapter addresses treatment and prevention of community-acquired pneumonia.

Goals of Therapy

- Assess severity of pneumonia. The pneumonia-specific severity of illness score guides the appropriate location for treatment, i.e., home, hospital ward or *intensive care unit* (Table 2). Alternatively, consider the functional status of the patient in the week or two prior to admission. For patients who are fully functional, walking with assistance, wheelchair bound and bedridden, the mortality rate is 4%, 5.6%, 20% and 25%, respectively[3]
- Eradicate infecting pathogen
- Relieve symptoms such as fever, cough, pleuritic chest pain, sputum production and/or dyspnea
- Promptly recognize and minimize complications such as metastatic infection (meningitis, purulent pericarditis, endocarditis, osteomyelitis), empyema, cavitation, pneumothorax, septic shock, respiratory failure and/or worsening of comorbid conditions (ischemic heart disease, diabetes mellitus)
- Provide compassionate end-of-life care if this emerges

Investigations

- History and physical examination with particular attention to:
  - symptoms: cough, shortness of breath, pleuritic chest pain, hemoptysis, sputum production, fever, chills, myalgia, headache, arthralgia, confusion (new onset may be common in the elderly)

    Check patients with ongoing fever (oral temperature > 37.5°C) for empyema. Perform drainage early. Drug fever should be kept in mind and the diagnosis reconsidered
  - history of recent travel and other risk factors for pneumonia such as tobacco smoking; excessive alcohol ingestion; hobbies such as exploring old caves; recent loss of consciousness; comorbid illnesses. Some of these risk factors may influence recovery from pneumonia
  - physical findings: general appearance, e.g., respiratory distress, well or chronically ill or acutely ill. Rales, crackles, wheezes, findings of consolidation of pulmonary tissue (dullness to percussion, increased tactile and vocal fremitus, bronchial breathing, whispered pectoriloquy), pleural friction rub, altered mental status
- Objective measurements:
  - vital signs: respiratory rate ≥ 30 breaths/min is the single most sensitive and specific sign of severe pneumonia in adults

- oxygenation status: measure oxygen saturation in all patients with CAP presenting to emergency. If oxygen saturation < 92% in a COPD patient, perform arterial blood gas
- chest radiograph: posterior-anterior and lateral views. Consider a CT scan of the chest in all those who have a negative chest radiograph but clinically suspect pneumonia

- Laboratory tests for patients presenting to emergency with CAP:
  - electrolytes, glucose, BUN, creatinine, CBC and differential white blood cell count
  - blood cultures: two samples drawn at separate sites. Anaerobic culture is generally not necessary
  - sputum for Gram stain and culture. Confirm sputum sample is from the lower respiratory tract (< 10 squamous epithelial cells/low power field). Special requests such as culture for *Mycobacterium tuberculosis*, Legionella, fungi such as *Blastomyces dermatiditis* or Cryptococcus are dictated by the clinical setting. A microbiologist should be consulted.
  - urine for Legionella antigen (will only detect serogroup 1 infections), if high clinical suspicion for Legionnaires' disease or for patients who require ICU admission because of progressive pneumonia. If available, use PCR test on sputum or other respiratory secretions that can amplify DNA of all Legionella species
  - consider rapid or culture tests for influenza
  - consider serologic studies as dictated by clinical setting, e.g., suspected *Mycoplasma pneumoniae* pneumonia. Obtain an acute or a 10- to 14-day convalescent phase serum sample. If Legionnaires' disease is suspected, collect a convalescent phase sample six weeks following acute phase sample. Hantavirus infection and Q fever (*Coxiella burnetii*) are best diagnosed serologically
  - for patients admitted to hospital and who undergo bronchoalveolar lavage in addition to routine testing samples, some laboratories have the capacity to use nucleic acid amplification tests to detect nucleic acid of Legionella spp, *M. pneumoniae*, Influenza A and B, respiratory syncytial virus, adenovirus, human metapneumovirus, parainfluenza viruses, coronaviruses, rhinoviruses

Treatment of Community-acquired Pneumonia

Therapeutic Choices

Pharmacologic Choices

Successful management of pneumonia (Figure 1) is based on an accurate assessment of illness severity (Table 2) and selection of the most appropriate site for treatment.[2]

Table 2: **Pneumonia-specific Severity of Illness (PSI) Score**

Patient characteristic	Points assigned
Males	age (years)
Females	age (years) minus 10
Nursing home resident	10
Comorbid illness	
Neoplastic disease	30
Liver disease	20
Congestive heart failure	10
Cerebrovascular disease	10
Renal disease	10
Physical examination findings	
Altered mental status	20
Respiratory rate ≥ 30 breaths/min	20
Systolic blood pressure < 90 mm Hg	20
Temperature < 35°C or ≥ 40°C	15
Pulse ≥ 125 beats/min	10
Laboratory findings	
Arterial pH < 7.35	30
Blood urea nitrogen > 11 mmol/L	20
Sodium < 130 mmol/L	20
Glucose ≥ 14 mmol/L	10
Hematocrit < 30%	10
Partial pressure of arterial oxygen < 60 mm Hg	10
Pleural effusion	10

Reproduced with permission from Fine MJ, Auble TE, Yealy DM et al. A prediction rule to identify low-risk patients with community-acquired pneumonia. *N Engl J Med* 1997;336(4):243-50. Copyright © 1997 Massachusetts Medical Society. All rights reserved.

The PSI score is designed to predict mortality rates among patients with CAP and is a validated tool for determining the need for admitting patients to hospital.[5,6] If the score is ≤ 90, treat as outpatient. Some patients in this category may require hospital admission (see Figure 1). If the PSI score is ≥ 91, treat in hospital. However, physician judgment is paramount in the assessment of any patient and should always override any scoring system.

Initial empiric antibiotic therapy is based on the likely causative pathogen after considering specific risk factors for each patient (e.g., COPD, smoking). Tailor the antibiotic therapy, once the etiology is established

(Table 3). Antibiotics used in the treatment of CAP are described in Table 4.

Table 3: Antibiotic Therapy for Community-acquired Pneumonia Caused by Specific Pathogens[2]

Streptococcus pneumoniae

Penicillin nonresistant (MIC < 2 mg/L)

Initial therapy: penicillin G, amoxicillin.

Alternatives: macrolide, **po** cephalosporins (cefprozil, cefuroxime), **iv** cephalosporins (cefuroxime, ceftriaxone, cefotaxime), clindamycin, doxycycline, respiratory fluoroquinolones[a]

Penicillin resistant (MIC ≥ 2 mg/L)

Initial therapy: cefotaxime, ceftriaxone, po or iv fluoroquinolone.

Alternatives: vancomycin, linezolid, high-dose amoxicillin (3 g/day for penicillin MIC ≤ 4 mg/L)

Haemophilus influenzae

2nd or 3rd generation cephalosporin or amoxicillin/clavulanate, fluoroquinolones, azithromycin, clarithromycin. Amoxicillin monotherapy if non-beta-lactamase producing.

Staphylococcus aureus

Methicillin-susceptible: cloxacillin, cefazolin, clindamycin

Methicillin-resistant: vancomycin, linezolid, sulfamethoxazole/trimethoprim

Legionella species (*Legionnaires' disease*)

Fluoroquinolones or azithromycin, or doxycycline (alternative)

Mycoplasma pneumoniae, Chlamydophila pneumoniae

Macrolides or tetracyclines, fluoroquinolones (alternative)

Coxiella burnetii (Q fever)

Doxycycline, fluoroquinolones, macrolides (alternative—although some strains may be resistant)

Aerobic gram-negative bacilli (e.g., *Escherichia coli*, *Enterobacter* spp., *Klebsiella* spp., *Serratia* spp, *Proteus* spp.)

2nd or 3rd generation cephalosporin, carbapenem[b] (some *Enterobacter* spp. and uncommon strains of *E. coli* and *Klebsiella* spp. produce cephalosporinases and initial therapy should be with cefoxitin or piperacillin/tazobactam)

Pseudomonas aeruginosa

Antipseudomonal beta-lactam[c] *plus* ciprofloxacin or levofloxacin (750 mg) or aminoglycoside, aminoglycoside *plus* ciprofloxacin or levofloxacin (750 mg)

[a] Respiratory fluoroquinolones: levofloxacin, moxifloxacin.
[b] Carbapenem: imipenem/cilastatin, meropenem, ertapenem.
[c] Antipseudomonal beta-lactam: ticarcillin, piperacillin, ceftazidime, cefepime, aztreonam, imipenem, meropenem.

Knowledge of local susceptibility patterns of bacteria (e.g., *S. pneumoniae*) aids in tailoring empiric antibiotic therapy. In 2005 in Canada, 15.1% of 2488 isolates of *S. pneumoniae* were not susceptible to penicillin; 10.5% were intermediate (MIC > 0.12 to 1 mg/L) and 4.6% of *S. pneumoniae* isolates were resistant (MIC ≥ 2 mg/L) compared to 6.5% in 2002.[4] Further, 19% of *S. pneumoniae* isolates were macrolide-resistant (versus 13.9% in 2002), 2.3% were resistant to ciprofloxacin (MIC ≥ 4 mg/L).[4] Knowledge of local epidemiologic patterns such as outbreaks or endemic foci of Legionella species, *Coxiella burnetii*, Hantavirus, *Cryptococcus neoformans* and dimorphic fungi such as Histoplasma, Blastomyces and Coccidiomyces is helpful in tailoring antibiotic and/or antifungal therapy.

Duration of Antibiotic Therapy

For patients who are well enough to be treated on an ambulatory basis, a minimum of a 5-day course of antibiotic therapy is usually adequate.[2] Patients who are hospitalized and who respond to treatment within 48 hours can be treated with 10 days of antibiotics.[1] In some patients, a 3-day course is as effective as an 8-day course.[7] Specific etiologies may require longer treatment such as 21 days for severe Legionnaires' disease, 14 days for bacteremic aerobic gram-negative bacilli pneumonia and up to 21 days for pneumonia caused by *Pseudomonas aeruginosa*.[1]

Aspiration Pneumonia

Aspiration pneumonia denotes two distinct clinical entities. The first is *aspiration pneumonitis*, which is aspiration of gastric contents (usually sterile as long as there is gastric acid present) into the lungs with a resultant inflammatory response. The second is pneumonia resulting from the aspiration of oropharyngeal flora into the lung with resultant bacterial infection. Risk factors for aspiration include altered level of consciousness, incompetent gastroesophageal junction, elevated intragastric pressure or volume, affected swallowing mechanisms secondary to neurologic diseases and interference of glottic closure because of neuromuscular diseases.

Younger patients, in general, aspirate due to altered level of consciousness (seizures, drugs, alcohol) and older patients aspirate due to neurologic diseases that affect the swallowing mechanism. Patients with aspiration pneumonia require admission to ICU more commonly than those with CAP due to other causes.

Aspiration pneumonitis does not require antibiotic therapy. Patients with aspiration pneumonia who have poor dental hygiene or putrid sputum or who are alcoholics (anaerobic infection suspected), should be treated with metronidazole, clindamycin, beta-lactam/beta-lactamase inhibitor combinations, carbapenems and fluoroquinolones with established anaerobic activity (e.g., moxifloxacin). Treat patients, without these specific risk factors for anaerobic infection, with standard antibiotics (Figure 1).

Methicillin-resistant Staphylococcus aureus (MRSA) Pneumonia[8]

Methicillin-resistant *S. aureus*, an uncommon yet emerging cause of CAP, accounts for 1 to 5% of cases. MRSA pneumonia is more common in patients with severe pneumonia who require treatment in an intensive care unit and among residents in long-term care facilities. *S. aureus*, both methicillin-sensitive (MSSA) and MRSA, is about the third most frequent cause of bacteremic pneumonia in the community. *S. aureus* pneumonia has classically been described as a secondary bacterial pathogen in the setting of a primary influenza virus upper respiratory tract infection.[9,10,11] In the setting of bacteremic *S. aureus* pneumonia, exclude endocarditis (often right sided), especially if multiple rounded opacities are present on the chest radiograph (septic emboli). More recently, community-acquired MRSA infections have been caused by strains producing the Panton-Valentine leukocidin, known to be associated with tissue necrosis. To date, PVL *S. aureus* infections including pneumonia have been more common in young patients.[12,13] **Vancomycin** and **linezolid** are effective choices.[14]

Prevention of Community-acquired Pneumonia

Smoking Cessation

Encourage smoking cessation. Tobacco smoking is associated with a two-fold increase in risk for invasive pneumococcal pneumonia.[15] It is likely that cessation of tobacco smoking will reduce the rate of pneumonia, but there are no data from clinical trials. Nevertheless, this recommendation is likely to have many benefits, including slowing the age-related decline in lung function and reducing the risk of lung cancer.

Vaccines

Influenza Vaccine[16,17]

Yearly influenza vaccination of the elderly reduces the rate of admission to hospital for both pneumonia and congestive heart failure.[18] Hospitalized patients with CAP demonstrated improved survival from prior vaccination.[19] Immunization of health care workers against influenza reduces mortality rate due to influenza in patients.[20] (see Chapter 97)

Pneumococcal Vaccine[21,22]

Currently, there is a 23-valent capsular polysaccharide vaccine available for use in adults. The most common capsular polysaccharide types of *S. pneumoniae* causing bacteremic pneumonia are represented in the vaccine. A booster dose is given five years after the first dose. A polysaccharide-protein conjugate vaccine is currently undergoing clinical trials, and may be more effective. A protein conjugate vaccine is available for use in children and its widespread use has resulted in a reduction in invasive pneumococcal disease amongst adults.

Prevention of Aspiration Pneumonia

For patients at risk of aspiration, the "chin down" posture has been found to reduce the occurrence of aspiration both before and during the swallow. This posture results in a posterior shift of the anterior pharyngeal structures, narrowing the laryngeal entrance while widening the angle of the epiglottis to the anterior tracheal wall. The end result is protection of the airway. Cleaning of the teeth and gingiva by caregivers after each meal reduced the latency time of the swallowing reflex and increased substance P in the saliva of patients with dysphagia due to cerebrovascular disease. Substance P stimulates the neural pathways to improve the swallowing reflex.

Therapeutic Tips

- Administer antibiotic therapy to patients presenting to emergency room with pneumonia *as soon as possible* after diagnosis. A significantly lower mortality was noted for patients ≥ 65 years who received antibiotics within 4–8 hours of presentation.[23,24]
- Administer an agent from a different therapeutic class if the patient has received antibiotics within the three months prior to diagnosis of CAP.
- Because of its lowered activity against *H. influenzae*, **erythromycin** *monotherapy* is not routinely recommended in patients with COPD.
- Switch patients from intravenous to an oral antibiotic when the following criteria are met:[2,25,26] GI tract is functioning normally (e.g., no vomiting, diarrhea or disorder compromising GI absorption); hemodynamically stable; two temperature readings are normal (oral temperature < 37.5°C) over 16 hours in previously febrile patients; normalized white blood cell count; subjective improvement in cough and shortness of breath; able to consume oral medications. If blood cultures are positive, the duration of intravenous therapy is dictated by the organism recovered from the blood.
- Discharge the patient when the following criteria are met in addition to those above: absence of complications from the pneumonia (e.g., empyema); absence of complications from comorbid illnesses (e.g., myocardial infarction); absence of complications from treatment (e.g., severe adverse drug reactions); physiological stability as indicated by an oxygen saturation of ≥ 92% while breathing room air at sea level for those who do not have COPD (for patients with COPD, a return to baseline status is desirable), pulse rate of < 100 beats/minute and respiratory rate ≤ 24 breaths/minute.[2]
- Prevent recurrent pneumonia in patients ≥ 65 years and in those suffering from recurrent episodes. A checklist that includes a search for causes of aspiration and measures to prevent recurrent aspiration may be useful.
- Review pneumococcal and influenza vaccine status and immunize if indicated.
- If a pleural effusion is > 1 cm on a decubitus chest film with the affected side down, aspirate and send for pH, culture (aerobes, anaerobes, *M. tuberculosis*), white cell count, LDH and protein. A pH < 7.2 suggests the need for prompt drainage to avoid loculation and fibrotic pleural disease.

- Perform follow-up chest radiographs for *all tobacco smokers over age 35* and *all patients over age 50*. Two per cent of all patients with CAP will have lung cancer and, in half of these, the cancer is not diagnosed on the initial radiograph. Do the follow-up chest radiograph at the time of the follow-up visit, usually within two weeks of presentation. If the pneumonia has not cleared, a repeat film should be done in eight weeks; if the pneumonic opacity is still present, further investigation such as bronchoscopy may be warranted.

Figure 1: **Initial Management of Community-acquired Pneumonia (CAP)**

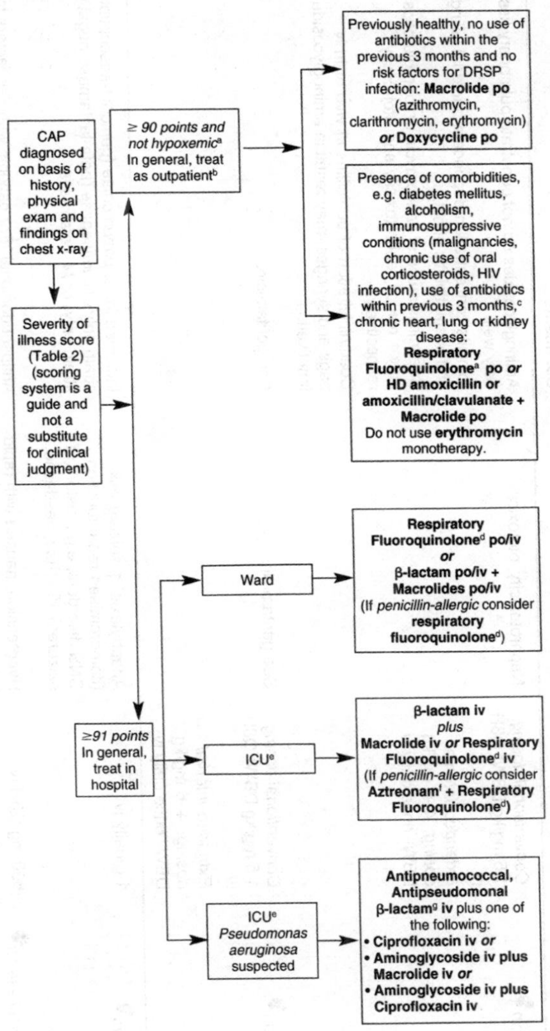

[a] Approximately 20% of patients in this category will require admission.[1]
[b] Psychosocial and medical factors, e.g., can reliably take oral medications, exacerbation of underlying disease (diabetes, COPD, heart failure), homelessness, may influence the decision to admit.
[c] For patients who have received an antibiotic within the past three months, use another class of antibiotics.
[d] Respiratory fluoroquinolone: moxifloxacin, levofloxacin. Gemifloxacin is currently not approved for CAP. For hospitalized patients, the dose of levofloxacin is 750 mg once daily for 5 to 7 days.
[e] Absolute indications for admittance into ICU: a) septic shock requiring vasopressors; b) acute respiratory failure requiring endotracheal intubation and mechanical ventilation.
[f] Aztreonam is available through the Special Access Programme, Therapeutic Products Directorate, Health Canada
[g] Cefepime, imipenem, meropenem, piperacillin/tazobactam.

Abbreviations: DRSP = drug-resistant *S. pneumoniae*; ICU = intensive care unit

Table 4: Antibiotics for the Treatment of Pneumonia

Drug Class	Drug	Dose	Adverse Effects	Comments	Cost[a]
Aminoglycosides	*gentamicin* generics	*Conventional dosing:* 1.5 mg/kg DBW[b] Q8H iv *Extended interval dosing:* 4–6 mg/kg DBW[b] once daily iv	Nephrotoxicity, ototoxicity.	Aminoglycosides *do not* penetrate pulmonary tissue very well. Exhibits concentration-dependent bacterial killing and postantibiotic effect. Coadministration of vancomycin or loop diuretics may ↑ risk of nephrotoxicity and ototoxicity, respectively. Coadministration of penicillins *in vivo* or in iv bags and syringes, may result in aminoglycoside inactivation.	$
	tobramycin generics	*Conventional dosing:* 1.5 mg/kg DBW[b] Q8H iv *Extended interval dosing:* 4–6 mg/kg DBW[b] once daily iv	See gentamicin.	See gentamicin.	$
Carbapenems	*ertapenem* Invanz	1 g daily iv	Anaphylaxis, ↑ seizure risk (compromised renal function, CNS disorders, e.g., history of seizures), diarrhea, headache.	Indicated for *S. pneumoniae* (penicillin-susceptible strain only), *H. influenzae* (beta-lactamase negative strain only) or *M. catarrhalis*.	$$$
	imipenem/ cilastatin Primaxin	500 mg Q6H iv	Hypotension, nausea with rapid infusion; seizure activity with high levels.	Antipseudomonal. For patients with risk factors for *P. aeruginosa*.	$$$$$

Drug Class	Drug	Dose	Adverse Effects	Comments	Cost[a]
	meropenem Merrem	1 g Q8H iv	Hypotension, nausea with rapid infusion; less likely than imipenem to cause seizures.	Antipseudomonal. For patients with risk factors for *P. aeruginosa*.	$$$$$
Cephalosporins, first-generation	*cefazolin* generics	1–2 g Q8H iv	Anaphylaxis, rash, gastrointestinal upset, renal and hepatic dysfunction, phlebitis and pain at site of im injection.		$-$$
Cephalosporins, second-generation	*cefaclor* generics	250 mg TID po	See cefazolin.		$
	cefprozil Cefzil, generics	500 mg BID po	See cefazolin.		$
	cefuroxime axetil Ceftin, generics	500 mg BID po	See cefazolin.	Do not use for treatment of penicillin-resistant *S. pneumoniae*.	$
	cefuroxime sodium Zinacef, generics	750 mg Q8H iv	See cefazolin.	Do not use for treatment of penicillin-resistant *S. pneumoniae*.	$
Cephalosporins, third-generation	*cefotaxime* Claforan	1–2 g Q8H iv	See cefazolin.	Can be used in hepatobiliary disease.	$$-$$$
	ceftazidime Ceftazidime for Injection USP, Fortaz	1–2 g Q8H iv	See cefazolin.		$$$-$$$$$
	ceftriaxone Rocephin	1–2 g Q24H iv	See cefazolin.		$$-$$$

(cont'd)

Table 4: **Antibiotics for the Treatment of Pneumonia** *(cont'd)*

Drug Class	Drug	Dose	Adverse Effects	Comments	Cost[a]
Cephalosporins, fourth-generation	*cefepime* Maxipime	1–2 g Q12H iv	See cefazolin.	Antipseudomonal; for patients with risk factors for *P. aeruginosa.*	$$$$
Fluoroquinolones	*ciprofloxacin* Cipro, generics	po: 500–750 mg BID iv: 400 mg Q12H	Gastrointestinal upset, headache, dizziness, photosensitivity, hepatitis. Cartilage toxicity: *avoid in children.*	Ciprofloxacin is *not* a first-line agent for CAP. Available as an oral suspension. Ciprofloxacin-resistant (MIC ≥ 4 mg/L) *S. pneumoniae* isolates in Canada in 2005 was 2.29%. Concomitant antacids, metal cations, sucralfate ↓ absorption of fluoroquinolones. Ciprofloxacin may ↓ theophylline or cyclosporine elimination; may prolong the INR if given with warfarin.	po: $ iv: $$$
	levofloxacin Levaquin, generics	po: 500 mg Q24H × 10 days *or* 750 mg Q24H × 5 days iv: 500 mg once daily	See ciprofloxacin.	Levofloxacin 750 mg daily for 5 days is equivalent to 500 mg daily for 10 days.[27] An alternative to β-lactam/macrolide combination for patients on hospital wards. Can switch from iv to po therapy while maintaining serum levels. Concomitant antacids, metal cations, sucralfate ↓ absorption of fluoroquinolones. May ↑ warfarin effect. Avoid in patients on Class Ia or III antiarrhythmics or with prolonged QT interval.	po: $ iv: $$

Drug Class	Drug	Dose	Adverse Effects	Comments	Cost[a]
	moxifloxacin Avelox	400 mg Q24H po/iv	See ciprofloxacin.	An alternative to β-lactam/macrolide combination for patients on hospital wards. Can switch from iv to po therapy while maintaining serum levels. Concomitant antacids, metal cations, sucralfate ↓ absorption of fluoroquinolones. Avoid in patients on Class Ia or III antiarrhythmics or with prolonged QT interval.	po: $ iv: $$$
Glycopeptides	*vancomycin* Vancocin, Vancomycin Hydrochloride USP Sterile, generics	1 g Q12H iv	Infusion-related adverse effects occur with shorter infusion times: intense flushing (red man or red neck syndrome), hypotension. Nephrotoxicity, ototoxicity.	For MRSA-pneumonia. Coadministration with aminoglycosides may ↑ risk of nephrotoxicity.	$$$$$
Ketolides	*telithromycin* Ketek	800 mg po daily × 7-10 days	Diarrhea, nausea, vomiting, elevated liver enzymes, hepatotoxicity.[28]	*Not considered first-line. Hepatotoxicity may be fatal.* ↑ telithromycin levels: atorvastatin, lovastatin, simvastatin, itraconazole, ketoconazole. ↑ digoxin levels Coadministration of pimozide and cisapride is contraindicated. Coadministration with ergot alkaloids is not recommended. Reports of exacerbation of myasthenia gravis with telithromycin,[29] therefore contraindicated.	$

(cont'd)

Table 4: **Antibiotics for the Treatment of Pneumonia** *(cont'd)*

Drug Class	Drug	Dose	Adverse Effects	Comments	Cost[a]
Lincosamides	*clindamycin* Dalacin C, Dalacin C Flavored Granules, Dalacin C Phosphate Solution Sterile, generics	300–450 mg Q6H po 600 mg Q8H iv	Abdominal pain, nausea, vomiting, diarrhea, *C. difficile* colitis.	Clindamycin-resistant *S. pneumoniae* isolates in Canada in 2005 was 8%.[4] For suspected aspiration; provides oral anaerobic coverage.	$
Macrolides	*azithromycin* Z-PAK, Zithromax, generics	po: 500 mg 1st day then 250 mg × 4 days iv: 500 mg daily × 7–10 days	Better tolerated than erythromycin. Gastrointestinal upset, rash, cholestatic hepatitis.	Oral azithromycin given daily × 5 days is equivalent to oral erythromycin QID × 10 days. A 5-day course of azithromycin is adequate for mild to moderate CAP. Azithromycin more active than clarithromycin for *H. influenzae*.	$
	clarithromycin Biaxin, Biaxin XL	Regular release: 500 mg BID po Extended release: 1000 mg po once daily	Better tolerated than erythromycin. Gastrointestinal upset, rash, cholestatic hepatitis.	Coadministration with pimozide is contraindicated. Rifampin: ↓ macrolide concentrations. May ↑ warfarin effect; ↑ concentrations of substrates of CYP3A4 (potent inhibitor) e.g., atorvastatin, carbamazepine, digoxin, lovastatin, simvastatin.	$
	erythromycin Erybid, Eryc, generics	500 mg QID po	Gastrointestinal upset, rash, cholestatic hepatitis.	See clarithromycin. Use cautiously with other drugs that cause QTc prolongation.	$
Nitroimidazoles	*metronidazole* Flagyl, generics	500 mg po/iv Q12H	Vertigo, headache, ataxia, gastrointestinal upset, taste alterations.	Concomitant intake of ethanol may lead to a disulfiram-like reaction; avoid alcohol until 48 hours after last dose of metronidazole.	$

Drug Class	Drug	Dose	Adverse Effects	Comments	Cost[a]
Oxazolidinones	*linezolid* Zyvoxam	600 mg Q12H po/iv	Gastrointestinal upset, headache, dose- and time-dependent bone marrow suppression, peripheral neuropathy, optic neuritis (rare).	Preferred agent for MRSA-pneumonia.[14,30] ↑ risk of serotonin toxicity with concomitant serotonergic drugs, e.g., selective serotonin reuptake inhibitors.[31,32]	$$$$$
Penicillins	*penicillin V potassium* generics	300 mg TID–QID po	Hypersensitivity reactions, rash, gastrointestinal upset, interstitial nephritis.		$
	penicillin G generics	2 million U Q4H iv	See penicillin V.		$
	amoxicillin generics	500 mg TID po	See penicillin V.	Consider high-dose amoxicillin if patient presents with drug-resistant *S. pneumoniae* risk factors.	$
	amoxicillin/ clavulanate Clavulin, generics	500/125 mg TID po *or* 875/125 mg BID	See penicillin V.	Consider high-dose amoxicillin/clavulanate if patient presents with drug-resistant *S. pneumoniae* risk factors.	$
	ampicillin generics	1 g Q6H iv	See penicillin V.		$
	cloxacillin generics	1 g Q6H iv	See penicillin V.		$
	piperacillin generics	3 g Q4H iv *or* 4 g Q6H iv	See penicillin V.		$$$$
	piperacillin/ tazobactam Tazocin	3 g/0.375 g Q6H iv	See penicillin V.	Antipseudomonal; for patients with risk factors for *P. aeruginosa.*	$$$$

(cont'd)

Table 4: **Antibiotics for the Treatment of Pneumonia** *(cont'd)*

Drug Class	Drug	Dose	Adverse Effects	Comments	Cost[a]
	ticarcillin/ clavulanate (renal adjustment symbol) Timentin	> 60 kg: 3.1 g Q4–6H iv < 60 kg: 200–300 mg/kg daily iv divided Q4–6H	Hypersensitivity, gastrointestinal upset.		$
Rifamycins	*rifampin* Rifadin, Rofact	300 mg BID po	Rash (petechial rash may suggest thrombocytopenia), orange discolouration of body fluids (contact lens staining), GI upset, liver toxicity, hematologic effects (e.g., thrombocytopenia).	*Should never be used as a single agent for CAP.* Induction of CYP isozymes resulting in many potential interactions. May ↓ levels of cyclosporine, tacrolimus, sirolimus, phenytoin, warfarin and oral contraceptives. Adjust dose of affected drug when rifampin is initiated or discontinued.	$
Sulfonamide Combinations	*sulfamethoxazole/ trimethoprim (SMX/TMP, cotrimoxazole)* (renal adjustment symbol) generics	800/160 mg BID po	Gastrointestinal upset, skin rash, Stevens-Johnson syndrome (rare).	May ↑ effect of sulfonylureas and warfarin. Use with caution in patients with G6PD deficiency, or impaired renal or hepatic function.	$
Tetracyclines	*doxycycline* Vibramycin, Vibra-tabs, generics	100 mg BID po 1st day then 100 mg daily	Gastrointestinal upset, photosensitivity.	Iron or antacids may ↓ doxycycline absorption. Alcohol, barbiturates, phenytoin, rifampin, carbamazepine may ↓ doxycycline levels.	$

[a] Cost of 1-day supply based on 6 foot male; includes drug cost only.

[b] In obese patients (> 30% ideal body weight [IBW]), use dosing body weight (DBW) instead of total body weight (TBW) to prevent overdosing. DBW = IBW + 0.4(TBW-IBW) where IBW (kg; males) = 50 + (2.3 × height in inches over 5 feet). IBW (kg; females) = 45.5 + (2.3 × height in inches over 5 feet).

(renal adjustment symbol) Dosage adjustment may be required in renal impairment; see Appendix I.

Legend: $ < $25 $-$$ < $25–50 $$ $25–50 $$-$$$ $25–75 $$$ $50–75 $$$$ $75–100 $$$-$$$$$ $50– >$100 $$$$$ > $100

Suggested Readings

Almirall J, Gonzalez CA, Balanzo X et al. Proportion of community-acquired pneumonia cases attributable to tobacco smoking. *Chest* 1999;116(2):375-9.

Mandell LA, Wunderink RG, Anzueto A et al. Infectious Diseases Society of America/American Thoracic Society consensus guidelines on the management of community-acquired pneumonia in adults. *Clin Infect Dis* 2007;44(Suppl 2):S27-72.

References

1. Marrie T, Campbell G, Walker D, Low D. Pneumonia. In: Kasper DL et al. *Harrison's principles of internal medicine*. 16th ed. New York (NY): McGraw-Hill; 2005. p.1528-41.
2. Mandell LA, Wunderink RG, Anzueto A et al. Infectious Diseases Society of America/American Thoracic Society consensus guidelines on the management of community-acquired pneumonia in adults. *Clin Infect Dis* 2007;44(Suppl 2):S27-72.
3. Marrie TJ, Wu L. Factors influencing in-hospital mortality in community-acquired pneumonia: a prospective study of patients not initially admitted to the ICU. *Chest* 2005;127(4):1260-70.
4. Canadian Bacterial Surveillance Network. *Annual report: 2005*. Toronto (ON): Mount Sinai Hospital, Department of Microbiology. Available from: http://microbiology.mtsinai.on.ca/research/cbsn/cbsnnews/cbsn-annual-report05.pdf Accessed April 4, 2007.
5. Lin CC, Lee CH, Chen CZ et al. Value of the pneumonia severity index in assessment of community-acquired pneumonia. *J Formos Med Assoc* 2005;104(3):164-7.
6. Renaud B, Coma E, Labarere J et al. Routine use of the Pneumonia Severity Index for guiding the site-of-treatment decision of patients with pneumonia in the emergency department: a multicenter, prospective, observational, controlled cohort study. *Clin Infect Dis* 2007;44(1):41-9.
7. el Moussaoui R, de Borgie CA, van den Broek P et al. Effectiveness of discontinuing antibiotic treatment after three days versus eight days in mild to moderate-severe community acquired pneumonia: randomised, double blind study. *BMJ* 2006;332(7554):1355.
8. Soderquist B, Berglund C, Stralin K. Community-acquired pneumonia and bacteremia caused by an unusual methicillin-resistant Staphylococcus aureus (MRSA) strain with sequence type 36, staphylococcal cassette chromosome mec type IV and Panton-Valentine leukocidin genes. *Eur J Clin Microbiol Infect Dis* 2006;25(9):604-6.
9. Adam H, McGeer A, Simor A. Fatal case of post-influenza, community-associated MRSA pneumonia in an Ontario teenager with subsequent familial transmission. *CCDR* 2007; 33(4):45-48.
10. Frazee BW, Salz TO, Lambert L et al. Fatal community-associated methicillin-resistant Staphylococcus aureus pneumonia in an immunocompetent young adult. *Ann Emerg Med* 2005;46(5):401-4.
11. Hageman J, Uyeki T, Francis J et al. Severe community-acquired pneumonia due to *Staphylococcus aureus*, 2003-2004 influenza season. *Emerg Infect Dis* 2006;12:894–899.
12. Gillet Y, Issartel B, Vanhems P et al. Association between Staphylococcus aureus strains carrying gene for Panton-Valentine leukocidin and highly lethal necrotising pneumonia in young immunocompetent patients. *Lancet* 2002; 359(9308):753-9.
13. Francis JS, Doherty MC, Lopatin U et al. Severe community-onset pneumonia in healthy adults caused by methicillin-resistant Staphylococcus aureus carrying the Panton-Valentine leukocidin genes. *Clin Infect Dis* 2005 Jan 1;40(1):100-7.
14. Barton M, Hawkes M, Moore D et al. Guidelines for the prevention and management of community-associated methicillin-resistant Staphylococcus aureus: a perspective for Canadian health care practitioners. *Can J Infect Dis Med Microbiol* 2006;17(Suppl C):4C-24C. Available from: http://www.pulsus.com/infdis/17_SC/Pdf/mrsa_ed.pdf Accessed April 4, 2007.
15. Nuorti JP, Butler JC, Farley MM et al. Cigarette smoking and invasive pneumococcal disease. Active Bacterial Core Surveillance Team. *N Engl J Med* 2000;342(10):681-9.
16. Voordouw BC, Sturkenboom MC, Dieleman JP et al. Annual influenza vaccination in community-dwelling elderly individuals and the risk of lower respiratory tract infections or pneumonia. *Arch Intern Med* 2006;166(18):1980-5.
17. National Advisory Committee on Immunization (NACI). Statement on influenza vaccination for the 2006-2007 season. An Advisory Committee Statement (ACS). *Can Commun Dis Rep* 2006;32(ACS-7):1-27.
18. Nichol KL, Nordin J, Mullooly J et al. Influenza vaccination and reduction in hospitalizations for cardiac disease and stroke among the elderly. *N Engl J Med* 2003;348(14):1322-32.
19. Spaude KA, Abrutyn E, Kirchner C et al. Influenza vaccination and risk of mortality among adults hospitalized with community-acquired pneumonia. *Arch Intern Med* 2007;167(1):53-9.

20. Carman WF, Elder AG, Wallace LA et al. Effects of influenza vaccination of health-care workers on mortality of elderly people in long-term care: a randomised controlled trial. *Lancet* 2000;355(9198):93-7.
21. Fisman DN, Abrutyn E, Spaude KA et al. Prior pneumococcal vaccination is associated with reduced death, complications, and length of stay among hospitalized adults with community-acquired pneumonia. *Clin Infect Dis* 2006;42(8):1093-101.
22. Sisk JE, Moskowitz AJ, Whang W et al. Cost-effectiveness of vaccination against pneumococcal bacteremia among elderly people. *JAMA* 1997;278(16):1333-9.
23. Houck PM, Bratzler DW, Nsa W et al. Timing of antibiotic administration and outcomes for Medicare patients hospitalized with community-acquired pneumonia. *Arch Intern Med* 2004;164(6):637-44.
24. Meehan TP, Fine MJ, Krumholz HM et al. Quality of care, process, and outcomes in elderly patients with pneumonia. *JAMA* 1997;278(23):2080-4.
25. Ramirez JA, Srinath L, Ahkee S et al. Early switch from intravenous to oral cephalosporins in the treatment of hospitalized patients with community-acquired pneumonia. *Arch Intern Med* 1995;155(12):1273-6.
26. Oosterheert JJ, Bonten MJ, Schneider MM et al. Effectiveness of early switch from intravenous to oral antibiotics in severe community acquired pneumonia: multicentre randomised trial. *BMJ* 2006;333(7580):1193.
27. Dunbar LM, Wunderink RG, Habib MP et al. High-dose, short-course levofloxacin for community-acquired pneumonia: a new treatment paradigm. *Clin Infect Dis* 2003;37(6):752-60.
28. Clay KD, Hanson JS, Pope SD et al. Brief communication: severe hepatotoxicity of telithromycin: three case reports and literature review. *Ann Intern Med* 2006;144(6):415-20.
29. Perrot X, Bernard N, Vial C et al. Myasthenia gravis exacerbation or unmasking associated with telithromycin treatment. *Neurology*. 2006;67(12):2256-8.
30. Wunderink RG, Rello J, Cammarata SK et al. Linezolid vs vancomycin: analysis of two double-blind studies of patients with methicillin-resistant Staphylococcus aureus nosocomial pneumonia. *Chest* 2003;124(5):1789-97.
31. Lawrence KR, Adra M, Gillman PK. Serotonin toxicity associated with the use of linezolid: a review of postmarketing data. *Clin Infect Dis* 2006;42(11):1578-83.
32. Clark DB, Andrus MR, Byrd DC. Drug interactions between linezolid and selective serotonin reuptake inhibitors: case report involving sertraline and review of the literature. *Pharmacotherapy* 2006;26(2):269-76.

CHAPTER 99 Tuberculosis

Victoria J. Cook, MD, FRCPC and
J. Mark FitzGerald, MD, FRCPC

Goals of Therapy

- Prevent latent infection from progressing to clinically active disease
- Prevent person-to-person transmission by early diagnosis, appropriate infection control and initiation of treatment
- Treat active disease by eradicating *Mycobacterium tuberculosis* from the affected organ(s) and relieve symptoms (fever, sweats, weight loss, cough)
- Achieve cure without relapse; prevent complications; prevent development of drug resistance and death

Investigations[1,2,3,4,5,6,7]

- Thorough history with special attention to:
  - risk factors for acquisition of tuberculosis (TB), e.g., country of birth/origin, occupation, TB exposure, travel
  - risk factors for reactivation of latent infection, e.g., HIV/AIDS, recent TB infection, skin test conversion—previous or ≤ two years, predisposing medical conditions such as organ transplantation, end-stage renal disease, diabetes mellitus, hematologic malignancies, malnutrition, use of immunosuppressants (e.g., systemic corticosteroids, cancer chemotherapy), tumor necrosis-alpha (TNF-α) inhibitors, abnormal chest x-ray or silicosis
  - risk factors for drug resistance, e.g., previous treatment or previous drug-resistant disease, especially if not on directly observed therapy (DOT), noncompliance, HIV/AIDS, alcohol abuse, travel to or residence in countries with high prevalence of TB disease or high incidence of drug-resistant disease (e.g., countries of the former Soviet Union), contact with a patient with drug-resistant disease
  - *Mycobacterium bovis* bacillus Calmette-Guérin (BCG) vaccination, previous Mantoux (recommended method for intradermal tuberculin skin test) history and details of previous TB treatment
- Physical examination with special attention to:
  - nutritional status, fever, choroid tubercles, abnormal breath sounds, meningeal signs, erythema nodosum, adenopathy
  - concomitant diseases that may affect treatment, e.g., HIV/AIDS, chronic liver disease, chronic renal insufficiency
  - often unrewarding, especially for pulmonary TB
- Investigations:
  - chest x-ray (compare to old films if available)

- obtain three sputum specimens (collected once daily in the morning on three consecutive days) for acid fast bacilli (AFB) smear *and* mycobacterial culture; negative sputum smears do not preclude a diagnosis of active pulmonary TB (50% of the patients with TB have negative sputum smears)
- first morning-voided midstream urine for smear (usually negative) and culture if renal TB suspected
- lumbar puncture with bacterial and AFB smear (usually negative) and mycobacterial cultures plus TB DNA polymerase chain reaction (PCR) of cerebrospinal fluid if available, plus glucose, protein, white cell count and differential if meningitis is suspected. In patients with HIV/AIDS, cryptococcal antigen studies, viral culture and Rapid Plasma Reagin (RPR)
- baseline platelet count, creatinine, AST, ALT, alkaline phosphatase, bilirubin[8]
- counselling and testing for HIV infection is strongly recommended for all patients; if a patient is HIV-positive, document CD4 count and viral load after acute illness
- in HIV-positive persons, blood cultures and stool samples for mycobacteria may yield positive cultures (for both tuberculous and nontuberculous mycobacteria)

- Special procedures:
  - serial or repeated sputum induction in an appropriately ventilated room has a higher yield than bronchoscopy, with a lower risk of nosocomial transmission
  - fibre optic bronchoscopy +/- transbronchial biopsy, especially if miliary TB is a concern. A rapid diagnosis is possible if caseating granulomas or AFB are found on biopsy
  - gastric washings (fasting morning sample) may be positive in patients unable to produce sputum (40% effective)[9]
  - aspiration of pleural effusions for AFB smear (usually negative) and culture (positive in < 25% of specimens), chemical and cytological analysis. Diagnosis often requires pleural biopsy for culture and histology (positive 60%) via needle biopsy or video-assisted thoracic surgery (VATS)
  - a combination of culture and pleural biopsy improves diagnostic yield of mycobacterial cultures to 90%
  - nucleic acid amplification methods are commercially available to identify mycobacteria directly from sputum specimens (95% sensitivity, 98% specificity if smear positive; 48 to 53% sensitivity, 95% specificity if smear negative, culture positive). Confirms the diagnosis of TB but does not replace the need for routine AFB smear and culture[10,11]

- PCR for detection of mycobacteria in body fluids is used in some laboratories. Major advantage is rapid diagnosis, generally < 48 h and it is most useful in diagnosing meningeal TB

- *Mantoux test* (tuberculin skin test or TST) has three uses: diagnosis of infection, diagnosis of disease and as an epidemiologic tool (Figure 2). It should not be performed on persons with previous severe blistering tuberculin reactions, documented active or prior history of TB, extensive burns or eczema or a history of infections or vaccinations with live virus vaccines in the past month, e.g., mumps or measles
  - 48 to 72 hours after intradermal inoculation, the widest transverse diameter of induration (not erythema) is measured; routine anergy screening is not recommended
  - false negative tests can occur in seriously ill patients, who are often anergic, or with inappropriate technique/reading (e.g., drawing tuberculin material up in syringes more than 20 minutes before administration, significant exposure of tuberculin to sunlight). Patients' recall of test results is not reliable. Test results may vary by 15% between arms and between observers. A negative skin test should not preclude consideration of the diagnosis of TB. False negatives can also occur at the extremes of age
  - false positive tests can occur in patients with a history of BCG vaccination or exposure to nontuberculous mycobacteria and with inappropriate technique/reading. In general, a positive Mantoux > 15 years after BCG vaccination or > 15 mm induration should not be attributed to the vaccine, especially if the vaccine is given in infancy.[12] BCG vaccination status should not preclude the diagnosis of latent TB infection in the event of contact
  - reactivity to tuberculin antigen can diminish to nonreactivity with age
  - repeat Mantoux may boost reactivity. Thus, it is important in populations who are going to have serial Mantoux (e.g., nursing home residents, health care workers) to perform an initial two-step test to determine those whose response has waned over time. A second dose is administered one to three weeks after the first. Repeated skin testing will not induce a false-positive reaction but the initial test may stimulate the patient's ability to react to subsequent testing.
  - an in vitro diagnostic test, QuantiFERON-TB Gold (QFT-G), a whole blood interferon γ release assay, is now available to identify persons with latent TB and active TB infection; guidelines for the use of QFT-G are now available;[13] the precise role in at-risk populations (e.g., young children, HIV/AIDS) requires further evaluation. The T SPOT-TB, an enzyme-linked immunospot assay, is under review

- Maintain a high index of suspicion for TB in *immunocompromised* patients as manifestations of TB are atypical. Miliary disease is common, and sputum smears are often negative

Therapeutic Choices

All patients with known or suspected TB (usually pulmonary) should be hospitalized in a single negative pressure room and placed on respiratory precautions or isolated at home without high risk or new contacts. Discontinue isolation when consecutive sputum smears are negative for AFB on three separate days *and* there is evidence of adherence to an appropriate treatment regimen for a minimum of two weeks with clinical and radiographic response. Continue isolation in patients with pulmonary or laryngeal multiple drug-resistant TB for duration of hospital stay or until cultures are negative.

Proper *masks* (which filter particles one micron in size, have a 95% filter efficiency when tested in the unloaded state and provide a tight facial seal) should be worn when caring for patients with known or suspected TB. Surgical masks do not prevent the inhalation of droplet nuclei but are appropriate for infectious TB patients. All patients with a chest x-ray consistent with TB should be *isolated* pending results of sputum smear for AFB. The radiographic appearance of TB is variable in patients with HIV and may be normal (12%).

Notify the local Department of Health for contact tracing. Close *follow-up* is mandatory (initially, monthly visits and regular chest radiographs with a final chest x-ray at completion of treatment). Sputum smears and cultures for AFB should be followed monthly to monitor response to treatment and determine appropriate duration of treatment. *Directly observed therapy* (DOT) should be instituted. Failure to comply with therapy is the major reason for the marked increase in cases of multidrug-resistant TB (MDR-TB).

Nonpharmacologic Choices[5,6,7]

- Adequate nutrition is necessary to enhance healing and limit the chances of relapse.[14]
- BCG vaccine is not in general use in Canada (used in First Nations people in some jurisdictions) but continues to be used as a preventive measure against TB globally.[7,12]
- Discourage drinking of alcohol as it is a cofactor in drug-induced hepatitis.

Pharmacologic Choices (Table 1 and Table 2)

Directly Observed Therapy (DOT)[15]

DOT is the standard of care in the treatment of tuberculosis and improves treatment completion rates. DOT requires health professionals or trained individuals to watch the patients swallow the anti-TB drugs. The directly observed treatment, short-course strategy, recommended by WHO is a national case-based strategy which consists of five components: commitment of governments to a national tuberculosis program; case detection by at least sputum smear microscopy among symptomatic patients; a standardized treatment regimen for confirmed sputum smear–positive cases, with DOT for at least the initial two months; a regular, uninterrupted supply of all essential anti-TB drugs; and a standardized recording and reporting system that enables assessment of treatment results. Successful treatment of active TB is the responsibility of the patient, clinician, local department of health and government.

Latent Infection (Figure 1)[16]

Patients with latent TB infection (LTBI) have low numbers of tubercle bacilli in their bodies but do not have active disease. Compared to patients with active TB, they are asymptomatic and noninfectious. However, the risk of active disease in certain patient groups is high (e.g., HIV/AIDS, recent TB exposure, organ transplant recipients). Treatment of LTBI with a single drug can greatly reduce this risk. Rule out active TB prior to the initiation of treatment.

In general, patients with LTBI have a 10% risk of developing TB, and **isoniazid** (INH) can reduce this risk by over 90% in compliant patients. Offer treatment of LTBI for contacts, HIV-infected persons, organ transplant recipients and individuals with abnormal chest radiographs (e.g., apical fibrosis or granuloma) who have a positive Mantoux skin test of ≥ 5 mm.[13]

For those who have a positive Mantoux test (≥ 10 mm) and are in a lower-risk group (Figure 1), the risk of adverse effects from INH must be weighed against its benefit in reducing the risk of active disease. The risk of significant hepatitis increases with age and history of pre-existing liver disease; however, the risks of INH-related hepatitis has been overestimated and is 1 to 3 per 1000 person years.[8,17] Asymptomatic liver enzyme abnormalities (i.e., minor rises in transaminases 2–3 times normal) are common. For those with risk factors for reactivating dormant infection, age should not preclude offering LTBI treatment.

Isoniazid daily or twice weekly for nine months is the regimen of choice. If the source case may have been INH resistant or if the patient is unable to take INH, **rifampin** for four months may be substituted.[13,18] Short-course daily prophylaxis with **rifampin** and **pyrazinamide** for eight weeks is no longer recommended due to high rates of hospitalization and death due to liver injury.[19,20,21,22,23] The rate of moderate to severe liver injury using this regimen is 7.3%.[19,20,21,22,23] Consultation with a TB expert is recommended if rifampin ± pyrazinamide is used in the event of contact with drug-resistant patients. Highly intermittent (once weekly) treatment of LTBI is under investigation (e.g., INH and rifapentine once weekly for three months) but cannot presently be recommended.[24]

Baseline and monthly testing of transaminases is recommended for persons at risk for liver disease (e.g., alcohol use, HIV/AIDS).

Active Tuberculosis (Figure 2)[7,25,26,27,28]

Treat active TB with multiple drugs using DOT. Treatment usually begins with an initial (bactericidal or intensive) phase of two months to rapidly eliminate the majority of organisms and prevent emergence of drug resistance, followed by a continuation (sterilizing) phase of four to seven months to eradicate dormant organisms (Table 1). Knowledge of the local epidemiology of resistance is essential to appropriate treatment. Adjust therapy when susceptibility results are available (usually one to two months into therapy). Dose adjustments may be required for some patients (e.g., low BMI, renal insufficiency). Single drug therapy must never be used for active TB, nor should a single drug ever be added to a failing regimen. **Rifampin**-based short-course treatment (Table 1) is the standard of care. Response to treatment is monitored by culture of monthly sputum specimens for AFB smear and culture, repeated until two consecutive samples are negative. Repeat sensitivity testing is suggested if cultures are persistently positive after three months.

Research into alternative treatment includes respiratory quinolones (e.g., moxifloxacin as a substitute for INH in the intensive phase of treatment) and linezolid.[29,30] Despite widespread use of quinolones for nontuberculous respiratory infections, there is no indication at this time of resistance in *M. tuberculosis* isolates.[31]

For patients infected with fully susceptible organisms, **isoniazid**, **rifampin**, and **pyrazinamide** should be given for the intensive phase of two months followed by isoniazid and rifampin for the continuation phase of four months. This is the standard short-course regimen to treat active TB. This regimen can be used for empiric therapy in areas where there is no INH resistance. Twice-weekly DOTS with a rifampin-containing regimen can be given after an initial daily intensive phase or after two weeks of intensive treatment in HIV-negative patients. In HIV-negative patients without cavitating disease or positive smears after intensive treatment, **rifapentine** (600 mg or 900 mg) and INH (900 mg or 15 mg/kg) once weekly for the continuation phase of treatment of drug-susceptible pulmonary TB is also safe and effective.[32,33] This regimen is not recommended for HIV-positive patients due to high rates of relapse with rifamycin monoresistant TB (four out of five patients relapsed in once-weekly regimen versus zero out of three cases of relapse in twice-weekly regimen).[34] Relapse/failure was associated with low plasma concentrations of INH.[31] The optimal dose of rifapentine is not known at this time. A longer period of treatment (minimum nine months) is recommended for patients with drug-susceptible, cavitary pulmonary TB whose sputum cultures remain positive after two months of treatment because of increased risk of relapse and treatment failure.[28] This may reflect poor drug penetration at the site of disease or high bacillary burden at the time of diagnosis.[32] Short-course treatment (e.g., six months) is only recommended in rifampin-based regimens containing PZA in the intensive phase of treatment.

Table 1: **Treatment Regimens for Tuberculosis**

State of TB	Regimen[a]	Frequency[b] and Duration[c]	Comment
Latent TB Infection	INH	Daily[d] or twice weekly for 9 mo	Regimen of choice
	Rifampin	Daily[d] for 4 mo	For INH-resistant strains or in patients unable to tolerate INH
Active TB Disease	INH + Rifampin + PZA + EM	1) daily[d] for 2 mo, then INH + Rifampin daily for 4 mo or 2) daily[d] for 2 mo, then INH + Rifampin 2 ×/wk for 4 mo or 3) 3 ×/wk for 6 mo	For areas with INH resistance ≥ 4%. In areas with INH resistance < 4%, INH, rifampin and PZA without EM can be used pending sensitivity results. Total duration 6 mo only if culture conversion at 2 mo, non-cavitary disease and fully sensitive organism. Extend continuation phase to 7 mo in patients with cavitation and positive culture at 2 mo as they are at a higher risk of relapse[28]
	INH + Rifampin + EM	Daily[d] for 2 mo, then INH + Rifampin daily for 7 mo	
	Rifampin + PZA + EM ± a quinolone or SM	Daily[d] for at least 6 mo	For INH-resistant disease
	INH + PZA + EM ± a quinolone or SM	Daily[d] for 9–12 mo	For rifampin-resistant disease

[a] Other second-line drugs are available in the event of intolerance or multiple drug-resistant TB: cycloserine, ethionamide, p-aminosalicylic acid, amikacin and capreomycin.
[b] DOT recommended for all regimens. Twice- and thrice-weekly regimens should only be used with a DOTS program.
[c] Completion of therapy is not determined by the duration of therapy but by the number of doses taken.[35]
[d] Daily = 7 doses/wk or 5 doses/wk DOT.[28]
Abbreviations: INH = isoniazid; SM = streptomycin; PZA = pyrazinamide; EM = ethambutol

Treatment interruptions > 14 days in the initial or intensive phase of management should lead to a complete re-start of therapy from the beginning. Treatment interruptions > 3 months in the continuation phase of management should lead to a re-start of a four-drug regimen from the beginning due to concerns for resistance. Consultation with a local TB expert is suggested when confronted with treatment interruptions, treatment failure or relapse, drug intolerances or adverse effects and multiple drug resistance.

Patients with multidrug-resistant TB (MDR-TB) are resistant to both isoniazid and rifampin. Patients with extensively (or extended) drug-resistant TB (XDR-TB) are resistant to INH, RIF and to ≥ 3 out of the 6 classes of second-line drugs.[36] XDR-TB is associated with high mortality. Patients with MDR-TB and XDR-TB should be referred to a TB specialist.

Antituberculous Drug-Induced Hepatotoxicity[37]

In LTBI, drug-induced hepatotoxicity is defined as aspartate aminotransferase (AST) level > 3 times the upper limit of normal in symptomatic patients (i.e, nausea, vomiting, abdominal pain, jaundice) or > 5 times the upper limit of normal in asymptomatic patients. Withhold all hepatotoxic drugs and consult a local TB specialist. For active TB disease, consider reinstituting a nonhepatotoxic regimen (e.g., ethambutol, streptomycin and a quinolone) when or as liver test results improve. Alcohol is the most important cofactor in INH-induced hepatitis.[38]

Tuberculosis in Special Populations

Treatment During Pregnancy and Lactation[7,28]

Treatment of pregnant women with anti-TB medications should not be withheld because of the risk of TB to the fetus. The preferred initial treatment regimen is **isoniazid**, **rifampin** and **ethambutol**. The risk of teratogenicity with **pyrazinamide** has not been determined though it is unlikely to be teratogenic.[28] Its use should be considered if resistance to one of the initial drugs is suspected and susceptibility to pyrazinamide is likely. Streptomycin has been associated with congenital deafness and should not be used. Therapy for nine months with isoniazid and rifampin should be adequate if ethambutol is substituted for pyrazinamide during the first two months and the organism is fully sensitive. Breast-feeding need not be discouraged since only small concentrations of anti-TB drugs appear in breast milk and they do not produce toxicity in the newborn.

Pediatric Tuberculosis

With rare exceptions (e.g., cavitary or laryngeal tuberculosis), children with TB are not contagious.[39,40] Untreated children < 5 years are at increased risk of developing severe forms of TB such as miliary or meningeal TB; treatment should be initiated promptly upon suspicion of TB. Dose anti-TB medications by weight (mg/kg) in children. Regimens recommended in children are similar to those used in adults, except ethambutol is not recommended in children who cannot be assessed effectively for visual toxicity. Children < 5 years who are exposed to an active case of TB and are TST negative are eligible for primary preventative therapy with INH until a repeat TST is performed in 8 to 12 weeks.[7]

Extrapulmonary Tuberculosis

The basic principles of management for extrapulmonary tuberculosis are similar to pulmonary TB. Prolonged treatment (> 12 months) is required for bone and meningeal TB. Prolonged treatment may be required in patients slow to respond. In general, corticosteroids are indicated only for meningeal and pericardial TB as they have been shown to decrease mortality.[41,42] Corticosteroids may have a role in adrenal TB, pleural TB and drug reactions.

HIV Infection

Principles of treatment of active TB in HIV-infected adults are similar to treatment of uninfected individuals except that once-weekly isoniazid and rifapentine should not be used.[34,43,44,45] Twice-weekly intermittent therapy (e.g., rifabutin and isoniazid in the continuation phase) is not recommended in patients with HIV infection and CD4 counts < 100 cells/mm^3 due to concerns that it may contribute to rifamycin resistance.[46,47] Daily or thrice weekly DOT is strongly recommended due to high risk of resistance and relapse of infection.[28]

Dose adjustments may be required for anti-TB and antiretroviral agents.[44] Rifamycins may substantially decrease the concentration of protease inhibitors (PIs) and non-nucleoside reverse transcriptase inhibitors (NNRTIs). Among the rifamycins, **rifabutin** is the least potent enzyme inducer and can be substituted for rifampin with similar efficacy though dose adjustments of rifabutin may still be required. It has been recommended that the initiation of antiretroviral therapy (ART) be delayed for at least four to eight weeks after the start of anti-TB therapy for those patients with advanced HIV disease (CD4 < 100 cells/mm^3) who are not already taking ART.[28] For patients already receiving antiretroviral therapy, treatment should be continued during anti-TB treatment, especially if ART has been considered successful. Monitor for signs and symptoms of immune reconstitution inflammatory syndrome (fever, malaise, local reactions in organs) if anti-TB therapy and ART are started at the same time.[48,49] Until there have been controlled trials evaluating the optimal time to initiate ART in patients with HIV-related TB, this decision is made on an individual basis.

Management of HIV-infected patients with TB requires health care workers with expertise in these areas. Consultation with a respirologist or TB expert with experience managing HIV-related TB is strongly recommended due to possible drug interactions and the risk of the immune reconstitution syndrome.

Therapeutic Tips

- Prescribe **pyridoxine** 25 to 50 mg/day to prevent peripheral neuropathy in all adult patients given INH.[50]
- Recommend DOT in the treatment of TB, especially in patients with a history of treatment failure, drug resistance, disease relapse, HIV infection, substance use or psychiatric illness and in homeless patients.
- Before splitting a dose or switching to a second-line agent, consider administering first-line anti-TB drugs with some food if patients experience stomach upset.[35] Evaluate patients with GI symptoms for drug-induced hepatitis.

Figure 1: **Diagnosis and Management of Latent *M. tuberculosis* Infection**

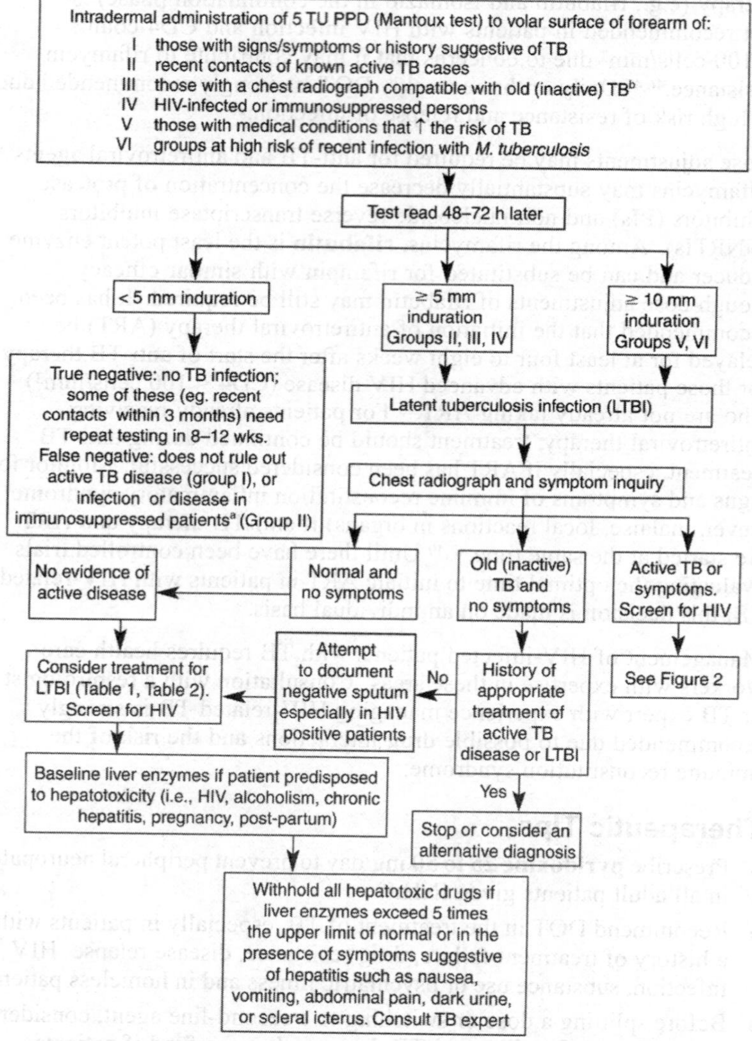

[a] Consider treatment for LTBI in HIV-positive patients with close contact with an active case of TB, a chest radiograph consistent with old (inactive) TB or a history of positive TST without a history of treatment for TB or LTBI. Consider primary preventive treatment in children ≤ 5 years who have had recent contact with an active case of TB, until repeat skin testing is available.

[b] If active TB disease is suspected, isolate the patient.

Abbreviations: LTBI = latent tuberculosis infection; PPD = purified protein derivative; TST = tuberculin skin test; TU = tuberculin units

Figure 2: **Diagnosis and Management of Pulmonary *M. tuberculosis* Disease**

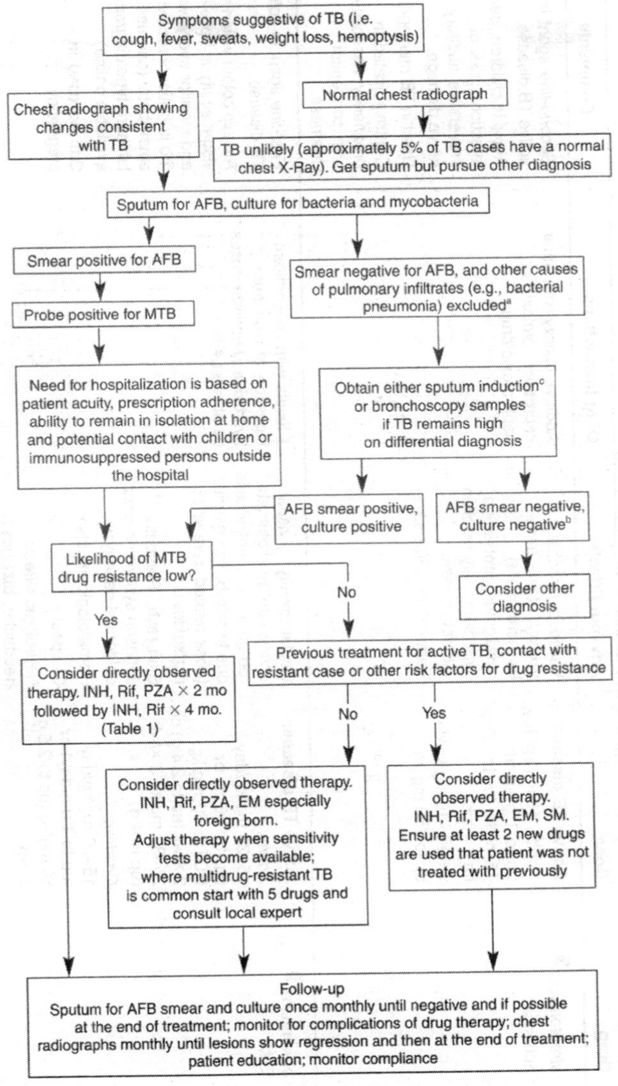

a 50% of pulmonary TB cases will be smear negative. Therefore, with suspicious chest radiograph and clinical scenario, consider initiating empiric antituberculosis therapy.

b 15% of pulmonary TB cases will be culture negative but diagnosis is based on clinical and radiographic response to therapy in the appropriate clinical setting.

c Induced sputum has higher yield, quicker turnaround and less risk to patients or health care workers than bronchoscopy.

Abbreviations: AFB = acid fast bacilli; INH = isoniazid; Rif = rifampin; SM = streptomycin; PZA = pyrazinamide; EM = ethambutol; MTB = Mycobacterium tuberculosis

Table 2: Antibiotics for the Treatment of *M. tuberculosis*

Class	Drug	Dose	Adverse Effects	Drug Interactions	Comments	Cost[a]
Aminoglycosides	*streptomycin* generics	**Active TB disease:** *Adults:* 15 mg/kg/day, up to 1 g im **or** 15 mg/kg (up to 1.5 g) im 3 ×/wk > 59 y: 10 mg/kg/day, up to 750 mg im	Vestibular/ cochlear toxicity, ataxia (may be permanent), nystagmus, proteinuria, hypersensitivity reaction with fever, rash. Hematologic effects.[b]	Additive toxicity with other neurotoxic, ototoxic or nephrotoxic drugs.	*Second-line* agent in active TB disease. Avoid in children: painful injections, risk of irreversible auditory nerve damage. Used in TB meningitis. Contraindicated in pregnancy; associated with congenital deafness.	$$$$$
Antimycobacterial Agents	*ethambutol* Etibi	**Active TB disease:** *Adults:* 15–25 mg/kg/day (up to 1.6 g) **or** DOTS: 50 mg/kg 2 ×/wk (up to 2.4 g) or 25–30 mg/kg 3 ×/wk (up to 4 g) *Children:* 15–20 mg/kg/day (up to 1.0 g/day) **or** 50 mg/kg (up to 2.5 g) 2 ×/wk	Ocular toxicity: ↓ visual acuity, central scotomata, red-green colour blindness due to retrobulbar neuritis (dose-related; rare at 15 mg/kg/day). Skin rash: Stevens-Johnson syndrome, toxic epidermal necrolysis. Hematologic effects.[b] GI upset.[c] Neurologic effects: headache, dizziness, confusion, hallucinations.	↓ levels with concomitant ingestion of aluminum hydroxide: separate doses by at least 4 h.	*First-line* agent in active TB disease. Assess colour vision and visual acuity at baseline and monitor every two mo in patients receiving ethambutol (can use Ishihara-type diagrams[7] available online). Can be used in pregnancy.	$

Class	Drug	Dose	Adverse Effects	Drug Interactions	Comments	Cost[a]
	isoniazid Isotamine, generics	**Latent TB infection:** *Adults:* 5 mg/kg/day (up to 300 mg/day) for 9 mo **or** DOTS: 900 mg 2 ×/wk for 9 mo *Children:* 10–15 mg/kg (up to 300 mg) for 9 mo **or** DOTS: 20–30 mg/kg (up to 900 mg) 2 ×/wk for 9 mo **Active TB disease:** *Adults:* 300 mg daily **or** DOTS: 15 mg/kg (up to 900 mg) 3 ×/wk *Children:* 10 mg/kg/day (up to 300 mg daily) **or** DOTS: 20–30 mg/kg (up to 900 mg) 2 ×/wk Consult expert in patients with severe liver disease	Asymptomatic ↑ hepatic transaminases and bilirubin (10–20%), clinical hepatitis (symptoms may occur within weeks to months), peripheral neuropathy (dose-related). Hematologic effects.[b] GI upset.[c] Gynecomastia, seizures, drowsiness, drug-induced lupus, toxic encephalopathy, fever, skin rash, mood changes, lymphadenopathy.	INH ↑ serum levels of carbamazepine, phenytoin, theophylline. ↑ hepatotoxicity of INH with rifampin, ethanol, acetaminophen. Cross-hepatotoxicity may occur between drugs that are chemically related (e.g., INH and pyrazinamide). Both agents should be avoided if a reaction to one of them occurs.	*First-line* agent in active TB disease. Educate patients on symptoms of hepatitis. Discontinue drug. Can be used in pregnancy. Prescribe pyridoxine 25–50 mg/day to prevent peripheral neuropathy.[50]	$

(cont'd)

Table 2: **Antibiotics for the Treatment of *M. tuberculosis*** *(cont'd)*

Class	Drug	Dose	Adverse Effects	Drug Interactions	Comments	Cost[a]
	pyrazinamide Tebrazid, generics	**Active TB disease:** *Adults:* 25 mg/kg/day (up to 2 g/day) **or** DOTS: 50 mg/kg (up to 4 g) 2 ×/wk or 35–40 mg/kg (up to 3 g) 3 ×/wk *Children:* 15–30 mg/kg/day (up to 2 g/day) **or** DOTS: 50 mg/kg (up to 2 g) 2 ×/wk	Hepatotoxicity (rare with 2 mo therapy), rash, arthralgia, ↑ uric acid (acute gout rarely seen), drug fever, GI upset. Hematologic effects.[b]	Rifampin and pyrazinamide: liver injury in patients with latent TB infection.[21] ↑ pyrazinamide levels: concomitant administration of allopurinol through inhibition of xanthine oxidase.	*First-line* agent in active TB disease.	$$$
Rifamycins	*rifabutin* Mycobutin	**Active TB disease:** *Adults:* 5 mg/kg/day (up to 300 mg/day) DOTS: 5 mg/kg (up to 300 mg) 2 or 3 ×/wk; in HIV patients, twice weekly rifabutin is not appropriate	Rash, orange discolouration of body fluids (contact lens staining), GI upset, liver toxicity, flu-like illness, neutropenia, leukopenia, myalgia.	Avoid in combination with saquinavir, delavirdine.[51] Protease inhibitors: ↓ clearance of rifamycins. Rifamycins: ↓ efficacy of protease inhibitors and NNRTIs. ↓ serum concentration of drugs due to hepatic enzyme induction, e.g., oral contraceptives, anticoagulants, antihyperglycemic agents, methadone. Adjust dose of affected drug when rifabutin is initiated or discontinued.	*First-line* agent in active TB disease.	$$$$$

Class	Drug	Dose	Adverse Effects	Drug Interactions	Comments	Cost[a]
	rifampin Rifadin, Rofact, generics	**Latent TB infection:** *Adults:* 10 mg/kg/day (up to 600 mg/day) for 4 mo *Children:* 10–20 mg/kg/day (up to 600 mg/day) for 4 mo **Active TB disease:** *Adults:* 10 mg/kg/day (up to 600 mg/day) **or** DOTS: 10 mg/kg (up to 600 mg/day) 2 or 3 ×/wk *Children:* 10–20 mg/kg/day (up to 600 mg/day) **or** DOTS: 10–20 mg/kg (up to 600 mg/day) 2 ×/wk Consult expert in patients with severe liver disease.	Rash (petechial rash may suggest thrombocytopenia), orange discolouration of body fluids (contact lens staining), GI upset, liver toxicity, flu-like illness, sub-clinical disseminated intravascular coagulation, diarrhea, urticaria, ataxia, confusion, visual disturbances, acute interstitial nephritis. Hematologic effects.[b]	Avoid in combination with amprenavir, fosamprenavir, atazanavir, indinavir, nelfinavir, saquinavir and delavirdine.[52] Lopinavir/ritonavir: ↑ ritonavir dose if used concomitantly with rifampin.[52] See rifabutin.	*First-line* agent in active TB disease. Can be used in pregnancy.	$$$
	rifapentine Priftin	**Active TB disease:** 10 mg/kg po weekly	Rash, orange discolouration of body fluids (contact lens staining), GI upset, liver toxicity, flu-like illness, hyperuricemia.	See rifampin.	*First-line* agent in active TB disease.	[d]

(cont'd)

Table 2: **Antibiotics for the Treatment of *M. tuberculosis*** *(cont'd)*

Class	Drug	Dose	Adverse Effects	Drug Interactions	Comments	Cost[a]
Fluoro-quinolones	*levofloxacin* Levaquin, generics	**Active TB disease:** *Adults:* 500–1000 mg po daily	Abdominal pain, nausea, vomiting, photosensitivity, dizziness, headache, drowsiness, insomnia, diarrhea, pseudomembranous colitis, eosinophilic meningitis, tendonitis and rupture.	↓ absorption of fluoroquinolones: concomitant iron, calcium, zinc, antacids, sucralfate, didanosine (buffered tablets). Separate doses by 2 h. Torsades de pointes in combination with drugs that prolong QT interval.	*Second-line* agent in active TB disease.	$$$$$
	moxifloxacin Avelox	**Active TB disease:** *Adults:* 400 mg po daily	See levofloxacin.	See levofloxacin.	*Second-line* agent in active TB disease.	$$$$$

[a] Cost of 30-day supply for adult dose; includes drug cost only.
[b] Hematologic effects may include any of eosinophilia, thrombocytopenia, transient leukopenia, hemolytic anemia, agranulocytosis, or sideroblastic or aplastic anemia.
[c] Gastrointestinal upset: nausea, vomiting, poor appetite, abdominal pain; common in the first few weeks of therapy—manage by administering with food or at bedtime; monitor AST to rule out hepatotoxicity.
[d] Not commercially available in Canada currently. Available as part of a study protocol and present in the American Thoracic Society guidelines.
Dosage adjustment may be required in renal impairment; see Appendix I.
Abbreviations: DOTS = directly observed therapy short-course; INH = isoniazid; NNRTI = non-nucleoside reverse transcriptase inhibitor
Legend: $ < $25 $$ $25–50 $$$ $50–75 $$$$ $75–100 $$$$$ > $100

Suggested Readings

American Thoracic Society; Centers for Disease Control and Prevention; Infectious Diseases Society of America. American Thoracic Society/Centers for Disease Control and Prevention/Infectious Diseases Society of America: controlling tuberculosis in the United States. *Am J Respir Crit Care Med* 2005;172(9):1169-227.

Blumberg HM, Burman WJ, Chaisson RE et al. American Thoracic Society/Centers for Disease Control and Prevention/Infectious Diseases Society of America: treatment of tuberculosis. *Am J Respir Crit Care Med* 2003;167(4):603-62.

Long R, editor. *Canadian tuberculosis standards.* 5th ed. Ottawa (ON): Canadian Lung Association; 2000. Available from: http://www.phac-aspc.gc.ca/publicat/cts-ncla00/pdf/cts00.pdf Accessed March 7, 2007.

World Health Organization. *Tuberculosis and air travel: guidelines for prevention and control.* 2nd edition. Geneva (CH): WHO; 2006. Available from: http://www.who.int/tb/publications/2006/who_htm_tb_2006_363.pdf Accessed March 7, 2007.

References

1. [No authors listed]. Targeted tuberculin testing and treatment of latent tuberculosis infection. This official statement of the American Thoracic Society was adopted by the ATS Board of Directors, July 1999. This is a Joint Statement of the American Thoracic Society (ATS) and the Centers for Disease Control and Prevention (CDC). This statement was endorsed by the Council of the Infectious Diseases Society of America. (IDSA), September 1999, and the sections of this statement. *Am J Respir Crit Care Med* 2000;161(4 Pt 2):S221-47.
2. [No authors listed]. Diagnostic Standards and Classification of Tuberculosis in Adults and Children. This official statement of the American Thoracic Society and the Centers for Disease Control and Prevention was adopted by the ATS Board of Directors, July 1999. This statement was endorsed by the Council of the Infectious Disease Society of America, September 1999. *Am J Respir Crit Care Med* 2000;161(4 Pt 1):1376-95.
3. Schluger NW. Changing approaches to the diagnosis of tuberculosis. *Am J Respir Crit Care Med* 2001;164(11):2020-4.
4. Greenaway C, Menzies D, Fanning A et al. Delay in diagnosis among hospitalized patients with active tuberculosis—predictors and outcomes. *Am J Respir Crit Care Med* 2002;165(7):927-33.
5. Menzies D, Fanning A, Yuan L et al. Hospital ventilation and risk for tuberculous infection in Canadian health care workers. Canadian Collaborative Group in Nosocomial Transmission of TB. *Ann Intern Med* 2000;133(10):779-89.
6. Menzies D, Fanning A, Yuan L et al. Factors associated with tuberculin conversion in Canadian microbiology and pathology workers. *Am J Respir Crit Care Med* 2003;167(4):599-602.
7. Long R, editor. *Canadian tuberculosis standards.* 5th ed. Ottawa (ON): Canadian Lung Association; 2000. Available from: http://www.phac-aspc.gc.ca/publicat/cts-ncla00/pdf/cts00.pdf Accessed March 7, 2007.
8. Nolan CM, Goldberg SV, Buskin SE. Hepatotoxicity associated with isoniazid preventive therapy: a 7-year survey from a public health tuberculosis clinic. *JAMA* 1999;281(11):1014-8.
9. Singh M, Moosa NV, Kumar L et al. Role of gastric lavage and broncho-alveolar lavage in the bacteriological diagnosis of childhood pulmonary tuberculosis. *Indian Pediatr* 2000;37(9):947-51.
10. Coll P, Garrigo M, Moreno C et al. Routine use of Gen-Probe Amplified Mycobacterium Tuberculosis Direct (MTD) test for detection of Mycobacterium tuberculosis with smear-positive and smear-negative specimens. *Int J Tuberc Lung Dis* 2003;7(9):886-91.
11. Brodie D, Schluger NW. The diagnosis of tuberculosis. *Clin Chest Med* 2005;26(2):247-71, vi.
12. Wang L, Turner MO, Elwood RK et al. A meta-analysis of the effect of Bacille Calmette Guerin vaccination on tuberculin skin test measurements. *Thorax* 2002;57(9):804-9.
13. Mazurek GH, Jereb J, Lobue P et al. Guidelines for using the QuantiFERON-TB Gold test for detecting Mycobacterium tuberculosis infection, United States. *MMWR Recomm Rep* 2005;54(RR-15):49-55.
14. Khan A, Sterling TR, Reves R et al. Lack of weight gain and relapse risk in a large tuberculosis treatment trial. *Am J Respir Crit Care Med* 2006;174(3):344-8.

15. Frieden TR, Munsiff SS. The DOTS strategy for controlling the global tuberculosis epidemic. *Clin Chest Med* 2005;26(2):197-205, v.
16. Blumberg HM, Leonard MK, Jasmer RM. Update on the treatment of tuberculosis and latent tuberculosis infection. *JAMA* 2005;293(22):2776-84.
17. LoBue PA, Moser KS. Use of isoniazid for latent tuberculosis infection in a public health clinic. *Am J Respir Crit Care Med* 2003;168(4):443-7.
18. Polesky A, Farber HW, Gottlieb DJ et al. Rifampin preventive therapy for tuberculosis in Boston's homeless. *Am J Respir Crit Care Med* 1996;154(5):1473-7.
19. Centers for Disease Control and Prevention (CDC). Fatal and severe hepatitis associated with rifampin and pyrazinamide for the treatment of latent tuberculosis infection--New York and Georgia, 2000. *MMWR Morb Mortal Wkly Rep* 2001;50(15):289-91.
20. Centers for Disease Control and Prevention (CDC). Update: fatal and severe liver injuries associated with rifampin and pyrazinamide for latent tuberculosis infection, and revisions in American Thoracic Society/CDC recommendations--United States, 2001. *MMWR Morb Mortal Wkly Rep* 2001;50(34):733-5.
21. Centers for Disease Control and Prevention (CDC). Update: fatal and severe liver injuries associated with rifampin and pyrazinamide treatment for latent tuberculosis infection. *MMWR Morb Mortal Wkly Rep* 2002;51(44):998-9.
22. Centers for Disease Control and Prevention (CDC); American Thoracic Society. Update: adverse event data and revised American Thoracic Society/CDC recommendations against the use of rifampin and pyrazinamide for treatment of latent tuberculosis infection—United States, 2003. *MMWR Morb Mortal Wkly Rep* 2003;52(31):735-9.
23. Ijaz K, Jereb JA, Lambert LA et al. Severe or fatal liver injury in 50 patients in the United States taking rifampin and pyrazinamide for latent tuberculosis infection. *Clin Infect Dis* 2006;42(3):346-55.
24. Schechter M, Zajdenverg R, Falco G et al. Weekly rifapentine/isoniazid or daily rifampin/pyrazinamide for latent tuberculosis in household contacts. *Am J Respir Crit Care Med* 2006;173(8):922-6.
25. Hershfield E. Tuberculosis: 9. Treatment. *CMAJ* 1999;161(4):405-11.
26. Park SK, Kim CT, Song SD. Outcome of chemotherapy in 107 patients with pulmonary tuberculosis resistant to isoniazid and rifampin. *Int J Tuberc Lung Dis* 1998;2(11):877-84.
27. Small PM, Fujiwara PI. Management of tuberculosis in the United States. *N Engl J Med* 2001;345(3):189-200.
28. Blumberg HM, Burman WJ, Chaisson RE et al. American Thoracic Society/Centers for Disease Control and Prevention/Infectious Diseases Society of America: treatment of tuberculosis. *Am J Respir Crit Care Med* 2003;167(4):603-62.
29. O'Brien RJ, Spigelman M. New drugs for tuberculosis: current status and future prospects. *Clin Chest Med*2005;26(2):327-40, vii.
30. Fortun J, Martin-Davila P, Navas E et al. Linezolid for the treatment of multidrug-resistant tuberculosis. *J Antimicrob Chemother* 2005;56(1):180-5.
31. Bozeman L, Burman W, Metchock B et al. Fluoroquinolone susceptibility among Mycobacterium tuberculosis isolates from the United States and Canada. *Clin Infect Dis* 2005;40(3):386-91.
32. Benator D, Bhattacharya M, Bozeman L et al. Rifapentine and isoniazid once a week versus rifampicin and isoniazid twice a week for treatment of drug-susceptible pulmonary tuberculosis in HIV-negative patients: a randomised clinical trial. *Lancet* 2002;360(9332):528-34.
33. Bock NN, Sterling TR, Hamilton CD et al. A prospective, randomized, double-blind study of the tolerability of rifapentine 600, 900, and 1,200 mg plus isoniazid in the continuation phase of tuberculosis treatment. *Am J Respir Crit Care Med* 2002;165(11):1526-30.
34. Vernon A, Burman W, Benator D et al. Acquired rifamycin monoresistance in patients with HIV-related tuberculosis treated with once-weekly rifapentine and isoniazid. Tuberculosis Trials Consortium. *Lancet* 1999;353(9167):1843-7.
35. American Thoracic Society; CDC; Infectious Diseases Society of America. Treatment of tuberculosis. *MMWR Recomm Rep* 2003;52(RR-11):1-77.
36. Centers for Disease Control and Prevention (CDC). Revised definition of extensively drug-resistant tuberculosis. *MMWR Morb Mortal Wkly Rep* 2006;55(43):1176. Available from: http://www.cdc.gov/mmwr/PDF/wk/mm5543.pdf Accessed March 7, 2007.
37. Saukkonen JJ, Cohn DL, Jasmer RM et al. An official ATS statement: hepatotoxicity of antituberculosis therapy. *Am J Respir Crit Care Med* 2006;174(8):935-52.
38. Kopanoff DE, Snider DE, Jr., Caras GJ. Isoniazid-related hepatitis: a U.S. Public Health Service cooperative surveillance study. *Am Rev Respir Dis* 1978;117(6):991-1001.
39. Curtis AB, Ridzon R, Vogel R et al. Extensive transmission of Mycobacterium tuberculosis from a child. *N Engl J Med* 1999;341(20):1491-5.
40. Pineda PR, Leung A, Muller NL et al. Intrathoracic paediatric tuberculosis: a report of 202 cases. *Tuber Lung Dis* 1993;74(4):261-6.
41. Dooley DP, Carpenter JL, Rademacher S. Adjunctive corticosteroid therapy for tuberculosis: a critical reappraisal of the literature. *Clin Infect Dis* 1997;25(4):872-87.

42. Thwaites GE, Nguyen DB, Nguyen HD et al. Dexamethasone for the treatment of tuberculous meningitis in adolescents and adults. *N Engl J Med* 2004;351(17):1741-51.
43. Burman WJ, Jones BE. Treatment of HIV-related tuberculosis in the era of effective antiretroviral therapy. *Am J Respir Crit Care Med* 2001;164(1):7-12.
44. Dean GL, Edwards SG, Ives NJ et al. Treatment of tuberculosis in HIV-infected persons in the era of highly active antiretroviral therapy. *AIDS* 2002;16(1):75-83.
45. FitzGerald JM, Houston S. Tuberculosis: 8. The disease in association with HIV infection. *CMAJ* 1999;61(1):47-51
46. Centers for Disease Control and Prevention (CDC). Acquired rifamycin resistance in persons with advanced HIV disease being treated for active tuberculosis with intermittent rifamycin-based regimens. *MMWR Morb Mortal Wkly Rep* 2002;51(10):214-5.
47. Burman W, Benator D, Vernon A et al. Acquired rifamycin resistance with twice-weekly treatment of HIV-related tuberculosis. *Am J Respir Crit Care Med* 2006;173(3):350-6.
48. Hammer SM, Saag MS, Schechter M et al. Treatment for adult HIV infection: 2006 recommendations of the International AIDS Society-USA panel. *JAMA* 2006;296(7):827-43.
49. Narita M, Ashkin D, Hollender ES et al. Paradoxical worsening of tuberculosis following antiretroviral therapy in patients with AIDS. *Am J Respir Crit Care Med* 1998;158(1):157-61.
50. Snider DE. Pyridoxine supplementation during isoniazid therapy. *Tubercle* 1980;61(4):191-6.
51. Centers for Disease Control and Prevention (CDC). Table 2. Recommendations for coadministering protease inhibitors and nonnucleoside reverse transcriptase inhibitors with rifabutin–United States, 2004. Atlanta (Ga): CDC; 2004. Available from: http://www.cdc.gov/nchstp/tb/TB_HIV_Drugs/Table2.htm Accessed March 7, 2007.
52. Centers for Disease Control and Prevention (CDC). *TB/HIV drug interactions: updated guidelines for the use of rifamycins for the treatment of tuberculosis among HIV-infected patients taking protease inhibitors or nonnucleoside reverse transcriptase inhibitors*. Atlanta (Ga): CDC; 2004. Available from: http://www.cdc.gov/nchstp/tb/tb_hiv_drugs/toc.htm Accessed March 7, 2007.

CHAPTER 100
Bacterial Meningitis

Alana Rosenthal, MD, FRCPC and
Lindy Samson, MD, FRCPC

Meningitis is described as inflammation of the cranial and spinal leptomeninges. *Bacterial meningitis* is characterized by bacterial invasion of the cranial and spinal leptomeninges. It most often develops following bacteremia but can also occur via extension from surrounding structures (mastoiditis, sinusitis) or direct inoculation during neurosurgery or open head trauma. The causative pathogens in bacterial meningitis depend on age and specific host and environmental factors (Table 1, Table 2).

Table 1: **Bacterial Meningitis: Probable Pathogens and Empiric Therapy Based on Age**

Age Group	Bacteria	Empiric Antibacterial Regimen
Infants < 6 wk	Group B streptococcus *E. coli* *L. monocytogenes* Other Enterobacteriaceae *Streptococcus pneumoniae* (rare) *Neisseria meningitidis* (rare)	Ampicillin + gentamicin *or* Ampicillin + cefotaxime[a]
Infants 6 wk–3 mo	*S. pneumoniae* (pneumococcus) *N. meningitidis* (meningococcus) Group B streptococcus *H. influenzae* type b[b] *E. coli* (rare) *L. monocytogenes* (rare) Other Enterobacteriaceae (rare)	Ceftriaxone or cefotaxime + Ampicillin + Vancomycin[c]
Infants > 3 mo, children and adults	*S. pneumoniae* *N. meningitidis* *H. influenzae* type b[b]	Ceftriaxone or cefotaxime + Vancomycin[c]
Elderly (> 50 y) or alcoholism	*E. coli* *S. pneumoniae* *N. meningitidis* *L. monocytogenes*	Ceftriaxone or cefotaxime + Ampicillin + Vancomycin[c]

[a] Cefotaxime is preferred over ceftriaxone in neonates because of the theoretical risk of displacement of bilirubin from albumin and therefore of possible hyperbilirubinemia.
[b] *H. influenzae* type b is rare since implementation of universal vaccination.
[c] Vancomycin is included in the initial antibacterial regimen due to increasing prevalence of resistant *S. pneumoniae*.

Table 2: **Bacterial Meningitis: Probable Pathogens and Empiric Therapy Based on Specific Host and Environmental Factors**

Risk Factor	Bacteria	Empiric Antibacterials
Cerebrospinal fluid leak	*S. pneumoniae* *S. pyogenes* *H. influenzae* type b	Ceftriaxone or cefotaxime + Vancomycin
Penetrating head trauma/neurosurgery[a]	*Staphylococcus* spp. *Streptococcus* spp. *E. coli* *Klebsiella* spp. *P. aeruginosa*	3rd generation cephalosporin[b] + Vancomycin[a]
Ventriculoperitoneal shunt	*S. epidermidis* *S. aureus* *S. pneumoniae* *N. meningitidis* *H. influenzae* type b Aerobic gram-negative bacilli (including *P. aeruginosa*) *Propionibacterium acnes*	3rd generation cephalosporin[b] + Vancomycin
Humoral immune deficiency states, e.g., agammaglobulinemia	*S. pneumoniae* *N. meningitidis* *H. influenzae* type b	Ceftriaxone or cefotaxime + Vancomycin
Cellular immune deficiency states, e.g., chemotherapy, HIV	*S. pneumoniae* *N. meningitidis* *L. monocytogenes* *H. influenzae* type b	Ceftriaxone or cefotaxime + Ampicillin + Vancomycin
Asplenia (anatomic or functional)	*S. pneumoniae* *N. meningitidis* *Salmonella* spp. *H. influenzae* type b	Ceftriaxone or cefotaxime + Vancomycin

[a] Consider adding anaerobic and antifungal coverage if the wound is contaminated.
[b] Ceftazidime is the cephalosporin of choice if there is a high suspicion of *P. aeruginosa* infection.

- There is still significant mortality and morbidity associated with bacterial meningitis. Acute complications may include but are not limited to:
  - subdural effusion or empyema
  - brain abscess
  - cerebritis or ventriculitis
  - venous sinus thrombosis
  - seizures
  - CNS infarction, resulting in hemiparesis, quadriparesis or spinal cord infarction
  - brain herniation

- shock and/or disseminated intravascular coagulopathy
- diabetes insipidus and/or the syndrome of inappropriate antidiuretic hormone release

- Neurologic *sequelae* may include but are not limited to:
  - sensorineural hearing loss
  - visual problems including cortical blindness
  - ataxia
  - hydrocephalus
  - behavioural difficulties
  - intellectual deficits
  - epilepsy

Goals of Therapy

- Eradicate bacteria from the CNS
- Decrease mortality
- Manage and minimize acute and chronic complications including permanent neurologic damage

Investigations

Clinical Presentation

- The clinical presentation varies and is related to age and developmental stage. It may be acute or insidious in onset.
  - *infants* may present with only a change in temperature (fever *or* hypothermia). Other signs are usually nonspecific and may include inconsolable crying, irritability, lethargy, seizures, poor feeding, vomiting, diarrhea, jaundice and/or a bulging anterior fontanelle. Signs of meningeal irritation such as a stiff neck are often absent and therefore, in infants, clinicians should have a low threshold for suspecting meningitis. A fever in a baby < 4 weeks of age warrants examination and culture of the cerebrospinal fluid (CSF) in all circumstances.
  - in *children and adults*, symptoms usually include fever, severe headache, stiff neck or back pain and/or photophobia. Patients often report feeling systemically unwell with associated vomiting. Neurologic signs may include loss of balance, seizures, disorientation, confusion, altered level of consciousness, stiff neck, positive Kernig's and Brudzinski's signs, cranial nerve palsies and/or other signs of increased intracranial pressure, e.g., papilledema. Signs of cerebral infarction may also be present.
  - patients of any age can present in septic shock. Other physical exam findings may include petechia or purpura, which are usually suggestive of meningococcal meningitis but can also be seen with *S. pneumoniae* and other bacterial pathogens.

Laboratory Investigations

CSF

- Examination of the CSF is essential for making the diagnosis and is warranted whenever meningitis is suspected. Lumbar puncture (LP) is contraindicated in the presence of increased intracranial pressure (ICP), papilledema, focal neurologic signs, deteriorating Glasgow Coma Score, shock, infection at the LP site and bleeding disorders.[1] Brain imaging may or may not be helpful in excluding increased ICP prior to lumbar puncture. If raised ICP is strongly suspected clinically, then the LP should be deferred. *Do not delay empiric antibacterial therapy* if an LP cannot be performed at the time of presentation.
- Examine the CSF for cell count and differential, culture and sensitivity, and glucose and protein concentrations. Findings consistent with bacterial meningitis include:
  - elevated CSF WBC count with a predominance of neutrophils is usually present; however, *initially* the CSF WBC count may be considerably less elevated. It is often not possible to differentiate bacterial from viral or other types of meningitis based purely on the CSF WBC
  - reduced CSF glucose (CSF-to-serum ratio < 0.6 for infants and < 0.4 for those over 2 months of age)[2]
  - normal or elevated CSF protein (range varies according to age)
  - CSF Gram stain is positive in up to 80 to 90% of hematogenously acquired meningitis,[3] but this varies according to the causative pathogen.[4]
- Culture is the gold standard for diagnosis, but may not be positive, particularly in those previously treated with antibacterials.
- Latex agglutination of the CSF in the setting of Gram stain and culture-negative meningitis is not routinely used because of poor sensitivity and specificity.[5,6]
- An elevated CSF lactate level (> 4 mmol/L) may be present in postoperative neurosurgical patients with bacterial meningitis.[7]
- A repeat LP is indicated in the following situations:
  - failure to improve clinically
  - immunocompromised patients
  - penicillin- or cephalosporin-resistant pneumococcal meningitis
  - meningitis caused by enteric gram-negative bacilli or other unusual pathogens
  - patients who received corticosteroids for prevention of complications due to meningitis (because corticosteroids may temporarily mask treatment failure)
  - meningitis caused by Group B streptococcus
  - some clinicians advocate a repeat LP in all cases of neonatal meningitis

Blood

- Complete blood count and differential; culture and sensitivity. Draw a blood glucose level at or near the time of the CSF glucose to enable comparison of the two values.

Imaging

- Imaging studies (CT or MRI of the head) are not routinely required but are indicated for those individuals with focal neurologic signs, clinical evidence of brain herniation, decreased/fluctuating level of consciousness, clinical deterioration, or persistent fever. In addition, some evidence suggests that CT scans should be done prior to LP in those with underlying neurologic conditions, immunodeficiency states or in individuals > 60 years of age.[8]

Therapeutic Choices

Pharmacologic Choices

Antibacterial Therapy

- Choice of empiric antibacterial therapy is based on the most likely causative organisms, host factors such as patient age (Table 1, Table 2) and local antimicrobial resistance patterns.
- Re-evaluate and modify antibacterial therapy when results of the CSF Gram stain, culture and then sensitivity become available (Table 3).
- The duration of therapy depends on host factors and the causative pathogen. General guidelines for duration of therapy for some common pathogens are shown in Table 3.
- Doses, most common adverse effects and drug interactions are shown in Table 4.
- Due to the increasing incidence of penicillin-resistant pneumococci and meningococci in Canada, penicillin G is no longer appropriate as empiric therapy.
- Use **vancomycin** and high-dose **ceftriaxone** or **cefotaxime** as empiric therapy for presumed pneumococcal meningitis in all individuals > 6 weeks of age. If an infant < 6 weeks of age has a Gram stain suggestive of pneumococcal meningitis, use vancomycin and cefotaxime, pending sensitivity results.[9]
- For penicillin and cephalosporin-resistant pneumococci, the use of cephalosporins alone, even in high doses, may be inadequate. The addition of vancomycin +/− **rifampin** to high-dose cephalosporins appears to enhance bacterial eradication in the CSF.[10,11]

Table 3: **Antibacterial Regimens for Specific Pathogens in Uncomplicated Bacterial Meningitis**

Pathogen	First-line	Alternative	Duration of Therapy[a]
S. pneumoniae (penicillin susceptible)	Penicillin G	Ceftriaxone or cefotaxime	10–14 days
S. pneumoniae (intermediate- or high-level resistance to penicillin, sensitive to cephalosporins)	Cefotaxime or ceftriaxone Consult infectious diseases specialist	Consult infectious diseases specialist	10–14 days
S. pneumoniae (intermediate- or high-level resistance to penicillin and 3rd generation cephalosporins)	Cefotaxime or ceftriaxone + Vancomycin +/– Rifampin Consult infectious diseases specialist	Consult infectious diseases specialist	10–14 days
N. meningitidis (penicillin-sensitive)	Penicillin G	Cefotaxime or ceftriaxone	5–7 days
N. meningitidis (penicillin-resistant)	Cefotaxime or ceftriaxone[b]		5–7 days
H. influenzae type b (beta-lactamase negative)	Ampicillin	Cefotaxime or ceftriaxone	7–10 days
H. influenzae type b (beta-lactamase positive)	Ceftriaxone or cefotaxime		7–10 days
Group B streptococcus	Penicillin + Gentamicin for synergy[c]	Ampicillin or cefotaxime	14–21 days
L. monocytogenes	Ampicillin + Gentamicin for synergy	Sulfamethoxazole/trimethoprim	At least 21 days
Enterobacteriaceae[d]	Ceftriaxone or cefotaxime[e] +/– Gentamicin[f]	Cefepime or meropenem[1]	21 days (Gentamicin for first 7–14 days)[1]

[a] These are general guidelines only; some cases may require a longer duration of therapy.
[b] Superiority over high-dose penicillin has not been proven.
[c] The addition of gentamicin provides in vitro and in vivo synergy. Gentamicin therapy should be continued for three to seven days, but may be longer in the case of delayed sterilization of the CSF.
[d] Therapy may be different depending on suspected pathogen and susceptibilities.
[e] Ampicillin can be used if organism is susceptible.
[f] Pediatric guidelines recommend addition of gentamicin; recommended in adults only when organism is *P. aeruginosa*.

Adjunctive Corticosteroids

The rationale behind adjunctive therapy with **dexamethasone** is that it will decrease the inflammatory response in the CNS, thereby limiting neurologic sequelae.

A theoretical concern regarding the use of dexamethasone in meningitis is the potential for delayed sterilization of the CSF (due to altered CSF drug penetration) in individuals treated with vancomycin for resistant *S. pneumoniae*. There are no large clinical studies to answer this question. The addition of **rifampin** to the antibacterial regimen should be strongly considered if resistant pneumococci are isolated in a patient who has received dexamethasone.[4,12]

The effect of dexamethasone on long-term cognitive function remains unclear. Therefore, careful follow-up of these patients is required.

Children

A meta-analysis of randomized controlled trials in children performed between 1988 and 1996 showed a beneficial effect of adjunctive dexamethasone therapy in reducing severe hearing loss in children with *H. influenzae* type b meningitis. In meningitis caused by *S. pneumoniae*, the use of dexamethasone showed a trend in protecting against hearing loss. If dexamethasone was given before or at the time of antibacterial administration, the benefit became significant.[13]

The use of adjunctive dexamethasone in children > 6 weeks of age with community-acquired bacterial meningitis may be considered after weighing the potential benefits and risks. Consultation with an infectious diseases specialist is warranted. The recommended dose for children is 0.6 mg/kg/day in four divided doses or 0.8 mg/kg/day in two divided doses, for two to four days.[9] This should be initiated either before or with the first dose of antibacterials.

Adults

A study in adults treated with dexamethasone did not show a significant beneficial effect on neurologic sequelae including hearing loss, but did demonstrate a reduction in unfavourable outcomes and mortality. The majority of these study patients had pneumococcal meningitis. Benefits were not seen in subgroups with meningitis caused by other bacteria, although patient numbers in those groups were small. In all groups, dexamethasone appeared to be the most beneficial in patients with moderate-to-severe disease on the Glasgow Coma Scale.[14] A systematic review of adjunctive steroid therapy in adults with acute bacterial meningitis showed that steroids significantly reduced mortality. However, the beneficial effect was statistically significant only in pneumococcal meningitis, where the number of deaths was greatest. There was a trend toward significant reduction in neurologic sequelae.[15]

For adults, the use of adjunctive dexamethasone is recommended in cases of community-acquired bacterial meningitis where *S. pneumoniae* is the known or suspected pathogen.[4] The dose for adults has been variable in published studies. A dose of 10 mg every six hours for four days has been used.[14] Practice guidelines from The Infectious Diseases Society of America recommend 0.15 mg/kg every six hours for two to four days, commencing either before or with the first dose of antibacterials.[4] Some experts recommend discontinuing corticosteroids if the pathogen is determined *not* to be *S. pneumoniae*;[4] however, this is controversial.[12]

Prevention

Vaccines

- With the implementation in Canada of universal infant immunization programs with conjugated *H. influenzae* type b, *S. pneumoniae* and *N. meningitidis* type C vaccines, the rates of bacterial meningitis have decreased significantly. There is also evidence of the development of herd immunity (protection of unvaccinated individuals extending from immunization of a majority of the population).
- The conjugated vaccine against *H. influenzae* type b has led to the virtual disappearance of meningitis due to this pathogen. The conjugated pneumococcal vaccine is > 95% effective in preventing invasive disease caused by the seven serotypes included in the vaccine.[16]
- The conjugated meningococcal vaccine against *N. meningitidis* type C has a reported efficacy of > 90% against invasive infection.[17] In 2006, a quadrivalent conjugate meningococcal vaccine against *N. meningitidis* types A,C,W,Y-135 became available in Canada for use in people over the age of 2 years. The impact of these vaccines on the incidence of meningococcal meningitis in older children and adults is not yet clear and will need to be evaluated if universal immunization programs are implemented.
- In individuals > 2 years of age, polysaccharide vaccines are safe and efficacious for the prevention of invasive pneumococcal and meningococcal infections. Certain high-risk individuals may benefit from receiving both conjugated and polysaccharide vaccines; consult the *Canadian Immunization Guide*, seventh edition, 2006 (see Suggested Readings).
- Vaccination to prevent meningitis is recommended in Canada for certain high-risk individuals. These recommendations are outlined in the *Canadian Immunization Guide*, seventh edition, 2006 (see Suggested Readings).

Intrapartum Prophylaxis

- The administration of intrapartum antibacterials to prevent mother-to-child transmission significantly reduces the incidence of early-onset invasive neonatal GBS infections.[18]

Post-exposure Prophylaxis[19,20]

- Those in close contact with individuals who have meningitis caused by either *H. influenzae* type b or *N. meningitidis* are at increased risk. Post-exposure prophylaxis is recommended, for close contacts only, to reduce the risk of transmission.
- The regimen following exposure to *H. influenzae* type b is **rifampin** 20 mg/kg (maximum dose 600 mg) orally once daily for four days.
- Following exposure to *N. meningitidis*, the prophylactic regimen for infants ≤ 1 month is **rifampin** 5 mg/kg orally every 12 hours for two days. Children > 1 month should receive rifampin 10 mg/kg (maximum 600 mg) every 12 hours for two days *or* a single dose of ceftriaxone 125 mg im. For adults, options include a single dose of **ciprofloxacin** 500 mg orally (if > 18 years), a single dose of ceftriaxone 250 mg im (if > 12 years) or rifampin 600 mg orally every 12 hours for two days.
- In pregnant women, ceftriaxone is recommended instead of rifampin or ciprofloxacin.
- In cases of meningitis involving either *N. meningitidis* or *H. influenzae*, the index patient should also receive prophylaxis prior to discharge to eradicate bacterial carriage, unless cefotaxime or ceftriaxone was used for treatment.

Therapeutic Tips

- In the case of empiric antimicrobial therapy consisting of vancomycin and a cephalosporin, give the cephalosporin first to ensure initial broad coverage and penetration into the CSF.
- With ventriculoperitoneal shunt–associated meningitis, successful treatment should include removal of the shunt with insertion of an external ventricular drain in addition to antimicrobial therapy.

Table 4: **Intravenous Antibacterial Therapy for Bacterial Meningitis** [4,19,21,21,22]

Class	Antibacterial	Dose	Adverse Effects	Drug Interactions	Cost[a]
Penicillins	*penicillin G* generics	**Neonates ≤ 7 days:** ≤ 2 kg: 100 000 U/kg/day divided Q12H > 2 kg: 150 000 U/kg/day divided Q8H Group B streptococcus: 250 000–450 000 U/kg/day divided Q8H **Neonates > 7 days:** < 1.2 kg: 100 000 U/kg/day divided Q12H 1.2–2 kg: 150 000 U/kg/day divided Q8H > 2 kg: 200 000 U/kg/day divided Q6H Group B streptococcus: 450 000 U/kg/day divided Q4–6H **Older infants and children:** 400 000 U/kg/day divided Q4–6H Max: 24 million U/day **Adults:** 20–24 million U/day divided Q4–6H	Rash, hypersensitivity, drug fever, hemolytic anemia, interstitial nephritis, seizures (with high doses).	Tetracycline, erythromycin may ↓ effectiveness.	$
	ampicillin generics	**Neonates ≤ 7 days:** ≤ 2 kg: 100 mg/kg/day divided Q12H > 2 kg: 150 mg/kg/day divided Q8H Group B streptococcus: 200 mg/kg/day divided Q8H	Rash, hypersensitivity, diarrhea, vomiting, drug fever, seizures (with high doses).	↑ incidence of rash with concurrent use of allopurinol.	$$$

(cont'd)

Table 4: **Intravenous Antibacterial Therapy for Bacterial Meningitis** [4,19,21,21,22] *(cont'd)*

Class	Antibacterial	Dose	Adverse Effects	Drug Interactions	Cost[a]
		Neonates > 7 days: < 1.2 kg: 100 mg/kg/day divided Q12H 1.2–2 kg: 150 mg/kg/day divided Q8H > 2 kg: 200 mg/kg/day divided Q6H Group B streptococcus: 300–400 mg/kg/day divided Q4–6H **Older infants and children:** 200–400 mg/kg/day divided Q4–6H **Adults:** 2 g Q4H Max: 12 g/day			
Cephalosporins	*cefotaxime* ◗ Claforan	**Neonates ≤ 7 days:** < 2 kg: 100 mg/kg/day divided Q12H ≥ 2 kg: 100–150 mg/kg/day divided Q8–12H **Neonates > 7 days:** 1.2–2 kg: 150 mg/kg/day divided Q8H > 2 kg: 150–200 mg/kg/day divided Q6–8H **6 wk–12 y:** 300 mg/kg/day divided Q6H[b] **> 12 y:** 2 g Q4–6H Max: 12 g/day	Hypersensitivity, phlebitis, diarrhea, pseudomembranous colitis, transient elevation in liver enzymes; leukopenia; neutropenia, eosinophilia; thrombocytopenia. Seizures, nephrotoxicity with large doses.		$$$$$

Class	Antibacterial	Dose	Adverse Effects	Drug Interactions	Cost[a]
	ceftriaxone Rocephin	**Infants and children:** 100 mg/kg Q12H × 3 doses, then Q24H **Adults:** 2 g Q12–24H Max: 4 g/day	See cefotaxime.		$$$$$
	ceftazidime Ceftazidime for Injection USP, Fortaz	**Neonates ≤ 7 days:** < 2 kg: 100 mg/kg/day divided Q12H ≥ 2 kg: 100–150 mg/kg/day divided Q8–12H **Infants > 7 days and children:** 150 mg/kg/day divided Q8H **Adults:** 2 g Q8H Max: 6 g/day	See cefotaxime.		$$$$$

(cont'd)

Table 4: **Intravenous Antibacterial Therapy for Bacterial Meningitis** [4,19,21,21,22] *(cont'd)*

Class	Antibacterial	Dose	Adverse Effects	Drug Interactions	Cost[a]
Aminoglycosides	*gentamicin* generics	**Neonates ≤ 7 days:** < 1.2 kg: 2.5 mg/kg Q12H **Neonates > 7 days and older children:** 1.2–2 kg: 2.5 mg/kg Q8–12H > 2 kg: 2.5 mg/kg Q8H **Adults:** 1–2 mg/kg Q8H	Nephrotoxicity: ↑ risk with ↑ dose and duration. Ototoxicity. Levels should be closely monitored to reduce incidence of toxicity.	↑ toxicity with use of amphotericin B, magnesium, cephalosporins, penicillins, loop diuretics, vancomycin, cisplatin, cyclosporin and indomethacin.	$$
Glycopeptides	*vancomycin* Vancocin, Vancomycin Hydrochloride USP, generics	**Neonates ≤ 7 days:** < 1.2 kg: 15 mg/kg Q24H 1.2–2 kg: 10–15 mg/kg Q12–18H > 2 kg: 10–15 mg/kg Q8–12H **Neonates > 7 days to 6 wk:** < 1.2 kg: 15 mg/kg Q24H 1.2–2 kg: 10–15 mg/kg Q8–12H > 2 kg: 10–15 mg/kg Q8H **Infants > 6 weeks and children:** 60 mg/kg/day divided Q6H **Adults:** 500 mg Q6H or 1 g Q12H Max: 4 g/day	Flushing, hypotension with rapid iv infusion; phlebitis.	May cause ototoxicity, nephrotoxicity if receiving other drugs with these effects.	$$$$$

[a] Cost per day based on 70 kg body weight; includes drug cost only.

[b] High-dose cefotaxime should be used for presumed resistant pneumococcal meningitis. Dose can be decreased to 200 mg/kg/day divided Q6H once it is known that the organism is susceptible to cephalosporins.

Dosage adjustment may be required in renal impairment; see Appendix I.

Legend: $ < $25 $$ $25–50 $$$ $50–75 $$$$ $75–100 $$$$$ $100–140

Suggested Readings

Infectious Diseases and Immunization Committee, Canadian Paediatric Society (CPS). Therapy of suspected bacterial meningitis in Canadian children six weeks of age and older. *Paediatr Child Health* 2001;6(3):147-52.

Kaplan SL. Clinical presentations, diagnosis, and prognostic factors of bacterial meningitis. *Infect Dis Clin North Am* 1999;13(3):579-94, vi-vii.

Kaplan SL, Mason EO. Mechanisms of pneumococcal antibacterial resistance and treatment of pneumococcal infections in 2002. *Pediatr Ann* 2002;31(4):250-60.

National Advisory Committee on Immunization. *Canadian immunization guide 2006*. 7th ed. Ottawa (ON): Public Health Agency of Canada, Infectious Disease and Emergency Preparedness Branch; 2006. Available from: http://www.phac-aspc.gc.ca/publicat/cig-gci/pdf/cig-gci-2006_e.pdf Accessed March 26 2007.

Quagliarello V, Scheld WM. Bacterial meningitis: pathogenesis, pathophysiology, and progress. *N Engl J Med* 1992;327(12):864-72.

Straus SE, Thorpe KE, Holroyd-Leduc J. How do I perform a lumbar puncture and analyze the results to diagnose bacterial meningitis? *JAMA* 2006;296(16):2012-22.

Tunkel AR, Hartman BJ, Kaplan SL et al. Practice guidelines for the management of bacterial meningitis. *Clin Infect Dis* 2004;39(9):1267-84.

References

1. Schaad UB. *Rev Med Microbiol* 1997;8:171-8.
2. Straus SE, Thorpe KE, Holroyd-Leduc J. How do I perform a lumbar puncture and analyze the results to diagnose bacterial meningitis? *JAMA* 2006;296(16):2012-22.
3. Saez-Llorens X et al. Acute bacterial meningitis beyond the newborn period. In: Long SS et al., editors. *Principles and practice of pediatric infectious diseases*. 2nd ed. New York (NY): Churchill Livingstone; 2003.
4. Tunkel AR, Hartman BJ, Kaplan SL et al. Practice guidelines for the management of bacterial meningitis. *Clin Infect Dis* 2004;39(9):1267-84.
5. Maxson S, Lewno MJ, Schutze GE. Clinical usefulness of cerebrospinal fluid bacterial antigen studies. *J Pediatr* 1994;125(2):235-8.
6. Tarafdar K, Rao S, Recco RA et al. Lack of sensitivity of the latex agglutination test to detect bacterial antigen in the cerebrospinal fluid of patients with culture-negative meningitis. *Clin Infect Dis* 2001;33(3):406-8.
7. Leib SL, Boscacci R, Gratzl O et al. Predictive value of cerebrospinal fluid (CSF) lactate level versus CSF/blood glucose ratio for the diagnosis of bacterial meningitis following neurosurgery. *Clin Infect Dis* 1999;29(1):69-74.
8. Hasbum R, Abrahams J, Jekel J et al. Computed tomography of the head before lumbar puncture in adults with suspected meningitis. *N Engl J Med* 2001;345(24):1727-33.
9. Infectious Diseases and Immunization Committee, Canadian Paediatric Society (CPS). Therapy of suspected bacterial meningitis in Canadian children six weeks of age and older. *Paediatr Child Health* 2001;6(3):147-52.
10. Doit C, Barre J, Cohen R et al. Bactericidal activity against intermediately cephalosporin-resistant Streptococcus pneumoniae in cerebrospinal fluid of children with bacterial meningitis treated with high doses of cefotaxime and vancomycin. *Antimicrob Agents Chemother* 1997;41(9):2050-2.
11. Klugman KP, Friedland IR, Bradley JS. Bactericidal activity against cephalosporin-resistant Streptococcus pneumoniae in cerebrospinal fluid of children with acute bacterial meningitis. *Antimicrob Agents Chemother* 1995;39(9):1988-92.
12. van de Beek D, de Gans J, Tunkel AR et al. Community-acquired bacterial meningitis in adults. *N Engl J Med* 2006;354(1):44-53.
13. McIntyre PB, Berkey CS, King SM et al. Dexamethasone as adjunctive therapy in bacterial meningitis. A meta-analysis of randomized clinical trials since 1988. *JAMA* 1997;278(11):925-31.

14. de Gans J, van de Beek D et al. Dexamethasone in adults with bacterial meningitis. *N Engl J Med* 2002;347(20):1549-56.
15. van de Beek D, de Gans J, McIntyre P et al. Steroids in adults with acute bacterial meningitis: a systematic review. *Lancet Infect Dis* 2004;4(3):139-43.
16. Black S, Shinefield H, Fireman B et al. Efficacy, safety and immunogenicity of heptavalent pneumococcal conjugate vaccine in children. Northern California Kaiser Permanente Vaccine Study Center Group. *Pediatr Infect Dis J* 2000;19(3):187-95.
17. Balmer P, Borrow R, Miller E. Impact of meningococcal C conjugate vaccine in the UK. *J Med Microbiol* 2002;51(9):717-22.
18. Schrag S, Gorwitz R, Fultz-Butts K et al. Prevention of perinatal group B streptococcal disease. Revised guidelines from CDC. *MMWR Recomm Rep* 2002;51(RR-11):1-22.
19. American Academy of Pediatrics. Meningococcal infections. In: Pickering LK, editor. *2000 Red book: report of the Committee on Infectious Diseases*. 25th ed. Elk Grove Village (IL): American Academy of Pediatrics; 2000.
20. American Academy of Pediatrics. Haemophilus influenzae infections. In: Pickering LK, editor. *2000 Red book: report of the Committee on Infectious Diseases*. 25th ed. Elk Grove Village (IL): American Academy of Pediatrics; 2000.
21. Taketomo CK. *Pediatric dosage handbook: including neonatal dosing, drug administration & extemporaneous preparations*. 9th ed. Hudson (OH): Lexi-Comp; 2002.
22. Wubbel L, McCracken GH. Management of bacterial meningitis: 1998. *Pediatr Rev* 1998;19(3):78-84.

CHAPTER 101
Acute Osteomyelitis

Simon Dobson, MD, FRCPC

Goals of Therapy

- Cure the acute infection
- Minimize morbidity, e.g., loss of limb function
- Prevent recurrence and progression to chronic osteomyelitis

Investigations

- History:
  - duration of symptoms: fever, pain, redness, swelling, limping or other loss of function or movement
  - any recent surgery, trauma or penetrating wound
  - vascular insufficiency
  - neuropathic ulcer of the diabetic foot
- Examination:
  - tenderness over affected bone (often exquisite).[1] No pain is elicited if advanced neuropathy of diabetic foot
  - range of movement in affected limb (any suggestion of septic arthritis?)
- Laboratory tests:
  - complete blood count and acute-phase reactants (erythrocyte sedimentation rate, C-reactive protein) as baseline[2]
  - blood culture before starting antibacterials (positive in 30 to 60%)
- Aspiration:
  - an organism can be obtained in up to 80% of cases of acute hematogenous osteomyelitis. This may become an increasingly important test as resistant organisms such as community-acquired methicillin-resistant *Staphylococcus aureus* (CA-MRSA) play a greater role in acute osteomyelitis.[3,4] Early consultation with an orthopedic surgeon is recommended
  - culture of superficial ulcer or draining sinus may be unreliable due to the possible presence of colonizing organisms. In addition, some true pathogens may be sufficiently fastidious that recovery from superficial culture is difficult (e.g., anaerobes). The best specimen is bone or periosteal aspirate, obtained surgically or by percutaneous biopsy through unaffected skin[5]
- Imaging:
  - x-ray may be normal initially; changes (e.g., periosteal reaction) are not evident for at least 10 days after onset

  - rarefaction of bone visible only when 50% loss of bone density (early in neonates, later in older children)
  - rarefaction of bone may be due to an adjacent chronic inflammatory lesion, which must be distinguished from lytic lesions of osteomyelitis
  - x-ray does not rule out diagnosis in diabetic foot. Chronic osteopathy may be present
- Bone scan:
  - imaging using technetium 99m-labelled methylene diphosphonate has improved early diagnosis. Early "blood pool images" should be taken, as well as later bone uptake images, to help differentiate cellulitis from bone infection
  - a negative bone scan does not rule out osteomyelitis.[6] In neonates an x-ray may be more reliable. Other causes of enhanced bone turnover (e.g., fracture or tumor) will also give a positive result
  - in the neuropathic foot, small stress fractures may be difficult to detect clinically or radiographically, but still show uptake on the bone scan. Vascular insufficiency may attenuate changes on the bone scan
  - *Note*: If the clinical findings suggest osteomyelitis, do not delay treatment until a bone scan is obtained
- Probe diabetic ulcer with sterile instrument. If bone can be reached, this has high specificity and positive predictive value for osteomyelitis (89%) but low sensitivity.[7] Best initial evaluation is x-ray plus a probe for bone.[5] If both are negative, treat for soft tissue infection but repeat x-ray in two weeks (Figure 2)

Therapeutic Choices (Figure 1)

Nonpharmacologic Choices

Surgical Drainage

Antibacterials do not penetrate well into collections of pus or into bone in which blood supply is compromised by infection. Surgical decompression and exploration are necessary when there has been a delay in presentation or diagnosis, when pus has been found on aspiration or when there is x-ray evidence of bone destruction. For early disease the role of immediate surgery has been controversial.[1,6] However, if swelling, pain, tenderness and fever do not resolve within days after starting antibacterials, consider surgical exploration, especially if initial empiric therapy did not cover MRSA. Suspicion of osteomyelitis secondary to a penetrating injury (e.g., to the calcaneus) requires bone exploration, débridement and culture. Osteomyelitis associated with diabetic foot infection often requires surgical débridement. This should be aggressive and may involve amputation of the infected bone.

Table 1: **Initial Empiric Antibacterial Therapy of Acute Osteomyelitis**[a]

Characteristics	Usual Causative Organisms	Empiric IV Antibacterials
Hematogenous Osteomyelitis		
Most common type Predominant in children Bloodborne bacteria lodge in bone as nidus of infection Possible in any bone but usually in long bones: femur 36%, tibia 33%, humerus 10% Vertebral osteomyelitis not uncommon in adults. Predisposing factors are iv drug abuse, trauma, other source of infection, e.g., urinary tract In neonates, septic arthritis often coexists	**Neonates:** group B streptococci, gram-negative enterics, *S. aureus* **Children:** *S. aureus* (MSSA & MRSA[b]), group A streptococci Rare: *H. influenzae*,[c] *S. pneumoniae*, gram-negative enterics **Adults:** *S. aureus*, gram-negative enterics	**Neonates:** if MRSA unlikely, cloxacillin[d] + cefotaxime (to cover gram-negative enteric bacilli); if MRSA possible, vancomycin + cefotaxime or ceftriaxone **Children:** if MRSA unlikely, cloxacillin;[d] if MRSA possible, vancomycin. Add cefotaxime (if not immunized against *H. influenzae*) **Adults:** cloxacillin[d] or cefazolin
Spread from Contiguous Sites[e]		
Spread from head/neck	*S. aureus*, anaerobes, gram-negative organisms, mixed infection	**Adults:** clindamycin ± gentamicin
Spread from soft tissue infection	*S. aureus*, streptococci	**Adults:** cloxacillin or cefazolin
Spread from genitourinary system	gram-negative enteric bacilli	**Adults:** fluoroquinolone or extended-spectrum beta-lactam (extended spectrum penicillin, carbapenem, 3rd generation cephalosporin)
	S. aureus, anaerobes, gram-negative organisms, mixed infection	**Adults:** clindamycin ± gentamicin
Penetrating Trauma (e.g., puncture wound of foot)		
	P. aeruginosa, *S. aureus*	**Children:** cloxacillin[d] + ceftazidime + gentamicin **Adults:** fluoroquinolone
Vascular Insufficiency		
Diabetic foot infection	*S. aureus*, streptococci, gram-negative bacilli, anaerobes	**Adults:** carbapenem *or* amoxicillin/clavulanate or piperacillin/tazobactam *or* moxifloxacin ± clindamycin or metronidazole

[a] The site and origin of infection and organism responsible are largely related to age.
[b] MRSA is increasing in importance as a cause of acute osteomyelitis.
[c] *H. influenzae* is of decreasing importance due to success of immunization.
[d] A semisynthetic, penicillinase-resistant penicillin (e.g., cloxacillin) provides coverage against *S. aureus* and streptococci.
[e] Common in elderly; predisposing factors include surgery, soft tissue infection
Abbreviations: MSSA = methicillin-sensitive *S. aureus*; MRSA = methicillin-resistant *S. aureus*

Pharmacologic Choices

Antibacterials

While cultures are pending, start empiric iv antibacterial therapy, based on the most likely infecting organism (Table 1) and on the prevalence in your geographical location of CA-MRSA as a cause of invasive staphylococcal infections.[8] A definitive choice can be made once the organism and sensitivities are identified (Table 2). The role of adjunctive antibacterials such as **fusidic acid** or **rifampin** has not been studied systematically. They cannot be used alone for staphylococcal infections because resistance develops rapidly.

Mild diabetic foot infection may be treated with appropriate wound care and an oral regimen of amoxicillin/clavulanate or ciprofloxacin plus clindamycin.[5]

Duration of antibacterial therapy should be a minimum of four weeks; many authorities recommend six weeks.[8] More severe initial presentation, extensive bone involvement, and slow resolution of systemic and local signs indicate a six-week course. In osteomyelitis following penetrating injury, 10 to 14 days of treatment is sufficient if adequate débridement has been performed. As home intravenous therapy programs have become more accessible to patients, this is an option to shorten hospital stay. The type of home iv pumps used in a particular program may limit specific treatment options, especially regarding dosing intervals. Choice of antibacterial therapy should not be compromised for the convenience of the local home iv program.

In diabetic foot infections, four to six weeks (or more) of therapy is required. If no débridement of bone occurs, a 10- to 12-week course has been curative. If all infected bone has been completely removed, two to three weeks may be sufficient.[5,9]

Sequential Intravenous–Oral Antibacterial Therapy

Since a long course is required, a switch from the iv to oral route has many advantages including shortened hospital stay and reduced complications from iv cannulae.[8] In children, continue iv antibacterials until the patient is systemically better, the temperature is normal and local signs of inflammation and tenderness are improved. This may take several days. Step-down oral antibacterial therapy may also be appropriate for adults.[10]

Switching to oral therapy can be undertaken with the following provisos:

- Patient is beyond neonatal age group and can be expected to attend for regular review
- No underlying immunocompromise present
- The dose of oral antibacterial is larger than that usually used for minor infections (Table 3)

- Compliance is vital. For children, the taste of the oral antibacterial is the most important factor. Cloxacillin liquid preparations are unpalatable; cephalexin has a more acceptable taste
- If no organism was isolated but the patient has recovered well on the empiric iv regimen, a switch to a comparable oral antibacterial therapy can still be made. Recurrence of symptoms while on oral step-down therapy demands immediate reassessment and resumption of iv antibacterials. Home iv therapy is recommended when oral step-down is not appropriate.
- Some infectious disease specialists suggest obtaining blood for serum inhibitory concentration testing, in order to assess the bioavailability of some drugs, particularly oral beta-lactams

Table 2: **Definitive Antibacterial Therapy for Acute Osteomyelitis**

Organism	Initial iv Antibacterials	Oral Antibacterials (for completion of course)
MSSA	Cloxacillin, cefazolin or clindamycin	Cloxacillin, cephalexin, clindamycin or amoxicillin-clavulanate
Streptococcus group A	Penicillin	Penicillin, amoxicillin or clindamycin
Streptococcus group B	Penicillin	In neonates, oral antibacterials are not appropriate
Enteric gram-negative bacilli	Cefotaxime	In neonates, oral antibacterials are not appropriate
P. aeruginosa	Ceftazidime + Gentamicin	Adults: ciprofloxacin No suitable oral preparation available for children. However, oral ciprofloxacin is sometimes used in children after careful consideration and discussion of potential risks with child's parents/guardians
MRSA	Vancomycin	CA-MRSA may be sensitive to clindamycin as an oral agent; otherwise use home iv therapy[a]
Mixed aerobic/anaerobic	Carbapenem, moxifloxacin, amoxicillin/clavulanate or piperacillin/tazobactam	Ciprofloxacin + clindamycin or amoxicillin/clavulanate

[a] The microbiology laboratory must do a test (usually a "D" test) of inducible clindamycin resistance in MRSA.
Abbreviations: MSSA = methicillin-sensitive *S. aureus*; MRSA = methicillin-resistant *S. aureus*; CA-MRSA = community-acquired methicillin-resistant *S. aureus*

Follow-up

Success of treatment is judged by careful follow-up of systemic signs (i.e., fever and well-being, local signs of decreasing inflammation and tenderness and return of full function). Erythrocyte sedimentation rate gradually returns to normal over several weeks. The C-reactive protein returns to normal in a matter of days.

Therapeutic Tips

- The consequences of treating osteomyelitis empirically with what turns out to be the wrong antibiotic can be dire. In an era of increasing incidence of CA-MRSA, persuading a surgeon to obtain pus by aspirating the bone at the time of presentation allows an accurate microbiologic diagnosis and tailored antibiotic therapy.
- Home iv therapy or oral step-down therapy can be appropriate for many patients, reducing hospital stay and still assuring cure.

Figure 1: **Management of Acute Osteomyelitis**

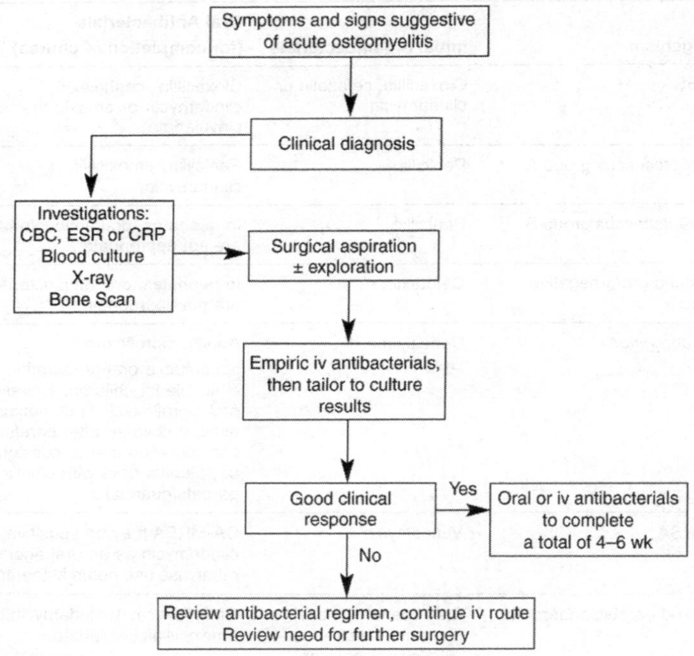

Figure 2: **Management of Diabetic Foot Osteomyelitis**

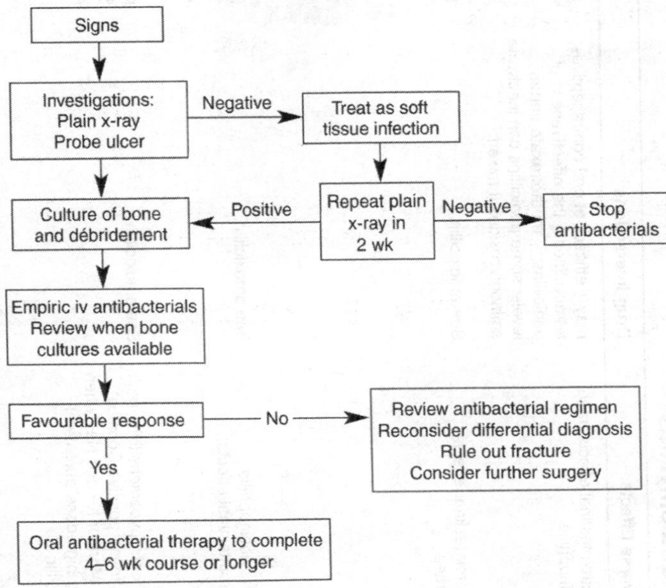

Table 3: Antibacterials Used for the Treatment of Acute Osteomyelitis[a]

Class	Antibacterial	Dose	Adverse Effects	Drug Interactions	Cost[b]
Penicillins	*amoxicillin* generics	Children: 100 mg/kg/day, po divided Q8H; max 3 g/day Adults: 0.5–1 g po Q8H	Gastrointestinal effects, rash, eosinophilia.	may ↓ efficacy of oral contraceptives; tetracyclines ↓ the effectiveness of penicillins; ↑ methotrexate serum levels; some penicillins can inactivate aminoglycosides if mixed.	$
	amoxicillin/ clavulanate Clavulin, generics	Children: 100 mg (amoxicillin)/kg/day po divided Q8H; max 1750 mg (amoxicillin)/day, given as amoxicillin 40 mg/mL + clavulanate 5.7 mg/mL suspension Adults: (amoxicillin) 500 mg po Q8H or 875 mg po Q12H	Gastrointestinal effects, diarrhea.	See amoxicillin.	$
	cloxacillin generics	Children: 200 mg/kg/day iv or 150–200 mg/kg/day po divided Q6H; max 6 g/day Adults: 2 g iv Q4H	Rash, eosinophilia, gastrointestinal effects.	See amoxicillin.	Pediatric: $ Adult: $$
	penicillin G generics	Children: 200 000 units/kg/day iv divided Q4–6H; max 20 million units/day Adults: 5–24 million units/day iv divided Q4–6H	GI effects, hypersensitivity, rash, drug fever, positive Coombs' test. Monitor K+ and Na+ when using high-dose parenteral penicillin G.	See amoxicillin.	Pediatric: $ Adult: $$

Class	Antibacterial	Dose	Adverse Effects	Drug Interactions	Cost[b]
	penicillin V Pen-Vee, generics	Children: 100 mg/kg/day po divided Q6H; max 3 g/day Adults: 0.75–1 g QID	GI effects, hypersensitivity, rash, drug fever, positive Coombs' test.	See amoxicillin.	$
	piperacillin/ tazobactam Tazocin	Children: 300 mg (piperacillin)/kg/day iv in divided doses Q6–8H; max (piperacillin) 4 g/dose, 12 g/day Adults: 3.375 g iv Q6H	Diarrhea, other GI effects, headache, rash, hypersensitivity, phlebitis.	See amoxicillin.	Pediatric: $$ Adult: $$$
Cephalosporins	*cefazolin* generics	Children: 100 mg/kg/day iv divided Q8H; max 6 g/day Adult: 2 g iv Q8H	GI effects, especially diarrhea.	↑ nephrotoxic effects of aminoglycosides; ↑ INR with warfarin.	Pediatric: $ Adult: $$
	cefotaxime Claforan	Children: 150 mg/kg/day iv divided Q8H; max 10 g/day Adults: 2 g iv Q4–8H	Phlebitis, hypersensitivity, positive Coombs' test.	See cefazolin.	Pediatric: $$ Adult: $$$
	ceftazidime Fortaz, generic	Children: 150 mg/kg/day iv divided Q8H; max 6 g/day Adults: 2 g iv Q8H	Phlebitis, eosinophilia, positive Coombs' test, ↑ AST, superinfections.	See cefazolin.	Pediatric: $$$ Adult: $$$$
	ceftriaxone Rocephin, generics	Children: 75 mg/kg/day iv divided Q12–24H; max 4 g/day Adults: 1–2 g/day in 1–2 divided doses; max 4 g/day	See ceftazidime.	See cefazolin.	$$

(cont'd)

Table 3: **Antibacterials Used for the Treatment of Acute Osteomyelitis**[a] *(cont'd)*

Class	Antibacterial	Dose	Adverse Effects	Drug Interactions	Cost[b]
	cephalexin generics	Pediatric: 100–150 mg/kg/day po divided Q6H; max 3 g/day Adults: 1–4 g/day divided Q6H	Gastrointestinal effects, rash, eosinophilia, leukopenia, positive Coombs' test, ↑ aspartate transaminase.	See cefazolin.	$
Fluoro-quinolones	*ciprofloxacin* Cipro, generics	Adults: 400 mg iv Q12H or 750 mg po Q12H Children (off-label): 30 mg/kg/day po divided Q12H; max 1500 mg/day po	Abdominal pain, nausea, vomiting, rash, dizziness, headache, drowsiness, diarrhea.	Absorption ↓ by antacids, iron salts, magnesium sucralfate; ↓ theophylline and caffeine elimination.	iv: $$$ po: $
	moxifloxacin Avelox	Adult: 400 mg po or iv Q24H	See ciprofloxacin.	Absorption ↓ by antacids, iron salts, magnesium sucralfate.	iv: $$$ po: $
Lincosamides	*clindamycin* Dalacin C, Dalacin C Flavored Granules, Dalacin C Phosphate Sterile Solution, generics	Children: 40 mg/kg/day iv divided Q6H or 30 mg/kg/day po divided Q8H; max 2 g/day Adults: 450–600 mg iv or po Q8H	Rash, neutropenia, ↑ aspartate transaminase and alkaline phosphatase, pseudomembranous colitis.	↓ absorption with aluminum salts; ↑ effects of anesthetic agents.	iv: $$ po: $
Aminoglyco-sides	*gentamicin* generics	Children: 6 mg/kg/day iv divided Q8H Adults: 5–7 mg/kg/day iv divided Q8H or once daily if renal function permits	Nephrotoxicity usually reversible, ↑ risk with dose, duration; ototoxicity often reversible.	↑ toxicity with other nephrotoxic or ototoxic drugs; ↑ effects of anesthetic agents.	Pediatric: $ Adult: $$
Carbapenems	*imipenem/cilastatin* Primaxin	Adults: 500 mg iv Q6H	Caution in beta-lactam sensitivity; risk of seizures if dose exceeded in renal failure.	May cause seizures with theophylline.	$$$$

Class	Antibacterial	Dose	Adverse Effects	Drug Interactions	Cost[b]
	meropenem Merrem	Adults: 500 mg iv Q6H	See imipenem/cilastatin.	May ↓ valproate levels.	$$$$
Glycopeptides	*vancomycin* Vancocin, Vancomycin , generics	Children: 40 mg/kg/day iv divided Q6H; max 4 g/day Adults: 1 g iv Q12H	Hypotension, flushing, red man syndrome, chills, drug fever, eosinophilia.	↑ toxicity with other nephrotoxic or ototoxic drugs.	Pediatric: $$ Adult: $$$$

[a] Therapy is initiated with iv antibacterials. Patients can be stepped down to oral antibacterials under certain conditions.
[b] Cost per day (pediatric dosage based on 20 kg and adult based on 70 kg body weights); includes drug cost only.
Dosage adjustment may be required in renal impairment; see Appendix I.
Legend: $ < $10 $$ $10–50 $$–$$$ $10–100 $$$ $50–100 $$$$ > $100

Suggested Readings

Carek PJ, Dickerson LM, Sack JL. Diagnosis and management of osteomyelitis. *Am Fam Physician* 2001;63(12):2413-20.

Cunha BA. Osteomyelitis in elderly patients. *Clin Infect Dis* 2002;35(3):287-93.

Raasch RH. Osteomyelitis/Septic arthritis. In: Koda-Kimble M, Young LY, editors. *Applied therapeutics: the clinical use of drugs.* 7th ed. Philadelphia (PA): Lippincott Williams & Wilkins; 2001. p.64.1-64.7.

References

1. Nade S. Acute haematogenous osteomyelitis in infancy and childhood. *J Bone Joint Surg Br* 1983;65(2):109-19.
2. Unkila-Kallio L, Kallio MJ, Eskola J et al. Serum C-reactive protein, erythrocyte sedimentation rate, and white blood cell count in acute hematogenous osteomyelitis of children. *Pediatrics* 1994;93(1):59-62.
3. Kaplan SL. Community-acquired methicillin-resistant Staphylococcus aureus infections in children. *Semin Pediatr Infect Dis* 2006;17(3):113-9.
4. Arnold SR, Elias D, Buckingham SC et al. Changing patterns of acute hematogenous osteomyelitis and septic arthritis: emergence of community-associated methicillin-resistant Staphylococcus aureus. *J Pediatr Orthop* 2006;26(6):703-8.
5. Caputo GM, Cavanagh PR, Ulbrecht JS et al. Assessment and management of foot disease in patients with diabetes. *N Engl J Med* 1994;331(13):854-60.
6. Lew DP, Waldvogel FA. Osteomyelitis. *N Engl J Med* 1997;336(14):999-1007.
7. Grayson ML, Gibbons GW, Balogh K et al. Probing to bone in infected pedal ulcers. A clinical sign of underlying osteomyelitis in diabetic patients. *JAMA* 1995;273(9):721-3.
8. Canadian Paediatric Society, Infectious Diseases and Immunization Committee. *Can J Infect Dis* 1994;4:10-2.
9. Eckman MH, Greenfield S, Mackey WC et al. Foot infections in diabetic patients. Decision and cost-effectiveness analyses. *JAMA* 1995;273(9):712-20.
10. Daver NG, Shelburne SA, Atmar RL et al. Oral step-down therapy is comparable to intravenous therapy for Staphylococcus aureus osteomyelitis. *J Infect* 2007;54(6):539-44.

CHAPTER 102
Sepsis and Septic Shock

Steven C. Reynolds, MD, FRCPC and
Anthony W. Chow, MD, FRCPC, FACP

Goals of Therapy

- Recognize sepsis early (Table 1)
- Promptly initiate goal-directed resuscitative efforts to restore tissue perfusion within the first six hours
- Eradicate causative pathogens (administer appropriate antibiotics within the first hour of recognizing sepsis)
- Establish *source control* (eliminate potential sources of infection) through measures such as:
  - débridement of infected necrotic tissue
  - drainage of abscesses
  - removal of potentially infected devices or foreign bodies
- Restore intravascular fluid volume
- Correct metabolic acidosis and coagulation defects
- Reduce oxygen demand
- Neutralize the biologic effects of exotoxins and/or endotoxins
- Manage complications, e.g., acute renal failure, acute respiratory distress syndrome, disseminated intravascular coagulation, multiple organ dysfunction syndrome
- Prevent nosocomial infections
- Prevent progression from sepsis to full septic shock

Investigations

- Thorough history with special attention to underlying disease, precipitating event and possible sites of infection
- Physical examination to determine the site and extent of infection, assess end-organ dysfunction and identify evidence of DIC or disseminated infection (e.g., skin rash, purpura, ecthyma gangrenosum, subcutaneous nodules)
- Clinical monitoring of vital signs, urine output, weight, level of consciousness
- Laboratory monitoring:
  - CBC and differential
  - arterial blood gases
  - electrolytes, plasma lactate, acid-base status
  - BUN and serum creatinine
  - liver function tests

- serum calcium and phosphate
- chest x-ray, ECG
- coagulation status
- stool for occult blood
- Gram stain and cultures of: blood drawn from two separate sites (peripheral and central lines), urine, sputum and other body sites as appropriate
- imaging studies to search for the locus of infection

- Additional investigations may be necessary to monitor cardiopulmonary status and to localize the site of infection
- Give serious consideration to insertion of a central venous catheter into the superior vena cava for the measurement of central venous oxygen saturation and central venous pressure in all patients with suspected sepsis. This facilitates rapid and appropriate resuscitation efforts

Classification of Sepsis and Septic Shock

Categorize patients into one of three syndromes (Table 1).

Table 1: **Classification of Sepsis, Severe Sepsis and Septic Shock**[1]

Clinical Staging	Diagnostic Criteria
Sepsis	Clinical evidence suggestive of infection *plus*: Signs of a systemic inflammatory response to infection (≥ 2 of the following): Tachypnea (> 20 breaths/min or $PaCO_2$ < 32 mm Hg [< 4.3 kPa]) Tachycardia (> 90 beats/min) Hyperthermia (> 38°C) or hypothermia (< 36°C) WBC > 12 × 10^9 cells/L, or < 4 × 10^9 cells/L, or > 10% immature (band) forms
Severe sepsis	Sepsis with hypotension (systolic blood pressure < 90 mm Hg or a 40 mm Hg decrease from baseline in the absence of other causes), organ dysfunction and perfusion abnormalities such as: Oliguria: < 0.5 mL/kg for at least 1 h in patients with urinary catheters ↑ plasma lactate (> normal upper limit) Altered mental status
Septic shock	Severe sepsis as defined above, despite adequate fluid resuscitation *Note*: patients who are on pressor agents may not be hypotensive

Therapeutic Choices (Figure 1)

Resuscitation and Monitoring

Meticulous monitoring of the patient's circulating volume and ventilatory status is essential, with immediate resuscitation if required. If simple measures do not quickly restore hemodynamic stability, consider intensive care with invasive hemodynamic monitoring and aggressive cardiovascular support.[2,3]

Early institution of *mechanical ventilation* and *sedation* helps to reduce oxygen demand and improve oxygen delivery and extraction at the tissue level.[4] *Neuromuscular blockade* should be avoided if at all possible due to the risk of prolonged muscular weakness. Sedation protocols should include a process of daily lightening of sedation with a careful clinical evaluation. *Adequate caloric intake* with trace element and vitamin supplements, preferably through the enteral route, is also important.[5]

A seminal study demonstrated a marked improvement in 28-day mortality in patients for whom the following goals of resuscitation were accomplished within six hours:[2]

- *central venous pressure*: 8-12 mm Hg (in a mechanically ventilated patient, the target central venous pressure should be 12–15 mm Hg, due to the increased intrathoracic pressure)
- *mean arterial pressure* ≥ 65 mm Hg
- *urine output* ≥ 0.5 mL/kg/hour
- central venous (superior vena cava) or mixed venous *oxygen saturation* ≥ 70%

If fluid resuscitation yields a central venous pressure of 8–12 mm Hg (or 12–15 mm Hg in a mechanically ventilated patient) but does not result in a mixed venous saturation of ≥ 70%, give a *packed red blood cell transfusion* to achieve a hematocrit of ≥ 30%. If the hematocrit is at or above this goal and the mixed venous saturation is not < 70%, initiate a **dobutamine** infusion to achieve the target saturation of ≥ 70%.

Transfusion Therapy

Maintain the hemoglobin above 70 to 80 g/L in septic shock. A higher concentration, 90 to 100 g/L, is recommended in patients with myocardial ischemia and low mixed venous oxygen saturation.[6]

Glucose Control

Despite conflicting results in recent studies, it is still prudent to maintain euglycemia in septic patients. Administration of intravenous **insulin** can be associated with hypoglycemic episodes, which can have significant morbidity; monitor blood sugar at hourly intervals. Although the original data supported a glycemic goal of 4.4 to 6.1 mmol/L, many clinicians relax this by providing an upper limit of approximately 8.3 mmol/L to avoid potential hypoglycemic episodes. Intravenous regular human insulin is given by continuous infusion with a glycemic check every hour.[7]

Localization and Evacuation of Loculated Infections

Plain radiographs and tomograms, ultrasonography, computed tomography and magnetic resonance imaging are invaluable for localizing the nidus of infection in the thorax, abdomen, pelvis or the central nervous system. Drain loculated abscesses and remove infected foreign bodies, as appropriate.[8]

Anticipation and Prevention of Complications

- *Acute renal failure*: avoid nephrotoxic drugs; monitor and dialyze as needed. Intermittent hemodialysis and continuous venovenous hemofiltration are equally effective, although the latter may be better tolerated from a hemodynamic and fluid balance perspective.
- *Acute respiratory distress syndrome (ARDS)*: anticipate and treat supportively (i.e., ventilatory support, **inhaled beta$_2$-agonists** and judicious use of **crystalloids** or **colloids**). Lung-protective ventilation strategies should be used to avoid ARDS. This includes the use of low tidal volumes (6 mL/kg) and a goal of maintaining end-inspiratory pressures < 30 cm of H_2O. Often, a moderate increase in arterial carbon dioxide tension ($PaCO_2$), i.e., permissive hypercapnia, is necessary to achieve these ventilator goals. Permissive hypercapnia may not be appropriate for patients with metabolic acidosis and is contraindicated in head injuries. Positive end-expiratory pressure (PEEP) should be used to minimize lung injury. The level of PEEP will vary from patient to patient but a reasonable starting point is 5–10 mm H_2O.
- *Aspiration*: whenever possible, raise the head of the patient's bed 45 degrees to minimize the risk of passive aspiration and ventilator-acquired pneumonia.
- *Electrolyte and acid-base status*: correct initial hyponatremia and acidosis; anticipate and correct hypocalcemia.
- *Edema, pericardial and pleural effusions*: maintain adequate intravascular volume before using **diuretics** to mobilize extravascular fluid. Drain empyemas as soon as possible with a large-bore chest tube. Maintain a high index of suspicion of a tamponade in a patient with a pericardial effusion.
- *Disseminated intravascular coagulation and thrombocytopenia*: when thrombosis is the major symptom, **heparin** anticoagulation is used. When the predominant manifestation is bleeding, administer fresh frozen plasma and platelets as required. Although heparin will theoretically prevent further consumption of clotting factors by reducing thrombin generation, its use in patients with bleeding is controversial.
- *Deep vein thrombosis*: **unfractionated heparin**, **low molecular weight heparins** or venous compression devices (see Chapter 42) are used to prevent deep vein thrombosis.[9] This practice may improve survival.[10]
- *Hepatic dysfunction*: If hepatic dysfunction occurs, avoid drugs requiring biotransformation in the liver.
- *Impaired gastrointestinal motility and stress ulcers:* impaired motility may manifest as abnormal gastric emptying or as an adynamic ileus.

Stress ulceration is another common complication in the acutely ill. If the patient is not being fed orally, prophylaxis with **H_2-receptor blockers** reduces bleeding and improves clinical outcome.[11] It is particularly indicated in those patients with prolonged mechanical ventilation, hypotension and coagulopathy. Enteral feeding, if feasible, is an effective means of ulcer prophylaxis.[9]

- *Central nervous system dysfunction*: anticipate irrational behaviour; manage seizures with anticonvulsants.
- *Nosocomial infections*: strict adherence to handwashing, aseptic technique and other infection control principles is required to minimize the development of nosocomial infections. Make every effort to reduce the number of invasive intravascular catheters. To prevent nosocomial sinusitis, avoid nasogastric and nasotracheal intubation. Weaning protocols should be in place, and patients should have daily spontaneous breathing trials whenever possible. This has been shown to minimize the number of days on mechanical ventilation and lower the risk of ventilator-acquired pneumonia.
- *Pneumothorax*: be vigilant in watching for pneumothoraces in patients who are mechanically ventilated.

Empiric Antimicrobial Therapy

Antimicrobial therapy remains the cornerstone of treatment for sepsis and septic shock. However, the underlying disease, comorbid conditions and development of complications (e.g., ARDS, multi-organ dysfunction) often dictate the eventual outcome of therapy. Source control (see Goals of Therapy) is critical for the adequate treatment of infections.

Broad-spectrum antibiotics should be administered immediately, with the first dose being ordered and administered "stat." There is good evidence that mortality increases dramatically with each hour that appropriate antibiotic administration is delayed in the septic patient.[12] Ideally, all samples for microbial identification should be acquired prior to the administration of antibiotics, although sometimes this is not feasible. Antibiotic administration *should not* be delayed in the critically ill patient for the sole purpose of maximizing the microbial yield.

Initial antimicrobial therapy is empiric because gram-positive, gram-negative, mycobacterial, fungal and viral sepsis are often clinically indistinguishable. Antibiotic selection is based on the most likely source/site of infection and hence the most likely causative microorganisms and their anticipated susceptibility profiles (Table 2, Table 3). The choice of antimicrobial agents, described in Table 4, may also be influenced by the presence of acute renal or hepatic failure, hypersensitivity reactions, need for fluid restriction, local antimicrobial susceptibility patterns, emergence of resistance and drug interactions.

Administer antibiotics intravenously in critically ill patients and reassess within 48 to 72 hours. Adjustments are guided by culture results, in vitro susceptibility patterns and clinical response.

Antifungal therapy is controversial in the intensive care unit (ICU) as approximately 50% of candidemias are recognized only at autopsy. In special at-risk populations such as neutropenic patients, empiric antifungal therapy should be considered. Other patients need to be considered on a case-by-case basis for empiric antifungal therapy. Risk factors for candidemia include multiple colonization sites, long-term broad spectrum antibiotic therapy, hollow viscus rupture or abdominal surgery, intravenous catheters, prolonged ICU stay and total parenteral nutrition.[13]

The most appropriate choice of empiric antifungal therapy is not entirely clear. Fluconazole, amphotericin B (liposomal or conventional) and caspofungin are all reasonable choices. Care must be taken to avoid and monitor for toxicities, such as renal failure with amphotericin B. Fluconazole should be avoided if the patient has received fluconazole in the recent past, is hemodynamically unstable, is neutropenic or if there is a high local incidence of *Candida glabrata* or *Candida krusei*.[14]

Table 2: **Empiric Antimicrobial Treatment of Sepsis and Septic Shock**

Source of Infection	Common Pathogens	Initial Antimicrobial Regimen
Oral cavity, lower respiratory tract	*Streptococcus viridans*, *Streptococcus pyogenes*, *Streptococcus pneumoniae*, *Haemophilus influenzae*, *Klebsiella pneumoniae*, *Peptostreptococcus* spp., *Bacteroides* spp., *Fusobacterium* spp., *Legionella pneumophila*	3rd generation cephalosporin ± metronidazole *or* extended-spectrum penicillin *or* carbapenem *or* extended-spectrum fluoroquinolone *or* macrolide
Gastrointestinal tract, female pelvis	Enteric gram-negative bacilli, *Bacteroides fragilis*, *Peptostreptococcus* spp., *Clostridia* spp., *Enterococcus* spp.	Extended spectrum beta-lactam (3rd or 4th generation cephalosporin, extended-spectrum penicillin or carbapenem) + aminoglycoside *or* ciprofloxacin
Urinary tract	*Escherichia coli*, *Pseudomonas aeruginosa*, other enteric gram-negative bacilli, *Staphylococcus saprophyticus*, *Enterococcus*spp.	Extended-spectrum beta-lactam ± ciprofloxacin *or* aminoglycoside

(cont'd)

Table 2: **Empiric Antimicrobial Treatment of Sepsis and Septic Shock** *(cont'd)*

Source of Infection	Common Pathogens	Initial Antimicrobial Regimen
Cardiac valves	*Staphylococcus aureus*, *S. viridans*, *Enterococcus* spp., *Corynebacterium* spp., *Coxiella burnetii*, HACEK group (*Haemophilus aphrophilus*, *Actinobacillus actinomycetemcomitans*, *Cardiobacterium hominis*, *Eikenella corrodens*, *Kingella* spp.).	Dependent upon acuity and presence or absence of prosthetic valve. Vancomycin ± cloxacillin ± 3rd generation cephalosporin
Central nervous system	*Neisseria meningitidis*, *H. influenzae*, *S. pneumoniae*, *S. aureus*, enteric gram-negative bacilli, *Bacteroides* spp., *Nocardia asteroides*, *Peptostreptococcus* spp.	3rd generation cephalosporin ± vancomycin ± ampicillin
Necrotizing skin and soft tissues	Group A streptococcus, *S. aureus*, enteric gram-negative bacilli, *B. fragilis*, *Clostridia* spp., Peptostreptococcus spp., mixed anaerobes. Gram-negative and anaerobic bacteria are prominent in perirectal/genital infections.	Extended spectrum beta-lactam + clindamycin ± vancomycin
Intravascular devices-associated	*S. aureus*, *Staphylococcus epidermidis*, *Staphylococcus haemolyticus*, enteric gram-negative bacilli, *Candida* spp.	Vancomycin

Table 3: **Antimicrobial Sensitivities of Common Pathogens in Sepsis and Septic Shock**

Pathogen	Activity	Antimicrobials[a]
Staphylococci	Excellent	cloxacillin (no activity against MRSA or coagulase-negative Staphylococcus but agent of choice for MSSA), vancomycin (including MRSA)
	Moderate	carbapenems, cefepime, levofloxacin, moxifloxacin, piperacillin/tazobactam
	Some	ceftriaxone, cefotaxime, ciprofloxacin, ticarcillin/clavulanate
	Negligible/none	aminoglycosides, ceftazidime

(cont'd)

Table 3: **Antimicrobial Sensitivities of Common Pathogens in Sepsis and Septic Shock** *(cont'd)*

Pathogen	Activity	Antimicrobials[a]
Streptococci	Excellent	carbapenems, ceftriaxone, cefotaxime, cefepime, extended-spectrum penicillins, moxifloxacin, vancomycin
	Moderate	ceftazidime, levofloxacin
	Some	ciprofloxacin
	Negligible/none	aminoglycosides
Enterococci	Excellent	ampicillin, piperacillin/tazobactam
	Moderate	aminoglycosides (synergy only), imipenem/cilastatin, vancomycin
	Negligible/none	meropenem, ticarcillin/clavulanate, fluoroquinolones
Haemophilus	Excellent	carbapenems, 3rd and 4th generation cephalosporins, extended-spectrum penicillins, moxifloxacin
	Moderate	ciprofloxacin, levofloxacin
	Negligible/none	aminoglycosides, vancomycin
Enteric gram-negative bacilli	Excellent	aminoglycosides, carbapenems, cefepime, ceftazidime, extended-spectrum penicillins
	Moderate	cefotaxime, ceftriaxone, fluoroquinolones
	Negligible/none	vancomycin
Pseudomonas, resistant gram-negative bacilli	Excellent	carbapenems, cefepime, ciprofloxacin
	Moderate	aminoglycosides (particularly tobramycin), ceftazidime, levofloxacin, piperacillin/tazobactam
	Some	moxifloxacin
	Negligible/none	cefotaxime, ceftriaxone, vancomycin
Anaerobes	Excellent (incl. *B. fragilis*)	carbapenems, metronidazole, piperacillin/tazobactam
	Moderate	moxifloxacin
	Some	ceftazidime, ceftriaxone
	Negligible/none	aminoglycosides, ciprofloxacin, levofloxacin, vancomycin

[a] Antimicrobials listed alphabetically, not in order of preference.
Abbreviations: MSSA = methicillin-sensitive *S. aureus*; MRSA = methicillin-resistant *S. aureus*.

Vasoactive Agents for Cardiovascular Support

Although rapid fluid administration alone may be sufficient to restore hemodynamic stability, vasopressors are often necessary to restore minimal tissue perfusion pressure and enhance myocardial contractility.

Dopamine (5 to 20 μg/kg/min) has positive chronotropic, inotropic and vasoconstrictive effects. It is not often chosen as a first-line agent due to its mixed clinical effects. Low-dose dopamine does not preserve renal function.[15] **Norepinephrine** (0.03 to 1.5 μg/kg/min) has peripheral vasoconstricting activity and may be superior to **dopamine** in septic shock by increasing peripheral resistance and improving splanchnic perfusion.[16,17] **Phenylephrine** (2 to 10 μg/kg/min) also has potent vasoconstricting properties and increases blood pressure. Its relative lack of chronotropy makes it useful in tachyarrhythmias. **Dobutamine** (2 to 25 μg/kg/min) is inotropic but does not effectively increase blood pressure due to its vasodilatory properties. When added to norepinephrine, it may improve splanchnic blood flow.[18]

Occasionally, low-dose **vasopressin** (0.02-0.04 μg/min) is used as an adjunctive or “rescue” vasopressor. This is based on animal studies; major clinical studies addressing the use of vasopressin are due to be published in the near future.[19]

Drotrecogin alfa

Drotrecogin alfa (activated protein C) is indicated for use in adult patients with severe sepsis and an Acute Physiology and Chronic Health Evaluation (APACHE II) score of > 25 or multiple acute organ dysfunction. Randomized, placebo-controlled trials show a 19% relative reduction in mortality.[20,21] It is administered as an iv infusion at a rate of 24 μg/kg/h for a total of 96 hours. The major risk is bleeding; hence, avoid in patients with prolonged PT or aPTT, thrombocytopenia (platelet count $< 30 \times 10^9$/L), bleeding at a noncompressible site, risk of intracranial hemorrhage or predisposing conditions such as gastrointestinal ulceration.

Corticosteroids

Corticosteroids at pharmacologic doses for one to two days have failed to demonstrate benefit in controlled trials.[22] In contrast, smaller replacement or stress doses of longer duration were beneficial in achieving seven-day shock reversal[23] and reduction of vasopressor use.[24] A large randomized, placebo-controlled trial of 300 adult patients with septic shock showed that a 7-day course of **hydrocortisone** (50 mg iv Q6H) and **fludrocortisone** (50 μg po daily) reduced the 28-day mortality from 63 to 53% (p=0.02) in those with relative adrenal insufficiency.[25] This regimen should be considered in patients with septic shock, particularly those who are refractory to vasoactive agents.

Many clinicians advocate performing a stimulation test with adrenocorticotropic hormone (ACTH) to determine adrenal reserves, and administrating hydrocortisone while awaiting the test results. Cortisol levels are measured before and 30–60 minutes after administration of ACTH. A failure to increase by ≥ 250 nmol/L indicates a relative adrenally deficient state. If the ACTH stimulation test must be delayed but relative adrenal insufficiency is suspected, a dose of **dexamethasone** may be given as it will not interfere with the cortisol assay.

There are conflicting results regarding the specific patient population that will best benefit from corticosteroids in septic shock. Pertinent studies are nearing completion and may shed more light on this question.

Immune Globulins

Immunotherapy to neutralize or remove specific exotoxins may be worthwhile if etiologic agents are identified (e.g., diphtheria, botulism, anthrax, clostridial septicotoxemia, toxic shock syndrome). However, as specific antisera are seldom available, immunoglobulins pooled from healthy donors are often used instead.

The use of polyclonal **iv immune globulins (IVIG)** is recommended in patients with hereditary or acquired immunodeficiency.[26,27] An observational study also suggested that IVIG at 2 g/kg for one to two doses would be useful in streptococcal toxic shock syndrome.[28] IVIG improves outcome in cases of necrotizing fasciitis due to group A streptococcus (*Streptococcus pyogenes*) at a dose of 1 g/kg on day one and then 0.5 g/kg on days two and three.[29] IVIG may also be useful in staphylococcal toxic shock syndrome.[30]

Currently there is clinical equipoise regarding the use of polyclonal IVIG in septic shock. There have been conflicting results in recent meta-analyses, and further well-designed, multicentre, randomized, placebo-controlled trials are needed to shed further light on this topic.[31,32]

Therapeutic Tips

- Empiric broad-spectrum antibiotic therapy primarily directed at enteric gram-negative bacilli must be initiated early in *neutropenic* patients (see Chapter 108).[33] The classic signs and symptoms of infection, other than fever, are often absent, making it much more difficult to localize the primary source of infection. Infections (especially gram-negative) in these patients tend to disseminate rapidly and widely and are associated with a high mortality rate. The clinical outcome is often dictated by the speed of bone marrow recovery and successful avoidance of complications (e.g., superinfections).
- *Persistent bacteremia,* despite appropriate antimicrobial therapy, suggests a valvular or endovascular infection, a loculated abscess with dissemination, or the emergence of resistant microorganisms.
- *Culture-negative infections* are particularly common among patients who have received partial antimicrobial therapy before cultures are obtained, and in immunocompromised patients undergoing bone marrow or solid organ transplants. The possibility of fastidious or culture-negative organisms, particularly *Legionella* spp., rickettsia, invasive fungi and viruses, should be seriously considered and appropriate investigations implemented.

Figure 1: **Early Management of Septic Shock**[34]

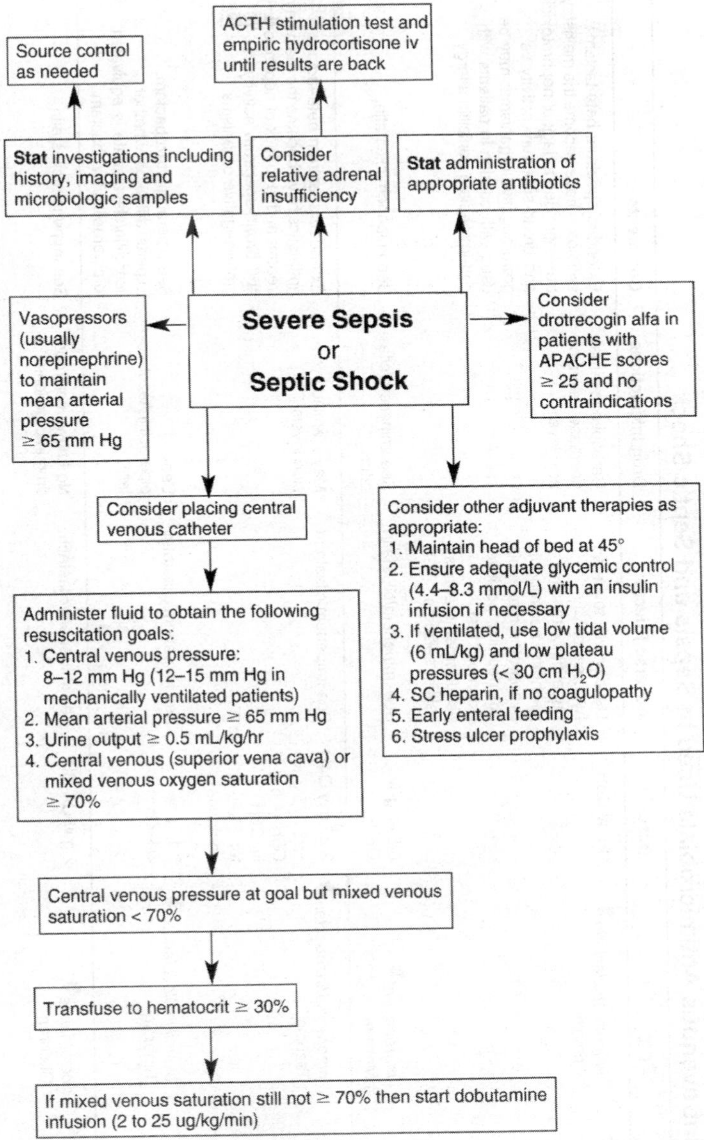

Abbreviations: ACTH = adrenocorticotropic hormone; APACHE = Acute Physiology and Chronic Health Evaluation

Table 4: Intravenous Antimicrobials Used in Sepsis and Septic Shock

Class	Drug	Dose	Adverse Effects	Drug Interactions	Comments	Cost[a]
Carbapenems	*imipenem/cilastatin* Primaxin	1 g iv Q6H	Usually well tolerated; hypersensitivity; hepatitis; interstitial nephritis; neutropenia, hypoprothrombinemia; eosinophilia; positive Coombs' test; pseudomembranous colitis; seizures.	Carbapenems may decrease valproic acid levels.	Extended spectrum beta-lactam antibiotics have become the mainstay of treatment due to lack of nephrotoxicity and broad-spectrum activity vs gram-negative organisms; may be used with caution in patients with non-immediate penicillin allergy.	$$$$$
	meropenem Merrem	0.5–1 g iv Q8H	See imipenem/cilastatin.	See imipenem/cilastatin.	See imipenem/cilastatin.	$$–$$$
Penicillins, Extended-spectrum	*piperacillin/tazobactam* Tazocin	2.25 g iv Q4H or 3.375 g iv Q6H (4.5 g iv Q6H for *Pseudomonas*)	See imipenem/cilastatin.	May ↓ aminoglycoside levels.	Extended spectrum beta-lactam antibiotics have become the mainstay of treatment due to lack of nephrotoxicity and broad-spectrum activity vs gram-negative organisms.	$$
	ticarcillin/clavulanate Timentin	3.1 g iv Q4–6H	See imipenem/cilastatin.	See piperacillin/tazobactam.	See piperacillin/tazobactam. Experts differ on whether ticarcillin/clavulanate is equivalent to piperacillin/tazobactam.	$-$$
Cephalosporins, 3rd generation	*cefotaxime* Claforan	2 g iv Q6–8H	See imipenem/cilastatin.	No known common drug interactions.	See imipenem/cilastatin.	$$

Class	Drug	Dose	Adverse Effects	Drug Interactions	Comments	Cost[a]
	ceftazidime Ceftazidime for Injection USP, Fortaz	2 g iv Q6H	See imipenem/cilastatin.	No known common drug interactions.	See imipenem/cilastatin. Good antipseudomonal activity, poor gram-positive coverage.	$$$$
	ceftriaxone Rocephin, generics	1–2 g iv Q24H	See imipenem/cilastatin.	Possible disulfiram-like reaction with ethanol.	See imipenem/cilastatin.	$$
Cephalosporins, 4th Generation	*cefepime* Maxipime	2 g iv Q12H	See imipenem/cilastatin. Associated with hemolytic anemia.	No known common drug interactions.	See imipenem/cilastatin. Excellent activity against many resistant gram-negative pathogens including *Pseudomonas*. Good activity against most gram-positive organisms.	$$$$$
Aminoglycosides	*amikacin* Amikin, generics	7.5 mg/kg iv Q12H or 15–20 mg/kg iv once daily	Nephrotoxicity, ototoxicity, neuromuscular blockade.	Penicillins may ↓ serum levels.	May be required in combination with beta-lactams for *Pseudomonas* or multiresistant gram-negative bacilli. Avoid in septic shock due to nephrotoxicity and ototoxicity; monitor serum drug levels to guide dosing and avoid toxicity. Desired peak 40 µg/mL; desired trough < 10 µg/mL.	$$
	gentamicin generics	1.5 mg/kg iv Q8H or 4–7 mg/kg iv once daily	See amikacin.	See amikacin.	See amikacin. Desired peak 10 µg/mL; desired trough < 2 µg/mL.	$

(cont'd)

Table 4: **Intravenous Antimicrobials Used in Sepsis and Septic Shock** *(cont'd)*

Class	Drug	Dose	Adverse Effects	Drug Interactions	Comments	Cost[a]
	tobramycin generics	1.5 mg/kg iv Q8H or 4–7 mg/kg iv once daily	See amikacin.	See amikacin.	See gentamicin. Desired peak 10 μg/mL; desired trough < 2 μg/mL.	$
Fluoroquinolones	*ciprofloxacin* Cipro	400 mg iv Q8–12H	GI upset, insomnia, headache, cartilage damage, rash, seizures (rare).	Inhibitor of CYP1A2; may ↑ theophylline (toxicity), ↑ caffeine levels; may cause nephrotoxicity with cyclosporine; may ↑ INR with warfarin.	Oral formulations available for step-down therapy; most appropriate fluoroquinolone for pseudomonal infections; emerging resistance worldwide; all fluoroquinolones effective against atypical pathogens of community-acquired pneumonia.	$-$$
	levofloxacin Levaquin, generics	500–750 mg iv Q24H	See ciprofloxacin. Hypo- or hyperglycemia.	May ↑ warfarin effect.	Oral formulations available for step-down therapy; all fluoroquinolones effective against atypical pathogens of community-acquired pneumonia.	$$
	moxifloxacin Avelox	400 mg iv Q24H	See ciprofloxacin.	Avoid in patients taking class Ia or III antiarrhythmics.	Oral formulations available for step-down therapy; improved activity against anaerobic bacteria as well as gram-positive cocci and enteric gram-negative bacilli; all fluoroquinolones effective against atypical pathogens of community-acquired pneumonia; associated with prolonged QTc interval and torsades de pointes. Caution with ↓ K^+, ↓ Mg^{++}, underlying cardiac disease and concomitant use of class Ia or III antiarrhythmics.	$$

Class	Drug	Dose	Adverse Effects	Drug Interactions	Comments	Cost[a]
Glycopeptides	*vancomycin* Vancocin, Vancomycin Hydrochloride USP, generics	1 g iv Q12H (monitor levels in a septic patient and vary dose accordingly)	Nephrotoxicity, ototoxicity, phlebitis; "red man syndrome" (flushing/rash, hypotension) if infused too rapidly (< 1 h).	Enhanced nephrotoxicity when used with aminoglycosides.	Desired serum levels: trough < 15 μg/mL. Useful if serious infection with enterococci or coagulase-negative staphylococci, or for methicillin-resistant *S. aureus*.	$$$
Lincosamides	*clindamycin* Dalacin C Phosphate Sterile Solution, generics	600–900 mg iv Q6H	Rash, thrombophlebitis, GI effects, pseudomembranous colitis,[b] blood dyscrasias, ↑ liver function tests.	May ↑ neuromuscular blocking action of other agents.	Often chosen to cover anaerobes in head/neck, intra-abdominal, female pelvic or necrotizing skin infections, but lack coverage against facultative gram-negative organisms (most often used with aminoglycosides or fluoroquinolones); may require dosage adjustment in hepatic failure; may decrease endotoxin production.	$$
Nitroimidazoles	*metronidazole* generics	500 mg iv Q8H	Rash; thrombophlebitis; GI effects; metallic taste; blood dyscrasias.	↑ lithium levels; ↑ INR with warfarin; disulfiram-like reaction with alcohol; acute psychosis and confusion with disulfiram.	See clindamycin.	$

(cont'd)

Table 4: **Intravenous Antimicrobials Used in Sepsis and Septic Shock** *(cont'd)*

Class	Drug	Dose	Adverse Effects	Drug Interactions	Comments	Cost[a]
Macrolides	*erythromycin* Erythrocin	15–20 mg/kg/day iv, divided Q6H	Venous irritation/thrombophlebitis; rarely, prolongation of QT interval; ventricular arrhythmias; ototoxicity.	↑ theophylline, carbamazepine, cyclosporine levels; ↑ INR with warfarin; inhibitor of CYP3A4 (potent) and CYP1A2; may increase serum concentrations of cardiac glycosides.	Caution if hepatic dysfunction; often included in initial empiric therapy if *Legionella* is suspected.	$
	azithromycin Zithromax	500 mg iv Q24H	See erythromycin.	May increase serum concentrations of cardiac glycosides.	Used for coverage of atypical pathogens in community-acquired pneumonia (not necessary if patient is taking a fluoroquinolone).	$
Glycylcyclines	*tigecycline* Tygacil	100 mg initially, then 50 mg iv Q12H	Nausea and vomiting relatively common; photosensitivity; pancreatitis; pseudotumor cerebri; induction of a catabolic state.	Decreases efficacy of oral contraceptives. Possible increased risk of pseudotumor cerebri in patients taking isotretinoin.	Broad spectrum; active against most gram-positive, gram-negative and anaerobic bacteria. No activity against *Pseudomonas*. Active against VRE and MRSA. Avoid in pregnant women.	$$$
Cyclic Lipopeptides	*daptomycin* Cubicin	Skin and soft tissue infections: 4 mg/kg iv daily Bacteremias: 6 mg/kg iv daily	Myalgias; occasionally, rhabdomyolysis.	No known significant drug interactions.	Effective against gram-positive organisms including MRSA and VRE. Should not be used in pneumonia, due to poor lung penetration.	[c]

Class	Drug	Dose	Adverse Effects	Drug Interactions	Comments	Cost[a]
Oxazolidinones	*linezolid* Zyvoxam	600 mg iv/po BID	Lactic acidosis; peripheral and optic neuropathy; possible serotonin syndrome, particularly in conjunction with MAOIs or SSRIs; myelosuppression.	Avoid tyramine-rich foods; may potentiate the pressor effect of adrenergic agents; possible serotonin syndrome when used with SSRIs or MAOIs.	Effective against gram-positive organisms; 100% oral bioavailability; may have better outcomes than vancomycin in MRSA-associated pneumonia.	$$$$$
Streptogramins	*quinupristin/dalfopristin* Synercid	7.5 mg/kg iv Q8–12H	Arthralgia/myalgia; pain at injection site.	Inhibitor of CYP3A4; use with caution in combination with substrates of CYP3A4 whose toxicity could be potentiated through decreased clearance (e.g., clozapine, lovastatin, meperidine, morphine, oxycodone, ritonavir, trazodone).	Active against most gram-positive pathogens including MRSA and most VRE; not active against *Enterococcus faecalis.*	$$$$$

[a] Cost of 7-day supply based on 70 kg body weight; includes drug cost only.
[b] Pseudomembranous colitis can occur with any antibiotic but is more common with clindamycin.
[c] Available through Special Access Programme, Therapeutic Products Directorate, Health Canada.
Dosage adjustment required in renal impairment; see Appendix I.
MAOI = monoamine oxidase inhibitor; MRSA = methicillin-resistant *S. aureus*; SSRI = selective serotonin reuptake inhibitor; VRE = vancomycin-resistant enterococci
Legend: $ < $300 $–$$ < $300–600 $$ $300–600 $$–$$$ $300–900 $$$ $600–900 $$$$ $900–1200 $$$$$ > $1200

Suggested Readings

Bernard GR, Vincent JL, Laterre PF et al. Efficacy and safety of recombinant human activated protein C for severe sepsis. *N Engl J Med* 2001;344(10):699-709.

Dellinger RP, Carlet JM, Masur H et al. Surviving Sepsis Campaign guidelines for management of severe sepsis and septic shock. *Crit Care Med* 2004;32(3):858-73.

Hotchkiss RS, Karl IE. The pathophysiology and treatment of sepsis. *N Engl J Med* 2003;348(2):138-50.

Rivers E, Nguyen B, Havstad S et al. Early goal-directed therapy in the treatment of severe sepsis and septic shock. *N Engl J Med* 2001;345(19):1368-77.

Van den Berghe G, Wouters P, Weekers F et al. Intensive insulin therapy in the critically ill patients. *N Engl J Med* 2001;345(19):1359-67.

References

1. [No authors listed]. American College of Chest Physicians/Society of Critical Care Medicine Consensus Conference: definitions for sepsis and organ failure and guidelines for the use of innovative therapies in sepsis. *Crit Care Med* 1992;20(6):864-74.
2. Rivers E, Nguyen B, Havstad S et al. Early goal-directed therapy in the treatment of severe sepsis and septic shock. *N Engl J Med* 2001;345(19):1368-77.
3. [No authors listed]. Practice parameters for hemodynamic support of sepsis in adult patients in sepsis. Task Force of the American College of Critical Care Medicine, Society of Critical Care Medicine. *Crit Care Med* 1999;27(3):639-60.
4. Manthous CA, Hall JB, Olson D et al. Effect of cooling on oxygen consumption in febrile critically ill patients. *Am J Respir Crit Care Med* 1995;151(1):10-4.
5. Cerra FB, Benitez MR, Blackburn GL et al. Applied nutrition in ICU patients. A consensus statement of the American College of Chest Physicians. *Chest* 1997;111(3):769-78.
6. Vincent JL. Hemodynamic support in septic shock. *Intensive Care Med* 2001;27(Suppl 1):S80-92.
7. Van den Berghe G, Wilmer A, Hermans G et al. Intensive insulin therapy in the medical ICU. *N Engl J Med* 2006;354(5):449-61.
8. Jimenez MF, Marshall JC; International Sepsis Forum. Source control in the management of sepsis. *Intensive Care Med* 2001;27(Suppl 1):S49-62.
9. Perez J, Dellinger RP; International Sepsis Forum. Other supportive therapies in sepsis. *Intensive Care Med* 2001;27(Suppl 1):S116-27.
10. Davidson BL, Geerts WH, Lensing AW. Low-dose heparin for severe sepsis. *N Engl J Med* 2002;347(13):1036-7.
11. Steinberg KP. Stress-related mucosal disease in the critically ill patient: risk factors and strategies to prevent stress-related bleeding in the intensive care unit. *Crit Care Med* 2002;30(6 Suppl):S362-4
12. Kumar A, Roberts D, Wood KE et al. Duration of hypotension before initiation of effective antimicrobial therapy is the critical determinant of survival in human septic shock. *Crit Care Med* 2006;34(6):1589-96.
13. Pappas PG, Rex JH, Sobel JD et al. Guidelines for treatment of candidiasis. *Clin Infect Dis* 2004; 38(2):161-89.
14. Ostrosky-Zeichner L, Pappas PG. Invasive candidiasis in the intensive care unit. *Crit Care Med* 2006:34(3):857-63.
15. Bellomo R, Chapman M, Finfer S et al. Low-dose dopamine in patients with early renal dysfunction: a placebo-controlled randomised trial. Australian and New Zealand Intensive Care Society (ANZICS) Clinical Trials Group. *Lancet* 2000;356(9248):2139-43.
16. Martin C, Papazian L, Perrin G et al. Norepinephrine or dopamine for the treatment of hyperdynamic septic shock? *Chest* 1993;103(6):1826-31.
17. Marik PE, Mohedin M. The contrasting effects of dopamine and norepinephrine on systemic and splanchnic oxygen utilization in hyperdynamic sepsis. *JAMA* 1994;272(17):1354-7.
18. Duranteau J, Sitbon P, Teboul JL et al. Effects of epinephrine, norepinephrine, or the combination of norepinephrine and dobutamine on gastric mucosa in septic shock. *Crit Care Med* 1999;27(5):893-900.
19. Sutherland AM, Gordon AC, Russell JA. Are vasopressin levels increased or decreased in septic shock? *Crit Care Med* 2006;34(2):542-3.
20. Siegel JP. Assessing the use of activated protein C in the treatment of severe sepsis. *N Engl J Med* 2002;347(13):1030-4.

21. Bernard GR, Vincent JL, Laterre PF et al. Efficacy and safety of recombinant human activated protein C for severe sepsis. *N Engl J Med* 2001;344(10):699-709.
22. Lefering R, Neugebauer EA. Steroid controversy in sepsis and septic shock: a meta-analysis. *Crit Care Med* 1995;23(7):1294-303.
23. Bollaert PE, Charpentier C, Levy B et al. Reversal of late septic shock with supraphysiologic doses of hydrocortisone. *Crit Care Med* 1998;26(4):645-50.
24. Briegel J, Forst H, Haller M et al. Stress doses of hydrocortisone reverse hyperdynamic septic shock: a prospective, randomized, double-blind, single-center study. *Crit Care Med* 1999;27(4):723-32.
25. Annane D, Sebille V, Charpentier C et al. Effect of treatment with low doses of hydrocortisone and fludrocortisone on mortality in patients with septic shock. *JAMA* 2002;288(7):862-71.
26. Schwartz SA. Intravenous immunoglobulin treatment of immunodeficiency disorders. *Pediatr Clin North Am* 2000;47(6):1355-69.
27. Spector SA, Gelber RD, McGrath N et al. A controlled trial of intravenous immune globulin for the prevention of serious bacterial infections in children receiving zidovudine for advanced human immunodeficiency virus infection. Pediatric AIDS Clinical Trials Group. *N Engl J Med* 1994;331(18):1181-7.
28. Kaul R, McGeer A, Norrby-Teglund A et al. Intravenous immunoglobulin therapy for streptococcal toxic shock syndrome—a comparative observational study. The Canadian Streptococcal Study Group. *Clin Infect Dis* 1999;28(4):800-7.
29. Darenberg J, Ihendyane N, Sjolin J et al. Intravenous immunoglobulin G therapy in streptococcal toxic shock syndrome: a European randomized, double-blind, placebo-controlled trial. *Clin Infect Dis* 2003;37(3):333-40.
30. Darenberg J, Soderquist B, Normark BH et al. Differences in potency of intravenous polyspecific immunoglobulin G against streptococcal and staphylococcal superantigens: implications for therapy of toxic shock syndrome. *Clin Infect Dis*2004;38(6):836-42.
31. Turgeon AF, Hutton B, Fergusson DA et al. Meta-analysis: intravenous immunoglobulin in critically ill adult patients with sepsis. *Ann Intern Med* 2007;146(3):193-203.
32. Pildal J, Gotzsche PC. Polyclonal immunoglobulin for treatment of bacterial sepsis: a systematic review. *Clin Infect Dis* 2004;39(1): 38-46.
33. Hughes WT, Armstrong D, Bodey GP et al. 2002 guidelines for the use of antimicrobial agents in neutropenic patients with cancer. *Clin Infect Dis* 2002;34(6):730-51.
34. Dellinger RP, Carlet JM, Masur H et al. Surviving Sepsis Campaign guidelines for management of severe sepsis and septic shock. *Crit Care Med* 2004;32(3):858-73.

CHAPTER 103
Urinary Tract Infection

Lindsay E. Nicolle, MD

Goals of Therapy

- Ameliorate symptoms in acute infection
- Prevent recurrent infection
- Prevent pyelonephritis in pregnancy

Investigations (Table 2)

Note: *Relapse* is recurrence of urinary tract infection (UTI) with the same organism due to persistence of the organism within the urinary tract, usually in the prostate or kidneys. *Reinfection* is recurrent UTI with a new organism; it generally follows ascension of microorganisms from the periurethral area into the bladder.

Therapeutic Choices (Figure 1, Table 1)

Pharmacologic Choices (Table 3)

Sulfamethoxazole/trimethoprim (SMX/TMP) and Trimethoprim (TMP)

SMX/TMP and **TMP** are the drugs of choice for most UTIs. Both may be used as three-day therapy for acute uncomplicated UTI. Resistance to SMX/TMP and TMP is increasing and must be considered in individuals who have failed empiric therapy or who have had recent prior therapy with these agents. Use of SMX/TMP is limited by sulfa allergy (TMP alone may be used in sulfa-allergic patients).

Nitrofurantoin

Nitrofurantoin, a urinary antiseptic, has been widely used to treat UTIs. It may not be as effective as SMX/TMP for three-day therapy in the treatment of acute uncomplicated UTI. It is not recommended for treatment of pyelonephritis and is contraindicated in renal failure (creatinine clearance < 60 mL/min). Pulmonary and hepatic toxicity may occur, usually with long-term use at full therapeutic doses. Nitrofurantoin *macrocrystals* may be better tolerated than the standard formulation.

Amoxicillin and Amoxicillin/Clavulanic Acid

Resistance of *E. coli* to amoxicillin limits its current use. It should be reserved for UTIs with streptococci or enterococci or when the infecting organism is known to be susceptible.

Amoxicillin is not recommended for empiric therapy of uncomplicated UTI as it will be about 20% less effective than SMX/TMP. **Amoxicillin with clavulanic acid** is an effective alternative for resistant organisms, but it is more expensive and is associated with substantial gastrointestinal (GI) side effects (10 to 25% incidence).

Fosfomycin Tromethamine[1,2]

Fosfomycin tromethamine does not show cross resistance with other antimicrobials, and most community-acquired strains are susceptible. It is prescribed as a single dose and indicated only for treatment of acute uncomplicated urinary infection. It has equivalent efficacy to nitrofurantoin, but is about 10% less effective than SMX/TMP or fluoroquinolones. It is safe for use in pregnancy.

Fluoroquinolones

The renally excreted fluoroquinolones (**norfloxacin, ciprofloxacin, ofloxacin** and **levofloxacin**) are as effective as SMX/TMP for three-day treatment of acute uncomplicated UTI due to susceptible organisms, but are generally second-line therapy due to cost and concerns about development of resistance. Gatifloxacin was voluntarily removed from the market in 2006 following reports of serious hypo- and hyperglycemic effects.

Single-dose therapy with fluoroquinolones is not reliable for *S. saprophyticus*.[3] In addition, single-dose therapy may have poor patient acceptance because symptoms persist for 48 to 72 hours. Fluoroquinolones are important agents in the treatment of *complicated* UTI, particularly for patients infected with resistant organisms. Ciprofloxacin for seven days is adequate therapy for less severe presentations of acute nonobstructive pyelonephritis.[4] Fluoroquinolones should not be used in children and pregnant women because of potential adverse effects on developing cartilage.

Use of the quinolone **nalidixic acid** is limited by development of resistance.

Cephalosporins

All the cephalosporins including **cephalexin, cefazolin, cefaclor, cefuroxime** and **cefixime** are effective for treatment of UTI. They are not as well studied as SMX/TMP or fluoroquinolones and are somewhat less effective for acute cystitis, especially with short courses of therapy. Cephalosporins may be associated with a greater likelihood of vulvovaginal candidiasis. Third-generation cephalosporins such as **ceftriaxone** and **cefotaxime** are effective agents for parenteral treatment of pyelonephritis.

Aminoglycosides

Aminoglycosides **(gentamicin, tobramycin** and **amikacin)** remain the therapy of choice for the treatment of acute pyelonephritis requiring parenteral therapy. Most gram-negative organisms, especially in patients with community-acquired infections, will remain susceptible to these agents. Initial parenteral therapy is switched to oral therapy as soon as symptoms and signs have settled (72 to 96 hours). With such short duration of therapy, ototoxicity and nephrotoxicity are unlikely. The aminoglycosides are usually interchangeable for the treatment of UTI; antimicrobial susceptibility and cost determine selection of an individual agent.

Table 1: **Recommended Empiric Treatment of UTI**

Condition	1st Line Therapy	2nd Line Therapy
Acute uncomplicated UTI[a]	SMX/TMP po × 3 days *or* Trimethoprim po × 3 days *or* Nitrofurantoin po × 7 days	Fluoroquinolone po × 3 days *or* Cephalexin po × 7 days *or* Fosfomycin tromethamine single dose
Pyelonephritis[b]		
Mild to moderate[c]	Fluoroquinolone po × 10–14 days	Amoxicillin/clavulanate po × 10–14 days *or* SMX/TMP po × 10–14 days*or* Trimethoprim po × 10–14 days
Severe[d]	Aminoglycoside iv ± ampicillin[e] iv × 10–14 days	Fluoroquinolone iv × 10–14 days *or* 3rd generation cephalosporin iv ± aminoglycoside iv × 10–14 days
Complicated UTI[b]		
Mild to moderate[c]	Fluoroquinolone po × 7–10 days *or* SMX/TMP po × 7–10 days *or* Trimethoprim po × 7–10 days *or* Nitrofurantoin po × 7–10 days	Amoxicillin/clavulanate po × 7–10 days
Severe[d]	Aminoglycoside iv ± ampicillin[e] iv × 10–14 days	Fluoroquinolone iv × 10–14 days *or* 3rd generation cephalosporin iv × 10–14 days
Prostatitis		
Acute	Aminoglycoside iv ± cloxacillin iv ± ampicillin iv[e]	Fluoroquinolone iv or po *or* SMX/TMP po
Chronic, bacterial	Fluoroquinolone po × 4–8 wk	SMX/TMP po × 4–6 wk *or* Trimethoprim po × 4–6 wk

[a] For postmenopausal women, women with recurrent infections in less than one month or women with symptoms persisting for more than a week, treatment should be for seven days.[5]

[b] Always obtain urine culture prior to initiating therapy, and use results to step down therapy or modify empiric therapy.

[c] Hemodynamically stable, no vomiting.

[d] High fever, sepsis, vomiting.

[e] Include ampicillin if *Enterococcus* is a concern.

Therapeutic Tips

- Whenever possible, base initial selection of antimicrobial therapy on urine culture results.
- Antimicrobial susceptibility in populations is dynamic.
- Base selection of empiric therapy in symptomatic patients on anticipated local antimicrobial susceptibilities and an individual patient's recent antimicrobial exposure and tolerance.
- Use parenteral therapy for patients who are septic, unable to tolerate oral medications, pregnant with pyelonephritis or those with resistant organisms requiring parenteral therapy.
- Consider prophylaxis for women with frequent recurrent uncomplicated UTI.
- Without microbiologic confirmation of a bacterial infection, symptoms of chronic prostatitis are not an indication for antimicrobial therapy.[6]

Figure 1: **Management of Recurrent Acute, Uncomplicated UTI**

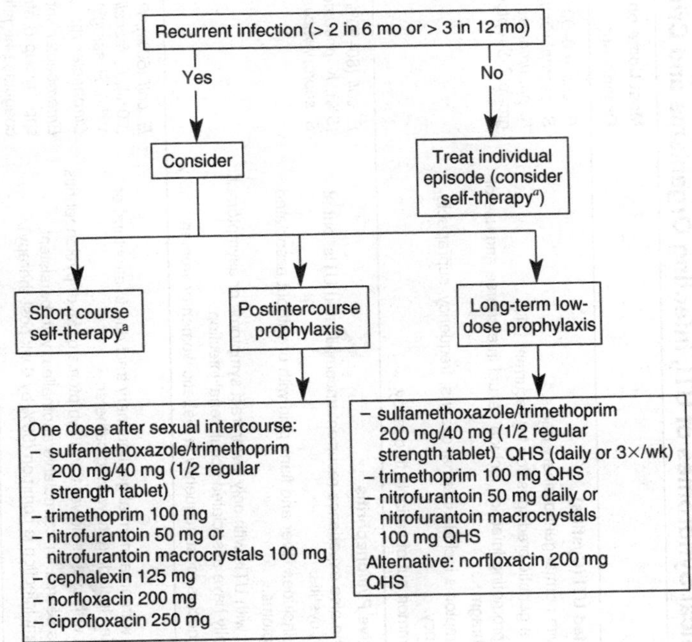

[a] Three-day course of treatment, self-administered on appearance of symptoms.

Table 2: Clinical Syndromes of UTI, Infecting Organisms and Criteria for Microbiologic Diagnosis

Syndrome	Most Common Infecting Organisms[a]	Microbiologic Diagnosis	Urine Culture
Acute Uncomplicated UTI (Cystitis) Occurs in females with normal genitourinary tracts. These women have a genetic predisposition for recurrent UTI. Behavioural factors promoting infection include sexual intercourse and use of spermicides or diaphragm. Usual presenting symptoms include internal dysuria, frequency, suprapubic discomfort and urgency. Recurrences are common but of variable frequency.	*E. coli* (80–90%), *S. saprophyticus* (5–10%), *K. pneumoniae*, *P. mirabilis*, group B *Streptococcus*	Presence of any quantitative count of a gram-negative organism or *S. saprophyticus* in a voided urine specimen with pyuria.	Generally not recommended. Culture if failure to respond to empiric therapy, early (< 1 mo) recurrence following therapy, diagnostic uncertainty or pregnant patient.
Acute Nonobstructive Pyelonephritis Occurs in women who also experience recurrent uncomplicated UTIs, but at lower frequency than cystitis. Classic presentation includes fever and flank pain with or without associated irritative urinary symptoms. Patients who present with UTIs with only lower tract symptoms or asymptomatic bacteriuria occasionally have associated occult renal infection. Bacteremic infection occurs most frequently in diabetic women or women > 65 y.	*E. coli* (80–90%), *P. mirabilis* (5%), *K. pneumoniae* (5%), *S. saprophyticus*	≥ 10^7 cfu/L[b] in voided specimen.	Always indicated. Obtain before initiating antimicrobials. Consider blood cultures.
Complicated UTI Occurs in individuals with an abnormal genitourinary tract due to structural or functional abnormalities including indwelling catheter. Patients may present with cystitis (lower tract) symptoms or fever/pyelonephritis. Management includes search for correctable anomalies; with persistent abnormalities, recurrent infection is common (50% by 6 wk post-therapy).	*E. coli* (50%), *P. mirabilis* (20%), *E. faecalis* (entercoccus; 10%), *P. aeruginosa*, *P. stuartii*, *Citrobacter* spp., *Enterobacter* spp., *Serratia* spp., group B streptococci, coagulase-negative staphylococci	≥ 10^8 cfu/L[b] in voided specimen or any quantitative count in catheterized specimen.	Always, before antimicrobial therapy.

Syndrome	Most Common Infecting Organisms[a]	Microbiologic Diagnosis	Urine Culture
Bacterial Prostatitis[c] **Acute:** infection usually due to *E. coli* or *S. aureus*. Symptoms include sudden chills, fever, perineal and low back pain, irritative and obstructive voiding. The prostate is tender, swollen, indurated and warm. Prostatic massage is not recommended because it may cause bacteremia.	*E. coli*, enterobacteriaceae, *P. aeruginosa, S. aureus*, others	Urine culture > 10^8 cfu/L[b]; blood cultures positive; aspirate prostate abscess.	Voided urine specimen before empiric therapy.
Chronic Bacterial: uncommon, ↑ with age. Intermittent, cystitis-like urinary symptoms; history of recurrent UTI. Prostate examination is usually normal.	*E. coli* (80%), *Klebsiella* spp, *P. aeruginosa*, *Proteus* spp	Meares-Stamey localization test (triple glass test; involves obtaining urine/prostate secretion samples before and after prostate massage).	Urine culture with acute symptoms.
Asymptomatic Bacteriuria Microbiologic evidence for UTI in the absence of associated symptoms. Asymptomatic bacteriuria is more common in women, ↑ with age. In pregnancy, screening should be performed for asymptomatic bacteriuria at 12–16 wk.	*E. coli* (60–70%), *P. mirabilis*, group B *streptococcus*, coagulase-negative staphylococci, others	≥ 10^8 cfu/L[b] in 2 consecutive specimens.	Screening of asymptomatic populations recommended only in pregnancy or before invasive genitourinary procedures.

a *E. coli* is the single most frequent organism causing UTI. Individuals with complicated UTI or recent exposure to antimicrobials are more likely to have organisms other than *E. coli* or organisms of increased antimicrobial resistance.

b 10^7 cfu/L = 10^4 cfu/mL; 10^8 cfu/L = 10^5 cfu/mL.

c Symptoms of chronic prostatitis are not considered attributable to infection in the absence of microbiologic documentation. Antimicrobial therapy does not improve these symptoms when compared to placebo.[6]

Abbreviations: cfu = colony-forming units

Table 3: **Antimicrobials for the Treatment of Urinary Tract Infection**

Class	Drug	Dose	Adverse Effects	Drug Interactions	Cost[a]
Penicillins	*amoxicillin* generics	500 mg TID po	Hypersensitivity reactions, rash, nausea, vomiting, pseudomembranous colitis, GI effects.	↓ efficacy of oral contraceptives; tetracyclines ↓ the effectiveness of penicillins; ↑ methotrexate serum levels.	$
	amoxicillin/clavulanate Clavulin, generics	500 mg TID po	See amoxicillin.	See amoxicillin.	$
	ampicillin generics	1 g Q6H iv	See amoxicillin.	See amoxicillin.	$$
	piperacillin generics	3 g Q6H iv	See amoxicillin.	See amoxicillin.	$$$$
	ticarcillin/clavulanate Timentin	3.1 g Q4–6H iv	See amoxicillin.	See amoxicillin.	$$$$$
Cephalosporins, first-generation	*cefazolin* generics	1 g Q8H iv	Hypersensitivity reactions, rash, nausea, vomiting, pseudomembranous colitis, renal and hepatic dysfunction.	↑ nephrotoxic effects of aminoglycosides; ↑ INR with warfarin.	$
	cephalexin generics	500 mg QID po	See cefazolin.	See cefazolin.	$
Cephalosporins, second-generation	*cefaclor* Ceclor, generics	250 mg TID po	See cefazolin.	See cefazolin.	$

Class	Drug	Dose	Adverse Effects	Drug Interactions	Cost[a]
	cefuroxime axetil Ceftin	250 mg BID po	See cefazolin.	See cefazolin.	$
	cefuroxime sodium Zinacef, generics	750 mg Q8H iv	See cefazolin.	See cefazolin.	$$$
Cephalosporins, third-generation	*cefixime* Suprax	400 mg/day po	See cefazolin.	See cefazolin.	$
	cefotaxime Claforan	1 g Q8H iv	See cefazolin. Safe in hepatobiliary disease.	See cefazolin.	$$$
	ceftazidime Ceftazidime for Injection USP, Fortaz, generics	1 g Q8H iv	See cefazolin.	See cefazolin.	$$$$
	ceftriaxone Rocephin	1 g Q24H iv	See cefazolin.	See cefazolin.	$$$
Fluoroquinolones	*ciprofloxacin* Cipro, Cipro XL generics	Oral: Immediate-release: 250–500 mg BID po Long-acting: 500–1000 mg daily po IV: 200–400 mg BID	Abdominal pain, nausea, vomiting, photosensitivity, dizziness, headache, drowsiness, insomnia, diarrhea, pseudomembranous colitis. Potential adverse effects on developing cartilage; avoid in children and in pregnancy.	Concomitant iron, antacids, sucralfate ↓ absorption of fluoroquinolones; ↑ INR with warfarin; may ↓ theophylline and caffeine elimination.	PO: $ IV: $$-$$$
	levofloxacin Levaquin, generics	250 mg/day po or 250 mg/day iv	See ciprofloxacin.	Iron, antacids, sucralfate ↓ absorption of quinolones; ↑ INR with warfarin.	PO: $ IV: $$

(cont'd)

Table 3: **Antimicrobials for the Treatment of Urinary Tract Infection** *(cont'd)*

Class	Drug	Dose	Adverse Effects	Drug Interactions	Cost[a]
	norfloxacin generics	400 mg BID po	See ciprofloxacin.	See ciprofloxacin.	$
	ofloxacin Floxin, generics	400 mg BID po	See ciprofloxacin.	See levofloxacin.	$
Aminoglycosides	*amikacin* Amikin	15 mg/kg/day iv	Nephrotoxicity, usually reversible, ↑ with dose and duration; ototoxicity, often reversible.	↑ ototoxicity with loop diuretics, ↑ nephrotoxicity with other nephrotoxic drugs; can be inactivated if mixed with some penicillins.	$$$[b]
	gentamicin generics	3–5 mg/kg/day iv	See amikacin.	See amikacin.	$$[b]
	tobramycin Tobramycin Injection USP, generics	3–5 mg/kg/day iv	See amikacin.	See amikacin.	$$[b]
Phosphoric Acid Derivatives	*fosfomycin tromethamine* Monurol	One 3 g sachet (single dose)	Diarrhea, headache, vaginitis, nausea.	Metoclopropamide, probenicid: ↓ fosfomycin levels.	$$
Sulfonamide Combinations	*sulfamethoxazole/trimethoprim* (SMX/TMP) generics	800/160 mg (2 regular-strength tablets or 1 DS tablet) BID po	Hypersensitivity reactions, nausea, vomiting, diarrhea, rash, false ↑ serum creatinine, renal impairment, neutropenia, thrombocytopenia, anemia, agranulocytosis.	↑ phenytoin levels, ↑ INR with warfarin, hypoglycemia with sulfonylureas, ↑ nephrotoxicity with cyclosporine.	$
Folate Antagonists	*trimethoprim* generics	100 mg BID po	Rash, pruritus.	↑ phenytoin levels; ↑ myelosuppression with methotrexate.	$

Class	Drug	Dose	Adverse Effects	Drug Interactions	Cost[a]
Nitrofuran Derivatives	*nitrofurantoin* Macrodantin, generics (kidney symbol)	50–100 mg QID po	Headache, nausea, flatulence, loss of appetite; pulmonary and hepatic toxicity with long-term use; rare acute pulmonary toxicity.	Antacids may ↓ absorption.	$
	nitrofurantoin monohydrate/nitrofurantoin macrocrystals (kidney symbol) MacroBID	100 mg BID po	See nitrofurantoin. Macrocrystal formulation better tolerated.	See nitrofurantoin.	$$

[a] Cost per day; includes drug costs only.
[b] Cost based on 70 kg body weight.
(kidney symbol) Dosage adjustment may be required in renal impairment; see Appendix I.
Abbreviations: GI = gastrointestinal; INR = International Normalized Ratio
Legend: $ < $10 $$ $10–25 $$-$$$ $10–50 $$$ $25–50 $$$$ $50–75 $$$$$ > $75

Suggested Readings

Habermacher GM, Chason JT, Schaeffer AJ. Prostatic/chronic pelvic pain syndrome. *Annu Rev Med* 2006;57:195-206.

Hooton TM, Stamm WE. Diagnosis and treatment of uncomplicated urinary tract infection. *Infect Dis Clin North Am* 1997;11(3):551-81.

Nicolle LE. Complicated urinary tract infection in adults. *Can J Infect Dis Med Micro* 2005;16:349-360.

Nicolle LE, Bradley S, Colgan R et al. Infectious Diseases Society of America guidelines for the diagnosis and treatment of asymptomatic bacteriuria in adults. *Clin Infect Dis* 2005;40(5):643-54.

Nicolle LE, Ronald AR. Recurrent urinary tract infection in adult women: diagnosis and treatment. *Infect Dis Clin North Am* 1987;1(4):793-806.

References

1. Hooton TM. Fluoroquinolones and resistance in the treatment of uncomplicated urinary tract infection. *Int J Antimicrob Agents* 2003;22(Suppl 2):65-72.
2. Patel SS, Balfour JA, Bryson HM. Fosfomycin tromethamine. A review of its antibacterial activity, pharmacokinetic properties and therapeutic efficacy as a single-dose oral treatment for acute uncomplicated lower urinary tract infections. *Drugs* 1997; 53(4):637-56.
3. Richard GA, Mathew CP, Kirstein JM et al. Single-dose fluoroquinolone therapy of acute uncomplicated urinary tract infection in women: results from a randomized, double-blind, multicenter trial comparing single-dose to 3-day fluoroquinolone regimens. *Urology* 2002;59(3):334-9.
4. Talan DA, Stamm WE, Hooton TM et al. Comparison of ciprofloxacin (7 days) and trimethoprim-sulfamethoxazole (14 days) for acute uncomplicated pyelonephritis pyelonephritis in women: a randomized trial. *JAMA* 2000;283(12):1583-90.
5. Vogel T, Verreault R, Gourdeau M et al. Optimal duration of antibiotic therapy for uncomplicated urinary tract infection in older women: a double-blind randomized controlled trial. *CMAJ* 2004; 170(4):469-73.
6. Alexander RB, Propert KJ, Schaeffer AJ et al. Ciprofloxacin or tamsulosin in men with chronic prostatitis/chronic pelvic pain syndrome: a randomized, double-blind trial. *Ann Intern Med* 2004;141(8):581-9.

CHAPTER 104

Sexually Transmitted Infections

Natasha Press, MD, FRCPC

Sexually transmitted infections (STIs) can be characterized according to whether the major initial manifestations are vaginal discharge, urethritis or cervicitis, or genital lesions. Anogenital warts and pelvic inflammatory disease, an infection of the upper genital tract, are discussed as well.

Goals of Therapy

- Treat the infection
- Abolish symptoms
- Decrease spread to sexual partners
- Decrease vertical transmission from mother to newborn
- Reduce transmission of HIV
- Decrease probability of complications, such as infertility, chronic pain, sepsis

Investigations[1,2]

- History:
  - duration of symptoms, if any
  - risk factors, e.g., sexual contact with person with known STI, recent new partner, more than two partners in past year, injection drug use, commercial sex workers
  - recent childbirth, intrauterine contraceptive device insertion
  - past history of STIs, therapy and response
- Physical:
  - search for systemic signs of STIs, e.g., syphilis, disseminated gonococcus
  - inspect mucocutaneous regions including pharynx and anus
  - inspect external genitalia for lesions, inflammation, discharge
  - consider a digital rectal exam and anoscopy if perianal warts are present or if patient has rectal symptoms or has practised receptive anal intercourse
  - palpate for inguinal lymphadenopathy
  - in women: perform speculum examination to visualize cervix and vaginal walls and to evaluate endocervical and vaginal discharges; bimanual pelvic exam to detect uterine or adnexal masses or tenderness

  - in men: search for signs of urethral discharge, palpate testicles/epididymides
- Laboratory tests:
  - for women: cervical swabs for chlamydia test, i.e., nucleic acid amplification tests (NAATs)[3] and gonorrhea culture (NAATs will not give information on antibiotic susceptibility); vaginal swab for pH test, Gram stain and trichomoniasis wet preparation slide; culture for trichomoniasis (more sensitive than wet mount microscopy); ultrasound if pelvic inflammatory disease (PID) suspected; consider beta-hCG to rule out ectopic pregnancy; rectal specimens for chlamydia and lymphogranuloma venereum (LGV), as indicated
  - for men: urethral swab for gonorrhea culture, first-void urine for chlamydia; scrotal ultrasound if epididymo-orchitis suspected, consider testing for LGV (culture, NAAT, serology); rectal specimens for chlamydia and LGV, as indicated
  - for external lesions: swabs for herpes (use viral media), bacteria, syphilis (send fluid from lesion for darkfield test or direct immunofluorescence test) as indicated
  - throat and rectal swabs for gonorrhea if indicated
  - consider serology for syphilis, HIV (see Chapter 106), hepatitis B (see Chapter 52), hepatitis C (see Chapter 52) as indicated

Infections Characterized by Vaginal Discharge

The three infections most frequently associated with vaginal discharge are *trichomoniasis* (caused by *Trichomonas vaginalis*), *bacterial vaginosis* (caused by a replacement of the normal vaginal flora by an overgrowth of anaerobic microorganisms, mycoplasmas and *Gardnerella vaginalis*) and *vulvovaginal candidiasis* (commonly caused by *Candida albicans*) (Table 1). There is an element of recurrence in these conditions. Recurrent vulvovaginal candidiasis (≥ 4 episodes/year) requires investigation and possibly referral. Address predisposing causes if present, e.g., use of systemic antibiotics, poorly controlled diabetes or HIV (consider testing).

Nonsexually transmitted causes of vaginitis are numerous, e.g., atrophic vaginitis, trauma, malignancy, detergents, contraceptive chemicals, allergy to latex condoms. Candidiasis and bacterial vaginosis are not usually considered sexually transmitted (Table 2).

Therapeutic Choices (Figure 1)

Pharmacologic Choices (Table 3, Table 4, Table 5)

Treatment of trichomoniasis is necessary for all nonpregnant women, including asymptomatic women.

Treatment of asymptomatic bacterial vaginosis is necessary in high-risk pregnancy (history of preterm birth) and prior to IUD insertion, gynecologic surgery, therapeutic abortion or upper tract instrumentation.

Uncomplicated vulvovaginal candidiasis (VVC) can be treated by a short course of topical antifungal formulations. Individualize therapy considering factors such as patient preference, cost, convenience, compliance, portability and history of response or side effects to prior treatments. Vaginal **nystatin** is less effective than topical **azoles**. Avoid oral agents in pregnancy. Consider prophylactic **fluconazole** at start of antibiotic treatment in women prone to recurrent VVC secondary to antibiotic use.

Table 1: **Differential Diagnosis of Vaginal Discharge**[1,2]

	Candidiasis	Trichomoniasis	Bacterial Vaginosis
Signs/symptoms:			
Pruritus	+	+	–
Odour	–	+	+ (fishy)
Discharge	white, clumpy & curdy	off-white or yellow, frothy	grey or milky, thin, copious
Inflammation	+	+	–
Simple tests:			
pH	< 4.5	> 4.5	> 4.5
"Whiff" test[a]	–	+/-	+
Microscopic findings:			
Specific	budding yeast, psuedohyphae	motile trichomonads	clue cells,[b] predominant Gram-negative curved bacilli and coccobacilli
PMNs	++	+++	–
Lactobacilli	+	–	–

[a] Malodour often intensified after addition of 10% potassium hydroxide (KOH).
[b] Clue cells are vaginal epithelial cells covered with numerous coccobacilli.
Abbreviations: PMNs = polymorphonucleocytes

Infections Characterized by Urethritis and Cervicitis

The two main causes of urethritis and cervicitis are *gonorrhea* (caused by *Neisseria gonorrhoeae*) and *chlamydia* (caused by *Chlamydia trachomatis* serovars D to K). Patients with gonorrhea are often infected with chlamydia and should receive presumptive treatment for both.[1,2] Test and treat sexual partners (Table 2). Because individuals may be asymptomatic, symptoms should not be a prerequisite for screening individuals at risk for STIs. HIV screening is recommended.

In men, symptoms include purulent discharge and severe dysuria ("drip and burn"). Complications of urethritis include epididymitis, seminal vesiculitis, prostatitis and disseminated infection (fever, skin and joint involvement). If epididymo-orchitis is due to sexual transmission, empiric therapy for both gonorrhea and chlamydia are required, but the antichlamydial regimen should be given for at least 10 days and until resolution occurs. Scrotal elevation, bedrest and analgesics are advisable. Epididymo-orchitis may require referral to rule out other diagnoses such as testicular torsion and abscess.

In women, symptoms include copious vaginal discharge, dysuria, intermenstrual uterine bleeding and menorrhagia. Chlamydia may be asymptomatic; therefore, high-risk women should be screened (e.g., young, sexually active women, women with multiple sex partners or new sex partners).[2] Screen all pregnant women at first prenatal visit. Complications of cervicitis include pelvic inflammatory disease, ectopic pregnancy and infertility.

Both men and women can acquire anorectal or pharyngeal gonococcal infection.

Therapeutic Choices (Figure 1, Figure 2)

Pharmacologic Choices (Table 6, Table 7)

A test of cure for chlamydia is recommended if noncompliant, if an alternative treatment has been used, in prepubertal children and in pregnancy when erythromycin or amoxicillin is used.[1,2] Current Canadian guidelines recommend repeat screening of individuals with chlamydia infection at six months.[1]

A test of cure is not required for gonorrhea; retesting 3–12 months after treatment is recommended. Gonococcal infections of the pharynx are more difficult to treat.[1,2] **Fluoroquinolones** should not be used in areas with fluoroquinolone-resistant *N. gonorrhoeae* (3–5%).

Infections Characterized by Genital Ulcers

Six STIs are associated with genital ulcers. The two most common in North America are *genital herpes* (see Chapter 105) and syphilis. *Syphilis* is caused by *Treponema pallidum*, a bacterium that penetrates broken skin or mucous membranes, usually through sexual contact. *Lympogranuloma venereum* has recently surfaced in Canada and is caused by *C. trachomatis* serovars L1, L2 and L3. These strains are more invasive; they preferentially affect the lymph tissue.[1,2] LGV is transmitted through vaginal, anal or oral sexual contact. Complications include colorectal fissures and secondary bacterial infections.[1,2] Test and treat sexual partners (Table 2). Individuals with genital ulcers are at an increased risk of acquiring and transmitting HIV.

Refer individuals with HIV and syphilis and those with suspected or proven tertiary syphilis.

Therapeutic Choices (Figure 3)

Pharmacologic Choices

After treatment for syphilis (Table 8), patients should be followed serologically for treatment failure. For LGV (Table 9), test of cure is performed 3–4 weeks after completion of treatment.

Azithromycin for early syphilis is not standard-of-care and is not recommended at this time.[5]

Management of Specific Infections

Anogenital warts are caused by the human papillomavirus (HPV). No definitive evidence suggests any of the available treatments to be superior to the others, and no single treatment is ideal for all patients or all warts. Warts may resolve with or without treatment; however, there is a frustratingly high recurrence rate (approximately 33%) of genital warts one year after apparent cure.

Patients with warts on their cervix or anal mucosa should be referred.

Therapeutic Choices (Figure 4)

Pharmacologic Choices

Imiquimod, podophyllum resin and **podofilox** (Table 10) are used to treat genital warts but should not be used during pregnancy.

For prevention of genital warts and cervical cancer, a quadrivalent **HPV vaccine**, has been approved for females aged 9–26 years (Table 11). Annual cytology screening (Pap smear) is required as the vaccine does not prevent all strains of HPV.[6]

Pelvic inflammatory disease (PID) includes endometritis, salpingitis and peritonitis. Patients with PID should be hospitalized if they are pregnant, do not respond to or do not tolerate outpatient antibiotics, are noncompliant, have a tubo-ovarian abscess or are very ill, e.g., vomiting, high fever.[1,2] Test and treat sexual partners (Table 2).

Therapeutic Choices (Figure 5)

Pharmacologic Choices (Table 12, Table 13)

Empiric antimicrobial therapy for PID should include coverage of the likely pathogens: *N. gonorrhoeae*, *C. trachomatis*, anaerobes, gram-negative facultative bacteria and streptococci.

Therapeutic Tips

- Treat sexual partner(s) (Table 2).

- Discuss consistent and correct use of latex or polyurethrane condoms for optimal risk reduction of STIs.[7,8,9,10,11]
- Recommend immunization against Hepatitis B, if not previously immunized.
- Discuss and counsel on HIV and STI risk of acquisition and transmission.[12]

Table 2: Treatment of Sexual Contacts[1,2]

Disease	Management of Partner
Anogenital warts (human papillomavirus)	Likelihood of transmission and duration of infectivity unknown, but condoms associated with decreased abnormal Pap smears in women
Bacterial vaginosis	No treatment
Chlamydia and gonorrhea	Refer all recent (< 60 days) partners for testing and empiric treatment. No sex for patient or partner until 1 wk after initiation of treatment
Genital herpes	Use condoms, be aware of asymptomatic shedding
Lymphogranuloma venereum	Refer all recent (< 60 days) partners for testing and empiric treatment
Pelvic inflammatory disease	Refer all recent male partners (< 60 days) for examination and treatment. Treat empirically for *C. trachomatis* and/or *N. gonorrhoeae*. No sex for patient or partner until 1 wk after initiation of treatment
Syphilis, late latent	Refer for testing all long-term partners and any of their children who were possibly exposed during pregnancy
Syphilis, primary, secondary and early latent	Refer partners for empiric treatment even if seronegative. Trace-back period for primary, secondary and early latent syphilis is 3 months, 6 months and 1 year, respectively. Refer partners > 3 months for empiric treatment and testing
Trichomoniasis	Treat partner. No sex until patient and partner finished treatment and are asymptomatic
Vulvovaginal candidiasis	No treatment. Consider treatment of sex partner(s) in women with recurrent infections

Figure 1: **Management of Vaginitis and Cervicitis**

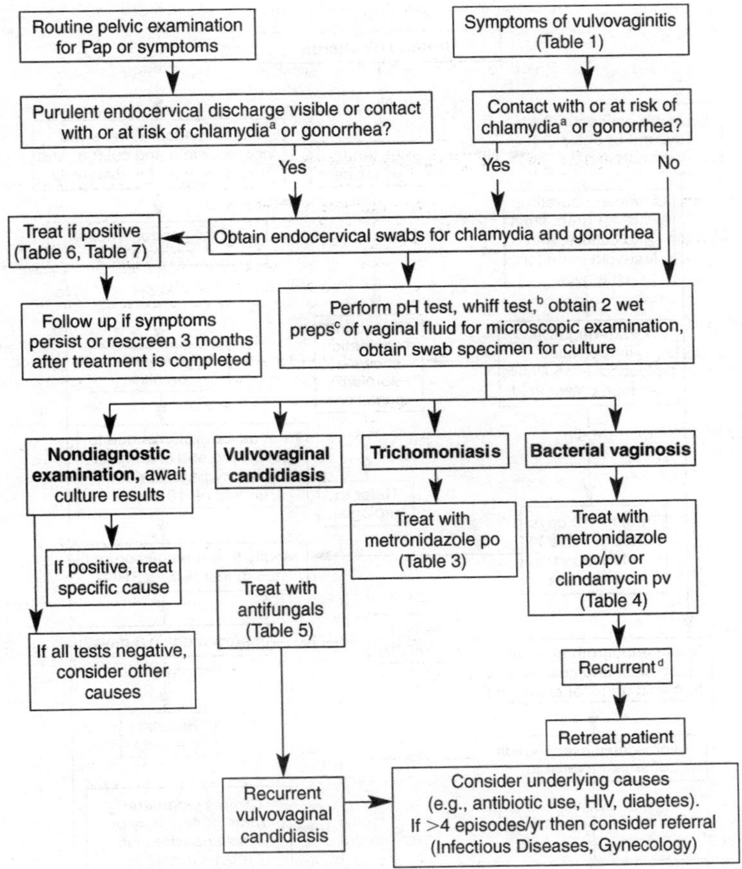

[a] Chlamydial nucleic acid amplification testing, e.g., PCR, of a first voided urine specimen is an option if vaginal examination is not possible.

[b] Malodour often intensified after addition of 10% potassium hydroxide (KOH).

[c] One sample mixed in a few drops of normal saline; second sample mixed with 10% KOH.

[d] Recurrent bacterial vaginosis may develop in ~15–30% of patients in the first 1–3 months of treatment.

Abbreviations: pv = intravaginally; po = orally

Figure 2: **Management of Urethritis and Epididymo-orchitis**

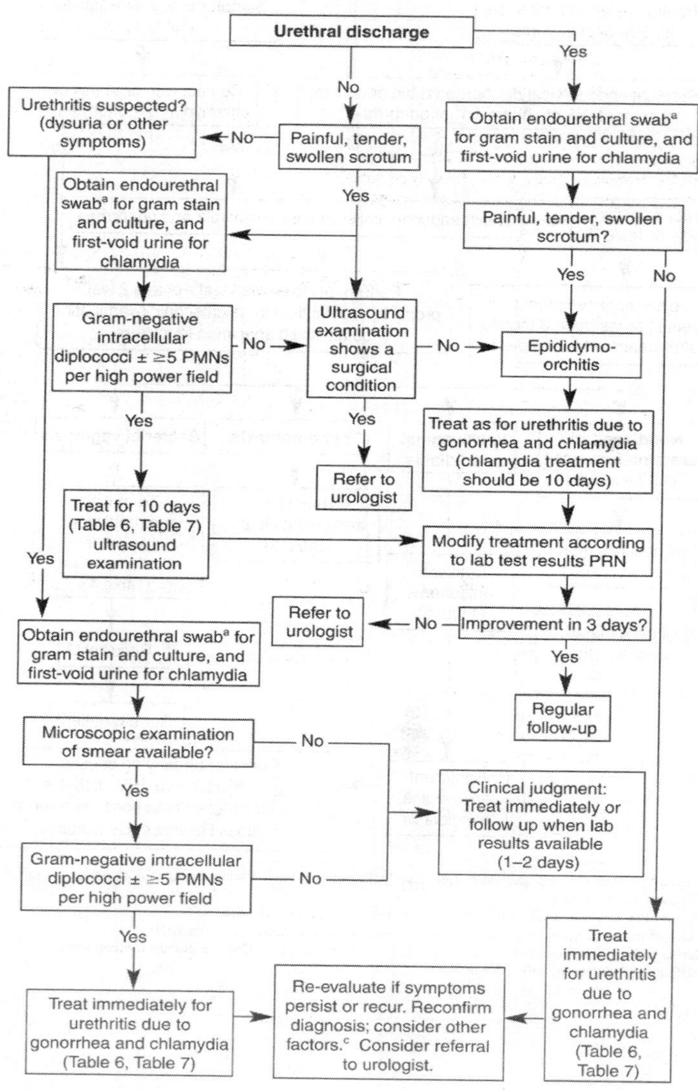

[a] Diagnosis of gonorrhea by culture, rather than nucleic acid amplification testing is preferred, in order to allow for antimicrobial susceptibility testing.

[b] Nucleic acid amplification testing, e.g., PCR, of a first voided urine specimen is accurate for chlamydia detection.

[c] Re-exposure; nonadherence; antimicrobial resistance; other etiologies such as urinary tract infections, prostatitis; other microorganisms such as *T. vaginalis*, *U. urealyticum*, *M. genitalium*.

Abbreviations: PMNs = polymorphonucleocytes; PRN = as needed

Figure 3: **Management of Genital Ulcers (Herpes, Lymphogranuloma Venereum, Syphilis)**

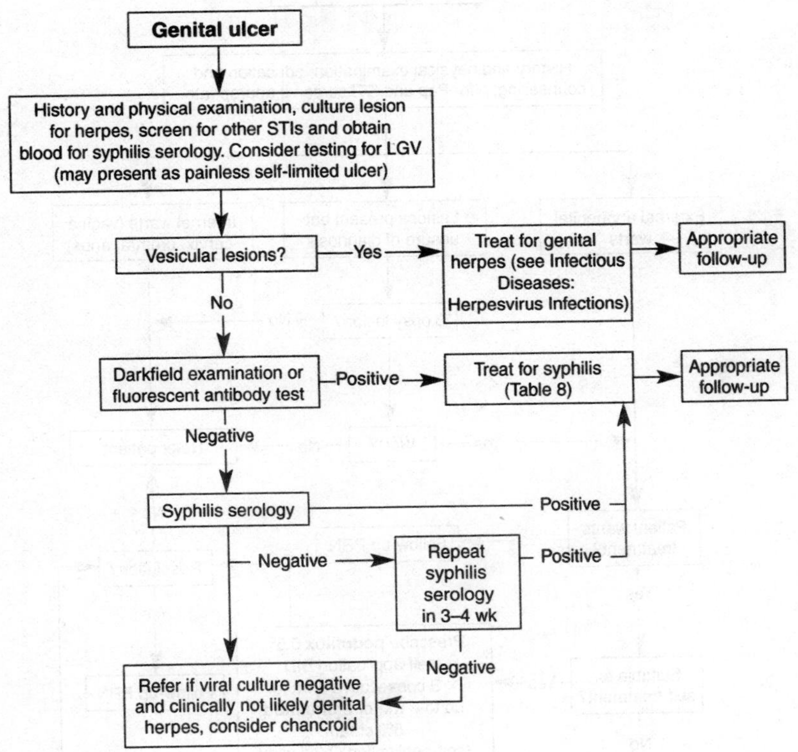

Figure 4: **Management of Anogenital Warts**

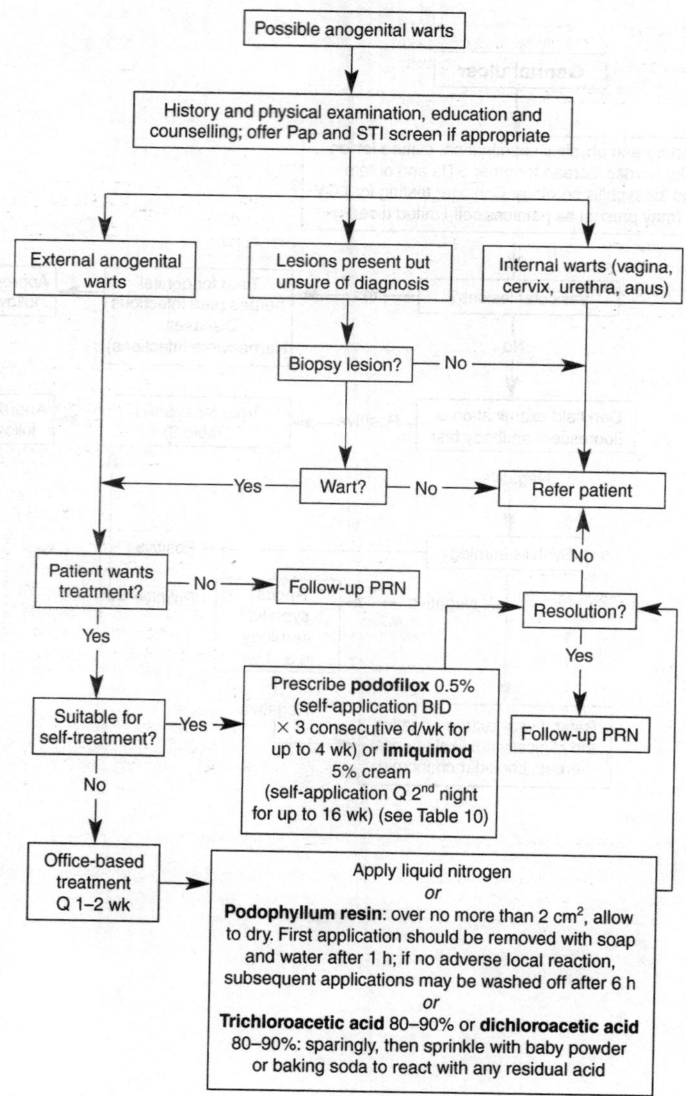

Figure 5: Management of Pelvic Inflammatory Disease

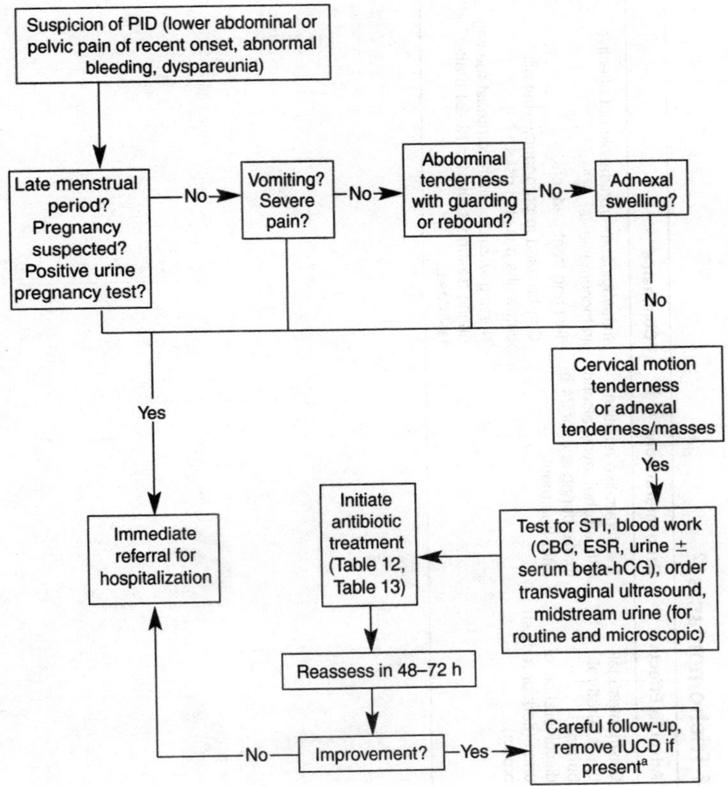

[a] If the patient has an IUCD in place, it should not be removed until after at least two doses of antimicrobial therapy have been given.

Abbreviations: CBC = complete blood count; ESR = erythrocyte sedimentation rate; hCG = human chorionic gonadotropin; IUCD = intrauterine contraceptive device

Table 3: Antibiotics for the Treatment of Trichomoniasis[1,2]

Class	Drug	Dose	Adverse Effects	Drug Interactions	Comments	Cost[a]
Nitroimidazoles	*metronidazole, oral* Flagyl, generics	2 g po × single dose ***or*** 500 mg po BID × 7 days	Gastrointestinal upset, urethral burning, discolouration of urine (dark or reddish brown).	Disulfiram-like reaction with alcohol: avoid alcohol intake during and for 24 h after treatment.	Intravaginal metronidazole not effective in trichomoniasis.[1,2,13] Test and treat partners. Can be used in pregnancy—benefit outweighs possible risks. Nursing women: withhold breast-feeding during treatment and for 12–24 h after last dose.	$

[a] Cost for specified duration of treatment; includes drug cost only.

Dosage adjustment required in renal impairment; see Appendix I.

Legend: $ < $10

Table 4: Antibiotics for the Treatment of Bacterial Vaginosis[1,2]

Class	Drug	Dose	Adverse Effects	Comments	Cost[a]
Lincosamides	*clindamycin, oral* Dalacin C, Dalacin C Flavored Granules, generics	300 mg po BID × 7 days	Gastrointestinal upset, *C. difficile* colitis, diarrhea.	*Alternative treatment to metronidazole.* Can be used in pregnant and nursing women; retest 1 mo after completion to ensure effective therapy. Treatment necessary in the following asymptomatic cases: high-risk pregnancy, i.e., history of preterm delivery; prior to insertion of intrauterine device; prior to gynecologic surgery, therapeutic abortion or upper tract instrumentation. Coadministration of kaolin ↓ clindamycin absorption.	$$
	clindamycin, vaginal cream Dalacin Vaginal Cream	2%: one applicatorful (5 g) once daily intravaginally QHS × 7 days	Vulvovaginitis.	Not recommended in pregnancy. Delay treatment until completion of menstrual period. Contains mineral oil—may weaken latex condoms and diaphragms.	$$$
Nitroimidazoles	*metronidazole, oral*[b] Flagyl, generics	Preferred dose: 500 mg po BID × 7 days Alternate dose: 2 g po × single dose Recurrent bacterial vaginosis: 500 mg po BID × 14 days	Gastrointestinal upset, urethral burning, dark or reddish brown discolouration of urine, metallic taste.	*Preferred treatment.* Can be used in pregnancy; nursing women: withhold breast-feeding during treatment and for 12–24 h after last dose; retest 1 mo after completion to ensure effective therapy. Treatment necessary in the following asymptomatic cases: high-risk pregnancy (i.e., history of preterm delivery); prior to insertion of intrauterine device; prior to gynecologic surgery, therapeutic abortion or upper tract instrumentation. Single dose metronidazole is associated with higher failure rate. Recurrent bacterial vaginosis: ≥ 3 episodes in previous y.	$

(cont'd)

Table 4: **Antibiotics for the Treatment of Bacterial Vaginosis[1,2]** *(cont'd)*

Class	Drug	Dose	Adverse Effects	Comments	Cost[a]
				Disulfiram-like reaction with alcohol—avoid alcohol intake during and for 24 h after treatment with oral metronidazole.	
	metronidazole, vaginal gel NidaGel, generics	Preferred dose: 0.75% gel: one applicatorful (5 g) once daily intravaginally × 7 days Recurrent BV: 0.75% gel: one applicatorful (5 g) once daily × 10 days followed by twice a wk × 4–6 mo	Vaginal discharge, yeast infection, vulva/ vaginal irritative symptoms, pain and discomfort.		$$

[a] Cost of preferred dose; includes drug cost only.
[b] Preferred treatment.
Dosage adjustment required in renal impairment; see Appendix I.
Legend: $ < $10 $$ $10–20 $$$ $20–30

Table 5: **Antifungals for the Treatment of Symptomatic Vulvovaginal Candidiasis**[1,2]

Class	Drug	Dose	Adverse Effects	Comments	Cost[a]
Polyenes	*nystatin* ratio-Nystatin, other generics	Vaginal cream 100 000 units/g: 1 g pv × 14 days	Local hypersensitivity.	Less effective than azoles. Follow-up required if symptoms persist despite treatment or recur within 2 mo of onset.	$
Azoles, oral	*fluconazole* Diflucan-150, generics	150 mg po × single dose[14] Recurrent vulvovaginal candidiasis: 150 mg po daily × 3 days then once weekly[15] (if > 4 episodes/y, consider referral)	Headache, nausea, abdominal pain, diarrhea, dyspepsia, dizziness.	Single dose may elevate prothrombin time in women with chronic warfarin therapy. Follow-up required if symptoms persist despite treatment or recur within 2 mo of onset.	$
Azoles, topical[b]	*clotrimazole* Canesten Vaginal, generics	200 mg/vaginal tablet: 1 tablet intravaginally × 3 days 1% vaginal cream: 1 applicatorful pv daily × 6 days	Local hypersensitivity.	Also comes in combination with external cream; available over the counter. Do not use in first trimester of pregnancy. Treat for 7–14 days in pregnancy. Follow-up required if symptoms persist despite treatment or recur within 2 mo of onset.	$$
	econazole Ecostatin	150 mg/vaginal ovule: 1 ovule pv × 3 days	Local hypersensitivity.	Contains hydrogenated vegetable oil; ↓ efficacy (weakens) of latex condoms or diaphragms. Do not use in first trimester of pregnancy. Follow-up required if symptoms persist despite treatment or recur within 2 mo of onset.	$$

(cont'd)

Table 5: **Antifungals for the Treatment of Symptomatic Vulvovaginal Candidiasis**[1,2] *(cont'd)*

Class	Drug	Dose	Adverse Effects	Comments	Cost[a]
	miconazole Monistat, generics	2% vaginal cream: 1 applicatorful pv daily × 7 days 4% vaginal cream: 1 applicatorful pv daily × 3 days 100 mg/ovule: 1 ovule pv × 7 days 400 mg/ovule: 1 ovule pv × 3 days 1200 mg/ovule: 1 ovule pv × single dose	Local hypersensitivity.	Also comes in combination with external cream; available over the counter. Ovules contain hydrogenated vegetable oil, mineral oil; ↓ efficacy of latex condoms or diaphragms. Treat for 7–14 days in pregnancy. Follow-up required if symptoms persist despite treatment or recur within 2 mo of onset.	$$
	butoconazole Gynazole-1	2% cream: 5 g pv × single dose	Local hypersensitivity.	Cream contains mineral oil; ↓ efficacy (weakens) of latex condoms or diaphragms. Though a 1-day treatment, it takes a few days for symptoms to resolve. Follow-up required if symptoms persist despite treatment or recur within 2 mo of onset.	$$
	terconazole Terazol, generics	0.4% vaginal cream: 1 applicatorful pv HS × 7 days 0.8% vaginal cream: 1 applicatorful pv HS × 3 days 80 mg/ovule: 1 ovule pv × 3 days	Local hypersensitivity.	Ovules contain hydrogenated vegetable oil; ↓ efficacy of latex condoms or diaphragms. Follow-up required if symptoms persist despite treatment or recur within 2 mo of onset.	$$$

[a] Cost of treatment; includes drug cost only.
[b] Preferred treatment.
Legend: $ < $10 $$ $10–20 $$$ $20–30

Table 6: **Antibiotics for the Treatment of Uncomplicated Chlamydia Infection**

Class	Drug	Dose	Adverse Effects	Drug Interactions	Comments	Cost[a]
Macrolides	*azithromycin* Zithromax, generics	Adults and children ≥ 45 kg: 1 g po × single dose	Gastrointestinal upset.	May ↑ digoxin levels.	*Preferred treatment*; may especially benefit situations in which poor compliance is expected. Test and treat partners. Initiate empiric gonorrhea therapy. Compared to doxycycline, azithromycin is more expensive; similar high cure rates. Can be used in pregnant and nursing women; test of cure indicated. Repeat dose if vomiting < 1 h post-administration.	$
	erythromycin Eryc, Erybid, PCE, generics	Adults: erythromycin base 500 mg po QID × 7 days; max 2 g/day. If tolerance is a concern: erythromycin base 250 mg po QID × 14 days *Chlamydia trachomatis in infants, ophthalmia neonatorum*: erythromycin base 12.5 mg/kg QID × 14 days, may need second course of treatment, follow-up	Gastrointestinal upset.	May ↑ levels of carbamazepine, digoxin, HMG CoA reductase inhibitors, e.g., simvastatin, protease inhibitors, sildenafil, theophylline, warfarin. Avoid use with pimozide, cisapride, disopyramide.	Alternative to doxycycline and azithromycin. Test and treat partners. Initiate empiric gonorrhea therapy. Can be used in pregnant and nursing women. Erythromycin estolate is not used during pregnancy due to reports of cholestatic hepatitis. Test of cure indicated. Conjunctivitis: use systemic therapy since topical treatment not adequate. Reports of infantile hypertrophic pyloric stenosis with erythromycin use in infants < 6 wk; monitor signs and symptoms.	$

(cont'd)

Table 6: **Antibiotics for the Treatment of Uncomplicated Chlamydia Infection** *(cont'd)*

Class	Drug	Dose	Adverse Effects	Drug Interactions	Comments	Cost[a]
Fluoro-quinolones	*levofloxacin* Levaquin, generics	500 mg po daily × 7 days	Gastrointestinal upset, headache.	↓ levels with concurrent antacids, iron or didanosine (buffered formulations). Monitor blood sugar in diabetics on oral antihyperglycemic agents when used concomitantly. ↑ risk of tendon rupture with concomitant corticosteroid use. Avoid use with QT_c prolonging agents, e.g., Class 1A, III antiarrhythmics—may result in arrhythmias.	Alternative to doxycycline and azithromycin. Should not be used in areas with fluoroquinolone-resistant *N. gonorrhoeae* (3–5%). Test and treat partners. Initiate empiric gonorrhea therapy. Contraindicated in pregnant and nursing women. Safety in children < 18 y not established.	$$
	ofloxacin Floxin, generics	300 mg po BID × 7 days	Gastrointestinal upset, headache.	See levofloxacin.	See levofloxacin. Similar high cure rate as doxycycline and azithromycin.	$$

Class	Drug	Dose	Adverse Effects	Drug Interactions	Comments	Cost[a]
Penicillins	*amoxicillin* generics	500 mg TID × 7 days	Rash, gastrointestinal upset.	May ↓ efficacy of oral contraceptives. Tetracyclines may ↓ amoxicillin effectiveness.	May be used in pregnant and nursing women; test of cure indicated. Test and treat partners.	$
Tetracy-clines	*doxycycline* Vibra-Tabs, generics	Adults and children ≥ 8 y: 100 mg po BID × 7 days	Gastrointestinal upset, rash, candidal vaginitis, photosensitivity.	↓ levels with antacids, iron, barbiturates, bismuth, carbamazepine, phenytoin. ↓ effectiveness of penicillins and oral contraceptives.	*Preferred treatment.* Test and treat partners. Initiate empiric gonorrhea therapy. Similar high cure rates to azithromycin. Contraindicated in pregnant and nursing women.	$

[a] Cost of treatment; includes drug cost only.

Dosage adjustment required in renal impairment; see Appendix I.

Legend: $ < $10 $$ $10–20

Table 7: **Antibiotics for the Treatment of Uncomplicated Gonorrhea Infection: Endocervical, Rectal, Urethral**[1,2]

Class	Drug	Dose	Adverse Effects	Comments	Cost[a]
Aminoglycosides	*spectinomycin*	2 g im × single dose Children < 9 y or < 45 kg: 40 mg/kg im × single dose; max 2 g	Pain at injection site.	*Not effective for pharyngeal infection; test of cure is recommended.* Alternative treatment if fluoroquinolones not recommended, cephalosporin allergy or immediate/ anaphylactic penicillin allergy. Test and treat partners. Initiate empiric chlamydia therapy. Can be used in pregnant and nursing women. Repeat screening recommended.	[b]
Cephalosporins, 3rd generation	*cefixime* Suprax	400 mg po × single dose Children < 9 y: 8 mg/kg po × single dose; max 400 mg, follow-up culture required	Gastrointestinal upset, hypersensitivity reactions.	*Preferred treatment.* Initiate empiric chlamydia therapy. Repeat screening recommended.	$
	ceftriaxone Rocephin	125 mg im × single dose Children < 9 y: 125 mg im × single dose; alternative to cefixime if follow-up not ensured *Ophthalmia neonatorum:* 25–50 mg/kg iv or im × single dose; max 125 mg	Gastrointestinal upset, hypersensitivity reactions.	*Preferred treatment*; cefixime costs less and is taken orally. Ophthalmia neonatorum: use systemic therapy since topical antibiotic is ineffective. An alternative to cefixime in pregnant and nursing women. May be mixed with 1–2 mL of 1% lidocaine, as it is irritating.	$$

Class	Drug	Dose	Adverse Effects	Comments	Cost[a]
Fluoroquinolones	*ciprofloxacin* ◗ Cipro, generics	500 mg po × single dose	Gastrointestinal upset, headache.	*Preferred treatment* except in men who have sex with men and in areas with increased rates of quinolone-resistant *N. gonorrhoeae* (> 3–5%) such as Australia, UK, Hawaii and some areas of Canada and USA. Please check with local public health officials for quinolone resistance in your area. Test and treat partners. Initiate empiric chlamydia therapy. Safety in children < 18 y not established. Contraindicated in pregnant and nursing women. Repeat screening recommended. ↑ levels with concurrent use of antacids, iron or with didanosine (buffered formulations). Monitor blood sugar levels in diabetics on oral antihyperglycemic agents when used concomitantly. ↑ risk of tendon rupture with concomitant corticosteroid use.	$
	ofloxacin ◗ Floxin, generics	400 mg po × single dose	See ciprofloxacin.	See ciprofloxacin.	$

[a] Cost of treatment; includes drug cost only.
[b] Available through Special Access Programme, Therapeutic Products Directorate.
◗ Dosage adjustment required in renal impairment; see Appendix I.
Legend: $ < $5 $$ $5–10

Table 8: **Antibiotics for the Treatment of Syphilis**[1,2]

Class	Drug	Dose	Adverse Effects	Comments	Cost[a]
Penicillins	*penicillin G benzathine* (renal dosage symbol) Bicillin	*Primary, secondary and early latent syphilis:* 2.4 million units im × single dose *Late latent syphilis, latent syphilis of unknown duration, cardiovascular syphilis, tertiary syphilis not involving CNS:* 2.4 million units im weekly × 3 doses *Secondary syphilis + > 20 weeks gestation:* 2.4 million units im weekly × 2 doses	Jarisch-Herxheimer reaction: *not a drug allergy*; may occur at any stage but prevalent during 2° syphilis; fever, chills, rigors, sweating may occur; resolves within 24 h.	*Preferred treatment.* Available through Special Access Programme through provincial/territorial Sexually Transmitted Disease Services. See penicillin G	[b]
	penicillin G (renal dosage symbol) generics	*Neurosyphilis:* 3–4 million units iv Q4–6H (16–24 million units daily) × 10–14 days	See penicillin G benzathine.	Can be used in pregnant and nursing women; consider penicillin desensitization in pregnant women who are allergic to penicillin. Test and treat partners. Tetracyclines may ↓ penicillin efficacy.	$$$$
Tetracyclines	*doxycycline* Vibra-Tabs, generics	*Primary, secondary and early latent syphilis:* 100 mg po BID × 14 days *Late latent syphilis, latent syphilis of unknown duration, cardiovascular syphilis, tertiary syphilis not involving CNS:* 100 mg po BID × 28 days	Gastrointestinal upset, rash, candidal vaginitis, photosensitivity.	Alternative treatment.[1,2,16] Test and treat partners. Contraindicated in pregnant and nursing women. ↓ levels with antacids, iron, barbiturates, bismuth, carbamazepine, phenytoin. ↓ efficacy of penicillins and oral contraceptives.	$$

[a] Cost for duration of treatment; includes drug cost only.
[b] Available through Special Access Programme, Therapeutic Products Directorate.
(renal dosage symbol) Dosage adjustment required in renal impairment; see Appendix I.
Legend: $ < $15 $$ $15–35 $$$ $35–250 $$$$ $250–300

Table 9: **Antibiotics for the Treatment of Lymphogranuloma Venereum[1,2]**

Class	Drug	Dose	Adverse Effects	Drug Interactions	Comments	Cost[a]
Macrolides	*azithromycin* Zithromax, generics	1 g once weekly po × 21 days; clinical data lacking Partners: 1 g po × single dose, optimum interval unknown	Gastrointestinal upset.	May ↑ levels of digoxin.	Alternative treatment to doxycycline. Test and treat partners. Test of cure performed 3–4 wk after completion of therapy; follow-up until chlamydial tests are negative. Can be used in pregnant and nursing women. Repeat dose if vomiting < 1 h post-administration.	$$
	erythromycin ◗ Eryc, PCE, generics	Erythromycin base: 500 mg po QID × 21 days	Gastrointestinal upset.	May ↑ levels of carbamazepine, digoxin, simvastatin, atorvastatin, lovastatin, protease inhibitors, sildenafil, theophylline. Avoid use with pimozide, cisapride, disopyramide, clindamycin.	Alternative treatment to doxycycline. Test and treat partners. Test of cure performed 3–4 wk after completion of therapy; follow-up until chlamydial tests are negative. Can be used in pregnant and nursing women. Erythromycin estolate is not used during pregnancy due to reports of cholestatic hepatitis.	$$$
Tetracyclines	*doxycycline* Vibra-Tabs, generics	100 mg po BID × 21 days	Gastrointestinal upset, rash, candidal vaginitis, photosensitivity.	↓ levels with antacids, iron, barbiturates, bismuth, carbamazepine, phenytoin. ↓ efficacy of penicillins and oral contraceptives.	*Preferred treatment.* Test and treat partners. Test of cure performed 3–4 wk after completion of therapy; follow-up until chlamydial tests are negative. Contraindicated in pregnant and nursing women.	$$

[a] Cost of treatment; includes drug cost only.
◗ Dosage adjustment required in renal impairment; see Appendix I.
Legend: $ < $20 $$ $20–30 $$$ $30–40

Table 10: **Topical Drugs for the Treatment of External Anogenital Warts**

Class	Drug	Dose	Adverse Effects	Comments	Cost
Antimitotic Agents	*podofilox* Condyline	*Self-applied* Apply to visible genital warts BID with a cotton swab × 3 days, followed by 4 days without therapy May repeat cycle up to 4 times Total wart areas should be ≤ 10 cm^2 Total daily volume is 0.5 mL	Local irritation, pain, inflammation, erosion, burning, bleeding, pruritus, dizziness, insomnia.	Perform initial application to demonstrate proper application and to identify warts that should be treated. Treatment does not eliminate HPV infection; may recur. May require up to 3 mo for response. Do not use in pregnancy.	$/3.5 mL bottle
	podophyllum resin Podofilm	*Office-based treatment* Apply, with a cotton applicator, over no more than 2 cm^2 and allow to dry. Remove first application with soap and water after 1 h. If no adverse local reaction, subsequent applications may be washed off after 6 h.	Systemic: urticaria, fever, paresthesia, polyneuritis, paralytic ileus, blood dyscrasias, coma, death. Local: severe necrosis, scarring, paraphimosis, pseudoepitheliomatous hyperplasia.	Protect normal skin adjacent to lesion with petrolatum. Can reapply at weekly intervals if necessary. Do not use in pregnancy.	$
	dichloroacetic acid (DCA)	*Office-based treatment* Apply DCA (80-90%) sparingly. Sprinkle after with baby powder or baking soda to react with any residual acid.	Inflammation, erosion, pain, burning, ulceration.	Can be used in pregnant and nursing women.	$

Class	Drug	Dose	Adverse Effects	Comments	Cost
	trichloroacetic acid (TCA)	*Office-based treatment* Apply TCA (80-90%) sparingly. Sprinkle after with baby powder or baking soda to react with any residual acid.	See dichloracetic acid.	See dichloracetic acid.	$
Immune Response Modifiers	*imiquimod* Aldara	*Self-applied* Apply 3 times per wk at HS for up to 16 wk; rub cream in until no longer visible Wash hands before and after treatment application Wash treatment area with soap and water 6–10 h after application	Local irritation, pain, mild to moderate erythema, burning.	Physicians: Perform initial application to demonstrate proper application and to identify warts that should be treated. Treatment does not eliminate HPV infection; may recur. May require up to 3 mo for response. Do not use in pregnancy.	$$$/12 packets

Legend: $ < $50 $$ $50–100 $$$ $100–150

Table 11: Vaccines for the Prevention of External Anogenital Warts

Class	Drug	Dose	Adverse Effects	Comments	Cost
Vaccines	*human papilloma quadrivalent vaccine* Gardasil	9–26 *y*: administered 0, 2, 6 mo im	Pain, swelling, erythema and pruritus at injection site, headache, fatigue.	Prevention of cervical dysplasia, cervical carcinoma, vulvar dysplastic lesions and external genital warts caused by HPV 6, 11, 16 and 18. Annual Pap smear is required as the vaccine does not protect against all HPV strains. Not recommended in pregnancy. Can be used in nursing mothers.	$$$/injection

Legend: $$$ $100–150

Table 12: **Antibiotic Combination Therapy for the Outpatient Management of Pelvic Inflammatory Disease (PID)[1,2]**

Class	Drug	Dose	Adverse Effects	Drug Interactions	Comments	Cost[a]
Fluoro-quinolones ± Nitroimidazoles	*levofloxacin* ± *metronidazole*	Levofloxacin: 500 mg po once daily × 14 days ± Metronidazole: 500 mg po BID × 14 days	*Levofloxacin:* gastrointestinal upset, headache. *Metronidazole:* gastrointestinal upset, urethral burning, dark or reddish brown discolouration of urine.	*Levofloxacin:* ↓ levels with concurrent use of antacids, iron or with didanosine (buffered formulations). Monitor blood sugar levels in diabetics on oral antihyperglycemic agents when used concomitantly. ↑ risk of tendon rupture with concomitant corticosteroid use. Caution with concomitant use of agents with QT_c prolongation, e.g., amiodarone; assess risks/benefits of therapy. *Metronidazole:* disulfiram-like reaction with alcohol—avoid alcohol intake during and for 24 h after treatment.	Initiate broad-spectrum antibiotics covering *N. gonorrhoeae*, *C. trachomatis*, anaerobic and mycoplasma bacteria due to multifactorial etiology of PID. Test and treat partners. Re-evaluate patients 2–3 days after initiation of therapy; if no improvement, parenteral therapy required. *Levofloxacin:* contraindicated in pregnant and nursing women; safety in children < 18 y not established; not to be used when patient or partner are from areas with increased rates of quinolone-resistant *N. gonorrhoeae* (>3–5%) such as Australia, UK, Hawaii and some areas of Canada and USA. Check with local public health officials for quinolone resistance in your area. *Metronidazole:* provides anaerobic coverage.	$$

(cont'd)

Table 12: **Antibiotic Combination Therapy for the Outpatient Management of Pelvic Inflammatory Disease (PID)[1,2]** *(cont'd)*

Class	Drug	Dose	Adverse Effects	Drug Interactions	Comments	Cost[a]
	ofloxacin ± *metronidazole*	Ofloxacin: 400 mg po once daily × 14 days ± Metronidazole: 500 mg po BID × 14 days	*Ofloxacin:* gastrointestinal upset, headache. *Metronidazole:* gastrointestinal upset, urethral burning, dark or reddish brown discolouration of urine.	See levofloxacin ± metronidazole.	See levofloxacin ± metronidazole. *Ofloxacin:* contraindicated in pregnant and nursing women; safety in children < 18 y not established; not to be used when patient or partner are from areas with increased rates of quinolone-resistant *N. gonorrhoeae* (>3–5%) such as Australia, UK, Hawaii and some areas of Canada and USA. Check with local public health officials for quinolone resistance in your area. *Metronidazole:* provides anaerobic coverage.	$

Class	Drug	Dose	Adverse Effects	Drug Interactions	Comments	Cost[a]
Cephalosporins + Tetracyclines ± Nitroimidazoles	*ceftriaxone* + *doxycycline* ± *metronidazole*	Ceftriaxone: 250 mg im × single dose + Doxycycline: 100 mg po BID × 14 days ± Metronidazole: 500 mg po BID × 14 days	*Ceftriaxone:* gastrointestinal upset, *C. difficile* colitis. *Doxycycline:* gastrointestinal upset, rash, candidal vaginitis, photosensitivity. *Metronidazole:* gastrointestinal upset, urethral burning, dark or reddish brown discolouration of urine.	*Ceftriaxone:* ↑ anticoagulant effect of warfarin. ↑ levels with probenecid. *Doxycycline:* ↓ levels with antacids, iron, barbiturates, bismuth, carbamazepine, phenytoin. ↓ efficacy of penicillins and oral contraceptives. *Metronidazole:* disulfiram-like reaction with alcohol—avoid alcohol intake during and for 24 h after treatment.	See levofloxacin ± metronidazole. *Doxycycline:* contraindicated in pregnant and nursing women. *Metronidazole:* provides anaerobic coverage.	$$$$$
	cefotaxime + *doxycycline* ± *metronidazole*	Cefotaxime: 1 g im × single dose + Doxycycline: 100 mg po BID × 14 days ± Metronidazole: 500 mg po BID × 14 days	*Cefotaxime:* pruritus, diarrhea, nausea, vomiting. *Doxycycline:* gastrointestinal upset, rash, candidal vaginitis, photosensitivity. *Metronidazole:* gastrointestinal upset, urethral burning, dark or reddish brown discolouration of urine.	*Cefotaxime:* ↑ risk of additive nephrotoxicity with aminoglycosides, furosemide. ↑ levels with probenecid. *Doxycycline:* ↓ levels with antacids, iron, barbiturates, bismuth, carbamazepine, phenytoin. ↓ efficacy of penicillins and oral contraceptives. *Metronidazole:* disulfiram-like reaction with alcohol—avoid alcohol intake during and for 24 h after treatment.	See levofloxacin ± metronidazole. *Doxycycline:* contraindicated in pregnant and nursing women. *Metronidazole:* provides anaerobic coverage.	$$$$$

(cont'd)

Table 12: **Antibiotic Combination Therapy for the Outpatient Management of Pelvic Inflammatory Disease (PID)**[1,2] *(cont'd)*

Class	Drug	Dose	Adverse Effects	Drug Interactions	Comments	Cost[a]
Cephalosporins + Uricosuric + Tetracyclines ± Nitroimidazoles	*cefoxitin* + *probenecid* + *doxycycline* ± *metronidazole*	Cefoxitin: 2 g im × single dose + Probenecid: 1 g po × single dose Doxycycline: 100 mg po BID × 14 days ± Metronidazole: 500 mg po BID × 14 days	*Cefoxitin:* diarrhea. *Doxycycline:* gastrointestinal upset, rash, candidal vaginitis, photosensitivity. *Metronidazole:* gastrointestinal upset, urethral burning, dark or reddish brown discolouration of urine.	*Cefoxitin:* ↑ risk of additive nephrotoxicity with aminoglycosides, furosemide. ↑ levels with probenecid. *Doxycycline:* ↓ levels with antacids, iron, barbiturates, bismuth, carbamazepine, phenytoin. ↓ efficacy of penicillins and oral contraceptives. *Metronidazole:* disulfiram-like reaction with alcohol—avoid alcohol intake during and for 24 h after treatment.	See levofloxacin ± metronidazole. *Doxycycline:* contraindicated in pregnant and nursing women. *Metronidazole:* provides anaerobic coverage. Probenecid not required if renal impairment is present.	$$

[a] Cost for duration of treatment; includes drug cost only.
Dosage adjustment required in renal impairment; see Appendix I.
Legend: $ < $25 $$ $25–50 $$$ $50–75 $$$$ $75-100 $$$$$ $100–125

Table 13: **Antibiotic Combination Therapy for Inpatient Management of Pelvic Inflammatory Disease (PID)**[1,2]

Class	Drug	Dose	Adverse Effects	Drug Interactions	Comments	Cost[a]
Cephalosporins + Tetracyclines	*cefoxitin* + *doxycycline*	Cefoxitin: 2 g iv Q6H + Doxycycline: 100 mg po or iv Q12H. Therapy is for 14 days	*Cefoxitin:* diarrhea. *Doxycycline:* gastrointestinal upset, rash, candidal vaginitis, photosensitivity.	*Cefoxitin:* ↑ risk of additive nephrotoxicity with aminoglycosides, furosemide. ↑ levels with probenecid. *Doxycycline:* ↓ levels with antacids, iron, barbiturates, bismuth, carbamazepine, phenytoin. ↓ efficacy of penicillins and oral contraceptives.	Initiate broad-spectrum antibiotics covering *N. gonorrhoeae*, *C. trachomatis*, anaerobic and mycoplasma bacteria due to multifactorial etiology of PID. Test and treat partners. Re-evaluate patients 2–3 days after initiation of therapy; if no improvement, parenteral therapy required. Consider discontinuation of iv therapy and po stepdown after demonstrated clinical improvement; total duration of treatment is 14 days. *Doxycycline:* contraindicated in pregnant and nursing women.	$$$$
Lincosamides + Amino-glycosides	*clindamycin* + *gentamicin*	Clindamycin: 900 mg iv Q8H, step down to 450 mg po QID. Therapy is for 14 days + Gentamicin: loading dose 2 mg/kg iv or im, then 1.5 mg/kg Q8H *or* 5 mg/kg iv Q24H	*Clindamycin:* *C. difficile* colitis, diarrhea. *Gentamicin:* ototoxicity, nephrotoxicity (monitor kidney function at baseline and during treatment).	*Clindamycin:* monitor kidney function with concomitant aminoglycoside. May ↓ therapeutic effect of live typhoid vaccine. Administer typhoid vaccine > 24 h after last dose of clindamycin. *Gentamicin:* Imidazoles ↓ levels	See cefoxitin + doxycycline.	$$$$ [b]

(cont'd)

Table 13: **Antibiotic Combination Therapy for Inpatient Management of Pelvic Inflammatory Disease (PID)**[1,2] *(cont'd)*

Class	Drug	Dose	Adverse Effects	Drug Interactions	Comments	Cost[a]
Fluoro-quinolones ± Nitroimidazoles	*levofloxacin* (renal symbol) ± *metronidazole* (renal symbol)	Levofloxacin: 500 mg iv once daily ± Metronidazole: 500 mg iv Q8H	*Metronidazole:* Gastrointestinal upset, urethral burning, dark or reddish brown discolouration of urine.	*Levofloxacin:* monitor blood sugar levels in diabetics on oral antihyperglycemic agents when used concomitantly. ↑ risk of tendon rupture with concomitant corticosteroid use. Caution with concomitant use of agents with QT_c prolongation, e.g., amiodarone; assess risks/benefits of therapy. *Metronidazole:* disulfiram-like reaction with alcohol—avoid alcohol intake during and for 24 h after treatment.	See cefoxitin + doxycycline. *Levofloxacin:* contraindicated in pregnant and nursing women; safety in children < 18 y not established; not to be used when patient or partner are from areas with increased rates of quinolone-resistant *N. gonorrhoeae* (>3–5%) such as Australia, UK, Hawaii and some areas of Canada and USA. Check with local public health officials for quinolone resistance in your area. *Metronidazole:* provides anaerobic coverage.	$$$

[a] Cost for 1-day supply; includes drug cost only.
[b] Cost based on dosage for 50 kg person.
(renal symbol) Dosage adjustment required in renal impairment; see Appendix I.
Legend: $ < $25 $$ $25–50 $$$ $50–75 $$$$ $75–100

Suggested Readings

Centers for Disease Control and Prevention. Sexually transmitted diseases treatment guidelines, 2006. *MMWR Recomm Rep* 2006;55(RR-11):1-94. Available from: http://www.cdc.gov/std/treatment/2006/rr5511.pdf Accessed February 6, 2007.

Expert Working Group on Canadian Guidelines for Sexually Transmitted Infections. *Canadian guidelines on sexually transmitted infections, 2006 edition.* Ottawa (ON): Public Health Agency of Canada; 2006. Available from: http://www.phac-aspc.gc.ca/std-mts/sti_2006/pdf/sti2006_e.pdf Accessed February 6, 2007.

Hollier LM, Workowski KW. Treatment of sexually transmitted infections in pregnancy. *Clin Perinatol* 2005;32(3):629-56.

van Schalkwyk J, Money DM. *Pregnancy.* Ottawa (ON): Public Health Agency of Canada; 2006. Available from: http://www.phac-aspc.gc.ca/std-mts/sti_2006/pdf/pregnancy_e.pdf Accessed February 6, 2007.

References

1. Expert Working Group on Canadian Guidelines for Sexually Transmitted Infections. *Canadian guidelines on sexually transmitted infections, 2006 edition.* Ottawa (ON): Public Health Agency of Canada; 2006. Available from: http://www.phac-aspc.gc.ca/std-mts/sti_2006/pdf/sti2006_e.pdf Accessed February 6, 2007.
2. Centers for Disease Control and Prevention. Sexually transmitted diseases treatment guidelines, 2006. *MMWR Recomm Rep* 2006;55(RR-11):1-94. Available from: http://www.cdc.gov/std/treatment/2006/rr5511.pdf Accessed February 6, 2007.
3. Cook RL, Hutchison SL, Ostergaard L et al. Systematic review: noninvasive testing for Chlamydia trachomatis and Neisseria gonorrhoeae. *Ann Intern Med* 2005;142(11):914-25.
4. Sena AC, Miller WC, Hobbs MM et al. Trichomonas vaginalis infection in male sexual partners: implications for diagnosis, treatment, and prevention. *Clin Infect Dis* 2007;44(1):13-22.
5. Riedner G, Rusizoka M, Todd J et al. Single-dose azithromycin versus penicillin G benzathine for the treatment of early syphilis. *N Engl J Med* 2005;353(12):1236-44.
6. Committee on Adolescent Health Care; ACOG Working Group on Immunization. ACOG Committee Opinion No. 344: Human papillomavirus vaccination. *Obstet Gynecol* 2006;108(3 Pt 1):699-705.
7. Warner L, Stone KM, Macaluso M et al. Condom use and risk of gonorrhea and Chlamydia: a systematic review of design and measurement factors assessed in epidemiologic studies. *Sex Transm Dis* 2006;33(1):36-51.
8. Winer RL, Hughes JP, Feng Q et al. Condom use and the risk of genital human papillomavirus infection in young women. *N Engl J Med* 2006;354(25):2645-54.
9. Wald A, Langenberg AG, Krantz E et al. The relationship between condom use and herpes simplex virus acquisition. *Ann Intern Med* 2005;143(10):707-13.
10. Hogewoning CJ, Bleeker MC, van den Brule AJ et al. Condom use promotes regression of cervical intraepithelial neoplasia and clearance of human papillomavirus: a randomized clinical trial. *Int J Cancer* 2003;107(5):811-6.
11. Bleeker MC, Hogewoning CJ, Voorhorst FJ et al. Condom use promotes regression of human papillomavirus-associated penile lesions in male sexual partners of women with cervical intraepithelial neoplasia. *Int J Cancer* 2003;107(5):804-10.
12. Kamb ML, Fishbein M, Douglas JM et al. Efficacy of risk-reduction counseling to prevent human immunodeficiency virus and sexually transmitted diseases: a randomized controlled trial. Project RESPECT Study Group. *JAMA* 1998;280(13):1161-7.
13. duBouchet L, McGregor JA, Ismail M et al. A pilot study of metronidazole vaginal gel versus oral metronidazole for the treatment of Trichomonas vaginalis vaginitis. *Sex Transm Dis* 1998;25(3):176-9.
14. Sobel JD, Brooker D, Stein GE et al. Single oral dose fluconazole compared with conventional clotrimazole topical therapy of Candida vaginitis. Fluconazole Vaginitis Study Group. *Am J Obstet Gynecol* 1995;172(4 Pt 1):1263-8.
15. Sobel JD, Wiesenfeld HC, Martens M et al. Maintenance fluconazole therapy for recurrent vulvovaginal candidiasis. *N Engl J Med* 2004;351(9):876-83.
16. Ghanem KG, Erbelding EJ, Cheng WW et al. Doxycycline compared with benzathine penicillin for the treatment of early syphilis. *Clin Infect Dis* 2006;42(6):e45-9.

CHAPTER 105
Herpesvirus Infections

Fred Y. Aoki, MD

This chapter addresses treatment of herpes simplex virus (HSV) and varicella-zoster virus (VZV) infections in immunocompetent and immunocompromised patients.

The characteristics of some herpesvirus infections, such as recurrent genital or orolabial herpes simplex virus infection, differ when caused by HSV type 1 or 2. However, knowledge of HSV type is not of practical value in guiding selection of drug therapy since both are similarly susceptible to available drugs. Drug choices can be based on the nature and severity of the disease and evidence from controlled clinical trials.

In immunocompromised patients, HSV and herpes VZV infections may be more severe and resolve less rapidly than in immunocompetent hosts. The recommended drugs are the same in both types of patients; however, dose regimens may be different.

Herpes Simplex Virus

Orolabial Infection

Goals of Therapy

- Improve symptoms
- Prevent outbreaks

Pharmacologic Choices (Table 1)

Primary HSV Gingivostomatitis

Primary HSV gingivostomatitis is commonly seen in children. If the child can swallow, treat mild to moderate gingivostomatitis with **acyclovir** oral suspension. Acyclovir 15 mg/kg five times per day for 7 days[1] or 600 mg/m^2 QID for 10 days[2] accelerates resolution of orolabial signs and symptoms and fever, and reduces the duration of viral shedding. Acyclovir is well tolerated. If the severity of disease precludes ingestion of medication, iv acyclovir in pediatric doses analogous to those which are effective and safe in adults with primary genital herpes (Table 1), can be inferred to be appropriate treatment, although no published data support this recommendation.

Recurrent Orolabial Herpes

Treat recurrent orolabial herpes in immunocompetent adults with oral antivirals (acyclovir, famciclovir and valacyclovir) for 4 to 5 days.

Oral **acyclovir** 400 mg five times per day for 5 days, initiated within 1 hour of onset, reduced the duration of pain by 0.9 days compared with

placebo although no other disease parameters, such as time to healing and duration of virus shedding, are altered.[3]

Valacyclovir is approved for 1-day treatment of cold sores in patients 12 years of age or older.[4] Valacyclovir 2 g BID × 2 doses, self-initiated an average of 2 hours after the earliest symptom of tingling, itching or burning, reduced the duration of the episode by about 1 day compared with placebo.[5] Valacyclovir is well tolerated.

Famciclovir 750 mg BID for 1 day or 1500 mg once, started within 1 hour of onset of cold sore prodromal symptoms, improved a number of lesional symptoms and signs, [6] reduced the duration of pain and tenderness and the median times to healing. Median times to normal skin were 5.7 to 4.5 days with treatment compared to 7.0 days with placebo. Famciclovir is well tolerated.

Topical antiviral creams are effective but require frequent applications and carry a risk of self-inoculation. Topical acyclovir ointment is not effective. **Acyclovir 5% cream**, self-initiated within 1 hour of the onset of a recurrent episode and applied five times daily for 4 days, reduced the duration of pain by about one-half day compared with placebo; however, acyclovir cream did not prevent progression to vesicles, ulcers and/or crusts.[7] **Penciclovir 1% cream** initiated within 1 hour and applied every 2 hours while awake for 4 consecutive days, accelerated healing of cold sores by an average of 0.7 days compared with placebo.[8] Provide patients with prescriptions for antivirals to enable them to self-initiate therapy at the onset of symptoms.

For healthy persons with recurrent cold sores (> 6 times per year) daily ingestion of oral antivirals can suppress recurrences during therapy of up to 4 months. Oral acyclovir 400 mg BID[9] or 200 mg QID[10] and oral valacyclovir 500 mg daily[11] are comparably effective and well tolerated as suppressive therapy. Once therapy is discontinued, however, cold sores tend to recur. The effectiveness of these regimens for periods greater than 4 months is unknown.

For individuals in whom orolabial herpes is reactivated by exposure to sunlight, oral acyclovir 400 mg BID begun 12 hours prior to sun exposure with frequent **sunscreen** use prevents attacks. Prophylaxis is continued for the duration of sun exposure.[12]

Otherwise healthy adults with a history of cold sores who undergo elective trigeminal nerve decompression to treat tic doloureux may be treated with oral acyclovir 400 mg BID started on the evening prior to surgery and continued for 5 days. This reduces the incidence of cold sore by 75%.[13]

Anogenital Infection

Goals of Therapy

- Improve symptoms
- Prevent outbreaks

- Prevent acquisition of infection

Pharmacologic Choices (Table 2)

Primary Episodes of Genital Herpes

First episodes of genital herpes in otherwise healthy individuals may range from inapparent to severe. Treatment is effective if initiated up to 7 days after onset.[16] For severe cases, use iv **acyclovir** 5 mg/kg every 8 hours for 5 to 10 days.[14] Oral acyclovir 200 mg five times daily for 5 to 10 days is also effective.[15] IV treatment is approximately 25% better than oral treatment overall with improved resolution of local and systemic symptoms and decreased time to healing but no difference in viral shedding.[16] **Famciclovir** 250 mg TID for 7 days[17] and **valacyclovir** 500 to 1000 mg BID for 10 days[18] have comparable efficacy and tolerance to oral acyclovir. The simplicity of the famciclovir and valacyclovir regimens is an advantage.

Recurrent Genital Herpes

Recurrent genital herpes in immunocompetent patients, traditionally treated for 5 to 7 days, can now be treated for 1 to 3 days using higher doses than those formerly recommended. Five days of treatment with oral **acyclovir** 200 mg five times daily[19], **famciclovir** 125 mg BID[20] or **valacyclovir** 500 mg BID[21] initiated within the first 12 hours after symptom onset, reduced median times to pain relief and lesion healing by 1 to 2 days.

Shorter courses of therapy (1 to 3 days) appear to be as effective as 5-day treatments for episodes of recurrent genital herpes in healthy individuals. Acyclovir 800 mg TID for 2 days was more effective than placebo[22]; the benefit was similar to that observed with 200 mg five times per day for 5 days.[19] Valacyclovir 500 mg BID for 3 days is as effective as the same dose given for 5 days.[23] Famciclovir 1000 mg × 2 doses beginning less than 6 hours after symptom onset reduced median duration of pain and median lesion healing time from 6.1 to 4.3 days.[24] Short courses of therapy are effective and well tolerated, though therapy needs to be initiated within hours of symptom onset.

For individuals with frequently recurring disease (≥ 6 episodes per year), *suppressive* therapy is more effective than *episodic* therapy. Initiate suppressive therapy in immunocompetent patients with acyclovir 200 mg TID. Acyclovir 200 mg five times per day[25], 400 mg BID[26] and 800 mg daily is effective.[27] If the response to acyclovir 200 mg TID is favourable, the dose may be reduced to BID and if unfavourable, increased to 200 mg five times daily or 400 mg BID. Famciclovir 250 mg BID[28] and valacyclovir 500 mg daily (for < 9 recurrences per year) or 1000 mg daily (for > 9 recurrences per year)[29] are approved for suppressive therapy of recurrent genital herpes in healthy adults. Valacyclovir, 500 or 1000 mg, is the only treatment approved for once-daily dosing. Valacyclovir 500 mg daily appeared better than famciclovir 250 mg BID for suppression

of genital herpes and associated HSV shedding.[30] The time to a first virologically confirmed recurrence was shorter among famciclovir recipients. Acyclovir 400 mg BID can also be used. The safety of all the drugs has been demonstrated in placebo-controlled trials up to one year and in the case of acyclovir, an uncontrolled study suggested it is safe for up to five years.[31] Suppression should be interrupted periodically to evaluate the need for continued treatment. One strategy is to stop every 3 to 6 months and to await two recurrences. Only if these two recurrences are close together (maximum of 2 months apart) would another 3- to 6-month course be appropriate. This strategy can be continued indefinitely.[32]

Transmission of symptomatic genital herpes disease was reduced by 77% with **valacyclovir** 500 mg daily in a placebo-controlled trial in monogamous couples discordant for genital herpes infection.[47] Transmission of infection, symptomatic disease as well as asymptomatic seroconversion, was reduced by 50%.

Herpes Proctitis

Herpes proctitis acquired by anal intercourse or through oral-anal contact refers to the inflammation of the rectal mucosa.[33] Symptoms include anorectal pain and mucopurulent or bloody rectal discharge.[33] Herpes proctitis can be treated using acyclovir. **Acyclovir** 400 mg five times per day initiated within 12 days of onset and continued for 10 days, reduces healing time for first-episode herpes proctitis from 14 to 5 days.[34]

Genital Herpes and HIV

In HIV-infected patients, first episodes of genital HSV infection may be more severe and prolonged than in non-HIV infected patients.[35] Although data from controlled trials are lacking, iv and oral regimens recommended for non-immunocompromised patients (*vide supra*) are likely to be effective in HIV-infected patients. Some experts, however, recommend higher doses.[36,37] Oral **acyclovir** 400 mg three to five times daily can be continued until healing is complete. The duration of therapy will generally exceed the 5 to 10 days used in HIV-negative patients.

Treat recurrent genital herpes in HIV-infected patients with **acyclovir** 200 to 400 mg five times per day, **famciclovir** 500 mg BID or **valacyclovir** 1000 mg BID for 5 to 7 days. Controlled trials have shown that **famciclovir** 500 mg BID for 7 days is as effective as acyclovir 400 mg five times per day for 7 days.[38] **Valacyclovir** 1000 mg BID was as effective as acyclovir 200 mg five times per day, both for 5 days.[39] Shorter 1- and 3-day courses have not been tested in HIV-infected patients.

In patients with frequently recurring episodes of genital herpes complicating HIV infection, valacyclovir 500 mg BID reduced recurrences,[40] was 20% more efficacious than 1000 mg daily and tended to be more efficacious than acyclovir 400 mg BID. Famciclovir 500 mg BID reduced recurrences by 69% compared with placebo.[41] All regimens are well tolerated.

There is a significant risk that drug-resistant HSV mutants will be selected by suppressive therapy in HIV-infected patients, especially among those who are severely immunocompromised.[42] Accordingly, it is important that optimal HAART therapy be coadministered if appropriate. If refractory mucocutaneous HSV infection appears, consultation with an infectious diseases expert is advised. Intravenous and topical **foscarnet**, topical **trifluorothymidine** alone or in combination with **interferon alfa** and **cidofovir** have all been reported to be effective.[43] (See Chapter 107)

Genital Herpes and Pregnancy

Genital herpes in the pregnant woman may result in neonatal herpes, a serious and potentially fatal infection.[44] Transmission occurs at parturition and is greater if the maternal infection develops late in pregnancy than if she has been infected prior to becoming pregnant.[45] **Acyclovir**, taken daily beginning at 36 weeks' gestation, reduces recurrences, asymptomatic shedding and the need for Caesarean section because herpetic lesions are less commonly observed in labour. Doses of acyclovir 200 mg QID to 400 mg TID are effective and safe.[46] In managing genital herpes in a pregnant woman, consultation with an infectious diseases specialist is recommended.

Eczema Herpeticum

Eczema herpeticum is an uncommon HSV infection of eczematous skin that can cause extensive disease (fever, malaise, lymphadenopathy), presumably arising from autoinoculation from a cold sore or virus shed asymptomatically in saliva. Complications include keratoconjunctivitis, viremia and multiorgan involvement with meningitis and encephalitis.

Pharmacologic Choices (Table 3)

Oral **acyclovir** 200 mg five times per day for 5 days shortened disease duration in 81% of patients in the acyclovir group compared to 43% in the placebo group.[51] Acyclovir treatment may be life saving.[48] In severe cases, iv acyclovir 5–10 mg/kg Q8H for 7 days is recommended for patients over 12 years of age.[49] For younger children, 750 mg/m^2 per dose intravenously TID for 7 days is recommended.

There are no published trials supporting the effectiveness and safety of valacyclovir and famciclovir in eczema herpeticum.[49]

Encephalitis

Herpes simplex encephalitis (HSE) is characterized by acute onset of fever plus focal neurologic symptoms and signs (behavioural changes, speech disturbances and, less frequently, seizures). A brain abscess is the principal differential diagnostic possibility and antibiotic therapy should be included in the initial treatments prescribed, preferably with the help of an infectious diseases consultant.

During therapy, diagnostic testing to demonstrate focal unilateral frontotemporal cerebritis (MRI, EEG, brain scan, CT) and HSV etiology (by detection of HSV in brain biopsy or of HSV DNA in CSF) should be rapidly effected. Culture of CSF for HSV is uniformly negative. Acute phase serum will contain no HSV antibody in one out of three patients. A rise in titre demonstrated in a convalescent phase serum sample in these patients indicates primary HSV infection.[50]

Goals of Therapy

- Prevent death
- Prevent long-term neurologic sequelae

Pharmacologic Choices (Table 4)

Initiate iv **acyclovir** as soon as the diagnosis of HSE is considered.[52] The dose is 10 mg/kg infused iv over not less than 60 minutes to obviate obstructive nephropathy caused by formation of acyclovir crystals in the renal tubular lumen. Repeat the dose at 8-hour intervals in persons with normal renal function. Because acyclovir is eliminated exclusively through renal excretion by filtration and tubular secretion, dose intervals should be increased in renal dysfunction (see Appendix I). Duration of treatment is usually 21 days. Rarely, relapse with virologically confirmed recrudescence occurs, necessitating prolonged therapy for 10 to 14 more days.

Valacyclovir and famciclovir have not been evaluated as treatment for HSE.

Keratoconjunctivitis

HSV can cause keratitis and/or conjunctivitis and uveitis. Because distinguishing HSV conjunctivitis from bacterial infection can be difficult, and because of the risk of visual impairment, consultation with an ophthalmologist is strongly advised if HSV infection is suspected. Consult with an ophthalmologist for all HSV eye infections, except typical dendritic keratitis.

Goals of Therapy

- Ameliorate symptoms
- Prevent corneal injury with vision impairment

Pharmacologic Choices (Table 5)

Topical **trifluridine** (Viroptic) and **idoxuridine** (Herplex-D) are similar in efficacy although idoxuridine is less well tolerated.[53,54]

The role of oral **acyclovir** is controversial. Oral acyclovir 400 mg BID for 12 months in immunocompetent patients reduced the rate of recurrent stromal keratitis, the most common serious form of HSV ocular disease, more effectively than placebo.[55]

Herpes Varicella-Zoster Virus

Chickenpox

Goals of Therapy

- Accelerate healing of skin lesions
- Prevent complications, e.g., pneumonia, encephalitis

Nonpharmacologic Choices

- Individuals who do not have a history of chickenpox should avoid patients with chickenpox. Herpes varicella-zoster virus (VZV) can be transmitted through the air and by direct contact from skin lesions. A person is infectious from a couple of days prior to the development of the rash until the last lesion has crusted.
- Closely crop nails and use astringent soaks to avoid secondary bacterial infection associated with scratching pruritic skin lesions.

Pharmacologic Choices (Table 3)

Antivirals

In healthy children[56], adolescents[57] and adults[58], the benefit of **acyclovir** therapy exceeds placebo effects, i.e., reduced number of lesions, total time to crusting and duration of fever, if initiated within 24 hours of rash onset. The American Academy of Pediatrics does not recommend routine use of acyclovir in healthy children.[59] Consider acyclovir in healthy patients who are at increased risk of moderate to severe varicella such as those ≥ 12 years, patients with chronic cutaneous or pulmonary disorders, patients receiving long-term salicylate treatment and in those receiving short, intermittent or aerosolized courses of corticosteroids.

Adjust the dose of acyclovir according to age for children[59]: 5 to 7 years of age, 20 mg/kg; 8 to 12 years, 15 mg/kg; 13 to 16 years, 10 mg/kg given QID for 5 to 7 days. For adults, oral acyclovir 800 mg five times daily for 5 days or iv acyclovir 10 mg/kg every 8 hours for 5 days accelerates healing and is well tolerated.[58] Rare complications such as varicella pneumonia are more common in adults than in children. It is not known whether acyclovir prevents complications, or whether famciclovir or valacyclovir is as effective as acyclovir in the treatment of chickenpox.

In immuncompromised patients, treat chickenpox even if more than 24 hours have elapsed since the rash began. Data regarding antiviral efficacy in immunocompromised patients are lacking.

Vaccines (Table 6)

One dose of **varicella virus vaccine** is recommended in healthy children 12 months to 12 years of age. Two doses of the vaccine given 4 to 8 weeks apart is recommended in adults and adolescents ≥ 13 years.[60] Vaccinate all susceptible adults. The varicella virus vaccine is not recommended in pregnancy.[60]

Acute Herpes Zoster (Shingles)

Goals of Therapy

- Stop viral replication
- Accelerate healing of skin lesions
- Relieve acute neuritis
- Prevent postherpetic neuralgia (see Chapter 15)

Nonpharmacologic Choices[61]

- Keep rash clean and dry to reduce risk of bacterial superinfection. Consult physician if fever is present.
- Avoid use of topical antibiotics and dressing with adhesives as these may cause irritation and delay rash healing.
- Use sterile wet dressing to relieve discomfort in some patients.

Pharmacologic Choices

Antivirals (Table 3)

Systemic antivirals (**acyclovir, famciclovir, valacyclovir**), initiated within 72 hours of rash onset, reduce the duration of viral shedding and acute pain and the appearance of new lesions and may reduce the risk of postherpetic neuralgia.[61,62,63,64] Topical antivirals are not effective in the treatment of herpes zoster.[61] To reduce the risk of postherpetic neuralgia and other complications, initiate systemic antiviral therapy ≤ 72 hours after rash onset. In patients with ocular zoster, treat even if the rash has been present for up to 7 days to prevent ocular complications. Advanced age (patients < 50 years rarely develop postherpetic neuralgia[65]), severe pain and extensive disease identify patient and zoster disease characteristics that correlate with an increased risk of postherpetic neuralgia.[61,65,66] Promptly refer patients with ocular complications to an ophthalmologist. Acyclovir, famciclovir and valacyclovir are well tolerated. Common adverse effects include nausea and headache. Famciclovir and valacyclovir may improve patient adherence because they can be given TID.

Corticosteroids, Analgesics and Opioids

Prevention of postherpetic neuralgia using antiviral therapy is not absolute. Analgesics, opioids, tramadol, gabapentin, pregabalin and corticosteroids may be used in the treatment of pain related to herpes zoster.[61] Corticosteroid therapy improves quality of life (resolution of acute neuritis, uninterrupted sleep and return to normal activity) but does not accelerate healing or reduce the incidence of postherpetic neuralgia compared to acyclovir alone.[67] For more information on acute and postherpetic neuralgia, see Chapter 15.

Vaccines (Table 6)

A live, attenuated **varicella zoster vaccine** (Zostavax) containing approximately 15 times more virus than varicella virus vaccines marketed in Canada, reduced the incidence of shingles and postherpetic neuralgia by 51% and 67%, respectively, compared with placebo, in healthy adults ≥ 60 years and was well tolerated.[68] While it may be valuable as an individual health measure, its cost-effectiveness as a public health measure is not clear, depending on cost of the vaccine and the effectiveness criteria used.[69]

Therapeutic Tips

- For orolabial and genital herpes virus infections, provide patients with prescriptions enabling them to self-initiate therapy at the onset of symptoms.
- For patients with mild to moderate pain secondary to herpes zoster, a constant level of analgesia may be more beneficial than PRN dosing.
- Famciclovir 125 mg BID is recommended for treating recurrences of genital herpes whereas famciclovir 250 mg BID is recommended for prevention and suppression of recurrences. Assess most appropriate dose case-by-case.

Figure 1: **Management of Herpes Zoster**

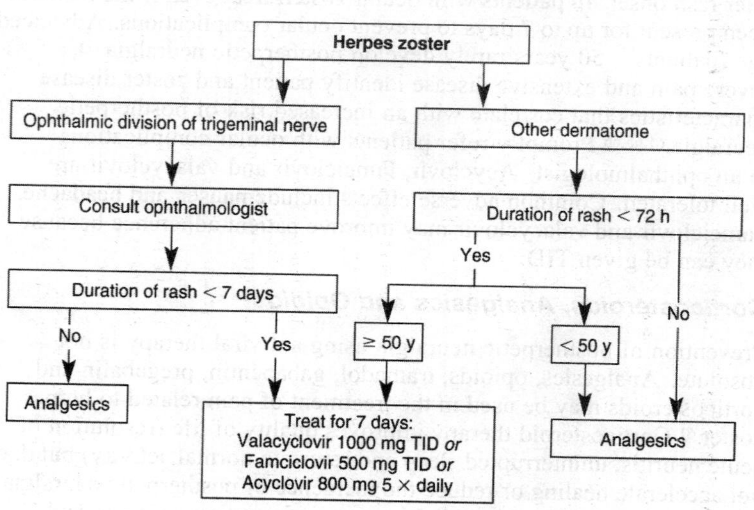

Table 1: Antivirals for Orolabial and Mouth HSV Infections

Class	Drug	Indication/ Dose	Adverse Effects	Cost[a]
Guanine Nucleoside Analogues	*acyclovir* Zovirax, generics	HSV gingivostomatitis in children: 15 mg/kg po 5 × daily × 7 days *or* 600 mg/m² po QID × 10 days 250 mg/m² Q8H iv × 5–10 days Recurrent orolabial HSV: *Treatment*: 400 mg po 5 × daily × 5 days *Prophylaxis*: 400 mg po BID 12 h prior to sun exposure × duration of exposure *Suppression*: 200 mg po QID or 400 mg BID up to 4 mo	Not different from placebo.	HSV gingivostomatitis in children: po:$$ iv[b]:$$$$ Recurrent orolabial HSV: Treatment: $ Prophylaxis: $$/30 day supply Suppression: $$$/30 day supply
	famciclovir Famvir, generics	Recurrent orolabial HSV: *Treatment*: 750 mg po BID × 1 day *or* 1500 mg po as a single dose	See acyclovir.	$$
	penciclovir Denavir	Recurrent orolabial HSV: *Topical Treatment:* Apply Q2H during waking hours × 4 days at earliest sign or symptom	Erythema (common).	$/2 g tube
	valacyclovir Valtrex	Recurrent orolabial HSV: *Treatment*: 2 g po BID × 1 day *or* 750 mg po BID × 1 day *or* 1500 mg po once *Suppression*: 500 mg po daily × 4 mo	See acyclovir.	Treatment: $ Suppression: $$$/30 day supply

[a] Cost per course of treatment unless otherwise specified; includes drug cost only. Cost of iv acyclovir assumes no wastage.
[b] Based on 20 kg body weight for children and 70 kg for adults.
Dosage adjustment may be required in renal impairment; see Appendix I.
Legend: $ < $50 $$ $50–100 $$$ $100–150 $$$$ > $150

Table 2: **Antivirals for Genital and Anal HSV Infections**

Class	Drug	Indication	Adverse Effects	Cost[a]
Guanine Nucleoside Analogues	*acyclovir* Zovirax, generics	Genital HSV infection, first episode: 5 mg/kg Q8H iv × 5–10 days 200 mg po 5 × daily × 5–10 days Recurrent genital HSV infection: *Treatment*: 200 mg po 5 × daily × 5–7 days *or* 800 mg po TID × 2 days *Suppression*: 200 mg po BID up to 5 × daily *or* 400 mg po BID *or* 800 mg po daily × 3–6 mo HSV proctitis: 400 mg po 5 × daily × 10 days	Not different from placebo.	Genital HSV infection, first episode: po:$ iv[b]:$$$$ Recurrent genital HSV infection: Treatment: $ Suppression: $$-$$$/30 day supply HSV proctitis: $$
	famciclovir Famvir, generics	Genital HSV infection, first episode: 250 mg po TID × 10 days Recurrent genital HSV infection: *Treatment*: 125 mg po BID × 5 days *or* 1000 mg po BID × 1 day *Suppression*: 250 mg po BID × 3–6 mo	See acyclovir.	Genital HSV infection, first episode: $$$ Recurrent genital HSV infection: Treatment: $ Suppression: $$$$/30 day supply
	valacyclovir Valtrex	Genital HSV infection, first episode: 1000 mg po BID × 10 days Recurrent genital HSV infection: *Treatment*: 500 mg po BID × 3–5 days *Suppression*: ≤ 9 recurrences: 500 mg po daily × 3–6 mo > 9 recurrences: 1000 mg po daily × 3–6 mo	See acyclovir	Genital HSV infection, first episode: $$ Recurrent genital HSV infection: Treatment: $ Suppression: $$$-$$$$/30 day supply Prevention of genital HSV infection transmission: $$$/30 day supply

Class	Drug	Indication	Adverse Effects	Cost[a]
		Prevention of genital HSV infection transmission: 500 mg po daily		

[a] Cost per course of treatment unless otherwise specified; includes drug cost only. Cost of iv acyclovir assumes no wastage.
[b] Based on 20 kg body weight for children and 70 kg for adults.
Dosage adjustment may be required in renal impairment; see Appendix I.
Legend: $ < $50 $$ $50–100 $$-$$$ $50–150 $$$ $100–150 $$$-$$$$ $100– >150 $$$$ > $150

Table 3: Antivirals for Herpesvirus Infections of the Skin

Class	Drug	Indication/Dose	Adverse Effects	Cost[a]
Guanine Nucleoside Analogues	*acyclovir* ◗ Zovirax, generics	Chickenpox: Children: 10–20 mg/kg po QID × 5–7 days Adults: 800 mg po 5 × daily × 5 days *or* 10 mg/kg iv Q8H × 5 days Eczema herpeticum: 200 mg po 5 × daily × 5 days Herpes zoster: 800 mg po 5 × daily × 7 days	Not different from placebo.	Chickenpox: Children[b]: $ Adults: po: $$; iv[b]: $$$$ Eczema herpeticum: $ Herpes zoster: $$
	famciclovir ◗ Famvir, generics	Herpes zoster: 500 mg po TID × 7 days	See acyclovir.	$$$
	valacyclovir ◗ Valtrex	Herpes zoster: 1000 mg po TID × 7 days	See acyclovir.	$$$

[a] Cost per course of treatment; includes drug cost only. Cost of iv acyclovir assumes no wastage.
[b] Based on 20 kg body weight for children and 70 kg for adults.
◗ Dosage adjustment may be required in renal impairment; see Appendix I.
Legend: $ < $50 $$ $50–100 $$$ $100–150 $$$$ > $150

Table 4: Antivirals for HSV Encephalitis

Class	Drug	Dose	Adverse Effects	Cost[a]
Guanine Nucleoside Analogues	*acyclovir* (renal symbol) Zovirax, generics	10 mg/kg iv Q8H × 21 days	GI upset, lightheadedness, redness at injection site.	$$$$[b]

[a] Cost per course of treatment; includes drug cost only. Cost of iv acyclovir assumes no wastage.
[b] Based on 20 kg body weight for children and 70 kg for adults.
(renal symbol) Dosage adjustment may be required in renal impairment; see Appendix I.
Legend: $$$$ > $150

Table 5: **Antivirals for HSV Keratoconjunctivitis**

Class	Drug	Indication/Dose	Adverse Effects	Cost[a]
Guanine Nucleoside Analogues	*acyclovir* [renal] Zovirax, generics	*Suppression of recurrent keratoconjunctivitis*: 400 mg po BID up to 12 mo	Not different from placebo.	$$$/30 day supply
	idoxuridine 0.1% Herplex, generic	*Treatment:* 1 drop Q1H while awake and Q2H at night continued until definite improvement. Continue treatment for 5–7 days after healing is complete to avoid recurrence (duration of treatment should not exceed 21 days)	Burning, stinging.	$/15 mL
	trifluridine Viroptic 1.0% solution, generic	*Treatment:* 1 drop Q2H onto cornea while awake (max 9 drops/ day) until complete re-epithelialization of cornea, then ↓ to 1 drop Q4H while awake (max 5 drops/day) × 7 days post re-epithelialization of the cornea Store under refrigeration	See idoxuridine.	$$$

[a] Cost per course of treatment unless otherwise specified; includes drug cost only. Cost of iv acyclovir assumes no wastage.

[renal] Dosage adjustment may be required in renal impairment; see Appendix I.

Legend: $ < $50 $$ $50–100 $$$ $100–150

Table 6: **Vaccines for Prevention of Varicella Virus Infection**

Class	Drug	Dose	Comments	Cost[a]
Vaccines, viral	*varicella virus vaccine, live attenuated* Varilix, Varivax III	12 mo–12 y: one dose ≥ 13 y: 2 doses of the vaccine given 4 to 8 weeks apart	Not recommended in pregnancy.[60] Common side effects: local pain, swelling, redness.	$55

[a] Cost of 1 dose; includes drug cost only.

Suggested Readings

Aoki FY. Contemporary antiviral drug regimens for the prevention and treatment of orolabial and anogenital herpes simplex virus infection in the normal host: four approved indications and 13 off-label uses. *Can J Infect Dis* 2003;14(1):17-27.

Aoki FY. Genital herpes simplex virus (HSV) infections. In: *Canadian guidelines on sexually transmitted infections*. 2006 edition. Ottawa (ON): Public Health Agency of Canada; 2006. Available from: http://www.phac-aspc.gc.ca/std-mts/sti_2006/pdf/sti2006_e.pdf Accessed June 12, 2007.

Corey L. Herpes simplex virus. In: Mandell GL, Bennett JE, Dolin R, editors. *Mandell, Douglas and Bennett's Principles and practice of infectious diseases*. 5th ed. Philadelphia (PA): Churchill Livingstone; 2000. p.1564-80.

Hyndiuk RA, Tabbara KF, editors. *Infections of the eye*. Boston (MA): Little, Brown; 1986.

Whitley RJ. Varicella-zoster virus. In: Mandell GL, Bennett JE, Dolin R, editors. *Mandell, Douglas and Bennett's Principles and practice of infectious diseases*. 5th ed. Philadelphia (PA): Churchill Livingstone; 2000. p.1580-86.

References

1. Amir J, Harel L, Smetana Z et al. Treatment of herpes simplex gingivostomatitis with aciclovir in children: a randomized, double blind, placebo controlled study. *BMJ* 1997:314(7097):1800-3.
2. Aoki FY et al. Acyclovir suspension for the treatment of acute HSV gingivostomatitis in children: a placebo-controlled, double-blind trial [abstract]. *33rd Interscience Conference on Antimicrobial Agents and Chemotherapy*; 1993 Oct 17-20; New Orleans (LA).
3. Spruance SL, Stewart JC, Rowe NH et al. Treatment of recurrent herpes simplex labialis with oral acyclovir.*J Infect Dis* 1990;161(2):185-90.
4. [No authors listed]. Valacyclovir (Valtrex) for herpes labialis. *Med Lett Drugs Ther* 2002;44(1143):95-6.
5. Spruance SL, Jones TM, Blatter MM et al. High dose, short-duration, early valacyclovir therapy for episodic treatment of cold sores: results of two randomized, placebo-controlled, multicenter studies. *Antimicrob Agents Chemother* 2003;47(3):1072-80.
6. Bodsworth N. Single-dose, patient-initiated famciclovir for episodic treatment of herpes labialis; expert opinions in new herpes data [abstract]. *Update from recent international congresses at 12th Annual Meeting of the IHMF*; 2005 Oct 28-30; Lisbon (PO).
7. Spruance SL, Nett R, Marbury R et al. Acyclovir cream for treatment of herpes simplex labialis: results of two randomized, double-blind, vehicle-controlled, multicenter clinical trials. *Antimicrob Agents Chemother* 2002;46(7):2238-43.
8. Spruance SL, Rea TL, Thoming C et al. Penciclovir cream for the treatment of herpes simplex labialis. A randomized, multi-center, double-blind, placebo-controlled trial. *JAMA* 1997;277(17):1374-9.
9. Rooney JF, Straus SE, Mannix ML et al. Oral acyclovir to suppress frequently recurrent herpes labialis. A double-blind, placebo-controlled trial. *Ann Intern Med* 1993;118(4):268-72.
10. Meyrick Thomas RH, Dodd HJ, Yeo JM et al. Oral acyclovir in the suppression of recurrent non-genital herpes simplex virus infection. *Br J Dermatol* 1985;113(6):731-5.
11. Baker DA et al. Valacyclovir effective for suppression of recurrent HSV-1 herpes labialis [abstract].*40th Interscience Conference on Antimicrobial Agents and Chemotherapy*; 2000 Sep 17-20; Toronto (ON).
12. Spruance SL, Hamill ML, Hoge WS et al. Acyclovir prevents reactivation of herpes simplex labialis in skiers. *JAMA* 1988;260:1597-99.
13. Schadelin J, Schilt HV, Rohner M. Preventive therapy of herpes labialis associated with trigeminal surgery. *Am J Med* 1988;85(2A):46-8.
14. Corey L, Fife KH, Benedetti JK et al. Intravenous acyclovir for the treatment of primary genital herpes. *Ann Int Med* 1983;98(6):914-21.
15. Mertz GJ, Critchlow CW, Benedetti J et al. Double-blind, placebo-controlled trial of oral acyclovir in first-episode genital herpes simplex virus infection. *JAMA* 1984;252(9):1147-51.

16. Corey L, Benedetti J, Critchlow CW et al. Treatment of primary first-episode genital herpes simplex virus infections with acyclovir: results of topical, intravenous and oral therapy. *J Antimicrob Chemother* 1983;12(Suppl B):79-88.
17. Loveless M, Harris JRW, Sacks SL. Famciclovir in the management of first-episode genital herpes. *Infect Dis Clin Prac* 1997;6(Suppl 1):S12-S16.
18. Fife KH, Barbarash RA, Rudolph T et al. Valaciclovir versus acyclovir in the treatment of first-episode genital herpes infection. Results of an international, multicenter, double-blind, randomized clinical trial. The Valaciclovir International Herpes Simplex Virus Study Group. *Sex Transm Dis* 1997;24(8):481-6.
19. Tyring SK, Douglas JM, Corey L et al. A randomized, placebo-controlled comparison of oral valacyclovir and acyclovir in immunocompetent patients with recurrent genital herpes infections. The Valaciclovir International Study Group. *Arch Dermatol* 1998;134(2):185-91.
20. Sacks SL, Aoki FY, Diaz-Mitoma F et al. Patient-initiated, twice-daily oral famciclovir for early recurrent genital herpes. A randomized, double-blind multicenter trial. Canadian Famciclovir Study Group. *JAMA* 1996;276(1):44-9.
21. Spruance SL, Tyring SK, DeGregorio B et al. A large-scale, placebo-controlled, dose-ranging trial of peroral valaciclovir for episodic treatment of recurrent herpes genitalis. Valaciclovir HSV Study Group. *Arch Intern Med* 1996;156(15):1729-35.
22. Wald A, Carrell D, Remington M et al. Two-day regimen of acyclovir for treatment of recurrent genital herpes simplex virus type 2 infection. *Clin Infect Dis* 2002;34(7):944-8.
23. Leone PA, Trottier S, Miller JM. Valacyclovir for episodic treatment of genital herpes: a shorter 3-day treatment course compared with 5-day treatment. *Clin Infect Dis* 2002;34(7):958-62.
24. Aoki FY, Tyring S, Diaz-Mitoma F et al. Single-day, patient-initiated famciclovir therapy for recurrent genital herpes: a randomized, double-blind, placebo-controlled trial. *Clin Infect Dis* 2006;42(1):8-13.
25. Douglas JM, Critchlow C, Benedetti J et al. A double-blind study of oral acyclovir for suppression of recurrences of genital herpes simplex virus infection. *N Engl J Med* 1984;310(24):1551-6.
26. Mertz GJ, Jones CC, Mills J et al. Long-term acyclovir suppression of frequently recurring genital herpes simplex virus infection. A multicenter double-blind trial. *JAMA* 1988;260(2):201-6.
27. Mostow SR, Mayfield JL, Marr JJ et al. Suppression of recurrent genital herpes by single daily dosages of acyclovir. *Am J Med* 1988; 85(2A):30-3.
28. Mertz GJ, Loveless MO, Levin MJ et al. Oral famciclovir for suppression of recurrent genital herpes simplex virus infection in women. A multicenter, double-blind, placebo-controlled trial. Collaborative Famciclovir Genital Herpes Research Group. *Arch Intern Med* 1997;157(3):343-9.
29. Reitano M, Tyring S, Lang W et al. Valaciclovir for the suppression of recurrent genital herpes simplex virus infection: a large-scale dose range-finding study. International Valaciclovir HSV Study Group. *J Infect Dis* 1998;178(3):603-10.
30. Wald A, Selke S, Warren T et al. Comparative efficacy of famciclovir and valacyclovir for suppression of recurrent genital herpes and viral shedding. *Sex Trans Dis* 2006;33(9):529-33.
31. Goldberg LH, Kaufman R, Kurtz TO et al. Long-term suppression of recurrent genital herpes with acyclovir. A 5-year benchmark. Acyclovir Study Group. *Arch Dermatol* 1993;129(5):582-7.
32. Aoki FY. Contemporary antiviral drug regimens for the prevention and treatment of orolabial and anogenital herpes simplex virus infection in the normal host: four approved indications and 13 off-label uses. *Can J Inf Dis* 2003;14(1):17-27.
33. Rompalo AM. Diagnosis and treatment of sexually acquired proctitis and proctocolitis: An update. *Clin Infect Dis* 1999;28(Suppl 1):S84-S90.
34. Rompalo AM, Mertz GJ, Davis LG et al. Oral acyclovir for treatment of first-episode herpes simplex virus proctitis. *JAMA* 1988;259(19):2879-81.
35. Maier JA, Bergman A, Ross MG. Acquired immunodeficiency syndrome manifested by chronic primary genital herpes. *Am J Obstet Gynecol* 1986;155(4):756-8.
36. Strick LB, Wald A, Celum C. Management of herpes simplex virus type 2 infection in HIV type-1 infected persons. *Clin Infect Dis* 2006;43(3):347-56.
37. Drew WL, Stempien MJ, Kheraj M et al. Management of herpesvirus infections (cytomegalovirus, herpes simplex virus and varicella-zoster virus). In: Sande MA, Volberding PA, editors. *The medical management of AIDS*. 6th ed. Philadelphia (PA): Saunders; 1999. p. 444.
38. Romanowski B, Aoki FY, Martel AY et al. Efficacy and safety of famciclovir for treating mucocutaneous herpes simplex infection in HIV-infected individuals. Collaborative Famciclovir HIV Study Group. *AIDS* 2000;14(9):1211-7.
39. Schacker T. The International Valaciclovir HSV Study Group. Valaciclovir as acute treatment for recurrent anogenital herpes in immunocompromised (HIV positive) individuals [abstract]. *International Society for Sexually Transmitted Diseases Research*; Denver (CO); 1999.
40. Warren T, Harris J, and Brennan CA. Efficacy and safety of valacyclovir for the suppression and episodic treatment of herpes simplex virus in patients with HIV. *Clin Infect Dis* 2004;39(Suppl 5):S258-66.
41. Schacker T, Hu HL, Koelle DM et al. Famciclovir for the suppression of symptomatic and asymptomatic herpes simplex virus reactivation in HIV-infected persons. A double-blind, placebo-controlled trial. *Ann Intern Med* 1998;128(1):21-8.

42. Levin MJ, Bacon TH, Leary JJ. Resistance of herpes simplex virus infections to nucleoside analogues in HIV-infected patients. *Clin Infect Dis* 2004;39(Suppl 5):S248-57.
43. Aoki FY. Management of genital herpes in HIV-infected patients. *Herpes* 2001;8(2):41-5.
44. Brown ZA, Wald A, Morrow RA et al. Effect of serologic status and cesarean delivery on transmission rates of herpes simplex virus from mother to infant. *JAMA* 2003;289(2);203-9.
45. Nahmias AJ, Josey WE, Naib ZM et al. Perinatal risk associated with maternal genital herpes simplex virus infection. *Am J Obstet Gynecol* 1971;110(6):825-37.
46. Aoki FY. Genital herpes simplex virus (HSV) infections. In: *Canadian guidelines on sexually transmitted infections*. 2006 ed. Ottawa (ON): Public Health Agency of Canada; 2006. Available from: http://www.phac-aspc.gc.ca/std-mts/sti_2006/pdf/sti2006_e.pdf Accessed June 12, 2007.
47. Corey L, Wald A, Patel R et al. Once daily valacyclovir reduces transmission of genital herpes. *N Engl J Med* 2004;350:11-20.
48. Sanderson IR, Brueton LA, Savage MO et al. Eczema herpeticum: a potentially fatal disease. *Br Med J (Clin Res Ed)* 1987;294(6573):693-4.
49. Wollenberg A, Wetzel S, Burgdorf WH et al. Viral infections in atopic dermatitis: pathogenic aspects and clinical management. *J Allergy Clin Immunol* 2003;112(4):667-74.
50. Whitley RJ, Lakeman F. Herpes simplex virus infection of the central nervous system: therapeutic and diagnostic considerations. *Clin Infect Dis* 1999;20(2):414-20.
51. Niimura M, Nishikawa T. Treatment of eczema herpeticum with oral acyclovir. *Am J Med* 1988;85(2A):49-52.
52. Whitley RJ, Alford CA, Hirsch MS et al. Vidarabine versus acyclovir therapy in herpes simplex encephalitis. *N Eng J Med* 1986;314(3):144-9.
53. Van Bijsterveld OP, Post H. Trifluorothmidine versus adenine arabinoside in the treatment of herpes simplex keratitis. *Br J Ophthalmol* 1908;64:33-6.
54. Pavan-Langston D. Major ocular viral infections. In: Galasso GH, Whitley RJ, Merigan TC, editors. *Antiviral agents and viral diseases of man*. New York (NY): Raven Press; 1999. p. 183-223.
55. [No authors listed]. Acyclovir for the prevention of recurrent herpes simplex virus eye disease. Herpetic Eye Disease Study Group*N Engl J Med* 1998;339(5):300-6.
56. Dunkle LM, Arvin AM, Whitley RJ et al. A controlled trial of acyclovir for chickenpox in normal children. *N Engl J Med* 1991;325(22)1539-44.
57. Balfour HH, Rothart HA, Feldman S et al. Acyclovir treatment of varicella in otherwise healthy adolescents. The Collaborative Acyclovir Varicella Study Group. *J Pediatr* 1992;120(4 Pt 1):627-33.
58. Wallace MR, Bowler WA, Murray NB et al. Treatment of adult varicella with oral acyclovir. A randomized, placebo-controlled trial. *Ann Intern Med* 1992;117(5):358-63.
59. American Academy of Pediatrics. Varicella-zoster infections. In: Pickering LK, Baker CJ, Long SS et al, editors. *Red book: 2006 report of the Committee on Infectious Diseases*. 27th edition. Elk Grove Village (IL): American Academy of Pediatrics; 2006. p. 711-25.
60. Public Health Agency of Canada. Canadian Immunization Guide. 2006, Ottawa, Canada.
61. Dworkin RH, Johnson RW, Breuer J et al. Recommendations for the management of herpes zoster. *Clin Infect Dis* 2007;44:(Suppl 1):S1-26.
62. Beutner KR, Friedman DJ, Forszpaniak C et al. Valacyclovir compared with acyclovir for improved therapy for herpes zoster in immunocompetent adults. *Antimicrob Agents Chemother* 1995;39(7):1546-53.
63. Degreef H. Famciclovir, a new oral anti herpes drug: results of the first controlled clinical study demonstrating its efficacy and safety in the treatment of uncomplicated herpes zoster in immunocompetent patients. *Int J Antimicrob Agents* 1994;4:241-6.
64. Wood, MJ, Kay R, Dworkin RH et al. Oral acyclovir accelerates pain resolution in herpes zoster: a meta-analysis of placebo-controlled trials. *Clin Infect Dis* 1996;22(2):341-7.
65. Choo PW, Galil K, Donahue JG et al. Risk factors for postherpetic neuralgia. *Arch Intern Med* 1997;157(11):1217-24.
66. Whitley RJ, Weiss WL, Zoong SJ et al. Herpes zoster: risk categories for persistent pain. *J Inf Dis* 1999;179:9-15.
67. Whitley RJ, Weiss H, Gnann JW et al. Acyclovir with and without prednisone for the treatment of herpes zoster. A randomized, placebo-controlled trial. The National Institute of Allergy and Infectious Diseases Collaborative Antiviral Study Group. *Ann Int Med* 1996;125(5):376-83.
68. Oxman MN, Levin MJ, Johnson GR et al. A vaccine to prevent herpes zoster and post-herpetic neuralgia in older adults. *N Engl J Med* 2005;352(22):2271-84.
69. Rothberg MB, Virapongse A, Smith KJ. Cost-effectiveness of a vaccine to prevent herpes zoster and postherpetic neuralgia in older adults. *Clin Infect Dis* 2007;44(10):1280-8.

CHAPTER 106
HIV Infection

Valentina Montessori, MD, FRCPC
Marianne Harris, MD, CCFP and
Julio S.G. Montaner, MD, FRCPC, FCCP

Goals of Therapy

- Prolong survival
- Slow disease progression
- Improve quality of life
- Decrease viral replication
- Prevent/reverse immunologic impairment
- Delay/prevent the emergence of HIV-resistant strains

Investigations

- Clinical history:
  - risk behaviours, social support and need for counselling
  - establish date of infection based on a review of past sexual contacts, period of needle sharing, receipt of blood or blood products, availability of a previous negative test or a history of possible seroconversion illness (i.e., mononucleosis or severe flu-like illness) shortly after a high-risk exposure
  - general indicators: anorexia, weight loss, fatigue or malaise, lymphadenopathy
  - symptoms of opportunistic infections, e.g., fever, night sweats, cough, dyspnea, diarrhea, headache or skin rashes
  - travel history
- Past medical history:
  - sexually transmitted diseases (gonorrhea, syphilis, chlamydia, granuloma inguinale, lymphogranuloma venereum, herpes simplex, genital warts, pubic lice)
  - past history or exposure to tuberculosis (TB), hepatitis B or C
  - conditions that may compromise future drug therapy, e.g., kidney dysfunction, peripheral neuropathy, liver disease, pancreatitis, cardiovascular disease, psychiatric disorders, substance abuse
  - allergies
  - immunization history
- Physical examination:
  - focus on signs of immune dysfunction and indications of opportunistic disease

  - direct specific attention to examination of the mental status, skin, visual fields, ocular fundi, oral cavity, lymph nodes, abdomen, rectal and genital exam (including cervical Pap smear in women and anal Pap smear in men with history of Human Papillomavirus infection)
- Laboratory investigations:
  - HIV antibody test (repeat to rule out lab error)
  - plasma HIV RNA level (also known as plasma viral load or pVL) is the best prognostic marker for progression to AIDS and survival.[1] Plasma viral load ranges vary according to the test employed. There is no "safe" level. The most sensitive plasma HIV-1 RNA assays currently available have a quantitation limit of 50 copies/mL
  - A baseline resistance test is also desirable, particularly in areas where the background level of primary resistance to antiretrovirals is unknown or ≥ 5%[2]
  - CD4 lymphocyte count and percentage is useful in determining where a patient lies in the continuum of HIV disease and the need for specific intervention (Table 1). Knowledge of the CD4 count can also help to narrow the differential diagnosis in a symptomatic HIV-infected patient. In adults, a CD4 count of 430 to 1360 cells/μL (0.43 to1.36 Giga/Litre or G/L) is considered normal in most laboratories
  - CBC, differential and platelet count
  - liver (AST, ALT, GGT, LDH, CPK, alkaline phosphatase, bilirubin, INR, albumin) and renal (BUN, creatinine, electrolytes, urinalysis) profiles
  - metabolic profiles (fasting glucose and lipids—total cholesterol, LDL, HDL, triglycerides)
  - hepatitis B, hepatitis C, syphilis, cytomegalovirus (CMV) and toxoplasmosis serologies
  - cultures and smears for sexually transmitted diseases as indicated
  - skin tests, sputum cultures and smears for mycobacteria as indicated
  - chest x-ray

Therapeutic Choices (Table 1)

Nonpharmacologic Choices

Counselling recommendations are included in Table 1.

Table 1: **Management of Patients with HIV Infection**

CD4 Count (cells/μL)	Action
At all levels	• General counselling (safer sex, nutrition, need for follow-up, importance of compliance, etc.) • History and physical examination every 3–6 mo • Plasma viral load and CD4 count at least every 3–4 mo • Herpes suppression if frequent recurrences (more than 4–6 episodes per year) • Syphilis serology • Pneumococcal vaccine; hepatitis A and B vaccines if appropriate; update diphtheria, tetanus and inactivated polio vaccines as needed; consider annual influenza vaccinations • TB skin test and isoniazid prophylaxis if indicated (consider repeating skin test yearly)
< 500	• Plasma viral load and CD4 count every 3–4 mo • Clinical evaluations and laboratory investigations at least bimonthly if symptomatic, diagnosed with AIDS, or on antiretroviral therapy
< 200	• Start prophylaxis for *Pneumocystis jirovecii* pneumonia (PJP)
< 100	• Start toxoplasmosis prophylaxis if seropositive and not on trimethoprim/sulfamethoxazole for PJP prophylaxis
< 75	• Consider MAC prophylaxis
< 50	• Screen by an ophthalmologist for early CMV retinitis (repeat at 3–6 mo intervals) or consider CMV prophylaxis

Abbreviations: CMV = cytomegalovirus.

Pharmacologic Choices (Table 2)

Antiretroviral Therapy

The goal of therapy is to suppress viral replication to prevent the *emergence of resistant* strains and therefore prolong the durability of the antiviral response. Long-term nonprogression of disease can be expected if the plasma viral load is maintained below the level of detection on a long-term basis. The goal of a plasma viral load < 50 copies/mL is recommended as this is the lower limit of quantitation common to all currently available assays (Figure 1). As newer, more sensitive assays become available, the goal may be revised.

An alternative approach is *partially suppressive therapy*. This is often the only option available to patients who have failed previous courses of therapy. Even short-term decreases in plasma viral load on the order of 0.5 to 1.5 log_{10} have been associated with substantial (two- to three-fold) reductions in disease progression and delayed mortality in clinical trials.[3]

Patients with CD4 counts between 250 and 350 cells/μL should be monitored closely given that rapid decreases in CD4 counts can occur, particularly among those with HIV RNA levels > 30 000 copies/μL. In such instances, more frequent monitoring may be appropriate (Figure 1).

Highly active antiretroviral therapy (HAART) is the standard of care and is defined as a combination of at least three drugs. HAART regimens recommended for first-line therapy consist of two nucleoside (or nucleotide) reverse transcriptase inhibitors plus either a non-nucleoside reverse transcriptase inhibitor or a ritonavir-boosted protease inhibitor (see Table 2). Other more recently introduced classes of drugs (fusion inhibitors, entry inhibitors, integrase inhibitors) are reserved for use in treatment-experienced patients with limited options due to drug resistance or intolerable adverse events.

Table 2: **Highly Active Antiretroviral Drug Regimens**

Regimen	Comment
2 N[t]RTIs + NNRTI	Favourable dosing schedule. As effective as PI-based regimens.
2 N[t]RTIs + PI + low-dose ritonavir	Daily or twice daily dosing, with minimal specific food requirements. Lower doses of PIs may decrease toxicity and side effects.

Abbreviations: N[t]RTI: nucleoside [or nucleotide] reverse transcriptase inhibitor; PI: protease inhibitor; NNRTI: non-nucleoside reverse transcriptase inhibitor.

Effective control of HIV infection with HAART reduces the incidence of opportunistic infections and certain cancers, and prolongs life.[4] Long-term treatment with HAART is associated with metabolic complications[5] and a small but significant increase in the incidence of cardiovascular events.[6]

When selecting the antiretroviral regimen, use agents with additive antiviral effects and avoid those with additive toxicities. Also consider issues of cross-resistance, compliance, convenience and cost (Table 3). Nonadherence to therapy promotes the emergence of drug-resistant HIV strains and is the single most important remaining challenge in the management of HIV infection.[7,8] Counselling and support are critical to ensure ongoing compliance.

A confirmed rebound towards baseline in plasma viral load implies *treatment failure*. The regimen should then be changed to a new three-drug regimen, avoiding cross-resistance with previous treatments.[9]

If a patient experiences drug toxicity, brief cessation of all medications is recommended. Avoid decreasing the dosage or stopping only one medication, as this will promote the development of resistance.[9,10]

The risk of opportunistic infections and death was higher in patients randomized to episodic treatment interruptions based on CD4 count as compared with continuous HAART in the SMART study.[11] For this reason, structured treatment interruptions ("drug holidays") are not recommended.[12]

Postexposure Prophylaxis

For recommendations on HIV postexposure prophylaxis, see "Management of Occupational Exposure to Bloodborne Pathogens" in the

current edition of the *Compendium of Pharmaceuticals and Specialties* (*CPS*).

HIV in Pregnancy

Optimal management of *HIV in pregnancy* requires referral to specialists. Monotherapy with AZT in the second and third trimesters decreases vertical transmission of HIV.[13] Studies of the safety and efficacy of combination antiretroviral therapy in pregnancy are ongoing. Although prevention of HIV in the infant and avoidance of teratogenicity are important considerations in the treatment of HIV-infected pregnant women, at the present time, optimal therapy of the mother should be the primary treatment goal.[9]

Breastfeeding by HIV-positive women is a recognized risk factor for HIV transmission to the infant and is strongly discouraged.

Therapeutic Tips

- Develop a long-term treatment strategy in advance to deal with drug intolerance and treatment failure due to resistance.
- *Poor compliance (or adherence)* is the single most critical determinant of therapeutic failure. Promote compliance by prescribing the simplest possible regimen.
- Nonquantifiable (“undetectable”) viral levels in plasma do not imply cure, eradication or a reason for complacency with safer sex practices or similar safety measures.
- The variability of the plasma viral load assays is approximately 0.3 to 0.5 $\log_{10}$. Hence, changes in plasma viral load of < 0.3 to 0.5 $\log_{10}$ are usually not regarded as clinically significant.[14]
- Intercurrent illnesses or vaccinations can transiently but substantially increase plasma viral load.[15]
- CD4 counts show diurnal variation, being lowest in the morning and highest in the evening.[16] Fluctuations of up to 30% may occur, which are not attributable to a change in disease status. Overall, it is important to monitor the trends in CD4 counts over time rather than placing too much emphasis on one specific reading.
- From a practical standpoint it is useful to consider the CD4 count as indicative of “the immunologic damage that has already occurred” and the plasma viral load as “the damage that is about to occur.”
- If the plasma viral load rebounds despite ongoing therapy, consider noncompliance and resistance as the most likely causes.[9]
- Some antiretroviral agents have variable pharmacokinetic profiles which may lead to suboptimal therapeutic responses even in a compliant patient.[9]

Figure 1: Approach to Antiretroviral Therapy

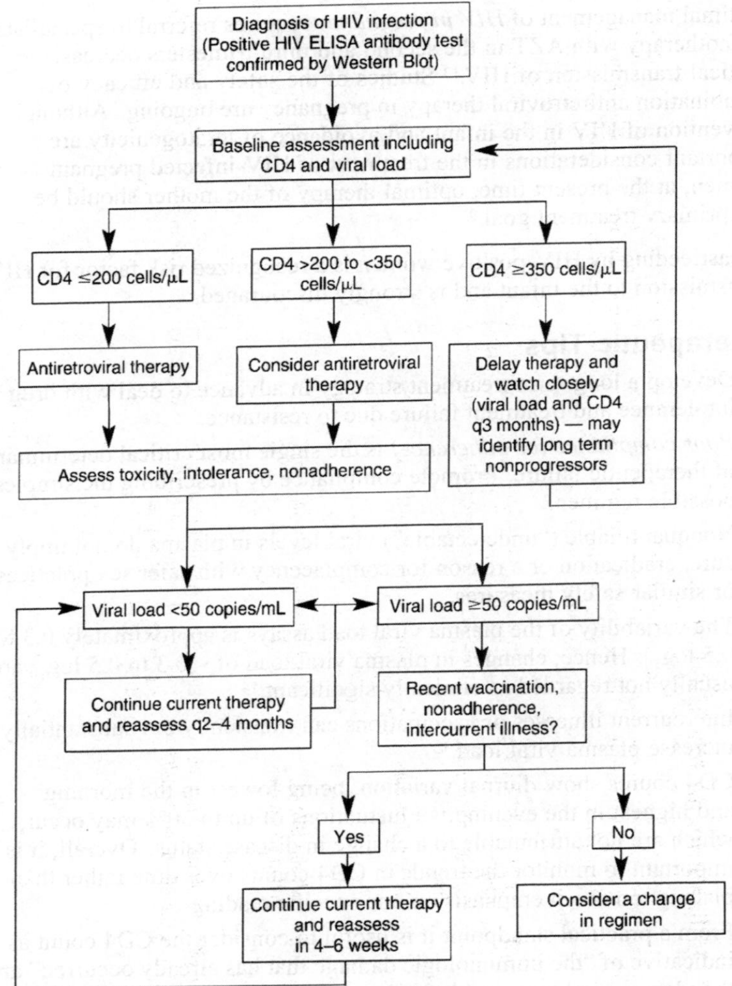

Table 3: Antiretroviral Medications for HIV Therapy

Class	Drug	Dose	Adverse Effects	Drug Interactions	Comments	Cost[a]
Nucleoside Reverse Transcriptase Inhibitors (NRTI)	*abacavir (ABC)* Ziagen	600 mg once daily or 300 mg BID	Hypersensitivity reactions in patients with a genetic predisposition (can be severe).[b]	Alcohol may ↑ abacavir plasma concentration.	Recommended first-line therapy. Close early clinical monitoring.	$$$$
	didanosine (ddI) Videx EC	< 60 kg: 250 mg once daily ≥ 60 kg: 400 mg once daily	GI intolerance, pancreatitis, gout, reversible peripheral neuropathy, ↑ lactic acid, hepatic steatosis.	Should not be combined with TDF. Avoid concurrent use with ribavirin.	Avoid combined use of ddI and d4T or TDF.	$$-$$$
	emtricitabine (FTC) Emtriva	200 mg once daily	Minimal toxicity, generally well tolerated.		Recommended first-line therapy. Avoid combined use of FTC and 3TC.	c
	lamivudine (3TC) 3TC	150 mg BID or 300 mg once daily	Minimal toxicity, generally well tolerated.		Recommended first-line therapy. Avoid combined use of 3TC and FTC.	$$
	stavudine (d4T) Zerit	< 60 kg: 30 mg BID ≥ 60 kg: 40 mg BID	Reversible peripheral neuropathy, ↑ lactic acid, hepatic steatosis, pancreatitis, lipoatrophy, dyslipidemia.	Should not be combined with AZT; ↑ toxicity with ddI.	Avoid combined use of d4T and AZT or ddI.	$$

(cont'd)

Table 3: **Antiretroviral Medications for HIV Therapy** *(cont'd)*

Class	Drug	Dose	Adverse Effects	Drug Interactions	Comments	Cost[a]
	zidovudine (AZT) Retrovir	300 mg BID or 200 mg TID	Nausea, headache, malaise, fatigue, rash, myositis, myocarditis, anemia, leukopenia, ↑ liver enzymes, ↑ lactic acid, hepatic steatosis, ↑ CK.	Additive hemotoxicity with other agents, e.g., anemia with ribavirin.	Avoid combined use of AZT and d4T.	$$$
Nucleotide Reverse Transcriptase Inhibitors (NtRTI)	*tenofovir (TDF)* Viread	300 mg once daily	Renal toxicity. Monitor renal function and serum phosphorous.	Do not use in combination with ddI.	Recommended first-line therapy.	$$$$$
Non-nucleoside Reverse Transcriptase Inhibitors (NNRTI)	*efavirenz (EFV)* Sustiva	600 mg once daily	CNS toxicity, drowsiness, rash, ↑ liver enzymes. Avoid in patients with a history of anxiety, depression or psychosis. Contraindicated in pregnancy (teratogenic in animals). Avoid in women of child-bearing potential.		Recommended first-line therapy.	$$$$
	nevirapine (NVP) Viramune	200 mg once daily for 2 wk then 200 mg BID Full daily dose can be given once a day	Rash (rare severe allergic reactions). ↑ liver enzymes (rare cases of fatal hepatitis). Not recommended in liver disease, if starting ABC, or if the baseline CD4 count is ≥ 250/µL in women or ≥ 400/µL in men.	Rifampin ↓ levels of NNRTIs.	Recommended first-line therapy.	$$$
	delavirdine (DLV) Rescriptor	400 mg TID	Rash, headache, ↑ liver enzymes.		Not for first-line therapy: inferior efficacy.	$$

Class	Drug	Dose	Adverse Effects	Drug Interactions	Comments	Cost[a]
	etravirine *(TMC-125)*	200 mg BID	Headache, diarrhea, rash.	TPV/RTV, NVP and EFV ↓ etravirine exposure (avoid combined use). Etravirine ↑ f-APV/RTV exposure.	Reserve for treatment-experienced patients with limited options. May be effective against NNRTI-resistant HIV.	[d]
Protease Inhibitors (PI)	*atazanavir (ATZ)* Reyataz	400 mg once daily *or* 300 mg + RTV 100 mg once daily	Hyperbilirubinemia in patients with a genetic predisposition.[e] Rash (rare).	PIs are not recommended in combination with lovastatin, simvastatin, rifampin, midazolam, triazolam, ergot alkaloids or St. John's wort. Do not use atazanvir with proton-pump inhibitors or H_2 antagonists.	Recommended first-line therapy.	$$$$$
	fosamprenavir *(f-APV)* Telzir	700 mg + RTV 100 mg BID *or* 1400 mg + RTV 200 mg once daily	Rash, GI upset.	See atazanavir	Recommended first-line therapy. Approved for use only with ritonavir.	$$$$
	darunavir *(TMC-114)* Prezista	600 mg + RTV 100 mg BID	Diarrhea, nausea, headache, rash (possible cross-sensitivity with sulfonamides).	See atazanavir	Approved for use only with ritonavir. Reserve for treatment-experienced patients with limited options.	$$$$$
	indinavir (IDV) Crixivan	800 mg TID *or* 800 mg + RTV 100 or 200 mg BID	Liver enzyme elevations, nephrolithiasis.	See atazanavir	Avoid because of adverse effects.	$$$$$

(cont'd)

Table 3: **Antiretroviral Medications for HIV Therapy** *(cont'd)*

Class	Drug	Dose	Adverse Effects	Drug Interactions	Comments	Cost[a]
	lopinavir/ritonavir (LPV/RTV) Kaletra	400/100 mg BID	GI upset, hyperlipidemia, liver enzyme elevations.	See atazanavir. EFV, NVP: ↓ levels.	Recommended first-line therapy.	$$$$$
	nelfinavir (NFV) Viracept	1250 mg BID *or* 750 mg TID	Diarrhea.	See atazanavir.	Not boosted by RTV to a significant extent.	$$$$$
	ritonavir (RTV) Norvir	600 mg BID (sole PI). As a PK booster, see atazanavir, darunavir, fosamprenavir, indinavir, saquinavir and tipranavir	GI upset, diarrhea, circumoral paresthesia, liver enzyme elevations, hyperlipidemia.	See atazanavir.	As a PK booster, low-dose RTV is a component of many regimens. Avoid unboosted RTV because of adverse effects.	$$$$$
	saquinavir (SQV) Invirase	1000 mg + RTV 100 mg BID	↑ liver enzymes, GI upset, headache.	See atazanavir.	Avoid unboosted SQV: inferior efficacy. Approved for use only with ritonavir.	$$$$$
	tipranavir (TPV) Aptivus	500 mg + RTV 200 mg BID	Hepatotoxicity, rash (possible cross-sensitivity with sulfonamides). Intracranial hemorrhage (rare).	See atazanavir.	Reserve for treatment-experienced patients with limited options.	$$$$$
Fusion Inhibitors	*enfuvirtide (T20)* Fuzeon	90 mg BID sc	Most patients experience injection site reactions (may be severe). Hypersensitivity reactions.	Does not interact with CYP isozymes.	Reserve for treatment-experienced patients with limited options.	$$$$$

Class	Drug	Dose	Adverse Effects	Drug Interactions	Comments	Cost[a]
Entry Inhibitors	*maraviroc* Celsentri	Usual: 300 mg BID 150 mg BID with CYP3A4 inhibitors See Drug Interactions 600 mg BID with CYP3A4 inducers See Drug Interactions	Diarrhea, nausea, fatigue, headache.	↓ levels with CYP3A4 inducers: efavirenz, nevirapine, rifampin, rifabutin ↑ levels with CYP3A4 inhibitors: protease inhibitors (except TPV, RTV), itraconazole, ketoconazole, clarithromycin, telithromycin	Phenotype test required prior to treatment: effective only in patients with CCR5 tropic HIV (not CXCR4 or mixed-tropic virus).	[d]
Integrase Inhibitors	*raltegravir* Isentress	400 mg BID	Diarrhea, nausea, fatigue, headache, itching.	Not a potent inhibitor or inducer of CYP isozymes.	Reserve for treatment-experienced patients with limited options.	[d]
RTI Combination Products	*abacavir/ lamivudine* Kivexa	600 mg/300 mg once daily	See abacavir. See lamivudine.	See abacavir.		$$$$$
	abacavir/ lamivudine/ zidovudine Trizivir	300 mg/150 mg/300 mg twice daily	See abacavir. See lamivudine. See zidovudine.	See abacavir. See zidovudine.		$$$$$
	lamivudine/ zidovudine Combivir	150 mg/300 mg twice daily	See lamivudine. See zidovudine.	See zidovudine.		$$$$$

(cont'd)

Table 3: **Antiretroviral Medications for HIV Therapy** *(cont'd)*

Class	Drug	Dose	Adverse Effects	Drug Interactions	Comments	Cost[a]
	emtricitabine/ tenofovir Truvada	200 mg/300 mg once daily	See emtricitabine. See tenofovir.	See tenofovir.		$$$$$
	efavirenz/ emtricitabine/ tenofovir Atripla	600 mg/200 mg/300 mg once daily	See efavirenz. See emtricitabine. See tenofovir.	See tenofovir.		c

[a] Cost of 30-day supply; includes drug cost only.
[b] Patients with the HLA-B*5701 allele, which is present in 5% to 8% of white patients but is rare in patients of African and Asian descent.[17]
[c] Approved by Health Canada, but not currently marketed in Canada.
[d] Available through the Special Access Programme, Therapeutic Products Directorate, Health Canada.
[e] Patients with a particular polymorphism in the multidrug resistance gene 1 have higher plasma levels of atazanavir and higher bilirubin levels during atazanavir therapy than those without this polymorphism. The risk of severe hyperbilirubinemia during atazanavir therapy is further increased by the presence of distinct variants in the gene coding for UDP-glucuronosyltransferase (UGT1A).[18,19]
Dosage adjustment may be required in renal impairment; see Appendix I.
Abbreviations: CK = creatine kinase; CCR5 = chemokine receptor 5; CYP = cytochrome P450; PK = pharmacokinetic
Legend: $ $100–200 $$ $200–300 $$-$$$ $200–400 $$$ $300–400 $$$$ $400–500 $$$$$ > $500

Suggested Readings

AIDS Education & Training Centers National Resource Center. *Clinical manual for management of the HIV-infected adult.* Newark (NJ): AETC National Resource Center; 2006. Available from: http://www.aids-ed.org/aetc/aetc?page=cm-00-00 Accessed December 12, 2006.

Hammer SM, Saag MS, Schechter M et al. Treatment for adult HIV infection: 2006 recommendations of the International AIDS Society-USA Panel. *JAMA* 2006;296(7):827-43.

Hatano H, Deeks SG. Drug resistant HIV. *BMJ* 2007;334(7604):1124-5.

Hogg RS, Yip B, Chan KJ et al. Rates of disease progression by baseline CD4 cell count and viral load after initiating triple-drug therapy. *JAMA* 2001;286(20):2568-77.

U.S. Department of Health and Human Services. AIDSinfo. *Guidelines for the use of antiretroviral agents in HIV-1-infected adults and adolescents.* Rockville (MD): AIDSinfo; 2006. Available from: http://AIDSinfo.nih.gov Accessed December 12, 2006.

Wood E, Hogg RS, Harrigan PR et al. When to initiate antiretroviral therapy in HIV-infected adults: a review for clinicians and patients. *Lancet Infect Dis* 2005;5(7):407-14.

References

1. Mellors JW, Kingsley LA, Rinaldo CR et al. Quantitation of HIV-1 RNA in plasma predicts outcome after seroconversion. *Ann Intern Med* 1995;122(8):573-9.
2. Weinstein MC, Goldie SJ, Losina E et al. Use of genotypic resistance testing to guide hiv therapy: clinical impact and cost-effectiveness. *Ann Intern Med* 2001;134(6):440-50.
3. Grabar S, Le Moing V, Goujard C et al. Clinical outcome of patients with HIV-1 infection according to immunologic and virologic response after 6 months of highly active antiretroviral therapy. *Ann Intern Med* 2000;133(6):401-10.
4. Palella FJ, Delaney KM, Moorman AC et al. Declining morbidity and mortality among patients with advanced human immunodeficiency virus infection. HIV Outpatient Study Investigators. *N Engl J Med* 1998;338(13):853-60.
5. Morse CG, Kovacs JA. Metabolic and skeletal complications of HIV infection: the price of success. *JAMA* 2006;296(7):844-54.
6. Friis-Moller N, Sabin CA, Weber R et al. Combination antiretroviral therapy and the risk of myocardial infarction. *N Engl J Med* 2003;349(21):1993-2003.
7. Condra JH, Schleif WA, Blahy OM et al. In vivo emergence of HIV-1 variants resistant to multiple protease inhibitors. *Nature* 1995;374(6522):569-71.
8. Descamps D, Flandre P, Calvez V et al. Mechanisms of virologic failure in previously untreated HIV-infected patients from a trial of induction-maintenance therapy. Trilege (Agence Nationale de Recherches sur le SIDA 072) Study Team). *JAMA* 2000;283(2):205-11.
9. Hammer SM, Saag MS, Schechter M et al. Treatment for adult HIV infection: 2006 recommendations of the International AIDS Society-USA panel. *JAMA* 2006;296(7):827-43.
10. Vanhove GF, Schapiro JM, Winters MA et al. Patient compliance and drug failure in protease inhibitor monotherapy. *JAMA* 1996;276(24):1955-6.
11. The Strategies for Management of Antiretroviral Therapy (SMART) Study Group. CD4+ count-guided interrruption of antiretroviral treatment. *N Engl J Med* 2006;355(22):2283-96.
12. Ananworanich J, Hirschel B. Intermittent therapy for the treatment of chronic HIV infection. *AIDS* 2007;21(2):123-34.
13. Connor EM, Sperling RS, Gelber R et al. Reduction of maternal-infant transmission of human immunodeficiency virus type 1 with zidovudine treatment. Pediatric AIDS Clinical Trials Group Protocol 076 Study Group. *N Engl J Med* 1994;331(18):1173-80.
14. Raboud JM, Montaner JS, Conway B et al. Variation in plasma RNA levels, CD4 cell counts, and p24 antigen levels in clinically stable men with human immunodeficiency virus infection. *J Infect Dis* 1996;174(1):191-4.
15. Staprans SI, Hamilton BL, Follansbee SE et al. Activation of virus replication after vaccination of HIV-1-infected individuals. *J Exp Med* 1995;182(6):1727-37.

16. Raboud JM, Haley L, Montaner JS et al. Quantification of the variation due to laboratory and physiologic sources in CD4 lymphocyte counts of clinically stable HIV-infected individuals. *J Acquir Immune Defic Syndr Hum Retrovirol* 1995;10(Suppl 2):S67-73.
17. Phillips EJ. Genetic screening to prevent abacavir hypersensitivity reaction: are we there yet? *Clin Infect Dis* 2006;43(1):103-5.
18. Lankisch TO, Moebius U, Wehmeier M et al. Gilbert's disease and atazanavir: from phenotype to UDP-glucuronosyltransferase haplotype. *Hepatology* 2006;44(5):1324-32.
19. Rodriguez-Novoa S, Martin-Carbonero L, Barreiro P et al. Genetic factors influencing atazanavir plasma concentrations and the risk of severe hyperbilirubinemia. *AIDS* 2007;21(1):41-6.

CHAPTER 107
Opportunistic Infections in HIV-positive Patients

Edward D. Ralph, BSc, MD, FRCPC

Opportunistic infections are a major cause of mortality and morbidity in HIV-positive patients and are often the first evidence of immunodeficiency that leads to the diagnosis of AIDS. Susceptibility to specific opportunistic infections increases as the CD4 (helper T-cell) count declines. This relationship is very useful in the differential diagnosis of various infectious syndromes, especially at CD4 counts < 200/μL.[1]

Goals of Therapy

- Prevent specific infections
- Treat established opportunistic infections
- Reduce drug burden by discontinuing chemoprophylactic regimens and maintenance therapy when appropriate

Investigations[2]

The initial investigations will be predicated on whether the patient is symptomatic. If a patient is symptomatic, the following tests establish a baseline for determining the susceptibility to various opportunistic infections. In general, latent infections can reactivate as the CD4 count declines.

- Complete blood count
- Lymphocyte flow cytometry—CD4 count and percentage, CD4/CD8 ratio
- HIV viral load
- Tuberculin skin test (the response is affected by CD4 count)
- Hepatitis A, B and C virus serology
- Herpes virus serology: varicella zoster virus (VZV), cytomegalovirus (CMV)
- Toxoplasma serology
- Syphilis serology (screening test)
- Chest x-ray
- Baseline biochemistry profile (prior to initiating drug therapy)
  - albumin
  - alkaline phosphatase
  - aminotransferases
  - bilirubin
  - blood urea nitrogen

- serum creatinine
- serum electrolytes
- serum amylase
- creatine kinase
- lactate dehydrogenase
- lipid profile (fasting)

- Glucose-6-phosphate dehydrogenase—in members of at-risk groups prior to treatment with oxidant medications (sulfonamides or dapsone)

If a patient has symptoms of a specific opportunistic infection, order appropriate investigations.

Therapeutic Choices

Nonpharmacologic Choices

Advise patients with HIV infection and immunosuppression that their risk of infections can be reduced by following good hygienic practices.

- Ensure thorough hand washing after contact with potentially contaminated substances (diapers, soil, uncooked meat and produce) or handling pets
- Avoid raw or uncooked meat and eggs, e.g., Caesar salad
- Drink from treated water sources only
- Avoid handling sick animals or pet (especially cat) litter
- Avoid cat scratches and do not allow cats to lick wounds
- Avoid contact with reptiles

Pharmacologic Choices

Preventive interventions are outlined in Table 1.

Clinical Syndromes

Respiratory Tract Syndromes

Most upper respiratory tract symptoms are caused by viruses, but bacterial superinfections (otitis media, sinusitis) are more common in HIV-infected patients and require antibiotic treatment. Patients with pneumonia (see Chapter 98) and CD4 counts > 200/μL can be treated for community-acquired pneumonia. As the CD4 count declines to < 200/μL, *Pneumocystis jirovecii* (formerly *P. carinii*) becomes an increasingly important pathogen. At counts < 100/μL, *Mycobacterium avium* complex (MAC), CMV, *Cryptococcus neoformans* and *Aspergillus* spp. are more frequently isolated. Empirical treatment for *P. jirovecii* is often started in patients in whom the diagnosis is suspected (fever, dyspnea, CXR findings). Bronchoscopy with bronchoalveolar lavage (BAL) and transbronchial biopsy is often required to confirm the diagnosis and may reveal the presence of other opportunistic pathogens.

Painful Mouth and Swallowing

Oral candidiasis is very common and can occur with CD4 counts > 200/µL. Treatment with azole antifungal agents is usually very effective, but with prolonged use, especially in those with low CD4 counts, resistance can develop. Discrete ulcerative lesions are usually caused by herpes simplex virus (HSV), CMV or aphthous ulcers. The same pathogens can cause odynophagia, but empirical treatment for candidiasis is instituted. Failure to respond after a week's treatment necessitates endoscopy with cultures and biopsy.

Table 1: **Preventive Interventions for HIV-positive Patients**[1]

Indications	Condition	Prophylactic Therapy
Independent of CD4 count	Routine immunizations	Update all vaccines (no live vaccines with the possible exception of MMR)
	Meningocococcal disease	Meningococcal vaccine
	Pneumococcal infection	23–valent polysaccharide pneumococcal vaccine, repeat once after 5 years
	Influenza	Annual influenza immunization
	Hepatitis	Hepatitis A vaccine Hepatitis B vaccine for nonimmune individuals
	Varicella	Post-exposure prophylaxis with IVIG for nonimmune adults
	Cervical cancer (HPV)	Cervical Pap smear twice in the first year after diagnosis of HIV infection, then annually if the results are normal. Refer women with atypical squamous cells for colposcopy
	Frequent oral or genital herpes simplex outbreaks	Suppressive therapy with acyclovir, famciclovir or valacyclovir[a]
	Sexually transmitted infections (STIs)	Patients on antiretroviral therapy can become infected with STIs including resistant HIV strains. Condom use for personal protection is recommended
Positive PPD (≥ 5 mm), independent of CD4 count	*Mycobacterium tuberculosis*	The preferred prophylactic therapy is isoniazid + pyridoxine for 9 months[a] Rifampin for 4 months is an alternative[a,b]
CD4 < 200 cells/µL or thrush	*Pneumocystis jirovecii* pneumonia	The preferred prophylactic therapy is SMX/TMP[a] Alternatives include dapsone (alone or combined with pyrimethamine + leucovorin); or atovaquone; or monthly inhaled pentamidine[a]

(cont'd)

Table 1: **Preventive Interventions for HIV-positive Patients**[1] *(cont'd)*

Indications	Condition	Prophylactic Therapy
CD4 < 100 cells/μL and positive *T. gondii* serology	*Toxoplasma gondii* encephalitis	The preferred prophylactic therapy is SMX/TMP[a] Alternatives include dapsone alone or combined with pyrimethamine + leucovorin, or atovaquone alone or combined with pyrimethamine + leucovorin[a]
CD4 < 50 cells/μL	*Mycobacterium avium* complex	The preferred prophylactic therapy is a macrolide (azithromycin once weekly or twice-daily clarithromycin)[a] Rifabutin is an alternative[a]
	Cytomegalovirus	Prophylaxis is not cost effective. The focus of therapy is restoration of the immune system
	Fungal infections	Fluconazole may be used for persons with recurrent thrush or prior esophageal candidiasis[a]

[a] Prophylactic treatment regimens are presented in Table 3 for herpes simplex virus, in Table 6 for MAC and in Table 7 for PJP and *T. gondii* infections.

[b] Rifampin significantly alters the pharmacokinetics of many drugs including antiretroviral agents and its use is contraindicated with some drugs. Therefore, the regimen must be carefully reviewed, and modified if necessary, before starting and stopping rifampin therapy.

Abbreviations: PPD = purified protein derivative (of tuberculin); IVIG = intravenous immune globulin; HPV = human papillomavirus

Central Nervous System Symptoms

HIV-infected patients are at increased risk for opportunistic infections of the CNS, especially as their CD4 counts decline to < 200/μL. At CD4 counts > 200/μL the usual bacterial, mycobacterial (*M. tuberculosis*) and viral causes should be suspected. Unusual causes of CNS infection, especially *C. neoformans* (meningitis) and *T. gondii* (focal lesions) are disproportionately more common as the CD4 count falls to < 200/μL (Figure 1). Progressive multifocal leukoencephalopathy (PML) is an opportunistic infection caused by JC virus for which there is no effective prophylaxis or treatment.

Fever of Unknown Origin (Figure 1)

Patients with low CD4 counts may present with fever and flu-like symptoms but no specific focal symptoms to suggest a source. Possible infectious causes to be investigated include hepatitis viruses, sinusitis, MAC, *M. tuberculosis,* CMV disease, *P. jirovecii* pneumonia (negative chest x-ray) and HIV viremia.

Diarrhea

Diarrhea is a very common symptom in HIV-positive patients, and infectious causes must be distinguished from noninfectious causes including adverse drug effects. Acute bacterial gastroenteritis caused by the usual enteric bacterial pathogens may be more severe, may result in bacteremia and may require prolonged antibiotic treatment. Long-term antibiotic prophylaxis and hospitalization predisposes patients to *C. difficile* infection. Chronic diarrheal syndromes in patients with CD4 counts < 150/µL may be associated with MAC or parasitic infections including giardiasis, cryptosporidiosis, cyclosporiasis and microsporidiosis.

Immune Reconstitution Inflammatory Syndromes

Patients initiating antiretroviral therapy, especially those with low initial CD4 counts, may experience worsening of opportunistic infections as their CD4 count improves, despite appropriate antimicrobial treatment.[3,4] The opportunistic infections most frequently encountered in this setting are mycobacterial (tuberculosis or MAC) or cryptococcal, although any opportunistic infection, as well as autoimmune conditions and malignancies, may be exacerbated by immune reconstitution. This phenomenon has been attributed to an enhanced inflammatory response at the site of infection. Both HAART (Highly Active Antiretroviral Therapy) and antimicrobial treatment are usually continued with the judicious use of steroids in select individuals.

Discontinuation of Prophylaxis

Prophylaxis for some infections can be discontinued as the immune system recovers during antiviral therapy (Table 2).[5,6,7,8,9,10,11]

Table 2: Criteria for Discontinuing Prophylaxis of Opportunistic Infections in HIV-positive Patients[1]

Pathogen	Type of Prophylaxis	Criteria for Discontinuing
P. jirovecii	Primary and secondary	CD4 > 200 cells/µL × ≥ 3 mo
T. gondii	Primary	CD4 > 200 cells/µL × ≥ 3 mo
	Secondary	CD4 > 200 cells/µL × ≥ 6 mo
M. avium complex	Primary	CD4 > 100 cells/µL × ≥ 3 mo
	Secondary	CD4 > 100 cells/µL × ≥ 6 mo
CMV retinitis	Secondary	CD4 > 150 cells/µL × ≥ 6 mo No active disease Regular ophthalmic examination
C. neoformans	Secondary	CD4 > 100–200 cells/µL × ≥ 6 mo

Management of Specific HIV-associated Infections[6,12,13]

Candida Species

The frequency of mucosal infection increases as the CD4 count decreases. Esophageal candidiasis is usually a later manifestation, but can occur in the absence of oral or vaginal disease. Severe discomfort or esophageal disease requires systemic therapy (see Table 4).

For *oral thrush*, use topical therapy initially. For example, use **nystatin** suspension (swish and swallow) or use **miconazole** or **clotrimazole** vaginal tablets/suppositories as oral lozenges (see Table 4).

For *vaginal candidiasis*, topical azole antifungal creams or tablets/suppositories are the first-line therapy (see Table 4). **Fluconazole** is the first line oral systemic therapy. **Itraconazole** and **ketoconazole** are alternatives. Higher doses of fluconazole are used for esophageal disease with tapering of the dose when symptoms improve. **Amphotericin B** suspension is an alternative for less advanced disease. Intravenous amphotericin B or **caspofungin** are used in patients who do not respond to oral therapy. Lipid-based preparations of amphotericin B are less toxic but more expensive than the conventional formulation.

Cryptococcus neoformans

C. neoformans is a major cause of meningitis in the later stages of HIV infection (10% of AIDS patients). The diagnosis requires culture of the organism or detection of cryptococcal antigen in blood or CSF.

Induction therapy usually involves 2 to 6 weeks of intravenous **amphotericin B** with or without **flucytosine**, then completion of a 12-week course of oral or intravenous **fluconazole** 400 mg/day (see Table 4). Fluconazole may be used exclusively for patients who are well and who are followed closely. *Maintenance therapy* consists of daily oral fluconazole.

Cytomegalovirus

CMV usually occurs in patients with CD4 counts < 50 cells/μL. Retinitis with visual disturbances is the most common manifestation; however, enteritis, colitis, pneumonitis, encephalitis, myelitis and/or neuritis can also occur. The prognosis is poor without therapy. Ganciclovir-resistant strains of CMV have emerged and CMV that is resistant to ganciclovir may be cross-resistant to cidofovir and foscarnet.

Induction therapy involves oral **valganciclovir** (a prodrug of ganciclovir), or intravenous **ganciclovir**, or intravenous **foscarnet** for 14 to 21 days (see Table 3). *Maintenance therapy* involves daily administration of oral valganciclovir, intravenous foscarnet or intravenous **cidofovir**.

Mycobacterium avium complex

MAC occurs in patients with CD4 counts < 100 cells/μL. Symptoms include fever, weight loss, fatigue, night sweats alone or with diarrhea, anemia, lymphadenopathy and/or hepatitis. The diagnosis is made primarily by mycobacterial blood culture or biopsy and culture of involved tissue.

Multidrug regimens are used to treat MAC (see Table 6), the basis of which is an oral macrolide (**clarithromycin** or **azithromycin**) plus **ethambutol**. Additional drugs such as **rifabutin** (or **rifampin**), **ciprofloxacin** or **levofloxacin**, or **amikacin** may also be used depending on the circumstances. Therapy is given for 2 to 4 months, followed by maintenance therapy. *Maintenance therapy* consisting of clarithromycin (or azithromycin) plus ethambutol with or without rifabutin is continued for life unless a patient has sustained immune recovery on HAART.

Pneumocystis jirovecii

P. jirovecii is the primary cause of pneumonia in patients with CD4 counts < 200 celis/μL. PJP commonly presents as a persistent fever with progressive shortness of breath and cough, often with a normal chest x-ray. The organism cannot be cultured. Definitive diagnosis requires histopathologic examination of induced sputum, bronchoalveolar lavage or lung biopsy.

Standard therapy is 21 days of oral or intravenous **sulfamethoxazole/trimethoprim** (SMX/TMP, cotrimoxazole) (see Table 7). For severe disease, intravenous **pentamidine** may be given for 21 days. Oral **dapsone** plus trimethoprim is better tolerated than SMX/TMP, but is suitable only for mild or moderate disease (there is no iv formulation). Other alternatives include oral **atovaquone**; **clindamycin** plus **primaquine**; and **trimetrexate** plus **leucovorin**. In patients with severe PJP, the addition of oral **prednisone** decreases morbidity and the side effects of SMX/TMP. Patients with paO_2 < 70 mm Hg on room air or an alveolar-arterial O_2 gradient > 35 mm Hg should receive adjunctive prednisone 40 mg twice daily for 5 days, then 20 mg twice daily for 5 days, then 20 mg daily to complete 21 days of treatment.

Toxoplasma gondii

Up to 50% of HIV-positive patients with antibodies to this parasite will develop toxoplasma encephalitis when their CD4 cell count decreases to < 200 cells/μL. Patients most commonly present with a fever and focal neurologic signs. A CT scan with contrast or MRI usually reveals multiple intracranial-enhancing lesions.

Patients should be treated empirically. A marked clinical response usually occurs within 7 days; if there is no response, referral to a specialty centre should be considered. *Standard therapy* is **pyrimethamine** plus **leucovorin** and **sulfadiazine** given for 4 to 8 weeks (see Table 7). Alternatives include pyrimethamine plus **leucovorin** and **clindamycin**; or oral or intravenous **SMX/TMP**. Patients with perilesional edema require **dexamethasone**. *Maintenance therapy* comprises pyrimethamine plus leucovorin and sulfadiazine; or pyrimethamine plus leucovorin and clindamycin.

Therapeutic Tips

- All practitioners caring for patients who are HIV-positive should be aware of and participate in preventive interventions.
- Treatment of opportunistic infections requires specialized expertise and should be done in centres experienced with the management of HIV-infected patients.

Figure 1: **Management of Fever and Neurologic Complaints in HIV-positive Patients**

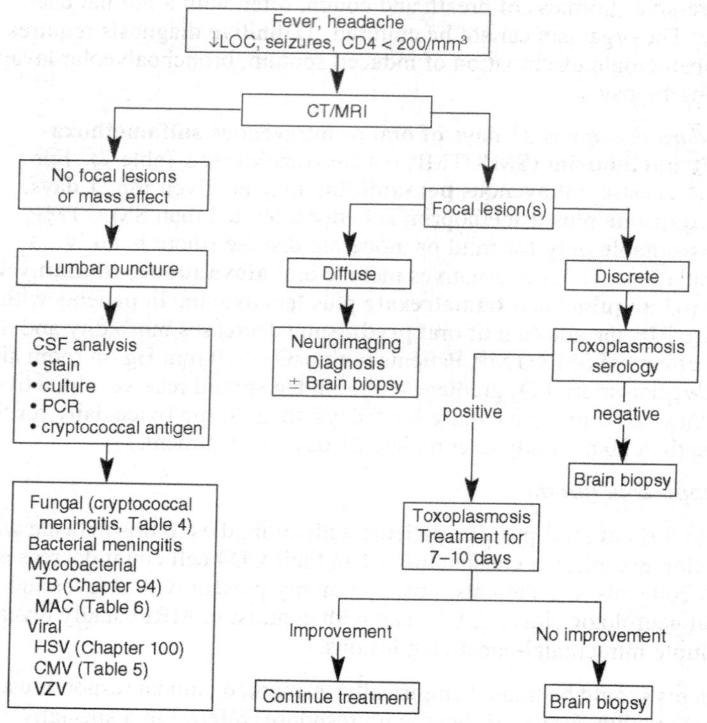

Abbreviations: CMV = cytomegalovirus; CT = computed tomography; HSV = herpes simplex virus; LOC = level of consciousness; MAC = mycobacterium avium complex; MRI = magnetic resonance imaging; TB = tuberculosis; VZV = varicella zoster virus.

Table 3: Drugs for Suppression of Frequent Oral or Genital Outbreaks of Herpes Simplex Virus

Class	Drug	Indication and Adult Dose[a]	Adverse Effects	Comments	Cost[b]
Guanine Nucleoside Analogue Antiviral Agents	*acyclovir* Zovirax Oral, generics	200 mg TID or 400 mg BID	Gastrointestinal, headache.	↑ CNS adverse effects when taken with AZT or probenecid. May impair renal excretion of tenofovir.	$
	famciclovir Famvir	250 mg BID	Gastrointestinal, headache.	Prodrug of penciclovir.	$
	valacyclovir Valtrex	500 mg BID	See acyclovir.	Prodrug of acyclovir. See acyclovir.	$

[a] Doses are oral unless indicated otherwise.
[b] Cost per day based on dosages in this table for a 50 kg person; includes drug cost only.
Dosage adjustment may be required in renal impairment; see Appendix I.
Abbreviations: AZT = zidovudine
Legend: $ < $10

Table 4: **Drugs for Prophylaxis and Treatment of *Candida* spp and *Cryptococcus neoformans* Infections**

Class	Drug	Indication and Adult Dose[a]	Adverse Effects	Comments	Cost[b]
Polyene Antifungal Agents	*amphotericin B* Fungizone	**Oral candidiasis treatment:** 300–500 mg po suspension QID swish and swallow **Esophageal candidiasis treatment:** 0.3–0.5 mg/kg/day iv × 2–3 wk then weekly after symptoms resolve ***C. neoformans* induction therapy:** 0.7 mg/kg/day iv × 2–6 wk ± flucytosine	**IV:** infusion reactions (fever, chills, nausea), hypotension, nephrotoxicity, electrolyte disturbances, anemia, myelosuppression.	↑ nephrotoxicity with other nephrotoxic drugs. ↑ hemotoxicity of AZT. Consider use of a liposomal preparation to reduce the incidence of nephrotoxicity.	iv:$$$$$ po:[c]
	amphotericin B lipid preparations Abelcet, AmBisome	AmBisome: 3–5 mg/kg/day iv Abelcet: 5 mg/kg/day iv	See amphotericin B.	Lipid preparations are better tolerated than standard amphotericin B.	$$$$$
	nystatin, generics	**Oral candidiasis treatment:** 500 000 U po suspension QID swish and swallow; or 100 000 U vaginal tab sucked QID	Gastrointestinal, local irritation.		$
Pyrimidine Antifungal Agents	*flucytosine*[c] Ancotil	***C. neoformans* induction therapy:** 100–150 mg/kg/day Q6H × 2 wk + amphotericin B	Gastrointestinal, neurological, myelosuppression (especially with high serum levels).	Amphotericin-induced nephrotoxicity predisposes patients to adverse effects. ↑ myelosuppression with other myelosuppressive agents (e.g. AZT, ganciclovir).	[c]
Echinocandin Antifungal Agents	*caspofungin* Cancidas	**Esophageal candidiasis treatment (alt):** 50 mg/day iv × 14 days	Headache, fever, elevated transaminase levels.	Rifampin and NNRTIs may ↓ caspofungin levels.	$$$$$

Class	Drug	Indication and Adult Dose[a]	Adverse Effects	Comments	Cost[b]
Azole Antifungal Agents	*fluconazole* (kidney symbol) Diflucan, generics	**Prophylaxis for frequent recurrence of oral or esophageal candidiasis:** 100–200 mg/day po or 400 mg/wk po **Oral, esophageal, or vaginal candidiasis:** 100–200 mg/day po × 7–14 days for oral lesions; up to 400 mg/day po or iv × 14–21 days for esophageal lesions ***C. neoformans* induction therapy:** 400 mg/day po or iv to complete 12 weeks of therapy after amphotericin B induction ***C. neoformans* maintenance therapy:** 200 mg/day po	Gastrointestinal, rash, elevated transaminase levels.	Inhibits CYP2C9 and 2C19. ↑ levels of cyclosporine, phenytoin, tacrolimus and warfarin, some HMG CoA reductase inhibitors (e.g., simvastatin) and some benzodiazepines. Metabolism induced by rifampin. Carbamazepine, phenytoin, and rifampin ↓ fluconazole levels.	po: $$ iv: $$$$
	itraconazole Sporanox Capsules, Sporanox Oral Solution	**Oral, esophageal or vaginal candidiasis:** 200 mg/day × 7–14 day for oral or vaginal lesions, × 14–21 days for esophageal lesions	Gastrointestinal, rash, headache, edema, hypokalemia.	Absorption requires gastric acid: ↓ absorption with ddI, antacids, H_2-blockers, PPIs. Inhibits CYP3A4 (many potential interactions). ↑ levels of cyclosporine, digoxin, warfarin, some HMG CoA reductase inhibitors (atorvastatin, lovastatin, simvastatin) and some benzodiazepines. Carbamazepine, isoniazid, phenytoin and rifampin ↓ itraconazole levels.	$
	ketoconazole generics	**Oral, esophageal or vaginal candidiasis:** 200–400 mg po once daily or BID	Gastrointestinal, elevated transaminase levels.	See itraconazole.	$

(cont'd)

Table 4: **Drugs for Prophylaxis and Treatment of *Candida* spp and *Cryptococcus neoformans* Infections** *(cont'd)*

Class	Drug	Indication and Adult Dose[a]	Adverse Effects	Comments	Cost[b]
	clotrimazole Canesten Vaginal, generics	**Oral candidiasis:** 100 mg vaginal tab sucked 5 times/day × 7–14 days **Topical therapy for vulvovaginal candidiasis:** 1% cream × 6 nights; or 2% cream and 200 mg vaginal tablet × 3 nights	Local irritation.		$
	econazole Ecostatin	**Topical therapy for vulvovaginal candidiasis:** 150 mg vaginal ovule × 3 nights	Local irritation.		$
	miconazole Monistat	**Topical therapy for vulvovaginal candidiasis:** 2% cream and/or 100 mg vaginal ovule × 7 nights; or 4% cream and/or 400 mg vaginal ovule × 3 nights	Local irritation.		$
	terconazole Terazol, generics	**Topical therapy for vulvovaginal candidiasis:** 0.4% cream × 7 nights; or 0.8% cream and/or 80 mg vaginal ovule × 3 nights	Local irritation.		$

[a] Doses are oral unless indicated otherwise.
[b] Cost per day based on dosages in this table for 50 kg person; includes drug cost only.
[c] Available through Special Access Programme, Therapeutic Products Directorate, Health Canada.
Dosage adjustment may be required in renal impairment; see Appendix I.
Abbreviations: Alt = alternative therapy; AZT = zidovudine; CYP = cytochrome P450; ddI = didanosine; NNRTI = non-nucleoside reverse transcriptase inhibitor; PPI = proton pump inhibitor
Legend: $ < $10 $$ $10–25 $$$ $25–50 $$$$ $50–100 $$$$$ > $100

Table 5: Drugs for Prophylaxis and Treatment of Cytomegalovirus Infection

Class	Drug	Indication and Adult Dose[a]	Adverse Effects	Comments	Cost[b]
Guanine Nucleoside Analogue Antiviral Agents	*ganciclovir* [renal] Cytovene	**CMV treatment:** 5 mg/kg iv Q12H × 14–21 days **CMV maintenance:** 5 mg/kg daily iv or 6 mg/kg iv 5–7 times/week or 1 g po Q8H	Fever, gastrointestinal, headache, confusion, pruritus, neuropathy, myelosuppression.	↑ AZT levels and hemotoxicity. ↓ renal excretion of tenofovir. G-CSF can be used for neutropenia; ganciclovir-resistant strains of CMV have emerged.	$$$
	valganciclovir [renal] Valcyte	**CMV treatment:** 900 mg po BID × 21 days **CMV maintenance:** 900 mg/day	See ganciclovir.	Prodrug of ganciclovir. See ganciclovir.	$$$$
Cytidine Nucleotide Analogue Antiviral Agents	*cidofovir*[c] [renal] Vistide	**CMV treatment (alt):** 5 mg/kg iv once/wk × 2 wk, then Q2wk Hydrate with NS. Give probenecid 2 g 3 h before, and 1 g 2 h and 8 h after each infusion	Gastrointestinal, myelosuppression, ocular hypotony, nephrotoxicity.	Avoid other nephrotoxins (additive nephrotoxicity).	c
Inorganic Pyrophosphate Analogue Antiviral Agents	*foscarnet*[c] [renal] Foscavir	**CMV induction (alt):** 60 mg/kg iv Q8H × 14–21 days **CMV maintenance (alt):** 90–120 mg/kg iv daily. Give 500 mL NS before and after each infusion	Gastrointestinal, fever, headache, electrolyte disturbances (may cause tetany, seizures), nephrotoxicity, anemia.	Prehydrate to ↓ nephrotoxicity. Avoid other nephrotoxins (additive nephrotoxicity). More difficult to administer and more toxic than ganciclovir, but may prolong survival. Ciprofloxacin ↑ seizure potential.	c

[a] Doses are oral unless indicated otherwise.
[b] Cost per day based on dosages in this table for 50 kg person; includes drug cost only.
[c] Available through Special Access Programme, Therapeutic Products Directorate, Health Canada.
[renal] Dosage adjustment may be required in renal impairment; see Appendix I.
Abbreviations: Alt = alternative therapy; AZT = zidovudine; CMV = cytomegalovirus; G-CSF = granulocyte colony-stimulating factor; NS = normal saline
Legend: $$$ $25–50 $$$$ $50–100

Table 6: Drugs for Prophylaxis and Treatment of *Mycobacterium avium* complex Infection and for Prophylaxis of *Mycobacterium tuberculosis* Infection

Class	Drug	Indication and Adult Dose[a]	Adverse Effects	Comments	Cost[b]
Macrolide Antibiotics	*azithromycin* Zithromax, generics	**MAC prophylaxis (1st choice):** 1200 mg once/wk **MAC treatment:** 500 mg/day + ethambutol ± 1–3 additional drugs (amikacin, ciprofloxacin or levofloxacin, rifabutin or rifampin) × 2–4 mo **MAC maintenance (alt):** 500 mg/day + ethambutol ± rifabutin	Gastrointestinal.	Interchangeable with clarithromycin for MAC therapy. May ↑ effect of digoxin, warfarin, theophylline.	$$
	clarithromycin Biaxin	**MAC prophylaxis (1st choice):** 500 mg BID **MAC treatment:** 500 mg BID + ethambutol ± 1–3 additional drugs (amikacin, ciprofloxacin or levofloxacin, rifabutin or rifampin) × 2–4 mo **MAC maintenance (1st choice):** 500 mg BID + ethambutol ± rifabutin	Gastrointestinal, abnormal taste. QTc prolongation (rare).	Interchangeable with azithromycin for MAC therapy. Substrate and inhibitor of CYP3A4 (many potential interactions). PIs may ↓ clearance of clarithromycin. May ↑ effects of carbamazepine, digoxin and warfarin. Use cautiously with other drugs that cause QTc prolongation.	$
Amino-glycoside Antibiotics	*amikacin* Amikin	**MAC treatment:** 10–15 mg/kg/day iv × 2–4 mo as an optional component in a regimen containing a macrolide + ethambutol	Nephrotoxicity, ototoxicity (auditory and vestibular).	↑ nephrotoxicity with other nephrotoxic drugs.	$$$$$

Class	Drug	Indication and Adult Dose[a]	Adverse Effects	Comments	Cost[b]
Rifamycin Antibiotics	*rifabutin* Mycobutin	**MAC prophylaxis (alt):** 300 mg/day **MAC treatment:** 300 mg/day × 2–4 mo as an optional component in a regimen containing a macrolide + ethambutol	Gastrointestinal, rash, pruritus, myelosuppression. Uveitis at doses > 300 mg/day. Hepatotoxicity is rare.	Substrate of CYP1A2 and 3A4; induces 3A4 (many potential interactions). Clinically significant drug interactions with PIs and NNRTIs: do not use in combination with ritonavir, saquinavir, delavirdine. Discolours body fluids and feces.	$
	rifampin Rifadin, Rofact	**MAC treatment:** 600 mg/day × 2–4 mo as an optional component in a regimen containing a macrolide + ethambutol **TB prophylaxis (alt):** 600 mg/day × 4–6 mo	Rash, pruritus, hepatitis (rare).	Broad-based induction of CYP isozymes (many potential interactions). Clinically significant drug interactions with many PIs and NNRTIs. Induces metabolism of AZT. Discolours body fluids and feces.	$
Fluoro-quinolone Antibiotics	*ciprofloxacin* ● Cipro, generics	**MAC treatment:** 500–750 mg BID × 2–4 mo as an optional component in a regimen containing a macrolide + ethambutol	Headache, gastrointestinal, tendon rupture (rare).	Absorption ↓ by antacids, calcium and iron (separate administration). Inhibits CYP1A2 and 3A4 (many potential interactions): markedly ↑ theophylline and tizanidine levels.	$
	levofloxacin ● Levaquin, Novo-Levofloxacin, other generics	**MAC treatment:** 500 mg/day × 2–4 mo as an optional component in a regimen containing a macrolide + ethambutol	See ciprofloxacin.	Absorption ↓ by antacids, calcium and iron (separate administration). Inhibits CYP1A2 (many potential interactions).	$

(cont'd)

Table 6: **Drugs for Prophylaxis and Treatment of *Mycobacterium avium* complex Infection and for Prophylaxis of *Mycobacterium tuberculosis* Infection** *(cont'd)*

Class	Drug	Indication and Adult Dose[a]	Adverse Effects	Comments	Cost[b]
Antimycobacterial Agents	*ethambutol* ➊ generics	**MAC treatment:** 15 mg/kg/day × 2–4 mo + clarithromycin or azithromycin ± 1–3 additional drugs (amikacin, ciprofloxacin or levofloxacin, rifabutin or rifampin) **MAC maintenance:** 15 mg/kg/day + clarithromycin or azithromycin ± rifabutin	Gastrointestinal, headache, confusion, peripheral neuritis, optic neuritis, rash, pruritus.	Absorption ↓ by aluminum salts (separate administration).	$
	isoniazid Isotamine, other generics	**TB prophylaxis (1st choice):** 300 mg/day or 900 mg twice/wk × 9 mo with pyridoxine 50 mg/day	Gastrointestinal, hepatotoxicity, peripheral neuropathy.	Absorption ↓ by antacids (administer separately). Inhibits metabolism of carbamazepine, phenytoin and theophylline.	$

[a] Doses are oral unless indicated otherwise.

[b] Cost per day based on dosages in this table for 50 kg person; includes drug cost only.

➊ Dosage adjustment may be required in renal impairment; see Appendix I.

Abbreviations: Alt = alternative therapy; AZT = zidovudine; CYP = cytochrome P450; ddI = didanosine; MAC = *Mycobacterium avium* complex; NNRTI = non-nucleoside reverse transcriptase inhibitor; PI = HIV protease inhibitor; TB = tuberculosis

Legend: $ < $10 $$ $10–25 $$$ $25–50 $$$$ $50–100 $$$$$ > $100

Table 7: Drugs for Prophylaxis and Treatment of *Pneumocystis jirovecii* and *Toxoplasma gondii* Infections

Class	Drug	Indication and Adult Dose[a]	Adverse Effects	Comments	Cost[b]
Sulfonamide Combinations	*sulfamethoxa-zole/trimetho-prim (SMX/TMP, cotrimoxazole)* Septra Injection, generics	**PJP, *T. gondii* prophylaxis (1st choice):** 1 DS tab/day (800/160 mg) is preferred; 1 SS tab/day (400/80 mg) or 1 DS tab M/W/F are alternatives **PJP treatment (1st choice):** 15–20 mg/kg/day (TMP) iv or po (divided Q6–8H) × 21 days ***T. gondii* treatment (alt):** 5–10 mg/kg/day (TMP) iv or po BID × 30 days	Adverse reactions are common, often requiring alternative agents. Nausea, vomiting and fever, hypersensitivity reactions (may be severe), myelosuppression, hyperkalemia with high (i.e., treatment) doses.	Use with caution in patients with G6PD deficiency, or impaired renal or hepatic function. May ↑ effect of sulfonylureas and warfarin. TMP ↓ excretion of dofetilide – avoid combination. ↑ hemotoxicity with AZT.	po: $ iv: $$$
Sulfonamide Antibiotics	*sulfadiazine*[c]	***T. gondii* treatment (1st choice):** 100–150 mg/kg (max 6g/day) Q6H + pyrimethamine + leucovorin × 4–8 wk ***T. gondii* maintenance (1st choice):** 1 g BID + pyrimethamine + leucovorin	Nausea, vomiting and fever, hypersensitivity reactions (may be severe), myelosuppression.	Use with caution in patients with G6PD deficiency, or impaired renal or hepatic function. May ↑ effect of sulfonylureas and warfarin. ↑ hemotoxicity with AZT.	[c]
Sulfone Antibiotics	*dapsone* Dapsone, generics	**PJP, *T. gondii* prophylaxis (alt):** 100 mg/day alone; or 50 or 200 mg/day + pyrimethamine + leucovorin **PJP treatment (alt):** 100 mg/d + TMP 15–20 mg/kg/d × 21 d	Hypersensitivity reactions (may be severe), myelosuppression, hemolytic anemia, methe-moglobinemia (more common in G6PD deficiency).	Better tolerated than SMX/TMP. Absorption ↓ by ddI. Clearance ↑ by rifampin. Excretion ↓ by probenecid. TMP + dapsone ↑ toxicity of both drugs. ↑ hemotoxicity with AZT, pyrimethamine, primaquine, TMP.	$

(cont'd)

Table 7: **Drugs for Prophylaxis and Treatment of *Pneumocystis jirovecii* and *Toxoplasma gondii* Infections** *(cont'd)*

Class	Drug	Indication and Adult Dose[a]	Adverse Effects	Comments	Cost[b]
Antiprotozoal Agents	*atovaquone* Mepron	**PJP prophylaxis (alt):** 1500 mg/day **PJP treatment (alt):** 750 mg BID	Gastrointestinal, headache, rash.	Less effective than SMX/TMP for treatment of mild-moderate PJP. High fat meal ↑ absorption. Clearance ↓ by rifabutin, rifampin. ↑ levels of AZT, rifabutin, rifampin.	$$$$$
	primaquine Primaquine, generics	**PJP treatment (alt):** 15–30 mg/day + clindamycin (300–450 mg Q6–8H or 600–900 mg iv Q8H)	Gastrointestinal, hemolytic anemia, methemoglobinemia.		$
	pyrimethamine Daraprim	**PJP prophylaxis (alt):** 50 or 75 mg once/wk + dapsone + leucovorin 25 mg/wk ***T. gondii* treatment (1st choice):** 100 mg Q12H × 2, then 50 mg/day (< 60 kg) or 75 mg/day (≥ 60 kg) + leucovorin 10–20 mg/day × 4–8 wk + sulfadiazine (or + clindamycin 600 mg iv or po Q6H rather than sulfadiazine) ***T. gondii* maintenance (1st choice):** 25–50 mg/day + leucovorin 10 mg/day + sulfadiazine (or with clindamycin 300 mg po Q6H rather than sulfadiazine)	Gastrointestinal, hypersensitivity reactions (may be severe), myelosuppression, anorexia, vomiting.	Leucovorin ↓ bone marrow toxicity. ↑ hemotoxicity with sulfonamides, AZT, ganciclovir.	$

Class	Drug	Indication and Adult Dose[a]	Adverse Effects	Comments	Cost[b]
	pentamidine (renal) generics	**PJP prophylaxis (alt):** aerosol 300 mg/mo **PJP treatment (alt for severe):** 4 mg/kg/day iv × 21 day	**Aerosol:** chest pain, rash, wheezing. **Injection:** anemia, arrhythmias, dysglycemia, hypotension, nephrotoxicity, myelosuppression, pancreatitis.	Aerosolized pentamidine is better tolerated but less effective than iv for PJP treatment. Give aerosol by Respirgard inhaler. Infuse over 1 h while monitoring BP. Caution with other drugs that cause QTc prolongation. ↑ nephrotoxicity with other nephrotoxic drugs.	$$$$
	trimetrexate, Neutrexin	**PJP treatment (alt):** 45 mg/m² or 1.2 mg/kg iv daily + leucovorin 0.5 mg/kg iv/po Q6H	Myelosuppression, elevated aminotransferases.	Leucovorin ↓ bone marrow toxicity. Continue leucovorin for 3 d after completing trimetrexate. ↑ hemotoxicity with AZT.	$$$$$

[a] Doses are oral unless indicated otherwise.
[b] Cost per day based on dosages in this table for 50 kg person; includes drug cost only.
[c] Available through Special Access Programme, Therapeutic Products Directorate, Health Canada.
(renal) Dosage adjustment may be required in renal impairment; see Appendix I.
Abbreviations: Alt = alternative therapy; AZT = zidovudine; CYP = cytochrome P450; ddI = didanosine; G6PD = glucose-6-phosphate dehydrogenase; PJP = *Pneumocystis jirovecii* pneumonia
Legend: $ < $10 $$ $10–25 $$$ $25–50 $$$$ $50–100 $$$$$ > $100

Suggested Readings

Aberg JA, Gallant JE, Anderson J et al. Primary care guidelines for the management of persons infected with human immunodeficiency virus: recommendations of the HIV Medicine Association of the Infectious Diseases Society of America. *Clin Infect Dis* 2004;39(5):609-29.

Bartlett JG, Gallant JE. *2005-2006 Medical management of HIV infection*. Baltimore (MD): Johns Hopkins University, Dept. of Infectious Diseases; 2005.

Lipman M, Breen R. Immune reconstitution inflammatory syndrome in HIV. *Curr Opin Infect Dis* 2006;19(1):20-5.

Masur H, Kaplan JE, Holmes KK. Guidelines for preventing opportunistic infections among HIV-infected persons–2002. Recommendations of the U.S. Public Health Service and the Infectious Diseases Society of America. *Ann Intern Med* 2002;137(5 Pt 2):435-78.

Mofenson LM, Oleske J, Serchuck L et al. Treating opportunistic infections among HIV-exposed and infected children: recommendations from CDC, the National Institutes of Health and the Infectious Diseases Society of America. *Clin Infect Dis* 2005:40(Suppl 1):S1-84.

References

1. Masur H, Kaplan JE, Holmes KK. Guidelines for preventing opportunistic infections among HIV-infected persons–2002. Recommendations of the U.S. Public Health Service and the Infectious Diseases Society of America. *Ann Intern Med* 2002;137(5 Pt 2):435-78.
2. Tessier D et al. *HIV care: a primer & resource guide for family physicians*. Mississauga (ON): College of Family Physicians of Canada; 2001. Available from: http://www.cfpc.ca/English/cfpc/programs/patient%20care/hiv%20primer/hivprimertoc/default.asp?s=1 Accessed October 10, 2006.
3. Battegay M, Nuesch R, Hirschel B et al. Immunological recovery and antiretroviral therapy in HIV-1 infection. *Lancet Infect Dis* 2006;6(5):280-87.
4. Lawn SD, Bekker LG, Miller RF. Immune reconstitution disease associated with mycobacterial infections in HIV-infected individuals receiving antiretrovirals. *Lancet Infect Dis* 2005;5(6):361-73.
5. Aberg JA, Williams PL, Liu T et al. A study of discontinuing maintenance therapy in human immunodeficiency virus-infected subjects with disseminated Mycobacterium avium complex: AIDS Clinical Trial Group 393 Study Team. *J Infect Dis* 2003;187(7):1046-52.
6. Benson CA, Kaplan JE, Masur H et al. Treating opportunistic infections among HIV-infected adults and adolescents: recommendations from CDC, the National Institutes of Health, and the HIV Medicine Association/Infectious Diseases Society of America. *MMWR Recomm Rep* 2004;53(RR-15):1-112. Available from: http://www.cdc.gov/mmwr/preview/mmwrhtml/rr5315a1.htm Accessed October 10, 2006.
7. Ledergerber B, Mocroft A, Reiss P et al. Discontinuation of secondary prophylaxis against Pneumocystis carinii pneumonia in patients with HIV infection who have a response to antiretroviral therapy. Eight European Study Groups. *N Engl J Med* 2001;344(3):168-74.
8. Lopez Bernaldo de Quiros JC, Miro JM, Pena JM et al. A randomized trial of the discontinuation of primary and secondary prophylaxis against Pneumocystis carinii pneumonia after highly active antiretroviral therapy in patients with HIV infection. Grupo de Estudio del SIDA 04/98. *N Engl J Med* 2001;344(3):159-67.
9. Miro JM, Lopez JC, Podzamczer D et al. Discontinuation of primary and secondary Toxoplasma gondii prophylaxis is safe in HIV-infected patients after immunological restoration with highly active antiretroviral therapy: results of an open, randomized, multicenter clinical trial. *Clin Infect Dis* 2006;43(1):79-89.
10. Tural C, Romeu J, Sirera G et al. Long-lasting remission of cytomegalovirus retinitis without maintenance therapy in human immunodeficiency virus-infected patients. *J Infect Dis* 1998;177(4):1080-3.
11. Vibhagool A, Sungkanuparph S, Mootsikapun P et al. Discontinuation of secondary prophylaxis for cryptococcal meningitis in human immunodeficiency virus-infected patients treated with highly active antiretroviral therapy: a prospective, multicenter, randomized study. *Clin Infect Dis* 2003;36(10):1329-31.
12. Bartlett JG, Gallant JE. *2005-2006 Medical management of HIV infection*. Baltimore (MD): Johns Hopkins University, Dept. of Infectious Diseases; 2005.

13. Sande MA, Eliopoulos GM, Moellering RC et al, editors. *The Sanford guide to HIV/AIDS therapy 2006-2007*. 15th edition. Hyde Park (VT): Antimicrobial Therapy; 2006.

CHAPTER 108
Infections in the Cancer Patient

Coleman Rotstein, MD, FRCPC, FACP, FIDSA

Infections are a significant cause of morbidity and mortality in cancer patients despite the progress that has been made in their recognition, therapy and prevention. The expanding armamentarium of antineoplastic chemotherapeutic agents, radiation therapy and immunotherapy has improved the survival of cancer patients, but has simultaneously rendered them more susceptible to infections.

Goals of Therapy

- Decrease morbidity associated with infection
- Minimize risk of death from infection
- Enhance the supportive care and quality of life of cancer patients by using prophylactic measures to prevent infection and outpatient antibiotic management when appropriate to facilitate care and reduce length of hospital stay

Investigations

- Thorough history with attention to:
  - the nature of the malignancy and associated defects in host defenses, e.g., neutropenia, B cell and/or T cell dysfunction
  - the effects of cytotoxic, myelosuppressive or immunosuppressive therapy employed to treat the patient's cancer; note day of onset of fever relative to the first day of the most recent cycle of chemotherapy
  - neutropenia (severity and expected duration)
  - iatrogenic procedures performed on the patient, e.g., splenectomy, placement of venous access devices or other surgical procedures
  - whether the nature of the malignancy suggests obstruction of natural body passages, e.g., bronchus, bowel, ureter, biliary tree
  - CNS dysfunction
  - occupational and travel history, and exposure to animals
- Complete physical examination with particular attention to venous access sites, wounds, skin, mouth, pharynx, sinuses, rectum and other possible sites of infection
- Laboratory tests:
  - CBC and differential to assess the total neutrophil count
  - biochemical profile with attention to renal and liver function

- at least two sets of blood cultures: ensure blood cultures are done from peripheral site as well as lumens of venous access devices.
- culture of any other suspected site of infection, e.g., urine, skin, sputum
- radiographic studies appropriate for suspected sites of infection, e.g., chest x-ray for pneumonia, CT scan of the head for encephalitis or cerebral abscess
- stool for *Clostridium difficile* and other potential pathogens (e.g., *Salmonella* spp., *Shigella* spp., *Campylobacter* spp., viruses and protozoa) if diarrhea is present
- serological tests (i.e., serology for cytomegalovirus, *Cryptococcus* spp., Epstein-Barr virus, hepatitis and *Toxoplasma* spp.) if indicated
- when appropriate, biopsy for pathology and culture of skin lesions suspected to be infectious

Therapeutic Choices

Nonpharmacologic Choices

- Infection control measures such as handwashing and use of high-efficiency particulate filtration rooms for profoundly neutropenic patients at high risk for filamentous fungal infections are mandatory.
- Use specialized infection control procedures (contact precautions) for patients colonized with multiple-resistant organisms, e.g., methicillin-resistant *Staphylococcus aureus* or vancomycin-resistant enterococci.
- For neutropenic patients, avoid ingesting raw fruits and vegetables, and avoid having fresh flowers and plants in the patient's room.

Pharmacologic Choices (Table 1)

Antibacterial Therapy

- Although neoplasms can cause fevers in cancer patients, an infectious etiology should be sought in all cases of elevated temperature. Fever is defined as a single oral temperature ≥ 38.3°C or a temperature of ≥ 38°C for ≥ 1-hour period in the absence of obvious environmental causes.[1]
- Most infections are caused by microorganisms that have colonized the patient at or near the site of infection, e.g., the skin, oropharynx, genitourinary tract or gastrointestinal tract.
- Bacteria are the principal pathogens causing infections in cancer patients, making up > 60% of initially documented episodes of infection.
- The choice of antibacterial agents in febrile cancer patients is predicated on the neutrophil count, the patient's clinical status and the site of infection (Figure 1). Neutropenia is defined as a neutrophil count ≤ 1.0×10^9/L. A more profound degree of neutropenia (< 0.5×10^9/L) confers a greater risk of developing more severe infection. In

addition, the risk of severe infection is directly related to the duration of neutropenia. Because of the high risk of life-threatening bacterial infection and the inability to reliably distinguish patients with bacterial infection from noninfected patients at presentation (particularly in neutropenic patients), prompt antibiotic therapy must be initiated by the intravenous route.

- In selecting the initial antibiotic regimen and the site of care (the inpatient or outpatient setting), consider concurrent comorbid medical illnesses (e.g., heart failure, renal disease, liver disease, bleeding disorders), the control of the cancer and presence of serious medical complications.[2,3,4] Outpatient antibiotic therapy may be employed not only for non-neutropenic patients, but also for low-risk neutropenic patients who do not have the aforementioned medical conditions or uncontrolled cancer (Figure 2).
- **Vancomycin** may be incorporated into the initial therapeutic regimen for patients with suspected venous access catheter-related infection, positive blood cultures for gram-positive bacteria in groups and chains, severe mucositis, known colonization with methicillin-resistant *S. aureus*, hypotension or other evidence of cardiovascular impairment.[1] Alternatively, vancomycin may be added later to the initial regimen once susceptibility testing has been completed. Vancomycin should be discontinued if the infecting organism is subsequently shown to be susceptible to other antibiotics.
- **Metronidazole** or **clindamycin** may be used as part of the initial antibiotic regimen for presumed anaerobic infection related to the gastrointestinal tract or skin.
- In neutropenic patients with a suspected bacterial infection, continue antibacterial therapy until they are no longer profoundly neutropenic (neutrophils $\geq 0.5 \times 10^9$/L) and are afebrile for $\geq$ 48 hours. For patients with microbiologically or clinically documented infection, continue antibacterial therapy for a minimum of 10 to 14 days and until patients are afebrile and no longer neutropenic (neutrophils $\geq 0.5 \times 10^9$/L).
- In non-neutropenic cancer patients with a suspected bacterial infection, continue antibiotic therapy for approximately 7 days and until the patient is afebrile for $\geq$ 48 hours. Alternatively, switch from intravenous antibiotic therapy to oral therapy to complete an appropriate course of therapy directed towards the site that is infected.

Antifungal Therapy

- Non-neutropenic patients who develop oral and or esophageal candidiasis may be treated with a topical agent such as **nystatin** or systemic oral agents such as **fluconazole, itraconazole, posaconazole** or **voriconazole**. Patients with extensive lesions may require parenteral therapy with **fluconazole**, an **amphotericin B** formulation, **caspofungin**, **micafungin** or **voriconazole**.

- Parenteral antifungal therapy should be initiated for *documented invasive or disseminated fungal infection* in non-neutropenic and neutropenic cancer patients.
- Treatment of a *documented or suspected fungal infection* in a neutropenic patient requires parenteral antifungal therapy with **amphotericin B**, most often, or with **caspofungin** or **fluconazole** in patients with renal dysfunction.[1]
- The **lipid-based preparations of amphotericin B** have equivalent efficacy but produce less nephrotoxicity and infusion reactions than conventional amphotericin B. They may be used as salvage therapy for patients with fungal infections that fail to respond to amphotericin B or for patients with amphotericin B toxicity or intolerance.[5]
- **Caspofungin** may be beneficial for the treatment of candidemia in neutropenic or non-neutropenic patients.[6]
- **Itraconazole**, which is only available in an oral formulation, has enhanced activity against *Aspergillus* spp. compared to fluconazole and is an alternative for oral step-down therapy after parenteral treatment for invasive aspergillosis.
- **Voriconazole**, available both in intravenous and oral formulations, has superior activity compared to **amphotericin B** when used as primary therapy for invasive aspergillosis,[7] and for infections caused by *Scedosporium* spp. and *Fusarium* spp.
- **Voriconazole** or **caspofungin**, alone or in combination or with a lipid-based formulation of **amphotericin B** may be used in the treatment of documented invasive aspergillosis.[8,9]
- **Posaconazole** may be used for refractory invasive fungal infections.[10]

Antiviral Therapy

- There is no indication for the empirical use of antiviral drugs in the treatment of cancer patients without evidence of viral disease.[1]
- Skin or mucous membrane lesions due to herpes simplex virus or varicella-zoster virus may be treated with oral or intravenous **acyclovir**. Oral **famciclovir** or **valacyclovir** are better absorbed from the gastrointestinal tract than acyclovir and are alternatives.[11]
- Intravenous **foscarnet** is available through the federal Special Access Programme for acyclovir-resistant herpesvirus infections.
- Cytomegalovirus infection in bone marrow transplant recipients may be treated with **ganciclovir**. **Valganciclovir** is used only when oral therapy is required.

Supportive Care Measures

- **Granulocyte (G-CSF)** and **granulocyte-macrophage (GM-CSF) colony-stimulating factors** may decrease the incidence and duration of neutropenia after chemotherapy. Their use is advocated for patients who remain profoundly neutropenic and have failed to respond to appropriate antimicrobial therapy for documented infection such as pneumonia, severe cellulitis or sinusitis.[1,12] Once neutrophil counts reach ≥ 1.0 × 10^9/L, colony-stimulating factor support should be discontinued.

Prevention of Infection in Cancer Patients

- For cancer patients with pronounced T cell dysfunction, prophylaxis with oral **sulfamethoxazole/trimethoprim** is recommended to prevent *Pneumocystis jirovecii* pneumonia. Alternative prophylactic agents are inhaled **pentamidine** and **dapsone**.
- Strategies designed to prevent bacterial infection in profoundly neutropenic cancer patients, such as those with acute leukemia, focus on eliminating indigenous microflora and preventing acquisition of new potential pathogens. Potential antimicrobial regimens are fluoroquinolones, sulfamethoxazole/trimethoprim or oral nonabsorbable antibiotics (**gentamicin**, **vancomycin** and **nystatin**). **Ciprofloxacin** or **levofloxacin** significantly decrease febrile morbidity, bacterial infections and mortality for patients with acute leukemia and those undergoing bone marrow transplantation.[13] Prophylaxis during the expected period of neutropenia in the first month of chemotherapy in patients with solid tumors or lymphoma (levofloxacin 500 mg for 7 days) also reduces the rate of febrile episodes.[14] There may be a predilection for gram-positive infection when ciprofloxacin is used prophylactically. This may be overcome by adding another antibiotic with good activity against gram-positive organisms (e.g., a penicillin or a macrolide).[15]
- Antifungal prophylaxis with oral **fluconazole** prevents invasive fungal infection in allogeneic bone marrow transplant recipients and patients with acute leukemia undergoing remission-induction chemotherapy.[16,17] **Itraconazole** prophylaxis may be preferred for individuals at greater risk of developing invasive aspergillosis.
- If fluconazole has been used prophylactically, it should not be used empirically or for documented fungal infections in neutropenic cancer patients. For these situations, a parenteral **amphotericin B** formulation or **caspofungin** are the drugs of choice.[8]

Therapeutic Tips

- Avoid **aminoglycosides** in patients with impaired renal function, particularly those receiving treatment with other nephrotoxic drugs such as cisplatin, cyclosporine or amphotericin B.
- In deciding on cost-effective empirical therapy, drug acquisition costs by themselves are of limited value. Consider the relative effectiveness, side effect profile and overall resource consumption of the available treatments as well.
- Monotherapy with an intravenous broad spectrum antipseudomonal beta-lactam (**ceftazidime, meropenem, imipenem/cilastatin** or **piperacillin/tazobactam**) is suitable for the treatment of febrile neutropenic episodes.

- Combination therapy for febrile neutropenia with a beta-lactam and an aminoglycoside is associated with more adverse events (i.e., a higher incidence of nephrotoxicity) than monotherapy with a beta-lactam.
- Identification of low-risk patients appropriate for outpatient antibiotic management may enhance the patient's quality of life and reduce costs.

Figure 1: **Approach to Fever in Cancer Patients**

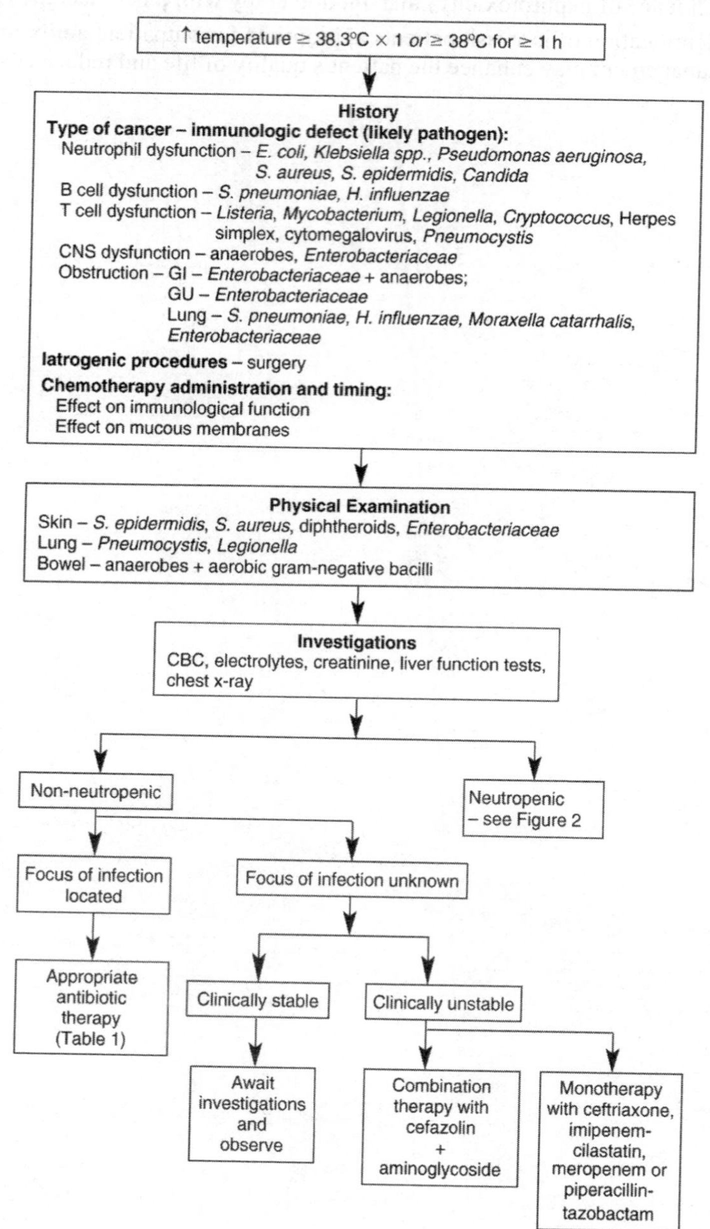

Figure 2: **Management of Infection in Febrile Neutropenic Cancer Patients**

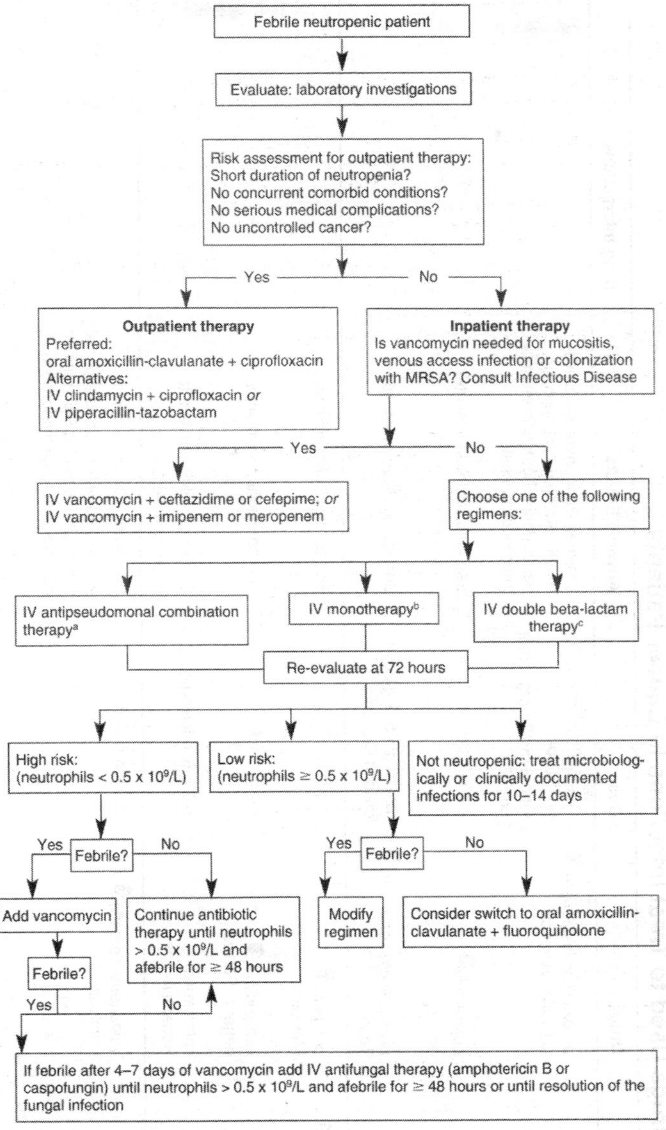

[a] Antipseudomonal combination therapy = a beta-lactam (piperacillin, piperacillin/tazobactam, ceftazidime, imipenem/cilastatin *or* meropenem) plus an aminoglycoside

[b] Cefepime, ceftazidime, imipenem/cilastatin *or* meropenem

[c] Double beta-lactam therapy = ceftazidime plus *either* piperacillin *or* piperacillin/tazobactam

Abbreviations: MRSA = methicillin-resistant *S. aureus*

Table 1: Drugs Used to Treat Infections in Cancer Patients

Class	Drug	Dose	Adverse Effects	Drug Interactions	Cost[a]
Penicillins	*amoxicillin/clavulanate* Clavulin, generics	One 500/125 mg tablet po TID **or** One 875/125 mg tablet po BID	Diarrhea, rash, hypersensitivity reactions, interstitial nephritis, neutropenia, hemolytic anemia; thrombocytopenia.		$
	piperacillin generics	4 g iv Q6H	See amoxicillin/clavulanate.		$$$$
	piperacillin/tazobactam Tazocin	12–16 g/1.5–2 g/day iv divided Q6–8H	See amoxicillin/clavulanate.		$$$–$$$$
Cephalosporins	*cefepime* Maxipime	2 g iv Q8H	See amoxicillin/clavulanate.		$$$$
	ceftazidime generic, Fortaz	2 g iv Q8H	See amoxicillin/clavulanate.		$$$$$
	ceftriaxone Rocephin	1–2 g iv once daily	See amoxicillin/clavulanate. Pseudocholelithiasis.		$$–$$$
Carbapenems	*imipenem/cilastatin* Primaxin	500 mg iv Q6H	See amoxicillin/clavulanate. Associated with seizures especially with high doses (1 g Q6H) and in patients with renal dysfunction.		$$$$$

Class	Drug	Dose	Adverse Effects	Drug Interactions	Cost[a]
	meropenem Merrem	1 g iv Q8H	Diarrhea, rash, nausea, hypersensitivity reactions: interstitial nephritis, neutropenia, hemolytic anemia; thrombocytopenia.		$$$$$
Aminoglycosides	*amikacin* generics	15–20 mg/kg once daily[b]	Ototoxicity (auditory and/or vestibular), nephrotoxicity, neuromuscular paralysis (rare).	Synergistic or additive toxicity if used with vancomycin and/or platinum-derived antineoplastics, amphotericin B and/or other nephrotoxic/ototoxic drugs.	$$$
	gentamicin generics	5–7 mg/kg once daily[b]	See amikacin.	See amikacin.	$
	tobramycin generics	5–7 mg/kg once daily[b]	See amikacin.	See amikacin.	$
Fluoroquinolones	*ciprofloxacin* Cipro, generics	500 or 750 mg po BID 400 mg iv Q12H	GI upset, rash, CNS toxicity.	Warfarin: ↑ INR. Binds with antacids, iron, sucralfate.	po:$ iv:$$$
	levofloxacin Levaquin, generics	500 mg po once daily 500 mg iv once daily	Nausea, diarrhea, headache, insomnia, dizziness.	Binds with antacids, sucralfate, metal cations.	po:$ iv:$$
	moxifloxacin Avelox	400 mg po once daily 400 mg iv once daily	Nausea, diarrhea, headache, insomnia, dizziness.	Binds with antacids, sucralfate, metal cations.	po:$ iv: $$$
	ofloxacin Floxin, generics	400 mg po BID	Nausea, vomiting, rash, headache insomnia, dizziness.	Warfarin: ↑ INR. Binds with antacids, iron, sucralfate.	$

(cont'd)

Table 1: **Drugs Used to Treat Infections in Cancer Patients** *(cont'd)*

Class	Drug	Dose	Adverse Effects	Drug Interactions	Cost[a]
Glycopeptides	*vancomycin* Vancocin, Vancomycin Hydrochloride USP Sterile, generics	15 mg/kg iv Q12H	Shock after rapid iv infusion (infuse over < 1 h), fever, chills, phlebitis, "red-neck" syndrome, tingling and flushing of head, neck, chest, rash, transient leukopenia or eosinophilia, ototoxicity.	Nephrotoxicity may be enhanced if given with aminoglycosides or other nephrotoxins.	$$$
Lincosamides	*clindamycin* Dalacin C Phosphate Sterile Solution, generics	600 mg iv Q8H	Diarrhea, minor reversible ↑ liver transaminases, reversible neutropenia, thrombocytopenia, pseudomembranous colitis.	May enhance action of neuromuscular blocking agents.	$$
Macrolides	*azithromycin* Zithromax	500 mg iv once daily	GI upset.	May ↑ bioavailability of digoxin.	$
	erythromycin Erythrocin, generics	1 g iv Q6H	Abdominal pain, nausea, vomiting, diarrhea; thrombophlebitis, transient hearing loss with high doses.	May interfere with metabolism of theophylline, warfarin, carbamazepine, cyclosporine, methylprednisolone.	$$$$
Nitroimidazoles	*metronidazole* generics	500 mg iv Q12H	GI upset, reversible neutropenia, seizures, peripheral neuropathy (rare), rash, metallic taste.	Disulfiram-like reaction with alcohol. Potentiation of warfarin effects and other oral coumarin-type anticoagulants.	$
Sulfonamide Combinations	*sulfamethoxazole/ trimethoprim* Septra Injection, generics	po/iv: trimethoprim 20 mg/kg/day and sulfamethoxazole 100 mg/kg/day divided QID	Nausea, vomiting, diarrhea; hypersensitivity reactions, leukopenia, thrombocytopenia, hepatitis (rare).	May ↑ effect of warfarin.	po: $ iv: $$

Class	Drug	Dose	Adverse Effects	Drug Interactions	Cost[a]
Polyene Antifungals	*amphotericin B* Fungizone	0.3–1.5 mg/kg iv Q24H	Rigors, renal dysfunction (azotemia), headache, hypokalemia, phlebitis, thrombocytopenia, anemia, leukopenia (rare), hypotension.	↑ azotemia when used with other nephrotoxic drugs.	$$–$$$
	amphotericin B lipid preparations Abelcet, AmBisome	3–5 mg/kg iv Q24H	Less nephrotoxicity than amphotericin B.		$$$$$
	nystatin, ratio-Nystatin, generics	3.6 million U po Q4H	Nausea, vomiting, diarrhea.		$
Triazole Antifungals	*fluconazole* Diflucan, generics	100–400 mg po Q24H 100–400 mg iv Q24H	Nausea, headache, skin rash, abdominal pain, vomiting, diarrhea.	May cause hepatotoxicity if used with other potentially hepatotoxic drugs. Sulfonylureas, phenytoin, cyclosporine, coumarin-like drugs may require dosage adjustment (monitor).	po:$ iv: $$-$$$
	itraconazole Sporanox	100–200 mg po daily–BID	Nausea, rash, headache, reversible ↑ hepatic enzymes.	Sulfonylureas, phenytoin, cyclosporine, coumarin-like drugs, digoxin may require dosage adjustment (monitor); didanosine, H_2-antagonists, rifampin, phenytoin, may ↓ itraconazole levels; itraconazole ↑ levels of statins.	$
	posaconazole Noxafil	Prophylaxis: 200 mg po TID Refractory invasive fungal infections: 400 mg po BID	Nausea, vomiting, fever, diarrhea, dry mouth, abdominal pain, headache.	Cyclosporine, tacrolimus, sirolimus, vinca alkaloids, midazolam and statins require dose adjustments (monitor). Rifabutin, phenytoin, cimetidine may ↓ posaconazole levels.	$$$$$

(cont'd)

Table 1: **Drugs Used to Treat Infections in Cancer Patients** *(cont'd)*

Class	Drug	Dose	Adverse Effects	Drug Interactions	Cost[a]
	voriconazole Vfend	200 mg po BID; 4–6 mg/kg iv Q12H	Visual disturbances, nausea, vomiting, rash, ↑ hepatic enzymes.	Sulfonylureas, cyclosporine, coumarin-like drugs may require dosage adjustment (monitor); rifampin, carbamazepine, barbiturates and phenytoin may ↓ voriconazole levels.	$$$$$
Echinocandin Antifungals	*caspofungin* Cancidas	70 mg iv loading dose, then 50 mg iv daily	Fever, rash, nausea, vomiting, phlebitis at the injection site	↑ LFTs with cyclosporine. Efavirenz, nelfinavir, phenytoin, dexamethasone, rifampin, carbamazepine ↓ caspofungin levels. Caspofungin ↓ levels of tacrolimus.	$$$$$
	micafungin Mycamine	50 mg iv daily as prophylaxis 150 mg iv daily for treatment of esophageal candidiasis	See caspofungin.	Micafungin increases serum levels of sirolimus and nifedipine	$$$$$
Antivirals	*acyclovir* generics	5–10 mg/kg iv Q8H	Phlebitis, rash, hypotension, headache, nausea, tremors, confusion, seizures (1%), renal dysfunction.	Probenecid ↓ renal clearance; may ↑ theophylline levels.	$$$$$
	famciclovir Famvir	500 mg po TID	Headache, nausea, pruritus.	Probenecid ↓ renal clearance.	$
	ganciclovir Cytovene	Induction: 5 mg/kg iv Q12H Maintenance: 6 mg/kg iv Q24H	Leukopenia, nausea, headache, behavioural changes.	Avoid use with zidovudine (↑ hematologic toxicity).	$$

Class	Drug	Dose	Adverse Effects	Drug Interactions	Cost[a]
	valganciclovir Valcyte	900 mg po daily	See ganciclovir.	Prodrug of ganciclovir. See ganciclovir.	$$
	valacyclovir (renal symbol) Valtrex	1 g po TID	Headache, nausea.	Probenecid ↓ renal clearance.	$

[a] Cost of 1-day supply based on 50 kg body weight; includes drug cost only.
[b] Administer in divided doses for patients with impaired renal function.
(renal symbol) Dosage adjustment may be required in renal impairment; see Appendix I.
Legend: $ < $25 $$ $25–50 $$–$$$ $25–75 $$$ $50–75 $$$–$$$$ $50–100 $$$$ $75–100 $$$$$ > $100

Suggested Readings

Hughes WT, Armstrong D, Bodey GP et al. 2002 guidelines for the use of antimicrobial agents in neutropenic patients with cancer. *Clin Infect Dis* 2002;34(6):730-51.

Paul M, Soares-Weiser K, Grozinsky S et al. Beta-lactam versus beta-lactam-aminoglycoside combination therapy in cancer patients with neutropenia. *Cochrane Database Syst Rev* 2003;(3):CD003038.

Rotstein C, Laverdiere M, Marciniak A et al. An economic evaluation of voriconazole for the treatment of invasive aspergillosis in Canada. *Can J Infect Dis Med Microbiol* 2004;15(5):277-84.

Rotstein C, Mandell LA, Goldberg N. Fluoroquinolone prophylaxis for profoundly neutropenic cancer patients: a meta-analysis. *Current Oncology* 1997;4(Suppl 2):S2-S7.

Yu DT, Seger DL, Peterson JF et al. Fluconazole for empiric antifungal therapy in cancer patients with fever and neutropenia. *BMC Infect Dis* 2006;6:173.

References

1. Hughes WT, Armstrong D, Bodey GP et al. 2002 guidelines for the use of antimicrobial agents in neutropenic patients with cancer. *Clin Infect Dis* 2002;34(6):730-51.
2. Talcott JA, Siegel RD, Finberg R et al. Risk assessment in cancer patients with fever and neutropenia: a prospective, two-center validation of a prediction rule. *J Clin Oncol* 1992;10(2):316-22.
3. Talcott JA, Whalen A, Clark J et al. Home antibiotic therapy for low-risk cancer patients with fever and neutropenia: a pilot study of 30 patients based on a validated prediction rule. *J Clin Oncol* 1994;12(1):107-14.
4. Paul M, Yahav D, Fraser A et al. Empirical antibiotic monotherapy for febrile neutropenia: systematic review and meta-analysis of randomized controlled trials. *J Antimicrob Chemother* 2006;57(2):176-89.
5. Walsh TJ, Finberg RW, Arndt C et al. Liposomal amphotericin B for empirical therapy in patients with persistent fever and neutropenia. National Institute of Allergy and Infectious Diseases Mycoses Study Group. *N Engl J Med* 1999;340(10):764-71.
6. Mora-Duarte J, Betts R, Rotstein C et al. Comparison of caspofungin and amphotericin B for invasive candidiasis. *N Engl J Med* 2002;347(25):2020-9.
7. Herbrecht R, Denning DW, Patterson TF et al. Voriconazole versus amphotericin B for primary therapy of invasive aspergillosis. *N Engl J Med* 2002;347(6):408-15.
8. Walsh TJ, Teppler H, Donowitz GR et al. Caspofungin versus liposomal amphotericin B for empirical antifungal therapy in patients with persistent fever and neutropenia. *N Engl J Med* 2004; 351(14):1391-402.
9. Marr KA, Boeckh M, Carter RA et al. Combination antifungal therapy for invasive aspergillosis. *Clin Infect Dis* 2004;39(6):797-802.
10. Walsh TJ, Raad I, Ratterson JF et al. Treatment of invasive aspergillosis with posaconazole in patients who are refractory or intolerant of conventional therapy: an externally controlled trial. *Clin Infect Dis* 2007;44(1):2-12.
11. [No authors listed]. Drugs for non-HIV viral infections.*Med Lett Drugs Ther* 2002;44(1123):9-16.
12. Ozer H, Armitage JO, Bennett CL et al. 2000 update of recommendations for the use of hematopoietic colony-stimulating factors: evidence-based, clinical practice guidelines. American Society of Clinical Oncology Growth Factors Expert Panel. *J Clin Oncol* 2000;18(20):3558-85.
13. Leibovici L, Paul M, Cullen M et al. Antibiotic prophylaxis in neutropenic patients: new evidence, practical decisions. *Cancer* 2006;107(8):1743-51.
14. Cullen M, Steven N, Billingham L et al. Antibacterial prophylaxis for solid tumors and lymphomas. *N Engl J Med* 2005;353(14):988-98.
15. Rotstein C, Mandell LA, Goldberg N. Fluoroquinolone prophylaxis for profoundly neutropenic cancer patients: a meta-analysis. *Current Oncology* 1997;4(Suppl 2):S2-S7.
16. Rotstein C, Bow EJ, Laverdiere M et al. Randomized placebo-controlled trial of fluconazole prophylaxis for neutropenic cancer patients: benefit based on purpose and intensity of cytotoxic therapy. *Clin Infect Dis* 1999;28(2):331-40.
17. Bow EJ, Laverdiere M, Lussier N et al. Antifungal prophylaxis for severely neutropenic chemotherapy recipients: a meta analysis of randomized-controlled clinical trials. *Cancer* 2002;94(12):3230-46.
18. Ullmann AJ, Lipton JH, Vesole DH et al. Posaconazole versus fluconazole or itraconazole prophylaxis in severe graft–versus–host disease. *N Engl J Med* 2007;356(4):335-47.

19. Cornely OA, Maertens J, Winston DJ et al. Posaconazole vs. fluconazole or itraconazole prophylaxis in patients with neutropenia. *N Engl J Med* 2007;356(4):348-59.
20. van Burik JA, Ratanatharathorn V, Stepan DE et al. Micafungin versus fluconazole for prophylaxis against fungal infections during neutropenia in patients undergoing hematopoietic stem cell transplantation. *Clin Infect Dis* 2004;39(10):1407-16.

CHAPTER 109 Travellers' Diarrhea

Laurence Green, MD, FRCPC and
J. Dick MacLean, MD, FRCPC

Travellers' diarrhea is defined as the passage of three or more unformed stools in a 24-hour period plus at least one symptom of enteric disease such as abdominal pain or cramps, nausea, vomiting, fever or tenesmus.[1] Diarrhea develops in 15–40% of travellers in less developed countries. In 10% of travellers, fever and/or bloody stools may occur.[2] Most cases in adults are caused by bacteria, predominantly enterotoxigenic *Escherichia coli* (ETEC) as well as *Campylobacter*, *Salmonella* and *Shigella*.[3] Other pathogens include viruses (norovirus, rotavirus) and protozoa, e.g., *Giardia intestinalis*. Recent studies suggest that enteroaggregative *E. coli* also plays a substantial role.[4] Incubation periods are short, and many patients develop diarrhea within the first week of travel.[5] Because of this and the frequent unavailability of reliable medical care, travellers must be prepared to institute self-therapy.

Goals of Therapy

- Reduce risk of infection in travellers
- Limit duration and severity of symptoms while travelling and during the immediate post-travel period

Investigations

- Counsel travellers about *self-diagnosis*
  - distinguish mild symptoms (abdominal cramps, malaise, nausea and frequent bowel movements) from the high fever and bloody and mucoid stools of more severe infection requiring urgent antibiotic therapy
- Patients developing symptoms after returning home or presenting with symptoms persisting more than two weeks after their return should be evaluated by:
  - history (e.g., destination and season of travel) and physical examination (signs of volume depletion, abdominal tenderness/guarding)
  - stool for occult blood
  - consider stool cultures especially in cases of dysentery, in food handlers and in health- and childcare workers
  - consider stool parasitology exams for diarrhea persisting more than two weeks after return

Prevention

Therapeutic Choices

Nonpharmacologic Choices

- "Boil it, cook it, peel it or forget it."
- Drink only boiled, bottled or carbonated beverages. Avoid bottled drinks if the cap is not sealed and intact.
- Boil clear water for one minute at altitudes under 2000 m (three minutes above 2000 m)[6] or sterilize water (five drops of 2% tincture of iodine per litre of clear water, or iodine water purification tablets or iodinizing resin filters).
- Avoid ice cubes unless made from safe water.
- Eat fruit (including tomatoes) only if it has been washed in safe water and peeled. Do not eat watermelon.
- Avoid salads and raw vegetables.
- Eat only thoroughly and recently cooked meats or fish.
- Avoid leftovers and condiments in open bottles.
- Avoid food from street vendors.
- Wash hands with soap and water before eating. Waterless hand sanitizers are also effective if hands are not visibly dirty.

Pharmacologic Choices (Table 1)

Bismuth Subsalicylate (BSS)

Prophylactic use of **bismuth subsalicylate (BSS)**, given QID with food, decreases attack rates of traveller's diarrhea from 40% to 14% when compared to placebo; twice-daily dosing is less effective.[7] BSS may have antibacterial activity as well as antisecretory and anti-inflammatory properties. Do not recommend BSS in travellers taking anticoagulants or salicylates or who are allergic to salicylates. Side effects are minimal with short-term use (less than three weeks) at recommended doses. Black stools produced by BSS may create diagnostic confusion by simulating melena.

Antibiotics

Give antibiotic prophylaxis only for short courses, i.e., less than three weeks, to those at increased health risk (e.g., the chronically ill or immunocompromised patient), or for persons who undertake critical travel (e.g., diplomatic missions) or get diarrhea every time they travel.

Fluoroquinolones (norfloxacin, ofloxacin, ciprofloxacin) effectively reduce attacks of travellers' diarrhea by up to 90% and are relatively safe, although bacterial resistance severely limits their use in Thailand,[8,9] India[10] and Nepal[11] and Indonesia. There is a risk, although low, of *Clostridium difficile*-associated diarrhea in travellers taking antibiotic prophylaxis or antibiotics for any purpose. **Sulfamethoxazole/trimethoprim** and

doxycycline are no longer recommended due to significant bacterial resistance.[1]

Rifaximin, a rifamycin-derived, nonabsorbable antibiotic, has shown good preventive efficacy relative to placebo (74% relative risk reduction).[12] Because it is not systemically absorbed, side effects are few and relatively mild. Rifaximin is not available in Canada.

Vaccines

An inactivated oral **cholera vaccine**, contains the B subunit of cholera toxin which has significant homology with the toxin of ETEC. It has protective efficacy of about 50% against ETEC and 25% against all travellers' diarrhea.[13] Because of its low efficacy and the rapid response to self-treatment, the inactivated oral cholera vaccine is not routinely recommended.[14] It is recommended for travellers at unusually high risk such as relief or aid workers, or health care professionals working in cholera risk zones.[15]

Probiotics

There is currently little evidence that probiotics such as *Lactobacillus* spp. or *Saccharomyces boulardii* are effective in the prevention of travellers' diarrhea.[16,17]

Self-Treatment

Therapeutic Choices (Figure 1)

Nonpharmacologic Choices

- Travellers with mild diarrhea may benefit from a clear fluid diet of carbonated, noncaffeinated beverages, canned fruit juices, safe water, clear salty soups and salted crackers.

Pharmacologic Choices (Table 1)

Oral Rehydration Salts (ORS)

Oral hydration, especially in infants, pregnant women and the frail elderly, is the cornerstone of all therapy. Commercially available sachets of **oral rehydration salts** (e.g., Gastrolyte, Pedialyte) are dissolved in safe water and the resulting liquid is consumed until thirst is quenched. The traveller should carry sufficient sachets to produce two to four litres of ORS.

If ORS is unavailable, an emergency but less ideal substitute can be prepared by adding 1 level teaspoon (5 mL) of table salt and 8 teaspoons (40 mL) of sugar to 1 litre of safe water.[16] Alternatively, 1/4 teaspoon (1 mL) of baking soda, 1/8 teaspoon (0.5 mL) of salt and 1/2 teaspoon (2.5 mL) of pasteurized honey can be added to 1 cup (240 mL) of fruit juice.[16] These ingredients may be harder to find.

Antimotility Agents

Do not use antimotility agents in children under three years of age (due to the risk of developing toxic megacolon and obscuring the severity of fluid loss) or in patients with bloody diarrhea and fever (temperature > 38.5°C). **Loperamide** provides relief for mild to moderate diarrhea (up to three to five loose stools per day and mild cramping pain) in adults and older children.[18] The combination of loperamide and an antibiotic is more effective than either alone in reducing the duration of diarrhea.[19,20] **Diphenoxylate with atropine** is not as effective as loperamide and has a less favourable side effect profile. It has been shown to prolong symptoms in infection secondary to *Shigella*.[21]

Antibiotics

Travellers' diarrhea (commonly caused by ETEC) is usually a mild, self-limited disease that responds promptly to appropriate therapy. Advise patients to take a one- to three-day course of antibiotics with them on their travels and to initiate therapy with the onset of symptoms, especially in the case of severe diarrhea with cramps, bloody diarrhea or high fever. Mild diarrhea can be managed with fluids and antimotility agents.

The **fluoroquinolones** (**ciprofloxacin**, **ofloxacin** or **norfloxacin**) effectively reduce the duration of diarrhea by more than 50% relative to placebo.[22,23] In Thailand, the most common cause of dysentery is *Campylobacter*. *Campylobacter* is generally fluoroquinolone-resistant, thus **azithromycin** has become the travellers' diarrhea antibiotic of choice.[24] Similar recommendations exist in India, Indonesia and Nepal due to the high frequency of fluoroquinolone-resistant *Campylobacter*. Despite lack of data, it is reasonable to extend this recommendation to other Southeast Asian and Indian subcontinent countries.

Sulfamethoxazole/trimethoprim is ineffective against *Campylobacter* and should be used only in areas with low rates of this infection, e.g., inland Mexico during summer.

Several clinical trials have shown the effectiveness of a single dose of antibiotic in the treatment of travellers' diarrhea (see Table 1 for recommended doses). The addition of loperamide to a single dose of antibiotic appears to be particularly effective.[16,19,25]

Travellers' Diarrhea in Children

The management of travellers' diarrhea in children and infants is difficult because of the increased risk and rapid onset of severe and life-threatening dehydration, different infectious agents (e.g., rotavirus in children under three) and more limited antibiotic choices (e.g., fluoroquinolones not recommended in children). Advise parents to travel with **oral rehydration salts** and educate them regarding their use. Seek medical help early. Do not use **loperamide** in children under three. Use loperamide sparingly, if at all, in older children. **Bismuth subsalicylate** (BSS) is contraindicated in children less than three years of age and should be used cautiously in older children. Use of **azithromycin** and **sulfamethoxazole/trimethoprim** in children is limited by the same resistance problems seen in adults. **Ciprofloxacin** has been avoided because of concern over its potential effects on cartilage development. However, studies in the past decade have not shown a problem with the short courses (one to three days) that are used to treat travellers' diarrhea.[26]

Therapeutic Tips

- Mild travellers' diarrhea usually resolves within 24 hours with antimotility agents and fluids.
- Discourage the use of over-the-counter drugs purchased abroad as they are ineffective for both prophylaxis and treatment. Some foreign products contain chloramphenicol, which may induce aplastic anemia, or iodochlorhydroxyquin, which can cause neurologic damage and optic atrophy with prolonged use.
- Investigate symptoms persisting more than two weeks after the return home (history, physical and stool parasitology as part of a first-line investigation). Irritable bowel disease is common. Also consider parasitic infection, antibiotic-associated colitis, disaccharidase deficiency and bowel carcinoma. Inflammatory bowel disease or celiac disease may be unmasked by an episode of travellers' diarrhea.
- Advise patients to seek medical attention if symptoms have not improved within 48 hours.

Figure 1: **Self-Management of Travellers' Diarrhea in Adults**

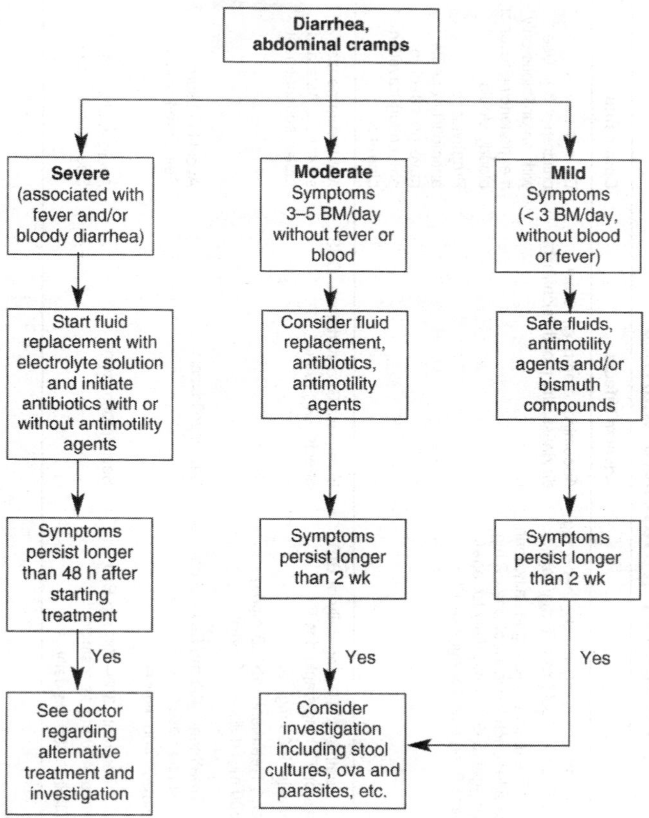

Abbreviations: BM = bowel movements

Table 1: **Drugs Used for the Treatment and Prevention of Travellers' Diarrhea**

Class	Drug	Dose	Adverse Effects	Comments	Cost[a]
Antiperistaltics	*loperamide* Imodium, Riva-Loperamide, generics	Adults: Treatment: 4 mg initially, then 2 mg after each loose stool (max 16 mg/day) Children: Treatment: 1–2 mg initially, then 1–2 mg after each loose stool (max 3 mg daily for ages 3–5 y, 4 mg daily for ages 5–8 y and 6 mg daily for ages 8–12 y)	Abdominal cramping, rarely dizziness, dry mouth, skin rash.	Do not use in children < 3 y. Use with an antibiotic only if experiencing fever or bloody stools. Prophylactic antimotility agents have no effect in preventing travellers' diarrhea.	$
Fluoroquinolones	*ciprofloxacin* Cipro, generics	Adults: Treatment: 500 mg daily or BID × 3 days or 750 mg single dose Prophylaxis:[b] 500 mg daily Children: Treatment: 15–20 mg/kg (max 500 mg) daily × 1–3 days	Infrequent GI disturbance, CNS effects, skin rash.	Not recommended in southeast Asia and Indian subcontinent.	$
	norfloxacin generics	Adults: Treatment: 400 mg BID × 3 days or 800 mg single dose Prophylaxis:[b] 400 mg/day	See ciprofloxacin.	Avoid in children. See ciprofloxacin.	$
	ofloxacin Floxin, generics	Adults: Treatment: 300–400 mg BID × 3 days or 400 mg as a single dose Prophylaxis:[b] 300 mg daily	See ciprofloxacin.	Avoid in children. See ciprofloxacin.	$

Class	Drug	Dose	Adverse Effects	Comments	Cost[a]
Intestinal Adsorbants	*bismuth subsalicylate* Pepto-Bismol, generics	Adults: Treatment: 524 mg (2 tablets) or 30 mL suspension Q30min (max 8 doses/day) Prophylaxis: 524 mg (2 tablets) or 30 mL suspension TID and QHS Children: Treatment: Give the following amounts of bismuth subsalicylate 17.6 mg/mL suspension Q30min (max 8 doses per 24 h): 10–14 y: 15 mL 5–9 y: 7.4 mL 3–4 y: 5 mL	Blackening of stools and tongue, mild tinnitus.	Avoid in patients taking therapeutic doses of salicylates or in whom salicylates are contraindicated (e.g., children and pregnant women). BID dosing is less effective than QID dosing in treating travellers' diarrhea. Avoid concomitant use with doxycycline: ↓ doxycycline absorption.	$
Macrolides	*azithromycin* Zithromax, generics	Adults: Treatment: 500 mg daily × 3 days or 1000 mg single dose Children: Treatment: 5–10 mg/kg (max 500 mg) daily × 1–3 days	GI disturbance infrequently.	Drug of choice for southeast Asia and Indian subcontinent. Can be used in children and in pregnancy. Available as suspension. Not recommended for prophylaxis.	$$

(cont'd)

Table 1: **Drugs Used for the Treatment and Prevention of Travellers' Diarrhea** *(cont'd)*

Class	Drug	Dose	Adverse Effects	Comments	Cost[a]
Sulfonamides	*sulfamethoxazole/ trimethoprim* [renal] generics	Adults: Treatment: 800/160 mg BID × 3 days or 1600/320 mg as a single dose Prophylaxis:[b] 800/160 mg daily Children ≤ 12 y: Treatment: sulfamethoxazole 20–25 mg/kg + trimethoprim 4–5 mg/kg (as pediatric suspension) BID × 3 days	GI disturbances, blood dyscrasias, skin reactions, Stevens-Johnson syndrome (rare).	Available as suspension. Only for regions where sulfamethoxazole/ trimethoprim resistance is uncommon (central Mexico in summer); not first choice in other geographic areas.	$
Vaccines	*Vibrio cholerae whole cell/B subunit vaccine* Dukoral	Prevention of enterotoxigenic *E. coli* diarrhea: Adults and children ≥ 2 y: Primary immunization: 2 doses. 2nd dose administered within 7–42 days after the 1st dose. Booster: 1 dose every 3 mo if the risk is continuous. Take orally on an empty stomach (do not take food or drink 1 h before or 1 h after administration of vaccine).		Variable protection for travellers' diarrhea. Not routinely recommended due to low efficacy rates. Limited protection against heat-labile enterotoxin-producing *E. coli*.	$$$/1 dose

[a] Cost of three-day treatment for adults unless otherwise specified; includes drug cost only.
[b] Prophylactic treatment should be started on the first day in the area of risk and continued for one or two days after return home, to a maximum of three weeks total.
[renal] Dosage adjustment may be required in renal impairment; see Appendix I.
Legend: $ < $10 $$ $10–20 $$$ $20–30

Suggested Readings

Adachi JA, Ostrosky-Zeichner L, DuPont HL et al. Empirical antimicrobial therapy for traveler's diarrhea. *Clin Infect Dis* 2000;31(4):1079-83.

Committee to Advise on Tropical Medicine and Travel (CATMAT). An Advisory Committee Statement (ACS). Statement on travellers' diarrhea. *Can Commun Dis Rep* 2001;27:1-12.

Diemert DJ Prevention and self-treatment of traveler's diarrhea. *Clin Microbiol Rev* 2006;19(3):583-94.

Plourde PJ. Travellers' diarrhea in children. *Paediatr Child Health* 2003;8(2):99-103.

References

1. Hill DR, Ericsson CD, Pearson RD et al. The practice of travel medicine: guidelines by the Infectious Diseases Society of America. *Clin Infect Dis* 2006;43(12):1499-539.
2. DuPont HL. New insights and directions in traveler's diarrhea. *Gastroenterol Clin North Am* 2006;35(2):337-53.
3. Black RE. Epidemiology of travelers' diarrhea and relative importance of various pathogens. *Rev Infect Dis* 1990;12(Suppl 1):S73-9.
4. Adachi JA, Jiang ZD, Mathewson JJ et al. Enteroaggregative Escherichia coli as a major etiologic agent in traveler's diarrhea in 3 regions of the world. *Clin Infect Dis* 2001;32(12):1706-9.
5. Steffen R, van der Linde F, Gyr K et al. Epidemiology of diarrhea in travelers. *JAMA* 1983;249(9):1176-80.
6. Centers for Disease Control and Prevention.*Travelers' health: yellow book. Health information for international travel, 2005-2006.* Atlanta (GA): CDC; 2006. Available from: http://www2.ncid.cdc.gov/travel/yb/utils/ybBrowseC.asp Accessed June 1, 2007.
7. DuPont HL, Ericsson CD, Johnson PC et al. Prevention of travelers' diarrhea by the tablet formulation of bismuth subsalicylate. *JAMA* 1987;257(10):1347-50.
8. Rademaker CM, Hoepelman IM, Wolfhagen MJ et al. Results of a double-blind placebo-controlled study using ciprofloxacin for prevention of travelers' diarrhea. *Eur J Clin Microbiol Infect Dis* 1989;8(8):690-4.
9. Wistrom J, Norrby SR, Burman LG et al. Norfloxacin versus placebo for prophylaxis against travellers' diarrhoea. *J Antimicrob Chemother* 1987;20(4):563-74.
10. Jain D, Sinha S, Prasad KN et al. Campylobacter species and drug resistance in a north Indian rural community. *Trans R Soc Trop Med Hyg* 2005;99(3):207-14.
11. Shlim DR. Update in traveler's diarrhea. *Infect Dis Clin North Am* 2005;9(1):137-49.
12. DuPont HL, Jiang ZD, Okhuysen PC et al. A randomized, double-blind, placebo-controlled trial of rifaximin to prevent travelers' diarrhea. *Ann Intern Med* 2005;142(10):805-12.
13. Peltola H, Siitonen A, Kyronseppa H et al. Prevention of travellers' diarrhoea by oral B-subunit/whole-cell cholera vaccine. *Lancet* 1991;338(8778):1285-9.
14. Committee to Advise on Tropical Medicine and Travel (CATMAT); National Advisory Committee on Immunization (NACI). Statement on new oral cholera and travellers' diarrhea vaccination. *Can Commun Dis Rep* 2005;31(ACS-7):1-11.
15. *Canadian immunization guide.* 7th edition. Ottawa (ON): Public Health Agency of Canada; 2006. Available from: http://www.phac-aspc.gc.ca/publicat/cig-gci/pdf/cig-gci-2006_e.pdf Accessed June 7, 2007.
16. Committee to Advise on Tropical Medicine and Travel (CATMAT). An Advisory Committee Statement (ACS). Statement on travellers' diarrhea. *Can Commun Dis Rep* 2001;27:1-12.
17. Adachi JA, Ostrosky-Zeichner L, DuPont HL et al. Empirical antimicrobial therapy for traveler's diarrhea. *Clin Infect Dis* 2000;31(4):1079-83.
18. Johnson PC, Ericsson CD, DuPont HL et al. Comparison of loperamide with bismuth subsalicylate for the treatment of acute travelers' diarrhea. *JAMA* 1986;255(6):757-60.
19. Ericsson CD, DuPont HL, Mathewson JJ et al. Treatment of traveler's diarrhea with sulfamethoxazole and trimethoprim and loperamide. *JAMA* 1990;263(2):257-61.
20. Taylor DN, Sanchez JL, Candler W et al. Treatment of travelers' diarrhea: ciprofloxacin plus loperamide compared with ciprofloxacin alone. A placebo-controlled, randomized trial. *Ann Intern Med* 1991;114(9):731-4.
21. DuPont HL, Hornick RB. Adverse effect of lomotil therapy in shigellosis. *JAMA* 1973;226(13):1525-8.
22. DuPont HL, Ericsson CD, Mathewson JJ et al. Five versus three days of ofloxacin therapy for traveler's diarrhea: a placebo-controlled study. *Antimicrob Agents Chemother* 1992;36(1):87-91.

23. Salam I, Katelaris P, Leigh-Smith S, et al. Randomised trial of single-dose ciprofloxacin for travellers' diarrhoea. *Lancet* 1994;344(8936):1537-9.
24. Kuschner RA, Trofa AF, Thomas RJ et al. Use of azithromycin for the treatment of Campylobacter enteritis in travelers to Thailand, an area where ciprofloxacin resistance is prevalent. *Clin Infect Dis* 1995;21(3):536-41.
25. Ericsson CD, DuPont HL, Mathewson JJ. Single dose ofloxacin plus loperamide compared with single dose or three days of ofloxacin in the treatment of traveler's diarrhea. *J Travel Med* 1997;4(1):3-7.
26. Grady R. Safety profile of quinolone antibiotics in the pediatric population. *Pediatr Infect Dis J* 2003;22(12):1128-32.

CHAPTER 110
Malaria Prevention

W.L. Wobeser, MD, FRCPC and
J.S. Keystone, MD, FRCPC

Malaria results in more than 1 million deaths worldwide each year. The risk of malaria for travellers is *greatest* in sub-Saharan Africa and Oceania, *intermediate* on the Indian subcontinent and Haiti and *lowest* in Southeast Asia and Latin America. There is regional and seasonal variation of risk within these areas. Each year in Canada 300–400 cases of malaria are reported along with several deaths. Since malaria is a potentially fatal disease, it is of utmost importance that travellers take appropriate measures to prevent this infection.

Goals of Therapy

- Assess risk of acquisition of malaria
- Provide safe and effective chemoprophylaxis

Therapeutic Choices (Figure 1)
Nonpharmacologic Choices

Malaria transmission by the anopheline mosquito mainly occurs between dusk and dawn. The following measures optimize protection during this time:

- Use **insect repellents** containing **diethyltoluamide** (DEET) before outdoor activity during the main hours of malarial transmission. DEET has been rarely associated with neurologic side effects in children exposed to high concentrations (> 35%) and prolonged use. The American Academy of Pediatrics now recommends that 30% DEET may be used in children as young as 2 months of age.[1]
- In standard formulations, 30% DEET is effective for four to six hours. Citronella is usually effective for less than one hour.[2,3]
- Use *bed nets*, preferably impregnated with **permethrin**.[4]
- Use *mosquito coils*, *aerosolized insecticides* or *electrically operated insecticide generators* containing **pyrethroids**.
- Wear clothes covering exposed skin, weather permitting. Sleep in an air-conditioned or screened room if possible.

Pharmacologic Choices (Table 1)
Principles of Chemoprophylaxis[5]

Determinants of acquisition risk include malaria endemicity, season, altitude, degree of rural travel and preventive measures for mosquito bites. Additional considerations in choosing chemoprophylaxis include antimalarial drug resistance, side effects, concurrent medications and illnesses, contraindications, pregnancy, age and allergies. All travellers to an endemic area require prophylaxis. Check an up-to-date source (e.g., Centers for Disease Control and Prevention at www.cdc.gov/travel or Public Health Agency of Canada at www.travelhealth.gc.ca) about the location and extent of drug-resistant Plasmodium species when counselling patients about malaria chemoprophylaxis, as recommendations may change periodically.

In Canada, **chloroquine** is recommended for prevention of malaria in areas where the parasite is still sensitive to this drug (i.e., Central America except Panama, Haiti and parts of the Dominican Republic and Middle East). In areas where chloroquine-resistant *P. falciparum* malaria exists, **mefloquine**, **doxycycline** or **atovaquone/proguanil** are the drugs of choice. **Primaquine** is an effective alternative. The combination of chloroquine and proguanil should not be used because it has limited efficacy in areas with chloroquine-resistant *P. falciparum*. Drugs that are effective in chloroquine-resistant areas may also be used in chloroquine-sensitive areas. Physicians without experience and expertise in malaria chemoprophylaxis should strongly consider referring patients to a well recognized travel medicine clinic.

Chloroquine and Hydroxychloroquine

Chloroquine is the drug of choice in areas where chloroquine-resistant *P. falciparum* malaria has not occurred. Hydroxychloroquine is an acceptable alternative to chloroquine and shares a similar side effect profile; however a different dose may be used. Chloroquine should be started one to two weeks before travelling to and continued until four weeks after leaving a malarious area.

Mefloquine[6,7,8]

Mefloquine is used to prevent malaria in travellers going to areas reporting chloroquine-resistant *P. falciparum*. However, resistance to mefloquine is clinically important along the Thai–Cambodian and Thai–Myanmar borders, Eastern Myanmar, Western Cambodia and South/Central Vietnam, and therefore it should not be used. Severe neuropsychiatric reactions (seizures and psychosis) occur in 1:13 000 patients who use the drug at appropriate prophylactic doses.[9,10] Less severe, disabling, neuropsychological side effects (e.g., anxiety, nightmares, depression, irritability) occur in about 1:250 to 500 users.[9,10] Mefloquine is contraindicated in those with a history of seizures, psychosis, depression or a recent anxiety disorder. Mefloquine should be started one to two weeks before travelling to and continued until four weeks after leaving a malarious area. Since most adverse events occur during the first three doses, many practitioners recommend starting the drug four weeks prior to departure to ensure tolerance. If a traveller does not have four weeks prior to departure, a loading dose may be given; one tablet is given daily for three days followed by weekly dosing thereafter. Should a dose be forgotten, the traveller can take the dose right away since mefloquine has a very long half life and, therefore, mefloquine blood levels have a lower chance of dropping below effective levels.

Doxycycline[7]

Doxycycline is recommended for those travelling to chloroquine-resistant areas who cannot take mefloquine and for those travelling to mefloquine-resistant areas. Unlike mefloquine, daily dosing is required. Users are advised to avoid prolonged sun exposure and to use a sunscreen that absorbs UVA radiation (see Chapter 79). Doxycycline should be taken with food and liberal amounts of fluids while in the upright position. Doxycycline chemoprophylaxis should begin one to two days before entry to the area and continue for four weeks after departure from the area. Doxycycline is contraindicated in pregnancy and children < 8 y.

Primaquine[11,12,13]

Primaquine is used for terminal prophylaxis, i.e., "radical cure," in long-term travellers returning from areas with *P. vivax* and *P. ovale*, both of which have dormant liver forms (hypnozoites). Hypnozoites are not affected by chloroquine or mefloquine. Primaquine may also be used as a prophylactic agent in areas of chloroquine-resistant *P. falciparum* malaria. It is a very effective prophylactic agent but must be taken daily. It is about 5–10% less effective than the drugs of choice (mefloquine, doxycycline, atovaquone/proguanil) for the prevention of chloroquine-resistant falciparum malaria. Primaquine should be started one to two days before entry to and continue for only three days after departure from the area. It is well tolerated and has few side effects when taken with food.

Primaquine is a potent oxidizing agent which can induce severe hemolytic anemia in those with G6PD deficiency. In risk groups for this enzyme deficiency (Blacks, Mediterraneans, Asians and Southeast Asians), a G6PD level is mandatory before primaquine is used. The drug is contraindicated in pregnancy.

Atovaquone/Proguanil[6,14,15,16]

Atovaquone/proguanil is better tolerated than mefloquine. Uncommon adverse effects include GI upset, headache, insomnia, cough and mouth ulcers. Atovaquone/proguanil should be taken daily with food, starting one to two days before entry to a malarious area and may be discontinued one week after departure from the area. The drug is not recommended in pregnancy or infants < 5 kg.[17,18]

Malaria Prevention in Special Populations

Pregnancy and Infancy

Pregnant women and young children should avoid travel to areas where chloroquine-resistant malaria is endemic. If travel is unavoidable, effective protection against mosquitoes and appropriate chemoprophylaxis is strongly recommended. Doxycycline, atovaquone/proguanil and primaquine are contraindicated in pregnancy.

Doxycycline is contraindicated in children < 8 years old or < 11 kg. In chloroquine-sensitive areas, chloroquine is recommended for pregnant women and young children. In chloroquine-resistant areas, mefloquine has been shown to be safe after the first trimester of pregnancy and can be used in children > 5 kg. Limited data suggest that mefloquine may also be safe in the first trimester.[19] Azithromycin is safe in pregnant women and young children but is suboptimally effective. There is no safe and effective chemoprophylaxis for pregnant women or children < 11 kg who travel to mefloquine-resistant areas.

Therapeutic Tips

- Mefloquine is not favoured as a prophylactic agent by some physicians in the United Kingdom and in developing countries. Travellers may be advised by physicians and travellers from these areas that they are on a dangerous drug. In general, such advice should be accepted politely and ignored.
- No currently available regimen of malaria chemoprophylaxis is ideal and completely effective. Adhering to the chemoprophylaxis regimen helps reduce the risk of malaria acquisition. Drug-resistant malaria continues to spread.
- Remind travellers in writing to continue taking their antimalarials even after their return from an endemic region. All travellers in whom fever develops within one year (particularly within three months) of return from a malaria-endemic area must be considered to have malaria, regardless of chemoprophylaxis. Consider this a medical emergency. Request thick and thin blood films to rule out malaria. If negative, repeat them twice over 48 hours.
- In sub-Saharan Africa, the rate of false positive blood films for malaria is at least 40%.[20] Travellers in this area should be warned that if they are taking an appropriate antimalarial regularly and are diagnosed with "malaria," they should follow the advice of local practitioners, but not stop their chemoprophylaxis.
- Travellers are advised to buy their full supply of medications before departure. The sale of poor quality and counterfeit antimalarials is rampant in the developing world.[21]

Figure 1: **Malaria Prophylaxis**

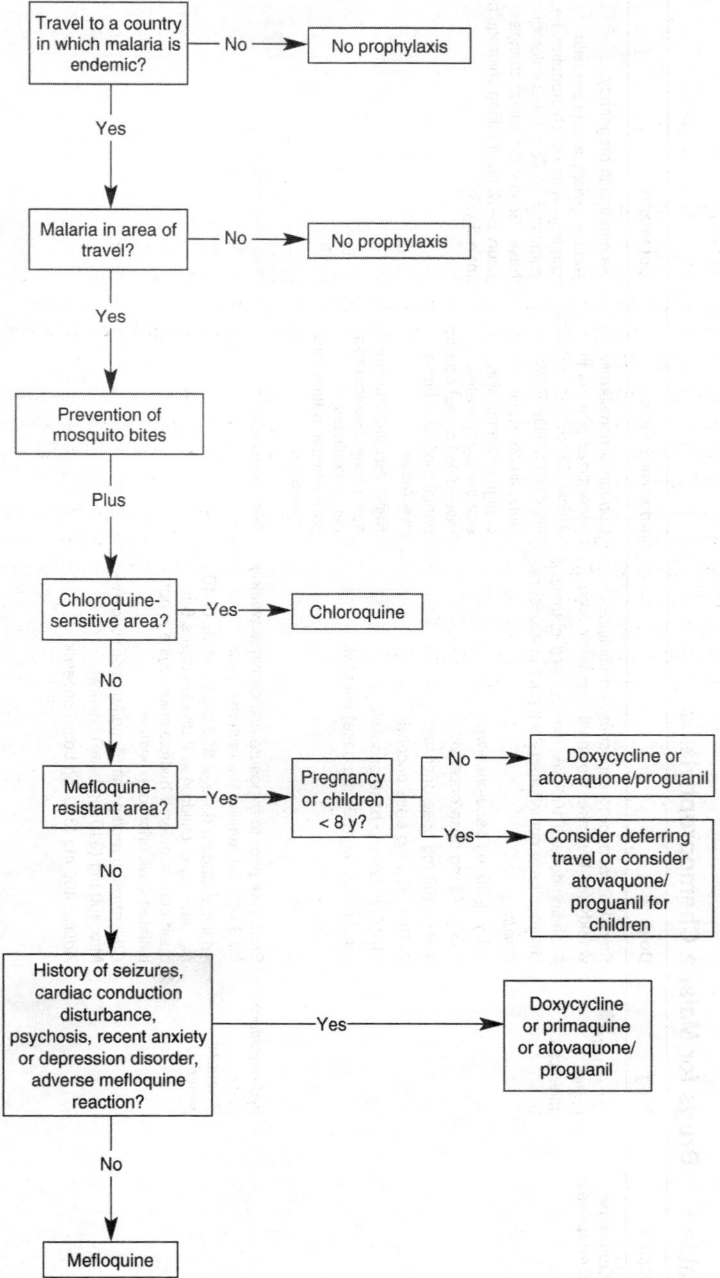

Table 1: Drugs for Malaria Chemoprophylaxis

Class	Drug	Dose	Adverse Effects	Comments	Cost[a]
Quinoline Derivatives	*chloroquine* Aralen, generics	Start 1–2 wk prior to exposure and continue **weekly** for 4 wk after leaving the endemic area A loading dose of 1000 mg can be used in adults if chloroquine is not initiated 2 wk prior to exposure. *Children:* < 1 y: 37.5 mg base once/wk 1–3 y: 75 mg base once/wk 4–6 y: 100 mg base once/wk 7–10 y: 150 mg base once/wk 11–16 y: 225 mg base once/wk *Adults:* 500 mg (300 mg base) once/wk	Common: nonallergic generalized pruritus in African Canadians, vomiting, headache, bitter taste. Uncommon: hair depigmentation, skin eruptions, myopathy, reversible corneal opacity, partial alopecia, blood dyscrasias. Rare: nail and mucous membrane discolouration, nerve deafness, photophobia, retinopathy, myopathy.	Safe to use in pregnancy. Retinal toxicity a concern with continuous use of chloroquine, i.e., cumulative dose > 100 g chloroquine base. Screen for retinal changes every 6–12 mo if taking chloroquine for > 5 y.[22,23]	$
	hydroxychloroquine Plaquenil, generics	Start 2 wk prior to exposure and continue **weekly** for 8 wk after leaving the endemic area. An initial loading dose of 800 mg to adults or 10 mg base/kg to children in 2 divided doses 6 h apart can be given if hydroxychloroquine is not initiated 2 wk prior to exposure *Children:* 6.5 mg/kg salt (5 mg/kg base) once/wk. Max 400 mg (310 mg base) once/wk *Adults*: 400 mg (310 mg base) once/wk	See chloroquine.	See chloroquine.	$$

Class	Drug	Dose	Adverse Effects	Comments	Cost[a]
	mefloquine Lariam	Start one wk prior to exposure, **weekly** during the stay in the region and weekly for 4 wk after leaving the endemic area Administer with a meal and with at least 240 mL of water *Children:* 5–9 kg: 31.25 mg base/wk 10–19 kg: 62.5 mg base/wk 20–30 kg: 125 mg base/wk 31–45 kg: 187.5 mg base/wk > 45 kg: adult dose *Adults:* 250 mg base once/wk Loading dose: 250 mg base once daily for 3 days, then 250 mg base weekly thereafter	Common: GI upset, dizziness, nausea, vomiting, diarrhea, headaches, sinus bradycardia, nightmares, insomnia, mood alteration, anxiety, irritability. Uncommon: hair loss, skin rash. Rare: seizures, psychosis, thrombotic-thrombocytopenia purpura.[24]	Used in regions of chloroquine-resistant *P. falciparum*; does not prevent multidrug-resistant *P. falciparum.* Contraindicated in patients with seizure disorders, active depression, recent history of depression episodes, anxiety disorders. Loading dose confers quicker attainment of steady state (4 days as opposed to 7–9 wk). Considered to be safe in 2nd and 3rd trimesters of pregnancy.	$$$$$
	primaquine Primaquine	Start one day prior to exposure, continue **daily** while in the malarial region and for 3 days after leaving the endemic area Administer with food *Children:* Prophylaxis: 0.5 mg base/kg/day. Max 30 mg base once/day Post-exposure: 0.5 mg base/kg/day × 14 days. Max 30 mg base once/day *Adults:* Prophylaxis: 52.6 mg (30 mg base) once/day; < 60 kg: 0.5 base/kg/day. Max 30 mg base once/day[25] Post-exposure: 52.6 mg (30 mg base) once/day × 14 days	Common: hemolysis with G6PD deficiency. Uncommon: GI upset (take with food). Rare: methemoglobinemia.	Used in regions of chloroquine-resistant *P. falciparum.* Determine G6PD deficiency in all individuals prior to administration. Contraindicated in pregnancy because of unknown G6PD status of infant and subsequent risk of hemolysis. Methemoglobinemia has been precipitated in HIV-infected patients who are being treated or are on prophylactic therapy for *P. jirovecii* pneumonia, especially if taken with dapsone.[25,26,27]	$$

(cont'd)

Table 1: **Drugs for Malaria Chemoprophylaxis** *(cont'd)*

Class	Drug	Dose	Adverse Effects	Comments	Cost[a]
Tetracyclines	*doxycycline* (renal symbol) Vibra-Tabs, generics	Start one day prior to exposure, continue **daily** while in the malarial region and for 4 wk after leaving the endemic area Administer with food and plenty of water. Important not to recline after administration. *Children:* ≥ 8 y: 2 mg/kg/day. Max 100 mg/day *Adults:* 100 mg once/day	Common: GI upset, photosensitivity, staining of teeth in children and fetuses, *candida vaginitis* (use fluconazole for self-treatment). Uncommon: azotemia in renal disease, enterocolitis. Rare: allergic reactions, blood dyscrasias, esophageal ulcerations.	Used in regions of chloroquine-resistant *P. falciparum*; can be used for prevention of multidrug-resistant *P. falciparum.* Contraindicated in pregnancy and children < 8 y. Because of the increased risk of photosensitivity, use sunscreens to block UV radiation.	$$$$$
Antimalarials, combination	*atovaquone/ proguanil* (renal symbol) Malarone, Malarone Pediatric	Start one day prior to exposure, continue **daily** while in the malarial region and for 1 wk after leaving the endemic area Administer with a meal *Children:* Use Malarone Pediatric (62.5 mg/25 mg) 5–8 kg:[17] 1/2 tab daily 9–10 kg:[17] 3/4 tab daily 11–20 kg: 1 tab daily 21–30 kg: 2 tabs daily 31–40 kg: 3 tabs daily > 40 kg: 250 mg/100 mg daily; use Malarone *Adults:* 250 mg/100 mg daily; use Malarone ClCr < 30 mL/min: Avoid	Common: GI upset, headache.	Used in regions of chloroquine-resistant *P. falciparum*; can be used for prevention of multidrug-resistant *P. falciparum.* Acts on pre-erythrocytic hepatic phase of malaria but it does not prevent the hypnozoite formation by *P. ovale* or *P. vivax.* Not recommended in pregnancy. Contraindicated in patients with renal insufficiency.	$$$$$

[a] Cost of two-week supply of adult dosage for 1 week of travel; includes drug cost only.
(renal symbol) Dosage adjustment may be required in renal impairment; see Appendix I.
Legend: $ < $5 $$ $5–10 $$$ $10–15 $$$$ $15–20 $$$$$ > $20

Suggested Readings

Baird JK, Fryauff DJ, Hoffman SL. Primaquine for prevention of malaria in travelers. *Clin Infect Dis* 2003;37(12):1659-67.

Chen LH, Keystone JS. New strategies for the prevention of malaria in travelers. *Infect Dis Clin North Am* 2005;19(1):185-210.

Fischer PR, Bialek R. Prevention of malaria in children. *Clin Infect Dis* 2002;34(4):493-8.

Fradin MS. Mosquitoes and mosquito repellents: a clinician's guide. *Ann Intern Med* 1998;128(11):931-40.

References

1. American Academy of Pediatrics. *West Nile Virus information. Follow safety precautions when using DEET on children.* Elk Grove Village (IL): American Academy of Pediatrics; 2003. Available from: http://www.aap.org/family/wnv-jun03.htm Accessed February 28, 2007.
2. Fradin MS, Day JF. Comparative efficacy of insect repellents against mosquito bites. *N Engl J Med* 2002;347(1):13-8.
3. Hill DR, Ericsson CD, Pearson RD et al. The practice of travel medicine: guidelines by the Infectious Diseases Society of America. *Clin Infect Dis* 2006;43(12):1499-539.
4. Nevill CG, Some ES, Mung'ala VO et al. Insecticide-treated bednets reduce mortality and severe morbidity from malaria among children on the Kenyan coast. *Trop Med Int Health* 1996;1(2):139-46.
5. Kain KC, Shanks GD, Keystone JS. Malaria chemoprophylaxis in the age of drug resistance. I. Currently recommended drug regimens. *Clin Infect Dis* 2001;33(2):226-34.
6. Nosten F, ter KF, Maelankiri L et al. Mefloquine prophylaxis prevents malaria during pregnancy: a double-blind, placebo-controlled study. *J Infect Dis* 1994;169(3):595-603.
7. Ohrt C, Richie TL, Widjaja H et al. Mefloquine compared with doxycycline for the prophylaxis of malaria in Indonesian soldiers. A randomized, double-blind, placebo-controlled trial. *Ann Intern Med* 1997;126(12):963-72.
8. Overbosch D, Schilthuis H, Bienzle U et al. Atovaquone-proguanil versus mefloquine for malaria prophylaxis in nonimmune travelers: results from a randomized, double-blind study. *Clin Infect Dis* 2001;33(7):1015-21.
9. Taylor WR, White NJ. Antimalarial drug toxicity: a review. *Drug Saf* 2004;27(1):25-61.
10. Palmer KJ, Holliday SM, Brogden RN. Mefloquine. A review of its antimalarial activity, pharmacokinetic properties and therapeutic efficacy. *Drugs* 1993;45(3):430-75.
11. Baird JK, Lacy MD, Basri H et al. Randomized, parallel placebo-controlled trial of primaquine for malaria prophylaxis in Papua, Indonesia. *Clin Infect Dis* 2001;33(12):1990-7.
12. Soto J, Toledo J, Rodriquez M et al. Primaquine prophylaxis against malaria in nonimmune Colombian soldiers: efficacy and toxicity. A randomized, double-blind, placebo-controlled trial. *Ann Intern Med* 1998;129(3):241-4.
13. Weiss WR, Oloo AJ, Johnson A et al. Daily primaquine is effective for prophylaxis against falciparum malaria in Kenya: comparison with mefloquine, doxycycline, and chloroquine plus proguanil. *J Infect Dis* 1995;171(6):1569-75.
14. Faucher JF, Binder R, Missinou MA et al. Efficacy of atovaquone/proguanil for malaria prophylaxis in children and its effect on the immunogenicity of live oral typhoid and cholera vaccines. *Clin Infect Dis* 2002;35(10):1147-54.
15. Ling J, Baird JK, Fryauff DJ et al. Randomized, placebo-controlled trial of atovaquone/proguanil for the prevention of Plasmodium falciparum or Plasmodium vivax malaria among migrants to Papua, Indonesia. *Clin Infect Dis* 2002;35(7):825-33.
16. Sukwa TY, Mulenga M, Chisdaka N et al.. A randomized, double-blind, placebo-controlled field trial to determine the efficacy and safety of Malarone (atovaquone/proguanil) for the prophylaxis of malaria in Zambia. *Am J Trop Med Hyg* 1999;60(4):521-5.
17. Boggild AK, Parise ME, Lewis LS et al. Atovaquone-proguanil: report from the CDC expert meeting on malaria chemoprophylaxis (II). *Am J Trop Med Hyg* 2007;76(2):208-223.
18. Borrmann S, Faucher JF, Bagaphou T et al. Atovaquone and proguanil versus amodiaquine for the treatment of *Plasmodium falciparum* malaria in African infants and young children. *Clin Infect Dis* 2003;37:1441-7.
19. Phillips-Howard PA, Steffen R, Kerr L et al. Safety of mefloquine and other antimalarial agents in the first trimester of pregnancy. *J Travel Med* 1998;5(3):121-6.
20. Reyburn H, Mbatia R, Drakeley C et al. Overdiagnosis of malaria in patients with severe febrile illness in Tanzania: a prospective study. *BMJ* 2004;329(7476):1212.
21. Dondorp AM, Newton PN, Mayxay M et al. Fake antimalarials in Southeast Asia are a major impediment to malaria control: multinational cross-sectional survey on the prevalence of fake antimalarials. *Trop Med Int Health* 2004;9(12):1241-6.

22. Chen LH, Wilson ME, Schlagenhauf P. Prevention of malaria in long-term travelers. *JAMA* 2006;296(18):2234-44.
23. Hughes C, Tucker R, Bannister B et al. Malaria prophylaxis for long-term travellers. *Commun Dis Public Health* 2003;6(3):200-8.
24. Fiaccadori E, Maggiore U, Rotelli C et al. Thrombotic-thrombocytopenic purpura following malaria prophylaxis with mefloquine. *J Antimicrob Chemother* 2006;57(1):160-1.
25. Hill DR, Baird JK, Parise ME et al. Primaquine: report from CDC expert meeting on malaria chemoprophylaxis I. *Am J Trop Med Hyg* 2006;75(3):402-15.
26. Sin DD, Shafran SD. Dapsone- and primaquine-induced methemoglobinemia in HIV-infected individuals. *J Acquir Immune Defic Syndr Hum Retrovirol* 1996;12(5):477-81.
27. Kantor GS. Primaquine-induced methemoglobinemia during treatment of Pneumocystis carinii pneumonia. *N Engl J Med* 1992;327(20):1461.

CHAPTER 111
Chemotherapy-induced Nausea and Vomiting

Lynne Nakashima, PharmD

Goals of Therapy

- Prevent or minimize *acute* (starting within 24 hours of chemotherapy), *delayed* (starting > 24 hours after chemotherapy) and *anticipatory* (starting before chemotherapy as a conditioned response) nausea and vomiting to help patient adherence with active treatment and to maintain quality of life
- Decrease incidence of nausea and vomiting (once it has occurred) and maintain patient comfort[1]
- Prevent complications such as esophageal tears, dehydration, anorexia, malnutrition, weight loss, pathological bone fractures, metabolic alkalosis, chloride and potassium depletion[1]

Investigations

- A thorough history including:
  - onset and duration of symptoms
  - timing of nausea and/or retching and/or vomiting
  - impact on the patient, e.g., weight loss, asthenia
  - description of the vomiting episodes
  - medications the patient is taking
- Physical examination with particular attention to:
  - orthostatic hypotension
  - abdominal pain, distention, constipation, hemorrhage
  - neurologic assessment including cranial nerves, vestibular and pupillary function, extrapyramidal signs
- Laboratory tests:
  - electrolytes: BUN, creatinine, sodium, potassium, chloride (to assess hydration status); calcium, albumin (to assess for hypercalcemia)
  - drug screening, such as for digoxin if suspected as a cause of nausea and vomiting

Although medication is the most likely cause of nausea and vomiting in a patient receiving chemotherapy, other potential causes (e.g., fluid/electrolyte abnormalities, bowel obstruction, CNS or hepatic metastases, infections and radiation therapy) should be ruled out. Other drugs (e.g., opioids, digoxin, antibiotics) may cause or exacerbate nausea and vomiting so a thorough medication history is essential.

Some chemotherapeutic agents are more likely to cause nausea and vomiting than others (Table 1). Therefore it is important to consider both the emetogenic potential and the expected pattern of emesis of the chemotherapy regimen when choosing antiemetics.[3,4,5,6,7]

Table 1: **Emetogenic Potential of Chemotherapy Agents**[a]

High (> 60%)		
carmustine cisplatin (> 50 mg/m²) cyclophosphamide (> 550 mg/m²)	cytarabine (> 500 mg/m²) dacarbazine dactinomycin (> 1.5 g/m²)	lomustine mechlorethamine streptozocin
Moderate (30–60%)		
capecitabine carboplatin daunorubicin doxorubicin	epirubicin ifosfamide irinotecan	methotrexate (dose-dependent) oxaliplatin procarbazine vinblastine
Low (< 30%)		
altretamine (hexamethylmelamine) amsacrine androgens aromatase inhibitors bevacizumab bleomycin bortezomib busulfan cetuximab chlorambucil docetaxel estramustine estrogens etoposide 5-fluorouracil	fludarabine gemcitabine hydroxyurea L-asparaginase melphalan mercaptopurine mitomycin mitoxantrone paclitaxel pemetrexed progestins ralitrexed	rituximab 6-thioguanine tamoxifen teniposide thiotepa topotecan trastuzumab vincristine vindesine vinorelbine

[a] Slowing infusion rate of certain chemotherapeutic agents (e.g., cisplatin) may decrease emesis.[2]

Patient-specific factors such as age less than 50 years, female gender, previous motion sickness or pregnancy-related nausea and vomiting, limited alcohol use and nausea and vomiting with previous chemotherapy regimens may predispose the patient to nausea and vomiting; therefore, antiemetic regimens must also be tailored to the individual patient.

Therapeutic Choices (Figure 1)

Nonpharmacologic Choices[1,8,9,10]

- Dietary adjustments
  - try small, light meals several times daily.
  - avoid foods high in fat or those with a heavy aroma.
  - try dry, starchy foods such as crackers.

  - if unable to tolerate solid foods, try ice chips and small sips of clear liquids.
  - avoid food preparation because the smell of food cooking often worsens nausea.
- Behavioural methods
  - relaxation techniques may help decrease physiologic arousal and anxiety.
  - individualized exercise programs may help decrease anxiety and depression.
  - systemic desensitization may be helpful for anticipatory nausea and vomiting.
- Other
  - keep movement to a minimum; rest in bed or a chair to avoid vestibular stimulation.
  - acupuncture and acupressure have been shown to have some effect on chemotherapy-induced emesis.[11]
  - sleep has been shown to protect against chemotherapy-induced nausea and vomiting.[12]

Pharmacologic Choices (Figure 1, Table 2)

Phenothiazines

The most commonly used is **prochlorperazine**. Considered moderately effective, it is usually used in low emetogenic regimens or as rescue medication.[3,13] The availability of a wide variety of dosage forms (tablet, suppository, injectable) facilitates prochlorperazine use, especially for outpatients.

Metoclopramide

Metoclopramide blocks the dopaminergic receptors in the chemoreceptor trigger zone and has serotonin antagonistic activity at higher doses. Low doses (10 to 20 mg) are generally as effective as prochlorperazine; however, in high doses (1 to 3 mg/kg), metoclopramide provides significantly higher antiemetic activity.[3,14] When metoclopramide is compared to serotonin antagonists for acute antiemetic efficacy against highly emetogenic chemotherapy, serotonin antagonists are superior and have fewer side effects.[15,16,17,18] For delayed nausea and vomiting, metoclopramide plus a corticosteroid are as effective as a serotonin antagonist plus a corticosteroid and are more cost effective.[15,19] A limitation to metoclopramide use is the development of extrapyramidal side effects.

Corticosteroids

Dexamethasone is the most commonly used corticosteroid, although several others including **methylprednisolone** have been studied.[20] The actual mechanism of action is unknown, but the efficacy of corticosteroids is documented. They appear to be effective as single agents, in combination with other antiemetics and for delayed nausea and vomiting.[20,21] Dexamethasone *in combination with* a **serotonin antagonist** is the most effective antiemetic regimen for *acute nausea and vomiting.*[19,22,23] Dexamethasone *alone or in combination with* **metoclopramide** appears to be the most effective regimen for *delayed nausea and vomiting.*[21,24,25,26] The optimal dose has not been identified; the usual range is from 6 to 60 mg daily.[20]

Serotonin Antagonists

The serotonin antagonists **dolasetron**, **granisetron** and **ondansetron** are equivalent in efficacy and toxicity.[27,28] Two newer serotonin antagonists are now available in the US: palonosetron and tropisetron.[29,30] Single agent efficacy is reported, but when used *in combination with* corticosteroids, efficacy is improved. The combination is recommended for the prevention of acute nausea and vomiting unless the patient has a contraindication to corticosteroids.[22,23] Serotonin antagonists plus corticosteroids are no more effective for delayed nausea and vomiting than metoclopramide plus corticosteroids or corticosteroids alone.[24,25] These drugs are well tolerated. At equivalent doses, oral formulations are equally effective and as safe as intravenous.[31] The major drawback to their use is cost. However, because of their superior efficacy, serotonin antagonists should be used for the prophylaxis of acute nausea and vomiting for moderately and highly emetogenic regimens. Choose serotonin antagonist based on cost.

Benzodiazepines

Benzodiazepines provide useful antianxiety, amnesic and sedating effects. **Lorazepam** and **alprazolam** are the most commonly used, and have been studied in cases of anticipatory nausea.[32,33] They are usually used in combination with other antiemetics.

Butyrophenones

Haloperidol has reported efficacy and is generally used as an alternative to high-dose metoclopramide or ondansetron in refractory nausea and vomiting.[34,35]

Cannabinoids

Nabilone and **dronabinol** are of limited use because they are available only as oral formulations and are associated with several side effects including mood alterations, hallucinations, delusions and increases in heart rate and blood pressure.[3,36,37,38] They are generally used in refractory nausea and vomiting or in combination with other antiemetics.[3,36]

Dimenhydrinate

An antihistamine useful for treating vomiting due to motion sickness, dimenhydrinate is considered no more effective than placebo against chemotherapy-induced nausea and vomiting.[39]

Scopolamine

Available as a transdermal system placed behind the ear, scopolamine can prevent vomiting related to motion sickness but is generally ineffective in managing nausea and vomiting associated with chemotherapy.[39,40]

Propofol

Propofol is an anesthetic agent with antiemetic properties.[5] Several studies suggest that a continuous infusion at low doses (1 mg/kg/hour) is effective in patients with cisplatin-induced nausea and vomiting that is refractory to serotonin antagonists combined with corticosteroids.[41,42,43] Its use is still considered investigational; however, propofol use may be considered in severe, refractory vomiting. Expertise in administration is required.

Neurokinin-1 Receptor Antagonists

Neurokinin-1 (NK1) receptor antagonists bind to substance P, found in the brainstem and GI tract. **Aprepitant** is the first in this class, and is available in the US. When added to a serotonin antagonist plus dexamethasone regimen for highly emetogenic chemotherapy, it improves prevention of acute and delayed emesis.[44,45] Aprepitant is a moderate inhibitor of CYP3A4, and interacts with corticosteroids. Therefore the dose of dexamethasone as an antiemetic in clinical trials was lowered. Aprepitant appears to be well tolerated, with asthenia/fatigue and hiccoughs being the most commonly reported side effects.[46]

Therapeutic Tips

- Prevention of acute nausea and vomiting is the best way to prevent delayed nausea and vomiting.
- Use antiemetic therapy to *prevent* anticipatory nausea and vomiting, which usually worsens with each cycle; up to 30% of patients refuse further chemotherapy because of intolerable nausea and vomiting.[3,4]
- *Regularly scheduled and administered* antiemetics (i.e., not PRN) are more effective at preventing nausea and vomiting.
- If the patient can tolerate oral antiemetics, this is the recommended route of administration. However, *rectally* administered antiemetics such as prochlorperazine are especially useful in patients who are vomiting or unable to take oral medications and who are at home. For hospitalized patients, the *iv route* of administration is recommended in patients who are vomiting.

Figure 1: **Management of Chemotherapy-induced Nausea and Vomiting (low emetogenic potential)**

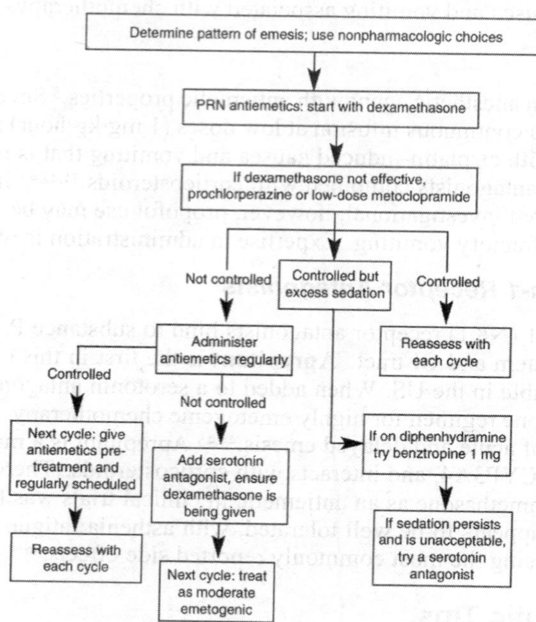

Figure 2: **Management of Chemotherapy-induced Nausea and Vomiting (moderate/high emetogenic potential)**

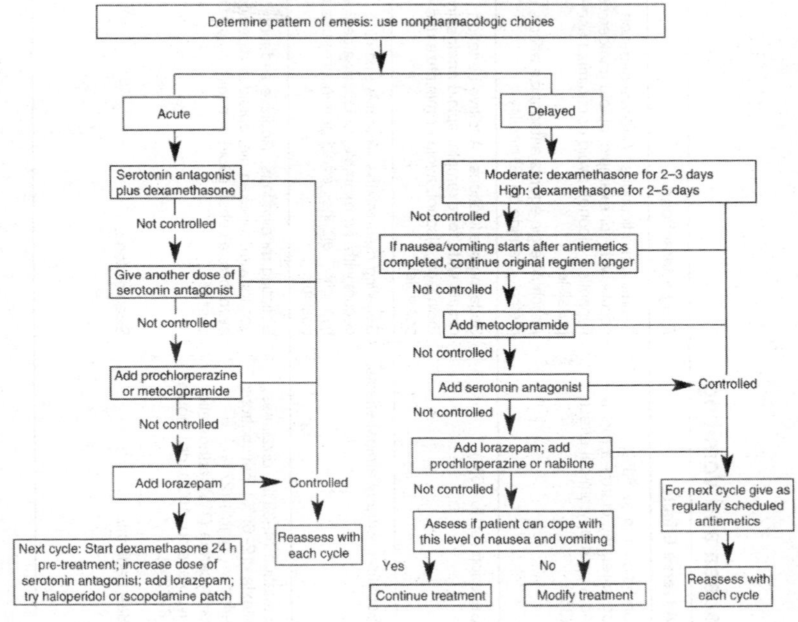

Table 2: **Drugs Used for Chemotherapy-induced Nausea and Vomiting**

Class	Drug	Dose	Adverse Effects	Drug Interactions	Cost[a]
Benzamides	*metoclopramide* generics	Low: 10–20 mg po Q6H High: 1–3 mg/kg po/iv Q3H	Sedation (up to 80%), dose-related diarrhea (up to 45%), extrapyramidal effects (3%).	Sedating medications. Additive sedation occurs with, for example, opioid analgesics, hypnotics, alcohol; avoid or minimize use if possible. Anticholinergic agents antagonize effects of metoclopramide on GI motility.	$–$$$$$
Benzodi-azepines	*lorazepam* Ativan, generics	1 mg po/sl prechemo, then 1–4 mg Q4H PRN	Sedation (up to 80%).	Sedating medications. Additive sedation occurs with, for example, opioid analgesics, hypnotics, alcohol; avoid or minimize use if possible.	$
Butyrophenones	*haloperidol* generics	1–2 mg po/im prechemo and Q8H	Sedation, extrapyramidal effects.	Sedating medications. Additive sedation occurs with, for example, opioid analgesics, hypnotics, alcohol; avoid or minimize use if possible.	$
Cannabinoids	*nabilone* Cesamet	1 mg po BID	Sedation (4–89%), dizziness, ataxia (12–65%), psychotropic effects ("high") (27%), tachycardia (7%), orthostatic hypotension (10%), dry mouth (6–62%).	Sedating medications. Additive sedation occurs with, for example, opioid analgesics, hypnotics, alcohol; avoid or minimize use if possible.	$
	dronabinol Marinol	5 mg/m² po Q2–4H Max 6 doses/day. May ↑ by 2.5 mg/m² to max 10 mg/m² per dose	See nabilone.	See nabilone.	$ [b]

Class	Drug	Dose	Adverse Effects	Drug Interactions	Cost[a]
Corticosteroids	*dexamethasone* Dexasone, generics	4–10 mg po prechemo and Q6–12H 8–20 mg iv prechemo and Q6–12H	Mood changes, increased appetite, GI irritation, ulceration, fluid retention, weight gain, may mask signs of infection.		$
	methylprednisolone Medrol, Solu-Medrol, generics	0.5–1 mg/kg po or iv prechemo and Q4 and 8H postchemo (max 4 mg/kg total dose) May also give as single 4 mg/kg dose 30 min prechemo	See dexamethasone.		$-$$
Phenothiazines	*prochlorperazine* Stemetil, generics	PO: 10 mg Q6–8H PR: 10 mg Q6–8H IM: 10 mg Q8–12H	Sedation, anticholinergic effects (dry mouth, blurred vision, constipation, nasal congestion, urinary retention), extrapyramidal effects, hypotension, hypersensitivity (1.4%), rare pancytopenia.	Sedating medications. Additive sedation occurs with, for example, opioid analgesics, hypnotics, alcohol; avoid or minimize use if possible.	$
Serotonin Antagonists	*dolasetron* Anzemet	1.8 mg/kg iv prechemo or 100 mg po prechemo	Headache (6–43%), constipation (4–19%), diarrhea (1–16%), sedation (4–10%), transient ↑ in LFTs (< 1–19%), bradycardia (4%), dizziness (3%). ECG interval changes have been reported.	Potential interaction with other drugs that prolong QTc intervals. Blood levels ↑ when coadministered with cimetidine and ↓ when coadministered with rifampin.	$-$$

(cont'd)

Table 2: **Drugs Used for Chemotherapy-induced Nausea and Vomiting** *(cont'd)*

Class	Drug	Dose	Adverse Effects	Drug Interactions	Cost[a]
	granisetron Kytril	10 µg/kg iv or 2 mg po prechemo or 1 mg prechemo and 12 h post	See dolasetron.		$$-$$$
	ondansetron Zofran, generics	8 mg po/iv prechemo	See dolasetron. Transient ECG changes have been reported.		$-$$

[a] Cost per day; includes drug cost only. Where doses are expressed in mg/kg, costs were calculated for a 50 kg person

[b] Cost for dronabinol based on 5 mg TID.

Dosage adjustment may be required in renal impairment; see Appendix I.

Abbreviations: LFTs = liver function tests

Legend: $ < $15 $–$$ < $15–30 $$ $15–30 $$–$$$ $15–45 $$$ $30–45 $$$$ $45–60 $–$$$$$ < $15–> 60 $$$$$ > $60

Suggested Readings

American Society of Clinical Oncology; Kris MG, Hesketh PJ et al. American Society of Clinical Oncology guideline for antiemetics in oncology: update 2006. *J Clin Oncol* 2006;24(18):2932-47.

ESMO recommendations for prophylaxis of chemotherapy-induced nausea and vomiting (NV). *Ann Oncol* 2001;12(8):1059-60.

Ioannidis JP, Hesketh PJ, Lau J. Contribution of dexamethasone to control of chemotherapy-induced nausea and vomiting: a meta-analysis of randomized evidence. *J Clin Oncol* 2000;18(19):3409-22.

Jordan K, Kasper C, Schmoll HJ. Chemotherapy-induced nausea and vomiting: current and new standards in the antiemetic prophylaxis and treatment. *Eur J Cancer* 2005;41(2):199-205.

References

1. Morrow GR, Rosenthal SN. Models, mechanisms and management of anticipatory nausea and emesis. *Oncology* 1996;53(Suppl 1):4-7.
2. Jordan NS, Schauer PK, Schauer A et al. The effect of administration rate on cisplatin-induced emesis. *J Clin Oncol* 1985;3(4):559-61.
3. Tortorice PV, O'Connell MB. Management of chemotherapy-induced nausea and vomiting. *Pharmacotherapy* 1990;10(2):129-45.
4. Lindley CM, Bernard S, Fields SM. Incidence and duration of chemotherapy-induced nausea and vomiting in the outpatient oncology population. *J Clin Oncol* 1989;7(8):1142-9.
5. Osoba D, Warr DG, Fitch MI et al. Guidelines for the optimal management of chemotherapy-induced nausea and vomiting: a consensus. *Can J Oncol* 1995;5(3):381-400
6. BC Cancer Agency. *Cancer management guidelines. Supportive care.* Available from: http://www.bccancer.bc.ca/HPI/CancerManagementGuidelines/SupportiveCare/default.htm Accessed March 27, 2007.
7. Cancer Care Ontario. *Nausea and vomiting. Management of chemotherapy-induced nausea and vomiting.* Revised April 2004. Available from : http://www.cancercare.on.ca/pdfchemo/NVguidelines.pdf Accessed March 27, 2007.
8. [No authors listed]. ASHP therapeutic guidelines on the pharmacologic management of nausea and vomiting in adult and pediatric patients receiving chemotherapy or radiation therapy or undergoing surgery. *Am J Health Syst Pharm* 1999;56(8):729-64.
9. Wickham R. Managing chemotherapy-related nausea and vomiting: the state of the art. *Oncol Nurs Forum* 1989;16(4):563-74.
10. McMillan C, Dundee JW, Abram WP. Enhancement of the antiemetic action of ondansetron by transcutaneous electrical stimulation of the P6 antiemetic point, in patients having highly emetic cytotoxic drugs. *Br J Cancer* 1991;64(5):971-2.
11. Kaptchuk TJ. Acupuncture: theory, efficacy, and practice. *Ann Intern Med* 2002;136(5):374-83.
12. Dominguez-Ortega L, Cubedo-Cervera R, Cortes-Funes H et al. Sleep protects against chemotherapy induced emesis. *Cancer* 1996;77(8):1566-70.
13. Wampler G. The pharmacology and clinical effectiveness of phenothiazines and related drugs for managing chemotherapy-induced emesis. *Drugs* 1983;25(Suppl 1):35-51.
14. Gralla RJ. Metoclopramide. A review of antiemetic trials. *Drugs* 1983;25(Suppl 1):63-73.
15. De Mulder PH, Seynaeve C, Vermorken JB et al. Ondansetron compared with high-dose metoclopramide in prophylaxis of acute and delayed cisplatin-induced nausea and vomiting. A multicenter, randomized, double-blind, crossover study. *Ann Intern Med* 1990;113(11):834-40.
16. Roila F. Ondansetron plus dexamethasone compared to the 'standard' metoclopramide combination. *Oncology* 1993;50(3):163-7.
17. Marty M, Pouillart P, Scholl S et al. Comparison of the 5-hydroxytryptamine3 (serotonin) antagonist ondansetron (GR 38032F) with high-dose metoclopramide in the control of cisplatin-induced emesis. *N Engl J Med* 1990;322(12):816-21.
18. [No authors listed]. Ondansetron versus granisetron, both combined with dexamethasone, in the prevention of cisplatin-induced emesis. Italian Group of Antiemetic Research. *Ann Oncol* 1995;6(8):805-10.
19. Mitchelson F. Pharmacological agents affecting emesis. A review (Part I). *Drugs* 1992;43(3):295-315.
20. Aapro MS. Corticosteroids as antiemetics. *Recent Results Cancer Res* 1988;108:102-11.
21. Ioannidis JP, Hesketh PJ, Lau J. Contribution of dexamethasone to control of chemotherapy-induced nausea and vomiting: a meta-analysis of randomized evidence. *J Clin Oncol* 2000;18(19):3409-22.
22. Roila F, Tonato M, Cognetti F et al. Prevention of cisplatin-induced emesis: a double-blind multicenter randomized crossover study comparing ondansetron and ondansetron plus dexamethasone. *J Clin Oncol* 1991;9(4):675-8.

23. Roila F, Tonato M, Basurto C et al. Ondansetron. *Eur J Cancer* 1993;29A(Suppl 1):S16-21.
24. Gebbia V, Testa A, Valenza R et al. Oral granisetron with or without methylprednisolone versus metoclopramide plus methylprednisolone in the management of delayed nausea and vomiting induced by cisplatin-based chemotherapy. A prospective randomized trial. *Cancer* 1995;76(10):1821-8.
25. [No authors listed]. Persistence of efficacy of three antiemetic regimens and prognostic factors in patients undergoing moderately emetogenic chemotherapy. Italian Group for Antiemetic Research. *J Clin Oncol* 1995;13(9):2417-26.
26. [No authors listed]. Dexamethasone alone or in combination with ondansetron for the prevention of delayed nausea and vomiting induced by chemotherapy. The Italian Group for Antiemetic Research. *N Engl J Med* 2000;342(21):1554-9.
27. Hesketh P, Navari R, Grote T et al. Double-blind, randomized comparison of the antiemetic efficacy of intravenous dolasetron mesylate and intravenous ondansetron in the prevention of acute cisplatin-induced emesis in patients with cancer. Dolasetron Comparative Chemotherapy-induced Emesis Prevention Group. *J Clin Oncol* 1996;14(8):2242-9.
28. del Giglio A, Soares HP, Caparroz C et al. Granisetron is equivalent to ondansetron for prophylaxis of chemotherapy-induced nausea and vomiting: results of a meta-analysis of randomized controlled trials. *Cancer* 2000;89(11):2301-8.
29. Gralla R, Lichinitser M, Van Der Vegt S et al. Palonosetron improves prevention of chemotherapy-induced nausea and vomiting following moderately emetogenic chemotherapy: results of a double-blind randomized phase III trial comparing single doses of palonsetron with ondansetron. *Ann Oncol* 2003;14(10):1570-7.
30. Eisenberg P, Figueroa-Vadillo J, Zamora R et al. Improved prevention of moderately emetogenic chemotherapy-induced nausea and vomiting with palonosetron, a pharmacologically novel 5 HT3 receptor antagonist: results of a phase III, single-dose trial versus dolasetron. *Cancer* 2003;98(11):2473-82.
31. American Society of Clinical Oncology; Kris MG, Hesketh PJ et al. American Society of Clinical Oncology guideline for antiemetics in oncology: update 2006. *J Clin Oncol* 2006;24(18):2932-47.
32. Malik IA, Khan WA, Qazilbash M et al. Clinical efficacy of lorazepam in prophylaxis of anticipatory acute and delayed nausea and vomiting induced by high doses of cisplatin. A prospective randomized trial. *Am J Clin Oncol*1995;18(2):170-5.
33. Razavi D, Delvaux N, Farvacques C et al. Prevention of adjustment disorders and anticipatory nausea secondary to adjuvant chemotherapy: a double-blind, placebo-controlled study assessing the usefulness of alprazolam. *J Clin Oncol* 1993;11(7):1384-90.
34. Plotkin DA, Plotkin D, Okun R. Haloperidol in the treatment of nausea and vomiting due to cytotoxic drug administration. *Curr Ther Res Clin Exp* 1973;15(9):599-602.
35. Tornetta FJ. Double-blind evaluation of haloperidol for antiemetic activity. *Anesth Analg* 1972;51(6):964-7.
36. Ward A, Holmes B. Nabilone. A preliminary review of its pharmacological properties and therapeutic use. *Drugs* 1985;30(2):127-44.
37. Vincent BJ, McQuiston DJ, Einhorn LH et al. Review of cannabinoids and their antiemetic effectiveness. *Drugs* 1983;25(Suppl 1):52-62.
38. Tramer MR, Carroll D, Campbell FA et al. Cannabinoids for control of chemotherapy induced nausea and vomiting: quantitative systematic review. *BMJ* 2001;323(7303):16-21.
39. Wood CD. Antimotion sickness and antiemetic drugs. *Drugs* 1979;17(6):471-9.
40. Longo DL, Wesley M, Howser D et al. Results of a randomized double-blind crossover trial of scopolamine versus placebo administered by transdermal patch for the control of cisplatin-induced emesis. *Cancer Treat Rep* 1982;66(11):1975-6.
41. Scher CS, Amar D, McDowall RH et al. Use of propofol for the prevention of chemotherapy-induced nausea and emesis in oncology patients. *Can J Anaesth* 1992;39(2):170-2.
42. Borgeat A, Wilder-Smith OH, Wilder-Smith CH et al. Propofol improves patient comfort during cisplatin chemotherapy. A pilot study. *Oncology* 1993;50(6):456-9.
43. Borgeat A, Wilder-Smith OH, Saiah M et al. Subhypnotic doses of propofol possess direct antiemetic properties. *Anesth Analg* 1992;74(4):539-41.
44. Hesketh PJ, Grunberg SM, Gralla RJ et al. The oral neurokinin-1 antagonist aprepitant for the prevention of chemotherapy-induced nausea and vomiting: a multinational, randomized, double-blind, placebo-controlled trial in patients receiving high-dose cisplatin-The Aprepitant Protocol 052 Study Group. *J Clin Oncol* 2003;21(22):4112-9.
45. Poli-Bigelli S, Rodrigues-Pereira J, Carides AD et al. Addition of the neurokinin 1 receptor antagonist aprepitant to standard antiemetic therapy improves control of chemotherapy-induced nausea and vomiting: results from a randomized, double-blind, placebo-controlled trial in Latin America. *Cancer* 2003;97(12):3090-8.
46. Dando TM, Perry CM. Aprepitant: a review of its use in the prevention of chemotherapy-induced nausea and vomiting. *Drugs* 2004;64(7):777-94.

CHAPTER 112

Management of Side Effects of Chemotherapy and Radiation Therapy

Pierre Fortin, MD, FACP, FRCPC

Cancer therapy encompasses three modalities of treatment: surgery, systemic therapies (chemotherapy, targeted agents, hormones) and radiation therapy. An initial decision regarding the goal of therapy has to be made: curative or palliative. Usually a combination of modalities is used in the treatment plan. Surgery remains the mainstay of curative treatments, with chemo- and/or radiotherapy reserved for neoadjuvant therapies to downstage the tumor before the surgery, or for adjuvant therapies in order to sterilize the surgical bed from suspected residual microscopic disease. If surgery is not feasible as in the case of hematologic malignancies, then chemotherapy with or without radiation is employed with curative or palliative intent.

If a decision is made to palliate the patient's symptoms, radiation is usually used to control the disease locally, while chemotherapy or other systemic agents are used to decrease the tumor burden throughout the whole body. Surgery can also be used with palliative intent. These therapies are less intense and the goal is an acceptable quality of life for the patient.

The following discussion will focus on managing the adverse effects of chemotherapy (Table 1 and Table 2) and radiation therapy (Table 3).[1] These tables outline treatments that are generally initiated by the oncology treatment team but include issues that may be encountered by generalists when following cancer patients.

Side Effects of Chemotherapy

Cancer cells grow and divide faster than normal cells. This difference is exploited when using chemotherapy. The drugs usually affect fast-growing cells during replication, killing more cancer cells than normal cells.

This characteristic also explains many of the side effects of chemotherapy. Fast-growing cells like the hematopoietic cells, the skin and its appendages and the epithelium of the intestine often suffer adverse effects of chemotherapy.

Table 1: **Acute Side Effects of Antineoplastic Drugs**

Acute Side Effect	**Management**	**Prevention**
Extravasation Vesicant drugs: **amsacrine** **bleomycin** **carmustine** **cisplatin** **dactinomycin** **daunorubicin** **doxorubicin** **epirubicin** **etoposide** **idarubicin** **mechlorethamine** **melphalan** **mitomycin** **mitoxantrone** **plicamycin** **streptozocin** **vinblastine** **vincristine** **vindesine** **vinorelbine**	Optimal management is unknown. Stop the infusion and aspirate any residual drug remaining in tissues. Local measures such as **topical dimethylsulfoxide (DMSO)**,[2,3] subcutaneous injections of **saline**, **steroids**, **hyaluronidase** or **sodium bicarbonate** may be helpful. There is weak evidence that ice packs may worsen the skin toxicity with vinca alkaloids. Severe cases may require plastic surgery intervention.	Take all possible precautions to ensure good blood return from and fluid flow into the iv line before injection. Be aware of potential damage to tendons. Avoid dorsum of the hand or cubital fossa.
Hypersensitivity Reactions Seen especially with **etoposide** and **taxanes**. Also seen with **rituximab**, **trastuzumab** and other biologics.	Stop chemotherapy infusion. Administer **antihistamines**, **steroids**, **vasoconstrictors**. Supportive care.	Premedicate with **antihistamines** (H_1- and H_2-blockers) and **corticosteroids**. Use slower infusion rates.
Tumor Lysis Syndrome	Rapid release of intracellular contents into the blood stream, resulting in hyperuricemia, hyperkalemia, hyperphosphatemia and hypocalcemia. Seen in diseases with large tumor burden and exquisitely sensitive to chemotherapy, e.g., leukemia, lymphomas.	IV hydration, **allopurinol** 300–600 mg/day until normal uric acid levels. Close monitoring of serum electrolytes with accordant adjustments of contents of iv fluids. **Rasburicase** is a uricolytic that may be used at a dose of 0.20 mg/kg/day for up to seven days in the treatment and prophylaxis of hyperuricemia. Since it is a protein it may induce allergic responses. When administered to patients with G-6-PD deficiency it can cause severe hemolysis.

Table 2: **Specific Side Effects of Antineoplastic Drugs**

Side Effect	Management	Prevention
Alopecia	Cosmetic intervention using wigs, hats or scarves. Hair usually begins regrowth 1–2 months after completion of chemotherapy.	Cryotherapy caps or scalp tourniquets are not effective and may be unsafe.
Anemia	Packed red blood cells given to patients with hemoglobin < 80 g/L, chest pain or shortness of breath with little exertion. Although these agents have significant potential for toxicity, in select patients erythropoetin as **epoetin alfa** or **darbepoetin** may reduce the need for transfusions. Hemoglobin targets of > 120 g/L were associated with increased risk of death and serious adverse events.[4]	Decrease doses of chemotherapy for subsequent cycles.
Cardiotoxicity **5-FU, capecitabine** cause coronary vasospasms, mimicking a myocardial infarct.	Treat symptomatically with **nitrates**. Discontinue therapy if necessary.	Avoid administration in patients with known coronary artery disease.
Trastuzumab can cause cardiac dysfunction including severe heart failure.	Left ventricular function should be evaluated at baseline and during therapy. Manage clinically significant cardiac dysfunction symptomatically. Discontinuation of trastuzumab usually recommended.	
Anthracyclines can cause acute inflammation (myocarditis/pericarditis syndrome). Chronically, a dose-dependent congestive myopathy may develop.	Perform ECG and serial ejection fractions. Treat symptomatically. Discontinue therapy if necessary.	Limit cumulative doses of anthracyclines. Consider discontinuing anthracyclines if serial ejection fraction is ↓ 25% from baseline. **Dexrazoxane** is a cardioprotective agent used at a dose of 500 mg/m² to reduce the incidence and severity of cardiotoxicity associated with doxorubicin. Dexrazoxane may add to the myelosuppressive effects caused by chemotherapeutic agents. As a result, blood counts and hepatic function tests should be performed regularly. Cardiac function should also be monitored.
Taxanes may cause bradycardia.	Observe patient. Treat symptomatically.	

(cont'd)

Table 2: **Specific Side Effects of Antineoplastic Drugs** *(cont'd)*

Side Effect	Management	Prevention
Carcinogenesis	Case specific.	Use the least amount of chemotherapy possible to control the disease.
Diarrhea Seen with **irinotecan, 5–FU, antimetabolites**.	IV hydration and supportive care if dehydration secondary to diarrhea. **Loperamide** and/or **diphenoxylate** PRN or **octreotide**.[5]	Decrease the dose of chemotherapy in subsequent cycles or change the chemotherapy regimen.
Gonadal Toxicity	Discuss assisted reproduction techniques with patients.	Sperm banking. Use chemotherapy with the least effect on spermatogenesis or ovarian function.
Hepatotoxicity Seen with **methotrexate, azathioprine, cytarabine, nitrosoureas, etoposide**.	Perform LFTs and bilirubin measurement. Discontinue chemotherapy depending on extent of damage.	Avoid offending agent or decrease doses.
Mucositis	Rule out infectious causes. Avoid "magic mouthwash" with topical steroids and antihistamines that can increase chances of fungal infection or sensitization. Combinations of xylocaine viscous, sucralfate, nystatin, fluconazole, antacids and sodium bicarbonate are used in local institutions. For severe mucositis in patients with hematologic malignancies receiving myelotoxic therapy and requiring stem cell support, the growth factor **palifermin** can be used at a dose of 60 μg/kg/day for 3 days before and 3 days after chemotherapy.[6] Adverse effects include mild to moderate taste alteration, mouth and tongue disorders, rash and edema.	Educate patients on basic oral hygiene. Treat pre-existing oral problems before starting chemotherapy. Avoid alcohol and spicy foods, which are irritating to the mucosa. Ice chips reduce the incidence and severity of 5-FU-induced mucositis.[7] Withhold offending agent until episode resolves.

(cont'd)

Table 2: **Specific Side Effects of Antineoplastic Drugs** *(cont'd)*

Side Effect	Management	Prevention
Myelosuppression/ Febrile Neutropenia	Start oral antibiotics in those at low risk of complications. **Ciprofloxacin** or **amoxicillin-clavulanate** are commonly used. Those at higher risk of complications include those with septic shock or signs of organ failure, neutropenia for > 6 days, signs of infections in lines, temperature ≥ 39°C and receiving bacterial/fungal prophylaxis.[8] These high-risk patients should receive broad gram-negative and antipseudomonal coverage with two agents. Add **vancomycin** if gram-positive infection suspected (see Chapter 108). Perform cultures and adjust antibiotics according to results.[8]	Growth factors such as **filgrastim** or **pegfilgrastim** used to increase the rate of neutrophil count recovery can be administered to allow chemotherapy to be given without delays or decreasing doses. It can improve quality of life and decrease hospitalization. CBC must be performed regularly during G-CSF (filgrastim) therapy. Bone pain related to these agents can generally be controlled with nonopioid analgesics. Serious allergic or anaphylactic reactions have occurred and require discontinuation of G-CSF.
Nausea/Vomiting	See Chapter 111	
Nephrotoxicity	IV hydration to achieve urine output of > 3 L/24 h while administering chemotherapy. Monitor creatinine, BUN and serum uric acid.	**Mesna** is a uroprotectant used to prevent hemorrhagic cystitis secondary to cyclophosphamide or ifosfamide. Most adverse effects of mesna are immediate and include nausea and vomiting, headache and urticaria. **Allopurinol** 300–600 mg/day po starting 24–48 h before chemotherapy for uric acid nephropathy.
Neurotoxicity Peripheral nerve damage is common with the **vinca alkaloids, platinum-based chemotherapy** and **taxanes**. It can be irreversible. Neurotoxicity can present as peripheral or central neuropathy, impotence, urinary retention. It can lead to muscle atrophy, motor weakness or loss of deep tendon reflexes. Autonomic neuropathy from vinca alkaloids presents with constipation and abdominal pain.	Dose reduction may be necessary with severe toxicity, or the drugs may have to be avoided altogether. Rule out other causes such as CNS metastases or leptomeningeal disease.	For vinca alkaloid constipation, use **stool softeners** or **stimulant laxatives** if necessary. Suggest increased physical activity and hydration if possible. Anticholinergic drugs may help.

(cont'd)

Table 2: **Specific Side Effects of Antineoplastic Drugs** *(cont'd)*

Side Effect	Management	Prevention
High-dose **methotrexate** may cause transient cerebral dysfunction.		
Ocular Blepharitis, epiphora, tear duct stenosis; conjunctivitis with **5-FU** and **taxanes**.	Discontinuation of the offending agent may be necessary.	For conjunctivitis, **corticosteroid eye drops** or **artificial tears** may be preventative.
Ototoxicity Seen with **platinum compounds**.	Can be irreversible. Reduce doses or avoid completely if possible.	Audiograms every 3–4 cycles.
Pulmonary Interstitial pneumonitis and fibrosis with **methotrexate, bleomycin, anthracyclines, vinca alkaloids, alkylating agents**. Acute respiratory distress syndrome with **gemcitabine**.	Rule out infectious causes. Withhold offending agent; supportive care, steroids (**prednisone** 50 mg/day with tapering doses). Ventilatory support may be necessary.	Avoid offending agent.
Teratogenicity	Contraception necessary while patient receiving chemotherapy.	Avoid pregnancy while on chemotherapy.

Side Effects of Radiation Therapy

Radiation treatment is used to control the disease locally, not unlike surgery. A target, whether the tumor itself or the surgical bed, is acquired with the help of a CT scan, and treatment fields are designed to encompass it. When the x-rays are delivered, they travel through the tissues from an entry point to an exit point. The enormous quantity of energy carried by the x-rays damage chromosomes either directly or indirectly by the production of free radicals in the neighbourhood of the chromosomes. As with chemotherapy, the cell cannot divide and dies. A normal inflammatory reaction ensues, producing the common side effects of radiation.

Contrary to chemotherapy, where the side effects are generally seen in a matter of minutes to days, the side effects of radiation are seen many days to weeks and even years after the treatment. Acute side effects in this context means within 30 days of the end of the treatments, subacute within 6 months and late side effects over 6 months after the completion of the therapy.

Side effects could be decreased by lowering the total radiation dose or its fractionation or keeping the field size as small as possible. However, the whole tumor has to be treated in order to control the disease appropriately.

Table 3: **Organ-specific Side Effects of Radiation Therapy**[9]

Organ/System	Side Effect	Management
CNS/Spinal Cord	Edema	Steroids, typically **dexamethasone** 4 mg po QID.
ENT/Esophagus	Mucositis/ esophagitis	Mouthwashes containing **nystatin, fluconazole, sucralfate, xylocaine viscous** may help symptoms. **Amifostine** is a cytoprotectant that may be used to reduce xerostomia. It may cause hypotension that can lead to dizziness or fainting. Monitor blood pressure and consider holding antihypertensives for 24 h prior to amifostine administration. Prophylactic serotonin antagonists may be used to reduce nausea and vomiting caused by amifostine. Systemic **analgesics** can be used for pain.
Heart	Pericarditis	**NSAIDs.**
Lungs	Pneumonitis	**Prednisone** (starting dose 1 mg/kg/day, to taper over weeks).
Skin	Desquamation/itchiness	If dry desquamation, use glaxal base or other moisturizers (e.g., Lubriderm, plain Keri Lotion) or vitamin E cream. If itchiness, use **hydrocortisone** 0.5% cream. If moist desquamation, use **silver sulfadiazine** cream.
Small Intestine/ Colon/Rectum	Enteritis/proctitis	Medical support: fluid replacement by po or iv route, **loperamide**, **diphenoxylate**. **Topical steroids** by enema or suppository. Antispasmodics such as **hyoscine butylbromide** (Buscopan) or **pinaverium** may provide symptomatic relief.
Stomach	Nausea	Antiemetics, e.g., **ondansetron, granisetron, dolasetron, dimenhydrinate, prochlorperazine, metoclopramide**.[10]

Suggested Readings

Schuchter LM, Hensley ML, Meropol NJ et al. 2002 update of recommendations for the use of chemotherapy and radiotherapy protectants: clinical practice guidelines of the American Society of Clinical Oncology. *J Clin Oncol* 2002;20(12):2895-903.

Smith TJ, Khatcheressian J, Lyman GH et al. 2006 update of recommendations for the use of white blood cell growth factors: an evidence-based clinical practice guideline. *J Clin Oncol* 2006;24(19):3187-205.

References

1. DeVita VT, Hellman S, Rosenberg SA, editors. *Cancer: principles and practice of oncology*. 7th ed. Philadelphia (PA): Lippincott, Williams & Wilkins; 2005.
2. Olver IN, Aisner J, Hament A et al. A prospective study of topical dimethylsulfoxide for treating anthracycline extravasation. *J Clin Oncol* 1988;6(11):1732–5.
3. Bertelli G, Gozza A, Forno GB et al. Topical dimethylsulfoxide for the prevention of soft tissue injury after extravasation of vesicant cytotoxic drugs: a prospective clinical study. *J Clin Oncol* 1995;13(11):2851–5.
4. *Health Canada endorsed important safety information on Erythropoiesis-Stimulating Agents (ESAs): Aranesp (darbepoetin alfa) and Eprex (epoetin alfa)*. Ottawa (ON): Health Canada, Drugs

& Health Products; 2007. Available from: http://www.hc-sc.gc.ca/dhp-mps/medeff/advisories-avis/prof/2007/aranesp_eprex_hpc-cps_e.html Accessed May 24, 2007.

5. Harris AG, O'Dorisio TM, Woltering EA et al. Consensus statement: octreotide dose titration in secretory diarrhea. Diarrhea Management Consensus Development Panel. *Dig Dis Sci* 1995;40:1464-73.
6. Rosen LS, Abdi E, Davis ID et al. Palifermin reduces the incidence of oral mucositis in patients with metastatic colorectal cancer treated with fluorouracil-based chemotherapy. *J Clin Oncol* 2006;24(33):5194-200.
7. Worthington HV, Clarkson JE, Eden OB. Interventions for preventing oral mucositis for patients with cancer receiving treatment. *Cochrane Database Syst Rev* 2006;(2):CD000978.
8. Hughes WT, Armstrong D, Bodey GP et al. 2002 guidelines for the use of antimicrobial agents in neutropenic patients with cancer. *Clin Infect Dis* 2002;34(6):730-51.
9. Perez CA, Brady LW, editors. *Principles and practice of radiation oncology*. 3rd ed. Philadelphia (PA): Lippincott-Raven; 1998.
10. Kris MG, Hesketh PJ, Somerfield MR et al. American Society of Clinical Oncology Guidelines for Antiemetics in Oncology: Update 2006. *J Clin Oncol* 24:2932–47.

CHAPTER 113

Nausea in Adults

C. MacLean, MD, CCFP, FCFP

Nausea is a common symptom that refers to the unpleasant sensation experienced prior to vomiting. It may be a "simple," transient symptom, secondary to a self-limited condition such as viral gastroenteritis, requiring only symptomatic relief. Nausea may also be a part of a more complex medical problem. Nausea is a symptom, not a diagnosis, and the underlying cause should be determined (Table 1). Approaches to nausea and its treatment are dependent on the associated diagnosis, for example, postoperative nausea and vomiting (PONV), chemotherapy-induced nausea, metabolic, gastrointestinal, vestibular or neurologic causes.[1] This chapter does not address nausea in children, management of nausea in pregnancy (see Table 3, Appendix II) or the issue of cancer chemotherapy or radiation therapy–induced nausea and vomiting (see Chapter 111).

Table 1: **Common Causes of Nausea**

N	*Neurologic:* cerebrovascular accident, increased intracranial pressure, migraine, neoplasm, pain, trauma and vestibular causes (e.g., labyrinthitis, Meniere's disease, motion sickness)
A	*Alcohol and other drugs:* drug-related adverse effects (e.g., antibiotics, cancer chemotherapy, hormones, opioids, NSAIDs, etc.); drug toxicity (e.g., anticonvulsants, digitalis); drug initiation and withdrawal (e.g., benzodiazepines, narcotics, SSRIs)
U	*Usually accompanies:* anesthesia, diabetic ketoacidosis, heart failure, hypercalcemia, hyponatremia, malignancy including metastasis, myocardial infarction, noxious odours, pain, PONV, pregnancy, radiation therapy, uremia
S	*Stress and psychiatric:* anxiety, depression, fear, grief, pain *Surgical:* including nasogastric tube placement
E	*Enteral:* constipation; diseases of the liver, gallbladder and pancreas; functional gastrointestinal disorders (chronic idiopathic nausea; chronic intestinal pseudo-obstruction, gastroparesis, IBS, nonulcer dyspepsia); gastroenteritis; gastroesophageal reflux; ingestion of irritants and food poisoning; motility disorders; obstruction *Endocrine:* Addison's disease
A	*Anticipatory nausea:* in patients on cancer chemotherapy or situations in which patients are conditioned by previous experience of nausea and vomiting

Goals of Therapy

- Diagnose and remove or treat the underlying cause of the nausea
- Control nausea and provide patient comfort (nausea can be more distressing to some patients than actual vomiting)
- Prevent the development of anticipatory nausea

- Balance the benefit of symptomatic treatment with possible adverse effects and cost of medications
- Avoid complications associated with vomiting, which include dehydration with associated fluid and electrolyte disturbance, acid-base abnormalities and compromised nutritional status
- Control nausea so patients can resume treatment of other conditions

Investigations[1]

- History
  - determine if the nausea is acute or chronic
  - ascertain the frequency and severity of nausea
  - explore possible underlying causes, simple versus complex
  - establish the onset, progression and temporal sequence of associated events, e.g., surgery
  - identify other symptoms, e.g., headache, pain, vertigo
  - clarify the relationship between nausea and vomiting (if present)
  - complete an appropriate GI functional inquiry
  - inquire about diet history including any new foods, food allergies, or intolerances
  - establish any exposure to, or other symptoms of, infection such as gastroenteritis
  - in all women of reproductive age, inquire about last menstrual period to rule out pregnancy
  - obtain a thorough medication history including use of prescription, nonprescription, herbal or recreational drugs and alcohol
  - inquire about recent changes to drug regimens (dose increases or withdrawal) and correlation with nausea
  - inquire about the patient's feelings, concerns, ideas, and functional impairment and expectations of treatment
  - inquire about past history of migraine headaches, endocrine disorders, malignancy
  - explore possible psychosocial stressors, conflicts, sources of emotional pain or loss
- Physical examination
  - vital signs including blood pressure, pulse, respiratory rate and temperature
  - determine severity and consequences of symptoms—assess hydration including JVP, mucous membranes, skin turgor and postural changes in blood pressure and heart rate
  - assess systems related to the probable underlying cause when apparent, e.g., perform neurologic exam for a migraine patient, examine for bowel obstruction if the patient has a malignancy or

is postsurgical, check for nystagmus in vertigo-associated nausea, inspect fundi for papilledema
  - if no specific cause is identified in the history, use the physical exam to rule out other potential causes, e.g., abdominal mass
- Other investigations
  - laboratory investigations are determined by the history and physical exam
  - electrolytes may be indicated if metabolic disturbances are suspected, e.g., test for hypercalcemia in a patient with a malignancy, ketoacidosis in a diabetic patient, hypokalemia or hyponatremia in a patient on diuretics
  - CBC if an infective cause is suspected
  - serum creatinine and BUN to determine if there is a renal cause and assess degree of dehydration
  - drug levels in select cases, e.g. digoxin
  - x-rays may also be indicated; an abdominal series if a bowel obstruction is suspected or an upper GI with motility studies if gastroesophageal reflux or gastroparesis is suspected
  - ultrasound of the liver, gallbladder or pancreas may be useful in some patients

Therapeutic Choices

Nonpharmacologic Choices

- Some forms of complementary therapies have been used, e.g., acupuncture, neurostimulation therapy at the wrist, hypnosis.[2]
- A Cochrane systematic review of studies of acupuncture point stimulation concluded that there was possible benefit for a variety of causes of nausea and vomiting.[3]
- Dietary interventions may be important for nausea associated with certain food intolerances.
- Recommend consumption of frequent small meals and snacks rather than large meals at infrequent intervals.
- Advise patients to avoid smells and foods that cause nausea.
- Recommend controlled breathing for motion sickness.
- Relaxation therapy and cognitive behaviour therapies may be useful in the treatment of nausea associated with irritable bowel syndrome and anticipatory nausea.[1]
- Gastric electric stimulation may be effective for refractory gastroparesis.[4]
- Engage the patient in the decisions around treatment. Not every patient will want treatment; watchful waiting is an alternative to medication for these individuals.

Pharmacologic Choices (Table 2)

Although antiemetics are widely prescribed, there is a paucity of randomized controlled trials examining their effectiveness, with the exception of serotonin (5-HT_3) antagonists for chemotherapy-induced nausea (see Chapter 111) and PONV. When selecting a drug, consider if the nausea is acute or chronic, review concurrent medications and attempt to identify the underlying cause of nausea (Figure 1). Many patients cannot tolerate oral medications when nauseated, and alternative routes of administration (im, sc, rectal or transdermal) may be more effective.

In an emergency room setting, iv **droperidol** 1.25 mg was significantly more effective 30 minutes after administration than iv **metoclopramide** 10 mg, iv **prochlorperazine** 10 mg or saline placebo for relief of moderate to severe nausea and/or vomiting of any etiology. Metoclopramide and prochlorperazine were not more effective than placebo in this randomized trial. Twenty-four hours after treatment, 70% of droperidol recipients reported experiencing anxiety or restlessness (vs. 24% of patients receiving other treatments).[5] Despite the differences in efficacy and tolerability, 95% of patients enrolled in the trial were satisfied with the treatment they received.

Ginger (*Zingiber officinale*) has been studied in controlled trials as a treatment for nausea and vomiting.[6,7,8] At doses > 1 g/day, ginger was significantly more effective than placebo[9] and vitamin B_6[10] for pregnancy-induced nausea and vomiting in randomized trials. However, ginger does not enhance the efficacy of standard antiemetic therapy in the setting of PONV[11] or cancer chemotherapy.[12] In the absence of trials comparing ginger with antiemetic drugs, it is not possible to make definitive conclusions about its place in therapy. Until such trials become available, ginger should be considered to be an alternative to drug therapy in patients unable to tolerate or unwilling to take antiemetic drugs.

A preventive approach may be appropriate in certain situations, for example, in the management of motion sickness.

If nausea is associated with gastroesophageal reflux (see Chapter 53) or peptic ulcer disease (see Chapter 54), treatment should address the underlying cause.

Therapeutic Tips

- Preemptive treatment may reduce nausea with certain procedures, for example, insertion of a nasogastric tube, or with certain medications.
- When a more complex cause is suspected, antiemetics may provide some symptomatic relief. However, when possible, determine and treat the underlying cause.[13]
- Start with a low dose and increase the dose slowly when prescribing for the elderly.
- Combination therapy may be required and has been found to be most useful in chemotherapy-induced nausea.

- If management of a nauseated patient fails to provide some symptomatic relief, reassess the patient and look for other causes.
- Know a few medications well. If one medication fails, try a different class of antinauseant or try an alternative route of administration.
- Consider the use of an alternative (i.e., non-oral) route of administration if drug absorption is likely to be delayed.
- Start with less expensive choices unless there is a preferred antiemetic for a specific disorder. For example, **ondansetron** is more effective than metoclopramide for nausea and vomiting in uremic patients.[14]

Figure 1: Management of Nausea

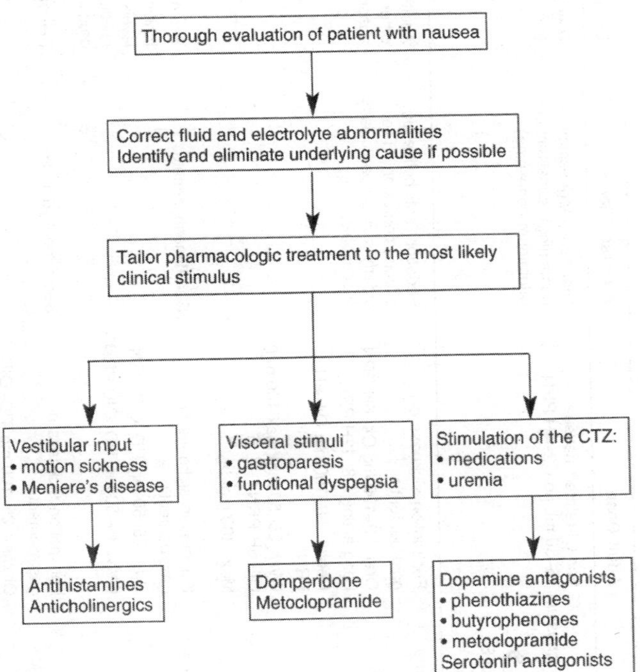

Abbreviations: CTZ = chemoreceptor trigger zone

Table 2: Drugs Used to Treat Nausea

Class	Drug	Adult Dose	Adverse Effects	Drug Interactions	Cost[a]
Antacids	*aluminum hydroxide/magnesium hydroxide combinations*[3] Diovol, Diovol Ex various others	For GI-related nausea 15–30 mL po Q2–4H PRN	Diarrhea (magnesium-containing), constipation (aluminum-containing).	May ↓ bioavailability of some drugs (e.g., digoxin); separate dosing by 2 h.	\$–\$\$
Antihistamines	*dimenhydrinate* Gravol Preparations, generics	For motion sickness or gastroenteritis Oral: 50–100 mg Q4–6H PRN; Long acting Q8–12H PRN Rectal: 50–100 mg Q4–6H PRN IM/iv: 25–50 mg (max 100 mg) Q4–6H PRN Max: 300 mg/day	Sedation, anticholinergic effects, confusion. The elderly may be particularly susceptible.	Additive sedation with alcohol or other sedating medications. May ↑ absorption of digoxin.	po: \$ rectal: \$\$ iv: \$-\$\$
	diphenhydramine Benadryl Preparations, generics	For motion sickness or gastroenteritis Oral: 25–50 mg TID–QID PRN IM/iv: 10–50 mg TID–QID PRN	See dimenhydrinate.	See dimenhydrinate. Inhibits CYP2D6 and can ↑ serum levels of many drugs including antidepressants and cardiovascular drugs.	po: \$ iv: \$\$
	hydroxyzine Atarax, generics	For motion sickness or gastroenteritis Oral/im: 25–100 mg TID–QID PRN	See dimenhydrinate.	See dimenhydrinate.	po: \$ iv: \$\$

Class	Drug	Adult Dose	Adverse Effects	Drug Interactions	Cost[a]
	meclizine Bonamine	For labyrinthitis Oral: 25–50 mg Q24H PRN	Sedation, anticholinergic effects.	Additive sedation with alcohol or other sedating medications.	$
Anticholinergics	*scopolamine* Transderm V	For motion sickness Transdermal: 1.5 mg (one patch) Q72H PRN	Constipation, dry mouth. Confusion (especially in the elderly).	Additive sedation with alcohol or other sedating medications.	$$
Benzamides	*domperidone* generics	For gastroparesis, functional dyspepsia Oral: 10 mg QID	Diarrhea, abdominal cramps and distention, headache, hyperprolactinemia.	See chlorpromazine.	$
	metoclopramide generics	For drug-induced nausea, migraine-related nausea, gastroparesis Oral/sc/iv: 10–20 mg TID–QID PRN	Diarrhea, abdominal cramps and distention, headache, hyperprolactinemia, drowsiness, fatigue, EPS.	See chlorpromazine.	po: $ iv: $$$$-$$$$$
Butyrophenones	*haloperidol* generics	For drug-induced nausea, PONV Oral/im/iv: 0.5–5 mg Q12H PRN	Sedation, extrapyramidal effects.	Additive sedation with alcohol or other CNS depressants.	po: $ iv: $$
	droperidol generics	IM/iv: 1–5 mg Q4–6H	See haloperidol.	See haloperidol.	iv: $$$$-$$$$$
Phenothiazines	*chlorpromazine* generics	For labyrinthitis Oral: 10–25 mg Q4–6H PRN IM/iv: 25–50 mg Q3–4H PRN	Sedation, anticholinergic effects, EPS. Hypotension with im/iv administration.	Additive sedation with alcohol or other CNS depressants.	po: $ iv: $$$$$

(cont'd)

Table 2: **Drugs Used to Treat Nausea** *(cont'd)*

Class	Drug	Adult Dose	Adverse Effects	Drug Interactions	Cost[a]
	perphenazine Trilafon, generics	For PONV Oral/im/iv: 2–4 mg Q8H PRN	Sedation, anticholinergic effects, EPS. Hypotension with im/iv administration.	See chlorpromazine.	$
	prochlorperazine Stemetil, generics	For drug-induced nausea, migraine-related nausea, PONV, vertigo-related nausea Oral/rectal: 5–10 mg TID–QID PRN IM/iv: 5–10 mg BID–TID PRN	Sedation, anticholinergic effects, EPS. Hypotension with im/iv administration.	See chlorpromazine.	po: $ rectal/iv: $$
	promethazine generics	For motion sickness or gastroenteritis 12.5–25 mg po/im/iv 4–6H PRN	See dimenhydrinate.	See dimenhydrinate.	$$
Serotonin Antagonists	*ondansetron* Zofran, generics	PONV; radiation and chemotherapy-induced nausea and vomiting 8 mg po/iv pre-procedure	Headache, constipation, diarrhea, sedation, bradycardia, dizziness. Transient ECG changes have been reported.		$$$$$

[a] Cost of 1-day supply; includes drug cost only.

Dosage adjustment may be required in renal impairment; see Appendix I.

Abbreviations: PONV = postoperative nausea and vomiting; EPS = extrapyramidal symptoms

Legend: $ < $2 $-$$ < $2–4 $$ $2–4 $$$ $4–6 $$$$ $6–8 $$$$-$$$$$ $6– >8 $$$$$ > $8

Suggested Readings

Flake ZA, Scalley RD, Bailey AG. Practical selection of antiemetics. *Am Fam Physician* 2004;69(5):1169-74.

Hasler WL, Chey WD. Nausea and vomiting. *Gastroenterology* 2003;125(6):1860-7.

Quigley EM, Hasler WL, Parkman HP. AGA technical review on nausea and vomiting. *Gastroenterology* 2001;120(1):263-86.

Tack J, Talley NJ, Camilleri M et al. Functional gastroduodenal disorders. *Gastroenterology* 2006;30(5):1466-79.

References

1. Quigley EM, Hasler WL, Parkman HP. AGA technical review on nausea and vomiting. *Gastroenterology* 2001;120(1):263-86.
2. Lee A, Done ML. Stimulation of the wrist acupuncture point P6 for preventing postoperative nausea and vomiting. *Cochrane Database Syst Rev* 2004;(3):CD003281.
3. Ezzo JM, Richardson MA, Vickers A et al. Acupuncture-point stimulation for chemotherapy-induced nausea or vomiting. *Cochrane Database Syst Rev* 2006;(2):CD002285.
4. Parkman HP. New advances in the diagnosis and management of nausea and vomiting. *Case Manager* 2002;13(2):83-6.
5. Braude D, Soliz T, Crandall C et al. Antiemetics in the ED: a randomized controlled trial comparing 3 common agents. *Am J Emerg Med* 2006;24(2):177-82.
6. Borrelli F, Capasso R, Aviello G, Pittler MH, Izzo AA. Effectiveness and safety of ginger in the treatment of pregnancy-induced nausea and vomiting. *Obstet Gynecol* 2005;105(4):849-56.
7. Chaiyakunapruk N, Kitikannakorn N, Nathisuwan S et al. The efficacy of ginger for the prevention of postoperative nausea and vomiting: a meta-analysis. *Am J Obstet Gynecol* 2006;194(1):95-9.
8. Morin AM, Betz O, Kranke P et al. [Is ginger a relevant antiemetic for postoperative nausea and vomiting?]. *Anasthesiol Intensivmed Notfallmed Schmerzther* 2004;39(5):281-5. German.
9. Willetts KE, Ekangaki A, Eden JA. Effect of a ginger extract on pregnancy-induced nausea: a randomised controlled trial. *Aust N Z J Obstet Gynaecol* 2003;43(2):139-44.
10. Smith C, Crowther C, Willson K et al. A randomized controlled trial of ginger to treat nausea and vomiting in pregnancy. *Obstet Gynecol* 2004;103(4):639-45.
11. Tavlan A, Tuncer S, Erol A et al. Prevention of postoperative nausea and vomiting after thyroidectomy: combined antiemetic treatment with dexamethasone and ginger versus dexamethasone alone. *Clin Drug Investig* 2006;26(4):209-14.
12. Manusirivithaya S, Sripramote M, Tangjitgamol S et al. Antiemetic effect of ginger in gynecologic oncology patients receiving cisplatin. *Int J Gynecol Cancer* 2004;14(6):1063-9.
13. Ozucelik DN, Karaca MA, Sivri B. Effectiveness of pre-emptive metoclopramide infusion in alleviating pain, discomfort and nausea associated with nasogastric tube insertion: a randomised, double-blind, placebo-controlled trial. *Int J Clin Pract* 2005;59(12):1422-7.
14. Ljutic D, Perkovic D, Rumboldt Z et al. Comparison of ondansetron with metoclopramide in the symptomatic relief of uremia-induced nausea and vomiting. *Kidney Blood Press Res* 2002;25(1):61-4.

CHAPTER 114

Constipation

Hugh Chaun, MA, BM, FRCP, FRCP(Ed), FRCPC, FACG

Constipation is a symptom, not a disease. Establishing the cause, if any, and correcting it is the primary objective of treatment.

Constipation may be defined on the basis of the frequency of defecation (< 3/week) and/or on the presence of other symptoms as outlined in Table 1.

Table 1: Diagnostic Criteria for Constipation[1]

The presence of 2 or more of the following symptoms for at least 12 weeks, which need not be consecutive, during the last 12 months :

- < 3 defecations per week
- Straining in > 25% of defecations
- Lumpy or hard stools in > 25% of defecations
- A sensation of incomplete evacuation in > 25% of defecations
- A sensation of anorectal obstruction or blockade in > 25% of defecations
- Manual manoeuvres to facilitate > 25% of defecations, e.g., digital evacuation, support of the pelvic floor

Loose stools are not present and the criteria for irritable bowel syndrome are not met (see Chapter 57)

Reprinted from Gastroenterology, 119, Locke et al. AGA technical review on constipation, Page 1767, Copyright (2000), with permission from American Gastroenterological Association[2]

Goals of Therapy

- Establish regular bowel function
- Abolish the need to strain and prevent the adverse effects of straining, e.g., hernia, coronary and cerebrovascular dysfunction in the elderly, gastroesophageal reflux
- Prevent complications, e.g., hemorrhoids, anal fissure, rectal prolapse, stercoral ulcer, fecal impaction, fecal incontinence
- Treat complications, e.g., fecal impaction, intestinal obstruction
- Use laxatives wisely and prevent adverse effects of laxative dependence, e.g., cathartic colon

Investigations

- Thorough history with special attention to:
  - duration of constipation
  - the most distressing features of constipation: infrequency, straining, hard stool, unusual toilet postures to facilitate stool expulsion,

digital manipulation, feeling of incomplete bowel evacuation, bloating, pain
- previous laxative use
- dietary fibre and fluid
- physical inactivity or immobilization
- drugs with constipating effects (see Table 2)
- neuropsychiatric disorders (including depression in the elderly)
- symptoms of obstructive disease (colonic neoplasm or stricture, anal stricture), painful hemorrhoid or fissure, pregnancy, neurologic disease, endocrine disorder (hypothyroidism, diabetes mellitus), collagen vascular disease (progressive systemic sclerosis)

Table 2: **Drugs with Constipating Effects**

Anticholinergic agents
Anticonvulsant agents
Antiparkinsonian agents
Antipsychotic agents
Antacids containing aluminum or calcium
Bismuth preparations
Calcium channel blockers (e.g. verapamil)
Diuretics that cause hypokalemia
Iron supplements
Opioids (codeine, morphine etc.)
Resins (e.g. cholestyramine, colestipol)
Sucralfate

- Physical examination:
  - abdominal/perineal/rectal examination looking for abdominal and rectal masses, rectal fissures and hemorrhoids
- Laboratory tests:
  - CBC
  - serum electrolytes and creatinine
  - thyroid-stimulating hormone
  - fecal occult blood
- Sigmoidoscopy
- Colonoscopy or double contrast barium enema if: recent onset in patients over 50 years old;[3] severe symptoms; symptoms do not resolve with simple measures; the cause of rectal bleeding is not demonstrated on sigmoidoscopy; alarm features are present (e.g., weight loss, anemia, unexplained positive fecal occult blood test);

family history of colorectal cancer. Routine use of colonoscopy is otherwise *not* recommended

- Psychological assessment when appropriate
- Transit studies (i.e., radiopaque markers,[4] defecography,[5] anorectal manometry[6]) and anorectal and pelvic floor tests in selected (usually < 5%) patients

Therapeutic Choices (Figure 1)

Nonpharmacologic Choices

- When possible, discontinue drugs with constipating effects (see Investigations).
- Encourage dietary fibre (20 to 30 g/day),[7,8] flax seed, unprocessed bran, whole grains, fruits and vegetables. The daily amount should be increased gradually to minimize side effects such as flatulence, bloating and unpleasant taste.
- Lactose-containing dairy products (milk, yogurt, young cheese) are an effective and natural cathartic in patients with lactase deficiency.[9]
- Increase fluid intake (at least 8 glasses of water or other liquids per day).
- Recommend prune juice, stewed prunes or figs.
- Encourage regular scheduled time for toilet use, for example, after breakfast, to develop a conditioned gastrocolic reflex.
- Advise patients not to ignore the urge to defecate.
- Avoid prolonged straining.
- Encourage physical exercise.[10]
- For constipation due to defecatory disorders, recommend relaxation exercises for the pelvic floor and external anal sphincter muscles in conjunction with biofeedback.[11,12]
- Digital manipulation of the anal sphincter may help in patients with motility problems, e.g., those with spina bifida.

Therapeutic Tips

Pharmacologic Choices (Table 3)

- In general, use drug therapy only when nonpharmacologic approaches have failed. Moreover, nonpharmacologic therapy should be continued and reinforced when drug therapy is initiated.
- Bulk-forming agents can be safely used for long-term therapy, but must be taken with adequate fluids.
- Use saline and stimulant laxatives as sparingly as possible to reduce side effects and avoid dependence[13] (i.e., short-term intermittent therapy, on an as-needed basis, once or twice weekly at most).
- At times, oral sodium phosphates or a more expensive agent such as a polyethylene glycol lavage solution is required.[14,15]

- Seek the patient's understanding and cooperation regarding general principles of therapy, and monitor laxative tolerance.
- To discontinue chronic laxative use, gradually reduce the frequency of use over three to four weeks, while optimizing nonpharmacologic approaches; use an osmotic laxative (e.g., lactulose) intermittently until bowel regularity is achieved.
- Patients with a narcotic prescription should be started on a stimulant laxative or lactulose at the same time to prevent opioid-induced constipation.

Figure 1: **Management of Constipation**

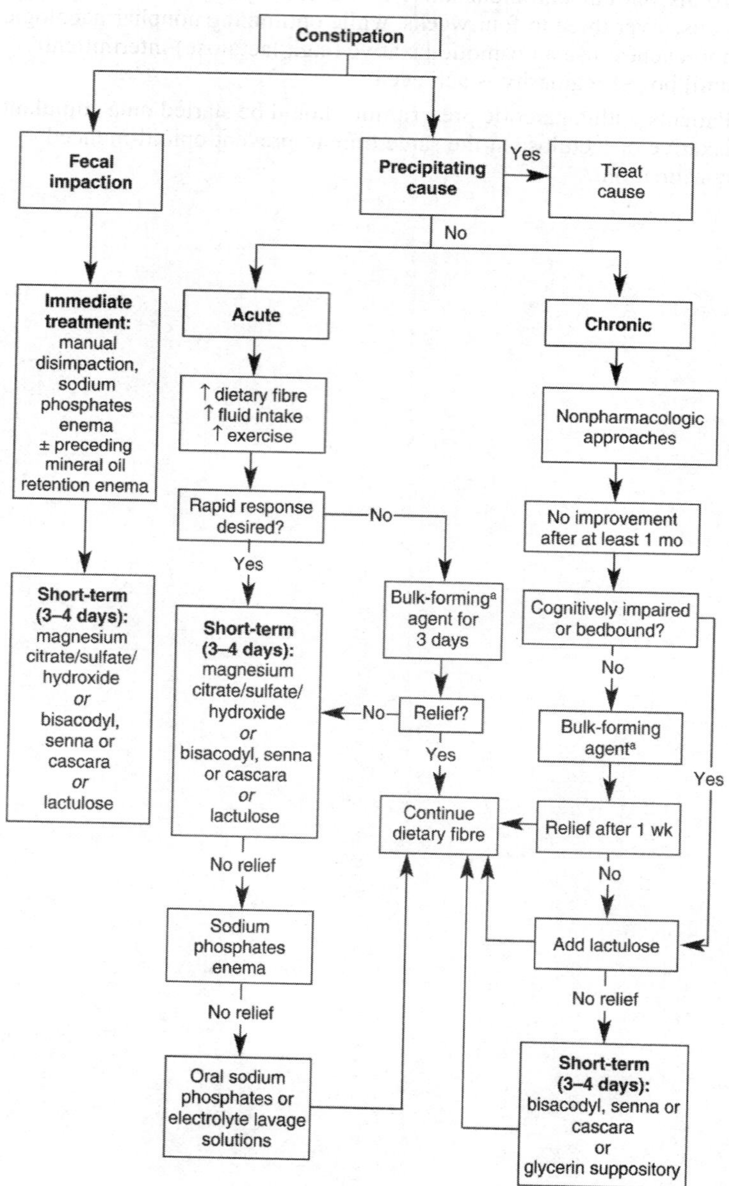

Table 3: **Drugs Used in Constipation**

Class	Drug	Adult Daily Dose (oral unless specified)	Adverse Effects	Comments	Cost[a]
Bulk-forming Agents	*psyllium hydrophilic mucilloid* Metamucil, Prodiem plain, generics	4.5–20 g (psyllium); onset: 12–72 h	Bloating, flatulence, abdominal discomfort, allergic reactions (rare), esophageal and colonic obstruction (rare).	Increases stool weight and consistency, decreases GI transit time and increases the frequency of defecation. Take with plenty of fluids. Can be used long term.	$
	sterculia gum Normacol	7–28 g; onset: 12–72 h	See psyllium.	See psyllium.	$
Hyperosmotic Agents	*glycerin* Glycerin Suppositories, generics	Suppository: 2.6 g; onset: 15 min–1 h	Rectal discomfort or burning.	Stimulates peristalsis.	$
	lactulose generics	15–60 mL (10–40 g); onset: 24–48 h	Bloating, flatulence, cramps, diarrhea.	Induces bowel water retention, improves stool consistency and increases the frequency of defecation.	$

(cont'd)

Table 3: **Drugs Used in Constipation** *(cont'd)*

Class	Drug	Adult Daily Dose (oral unless specified)	Adverse Effects	Comments	Cost[a]
Lubricants	*mineral oil* Fleet Enema Mineral Oil, Lansoyl, generics	15–45 mL; onset: 6–8 h Enema: 120 mL; onset: 2–15 min	Lipoid pneumonia if aspirated. Seepage from rectum causing pruritus and irritation.	Use the oral dosage form with extreme caution because of the risk of aspiration pneumonia. Stool softeners increase absorption of mineral oil (do not use together). Use only for short periods. ↓ absorption of fat-soluble vitamins.	po:$; enema:$$$$
Osmotic/Saline Agents	*magnesium citrate* Citro-Mag (15 g/300 mL)	4–15 g; onset: 30 min–6 h	Hypermagnesemia in renal dysfunction (Mg^{++} salts).	*Osmotic/saline agents*: stimulate peristalsis. Useful for rapid response (e.g., colonoscopy, preoperatively). *Magnesium-containing agents*: avoid in renal failure (risk of hypermagnesemia); ↓ absorption of quinolones and tetracyclines (separate administration).	$-$$$
	magnesium hydroxide Milk of Magnesia, generics	2.4–4.8 g; onset: 30 min–6 h	See magnesium citrate.	See osmotic/saline agents. See magnesium-containing agents.	$
	magnesium sulfate Epsom Salts, generics	10–30 g; onset: 30 min–6 h	See magnesium citrate.	See osmotic/saline agents. See magnesium-containing agents.	$
	sodium phosphates enema Fleet Enema, generics	120 mL (26.4 g); onset: 2–15 min	Hyperphosphatemia in patients with renal dysfunction.	See osmotic/saline agents. Avoid in renal failure (risk of hyperphosphatemia).	$

Class	Drug	Adult Daily Dose (oral unless specified)	Adverse Effects	Comments	Cost[a]
	sodium phosphates oral Fleet Phospho-Soda, Phosphates Solution	20 mL for laxative effect; 45 mL for purgative effect; onset: 30 min–6 h	Hyperphosphatemia in patients with renal dysfunction. Risk of arrhythmias if exceed recommended daily dosage.	See osmotic/saline agents Avoid in renal failure (risk of hyperphosphatemia).	$$$$

Stimulant Agents	*bisacodyl*
	Dulcolax, Carters Little Pills, Gentlax, generics
		Tablet: 5–15 mg; onset: 6–12 h
		Suppository: 10 mg; onset: 15 min–1 h
		Micro-enema: 10 mg; onset: 15 min–1 h
			Abdominal pain, cramps, cathartic colon.
			Rectal microscopic mucosal changes with suppository and enema.
				Stimulate colonic peristalsis.
				The most potent purgatives.
				Usually short term use only, but long-term use may be necessary and is suitable in patients on long-term opioid therapy (e.g., cancer patients).
					$ tablet
					$ suppos
					$$ micro-enema

	castor oil generics	15–60 mL; onset: 1–3 h	Abdominal pain, cramps.	See bisacodyl.	$-$$
	senna Senokot Preparations, others	15–30 mg (sennosides); onset: 6–12 h	Abdominal pain, cramps, cathartic colon. Melanosis coli (anthraquinone derivatives). Some senna preparations have high sugar content.	See bisacodyl.	$
Stool Softeners	*docusate sodium* Colace, generics	100–200 mg; onset: 12–72 h		Act as surfactants. Often used as 'stool softeners' after rectal surgery and in long-term opioid users, but there are no documented beneficial effects.	$

(cont'd)

Table 3: **Drugs Used in Constipation** *(cont'd)*

Class	Drug	Adult Daily Dose (oral unless specified)	Adverse Effects	Comments	Cost[a]
	docusate calcium generics	240 mg; onset: 12–72 h		See docusate sodium.	$
Lavage Solutions	*electrolyte solutions* PegLyte, Colyte, Klean-Prep, generics	1000–4000 mL; onset: 30 min–1 h	Retching, nausea, abdominal fullness and bloating.	Contain mainly sodium sulfate and polyethylene glycol. Excellent cleansing for colonoscopy. Klean-Prep is available as 4 × 1 L sachets.	$$$$

[a] Cost per day; includes drug cost only.
Legend: $ < $1 $-$$ < $1–2 $$ $1–2 $-$$$ < $1–3 $$$ $2–3 $$$$ > $3

Suggested Readings

American College of Gastroenterology Chronic Constipation Task Force. An evidence-based approach to the management of chronic constipation in North America. *Am J Gastroenterol* 2005;100(Suppl 1):S1-4.

Brandt LJ, Prather CM, Quigley EM et al. Systematic review on the management of chronic constipation in North America. *Am J Gastroenterol* 2005;100(Suppl 1):S5-21.

Lembo A, Camilleri M. Chronic constipation. *N Engl J Med* 2003;349(14):1360-8.

Wilson JA. Constipation in the elderly. *Clin Geriatr Med* 1999;15(3):499-510.

References

1. Thompson WG, Longstreth GF, Drossman DA et al. Functional bowel disorders and functional abdominal pain. *Gut* 1999;45(Suppl 2):II43-7.
2. Locke GR, Pemberton JH,.Phillips SF. AGA technical review on constipation. American Gastroenterological Association. *Gastroenterology* 2000;119(6):1766-78.
3. Locke GR, Pemberton JH, Phillips SF. American Gastroenterological Association medical position statement: guidelines on constipation. *Gastroenterology* 2000;119(6):1761-6.
4. Hinton JM, Lennard-Jones JE, Young AC. A new method for studying gut transit times using radioopaque markers. *Gut* 1969;10(10):842-7.
5. Shorvon PJ, McHugh S, Diamant NE et al. Defecography in normal volunteers: results and implications. *Gut* 1989;30(12):1737-49.
6. Barnett JL, Hasler WL, Camilleri M. American Gastroenterological Association medical position statement on anorectal testing techniques. American Gastroenterological Association. *Gastroenterology* 1999;116(3):732-60.
7. Cummings JH. Constipation, dietary fibre and the control of large bowel function. *Postgrad Med J* 1984;60(709):811-9.
8. Badiali D, Corazziari E, Habib FI et al. Effect of wheat bran in treatment of chronic nonorganic constipation. A double-blind controlled trial. *Dig Dis Sci* 1995;40(2):349-56.
9. Adolfsson O, Meydani SN,.Russell RM. Yogurt and gut function. *Am J Clin Nutr* 2004;80(2):245-56.
10. De Schryver AM, Keulemans YC, Peters HP et al. Effects of regular physical activity on defecation pattern in middle-aged patients complaining of chronic constipation. *Scand J Gastroenterol* 2005;40(4):422-9.
11. Chiarioni G, Salandini L, Whitehead WE. Biofeedback benefits only patients with outlet dysfunction, not patients with isolated slow transit constipation. *Gastroenterology* 2005;129(1):86-97.
12. Chiarioni G, Whitehead WE, Pezza V et al. Biofeedback is superior to laxatives for normal transit constipation due to pelvic floor dyssynergia. *Gastroenterology* 2006;130(3):657-64.
13. Velio P, Bassotti G. Chronic idiopathic constipation: pathophysiology and treatment. *J Clin Gastroenterol* 1996;22(3):190-6.
14. Andorsky RI, Goldner F. Colonic lavage solution (polyethylene glycol electrolyte lavage solution) as a treatment for chronic constipation: a double-blind, placebo-controlled study. *Am J Gastroenterol* 1990;85(3):261-5.
15. Corazziari E, Badiali D, Habib FI et al. Small volume isosmotic polyethylene glycol electrolyte balanced solution (PMF-100) in treatment of chronic nonorganic constipation. *Dig Dis Sci* 1996;41(8):1636-42.

Pharmacoeconomic Considerations: Constipation

Nicole Mittmann, MSc, PhD

Epidemiology	
Country (Year)	**Prevalence (%)**
Canada (2000)[1]	27.2% of adults self-reported constipation within the previous 3 months. Prevalence in women was twice that in men.
Canada, United Kingdom, United States[2]	10–15% 30–40% of those aged > 65 years

Cost of Illness Data		
Country and Year of Estimate	**Direct Costs[a]**	**Indirect Costs[b]**
United States[4]	Not reported	13.7 million days of restricted activity 3.42 million days of bed disability
United States[6]	US $2253 per nursing home resident	Not reported

Commentary

Constipation is an economic burden for patients, health care providers and society. Constipation is more common in females,[1] and increases in prevalence with increasing age (30–40% in those over age 65).[3,4] Direct costs are largely those associated with over-the-counter and prescription drugs and physician consultations. Indirect costs of constipation are associated with days of restricted activity and bed disability days.[4] In long-term care or nursing homes, reductions in the frequency and severity of complications of constipation can lead to a decrease in pharmacy expenditures.[7] Complications of constipation (impaction, pain, incontinence and perforation) may incur direct and indirect medical costs.

Quality of life is impaired in patients with constipation when compared to nonconstipated individuals. Drug treatments for constipation improve quality of life.[2] Medications for constipation are typically not the largest cost drivers.

There have been few formal economic analyses published for treatments associated with the care of constipation.[8,9,10] All studies

(cont'd)

Commentary
showed that the cost drivers for the studies were not medications but rather the cost of physician consultations or visits.

[a] Direct costs include those associated with physician services, nursing care, diagnostic procedures, drugs and hospitalization.
[b] Indirect costs include those associated with lost productivity and days off work due to morbidity or premature mortality.

References

1. Pare P, Ferrazzi S, Thompson WG et al. An epidemiological survey of constipation in Canada: definitions, rates, demographics and predictors of health care seeking. *Am J Gastroenterol* 2001;96(11):3130-7.
2. Dennison C, Prasad M, Lloyd A et al. The health-related quality of life and economic burden of constipation. *Pharmacoeconomics* 2005;23(5):461-76.
3. Stewart RB, Moore MT, Marks RG et al. Correlates of constipation in an ambulatory elderly population. *Am J Gastroenterol* 1992;87(7):859-64.
4. Sonnenberg A, Koch TR. Epidemiology of constipation in the United States. *Dis Colon Rectum* 1989;32(1):1-8.
5. Passmore AP. Economic aspects of pharmacotherapy for chronic constipation. *Pharmacoeconomics* 1995;7(1):14-24.
6. Frank L, Schmier J, Kleinman L et al. Time and economic cost of constipation in nursing homes. *J Am Med Dir Assoc* 2002;3(4):215-23.
7. Hull C, Greco RS, Brooks DL. Alleviation of constipation in the elderly by dietary fiber supplementation. *J Am Geriatr Soc* 1980;28(9):410-4.
8. Christie AH, Culbert P, Guest JF. Economic impact of low dose polyethylene glycol 3350 plus electrolytes compared with lactulose in the management of idiopathic constipation in the UK. *Pharmacoeconomics* 2002;20(1):49-60.
9. Lederle FA, Busch DL, Mattox KM et al. Cost-effective treatment of constipation in the elderly: a randomized double-blind comparison of sorbitol and lactulose. *Am J Med* 1990;89(5):597-601.
10. Passmore AP, Wilson-Davies K, Stoker C et al. Chronic constipation in long stay elderly patients: a comparison of lactulose and a senna-fibre combination. *BMJ* 1993;307(6907):769-71.

CHAPTER 115
Diarrhea

Richard N. Fedorak, MD, FRCPC and
Anna M. Borowiec, MD

Diarrhea is physiologically defined as the excretion of fecal matter at a rate greater than 200 g/24 hours, with increased loss of fecal water and electrolytes. Clinically, diarrhea is present when an alteration in a normal bowel habit occurs, characterized by a decrease in consistency to soft or liquid and an increase in frequency to ≥ 3 stools/day. *Acute diarrhea* is an episode of diarrhea of < 14 days in duration. *Persistent diarrhea* is diarrhea of > 14 days in duration. *Chronic diarrhea* is diarrhea that lasts > 30 days.

Goals of Therapy

- Provide interventions that will reduce symptoms and re-establish normal fecal weight (volume)
- Prevent and treat complications, i.e., dehydration, electrolyte depletion, nutrient malabsorption, hemorrhoids, rectal prolapse
- Remove or eradicate the cause of diarrhea where applicable

Investigations[1,2,3]

Establish a cause and make an early diagnosis of an acute episode of diarrhea.

Prior to the initiation of therapy, three key questions must be addressed:

- What is the patient's history? Obtain a thorough history that includes the following clinical and epidemiologic features:
  - when and how the illness began (duration of symptoms; abrupt or gradual onset)
  - stool characteristics (watery, bloody, mucousy, greasy)
  - frequency of bowel movements and quantity of stool produced
  - symptoms of volume depletion (thirst, tachycardia, orthostatic hypotension, decreased urination, lethargy, decreased skin turgor)
  - associated systemic symptoms and their frequency and intensity (nausea, vomiting, abdominal pain, cramps, headache, fever, myalgias, altered sensorium)
  - changes in diet
  - medication history including use of prescription and over-the-counter drugs, herbal or "natural" products and dietary supplements
  - recent travel history, locale of employment and residence and other family members or co-workers that have a similar illness

- Is this true diarrhea? Many people who complain of diarrhea actually have a motility disturbance (i.e., irritable bowel syndrome). They experience an increased frequency of very small bowel movements, but the 24-hour stool weight does not exceed normal amounts. Measuring fecal fat, osmolarity and bile acid levels can also help determine specific etiologies.
- Is the diarrhea acute or chronic? In the absence of fever, dehydration or bloody stools, the management of acute diarrhea should alleviate symptoms rather than provide a specific diagnosis or therapy. Acute diarrhea (Figure 1, Table 1) is frequently caused by viral agents, drugs or food toxins for which there is no specific therapy, and usually remits spontaneously within less than one week. Acute infectious diarrhea of a bacterial or parasitic etiology should be identified early to permit early successful intervention. Evaluate chronic diarrhea as in Figure 2.

Table 1: **Etiology of Acute Diarrhea**

Etiology		**Examples**
Infectious	Bacterial	*Shigella*, *Salmonella* (*typhi*, *enteritidis*), *Campylobacter*, *Yersinia*, *Escherichia coli* (EHEC 0157:H7, ETEC, EPEC), *Clostridium* (*difficile*, *perfringens*) *Vibrio* (*cholerae*, *parahaemolyticus*), *Staphylococcus aureus*, *Bacillus cereus*
	Viral	Norovirus (Norwalk virus), rotavirus, adenovirus, cytomegalovirus, herpes simplex virus
	Parasitic	*Cryptosporidium*, Microsporidia, *Entamoeba histolytica*, *Giardia lamblia*, *Cyclospora*
Medications		Antibiotics, colchicine, laxatives, Mg-containing antacids
Food intolerance		Lactose
Intestinal disease (acute episode)		Celiac disease, inflammatory bowel disease (ulcerative colitis, Crohn's disease)
Other		Thyrotoxicosis, carcinoid syndrome

Specific issues relating to diagnosis of an acute infectious etiology of the diarrhea are:[3]

- Proctitis can be diagnosed with sigmoidoscopy. Involvement of only the distal 15 cm suggests herpesvirus, gonococcal, chlamydial or syphilitic infection. Colitis extending more proximally suggests *Campylobacter*, *Shigella*, *Clostridium difficile* or chlamydial (LGV serotype) infection
- An inflammatory etiology (e.g., invasive colitis due to *Salmonella*, *Shigella* or *Campylobacter*; *C. difficile* colitis, inflammatory bowel disease) can be suspected on the basis of fever, tenesmus or bloody stools. Microscopy for fecal leukocytes or fecal lactoferrin testing may confirm inflammation. A meta-analysis and a recent review of the diagnostic test accuracy for fecal leukocytes demonstrated a sensitivity of only 70% and a specificity ranging from 50% to 84%.[1,3] Fecal

lactoferrin has a higher sensitivity and specificity of 90% and 79%, respectively, but is not widely available[4]

- Consider tests for parasitic causes of diarrhea to include fluorescence and enzyme immunoassay for *Giardia* and *Cryptosporidium* and acid-fast stains for *Cryptosporidium*, *Cyclospora*, *Isospora* or *Mycobacterium* species
- Any diarrheal illness accompanied by fever, bloody stools, systemic illness, recent use of antibiotics, daycare centre attendance, hospitalization or dehydration should prompt evaluation of a fecal specimen, including stool cultures plus other investigations as noted below and in Figure 1.
- In patients who do not appear unwell or do not have the above symptoms, the necessity of documenting a pathogen is not always clear, since acute diarrheal episodes are generally self-limiting and resolve within several days
- Selective fecal testing can improve the yield and usefulness of stool testing and should be adopted whenever possible using the following guidelines:
  - consider *E. coli* 0157 in persons with a history of undercooked red meat ingestion and acute bloody diarrhea or hemolytic uremic syndrome, as well as those with marked abdominal pain and bloody diarrhea but without high fever
  - consider *Vibrio* species in persons who have ingested shellfish within the three days before the illness began
  - consider *Yersinia enterocolitica* in fall or winter and in certain at-risk populations (e.g., Asians and African–American infants), as well as those with persistent abdominal pain and fever
  - consider a *C. difficile* toxin assay in hospitalized patients and those who have taken antimicrobial agents within the last eight weeks
  - immunocompromised patients or those with significant comorbidities that increase the risk for complications
  - patients with inflammatory bowel disease in whom distinction between a flare and superimposed infection is critical
  - fecal specimens from patients with diarrhea that develops after three days of hospitalization have a very low yield when cultured for standard bacterial pathogens (*Campylobacter*, *Salmonella*, *Shigella*, etc.) or examined for ova and parasites
  - consider Norwalk virus (a norovirus) in patients with nausea, vomiting, intense cramping and watery diarrhea. The disease is self-limited and usually lasts 48 to 72 hours. The virus is spread by ingestion of feces-contaminated water (including that in swimming pools) or food, contact with contaminated environments or individuals with the illness. The virus is shed in vomitus and the stool for at least 24 to 48 hours after the onset of illness. Given the classic clinical presentation and rapid recovery, the specific viral diagnosis is not necessary in adult gastroenteritis. In the case of

Norwalk virus, identifying the causative agent allows for institution of appropriate control measures:
  - frequent hand washing with soap
  - wearing of protective barriers such as gloves
  - careful washing of all fruits and vegetables
  - appropriate disposal of vomitus (in toilet) and disinfection of potentially contaminated surfaces
  - infected persons should not prepare foods while they are symptomatic and for 3 days after they have recovered

- Ask patients about potential epidemiologic risk factors for particular diarrheal diseases or for their spread:
  - travel to a developing country
  - daycare centre attendance or employment
  - visitation or employment in acute-care or long-term care facilities
  - ingestion of unsafe foods (e.g., raw meats, eggs or shellfish; unpasteurized milk or juices)
  - swimming in or drinking untreated water
  - visiting a farm or petting zoo or having contact with pets with diarrhea
  - knowledge of other ill family members or co-workers
  - recent antibiotic use
  - underlying medical conditions predisposing to infectious diarrhea (e.g., AIDS, immunosuppressive therapies, previous gastrectomy, extremes of age)
  - where appropriate, receptive anal intercourse or oral-anal sexual contact
  - occupation as a food-handler or caregiver

For persons with AIDS, a modified algorithm for the investigation and management of diarrhea is available.[3]

Public Health Considerations

Diagnostic testing of fecal specimens is indicated for certain groups.

- Food-handlers in the food service industry and health care workers with direct patient contact and diarrhea should be tested for parasitic and bacterial pathogens due to their potential to transmit the infections to large numbers of persons
- Similarly, daycare attendees and employees, or residents of an institutional facility (i.e., nursing home, psychiatric hospital, prison) with diarrhea should be tested for bacterial, parasitic or viral pathogens since the diarrhea may be an indicator of an endemic outbreak

Physicians who suspect an endemic diarrheal disease outbreak should report the concern to public health authorities and, in conjunction with these authorities, initiate appropriate diagnostic testing to facilitate identification of the pathogenic agent and to define the extent of the outbreak.

Follow-up Fecal Culture

Follow-up testing is not generally recommended. However, since food-handlers and health care workers can transmit bacterial and parasitic diseases even if they are asymptomatic, it is recommended that before returning to their jobs these persons have two consecutive negative stool samples taken 24 hours apart and at least 48 hours after resolution of symptoms.

Therapeutic Choices

Nonpharmacologic Choices[2]

- Discontinue medications that cause diarrhea (e.g., laxatives, antacids containing magnesium, antibiotics, diuretics, theophylline, cholinergic drugs, promotility agents, prostaglandins, acarbose, orlistat).
- Stop ingestion of poorly absorbed carbohydrates (e.g., dietetic candies and jams containing sorbitol, mannitol or xylitol, beverages and foods containing fructose, or lactose-containing dairy products). If the history is compatible with lactose intolerance, a two-week trial of a lactose-restricted diet can avoid costly diagnostic work-ups.
- Reduce food intake for 12 to 24 hours. This will improve the symptoms of acute diarrhea. Maintenance of adequate fluid and electrolyte intake is important and a bland diet (low fat, low carbohydrate, including for example, bananas, rice, unsweetened applesauce, clear soup) can be reintroduced once bowel motions have subsided.

Pharmacologic Choices (Table 2)

Oral Rehydration Therapy

Oral rehydration therapy (ORT, see Chapter 88) prevents dehydration and electrolyte loss in both acute and chronic diarrhea. Oral rehydration solutions should have a balanced sodium-to-glucose ratio. Excess glucose, for example in Jell-O and soda pop, or excess sodium, for example in Gatorade or other "sports drinks," may aggravate diarrhea as a consequence of their osmotic effect. Early use of ORT is essential for young children and the elderly.

Balanced electrolyte oral rehydration solutions are available commercially without prescription (e.g., Gastrolyte, Pedialyte). If necessary, a similar solution can be made by adding one level teaspoon (5 mL) of salt and eight teaspoons (40 mL) of sugar to one litre of water.[5]

Empiric Antibiotics

Aside from travellers' diarrhea, empiric antibiotic treatment is not generally recommended for acute diarrhea because of the self-limiting nature of most illnesses, the cost of treatment, the potential for promoting antimicrobial resistance and the possibility of adverse drug reactions.[5,6]

Bismuth

Bismuth subsalicylate has been shown to be effective, in small cohort studies, in the treatment of idiopathic diarrhea and diarrhea caused by microscopic colitis. Although frequently used in acute diarrheas, there is no firm evidence for its efficacy. The salicylate component can cause gastric and duodenal mucosal damage, particularly in patients who are also using ASA or NSAIDs. At high doses, the calcium carbonate in the tablet formation can cause hypercalcemia, hypercalciuria and associated metabolic symptoms. Bismuth-related encephalopathy can result from the use of doses 10 times those recommended, or after years of use. Black stools due to bismuth may be confused with melena.

Hydrophilic Bulking Agents

Psyllium is a hydrophilic agent that increases fecal water-holding capacity and may reduce nonspecific diarrheal symptoms. In some cases it has been used to bind bacterial-mediated toxins (i.e., *C. difficile* toxin), but its role in the management of diarrhea is limited. Many psyllium-containing products are mixed with laxatives; these products must be avoided in patients with diarrhea.

Cholestyramine resin, in addition to its hydrophilic action, has the ability to bind bile acids. Thus, it is useful in treating bile acid–induced diarrhea due to malabsorption of bile acids in diseased ileum (e.g., Crohn's disease) or in some cases of IBS where rapid transit results in loss of bile acids into the colon. Cholestyramine's ability to bind luminal bacterial toxins has led to adjunctive use in toxin-induced diarrhea (e.g., *C. difficile*).

Opioids

Available opioids include naturally occurring preparations (**paregoric** and **opium alkaloids**) and synthetic preparations (**codeine**, **diphenoxylate** and **loperamide**). These agents are very effective for symptomatic use in both acute and chronic diarrhea; however, side effects limit their acute use and tolerance usually occurs with chronic use. Antimotility effects are not desired if the diarrhea is caused by microorganisms because gastrointestinal stasis may enhance their invasion.[5,7] Diphenoxylate and loperamide have fewer CNS side effects than other opioids. Diphenoxylate is combined with atropine to limit its potential for abuse. Loperamide has the lowest incidence of side effects and abuse potential, is available without prescription and is effective in patients with radiotherapy- and chemotherapy-induced diarrhea and in patients with ileo-rectal pouch incontinence. Combining loperamide with simethicone provides faster and more complete relief of acute diarrhea associated with gas-related abdominal discomfort. Consider codeine if sedation or analgesia is also desired.

Alpha$_2$-adrenergic Agonists

Clonidine is effective against opioid-withdrawal diarrhea and diarrhea associated with diabetic autonomic neuropathy. Unfortunately, the dose required to achieve an antidiarrheal effect is often associated with sedation, dry mouth and symptomatic orthostatic hypotension.

Somatostatin Analogues

Somatostatin analogues can be administered sc daily **(octreotide)** or by im injection monthly (**octreotide acetate**, **lanreotide acetate**). These have been used to control diarrhea caused by neuroendocrine tumors (VIPoma, carcinoid, medullary carcinoma of the thyroid). Octreotide has also been shown to limit idiopathic and infant secretory diarrhea, as well as diarrhea associated with ileostomy, short bowel syndrome, diabetic neuropathy, chemotherapy, bone marrow transplant, cryptosporidia, graft versus host disease and HIV disease.

Somatostatin has a short half-life and requires continuous iv infusion, which limits its role in the management of diarrhea.

Probiotics (Table 3)

Probiotics are nonpathogenic bacteria that colonize the gut and improve intestinal microbial balance. Multiple clinical trials have looked at the use of probiotics in the prevention and treatment of gastrointestinal infections in adults and children. *Lactobacillus* GG and *Saccharomyces boulardii* are effective in preventing antibiotic-associated diarrhea among adults and children, including recurrent *C. difficile* infections.[8] Furthermore, in children, probiotics are effective in reducing the severity and duration of acute rotavirus-induced diarrhea.[9] There is no conclusive evidence for the effectiveness of probiotics in the management of traveller's diarrhea. Currently probiotics have no role in induction or remission maintenance in Crohn's disease; however, in acute ulcerative colitis certain preparations (*E. coli* Nissle) have been shown to be equivalent to low-dose 5-aminosalicylic acid. In small open trials, certain probiotic preparations (VSL#3) have been shown to decrease the occurrence and severity of post-radiation diarrhea.[10]

Therapeutic Tips

All patients and caregivers need to be made aware of the following issues:

- Infectious diarrhea can be prevented by following simple rules of personal hygiene and safe food preparation. Handwashing with soap is an effective step in preventing spread of the illness and should be emphasized for both patients and their caregivers.
- The importance of a balanced electrolyte oral rehydration solution in preventing dehydration and the inability of nonbalanced electrolyte solutions to achieve rehydration is critical for patients to understand.
- Repeated diarrheal illnesses in young children can lead to malnutrition and physical and cognitive growth impairment.

- Notify public health surveillance programs of pathogen-specific diagnoses to lower rates of transmission and control outbreaks.
- Specific vaccines are available for prevention of diarrhea due to cholera (*V. cholerae*) and enterotoxigenic *E. coli* in adults and children (see Chapter 109), typhoid fever (*S. typhi*) in adults and children, and rotavirus in infants.

Figure 1: **Evaluation of Acute Diarrhea**

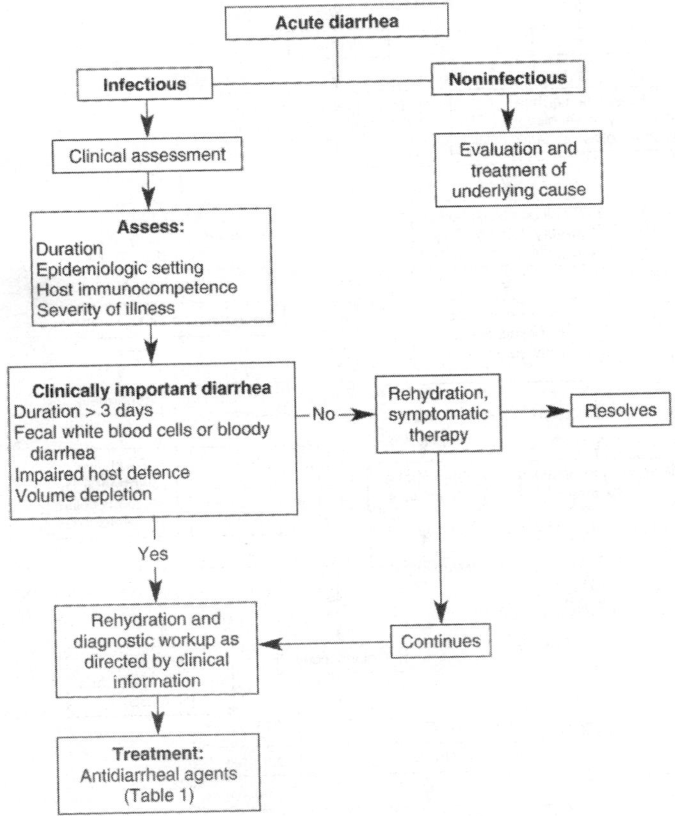

Figure 2: **Evaluation of Chronic Diarrhea**

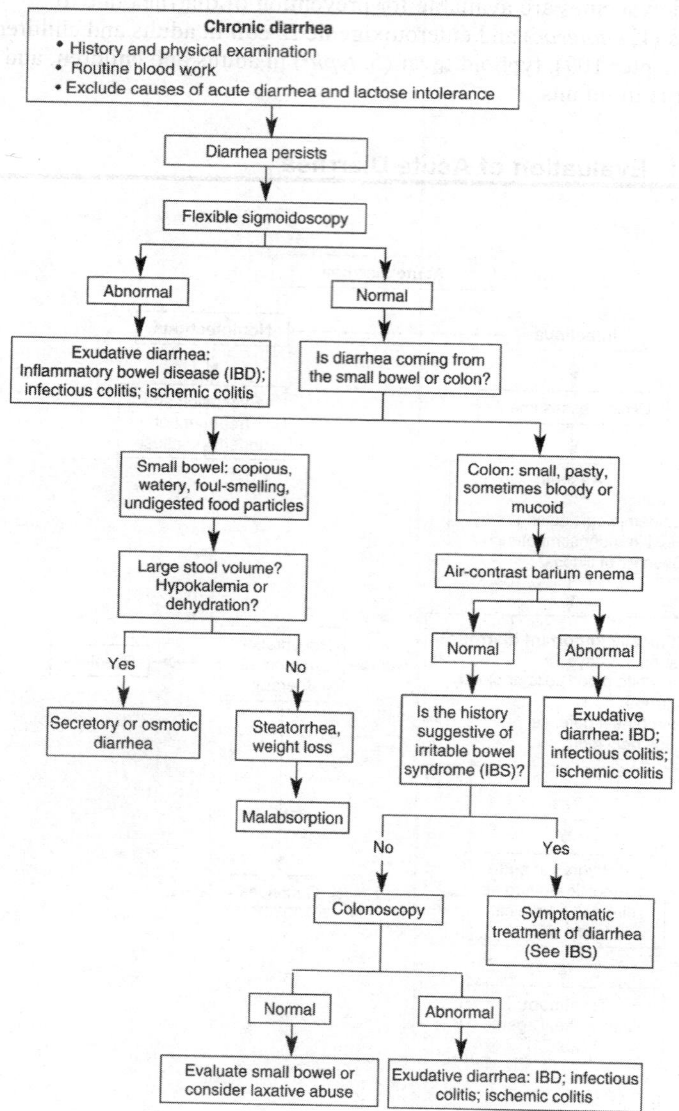

Table 2: **Drugs Used to Treat Diarrhea**

Class	Drug	Dose	Adverse Effects	Drug Interactions	Comments	Cost[a]
Bismuth	*bismuth subsalicylate* Pepto-Bismol liquid, generics	30 mL (17.6 mg BSS/mL) Q30 min to a max of 8 doses/day	Salicylate toxicity, black tongue, black stool, bismuth-induced encephalopathy.	↓ absorption of doxycycline and tetracycline.		$
	bismuth subsalicylate with calcium carbonate Pepto-Bismol chewables	2 tablets (262 mg BSS/tab) Q30 min to a max of 8 doses/day	See bismuth subsalicylate. Hypercalcemia, hypercalciuria.	See bismuth subsalicylate.		$
Hydrophilic Bulking Agents	*psyllium hydrophilic mucilloid* Metamucil Preparations, generics	1 teaspoon (5–6 g) Q12H	Inhalation of psyllium powder may cause allergic reactions.		Avoid combinations with laxatives.	$
	cholestyramine resin generics	4 g Q12H	Nausea, fat soluble vitamin deficiency with long-term use, constipation.	May bind other drugs in GI tract; do not take within 1 h before or 4–6 h after other medications.		$
Opioids	*loperamide* Imodium, Riva-Loperamide, generics	2 mg after each loose bowel movement (max of 16 mg/day)	Sedation, nausea, abdominal cramps. Lowest addiction potential of all opioids.			$

(cont'd)

Table 2: **Drugs Used to Treat Diarrhea** *(cont'd)*

Class	Drug	Dose	Adverse Effects	Drug Interactions	Comments	Cost[a]
	diphenoxylate with atropine sulfate Lomotil, generics	5 mg initially then 2.5 mg after each loose bowel movement (max of 20 mg/day)	Sedation, nausea, abdominal cramps, dry skin and mucous membranes (from atropine), some addiction potential.	Additive anticholinergic effects with other anticholinergic agents.	The elderly are particularly susceptible to the anticholinergic effects of atropine.	$
	codeine generics	30–60 mg Q4H PRN	Sedation, nausea, tolerance, potentially addictive.	Additive CNS depression with CNS depressants.		$
Alpha$_2$-adrenergic Agonists	*clonidine* Catapres, Dixarit, generics	0.1–0.6 mg Q12H	Centrally mediated sedation and hypotension.	Additive effects with drugs that cause hypotension. May ↑ cyclosporine concentrations.		$
Somatostatin Analogues	*octreotide* Sandostatin, generics	50–500 µg sc Q12H	Pain at injection site, nausea, mild diarrhea.			$$$
	octreotide acetate Sandostatin LAR	10–30 mg im monthly	See octreotide.			$1250–$2100/mo
	lanreotide acetate Somatuline autogel	60 mg im monthly	See octreotide.			[b]

[a] Cost of 1-day supply except Sandostatin LAR; includes drug cost only.
[b] Approved by Health Canada, but not currently marketed in Canada.
Abbreviations: BM = bowel movement; BSS = bismuth subsalicylate; IBS = irritable bowel syndrome; LAR = long-acting release
Legend: $ < $5 $$ $5–15 $$$ $10–90

Table 3: Select Probiotic Products Used to Treat Diarrhea

Class	Drug	Dose	Adverse Effects	Drug Interactions	Comments	Cost[a]
Probiotics	*Saccharomyces boulardii* Flurastar	1 capsule bid for 3 to 5 days per day (3 billion CFU), max 3 capsules per day	Constipation, bloating.	A yeast; therefore, do not administer with antifungal agents.		$$
	Lactobacillus GG Culturelle[b]	Adults: 1–2 40 mg capsules/day; children: ½ –1 capsule/day (1 cap = ≥10 billion CFU)	~2% of patients report bloating and gas for a few days.	A bacterium; therefore, do not administer with antibiotics.	May contain traces of casein or whey. Does not ferment lactose; unhelpful for lactose intolerance.	$$
	lactic acid bacterial mixture VSL#3[c]	The dose is based on the frequency of BM: Adults 1–2 packets/day if < 5 BM; 2–4 packets/day if 5–8 BM; 4 packets/day if > 8 BM	No evidence of adverse health effects.	A mixture of bacteria; therefore, do not administer with antibiotics.	Has been studied in patients with radiation-induced diarrhea, Crohn's disease, ulcerative colitis, ileal pouch anastomosis and IBS.	$$

[a] Cost of 1-day supply.
[b] Capsule contain at least 10 x 10^9 colony-forming units of *Lactobacillus rhamnosus* GG.
[c] Packets contain 450 x 10^9 freeze-dried lactic acid bacteria (*Bifidobacterium breve*, *B. longum*, *B. infantis*, *L. acidophilus*, *L. plantarum*, *L. casei*, *L. bulgaricus*, *Streptococcus thermophilus*) in a defined ratio.

Abbreviations: BM = bowel movement; CFU = colony-forming unit; IBS = irritable bowel syndrome

Legend: $ < $5 $$ $5–15

Suggested Readings

Aranda-Michel J, Giannella RA. Acute diarrhea: a practical review. *Am J Med* 1999;106(6):670-6.

Fedorak RN. Anti-diarrheal therapy. In: Friedman G, Jacobson ED, McCallum RW, editors. *Gastrointestinal pharmacology and therapeutics*. Philadelphia (PA): Lippincott-Raven; 1997. p. 175-93.

Fine KD, Schiller LR. AGA technical review on the evaluation and management of chronic diarrhea. *Gastroenterology* 1999;116(6):1464-86.

Thielman NM, Guerrant RL. Clinical practice. Acute infectious diarrhea. *N Engl J Med* 2004;350(1):38-47.

Theilman NM, Guerrant RL. An algorithmic approach to the workup and management of HIV-related diarrhea. *J Clin Outcomes Manag* 1997;4:36-47.

References

1. DuPont HL. Guidelines on acute infectious diarrhea in adults. The Practice Parameters Committee of the American College of Gastroenterology. *Am J Gastroenterol* 1997;92(11):1962-75.
2. Schiller LR. Chronic diarrhea. *Gastroenterology* 2004;127(1):287-93.
3. Thielman NM, Guerrant RL. Clinical practice. Acute infectious diarrhea. *N Engl J Med* 2004;350(1):38-47.
4. Kane SV, Sandborn WJ, Rufo PA et al. Fecal lactoferrin is a sensitive and specific marker in identifying intestinal inflammation. *Am J Gastroenterol* 2003;98(6):1309-14.
5. Committee to Advise on Tropical Medicine and Travel (CATMAT). Statement on travellers' diarrhea. *Can Commun Dis Rep* 2001;27(ACS-3):1-12. Available from: http://www.phac-aspc.gc.ca/publicat/ccdr-rmtc/01vol27/27sup/acs3.html Accessed March 22, 2007.
6. Sirinavin S, Garner P. Antibiotics for treating salmonella gut infections. *Cochrane Database Syst Rev* 2000;(2):CD001167.
7. Molbak K, Mead PS, Griffin PM. Antimicrobial therapy in patients with Escherichia coli O157:H7 infection. *JAMA* 2002;288(8):1014-6.
8. Huebner ES, Surawicz CM. Probiotics in the prevention and treatment of gastrointestinal infections. *Gastroenterol Clin North Am* 2006;35(2):355-65.
9. NASPGHAN Nutrition Report Committee; Michail S, Sylvester F et al. Clinical efficacy of probiotics: review of the evidence with focus on children. *J Pediatr Gastroenterol Nutr* 2006;43(4):550-7.
10. Delia P, Sansotta G, Donato V et al. Prevention of radiation-induced diarrhea with the use of VSL#3, a new high-potency probiotic preparation. *Am J Gastroenterol* 2002;97(8):2150-2.

CHAPTER 116
Fever in Children

Joanne M. Langley, MD, MSc, FRCPC

Fever is a regulated physiologic response in which a new set-point for body temperature is established. It is defined by a temperature consistently over 38°C (rectal or rectal equivalent).[1] The most common cause of fever in children is infection.[2] The body establishes a new balance of heat loss and production to maintain homeostasis. The febrile response rarely exceeds 41°C to 42°C. Normal body temperature varies throughout the day.

Temperature measurement from the rectum, mouth or tympanic membrane reflects core temperature. Axillary temperatures are lower than core, difficult to measure accurately and thus are only recommended for screening low-risk children. Although measurement error can occur with any method, rectal thermometry is, in general, regarded as the gold standard for definitive measurement of temperature in children < 5 years.[3] For children > 5 years, oral thermometry is recommended for confirmation of fever. Tympanic or axillary temperature measurement can be used as a screening tool for low-risk children.[4]

Fever itself is not harmful. Some host defense mechanisms may be enhanced by fever. Temperature greater than 41°C is rare with fever. Fever is a different state than disorders of thermoregulation, in which heat production exceeds heat loss (see Chapter 117).

Goals of Therapy

- Provide patient comfort
- Relieve parental anxiety
- Avoid potentially harmful secondary effects due to metabolic demands in those with cardiac or pulmonary disorders

There is little evidence that antipyretic therapy is beneficial to the child. In particular, it does not seem to prevent febrile seizures.[5]

Investigations

Fever is a symptom/sign, not a diagnosis, and most commonly is an adaptive response to an infection. Fever may also occur in malignancy, rheumatologic or immunologic diseases.

- History and physical examination to ascertain associated symptoms and source of the fever
- Clinical judgment determines if the underlying process is benign (e.g., viral respiratory tract infection) or life-threatening (e.g., bacterial meningitis)

- Bacteremia is more likely if the temperature is greater than 41.1°C in young children,[6,7] therefore blood cultures may be warranted
- Aggressiveness of the laboratory evaluation depends on the clinical assessment of the severity of illness, the child's age (especially if < 3 months) and immune status[8]
  - may include culture of suspected sources of infection (e.g., urine, blood, cerebrospinal fluid) or imaging studies (e.g., chest radiograph)
  - nonspecific tests such as the WBC and/or differential or C-reactive protein are not sufficiently sensitive or specific to be useful in initial management of the febrile child[1,9]

Therapeutic Choices

Nonpharmacologic Choices

Physical methods for heat reduction use convection, evaporation or conduction to overwhelm the body's attempt to maintain a higher temperature set-point. The body aggressively opposes physical cooling by attempting to re-establish a high temperature by shivering and vasoconstriction, both of which cause patient discomfort.[10] Pharmacologic methods are preferred because they lower the hypothalamic set-point.

In the rare instance where core temperatures exceed 41°C to 42°C or where the metabolic demands of fever are a consideration, physical methods may be used in addition to pharmacologic methods.

- *Sponging* with water uses evaporation to dissipate body heat. The colder the water used, the more uncomfortable the patient. Alcohol is not recommended as it may be absorbed through the skin, inhaled or accidentally ingested by the child.
- *Ice packs or cooling (hypothermia) blankets* may be applied to the skin to lower body temperature by conduction. In adult patients in the intensive care unit, this method is associated with greater temperature fluctuations and more rebound hyperthermia.[11]
- *Circulating fans*, sometimes directed over ice before reaching the patient, use convection to transfer heat away from the skin surface.

Pharmacologic Choices (Table 1)

Acetaminophen and **ibuprofen** are the only therapeutic choices available for managing fever in children. They have been well studied in large populations and are safe in therapeutic doses. Both medications have antipyretic and analgesic properties; ibuprofen has anti-inflammatory effects. Because acetaminophen has a larger body of safety data it is recommended over ibuprofen, which is reserved for second-line therapy.[12]

ASA is not recommended in children under 15 years of age because of the possible enhanced risk of Reye's syndrome.[14] A response to antipyretic therapy does not exclude the possibility that serious underlying illness is present. Clinical decision-making should not be based on response to fever treatment.[15]

Therapeutic Tips

- Use doses of acetaminophen and ibuprofen based on the child's weight, not on age. Maximum dose per day should be specified.
- There is insufficient evidence to support the practice of alternating acetaminophen and ibuprofen.[13]
- Acetaminophen is the most common cause of analgesic overdose in children under 6 years old. Store antipyretics in locked cabinets to prevent inappropriate access. Instruct parents to use a calibrated measuring device, and educate them about the many formulations available and the potential for error with substitution.

Table 1: **Antipyretic Medications for Children**

Class	Drug	Dose	Adverse Effects	Comments	Cost[a]
Para-aminophenol Derivatives	*acetaminophen* Atasol Preparations, Tempra, Tylenol, generics	10–15 mg/kg/dose Q4–6H as needed for symptom management; max 75 mg/kg/day or 4 g/day, whichever is less	Uncommon. Hypersensitivity, agranulocytosis and anemia (rare). Chronic use and overdose associated with hepatotoxicity, nephropathy. Potential for toxicity enhanced if concurrent dehydration, prolonged fasting, diabetes mellitus, obesity, concomitant viral infection or family history of hepatotoxic reaction.[16]	Rectal administration results in erratic absorption and should be used under health care provider supervision.[16] Available as oral drops, tablets, chewtabs, suppositories and suspension.	$
NSAIDs	*ibuprofen* Advil, Motrin (Children's), Motrin IB, generics	5–10 mg/kg Q6–8H as needed for symptom management; max 40 mg/kg/day or 2400 mg/day	Uncommon. GI intolerance and bleeding, allergic reactions, tinnitus, visual disturbances, nephropathy. Dehydration enhances risk of renal toxicity.	Limited data exists for the use of ibuprofen in children < 2 months. Do not give if dehydration is present. Available as tablets and suspension.	$

[a] Cost of 1-day supply; available without prescription.
Dosage adjustment may be required in renal impairment; see Appendix I.
Legend: $ < $2

Suggested Readings

Ishimine P. Fever without source in children 0 to 36 months of age. *Pediatr Clin North Am* 2006;53(2):167-94.

Kramer MS, Naimark L, Leduc DG. Parental fever phobia and its correlates. *Pediatrics* 1985;75(6):1110-3.

Mackowiak PA, Boulant JA. Fever's glass ceiling. *Clin Infect Dis* 1996;22(3):525-36.

McCullough HN. Acetaminophen and ibuprofen in the management of fever and mild to moderate pain in children. *Paediatr Child Health* 1998;3(4):246-51.

References

1. Baraff LJ, Bass JW, Fleisher GR et al. Practice guideline for the management of infants and children 0 to 36 months of age with fever without source. Agency for Health Care Policy and Research. *Ann Emerg Med* 1993;22(7):1198-210.
2. Ezzati T. Ambulatory care utilization patterns of children and young adults: National Ambulatory Medical Care Survey United States, January-December 1975. *Vital Health Stat 13* 1978;(39):1-43.
3. Community Pediatrics Committee, *Temperature measurement in paediatrics*. Ottawa (ON): Canadian Paediatric Society; 2006. Available from: http://www.cps.ca/english/statements/CP/cp00-01.htm Accessed March 8, 2007.
4. Kresch MJ. Axillary temperature as a screening test for fever in children. *J Pediatr* 1984;104(4):596-9.
5. El-Radhi AS, Barry W. Do antipyretics prevent febrile convulsions? *Arch Dis Child* 2003;88(7):641-2.
6. McCarthy PL, Dolan TF. Hyperpyrexia in children. Eight-year emergency room experience. *Am J Dis Child* 1976;130(8):849-51.
7. Press S, Fawcett NP. Association of temperature greater than 41.1 degrees C (106 degrees F) with serious illness. *Clin Pediatr (Phila)* 1985;24(1):21-5.
8. Ishimine P. Fever without source in children 0 to 36 months of age. *Pediatr Clin North Am* 2006;53(2):167-94.
9. Kramer MS, Tange SM, Mills EL et al. Role of the complete blood count in detecting occult focal bacterial infection in the young febrile child. *J Clin Epidemiol* 1993;46(4):349-57.
10. Meremikwu M, Oyo-Ita A. Physical methods for treating fever in children. *Cochrane Database Syst Rev* 2003;(2):CD004264.
11. O'Donnell J, Axelrod P, Fisher C et al. Use and effectiveness of hypothermia blankets for febrile patients in the intensive care unit. *Clin Infect Dis* 1997;24(6):1208-13.
12. Drug Therapy and Hazardous Substances Committee, Canadian Paediatric Society (CPS). *Acetaminophen and ibuprofen in the management of fever and mild to moderate pain in children*. Ottawa (ON): Canadian Paediatric Society; 1998. Available from: http://www.cps.ca/english/statements/DT/dt98-01.htm Accessed March 8, 2007.
13. Erlewyn-Lajeunesse MD, Coppens K, Hunt LP et al. Randomised controlled trial of combined paracetamol and ibuprofen for fever. *Arch Dis Child* 2006;91(5):414-6.
14. Belay ED, Bresee JS, Holman RC et al. Reye's syndrome in the United States from 1981 through 1997. *N Engl J Med* 1999;340(18):1377-82.
15. American College of Emergency Physicians Clinical Policies Committee; American College of Emergency Physicians Clinical Policies Subcommittee on Pediatric Fever. Clinical policy for children younger than three years presenting to the emergency department with fever. *Ann Emerg Med* 2003;42(4):530-45.
16. American Academy of Pediatrics. Committee on Drugs. Acetaminophen toxicity in children. *Pediatrics* 2001;108(4):1020-24.

CHAPTER 117
Thermoregulatory Disorders in Adults

Mathieu Simon, MD, FRCPC

Body temperature is maintained within a very narrow range to allow for normal metabolism. Disorders of thermoregulation can therefore produce a wide variety of symptoms ranging from minor discomfort to life-threatening emergencies.

Hyperthermia refers to a symptomatic increase in core body temperature above 38.2°C.[1] Hyperthermia may occur in vulnerable populations (extreme of ages, chronic diseases), with prescription drugs (e.g., anticholinergics, tricyclic antidepressants, sympathomimetics, salicylates, beta-lactams, succinylcholine, antipsychotics) that interfere with normal heat dissipation mechanisms or in healthy individuals exercising or working in extreme heat conditions. Clinical manifestations represent the adverse effects of increased body temperature and the secondary activation of inflammatory and coagulation cascades on various organ systems.[2]

Fever is most often the sign of an underlying infectious or inflammatory process. (See Chapter 116) Unlike fever, hyperthermia is not mediated by the hypothalamus. The distinction between fever and hyperthermia relies on findings from medical history such as hyperthermia resulting from environmental or toxic exposures and fever accompanying infectious, inflammatory or cancerous diseases. *Hyperpyrexia*, a fever of > 41.5°C, results from impairment of both heat loss mechanisms and hypothalamic thermostat set point. It is most often a sign of an overwhelming infection.

Hypothermia, a very common but often unrecognized problem, is defined as a core body temperature < 35°C.[3] Core temperature below 32°C predisposes patients to ventricular fibrillation, which could be preceded by ECG changes such as QT-interval prolongation, T-wave inversion and atrial fibrillation.[4] Drugs such as clonidine[5] and atypical antipsychotics[6] may increase the risk of accidental hypothermia.

In treating thermoregulatory disorders, focus on the cause of the temperature variance rather than the absolute thermometer reading. There is limited evidence to support the optimal treatment of patients with either hyperthermia or hypothermia.

Goals of Therapy

- Treat underlying cause
- Restore normal body temperature by cooling in hyperthermia and warming in hypothermia
- Prevent, diagnose and treat uncommon but lethal complications

- Avoid unnecessary, ineffective or dangerous interventions

Investigations (Table 1)

Hyperthermia and hypothermia are more commonly signs of an underlying illness than primary problems. Establish the appropriate diagnosis and institute definitive therapy.

- History:
  - environmental exposure and the context in which the symptoms developed, e.g., exposure to different types of medications (see Table 1)

    Urban hypothermia is often associated with alcohol/drug intoxication. Hypothermia in this setting may also result from prolonged immobilization of an elderly patient, even at normal room temperature, in association with loss of consciousness, a fall, stroke or fracture. Hypothyroidism may also play a significant role
  - consider thermoregulation disorders in the differential diagnosis of confusion and coma
  - hyperthermia: exclude infection, assess hydration status. Inquire about the use of medications (antipsychotics, anticholinergics, volatile anaesthetics), recreational drugs (cocaine, amphetamines, phencyclidine) and consider intoxication (ASA, tricyclic antidepressants overdose, organophosphates). Endocrinopathies (thyrotoxicosis, pheochromocytoma) may also present with hyperthermia
- Objective measurements:
  - accurate measurement of core body temperature

    Use electronic devices. Standard glass/mercury thermometers will not record temperature below 32°C or above 42°C. Frequent calibration of electronic instruments is mandatory. Tympanic thermometers are not recommended in extreme temperature disorders as they may provide inaccurate readings[7]
  - assess vital signs: pulse, respiration
  - order tests according to the clinical setting:

    Blood glucose, electrolytes (sodium, calcium, potassium), renal profile, CBC, CK, coagulation panel (INR, PTT), blood gases, ECG, blood or urine cultures, liver enzymes, urine myoglobin (only helpful if positive), thyroid function tests, toxicology screen

Table 1: **Clinical Characteristics of Hyperthermia Syndromes**

Diagnosis	Characteristics
Heat Cramps	• Core body temperature is normal, skin is moist and cool • Occurs in muscles following vigorous exercise in the heat • Caused by salt depletion from excess sweating combined with hypotonic fluid replacement, resulting in dilutional hyponatremia[8]
Heat Exhaustion	• Core body temperature is minimally increased and is between 37°C and 40°C[3] • Consequence of salt and water losses • Symptoms: muscle cramps, diaphoresis, headache, nausea, vomiting, orthostatic syncope[3]
Heat Stroke	• Core body temperature ≥ 40.6°C[3] • *Classic:* develops over several days during heat waves and affects primarily the elderly or those suffering from chronic illness[9] • *Exertional:* occurs acutely with workers, endurance athletes or soldiers submitted to conditions of high heat and humidity without appropriate access to salt and water[10,11,12] • Signs and symptoms: dehydration, central nervous system dysfunction (delirium, seizure, coma) and hot, dry skin[3,13] • Complications such as disseminated intravascular coagulation, rhabdomyolysis, renal failure, seizures and permanent neurologic damage can result[14,15]
Malignant Hyperthermia	• Drug-induced reaction characterized by genetic susceptibility to generalized and sustained skeletal muscle contraction after exposure to depolarizing muscle relaxants such as succinylcholine or volatile anesthetic agents, such as halothane or isoflurane[16,17] • Sustained muscle contraction and increased metabolism result in hyperthermia, metabolic acidosis, increased serum creatine kinase (CK) • Duchenne disease and myotonic muscular dystrophy have been associated with an increased incidence of malignant hyperthermia[18]
Neuroleptic Malignant Syndrome (NMS)	• Drug-induced idiosyncratic reaction characterized by hyperthermia, altered mentation, muscle rigidity[19] and autonomic instability, e.g., cardiac arrhythmias • Drugs implicated are most often phenothiazines (e.g., chlorpromazine) and butyrophenones (e.g., haloperidol) or withdrawal of a dopaminergic agent (e.g., levodopa) resulting in reduced central dopamine neurotransmission

Hyperthermia

Therapeutic Choices

Nonpharmacologic Choices (Table 2)

Therapy is directed toward reducing heat production and increasing thermal dissipation.

- Ensure adequate airway, breathing and circulation (ABC).

- Rest, cooling (icepacks, cooling blankets) and rehydration (intravenous electrolytes) is the mainstay of treatment.
- Monitor core body temperature continuously.[20] Discontinue cooling when core body temperature normalizes to prevent risk of iatrogenic hypothermia.

Table 2: **Nonpharmacologic Management of Heat Cramps, Heat Exhaustion and Heat Stroke**

Cause	Treatment
Heat Cramps	• Rest and oral rehydration with a salt-containing solution, e.g., 1 teaspoonful (5 mL) of salt in 500 mL of water • Normal saline iv (e.g., 2–3 L over 4–6 hours) is infrequently indicated[21]
Heat Exhaustion	• Rest in a cool environment • External cooling with fan and rehydration • Avoid strenuous exercise for 2–3 days[14]
Heat Stroke	• Primary objective: rapid lowering of core temperature below 39.4°C • Rehydration and immediate cooling; ideal approach is tepid (20°C) water misting enhanced by fan evaporation. Definitive studies on the optimal cooling method are lacking and optimal management is controversial. Despite this, cooling should not be delayed.[22] Ice-packs, wrapped in towels to avoid skin injury, and tepid water sponging are alternative approaches. Cooling should not be too intense since it could trigger shivering and increase heat generation • Cold-water immersion is not recommended when the patient has reached the hospital because it induces peripheral vasoconstriction, which is counterproductive, and does not permit close monitoring of the patient. In the field, priority should be given to rapidly reducing body temperature, and cold-water immersion remains a valid and possible life-saving option in this setting[23]

Pharmacologic Choices

Antipyretics are ineffective in treating hyperthermia since the hypothalamic thermostat set point is normal.[24] Malignant hyperthermia and neuroleptic malignant syndrome require expeditious pharmacologic therapy and demand special attention. Clinical characteristics of both conditions are listed in Table 1.

Malignant Hyperthermia

To reverse this potentially lethal condition, prompt recognition of malignant hyperthermia, interruption of the surgery, cessation of the offending drug, external cooling and administration of a muscle relaxant, **dantrolene** (2 mg/kg iv every 5 minutes up to 10 mg/kg), is necessary.[20,25] Some experts suggest prevention of recurrence by continuing dantrolene on an oral dosing regimen of 2 to 4 mg/kg/day for 2 to 3 days after an episode of malignant hyperthermia.[26]

Neuroleptic Malignant Syndrome

Treatment of neuroleptic malignant syndrome involves prompt cessation of the offending agent and nonspecific supportive therapy (hydration, cooling). Limited evidence exists to support administration of dopaminergic agonists (**bromocriptine** 2.5 to 20 mg po or through a nasogastric tube TID), and possibly the use of a **muscle relaxant** (nondepolarizing neuromuscular blockers or **dantrolene**).[20,25,27] Experience in the treatment of this uncommon condition remains limited.

Hypothermia

Nonpharmacologic Choices (Figure 1, Table 3)

Resuscitation and rewarming are the mainstay of treatment of hypothermia. In resuscitating a patient, ensure adequate airway, breathing and circulation. Resuscitate patient until temperature is between 32°C and 35°C. Assess vital signs carefully as severe hypothermia may result in barely perceptible pulse and respiration. Rewarming takes precedence once initial resuscitation has been initiated. The three progressive modalities of rewarming are *passive external rewarming*, *active external rewarming* and *active core rewarming* (Table 3). Monitor core body temperature continuously through a rectal or esophageal probe. Discontinue warming when core body temperature normalizes to prevent risk of iatrogenic hyperthermia.

Electrical defibrillation for ventricular fibrillation is less effective at core temperatures below 30°C but should be attempted. If one shock (120 to 200 J and 360 J respectively for biphasic and monophasic defibrillators)[28] is unsuccessful in restoring normal sinus rhythm, attention should be switched to aggressive rewarming while continuing advanced cardiac life support (ACLS) until body temperature reaches 30°C, when defibrillation attempts are more likely to be successful (see Figure 1).[29,30] Trivial manoeuvres such as endotracheal intubation or simply moving the patient could be sufficient triggers for ventricular fibrillation[31] but this should not discourage initial in-field stabilization and evacuation.

Favourable outcomes following prolonged resuscitation are well described, especially in children. Hypothermia victims should not be pronounced dead until rewarmed to a near normal core temperature.[3,28] This is especially true of near-drowning victims because immersion in cold water results in rapid cooling of the entire body that may provide some survival advantages such as protecting the brain and organs.

Controversies still exist about the utility of temperature-corrected arterial pH and blood gases relative to the hypothermia. Most literature now suggests that uncorrected pH, pO_2 and pCO_2 values are more physiologic and more valuable to the clinician in guiding the therapeutic interventions.[32]

Table 3: **Hypothermia: Rewarming Modalities**

Rewarming Modality	Characteristics
Passive external rewarming	• Minimize heat loss by removing wet or frozen clothing and keep the patient dry and covered with warm blankets. • Relies on the patient's ability to shiver, which is lost below 32°C. It is an essential first line intervention but additional steps should be taken in more severe hypothermia.
Active external rewarming	• Refers to the use of warming blankets or warm water immersion. • Use in stable patients with minimal metabolic abnormalities, since paradoxical acidosis and worsening of core hypothermia may result due to peripheral vasodilatation induced by external rewarming while thoracic and abdominal organs remain cold. If used, active external rewarming should be limited to the trunk.[33]
Active core rewarming	• Favoured approach in severe hypothermia. • Heated iv normal saline (40°C to 43°C) should be administered through a peripheral line. Using a central line allows for faster rewarming, but insertion may be complicated by malignant arrhythmia and significant bleeding secondary to coagulopathy. If a blood warmer is not available, iv solutions could be heated in a microwave oven but only if they do not contain dextrose and the temperature is monitored before administration.[34] Blood cannot be heated in a microwave because of its high cellular and protein content. • Mechanical ventilation using heated gases (40°C to 45°C) is another simple and effective technique.[35] Heated peritoneal lavage through a temporary dialysis catheter using 2000 mL of dialysate at 44°C exchanged every 20 minutes can increase core temperature by up to 2°C/hour. Disseminated intravascular coagulation, intra-abdominal bleeding and electrolyte imbalance are the most common complications.[36] Heated enemas, nasogastric lavage, bladder irrigation[36,37] and open and closed thoracic lavage[38] have all been attempted with mixed results. • Heated cardiopulmonary bypass provides the fastest and most physiologic means of active core rewarming. This technique is usually limited to the management of patients suffering cardiac arrest or those with unstable hemodynamics and arrhythmias.[29,37] Transfer of severely hypothermic patients to a hospital where the technique is available should be considered but is often impossible considering the extreme risks involved in the transport of these patients.

Pharmacologic Choices

Since hypothermia is often associated with alcohol intoxication, **thiamine** supplementation is part of the supportive therapy. **Glucose** and **naloxone** (if opioid overdose is suspected) should be administered. Consider other sources of intoxication and their therapy.

Prophylactic antibiotics are controversial. Some advocate wide-spectrum antibiotic coverage for the first three days but there are no clinical trial data to support this recommendation. Routine use of barbiturates or steroids is discouraged.

Hypothermic patients will usually require fluid resuscitation with warm isotonic solutions. Vasopressors should be avoided since they are usually ineffective and could precipitate arrhythmia.[39]

Pharmacologic management of cardiac arrest in hypothermic patients is difficult, and clinical experience is scarce. Most antiarrhythmic agents, with the exception of bretylium,[40] have been considered ineffective until rewarming. Only animal studies support the use of bretylium in hypothermic arrest and, since it has been removed from most ACLS protocols, availability is an issue. Recent evidence derived from animal models of hypothermic arrest suggest that American Heart Association (AHA) algorithms could be used safely and effectively in hypothermic patients. Avoid procainamide.[41,42] Withholding drugs until core temperature reaches 30°C and then applying appropriate ACLS algorithms, but using longer intervals between drug doses, is generally advocated.[28]

Therapeutic Tips

- Nonpharmacologic management is the basis for therapy of true thermoregulation disorders.
- Hypothermic patients are prone to cardiac arrhythmia. ECG monitoring is mandatory. Aggressive resuscitation and rewarming are warranted.
- The effectiveness of most medications is temperature dependent. Overmedication of the hypothermic patient could cause toxicity during rewarming.
- While treating severe hypothermia, close monitoring of serum K^+ is important. Rapid rewarming may induce severe hyperkalemia.
- Avoid alpha-adrenergic agonists in hyperthermia as they may decrease heat dissipation through vasoconstriction.
- Dantrolene is not effective in heat stroke.[43]

Figure 1: **Hypothermia Treatment**

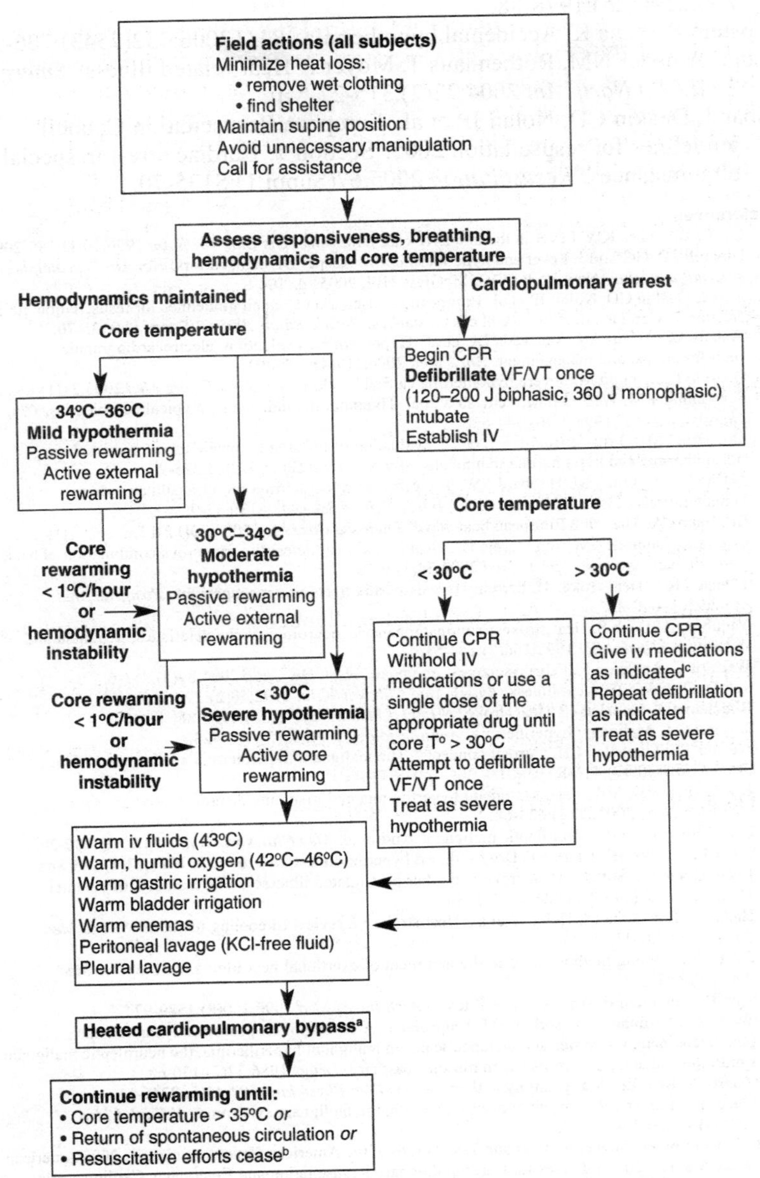

[a] Cardiac arrest and hemodynamic collapse are seen as the two usual indications for cardiopulmonary bypass in the setting of severe hypothermia.

[b] Successful resuscitations after prolonged ACLS, although unusual, have been reported, most of them in the pediatric literature. ACLS and active rewarming should, in most cases, be continued until the core temperature reaches 35°C.

[c] Use longer than standard intervals between doses.

Adapted with permission from Advanced Challenges in Resuscitation. Circulation 2000;102 (suppl 1): I-230.

Suggested Readings

Bouchama A, Knochel JP. Heat stroke. *N Engl J Med* 2002;346(25):1978-88.

Epstein E, Anna K. Accidental hypothermia. *BMJ* 2006;332(7543):706-9.

Lugo-Amador NM, Rothenhaus T, Moyer P. Heat-related illness. *Emerg Med Clin North Am* 2004;22(2):315-27, viii.

Soar J, Deakin CD, Nolan JP et al. European Resuscitation Council guidelines for resuscitation 2005. Section 7. Cardiac arrest in special circumstances. *Resuscitation* 2005;67(Suppl 1):S135-70.

References

1. Cunha BA, Shea KW. Fever in the intensive care unit. *Infect Dis Clin North Am* 1996;10(1):185-209.
2. Dinarello C, Gelfand J. Fever and hyperthermia. In: Kasper DL et al, editors. *Harrison's principles of internal medicine*. New York (NY): McGraw-Hill; 2005. p. 104-8.
3. Soar J, Deakin CD, Nolan JP et al. European Resuscitation Council guidelines for resuscitation 2005. Section 7. Cardiac arrest in special circumstances. *Resuscitation* 2005;67(Suppl 1):S135-70.
4. Aslam AF, Aslam AK, Vasavada BC et al. Hypothermia: evaluation, electrocardiographic manifestations, and management. *Am J Med* 2006;119(4):297-301.
5. Quail MT, Shannon M. Severe hypothermia caused by clonidine. *Am J Emerg Med* 2003;21(1):86.
6. Schwaninger M, Weisbrod M, Schwab S et al. Hypothermia induced by atypical neuroleptics. *Clin Neuropharmacol* 1998;21(6):344-6.
7. Ducharme MB, Frim J, Bourdon L et al. Evaluation of infrared tympanic thermometers during normothermia and hypothermia in humans. *Ann N Y Acad Sci* 1997;813:225-9.
8. Gaffin SL, Koratich M, Hubbard RW. The effect of hyperthermia on intracellular sodium concentrations of isolated human cells. *Ann N Y Acad Sci* 1997;813:637-9.
9. Bouchama A. The 2003 European heat wave. *Intensive Care Med* 2004;30(1):1-3.
10. Coris EE, Ramirez AM, Van Durme DJ. Heat illness in athletes: the dangerous combination of heat, humidity and exercise. *Sports Med* 2004;34(1):9-16.
11. Delaney KA. Heatstroke. Underlying processes and lifesaving management. *Postgrad Med* 1992;91(4):379-88.
12. Yaqub B, Al Deeb S. Heat strokes: aetiopathogenesis, neurological characteristics, treatment and outcome. *J Neurol Sci* 1998;156(2):144-51.
13. Waruiru C, Appleton R. Febrile seizures: an update. *Arch Dis Child* 2004;89(8):751-6.
14. Tek D, Olshaker JS. Heat illness. *Emerg Med Clin North Am* 1992;10(2):299-310.
15. Bouchama A, Knochel JP. Heat stroke. *N Engl J Med* 2002;346(25):1978-88.
16. Gronert GA. Malignant hyperthermia. *Anesthesiology* 1980;53(5):395-423.
17. Nelson TE, Flewellen EH. Current concepts. The malignant hyperthermia syndrome. *N Engl J Med* 1983;309(7):416-8.
18. Rosenbaum HK, Miller JD. Malignant hyperthermia and myotonic disorders. *Anesthesiol Clin North America* 2002;20(3):623-64.
19. Caroff SN, Mann SC. Neuroleptic malignant syndrome. *Med Clin North Am* 1993;77(1):185-202.
20. Chan TC, Evans SD, Clark RF. Drug-induced hyperthermia. *Crit Care Clin* 1997;13(4):785-808.
21. Lee-Chiong TL, Stitt JT. Heatstroke and other heat-related illnesses. The maladies of summer. *Postgrad Med* 1995;98(1):26-8, 31-3, 36.
22. Hadad E, Rav-Acha M, Heled Y et al. Heat stroke : a review of cooling methods. *Sports Med* 2004;34(8):501-11.
23. Smith JE. Cooling methods used in the treatment of exertional heat illness. *Br J Sports Med* 2005;39(8):503-7.
24. Styrt B, Sugarman B. Antipyresis and fever. *Arch Intern Med* 1990;150(8):1589-97.
25. Ward A, Chaffman MO, Sorkin EM. Dantrolene. A review of its pharmacodynamic and pharmacokinetic properties and therapeutic use in malignant hyperthermia, the neuroleptic malignant syndrome and an update of its use in muscle spasticity. *Drugs* 1986;32(2):130-68.
26. Moore JL, Rice EL. Malignant hyperthermia. *Am Fam Physician* 1992;45(5):2245-51.
27. Guze BH, Baxter LR. Current concepts. Neuroleptic malignant syndrome. *N Engl J Med* 1985;313(3):163-6.
28. ECC Committee, Subcommittees and Task Forces of the American Heart Association. 2005 American Heart Association Guidelines for Cardiopulmonary Resuscitation and Emergency Cardiovascular Care. *Circulation* 2005;112(24 Suppl):IV1-203.
29. Cummins RO, editor. *Advanced cardiac life support*. 2nd ed. Dallas (TX): American Heart Association; 1997.
30. Jolly BT, Ghezzi KT. Accidental hypothermia. *Emerg Med Clin North Am* 1992;10(2):311-27.
31. Lloyd EL. The cause of death after rescue. *Int J Sports Med* 1992;13(Suppl 1):S196-9.

32. Danzl DF, Pozos RS, Auerbach PS et al. Multicenter hypothermia survey. *Ann Emerg Med* 1987;16(9):1042-55.
33. Harnett RM, Pruitt JR, Sias FR. A review of the literature concerning resuscitation from hypothermia: Part I--the problem and general approaches. *Aviat Space Environ Med* 1983;54(5):425-34.
34. Anshus JS, Endahl GL, Mottley JL. Microwave heating of intravenous fluids. *Am J Emerg Med* 1985;3(4):316-9.
35. Morrison JB, Conn ML, Hayward JS. Thermal increment provided by inhalation rewarming from hypothermia. *J Appl Physiol* 1979;46(6):1061-5.
36. Reuler JB, Parker RA. Peritoneal dialysis in the management of hypothermia. *JAMA* 1978;240(21):2289-90.
37. Maresca L, Vasko JS. Treatment of hypothermia by extracorporeal circulation and internal rewarming. *J Trauma* 1987; 27(1):89-90.
38. Hall KN, Syverud SA. Closed thoracic cavity lavage in the treatment of severe hypothermia in human beings. *Ann Emerg Med* 1990;19(2):204-6.
39. Rankin AC, Rae AP. Cardiac arrhythmias during rewarming of patients with accidental hypothermia. *Br Med J (Clin Res Ed)* 1984;289(6449):874-7.
40. Cohen DJ, Cline JR, Lepinski SM et al. Resuscitation of the hypothermic patient. *Am J Emerg Med* 1988;6(5):475-8.
41. Wira C, Martin G, Stoner J et al. Application of normothermic cardiac arrest algorithms to hypothermic cardiac arrest in a canine model. *Resuscitation* 2006;69(3):509-16.
42. Danzl DF, Sowers MB, Vicario SJ et al. Chemical ventricular defibrillation in severe accidental hypothermia. *Ann Emerg Med* 1982;11(12):698-9.
43. Bouchama A, Cafege A, Devol EB et al. Seraj M. Ineffectiveness of dantrolene sodium in the treatment of heatstroke. *Crit Care Med* 1991;19(2):176-80.

CHAPTER 118
Chronic Cough in Adults

Pearce Wilcox, MD

Chronic cough is multifactorial in up to 90% of cases.[1,2,3,4] Consider upper airway cough syndrome (UACS, formerly known as postnasal drip syndrome), asthma, gastroesophageal reflux disease (GERD) or nonasthmatic eosinophilic bronchitis[1,3,4] in nonsmokers with chronic cough (present for > 8 weeks) (Table 1). Psychogenic cough is an uncommon diagnosis and is one of exclusion.

Acute cough is most often infectious, contributes to clearing secretions and does not generally require antitussive therapy.[1,3,4] Postinfectious cough is a persistent cough which lasts > 3 weeks after experiencing acute symptoms of an upper respiratory tract infection (e.g., *Mycoplasma pneumoniae*, *Bordetella pertussis*). Postinfectious cough does not usually last for > 8 weeks.[5] The cough is self-limited and resolves on its own.[5]

Goals of Therapy

- Choose appropriate and effective therapy based on cough etiology
- Resist nonspecific cough suppression therapy, which may delay diagnosis of a curative cause
- Prevent complications attributable to cough, e.g., rib fractures, syncope, loss of sleep

Investigations

A standardized approach will lead to identifiable cause(s) of cough in > 90% of patients.[6] (Figure 1). More detailed testing in nonsmokers (e.g., CT scan, bronchoscopy) should be reserved for those with no overt cause detected on initial evaluation and cough refractory to empiric therapeutic trials for the most common etiologies.

- History and physical exam, with special attention to:
  - duration of cough (variation in cough over the day), history of smoking (cigarette, cigar, pipe) and medication use, signs and symptoms of asthma, upper airway symptoms, GERD. Examine nasal cavities, oropharynx and otic canals
  - consider occupational and environmental causes, e.g., pollution
  - personal or family history of atopy/asthma
- Objective measurements needed to confirm diagnosis:
  - chest x-ray (CXR)
  - spirometry to evaluate for COPD if the patient has a smoking history (see Chapter 49)
  - nonasthmatic eosinophilic bronchitis: consider in patients with normal spirometry, normal CXR, negative methacholine challenge

and sputum eosinophilia or a response to inhaled corticosteroids (Table 1). No evidence of variable airflow obstruction or airway hyperresponsiveness

- investigation of less common causes of cough, e.g., carcinoma of respiratory tract, chronic lung infection, interstitial lung disease, occult left heart failure, irritable larynx syndrome, bronchiectasis; include CT and bronchoscopy
- if hemoptysis is present, consider bronchiectasis, chronic bronchitis, chronic infection, malignancy or causes of pulmonary hemorrhage. Investigations would include sputum for acid fast staining and culture, sputum cytology, CXR, CT scan of the chest and referral to a respirologist for fibre optic bronchoscopy

Table 1: **Chronic Cough: Common Causes, Clinical Features and Investigations**

Common Causes	Clinical Features	Investigations
Upper airway cough syndrome	Postnasal drainage; cobblestoning and mucus in oropharynx Nasal discharge Throat clearing	Sinus x-rays CT scan of paranasal sinuses
Asthma	Typical features of asthma, such as wheezing, often absent	Spirometry pre-/post-bronchodilator Methacholine challenge
Gastroesophageal reflux disease	Consider after exclusion of other etiologies Approximately 75% of cases not associated with other reflux symptoms[7,8]	Therapeutic trial of H_2-receptor blocker or a proton pump inhibitor (PPI) × 3 mo Upper GI series (limited sensitivity) pH monitoring (high sensitivity, moderate specificity) Endoscopy an option if pH monitoring not available (less sensitive)
ACE inhibitor[9]	Dry, nonproductive cough Onset hours-months post-initiation No predisposing factors Class effect of ACE inhibitors	Drug withdrawal; resolution or marked improvement of symptoms within 4 weeks
Nonasthmatic eosinophilic bronchitis[10]	Often prolonged in postinfectious setting	Normal spirometry and chest x-ray, negative challenge testing, sputum eosinophilia (if available)

Abbreviations: ACE = angiotensin converting enzyme

Pertussis, a highly contagious infection, leads to severe paroxysms of cough with frequent complications. Early administration of antibiotics is crucial. Clinical features include a two-week virus-like illness with symptoms such as conjunctivitis, rhinorrhea, fever and malaise. Later, cough is followed by the paroxysmal phase characterized by worsening cough associated with posttussive emesis and/or inspiratory whooping sound.[5] Nasopharyngeal swab is used for culture to confirm pertussis and if available, polymerase chain reaction.[5]

Therapeutic Choices

Nonpharmacologic Choices

- Advise on smoking cessation (see Chapter 10).
- Avoid exposure to allergens.

Pharmacologic Choices (Table 2)

Therapy of chronic cough is directed at the cause, once identified (Figure 1).

- Nonallergic rhinitis: **first-generation antihistamine** (e.g., chlorpheniramine) and **decongestant** (e.g., pseudoephedrine) for one to two weeks ± intranasal **ipratropium.**[11]
- Allergic rhinitis: appropriate therapy may include **antihistamines** or **intranasal corticosteroids** (see Chapter 45).
- Chronic sinusitis: **antibiotics** and **decongestants**[11] (see Chapter 95).
- Asthma: appropriate therapy includes **short-acting beta-agonist** PRN and inhaled **corticosteroids**. If asthma is not well controlled, consider adding **long-acting beta agonists, leukotriene receptor antagonists** or a one- to two-week pulse of **oral corticosteroids** (see Chapter 47).
- GERD: consider nonpharmacologic (dietary and lifestyle) approaches first. If nonpharmacologic therapy fails, consider an **H_2-receptor blocker** or **PPI ± prokinetic agent** (see Chapter 53). Although recommended in guidelines,[4] a Cochrane systematic review concludes that there are no benefits to using H_2-receptor blockers and PPIs in adults with GERD who have chronic cough.[12]
- ACE inhibitor-induced cough: stop ACE inhibitor.[13] The median time to resolution is four weeks. Depending on the indication and patient history, an angiotensin receptor blocker (ARB) may be an appropriate substitution and is generally not associated with cough.
- Pertussis: if probable or confirmed pertussis, isolate patients for five days and treat with macrolide antibiotics.[5,14] Administer booster pertussis vaccine every 10 years to all adults.[15]

Antitussives have a limited, if any, role to play in the management of chronic cough. However, they may sometimes be used to enable sleep or in certain social settings (e.g., live theatre) if the cough cannot be controlled by measures targeted at a specific diagnosis. Use caution when cough is productive.

Therapeutic Tips

- Consider cough due to ACE inhibitor whatever the temporal onset. Resolution most often occurs within one to four weeks but occasionally requires up to three months post-cessation.

- More than one cause of cough frequently occurs in the same individual. Therapy that has produced an improvement, but not resolution, of a cough should continue while investigations for other causes are pursued.
- Older antihistamines are usually more effective than newer agents for cough related to postnasal drip.[4]
- Mucolytics have no proven role in the treatment of cough.[4]
- Consider inhaled **ipratropium** for cough due to upper respiratory infection or chronic bronchitis[4] (see Chapter 49).
- **Nonsedating antihistamines** (e.g., loratadine) may be more effective in managing chronic cough due to allergic rhinitis. First-generation antihistamines, because of their anticholinergic effects, in combination with a decongestant benefit patients with nonallergic rhinitis.[11]

Figure 1: **Management of Chronic Cough**

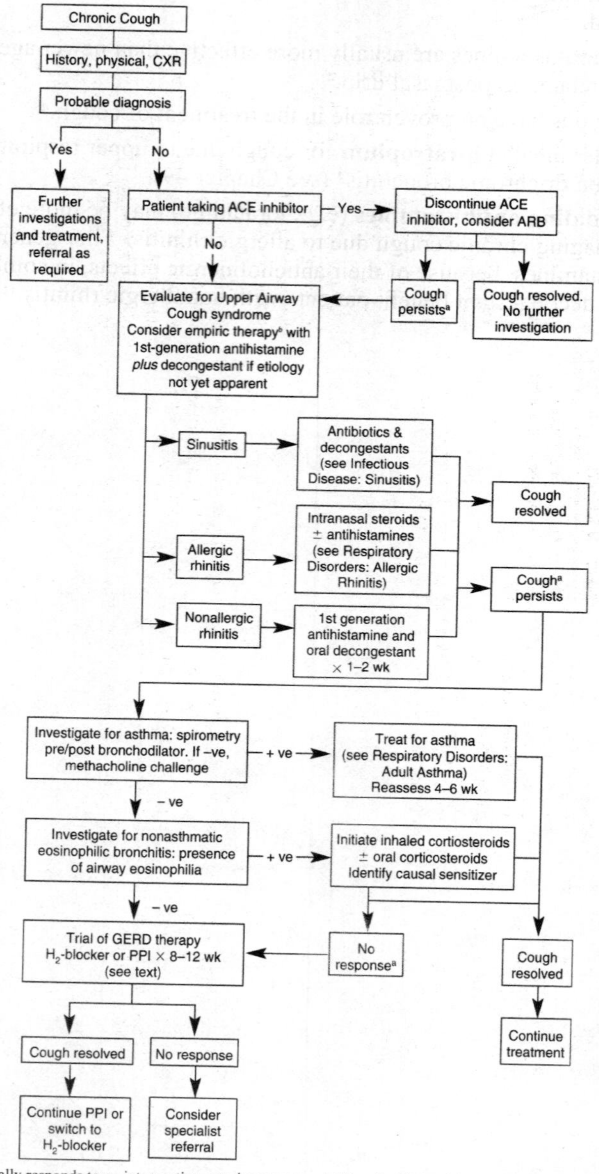

[a] If cough partially responds to an intervention, continue treatment (if applicable) and investigate other contributory causes, e.g., smoking (see Chapter 10).

[b] Consider sinus imaging if patient does not respond to empiric therapy with first-generation antihistamine plus decongestant.

Abbreviations: ACE = angiotensin converting enzyme; ARB = angiotensin receptor blocker; CXR = chest x-ray; GERD = gastroesophageal reflux disease; PPI = proton pump inhibitor; +ve = positive; -ve = negative

Table 2: **Drugs for Cough Suppression**

Class	Drug	Dose	Adverse Effects	Comments	Cost[a]
Anticholinergic Agents	*ipratropium bromide* Atrovent Nasal Spray, Atrovent HFA	Nasal spray (0.03%): 2 sprays in each nostril BID-TID. Dose is individualized. pMDI: 2–4 puffs QID	Nosebleeds, nasal dryness, dry mouth or throat, metallic taste.	Avoid accidental release of nasal spray into eyes. pMDI: For cough due to upper respiratory infection or chronic bronchitis.	$$$$$/nasal spray $$$$/inhaler
Antitussives	*codeine* generics	5–20 mg po Q4–8H	Constipation, drowsiness, nausea.	May be used if analgesia and sedation desired. Short-term symptomatic relief of coughing. For patients with upper respiratory infections or chronic bronchitis. Not recommended for ACE inhibitor–induced cough.	$
	dextromethorphan Benylin DM, Delsym (sustained-release), Formula 44, Robitussin Children's, others	*immediate-release*: 15–30 mg po Q6–8H *sustained-release:* 60 mg po Q12H	Drowsiness, GI upset, blurred vision and urinary hesitancy in patients who metabolize DM slowly.	May be used if analgesia and sedation desired. For patients with upper respiratory infections or chronic bronchitis. Not recommended for ACE inhibitor–induced cough.	$$[b]

(cont'd)

Table 2: **Drugs for Cough Suppression** *(cont'd)*

Class	Drug	Dose	Adverse Effects	Comments	Cost[a]
	hydrocodone Hycodan	5 mg po PRN; > 4 h between doses if need Administer after meals and/or at bedtime with food or a glass of milk Max 30 mg/24 h	See codeine.	May be used if analgesia and sedation desired. Short-term symptomatic relief of coughing. For patients with upper respiratory infections or chronic bronchitis. Not recommended for ACE inhibitor–induced cough.	$$
Antihistamines, first-generation	*chlorpheniramine* Chlor-Tripolon, generics	4–8 mg po HS	Sedation, anticholinergic effects.	For cough associated with nonallergic rhinitis, used in combination with a decongestant.	$[b]
Antihistamines, second-generation	*loratadine* Claritin, generics	10 mg po daily	Little to no sedation or anticholinergic effects.	For cough associated with allergic rhinitis.	$$[b]
Decongestants	*pseudoephedrine* Sudafed, generics	Adults and children ≥ 12 y: 60 mg Q4–6H or 120 mg SR Q12H or 240 mg CR Q24H; max 240 mg/24 h	Insomnia, tremor, irritability, headache, palpitations, tachycardia, urinary retention.	For cough associated with nonallergic rhinitis, used in combination with a 1st generation antihistamine.	$[b]

[a] Cost of 100 mL or 15 tablets unless otherwise specified; includes drug cost only.
[b] Available without prescription; retail mark-up may vary.
Abbreviations: HFA = hydrofluoroalkane; pMDI = pressurized metered dose inhaler
Legend: $ < $5 $$ $5–10 $$$ $10–15 $$$$ $15–20 $$$$$ > $20

Suggested Readings

Irwin RS, Baumann MH, Bolser DC et al. Diagnosis and management of cough: ACCP evidence-based clinical practice guidelines. *Chest* 2006;129(1 Suppl):1-287S.

Irwin RS, Madison JM. The persistently troublesome cough. *Am J Respir Crit Care Med* 2002;165(11):1469-74.

Morice AH, Fontana GA, Sovijarvi AR et al The diagnosis and management of chronic cough. *Eur Respir J* 2004;24(3):481-92.

Simpson CB, Amin MR. Chronic cough: state-of-the-art review. *Otolaryngol Head Neck Surg* 2006;134(4):693-700.

References

1. Carney IK, Gibson PG, Murree-Allen K et al. A systematic evaluation of mechanisms in chronic cough. *Am J Respir Crit Care Med* 1997;156(1):211-6.
2. Morice AH, Kastelik JA. Cough. 1: Chronic cough in adults. *Thorax* 2003;58(10):901-7.
3. Irwin RS, Madison JM. The persistently troublesome cough. *Am J Respir Crit Care Med* 2002;165(11):1469-74.
4. Irwin RS, Baumann MH, Bolser DC et al. Diagnosis and management of cough executive summary: ACCP evidence-based clinical practice guidelines. *Chest* 2006;129(1 Suppl):1S-23S.
5. Braman SS. Postinfectious cough: ACCP evidence-based clinical practice guidelines. *Chest* 2006;129(1 Suppl):138S-146S.
6. Irwin RS, Zawacki JK. Accurately diagnosing and successfully treating chronic cough due to gastroesophageal reflux disease can be difficult. *Am J Gastroenterol* 1999;94(11):3095-8.
7. Poe RH, Kallay MC. Chronic cough and gastroesophageal reflux disease: experience with specific therapy for diagnosis and treatment. *Chest* 2003;123(3):679-84.
8. Ing AJ, Ngu MC, Breslin AB. Chronic persistent cough and clearance of esophageal acid. *Chest* 1992;102(6):1668-71.
9. Dykewicz MS. Cough and angioedema from angiotensin-converting enzyme inhibitors: new insights into mechanisms and management. *Curr Opin Allergy Clin Immunol* 2004;4(4):267-70.
10. Gibson PG, Fujimura M, Niimi A. Eosinophilic bronchitis: clinical manifestations and implications for treatment. *Thorax* 2002;57(2):178-82.
11. Pratter MR. Chronic upper airway cough syndrome secondary to rhinosinus diseases (previously referred to as postnasal drip syndrome): ACCP evidence-based clinical practice guidelines. *Chest* 2006;129(1 Suppl):63S-71S.
12. Chang AB, Lasserson TJ, Gaffney J et al. Gastro-oesophageal reflux treatment for prolonged non-specific cough in children and adults. *Cochrane Database Syst Rev* 2005;(2):CD004823.
13. Irwin RS, Boulet LP, Cloutier MM et al. Managing cough as a defense mechanism and as a symptom. A consensus panel report of the American College of Chest Physicians. *Chest* 1998;114(2 Suppl Managing):133S-181S.
14. Hewlett EL, Edwards KM. Clinical practice. Pertussis—not just for kids. *N Engl J Med* 2005;352(12):1215-22.
15. National Advisory Committee on Immunization. *Canada immunization guide*. 7th ed. Ottawa (ON): Public Health Agency of Canada; 2006. Available from: http://www.phac-aspc.gc.ca/publicat/cig-gci/pdf/cig-gci-2006_e.pdf Accessed April 4, 2007.

CHAPTER 119
Persistent Hiccoughs

James M. Wright, MD, PhD, FRCPC

Persistent (2 to 60 days) or intractable (> 2 months) hiccoughs are unusual but distressing. They may cause insomnia, weight loss or depression and are associated with metabolic causes and abnormalities of the CNS, ear, throat, diaphragm, thorax and abdomen.

Goals of Therapy

- Stop or decrease frequency or intensity of hiccoughs
- Prevent recurrence

Investigations

- Complete history (including medication and alcohol use) and physical examination to provide clues for further investigations. If no abnormalities are identified, it is reasonable to do a CBC, electrolytes, creatinine and chest x-ray
  - drug-induced persistent hiccoughs are uncommon; alcohol, corticosteroids and benzodiazepines are the drugs most frequently implicated[1]
- Further investigations depend on findings from the history, physical and baseline investigations (e.g., upper GI tract endoscopy, CT brain, abdominal ultrasound)

If all investigations are negative or etiologic treatment is impossible, a therapeutic trial to stop the hiccoughs is warranted.

Therapeutic Choices

Nonpharmacologic Choices

- Vagal stimulation (e.g., posterior pharyngeal wall stimulation with a finger, forced expiration against a closed glottis for 10 seconds in the sitting position) is worth trying.
- If gastric distention is identified as the cause, gastric aspiration is effective.
- Acupuncture therapy has been associated with temporary or permanent relief in two patients.[2]
- Phrenic nerve disruption is reserved for cases where all else has failed.

Pharmacologic Choices (Table 1)

The condition is rare; one randomized, controlled trial — a cross-over trial comparing baclofen with placebo (see below) — was identified.[3] Most treatment recommendations are based on case reports or open trials in small numbers of patients.

Dopamine Antagonists

Chlorpromazine historically has been the drug of choice.[4] It has been used iv (25 to 50 mg over 0.5 to 1 hour) in the emergency room. A trial of 50 to 100 mg po daily for two to three days is also reasonable. **Haloperidol**, 2 to 5 mg im or 5 to 15 mg po, has also been effective in some cases. **Metoclopramide**, 10 mg iv or im followed by 10 to 20 mg QID po, has been successful. It may act as a dopamine antagonist or by enhancing gastric emptying. Adverse effects of dopamine antagonists include acute dystonia and postural hypotension. If chronic therapy is required, use back-titration to find the lowest effective dose taken once daily.

Baclofen

Baclofen has been effective in intractable hiccoughs, with maintenance therapy required in at least 50% of cases. A randomized, double blind, cross-over trial in four patients with intractable hiccoughs demonstrated that baclofen was unable to eliminate the hiccoughs, but did increase hiccough-free periods and decrease hiccough severity.[3] Starting with 5 mg BID, the dose is increased gradually every two to three days to a maximum daily dose of 75 mg. If effective, baclofen should not be discontinued suddenly. The minimum maintenance dose can be determined by gradually reducing the dose over time. Since baclofen is excreted by the kidney, much lower doses are required in the presence of renal failure (2.5 mg BID was effective in hemodialysis patients[5]). Side effects (drowsiness, weakness, nausea and fatigue) are relatively frequent.

Other drugs

In case reports or case series, many other drugs, including amitriptyline, carbamazepine, gabapentin, nifedipine and valproic acid, have been reported effective.

Therapeutic Tips

- Since this is a chronic condition, oral dosage forms are preferable to parenteral ones.
- When a drug is effective, hiccoughs generally stop abruptly within a few hours; in some cases, the frequency and severity may slowly decrease.
- Attempt to withdraw treatments gradually; maintenance therapy may be required in some cases.
- Avoid benzodiazepines, as worsening of hiccoughs has been reported.
- When a drug is ineffective, there is no need to continue treatment for more than three days.

Table 1: Drugs Used in Persistent or Intractable Hiccoughs

Class	Drug	Dose	Adverse Effects	Drug Interactions	Cost[a]
Dopamine Antagonists[b]	*chlorpromazine* generics	ER: 25–50 mg iv over 30–60 min Oral: 50–100 mg daily × 2–3 days	Anticholinergic effects, extrapyramidal effects, hypotension, sedation.	Additive sedative effects with CNS depressants, including alcohol.	$
	haloperidol generics	ER: 2–5 mg im Oral: 2–10 mg daily × 2–3 days	Sedation, extrapyramidal effects.	Additive sedative effects with CNS depressants, including alcohol.	$
	metoclopramide (renal) generics	ER: 10 mg iv or im Oral: 5–10 mg TID-QID × 2–3 days	Diarrhea, abdominal cramps, hyperprolactinemia, sedation, extrapyramidal effects, headache.	Additive sedative effects with CNS depressants, including alcohol.	$
Muscle Relaxants[b]	*baclofen* (renal) Lioresal Oral, generics	Start with 5 mg po BID; increase gradually every 2–3 days to a maximum of 75 mg per day	Sedation, muscle weakness, nausea, dizziness, lowered seizure threshold.	Additive sedative effects with CNS depressants, including alcohol.	$-$$

[a] Cost per day for oral therapy, unless otherwise specified; includes drug cost only.
[b] If chronic therapy required, establish lowest effective dose using gradual back-titration.
(renal symbol) Dosage adjustment may be required in renal impairment; see Appendix I.
Abbreviations: ER = emergency room
Legend: $ < $1 $-$$ < $1–3 $$ $1–3

Suggested Readings

Friedman NL. Hiccups: a treatment review. *Pharmacotherapy* 1996;16(6):986-95.

Smith HS, Busracamwongs A. Management of hiccups in the palliative care population.*Am J Hosp Palliat Care* 2003;20(2):149-54.

Walker P, Watanabe S, Bruera E. Baclofen, a treatment for chronic hiccup. *J Pain Symptom Manage* 1998;16(2):125-32.

References

1. [No authors listed]. Drug-induced hiccups. *Prescrire Int* 1999;8(39):23.
2. Schiff E, River Y, Oliven A et al. Acupuncture therapy for persistent hiccups. *Am J Med Sci* 2002;323(3):166-8.
3. Ramirez FC, Graham DY. Treatment of intractable hiccup with baclofen: results of a double-blind randomized, controlled, cross-over study. *Am J Gastroenterol* 1992;87(12):1789-91.
4. Friedgood CE, Ripstein CB. Chlorpromazine (thorazine) in the treatment of intractable hiccups. *J Am Med Assoc* 1955;157(4):309-10.
5. Hadjiyannacos D, Vlassopoulos D, Hadjiconstantinou V. Treatment of intractable hiccup in haemodialysis patients with baclofen. *Am J Nephrol* 2001;21(5):427-8.

CHAPTER 120
Palliative Care

David Duperé, MD, FRCP(C)

Symptoms confronted at the end of life (Table 1) require a team approach. This chapter is based on the *palliative medicine toolbox* (Table 4) containing medications selected by the experienced palliative care team to carry to the home setting.

Table 1: **Symptoms at the End of Life[1,a]**

Symptom	Incidence (%)
Noisy and moist breathing	56
Urinary dysfunction	53
Pain	51
Restlessness and agitation	42
Dyspnea	22
Nausea and vomiting	14
Sweating	14
Jerking, twitching	12

[a] End of life refers to the final 48 hours of life.

Goals of Therapy

- Limit physical and emotional suffering by adequately managing pain and other symptoms
- Support the ability to enjoy remaining life while avoiding inappropriate prolongation of death

Investigations

- History and physical to determine the nature and severity of symptoms
- Detailed medication history including nonprescription medications, herbals, vitamins and other natural therapies. Knowledge of prior experience of treatment benefit or intolerance saves time
- Minimal diagnostic testing will help preserve quality of life. Avoid invasive investigations whenever possible

Therapeutic Choices

Four rules are essential for optimal symptom management in the palliative setting:

- Any symptom is as distressing as a patient claims it to be.
- Treatment risks, benefits and alternatives need to be discussed in the context of the dying patient's values, culture, goals and fears.
- Individualize choice and dose of medication—preset recipes are not adequate.

- Cause of symptoms is irrelevant and investigation pointless when disease is advanced and death very near, unless detection would direct a useful change in symptomatic treatment.

Dyspnea

- The uncomfortable awareness of one's own breathing is completely subjective and easily misinterpreted; therefore, observer opinion or objective measurements are irrelevant.
- Management based on the symptom's impact on activities of daily living makes for more effective therapeutic choices. Treat reversible causes or components when appropriate. Associated anxiety requires special management.

Nonpharmacologic Choices

- Oxygen is a potent symbol of medical care that clearly has a role in the hypoxic patient.[2] Carefully consider oxygen use in the hypoxic patient who senses no benefit or the nonhypoxic patient who does sense benefit, e.g., try it on a continuous or as-needed basis and ask the patient if it helps. Similarly, let the patient choose the flow rate. Sometimes a mask with compressed air flow provides a sense of security.
- Relaxation therapies.
- Physical therapies, e.g., exercise program to avoid deconditioning.
- Electric fan for cool air flow to face.
- Open window; allow clear line of sight to the outside if bedbound.

Pharmacologic Choices (Table 4)

Respiratory Sedatives

Opioids

Morphine and **hydromorphone** can be highly effective in relieving dyspnea.[3,4] The acute situation may require frequent parenteral dosing (e.g., morphine 5 to 10 mg sc or iv Q30 minutes until settled). Otherwise Q4H dosing with appropriate Q1H breakthrough doses is usually indicated. Intermittent dyspnea can be treated with intermittent opioid. Tolerance to the respiratory depressant effects of opioids develops quickly. If titrated to control dyspnea, opioids will not hasten death. Increases in carbon dioxide partial pressure (pCO_2) and significant hypoventilation are dependent on previous exposure to opioids, the rate of increase of opioid dose and perhaps the route of administration. At present there is no clear evidence for the role of nebulized opioids.[5]

Fentanyl administered sublingually can also be beneficial for dyspnea in the home setting when parenteral or subcutaneous access may be limited. Starting doses of 0.5 to 1 ml (25 to 50 μg) sublingually are well tolerated. Onset is quick but duration of effect is only about 40 to 60 minutes.[6]

Nonopioids

Benzodiazepines (e.g., clonazepam, lorazepam, midazolam): Diazepam use in COPD has limited benefit in dyspnea.[7] Although their use is not validated, benzodiazepines may improve control of dyspnea in terms of duration of action, potency and reduced adverse effects, especially in the absence of pain or when there is a clear component of anxiety.

Phenothiazines (e.g., promethazine, chlorpromazine) can be effective at relieving refractory cases of dyspnea without causing respiratory depression.[8]

Corticosteroids have a specific role in the management of dyspnea resulting from obstructive lesions, lymphangitic carcinomatosis or COPD. CNS adverse effects may limit their utility.

Pain

- Determine the cause. Differentiate a nociceptive (somatic, visceral) pain from neuropathic (dysesthetic, neuralgic) to facilitate the choice of treatment options (see Chapter 15).
- Measure the intensity. A report of quantity of pain on a 0 to 10 scale (0 being no pain) is easy to use and reproducible.
- Review multidimensional aspects of pain. Address response and adverse effects to previously used analgesics, coping skills, past drug/alcohol abuse and concerns about addiction, metabolic abnormalities, cognitive impairment and finances.

Pharmacologic Choices (Table 4)

A step-wise approach to pain management is mandated in all cases (see Chapter 14 and Chapter 15 for discussions of acute pain and neuropathic pain). For mild pain, **nonopioid analgesics** can be tried (e.g., acetaminophen, NSAIDs or ASA) with or without codeine. In the acute palliative care setting the mainstays of therapy are usually the **opioids** (e.g., morphine and hydromorphone).

- The goal is opioid titration to achieve adequate pain control without opioid toxicity.
- Q4H dosing (po/sc/iv/pr) is best for dose titration. The acute situation may require more frequent parenteral dosing (e.g., morphine 5 to 10 mg sc or iv Q30min until settled).
- There are no maximum doses as responses to opioids vary greatly and can reach hundreds of milligrams Q4H.
- Providing a breakthrough dose (estimated as 10% of the total 24-hour dose) ordered as Q1H PRN allows for control of interdose pain and provides the essential dosing information required for opioid titration.

Therefore, the new Q4H dose = (all Q4H + all PRN doses in previous 24 hours)/6.

- Adjuvant drugs may be useful in particular pain syndromes (e.g., corticosteroids in bone pain, hepatic capsular pain) (Table 2).
- Anticipate and educate patient and caregivers about side effects of opioid use (Table 3).
- Opioid toxicity resulting from altered opioid metabolism (e.g., dehydration, renal failure) may respond to dose reduction and correction of the altered metabolism when possible. The presence of significant toxicity requires a switch to another opioid at 50 to 75% of the equianalgesic dose. Avoid meperidine as its neurotoxic metabolite can accumulate in patients with reduced renal function, possibly causing seizures.

Table 2: Adjuvant Analgesics

Type/Description of Pain	Suggested Drug Treatment
Bone Pain	**NSAID** with cytoprotection (e.g., **naproxen**➔ 500 mg po/pr BID with **misoprostol** 200 μg po BID or **omeprazole** 20 mg po daily[9]) Severe cases: **dexamethasone** 4 mg po/sc/iv TID-QID; high doses sometimes required (e.g., 24–32 mg/day)
Closed space pain	**Dexamethasone** as for bone pain
Pleuritic pain	**NSAID** as for bone pain
Neuropathic pain	See Chapter 15
Burning/dysesthetic	Add TCA[a] (e.g., **amitriptyline** or **imipramine**) 25 mg po BID-TID; increase gradually up to 150 mg/day if necessary
Shock-like/lancinating	Add **gabapentin**➔ 300 mg po QHS; increase gradually up to 1200 mg TID if necessary Severe cases: **dexamethasone** as above for severe bone pain

[a] Decrease doses of TCAs by 50% in the presence of hepatic or renal impairment or in the frail elderly.
➔ Dosage adjustment may be required in renal impairment; see Appendix I.

Table 3: Management of Adverse Effects of Opioids

General	Comments	Management
Nausea	Very common, tolerance develops in 2–3 days	Dimenhydrinate/metoclopramide PRN
Constipation	Ongoing treatment is mandatory	Daily laxatives (softener & stimulant)

(cont'd)

Table 3: **Management of Adverse Effects of Opioids** *(cont'd)*

General	Comments	Management
Somnolence	Very common, tolerance develops in 2–3 days	Reassure patient
Pruritus	Less common	May require change of opioid, antihistamines
Dry Mouth	Less common	Chew gum; suck on hard candy
Neurotoxic		
Myoclonus	Uncommon in early titrated opioid use	May require change of opioid
Delirium	See myoclonus	May require change of opioid
Visual hallucinations	See myoclonus	May require change of opioid

Terminal Delirium and Agitation

- With progressive multi-organ failure, patients often develop increasing confusion, drowsiness and/or restlessness and moaning.
- Search for reversible causes (e.g., dehydration, visual or hearing impairment)[10] although this is rarely successful.
- Never give opioids as sedatives.
- Terminal sedation: in the event of a severe symptom (e.g., pain, dyspnea, restlessness, hemorrhage) where adequate interventions have not resulted in an acceptable level of comfort, heavy sedation may be considered to render the patient unaware of the symptom. Commonly used agents are **midazolam** and **methotrimeprazine**. Review the option with the patient and/or caregivers and provide an understanding that this usually involves cessation of nutrition and hydration.

Nonpharmacologic Choices

- Reassure and educate the caregivers about the possibility of delirium and agitation.

Pharmacologic Choices (Table 4)

- Review present medications for adjustment of dosages or discontinuation (e.g., sedatives).
- **Haloperidol** is the mainstay of treatment. If ineffective at doses of greater than 20 mg/day, consider more sedating agents such as **methotrimeprazine** or **midazolam** in regular doses or as a continuous infusion if necessary.

Respiratory Secretions

- Pooling of secretions is common with decreased levels of consciousness.
- This symptom (unfortunately named "death rattle") is usually of no consequence to the patient but can be quite distressing to the caregivers.

Nonpharmacologic Choices

- Educate the caregivers that the patient is unaware of the distressful breathing sounds and that it is not a source of suffering.
- Position patient semi-prone if possible.
- Swab directly if possible and not too distressing for the patient.

Pharmacologic Choices (Table 4)

- Anticholinergics will not dry out built-up secretions, so use medications regularly at the very onset of excessive secretions.
- **Hyoscine** is the usual choice but has sedative effects. To avoid sedation, **glycopyrrolate** may be given.[11]

Therapeutic Tips

- With the approach of end of life, focus the goals of care on achieving patient comfort. Discontinue interventions not playing a role in supporting comfort (e.g., blood work, vital signs, blood glucose monitoring). The routine medical approach (e.g., iv fluid rehydration) often is best replaced by what the patient truly needs to be kept comfortable (e.g., good mouth care to control thirst).
- Choose medications with the goal of providing comfort. Most medications used for the treatment of chronic diseases (e.g., anti-anginals) rarely have a role at end of life and should be discontinued. Opioids and medications with sedating properties are frequently required and their use should be guided solely by any ongoing need to control symptoms.
- Successful end-of-life care in the home requires 24-hour access to a supportive multidisciplinary team ready to deal rapidly with issues as they arise.

Table 4: **Drugs in the "Palliative Medicine Toolbox"**

Class	Drug	Indication	Starting Doses	Adverse Effects	Comments	Cost[a]
Analgesics	*morphine* M.O.S., MS-IR, generics	Pain, dyspnea	PO: 5–10 mg Q4–6H po + appropriate PRN IV/SC: 2.5–5 mg Q4-6H + appropriate PRN	Nausea, vomiting, constipation, sedation, drowsiness, confusion, respiratory depression, urinary retention, dry mouth, myoclonus.	Highly individual dosing requirements. Dose escalation based on pain relief and adverse effects.	PO:$ IV/SC:$$
	hydromorphone Dilaudid, Hydromorph IR, generics	Pain, dyspnea	PO: 2–4 mg Q4–6H + appropriate PRN IV/SC: 1–2 mg Q4–6H + appropriate PRN	See morphine.	See morphine.	PO:$$ IV/SC: $$$
	fentanyl generics	Dyspnea	PO: 25–50 μg Q1H PRN	See morphine.	See morphine.	$$$$
Antiemetics	*dimenhydrinate*[b] Gravol Preparations, generics	Nausea, vomiting	PO/IM/PR: 25–50 mg Q4-6H PRN	Sedation, anticholinergic effects, confusion. The elderly may be particularly susceptible.	Additive sedation with other sedating medications.	PO:$ IM/PR:$$
	metoclopramide generics	Nausea, vomiting	PO/SC: 5–10 mg Q4-6H PRN	Diarrhea, abdominal cramps and distention, headache, hyperprolactinemia, drowsiness, fatigue, EPS.	See dimenhydrinate.	PO:$ SC: $$$

Class	Drug	Indication	Starting Doses	Adverse Effects	Comments	Cost[a]
	prochlorperazine Stemetil, generics	Nausea, vomiting	PO/IM/PR: 5–10 mg Q4-6H PRN	Sedation, anticholinergic effects (dry mouth, blurred vision, constipation, nasal congestion, urinary retention), extrapyramidal effects, hypotension, hypersensitivity; pancytopenia (rare).	See dimenhydrinate.	PO:$ IM: $$$ PR:$$
Antipsychotics	*haloperidol* generics	Agitation, nausea	PO/SC: 0.5–2 mg Q4-8H PRN	Sedation, extrapyramidal effects.	Usual drug of choice.	PO:$ SC:$$$
	methotrimeprazine Nozinan, generics	Agitation, nausea, adjuvant analgesia	PO/SC: 5–10 mg Q4-6H PRN	See haloperidol.		PO:$ SC:$$
	chlorpromazine generics	Dyspnea, nausea	PO/SC: 10 mg Q6H	See haloperidol. Hypotension with im/iv administration.		PO:$ SC:$$
Benzodiazepines	*midazolam* generics	Agitation, dyspnea	SC: 1–2 mg Q30min to Q1H PRN	Sedation, hypotension, transient apnea.		$$$$
	lorazepam Ativan, generics	Agitation, dyspnea	PO/SL: 1–2 mg Q6-8H PRN	Sedation (up to 80%), dizziness.		$
	clonazepam Rivotril, generics	Agitation, dyspnea	PO: 0.25–0.5 mg Q8-12H PRN	Sedation, dizziness.		$

(cont'd)

Table 4: **Drugs in the "Palliative Medicine Toolbox"** *(cont'd)*

Class	Drug	Indication	Starting Doses	Adverse Effects	Comments	Cost[a]
Corticosteroids	*dexamethasone* Dexasone, generics	Nausea, dyspnea, adjuvant analgesia	PO/SC: 4 mg Q6-8H	Mood changes, increased appetite, GI irritation, ulceration, fluid retention, weight gain, may mask signs of infection.		PO:$$ SC:$$$
Antimuscarinics	*glycopyrrolate* Glycopyrrolate Injection USP	Respiratory secretions	SC: 0.2–0.6 mg Q2-4H PRN (or Q4-8H PRN)	Dizziness, blurred vision, dry mouth, urinary retention.	Rarely causes sedation or delirium.	$$$$
	hyoscine hydrobromide (scopolamine)[b] generics	Respiratory secretions	SC: 0.3–0.8 mg Q2-4H PRN (or Q4-8H PRN)	Sedation, dizziness, blurred vision, dry mouth, urinary retention.		$$$$

[a] Cost of 1-day supply; includes drug cost only.
[b] Available without a prescription.
Dosage adjustment may be required in renal impairment; see Appendix I.
Legend: $ < $1 $$ $1–5 $$$ $5–10 $$$$ >$10

Suggested Readings

Lo B, Rubenfeld G. Palliative sedation in dying patients: "we turn to it when everything else hasn't worked". *JAMA* 2005;294(14):1810-6.

Morrison RS, Meier DE. Clinical practice. Palliative care. *N Engl J Med* 2004;350(25):2582-90.

Quigley C. The role of opioids in cancer pain. *BMJ* 2005;331(7520):825-9.

Stevenson J, Abernethy AP, Miller C et al. Managing comorbidities in patients at the end of life. *BMJ* 2004;329(7471):909-12.

University of Toronto, Faculty of Medicine, Continuing Education. *Ian Anderson continuing education program in end-of-life care*. Toronto (ON): University of Toronto. Available from: http://www.cme.utoronto.ca/endoflife/ Accessed January 30, 2007.

References

1. Lichter I, Hunt E. The last 48 hours of life. *J Palliat Care* 1990;6(4):7-15.
2. Bruera E, de Stoutz N, Velasco-Leiva A et al. Effects of oxygen on dyspnoea in hypoxaemic terminal-cancer patients. *Lancet* 1993;342(8862):13-4.
3. Bruera E, Macmillan K, Pither J et al. Effects of morphine on the dyspnea of terminal cancer patients. *J Pain Symptom Manage* 1990;5(6):341-4.
4. Robin ED, Burke CM. Single-patient randomized clinical trial. Opiates for intractable dyspnea. *Chest* 1986;90(6):888-92.
5. Jennings AL, Davies AN, Higgins JP et al. A systematic review of the use of opioids in the management of dyspnoea. *Thorax* 2002;57(11):939-44.
6. Zhang H, Zhang J, Streisand JB. Oral mucosal delivery: clinical pharmacokinetics and therapeutic applications. *Clin Pharmacokinet* 2002;41(9):661-80.
7. Wedzicha JA, Wallis PJ, Ingram DA et al. Effect of diazepam on sleep in patients with chronic airflow obstruction. *Thorax* 1988;43(9):729-30.
8. O'Neill PA, Morton PB, Stark RD. Chlorpromazine--a specific effect on breathlessness? *Br J Clin Pharmacol* 1985;19(6):793-7.
9. Singh G, Triadafilopoulos G. Appropriate choice of proton pump inhibitor therapy in the prevention and management of NSAID-related gastrointestinal damage. *Int J Clin Pract* 2005;59(10):1210-7.
10. Casarett DJ, Inouye S.C. et al. Diagnosis and management of delirium near the end of life. *Ann Intern Med* 2001;135(1):32-40.
11. Wildiers H, Menten J. Death rattle: prevalence, prevention and treatment. *J Pain Symptom Manage* 2002;23(4):310-7.

APPENDIX I

Dosage Adjustment in Renal Impairment

James McCormack, BSc(Pharm), PharmD
Bruce Carleton, BPharm, PharmD and
Piera Calissi, BSc(Pharm), PharmD

Careful dosage adjustment may reduce the risk of drug toxicity in patients with impaired renal function. The following is an approach to empiric dosage adjustments (dose and/or interval) in adult patients based on an estimate of renal function (Figure 1, Table 1). This approach does not apply to patients on dialysis (consult specialized references).

Patient/Drug Considerations

The following questions should be answered prior to making empiric dosage adjustments. Table 2 provides drug-specific information.

Is the patient's renal function impaired?

Use the following formula[1] to estimate the *weight-corrected creatinine clearance* (ClCr) and to guide empiric dosage adjustments:

$$\text{Males: ClCr (mL/s/70 kg)} = \frac{(140 - \text{age}) \times 1.5}{\text{serum creatinine } (\mu\text{mol/L})}$$

Females: ClCr (mL/s/70 kg) = 0.85 × above equation

Many clinicians may be more familiar with a ClCr formula that includes weight. When using formulas to estimate ClCr, first identify the reason for the ClCr determination. If an estimate of the patient's true ClCr (in mL/second) is needed, then use a ClCr formula that includes weight. However, if the estimate of the degree of renal impairment is to guide dosage adjustments, use a weight-corrected estimate of ClCr rather than the patient's actual ClCr. This weight-corrected estimate is then compared to a "normal" ClCr for a 70 kg male (1.8 to 2 mL/s) to approximate the degree of renal dysfunction. Charts that suggest empiric dosage adjustments are usually based on the assumption that the baseline or normal ClCr is 1.8 to 2 mL/s. In addition, a weight-corrected ClCr is easier to calculate.

Elderly (> 65 years) or malnourished patients may have relatively low muscle mass and therefore produce less creatinine. If the actual serum creatinine for such patients is used, the formula can often overestimate renal function. A rule of thumb in such patients is not to use a serum creatinine < 100 µmol/L in the above formula.

Over the last few years, a new equation (Modification of Diet in Renal Disease—MDRD) to estimate the glomerular filtration rate (GFR) has found its way into clinical use. The MDRD is recommended for staging chronic kidney disease because it has improved predictive performance over the Cockcroft and Gault equation in estimating the GFR. Some clinicians also use the MDRD to estimate the GFR in order to adjust medication doses in patients with renal impairment. However, in adjusting drug doses in patients with renal impairment, the improved accuracy of the MDRD equation to predict the GFR will not, in most cases, result in measurably improved outcomes such as enhanced medication safety or efficacy. This is because most recommendations for drug dosing in patients with renal impairment are not based on specific pharmacokinetic or pharmacodynamic outcome data. Instead, the dosage recommendations are based on somewhat broad and arbitrary GFR cut-off points. Given this, both the Cockcroft and Gault and MDRD equations provide sufficiently accurate estimates of renal function for use in drug dosage adjustment. Clinicians should likely choose the equation that is easiest to use or the one with which they are most familiar. Most importantly, clinicians need to determine rational starting doses using not only these equations, but also based on the urgency of the need for a response to drug therapy. All these issues make the current debate about which formula to use to estimate renal function somewhat irrelevant. However, regardless of the method used there is a critical next step: titrate the dose whenever possible, and determine the correct dose by monitoring a patient's response to the dose chosen.

In general, if ClCr estimates are > 1 mL/s/70 kg, empiric dosage adjustments are not required because changes in ClCr from 2 to 1 mL/s/70 kg are associated with relatively small changes in the half-life of a drug or its active metabolite. However, as ClCr falls below 1 mL/s/70 kg, empiric dosage adjustments should be based on the following questions.

Is the drug effective/safe in patients with renal impairment? (Table 2, Comments column)

Some drugs are ineffective or potentially toxic in patients with clinically important renal dysfunction (ClCr < 0.5 mL/s/70 kg) and should be avoided.

Is the drug nephrotoxic? (Table 2, Comments column)

A number of drugs have the potential to worsen renal function and an alternative non-nephrotoxic agent should be used if possible.

Is an immediate clinical effect required?

When failure to elicit an immediate response (e.g., life-threatening conditions or severe pain) poses a clinically important risk of mortality or morbidity, drug dosing should be aimed at obtaining a therapeutic response within minutes or hours irrespective of renal function. In an attempt to achieve a rapid response, usual initial doses should be used, followed by empiric dosage adjustments once the patient has responded.

If an immediate effect is not required can the dose be titrated?

Many conditions do not require an immediate or maximal effect, and dose titration can often be used to determine the lowest effective dose. To identify the correct dose for any patient, but particularly in patients with renal impairment, start with a low dose (e.g., one-quarter or one-half of the typically recommended dose), and titrate up to a clinical effect.

Is the drug > 50% renally eliminated or does it have active or toxic metabolites? (Table 2)

Drugs that are primarily eliminated by the kidney (> 50%) require empiric dosage adjustments based on an estimate of renal function. In addition, some drugs are metabolized to active or toxic metabolites which may be excreted by the kidney and may need dosage adjustments. Some drugs should be avoided in patients with compromised renal function if toxic metabolites can accumulate (e.g., meperidine).

Approach to Empiric Dosage Adjustments

When dose titration is not possible or desired, base empiric dosage adjustments on estimates of renal function.

Interval versus Dose Adjustment

For drugs given intermittently, the dose or the dosing interval can be adjusted based on the desired goal. Often a combination of extending the interval and reducing the dose is effective and convenient. If the aim is to achieve steady-state maximum/peak and minimum/trough concentrations (e.g., aminoglycosides) similar to those seen in patients with normal renal function, extend the interval between doses. If a relatively constant steady-state concentration is desired (e.g., antihypertensives), reduce the dose.

Drugs Eliminated ≥ 75% by the Kidney (Table 2)

Table 1 provides guidelines for the dosage of these drugs based on the usual dosing interval. For frequently administered drugs (e.g., Q4H–Q12H), extending the interval may decrease the cost of administration or adherence problems.

Drugs Eliminated 50 to < 75% by the Kidney (Table 2)

These drugs have a clinically important proportion of nonrenal clearance and therefore empiric dosage adjustments are generally not required until renal function estimates are < 0.75 mL/s/70 kg (Table 1).

Drugs Eliminated < 50% by the Kidney (Table 2)

For drugs eliminated < 50% by the kidneys, empiric dosage adjustments are generally not required, assuming the drug has no active or toxic metabolites. However, these drugs may require dosage adjustment in patients with clinically important liver dysfunction.

Drugs with Active or Toxic Metabolites (Table 2, Comments column)

Empiric dosage adjustments for drugs with active or toxic metabolites which are dependent on renal elimination should be made as though the drug were 75 to 100% renally eliminated.

Further Dosage Adjustments Based on Clinical Response

All of the above recommendations are for empiric dosage adjustments, and further dosage changes must always be made based on a patient-specific assessment of efficacy and toxicity. Serum drug concentration monitoring may guide dosage adjustments for certain drugs (Table 2, Comments column).

Suggested Readings

McCormack JP Cooper J, Carleton B. Simple approach to dosage adjustment in patients with renal impairment. *Am J Health Syst Pharm* 1997;54(21):2505–9.

Vidal L, Shavit M. Systematic comparison of four sources of drug information regarding adjustment of dose for renal function. *BMJ* 2005; 331(7511):263-6.

Figure 1: **Empiric Dosage Adjustment Based on Renal Function (Adults)**

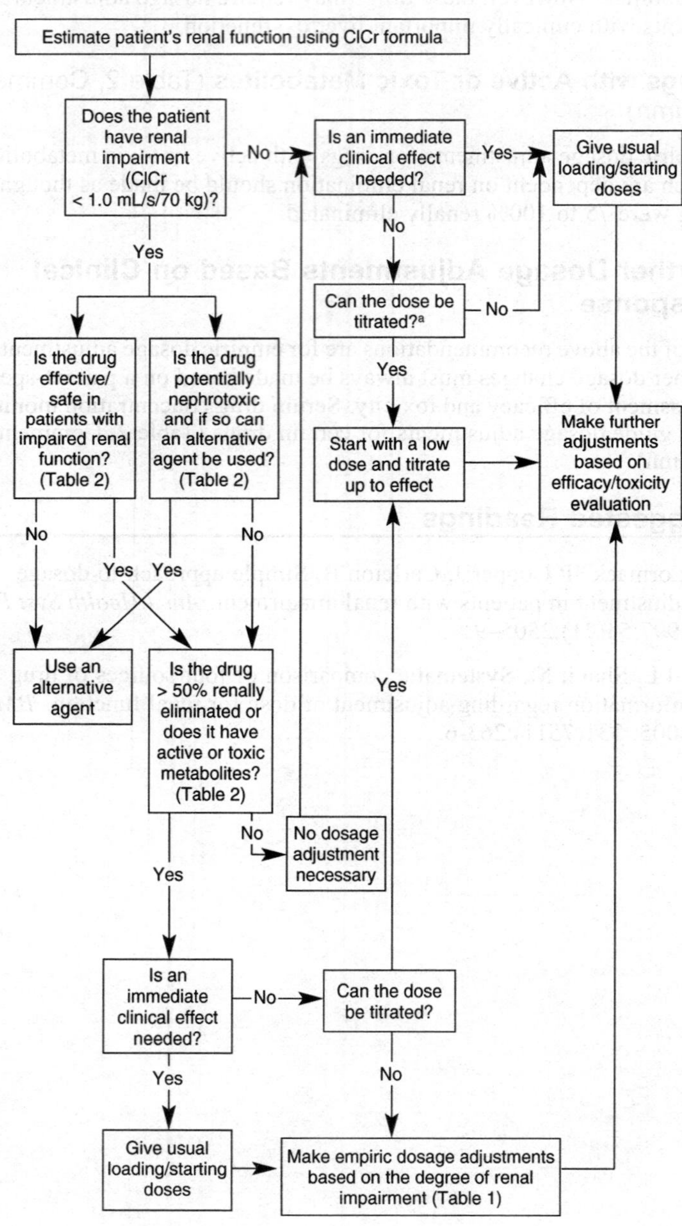

[a] For example, antihypertensives, antihyperglycemics, antidepressants.

Table 1: Suggested Empiric Dosage Adjustments in Adults for Drugs Primarily Renally Eliminated based on percentage renal elimination and estimated creatinine clearance (normal ClCr = 2.0 mL/s/70 kg)

How to Use Table 1:

1. Estimate renal function (ClCr), *e.g., a patient with an estimated ClCr of 0.42 mL/s/70 kg is receiving iv ampicillin.*
2. Determine percentage renal elimination of drug (Table 2), *e.g., ampicillin is 75–100% renally eliminated, according to Table 2.*
3. Determine normal dosing interval, *e.g., usual dosing interval for ampicillin is Q6H*
4. Using above information, determine empiric dosage adjustment, *e.g., the patient's ClCr is between 0.25–0.5 mL/s/70 kg. Therefore, the empiric dosing adjustment is to administer the ampicillin Q12H.*

			Normal Dosing Interval				
% Renal Elimination of Drug:	**75–100%**	**50–74%**	**Q4H**	**Q6H**	**Q8H**	**Q12H**	**Q24H**
	> 1.0	> 0.75	None	None	None	None	None
Estimated ClCr (mL/s/70 kg)	0.5–1.0	0.33–0.75	Q6H	Q8H	Q12H	Q24H	↓D 25%[a]
	0.25–0.5	0.16–0.33	Q8H	Q12H	Q24H	Q24H and ↓D 25%[a]	↓D 50%[a]
	< 0.25	< 0.16	Q12H	Q24H	Q24H and ↓D 25%[a]	Q24H and ↓D 50%[a]	↓D 75%[a]

[a] For certain drugs, decreasing the dose is not appropriate, or one may need to extend interval > Q24H if available dosage forms do not permit specific dose reductions.
None = no dosage adjustment necessary; ↓D = decrease usual dose by indicated percentage.

Table 2: **Dosage Adjustment in Renal Impairment—Adults**[a]

Drug	% Renal Elimination			Comments
	<50	50–74	≥75	
abacavir	•			
abatacept	•			
acarbose	•			
acebutolol		•		Active metabolite; assume ≥ 75% renal elimination for dosage adjustment
acetaminophen	•			
acetazolamide			•	Avoid; ineffective in severe impairment
acitretin	•			
acyclovir			•	
adalimumab	•			
adefovir dipivoxil	•			Nephrotoxic. Active metabolite; assume ≥ 75% renal elimination for dosage adjustment
adenosine	•			
alefacept	•			
alendronate	•			Avoid
alfuzosin	•			
allopurinol	•			Active metabolite; assume ≥ 75% renal elimination for dosage adjustment
almotriptan			•	
alprazolam	•			
alteplase	•			
amantadine			•	
amikacin			•	Nephrotoxic; monitor serum drug concentrations
amiloride		•		Avoid
5-aminosalicylic acid	•			
aminophylline	•			
amiodarone	•			Active metabolite but no dosage adjustment required
amitriptyline	•			Active metabolite but no dosage adjustment required
amlodipine	•			

[a]*Omission of a drug from this table does not imply that dosage adjustment is NOT required in renal impairment. Refer to specific references for dosing in dialysis.*

Table 2: Dosage Adjustment in Renal Impairment—Adults[a] *(cont'd)*

Drug	% Renal Elimination			Comments
	<50	50–74	≥75	
amoxicillin		•		
amoxicillin/clavulanate		•		
amphotericin	•			Nephrotoxic
ampicillin			•	
anakinra			•	
antacids: Al^{++}/Mg^{++}	•			Avoid; Al^{++} and/or Mg^{++} may accumulate
ASA	•			Nephrotoxic
atazanavir	•			
atenolol			•	
atomoxetine	•			
atorvastatin	•			Active metabolite but no dosage adjustment required
atovaquone	•			
atropine	•			
auranofin			•	Avoid; nephrotoxic
azatadine	•			
azathioprine	•			Active metabolite; assume ≥ 75% renal elimination for dosage adjustment
azithromycin	•			
baclofen			•	
benazepril	•			
benztropine	•			
bezafibrate		•		Avoid
bisacodyl	•			Active metabolite but no dosage adjustment required
bismuth subsalicylate	•			
bisoprolol		•		
bretylium			•	Active metabolite; assume ≥ 75% renal elimination for dosage adjustment
bromocriptine	•			
brompheniramine	•			

[a] *Omission of a drug from this table does not imply that dosage adjustment is NOT required in renal impairment. Refer to specific references for dosing in dialysis.*

Table 2: **Dosage Adjustment in Renal Impairment—Adults**[a] *(cont'd)*

Drug	% Renal Elimination			Comments
	<50	50–74	≥75	
bumetanide	•			Larger doses may be required In severe renal impairment
bupropion	•			Active metabolite; assume ≥ 75% renal elimination for dosage adjustment
buserelin	•			
buspirone	•			
butalbital	•			Active metabolite; assume ≥ 75% renal elimination for dosage adjustment
calcitonin	•			
candesartan	•			
captopril		•		
carbamazepine	•			Active metabolite but no dosage adjustment required
carvedilol	•			Active metabolite but no dosage adjustment required
caspofungin	•			
cefaclor		•		
cefadroxil			•	
cefazolin			•	
cefepime			•	
cefixime		•		
cefotaxime		•		Active metabolite; assume ≥ 75% renal elimination for dosage adjustment
cefoxitin			•	
cefprozil		•		
ceftazidime			•	
ceftriaxone	•			
cefuroxime			•	
celecoxib	•			Nephrotoxic
cephalexin			•	
cetirizine		•		
chloral hydrate	•			Avoid. Active metabolite; assume ≥ 75% renal elimination for dosage adjustment

[a]*Omission of a drug from this table does not imply that dosage adjustment is NOT required in renal impairment. Refer to specific references for dosing in dialysis.*

Table 2: **Dosage Adjustment in Renal Impairment—Adults**[a] *(cont'd)*

Drug	% Renal Elimination			Comments
	<50	50–74	≥75	
chlordiazepoxide	•			Active metabolite; assume ≥ 75% renal elimination for dosage adjustment
chloroquine		•		
chlorpheniramine	•			
chlorpromazine	•			Active metabolite but no dosage adjustment required
chlorpropamide	•			Avoid. Active metabolite; assume ≥ 75% renal elimination for dosage adjustment
chlorthalidone		•		Avoid; ineffective at low ClCr
cholestyramine	•			
cidofovir			•	Avoid; nephrotoxic. Active metabolite; assume ≥ 75% renal elimination for dosage adjustment
cilazapril	•			Active metabolite; assume ≥ 75% renal elimination for dosage adjustment
cimetidine		•		
cinacalcet	•			
ciprofloxacin		•		
citalopram	•			
clarithromycin	•			Active metabolite; assume ≥ 75% renal elimination for dosage adjustment
clemastine	•			
clindamycin	•			
clobazam	•			
clodronate			•	Avoid; nephrotoxic
clomiphene	•			
clomipramine	•			Active metabolite but no dosage adjustment required
clonazepam	•			
clonidine	•			
clopidogrel	•			
cloxacillin	•			
clozapine	•			Active metabolite but no dosage adjustment required

[a]*Omission of a drug from this table does not imply that dosage adjustment is NOT required in renal impairment. Refer to specific references for dosing in dialysis.*

Table 2: **Dosage Adjustment in Renal Impairment—Adults**[a] *(cont'd)*

Drug	% Renal Elimination <50	50–74	≥75	Comments
codeine	•			
colestipol	•			
colchicine	•			Avoid
cyclosporine	•			Nephrotoxic; monitor serum drug concentrations
cyproheptadine	•			
cyproterone acetate	•			
dalteparin			•	
danazol	•			
dantrolene	•			
dapsone	•			
daptomycin			•	
darbepoetin alfa	•			
darifenacin	•			
darunavir	•			
delavirdine	•			
desipramine	•			Active metabolite but no dosage adjustment required
desloratadine	•			Active metabolite; assume ≥ 75% renal elimination for dosage adjustment
dexamethasone	•			
dextroamphetamine		•		Active metabolite but no dosage adjustment required
dextromethorphan	•			Active metabolite; assume ≥ 75% renal elimination for dosage adjustment
diazepam	•			Active metabolite but no dosage adjustment required
diclofenac	•			Nephrotoxic
dicyclomine			•	
didanosine	•			Active metabolite; assume ≥ 75% renal elimination for dosage adjustment
diethylpropion	•			Active metabolite but no dosage adjustment required
diflunisal	•			Nephrotoxic

[a]*Omission of a drug from this table does not imply that dosage adjustment is NOT required in renal impairment. Refer to specific references for dosing in dialysis.*

Table 2: **Dosage Adjustment in Renal Impairment—Adultsª**
(cont'd)

Drug	% Renal Elimination			Comments
	<50	50–74	≥75	
digoxin			•	Monitoring serum concentrations
dihydroergotamine	•			Active metabolite
diltiazem	•			Active metabolite but no dosage adjustment required
dimenhydrinate	•			
diphenhydramine	•			
diphenoxylate	•			Active metabolite
dipyridamole	•			
disopyramide		•		
divalproex	•			
docusate	•			
dofetilide			•	
dolasetron	•			Active metabolite but no dosage adjustment required. Avoid in severe renal impairment
domperidone	•			
donepezil	•			Active metabolite but no dosage adjustment required
doxazosin	•			
doxepin	•			Active metabolite but no dosage adjustment required
doxycycline	•			
dronabinol	•			
drotrecogin alfa	•			
dutasteride	•			
efalizumab	•			
efavirenz	•			
eletriptan	•			
emtricitabine			•	
enalapril	•			Active metabolite; assume ≥ 75% renal elimination for dosage adjustment
enoxaparin			•	
entacapone	•			

ªOmission of a drug from this table does not imply that dosage adjustment is NOT required in renal impairment. Refer to specific references for dosing in dialysis.

Table 2: **Dosage Adjustment in Renal Impairment—Adults**[a]
(cont'd)

Drug	% Renal Elimination <50	% Renal Elimination 50–74	% Renal Elimination ≥75	Comments
entecavir		•		
eprosartan	•			
eptifibatide	•			Dosage adjustment recommended for patients with renal dysfunction
ergotamine	•			Avoid
ertapenem			•	
erythromycin	•			
escitalopram	•			Active metabolite but no dosage adjustment required
esmolol	•			
esomeprazole	•			
estrogens	•			
etanercept	•			
ethacrynic acid	•			Avoid in severe renal impairment
ethambutol		•		
ethopropazine				Route of elimination unknown
ethosuximide	•			
etidronate		•		Nephrotoxic
etodolac	•			Nephrotoxic
ezetimibe	•			
famciclovir	•			Active metabolite; assume ≥ 75% renal elimination for dosage adjustment
famotidine			•	
felodipine	•			
fenofibrate	•			Active metabolite; assume ≥ 75% renal elimination for dosage adjustment
fentanyl	•			
fexofenadine	•			Active metabolite; assume ≥ 75% renal elimination for dosage adjustment
finasteride	•			
flavoxate	•			
flecainide	•			Active metabolite; assume ≥ 75% renal elimination for dosage adjustment

[a] *Omission of a drug from this table does not imply that dosage adjustment is NOT required in renal impairment. Refer to specific references for dosing in dialysis.*

Table 2: **Dosage Adjustment in Renal Impairment—Adults**[a] *(cont'd)*

Drug	% Renal Elimination <50	50–74	≥75	Comments
fluconazole		•		
fludrocortisone	•			
flucytosine			•	
flunarizine	•			
flupenthixol	•			
fluphenazine	•			
fluoxetine	•			Active metabolite but no dosage adjustment required
flurazepam	•			Active metabolite but no dosage adjustment required
flurbiprofen	•			Nephrotoxic
fluvastatin	•			
fluvoxamine	•			
fondaparinux			•	
fosamprenavir	•			
foscarnet			•	Avoid; nephrotoxic
fosfomycin			•	
fosinopril	•			Active metabolite but no dosage adjustment required
furosemide		•		Larger doses may be required In severe renal impairment
gabapentin			•	
galantamine	•			
ganciclovir			•	
gemifloxacin	•			< 50% renal elimination but the manufacturer recommends dosage adjustment if ClCr < 0.5 mL/sec
gemfibrozil	•			Active metabolite; assume ≥ 75% renal elimination for dosage adjustment
gentamicin			•	Nephrotoxic; monitor serum drug concentrations
gliclazide	•			
glimepiride	•			Active metabolite; assume ≥ 75% renal elimination for dosage adjustment

[a] *Omission of a drug from this table does not imply that dosage adjustment is NOT required in renal impairment. Refer to specific references for dosing in dialysis.*

Table 2: **Dosage Adjustment in Renal Impairment—Adults**[a] *(cont'd)*

Drug	**% Renal Elimination** <50	50–74	≥75	**Comments**
glucosamine	•			
glyburide	•			Avoid. Active metabolite but no dosage adjustment required
glycopyrrolate	•			
goserelin	•			
granisetron	•			
haloperidol	•			
heparin	•			
hydralazine	•			
hydrochlorothiazide			•	Avoid; ineffective at low ClCr
hydrocodone	•			Active metabolite; assume ≥ 75% renal elimination for dosage adjustment
hydrocortisone	•			
hydromorphone	•			
hydroxychloroquine	•			
hydroxyzine	•			Active metabolite but no dosage adjustment required
hyoscine	•			
ibuprofen	•			Nephrotoxic
imipenem/cilastatin		•		
imipramine	•			Active metabolite but no dosage adjustment required
indapamide	•			Avoid; ineffective at low ClCr
indinavir	•			
indomethacin	•			Nephrotoxic
infliximab	•			
insulin	•			
interferon alfa	•			
irbesartan	•			
isoniazid	•			
isosorbide dinitrate or 5-mononitrate	•			Active metabolite but no dosage adjustment required

[a] *Omission of a drug from this table does not imply that dosage adjustment is NOT required in renal impairment. Refer to specific references for dosing in dialysis.*

Table 2: **Dosage Adjustment in Renal Impairment—Adults**[a]
(cont'd)

Drug	% Renal Elimination			Comments
	<50	50–74	≥75	
isotretinoin	•			Avoid
itraconazole	•			
ketoconazole	•			
ketoprofen	•			Nephrotoxic
ketorolac			•	Nephrotoxic
ketotifen		•		
labetalol	•			
lamivudine		•		Active metabolite; assume ≥ 75% renal elimination for dosage adjustment
lamotrigine	•			
lansoprazole	•			
leflunomide	•			Active metabolite; assume ≥ 75% renal elimination for dosage adjustment
leuprolide	•			
levetiracetam		•		
levodopa	•			Active metabolite but no dosage adjustment required
levofloxacin			•	
levonorgestrel	•			
levothyroxine	•			
lidocaine	•			Active metabolite but no dosage adjustment required
linezolid	•			
liothyronine				No data on elimination
lisinopril			•	
lithium			•	Nephrotoxic; monitor serum drug concentrations
loperamide	•			
lopinavir/ritonavir	•			
loratadine	•			Active metabolite but no dosage adjustment required
lorazepam	•			

[a]*Omission of a drug from this table does not imply that dosage adjustment is NOT required in renal impairment. Refer to specific references for dosing in dialysis.*

Table 2: **Dosage Adjustment in Renal Impairment—Adults**[a] *(cont'd)*

Drug	% Renal Elimination			Comments
	<50	50–74	≥75	
losartan	•			Active metabolite but no dosage adjustment required
lovastatin	•			
loxapine	•			
lumiracoxib	•			Nephrotoxic
maprotiline	•			Active metabolite but no dosage adjustment required
medroxyprogesterone	•			
mefenamic acid	•			Nephrotoxic
mefloquine	•			
megestrol	•			
meloxicam	•			Nephrotoxic
memantine			•	
meperidine	•			Active metabolite; assume ≥ 75% renal elimination for dosage adjustment
mercaptopurine	•			Active metabolite; assume ≥ 75% renal elimination for dosage adjustment
meropenem		•		
metformin			•	Avoid
methadone	•			
methazolamide	•			Avoid; ineffective in severe impairment
methimazole	•			
methotrexate			•	Avoid; nephrotoxic
methotrimeprazine	•			Active metabolite but no dosage adjustment required
methoxsalen	•			
methyldopa	•			Active metabolite; assume ≥ 75% renal elimination for dosage adjustment
methylphenidate	•			
methylprednisolone	•			
methysergide	•			Avoid
metoclopramide	•		•	

[a]*Omission of a drug from this table does not imply that dosage adjustment is NOT required in renal impairment. Refer to specific references for dosing in dialysis.*

Table 2: **Dosage Adjustment in Renal Impairment—Adults**[a]
(cont'd)

Drug	% Renal Elimination			Comments
	<50	50–74	≥75	
metolazone		•		Dosage reduction not necessary in renal impairment
metoprolol	•			
metronidazole	•			Active metabolite but no dosage adjustment required
mexiletine	•			Active metabolite but no dosage adjustment required
micafungin	•			
midazolam	•			
midodrine	•			Active metabolite; assume ≥ 75% renal elimination for dosage adjustment
minocycline	•			
mirtazapine			•	
misoprostol	•			
mixed salts amphetamine		•		Active metabolite but no dosage adjustment required
moclobemide	•			
montelukast	•			
morphine	•			Active metabolite; assume ≥ 75% renal elimination for dosage adjustment
moxifloxacin	•			
nabilone	•			
nabumetone	•			Nephrotoxic. Active metabolite; assume ≥ 75% renal elimination for dosage adjustment
nadolol			•	
nadroparin			•	
nafarelin	•			
nafcillin	•			
naltrexone	•			Active metabolite but no dosage adjustment required
naproxen	•			Nephrotoxic
naratriptan		•		
nateglinide	•			

[a]*Omission of a drug from this table does not imply that dosage adjustment is NOT required in renal impairment. Refer to specific references for dosing in dialysis.*

Table 2: **Dosage Adjustment in Renal Impairment—Adults**[a] *(cont'd)*

Drug	% Renal Elimination			Comments
	<50	50–74	≥75	
nelfinavir	•			Active metabolite but no dosage adjustment required
nevirapine	•			
niacin	•			
nicoumalone	•			
nifedipine	•			
nitrofurantoin	•			Avoid
nitroglycerin	•			
nizatidine		•		
norethindrone	•			
norfloxacin			•	
nortriptyline	•			Active metabolite but no dosage adjustment required
octreotide	•			Reduce dose in severe impairment
ofloxacin			•	
olanzapine	•			
olsalazine	•			
omalizumab	•			
omeprazole	•			
ondansetron	•			
orlistat	•			
oseltamivir	•			Active metabolite but no dosage adjustment required
oxaprozin	•			Nephrotoxic
oxazepam	•			
oxcarbazepine	•			Active metabolite; assume ≥ 75% renal elimination for dosage adjustment
oxprenolol	•			
oxtriphylline	•			
oxybutynin	•			Active metabolite but no dosage adjustment required
oxycodone	•			

[a]*Omission of a drug from this table does not imply that dosage adjustment is NOT required in renal impairment. Refer to specific references for dosing in dialysis.*

Table 2: **Dosage Adjustment in Renal Impairment—Adults**[a]

(cont'd)

Drug	% Renal Elimination			Comments
	<50	50–74	≥75	
pamidronate		•		Nephrotoxic
pantoprazole	•			
paroxetine	•			
peginterferon alfa	•			
penicillamine	•			Avoid; nephrotoxic
penicillin G/V		•		
pentamidine	•			Nephrotoxic when given iv
pentazocine	•			
pentoxifylline	•			
pergolide	•			
perindopril	•			Active metabolite; assume ≥ 75% renal elimination for dosage adjustment
perphenazine	•			
phenelzine	•			
phenobarbital	•			Active metabolite but no dosage adjustment required
phentermine			•	
phenylbutazone	•			Nephrotoxic
phenylephrine	•			
phenytoin	•			
pimozide	•			
pinaverium bromide	•			
pindolol	•			
pioglitazone	•			
piperacillin			•	
piperacillin/tazobactam			•	
piroxicam	•			Nephrotoxic
pivampicillin		•		
pivmecillinam		•		
pizotifen	•			
posaconazole	•			

[a]*Omission of a drug from this table does not imply that dosage adjustment is NOT required in renal impairment. Refer to specific references for dosing in dialysis.*

Table 2: **Dosage Adjustment in Renal Impairment—Adults**[a] *(cont'd)*

Drug	% Renal Elimination <50	% Renal Elimination 50–74	% Renal Elimination ≥75	Comments
pramipexole			•	
pravastatin	•			
prazosin	•			
prednisone	•			
pregabalin			•	
primaquine	•			
primidone	•			Active metabolite but no dosage adjustment required
probenecid	•			Avoid; ineffective in renal impairment
procainamide		•		Active metabolite; assume ≥ 75% renal elimination for dosage adjustment
prochlorperazine	•			Active metabolite; assume ≥ 75% renal elimination for dosage adjustment
procyclidine	•			Active metabolite; assume ≥ 75% renal elimination for dosage adjustment
progesterone	•			
proguanil	•			Active metabolite but no dosage adjustment required
promethazine	•			
propafenone	•			
propoxyphene	•			Avoid. Active metabolite
propranolol	•			
propylthiouracil	•			
pseudoephedrine			•	
pyrazinamide	•			Avoid
pyrimethamine	•			
quetiapine	•			
quinapril	•			Active metabolite; assume ≥ 75% renal elimination for dosage adjustment
quinidine	•			Active metabolite but no dosage adjustment required
quinine	•			
quinupristin/ dalfopristin	•			Active metabolite but no dosage adjustment required

[a]*Omission of a drug from this table does not imply that dosage adjustment is NOT required in renal impairment. Refer to specific references for dosing in dialysis.*

Table 2: Dosage Adjustment in Renal Impairment—Adults[a]
(cont'd)

	% Renal Elimination			
Drug	**<50**	**50–74**	**≥75**	**Comments**
rabeprazole	•			
raloxifene	•			
ramipril	•			Active metabolite; assume ≥ 75% renal elimination for dosage adjustment
ranitidine		•		
repaglinide	•			
rasagiline	•			Conclusive data are not available for renally impaired patients
reteplase			•	Dosage adjustment is not recommended
ribavirin	•			Avoid
rifabutin	•			Active metabolite but no dosage adjustment required
rifampin	•			Active metabolite but no dosage adjustment required
risedronate			•	Avoid
risperidone	•			Active metabolite; assume ≥ 75% renal elimination for dosage adjustment
ritonavir	•			Active metabolite but no dosage adjustment required
rituximab	•			Nephrotoxic
rivastigmine	•			
rizatriptan	•			Active metabolite but no dosage adjustment required
ropinirole	•			
rosiglitazone	•			
rosuvastatin	•			
saquinavir	•			
selegiline	•			Active metabolite but no dosage adjustment required
senna				% renally eliminated unknown
sertraline	•			
sibutramine	•			Active metabolite but no dosage adjustment required
sildenafil	•			

[a]*Omission of a drug from this table does not imply that dosage adjustment is NOT required in renal impairment. Refer to specific references for dosing in dialysis.*

Table 2: **Dosage Adjustment in Renal Impairment—Adults**[a] *(cont'd)*

Drug	% Renal Elimination			Comments
	<50	**50–74**	**≥75**	
simvastatin	•			
sodium aurothiomalate			•	Avoid; nephrotoxic
solifenacin		•		Active metabolite
sotalol		•		
spectinomycin			•	Dosage adjustment unnecessary
spironolactone	•			Avoid. Active metabolite; assume ≥ 75% renal elimination for dosage adjustment
stavudine	•			Active metabolite; assume ≥ 75% renal elimination for dosage adjustment
streptokinase	•			
streptomycin			•	Nephrotoxic; monitor serum drug concentrations
sucralfate	•			Al^{++} may accumulate
sulfadiazine		•		Nephrotoxic
sulfamethoxazole/ trimethoprim		•		
sulfasalazine	•			Active metabolite but no dosage adjustment required
sulfinpyrazone	•			Avoid; neprotoxic
sulindac	•			Nephrotoxic. Active metabolite but no dosage adjustment required
sumatriptan	•			
tadalafil	•			Active metabolite; assume ≥ 75% renal elimination for dosage adjustment
tamsulosin	•			
telbivudine			•	
telithromycin	•			
telmisartan	•			
temazepam	•			
tenecteplase	•			
tenofovir			•	Nephrotoxic
tenoxicam	•			Nephrotoxic
terazosin	•			

[a]*Omission of a drug from this table does not imply that dosage adjustment is NOT required in renal impairment. Refer to specific references for dosing in dialysis.*

Table 2: Dosage Adjustment in Renal Impairment—Adults[a] *(cont'd)*

Drug	% Renal Elimination			Comments
	<50	50–74	≥75	
teriparatide	•			Do not use if ClCr < 0.5 mL/sec
tetracycline		•		Nephrotoxic
theophylline	•			
thiothixene	•			
tiaprofenic acid			•	Nephrotoxic
ticarcillin			•	
ticarcillin/clavulanate		•		
ticlopidine	•			
tigecycline	•			
timolol	•			
tinzaparin			•	
tipranavir	•			
tirofiban		•		
tizanidine	•			
tobramycin			•	Nephrotoxic; monitor serum drug concentrations
tolbutamide	•			
tolcapone	•			
tolmetin	•			
tolterodine	•			
topiramate			•	
torsemide	•			
tramadol	•			Active metabolite; assume ≥ 75% renal elimination for dosage adjustment
trandolapril	•			Active metabolite; assume ≥ 75% renal elimination for dosage adjustment
tranylcypromine	•			Active metabolite; assume ≥ 75% renal elimination for dosage adjustment
trazodone	•			
triamterene	•			Avoid. Nephrotoxic. Active metabolite but no dosage adjustment required
triazolam	•			

[a] *Omission of a drug from this table does not imply that dosage adjustment is NOT required in renal impairment. Refer to specific references for dosing in dialysis.*

Table 2: **Dosage Adjustment in Renal Impairment—Adults**[a] *(cont'd)*

Drug	% Renal Elimination <50	50–74	≥75	Comments
trifluoperazine	•			
trihexyphenidyl			•	
trimeprazine	•			
trimethoprim			•	
trimetrexate	•			Conclusive data are not available for renally impaired patients
trimipramine	•			
triprolidine	•			
triptorelin	•			Conclusive data are not available for renally impaired patients but dosage adjustment may be required
trospium	•			Conclusive data are not available for renally impaired patients but dosage adjustment may be required
L-tryptophan	•			
valacyclovir	•			Active metabolite; assume ≥ 75% renal elimination for dosage adjustment
valganciclovir		•		Nephrotoxic. Active metabolite; assume ≥ 75% renal elimination for dosage adjustment
valproic acid	•			
valsartan	•			
vancomycin			•	Nephrotoxic; monitor serum drug concentrations
vardenafil	•			
varenicline			•	
vasopressin	•			
venlafaxine	•			Active metabolite; assume ≥ 75% renal elimination for dosage adjustment
verapamil	•			Active metabolite but no dosage adjustment required
verteporfin	•			
vigabatrin			•	
vitamin C			•	
vitamin E	•			

[a]*Omission of a drug from this table does not imply that dosage adjustment is NOT required in renal impairment. Refer to specific references for dosing in dialysis.*

Table 2: **Dosage Adjustment in Renal Impairment—Adults**[a]

(cont'd)

Drug	% Renal Elimination			Comments
	<50	50–74	≥75	
voriconazole	•			Avoid iv formulation in renal impairment; nephrotoxic vehicle
warfarin	•			
yohimbine				Avoid. Route of elimination unknown
zafirlukast	•			
zalcitabine		•		Active metabolite; assume ≥ 75% renal elimination for dosage adjustment
zanamivir	•			
zidovudine	•			
zoledronic acid			•	
zolmitriptan	•			Active metabolite but no dosage adjustment required
zopiclone	•			
zuclopenthixol	•			

[a]*Omission of a drug from this table does not imply that dosage adjustment is NOT required in renal impairment. Refer to specific references for dosing in dialysis.*

APPENDIX II

Drug Exposure During Pregnancy and Lactation

Orna Diav-Citrin, MD and
Gideon Koren, MD, FRCPC

Many pregnant women are exposed to a variety of medications that may exert therapeutic, toxic or teratogenic effects on the fetus. Since the thalidomide disaster, many physicians and pregnant women tend to withhold any medication during pregnancy, although the risk of teratogenic effect from most drugs in therapeutic doses is nonexistent. Major congenital defects occur in 1 to 3% of the general population at birth. Of the major defects, about 25% are of genetic origin (genetically inherited diseases, new mutations and chromosomal abnormalities) and 65% are of unknown etiology (multifactorial, polygenic, spontaneous errors of development and synergistic interactions of teratogens). Only 2 to 3% of malformations are thought to be associated with drug treatment. The remaining defects are related to other environmental exposures including infectious agents, maternal disease states, mechanical problems and irradiation.[1]

Proper prescribing in pregnancy is a challenge and should provide maximal safety to the fetus as well as therapeutic benefit to the mother. To date, very few drugs are proven teratogens in humans. However, drug-induced malformations are important because they are potentially preventable.

Maternal physiologic changes during pregnancy may alter the pharmacokinetics of drugs. Clearance rates of many drugs increase during late pregnancy due to increases in both renal and hepatic elimination (e.g., digoxin, phenytoin), while in others the clearance rate decreases (e.g., theophylline). Generally, little is known about the relationship between maternal serum drug concentration and risk of teratogenicity.

The importance of *timing of drug exposure* is better understood; the effect produced by a teratogenic agent depends upon the developmental stage in which the conceptus is exposed. Several important phases in human development are recognized:

- The *"all or none" period*, the time from conception until somite formation. Insults to the embryo in this phase are likely to result in death and miscarriage or intact survival. The embryo is undifferentiated, and repair and recovery are possible through multiplication of the still totipotential cells. Exposure to teratogens during the presomitic stage usually does not cause congenital malformations unless the agent persists in the body beyond this period.
- The *embryonic period*, from 18 to 60 days after conception when the basic steps in organogenesis occur. This is the period of maximum

sensitivity to teratogenicity since tissues are differentiating rapidly and damage becomes irreparable. Exposure to teratogenic agents during this period has the greatest likelihood of causing a structural anomaly. The pattern of anomalies produced depends on which systems are differentiating at the time of teratogenic exposure.

- The *fetal phase*, from the end of the embryonic stage to term, when growth and functional maturation of formed organs and systems occurs. Teratogen exposure in this period will affect fetal growth (e.g., intrauterine growth restriction) and the size or function of an organ, rather than cause gross structural anomalies. The term *fetal toxicity* is commonly used to describe such an effect. The potential effect of psychoactive agents (e.g., antidepressants, antiepileptics, alcohol and other drugs of abuse) on the developing central nervous system has led to a new field of behavioural teratology.

Many organ systems continue structural and functional maturation long after birth. Most of the adenocarcinomas associated with first trimester exposure to diethylstilbestrol occurred many years later.

Teratogens must reach the developing conceptus in sufficient amounts to cause their effects. Large molecules with a molecular weight greater than 1000 (e.g., heparin) do not easily cross the placenta into the embryonic-fetal bloodstream. Other factors influencing the rate and extent of placental transfer of drugs include polarity, lipid solubility and the existence of a specific protein carrier (e.g., P-glycoprotein).

In an attempt to provide the practitioner with a better assessment of fetal risk, the US Food and Drug Administration (FDA) developed a classification of fetal risk in 1979.[2] These categories initially appeared logical but were not found to be very helpful in counselling individual patients. Drug manufacturers may have legal rather than scientific reasons for assigning particular designations. The classification frequently results in ambiguity and even false alarm. For example, oral contraceptives are denoted as X (i.e., contraindicated in pregnancy), despite failure of two meta-analyses to show increased teratogenic risk. In 1994 the Teratology Society stated that the FDA ratings are inappropriate and should be replaced by narrative statements that summarize and interpret available data regarding hazards of developmental toxicity and provide estimates of teratogenic risk. During the last few years the FDA has begun a process to change the present system.

Teratology Counselling[3]

- Ascertain the clinical facts regarding the nature of the exposure: the length, dosage and timing during pregnancy, as well as other exposures of concern (e.g., alcohol, cigarette smoking, herbal remedies).
- Collect all available current data regarding the agent and the risk of exposure.
- Counselling should include background human baseline risk for major malformations, whether the fetus is at increased risk, which anomaly

has been associated with the agent in question, a risk assessment, methods of prenatal detection when available, limitations in our knowledge and limitations of prenatal diagnostic capabilities.

- Additional considerations include the potential risk of the medical condition for which a drug is prescribed, known interactions between the disease state and the pregnancy, and preventive measures when applicable (e.g., folic acid supplementation in carbamazepine exposure).
- Because more than 50% of pregnancies are unplanned, teratogenic risk assessment should be started prior to pregnancy.

Table 1: **Possible Teratogenic Drugs in Humans**[4,a]

Drug	Adverse Effects
Diazepam	A questionable small increase in the incidence of cleft lip and palate (small studies). Larger studies did not confirm the association.
Fluconazole	High-dose treatment: multiple synostosis, congenital heart defects, skeletal anomalies, and recognizable dysmorphic facial features (case reports).
HMG-CoA Reductase Inhibitors (statins)	A questionable increase in the risk of CNS and limb anomalies (retrospective data).
Lamotrigine	A questionable increase in the risk of isolated oral clefts (< 1%).
Methimazole	Scalp defects such as aplasia cutis congenita suggested through case reports and an epidemiological study in which methimazole had been added to animal feeds as a weight enhancer; methimazole embryopathy (choanal and esophageal atresia, scalp defects, minor facial anomalies and psychomotor delay).
Paroxetine	A questionable increase in the risk of cardiac malformations.
Penicillamine	High-dose treatment: connective tissue disorders (cutis laxa) (case reports).

[a] This list is not exhaustive.

Table 1 lists possible teratogenic drugs with insufficient evidence as yet for teratogenicity in humans. Table 2 lists drugs with sufficient evidence to prove their teratogenic effect in humans. Use an alternative in pregnancy when possible. Table 3 presents drugs of choice during gestation for common maternal conditions.

Note: Antenatal drug/chemical risk counselling or information on safety of drug use during lactation is available from the Motherisk Program, Hospital for Sick Children, Toronto, Ontario. Tel.: (416) 813-6780; email: momrisk@sickkids.on.ca; web site: www.motherisk.org

Table 2: **Proven Teratogenic Drugs in Humans**[3]

Drug	Adverse Effects
Angiotensin Converting Enzyme Inhibitors (ACEI) and Angiotensin II Antagonists	Adverse effects related to hemodynamic effects of ACEI and angiotensin II antagonists on the fetus. In late pregnancy, ACEI fetopathy: intrauterine renal insufficiency, neonatal hypotension, oliguria with renal failure, hyperkalemia, complications of oligohydramnios (i.e., fetal limb contractures, lung hypoplasia, and craniofacial anomalies), prematurity, intrauterine growth restriction and fetal death. Questionable teratogenic risk with first trimester exposure of cardiovascular and CNS malformations.[5]
Antineoplastic Agents	A significant increase in the incidence of various fetal malformations and early miscarriages following 1st trimester exposure.
Carbamazepine	1st trimester exposure: 1% risk of neural tube defects (10× baseline risk) and an increased risk of cardiovascular malformations. A pattern of malformations similar to the fetal hydantoin syndrome has also been associated.
Cocaine	Abruptio placenta, prematurity, fetal loss, decreased birth weight, microcephaly, limb defects, urinary tract malformations, and poorer neurodevelopmental performance. Methodological problems make the findings difficult to interpret. Cocaine abuse is often associated with poly-drug abuse, alcohol consumption, smoking, malnutrition and poor prenatal care. Human epidemiology indicates the risk of major malformation from cocaine is probably low, but the anomalies may be severe.
Corticosteroids (systemic)	Increased risk of oral cleft.
Coumarin Anticoagulants	1st trimester exposure (6–9 wk gestation): fetal warfarin syndrome (nasal hypoplasia and calcific stippling of the epiphyses). Intrauterine growth restriction and developmental delay (CNS damage), eye defects and hearing loss. Warfarin embryopathy is found in up to ⅓ of the cases where a coumarin derivative was given throughout pregnancy. Associated with high rate of miscarriage. Risk of CNS damage due to hemorrhage after the 1st trimester.
Diethylstilbestrol	Vaginal clear cell adenocarcinoma in offspring exposed in utero before 18th wk (> 90% of the cancers occurred after 14 y of age). High incidence of benign vaginal adenosis. Increased miscarriage rate and preterm delivery. In males exposed in utero: no signs of malignancy but genital lesions in 27% and pathologic changes in spermatozoa in 29%. The drug is not currently available in Canada.
Ethanol	Fetal alcohol syndrome: growth impairment, developmental delay and dysmorphic facies. Cleft palate and cardiac anomalies may occur. Full expression of the syndrome occurs with chronic daily ingestion of 2 g alcohol per kg (8 drinks/day) in about ⅓ and partial effects in ¾ of offspring.
Folic Acid Antagonists: aminopterin and methotrexate	Fetal aminopterin-methotrexate syndrome: CNS defects, craniofacial anomalies, abnormal cranial ossification, abnormalities in first branchial arch derivatives, intrauterine growth restriction and mental retardation after first trimester exposure. Maternal dose of methotrexate needed to induce defects is probably above 10 mg/wk with a critical period of 6–8 wk postconception.

(cont'd)

Table 2: **Proven Teratogenic Drugs in Humans**[3] *(cont'd)*

Drug	Adverse Effects
Hydantoins (phenytoin)	Fetal hydantoin syndrome: craniofacial dysmorphology, anomalies and hypoplasia of distal phalanges and nails, growth restriction, mental deficiency and cardiac defects.
Lithium	Small increase in risk for cardiac teratogenesis in early gestation (1%). The risk of Ebstein's anomaly exceeds spontaneous rate of occurrence. Fetal echocardiography if exposed in 1st trimester.
Misoprostol	1st trimester exposure: limb defects and Moebius sequence. Absolute teratogenic risk: probably low. Uterine contraction inducing activity.
Retinoids (acitretin, isotretinoin) and megadoses of Vitamin A	Systemic exposure: potent human general and behavioural teratogen. Retinoic acid embryopathy: craniofacial anomalies, cardiac defects, abnormalities in thymic development and alterations in CNS development. Risk for associated miscarriage: 40%.
Tetracyclines	Discolouration of the teeth after 17 wk gestation when deciduous teeth begin to calcify. Close to term: crowns of permanent teeth may be stained. Oxytetracycline and doxycycline associated with a lower incidence of enamel staining.
Thalidomide	Malformations limited to tissues of mesodermal origin, primarily limbs (reduction defects), ears, cardiovascular system and gut musculature. Critical period: 34–50th day after the beginning of the last menstrual period. A single dose of < 1 mg/kg has produced the syndrome. Embryopathy found in about 20% of pregnancies exposed in the critical period.
Valproic Acid	1st trimester exposure: neural tube defects with 1–2% risk of meningomyelocele, primarily lumbar or lumbosacral, cardiovascular malformations and hypospadias. Fetal valproate syndrome: craniofacial dysmorphology, cardiovascular defects, long fingers and toes, hyperconvex fingernails and cleft lip, has been delineated by some investigations. Neurobehavioural teratogen.

Drug Use During Lactation

The extent of drug exposure in the infant depends on several factors: the pharmacokinetic properties of the drug in the infant and mother, milk composition, the amount of milk consumed, timing of drug intake compared to timing of breastfeeding, the physiology of the breast and the infant's suckling pattern. The susceptibility of an infant to adverse effects from drugs depends on the extent of exposure and the infant's sensitivity. Adverse drug reactions can be dose related and reflect the pharmacologic effect of the drug, or idiosyncratic (rarely).

Most drugs taken by the breastfeeding mother are excreted into the milk. The amount of drug consumed by the infant is usually less than 5% of the maternal dose (weight adjusted). When maternal drug therapy is indicated, choose the agent with minimal risk to the infant. Monitor the infant for potential adverse effects. When toxicity is likely, drug concentration in the milk and infant's plasma may sometimes be measured.

Drugs to be Used with Caution During Lactation[6]

- **Antineoplastic drugs:** potential risk for toxicity.
- **Drugs of abuse:** potential hazard to nursing infant and concern that a mother using these substances may not be capable of proper infant care. However, there is increased morbidity and mortality with bottle-feeding, especially in low socioeconomic classes. Consider social factors in risk estimation.[6]
- **Ergot alkaloids** (ergotamine, bromocriptine): potential risk of suppression of lactation and adverse effects in infant.
- **Gold:** potential adverse effects and long half-life in infant. However, convincing cases of toxicity have not been reported.[7]
- **Iodine-containing compounds** (e.g., amiodarone): iodine is transported into breast milk and may induce goitre and hypothyroidism.
- **Lithium:** may cause one-third to one-half therapeutic blood concentration in infant; measurements in milk and baby are encouraged to calculate the specific individual risk.
- **Oral contraceptives:** not recommended in early lactation; may change milk composition and decrease yield. Progestin-only formulations are preferred.
- **Phenobarbital:** large amounts in milk.
- **Radioactive compounds:** potential exposure of the nursing infant to excessive radioactivity. Length of risk depends on isotope's half-life.

Table 3: **Drugs of Choice for Select Conditions During Pregnancy**[3]

Condition	Drugs of Choice	Alternative	Comments
Allergy	Antihistamines: chlorpheniramine, diphenhydramine, dimenhydrinate	Intranasal preparations of sodium cromoglycate, beclomethasone, budesonide; loratadine	
Anticoagulation	Heparin and low molecular weight heparins	An alternative may be heparin in the first trimester followed by warfarin in the 2nd and 3rd trimesters with heparin again at term	
Anxiety	Benzodiazepines		Watch neonate for possible withdrawal or "floppy" infant when high doses used close to term. For diazepam, there is a questionable small increase in the incidence of cleft lip and palate (small studies). Larger studies did not confirm the association.
Asthma	Inhaled bronchodilators (salbutamol, terbutaline or ipratropium bromide) and inhaled corticosteroids (beclomethasone, budesonide)	Systemic corticosteroids and theophylline	
Bacterial infections	Penicillins, cephalosporins	Aminoglycosides, quinolones	
Bipolar disorder	Lithium	Lamotrigine, carbamazepine, valproic acid	With lithium, monitor using fetal echocardiography. With carbamazepine and valproic acid, prescribe periconceptional folate supplementation and monitor using level II ultrasound for NTD prevention.

Condition	Drugs of Choice	Alternative	Comments
Constipation	Bulk-forming agents (e.g., methylcellulose, psyllium hydrophilic mucilloid)	Lubricants (e.g., paraffin oil, glycerin) or osmotic agents (e.g., magnesium salts, lactulose)	
Cough	Antihistamines, codeine (when indicated)		Avoid high doses of codeine close to term (risk of neonatal opioid withdrawal).
Depression	Tricyclic antidepressants, fluoxetine, citalopram, sertraline	Other selective serotonin reuptake inhibitors	Neonatal withdrawal may occur when used in 3rd trimester.
Diabetes mellitus	Human insulin	Metformin in gestational diabetes in 3rd trimester	Important to achieve strict glycemic control before conception and during the 1st trimester.
Diarrhea	Bulk-forming agents (e.g., methylcellulose, psyllium hydrophilic mucilloid), kaolin pectin	Loperamide	
Dyspepsia	Alginic acid compound — Gaviscon; antacids — numerous aluminum hydroxide combinations	H_2-antagonists, omeprazole	
Epilepsy	Carbamazepine	Benzodiazepines (see Anxiety), lamotrigine, valproic acid	With carbamazepine and valproic acid, prescribe periconceptional folate supplementation and monitor using level II ultrasound for NTD prevention.
Fever and pain	Acetaminophen	ASA, NSAIDs	Avoid full anti-inflammatory dose of NSAIDs in 3rd trimester.
Herpetic infections	Acyclovir	Valacyclovir	
Hypertension	Methyldopa, hydralazine	Calcium channel blockers, beta-blockers	With beta-blockers, reduced birth weight and persistent beta-blockade possible in newborn.

(cont'd)

Table 3: **Drugs of Choice for Select Conditions During Pregnancy**[3] *(cont'd)*

Condition	Drugs of Choice	Alternative	Comments
Hyperthyroidism	Propylthiouracil		Perform fetal ultrasound near term for goitre detection.
Migraine	Acetaminophen	ASA, NSAIDs, sumatriptan	Avoid full anti-inflammatory dose of NSAIDs in 3rd trimester.
Nausea/vomiting	Doxylamine/pyridoxine — Diclectin	Dimenhydrinate, metoclopramide	
Schizophrenia	Phenothiazines	Haloperidol, risperidone	Watch neonate for possible adverse effects if taken close to term.
Vaginal candidiasis	Vaginal: miconazole, clotrimazole, nystatin Topical azoles are preferred.[8,9]	Fluconazole: single systemic dose of 150 mg	

Abbreviations: NTD = neural tube defects

Suggested Readings

American Academy of Pediatrics Committee on Drugs. Transfer of drugs and other chemicals into human milk. *Pediatrics* 2001;108(3):776-89.

Briggs GG, Freeman RK, Yaffe SJ. *Drugs in pregnancy and lactation: a reference guide to fetal and neonatal risk.* 7th ed. Philadelphia (PA): Lippincott Williams & Wilkins; 2005.

Ito S. Drug therapy for breast-feeding women. *N Engl J Med* 2000;343(2):118-26.

Koren G. *Medication safety in pregnancy and breastfeeding: the evidence-based, A to Z clinician's pocket guide.* New York (NY): McGraw-Hill; 2007.

Moretti ME, Lee A, Ito S. Which drugs are contraindicated during breastfeeding? Practice guidelines. *Can Fam Physician* 2000;46:1753-7.

References

1. Koren G, Pastuszak A, Ito S. Drugs in pregnancy. *N Engl J Med* 1998;338(16):1128-37.
2. Briggs GG, Freeman RK, Yaffe SJ. *Drugs in pregnancy and lactation: a reference guide to fetal and neonatal risk.* 7th ed. Philadelphia (PA): Lippincott Williams & Wilkins; 2005.
3. Koren G, editor. *Maternal-fetal toxicology: a clinician's guide.* 4th ed. New York (NY): Marcel Dekker; 2007.
4. Motherisk.org. Toronto (ON): Hospital for Sick Children. Available from: http://www.motherisk.org Accessed January 18, 2007.
5. Cooper WO, Hernandez-Diaz S, Arbogast PG et al. Major congenital malformations after first-trimester exposure to ACE inhibitors. *N Engl J Med* 2006;354(23):2443-51.
6. Ito S. Drug therapy for breast-feeding women. *N Engl J Med* 2000;343(2):118-26.
7. toxnet.nlm.nih.org. Bethesda (MD): National Library of Medicine, Toxnet Toxicology Data Network. Available from: http://toxnet.nlm.nih.gov Accessed January 18, 2007.
8. Expert Working Group on Canadian Guidelines for Sexually Transmitted Infections. *Canadian guidelines on sexually transmitted infections, 2006 edition.* Ottawa (ON): Public Health Agency of Canada; 2006. Available from: http://www.phac-aspc.gc.ca/std-mts/sti_2006_e.pdf Accessed February 6, 2007.
9. Young GL, Jewell D. Topical treatment for vaginal candidiasis (thrush) in pregnancy. Cochrane Database Syst Rev 2001;(4):CD000225.

APPENDIX III

Pharmacoeconomic Considerations

Jeffrey A. Johnson, PhD

The economic impact of the choices made in a therapeutic area is an increasingly important consideration for health care systems and for individual clinicians. *Pharmacoeconomics* is the application of economic evaluation techniques in the study of drug therapy. Increasingly, studies are published incorporating economic evaluations of therapeutic choices for a variety of conditions. Where such evidence is available, some of the chapters in this edition provide information regarding the pharmacoeconomic considerations for that therapeutic area. This Appendix provides some general guidance when considering the pharmacoeconomic impact of your therapeutic choices.

Pharmacoeconomic evaluations are concerned with comparing the dollars spent on treatment alternatives for the outcomes achieved. It is important to remember that in choosing among many alternatives in a therapeutic area, both sides of the equation must be considered. Drug acquisition costs, while an important component, only provide one side of the cost-outcome story and only a part of that side. At the end of most chapters in this edition a summary table indicates the relative cost of each therapeutic choice. It is also important to consider the relative effectiveness of each choice.

Consider the following hypothetical example. There are three drug choices in a given therapeutic area, Drugs X, Y and Z. Drugs X and Y are older and are less expensive; Drug Z is newer and provides improved clinical outcomes, but is also more expensive.

Drug	Cost	Outcomes
X	$$	+
Y	$$	+
Z	$$$	+++

Although Drug Z costs $$$, it provides +++ level of outcomes, whereas Drug X costs $$ but provides only + level of outcomes. This would imply that, in general, Drug Z is more cost effective than Drug X.

However, defining what is a meaningful outcome is often difficult as *outcomes* have taken on many different forms. For this edition of *Therapeutic Choices*, it was not possible to reconcile all different outcome measures and provide a relative ranking for all therapeutic areas. Instead, we have attempted to draw attention to the issue and remind the reader to consider all possible and relevant treatment costs, not just drug acquisition costs, and also to consider the relative effectiveness of the choices where such information is available.

Cost Issues

Direct Costs

When considering the cost of drug therapy, it is important to recognize the impact of drug therapy choices on *downstream* costs. Such costs are often outside the drug budget, and may include additional laboratory tests required to monitor for adverse side effects, but may also include reduced costs for physician visits or hospitalizations for conditions that were not adequately controlled on previous therapeutic choices. Cost of resources used in the treatment of diseases or conditions is referred to as *direct medical costs*.

The following health care resources are all associated with direct medical costs. Any number of these resources may be important to consider when any therapeutic choice is made. That is, when one drug is chosen over another, it is important to consider what impact that treatment may have on any or all of:

- Hospitalizations
- Laboratory/radiologic tests
- Emergency room/medical centre visits
- Drug therapy
- Home care services
- Long-term care

Indirect Costs

Important cost considerations may also include *downstream* costs to society as a result of disease or medical interventions that are outside of the health care system and health care budgets. Such costs include lost or reduced productivity in the workplace due to death or illness. For example, if a drug therapy for migraine headaches is able to reduce the frequency of headaches and consequently reduce the number of days of work missed, this has a positive impact on the overall productivity of the employer and therefore society in general. These costs are referred to as *indirect costs*. The impact of health care on indirect costs is often difficult to quantify and may not always be included in economic evaluations, but is also an important consideration in making therapeutic choices.

Perspective on Costs

The perspective used in determining the important and relevant costs is also important. Who would be burdened with what costs? Pharmacoeconomic evaluations may assume the viewpoint of a single provider, an insurer, the provincial health care system, or society as a whole. Depending on the perspective, the total *costs* of a therapeutic choice may differ.

Consider a patient who moves through various levels of care from a hospital, to an extended care facility, to home. In the hospital's view, its relevant costs are those incurred during the hospital stay. For instance, the hospital would welcome any therapeutic choice that reduces the length of stay and/or other services during the stay. An earlier discharge, however, may mean that more intensive and more costly nursing home care is required. This is relevant from the perspective of the nursing home and the provincial or regional health care system; it is irrelevant to the hospital. Finally, when the patient is transferred home, a family member may assume the role of caregiver. From society's perspective, the caregiver's time is a cost; however, this cost is outside the realm of the health care system and outside the coverage of provincial health plans.

Outcomes

The bottom line in pharmacoeconomic considerations is the ratio of net dollars spent per outcome achieved. Outcomes or consequences of drug therapy can be valued in a number of different ways. The choice of which outcome is best depends on the information available and the condition being evaluated. Some commonly used approaches in pharmacoeconomic evaluations are discussed below.

Dollars spent per clinical outcome

- Outcomes are some recognized unit of clinical effect (e.g., cost per year of life saved; cost per case of nephrotoxicity avoided)
- Referred to as a *cost-effectiveness analysis*
- This approach is probably the most commonly used in pharmacoeconomic evaluations

Dollars spent for dollars saved

- Outcomes given a dollar value
- Referred to as a *cost-benefit analysis*
- This approach often requires the economic valuation of a human life, which presents many difficulties, methodological and philosophical

Dollars spent for quality of life outcomes

- Outcomes are measured as Quality Adjusted Life Years (QALYs) gained
- Referred to as a *cost-utility analysis*
- This approach is used when the impact on health-related quality of life is an important outcome of the condition or its treatment
- Theoretically, the use of a common outcome measure such as QALYs gained would allow for comparison of cost-outcome relationships across different therapeutic areas (see Laupacis et al., 1992). However, because of differences in study methodologies, this is not always possible

Patient Risk and Pharmacoeconomic Considerations

In assessing the economic impact of therapeutic choices, it is also important to consider the selection of patients in terms of level of risk. The economic benefits of drug therapies follow on the clinical benefits. A drug has to be clinically effective to be cost effective and the more effective a drug is, the more cost effective it is likely to be. As with clinical considerations, the economic impact of a treatment is likely to improve for patients who are at greater risk. The same therapeutic choice is not necessarily cost effective in all patients. This information is not always available when economic evaluations are based on clinical trials.

Suggested Readings

Destky AS, Naglie IG. A clinician's guide to cost-effectiveness analysis. *Ann Intern Med* 1990;113:147–154.

Laupacis A, Feeny D, Detsky AS, Tugwell PX. How attractive does a new technology have to be to warrant adoption and utilization? Tentative guidelines for using clinical and economic evaluations. *Can Med Assoc J* 1992;146:473–481.

Index

B

E

F

H

M

O

S

T

U